Biotechnology of Antibiotics

DRUGS AND THE PHARMACEUTICAL SCIENCES

DRUGS AND THE PHARMACEUTICAL SCIENCES

A Series of Textbooks and Monographs

1. Pharmacokinetics, *Milo Gibaldi and Donald Perrier*
2. Good Manufacturing Practices for Pharmaceuticals: A Plan for Total Quality Control, *Sidney H. Willig, Murray M. Tuckerman, and William S. Hitchings IV*
3. Microencapsulation, *edited by J. R. Nixon*
4. Drug Metabolism: Chemical and Biochemical Aspects, *Bernard Testa and Peter Jenner*
5. New Drugs: Discovery and Development, *edited by Alan A. Rubin*
6. Sustained and Controlled Release Drug Delivery Systems, *edited by Joseph R. Robinson*
7. Modern Pharmaceutics, *edited by Gilbert S. Banker and Christopher T. Rhodes*
8. Prescription Drugs in Short Supply: Case Histories, *Michael A. Schwartz*
9. Activated Charcoal: Antidotal and Other Medical Uses, *David O. Cooney*
10. Concepts in Drug Metabolism (in two parts), *edited by Peter Jenner and Bernard Testa*
11. Pharmaceutical Analysis: Modern Methods (in two parts), *edited by James W. Munson*
12. Techniques of Solubilization of Drugs, *edited by Samuel H. Yalkowsky*
13. Orphan Drugs, *edited by Fred E. Karch*
14. Novel Drug Delivery Systems: Fundamentals, Developmental Concepts, Biomedical Assessments, *Yie W. Chien*
15. Pharmacokinetics: Second Edition, Revised and Expanded, *Milo Gibaldi and Donald Perrier*
16. Good Manufacturing Practices for Pharmaceuticals: A Plan for Total Quality Control, Second Edition, Revised and Expanded, *Sidney H. Willig, Murray M. Tuckerman, and William S. Hitchings IV*
17. Formulation of Veterinary Dosage Forms, *edited by Jack Blodinger*
18. Dermatological Formulations: Percutaneous Absorption, *Brian W. Barry*
19. The Clinical Research Process in the Pharmaceutical Industry, *edited by Gary M. Matoren*
20. Microencapsulation and Related Drug Processes, *Patrick B. Deasy*
21. Drugs and Nutrients: The Interactive Effects, *edited by Daphne A. Roe and T. Colin Campbell*
22. Biotechnology of Industrial Antibiotics, *Erick J. Vandamme*
23. Pharmaceutical Process Validation, *edited by Bernard T. Loftus and Robert A. Nash*
24. Anticancer and Interferon Agents: Synthesis and Properties, *edited by Raphael M. Ottenbrite and George B. Butler*
25. Pharmaceutical Statistics: Practical and Clinical Applications, *Sanford Bolton*
26. Drug Dynamics for Analytical, Clinical, and Biological Chemists, *Benjamin J. Gudzinowicz, Burrows T. Younkin, Jr., and Michael J. Gudzinowicz*
27. Modern Analysis of Antibiotics, *edited by Adjoran Aszalos*
28. Solubility and Related Properties, *Kenneth C. James*
29. Controlled Drug Delivery: Fundamentals and Applications, Second Edition, Revised and Expanded, *edited by Joseph R. Robinson and Vincent H. Lee*

30. New Drug Approval Process: Clinical and Regulatory Management, *edited by Richard A. Guarino*

31. Transdermal Controlled Systemic Medications, *edited by Yie W. Chien*

32. Drug Delivery Devices: Fundamentals and Applications, *edited by Praveen Tyle*

33. Pharmacokinetics: Regulatory • Industrial • Academic Perspectives, *edited by Peter G. Welling and Francis L. S. Tse*

34. Clinical Drug Trials and Tribulations, *edited by Allen E. Cato*

35. Transdermal Drug Delivery: Developmental Issues and Research Initiatives, *edited by Jonathan Hadgraft and Richard H. Guy*

36. Aqueous Polymeric Coatings for Pharmaceutical Dosage Forms, *edited by James W. McGinity*

37. Pharmaceutical Pelletization Technology, *edited by Isaac GhebreSellassie*

38. Good Laboratory Practice Regulations, *edited by Allen F. Hirsch*

39. Nasal Systemic Drug Delivery, *Yie W. Chien, Kenneth S. E. Su, and Shyi-Feu Chang*

40. Modern Pharmaceutics: Second Edition, Revised and Expanded, *edited by Gilbert S. Banker and Christopher T. Rhodes*

41. Specialized Drug Delivery Systems: Manufacturing and Production Technology, *edited by Praveen Tyle*

42. Topical Drug Delivery Formulations, *edited by David W. Osborne and Anton H. Amann*

43. Drug Stability: Principles and Practices, *Jens T. Carstensen*

44. Pharmaceutical Statistics: Practical and Clinical Applications, Second Edition, Revised and Expanded, *Sanford Bolton*

45. Biodegradable Polymers as Drug Delivery Systems, *edited by Mark Chasin and Robert Langer*

46. Preclinical Drug Disposition: A Laboratory Handbook, *Francis L. S. Tse and James J. Jaffe*

47. HPLC in the Pharmaceutical Industry, *edited by Godwin W. Fong and Stanley K. Lam*

48. Pharmaceutical Bioequivalence, *edited by Peter G. Welling, Francis L. S. Tse, and Shrikant V. Dinghe*

49. Pharmaceutical Dissolution Testing, *Umesh V. Banakar*

50. Novel Drug Delivery Systems: Second Edition, Revised and Expanded, *Yie W. Chien*

51. Managing the Clinical Drug Development Process, *David M. Cocchetto and Ronald V. Nardi*

52. Good Manufacturing Practices for Pharmaceuticals: A Plan for Total Quality Control, Third Edition, *edited by Sidney H. Willig and James R. Stoker*

53. Prodrugs: Topical and Ocular Drug Delivery, *edited by Kenneth B. Sloan*

54. Pharmaceutical Inhalation Aerosol Technology, *edited by Anthony J. Hickey*

55. Radiopharmaceuticals: Chemistry and Pharmacology, *edited by Adrian D. Nunn*

56. New Drug Approval Process: Second Edition, Revised and Expanded, *edited by Richard A. Guarino*

57. Pharmaceutical Process Validation: Second Edition, Revised and Expanded, *edited by Ira R. Berry and Robert A. Nash*

58. Ophthalmic Drug Delivery Systems, *edited by Ashim K. Mitra*

59. Pharmaceutical Skin Penetration Enhancement, *edited by Kenneth A. Walters and Jonathan Hadgraft*

60. Colonic Drug Absorption and Metabolism, *edited by Peter R. Bieck*

61. Pharmaceutical Particulate Carriers: Therapeutic Applications, *edited by Alain Rolland*
62. Drug Permeation Enhancement: Theory and Applications, *edited by Dean S. Hsieh*
63. Glycopeptide Antibiotics, *edited by Ramakrishnan Nagarajan*
64. Achieving Sterility in Medical and Pharmaceutical Products, *Nigel A. Halls*
65. Multiparticulate Oral Drug Delivery, *edited by Isaac Ghebre-Sellassie*
66. Colloidal Drug Delivery Systems, *edited by Jörg Kreuter*
67. Pharmacokinetics: Regulatory • Industrial • Academic Perspectives, Second Edition, *edited by Peter G. Welling and Francis L. S. Tse*
68. Drug Stability: Principles and Practices, Second Edition, Revised and Expanded, *Jens T. Carstensen*
69. Good Laboratory Practice Regulations: Second Edition, Revised and Expanded, *edited by Sandy Weinberg*
70. Physical Characterization of Pharmaceutical Solids, *edited by Harry G. Brittain*
71. Pharmaceutical Powder Compaction Technology, *edited by Göran Alderborn and Christer Nyström*
72. Modern Pharmaceutics: Third Edition, Revised and Expanded, *edited by Gilbert S. Banker and Christopher T. Rhodes*
73. Microencapsulation: Methods and Industrial Applications, *edited by Simon Benita*
74. Oral Mucosal Drug Delivery, *edited by Michael J. Rathbone*
75. Clinical Research in Pharmaceutical Development, *edited by Barry Bleidt and Michael Montagne*
76. The Drug Development Process: Increasing Efficiency and CostEffectiveness, *edited by Peter G. Welling, Louis Lasagna, and Umesh V. Banakar*
77. Microparticulate Systems for the Delivery of Proteins and Vaccines, *edited by Smadar Cohen and Howard Bernstein*
78. Good Manufacturing Practices for Pharmaceuticals: A Plan for Total Quality Control, Fourth Edition, Revised and Expanded, *Sidney H. Willig and James R. Stoker*
79. Aqueous Polymeric Coatings for Pharmaceutical Dosage Forms: Second Edition, Revised and Expanded, *edited by James W. McGinity*
80. Pharmaceutical Statistics: Practical and Clinical Applications, Third Edition, *Sanford Bolton*
81. Handbook of Pharmaceutical Granulation Technology, *edited by Dilip M. Parikh*
82. Biotechnology of Antibiotics: Second Edition, Revised and Expanded, *edited by William R. Strohl*
83. Mechanisms of Transdermal Drug Delivery, *edited by Russell O. Potts and Richard H. Guy*
84. Pharmaceutical Enzymes, *edited by Albert Lauwers and Simon Scharpé*
85. Development of Biopharmaceutical Parenteral Dosage Forms, *edited by John A. Bontempo*

ADDITIONAL VOLUMES IN PREPARATION

Pharmaceutical Project Management, *edited by Anthony Kennedy*

Drug Products for Clinical Trials: An International Guide to Formulation • Production • Quality Control, *edited by Christopher T. Rhodes and Donald C. Monkhouse*

Automation and Validation of Information in Pharmaceutical Processing, *edited by Joseph deSpautz*

Development and Formulation of Veterinary Dosage Forms, *edited by Gregory E. Hardee and J. Desmond Baggot*

Biotechnology of Antibiotics

Second Edition, Revised and Expanded

edited by

William R. Strohl

The Ohio State University
Columbus, Ohio

MARCEL DEKKER, INC.   NEW YORK · BASEL · HONG KONG

ISBN: 0-8247-9867-8

The publisher offers discounts on this book when ordered in bulk quantities. For more information, write to Special Sales/Professional Marketing at the address below.

This book is printed on acid-free paper.

MARCEL DEKKER, INC.
270 Madison Avenue, New York, New York 10016
http://www.dekker.com

Current printing (last digit):
10 9 8 7 6 5 4 3 2 1

PRINTED IN THE UNITED STATES OF AMERICA

PREFACE

In the preface to the first edition, Professor Erick Vandamme indicated that the book originated in part from frustration, in the attempt to keep abreast of current literature and recent advancements in the field of antibiotics. He began his Preface by listing many of the processes in which microorganisms are used to produce chemicals of vital use to mankind. Professor Vandamme included the production of antibiotics, antitumor agents, vitamins, biopolymers, vaccines, and amino acids, as well as the bioconversion of steroids, antibiotics, vitamins, amino acids, and carbohydrates. Yet these cover only a small, albeit important, fraction of the vast biotechnological processes in which microorganisms are used to produce economically important molecules. The same applies to this second edition, as we can focus on only a small fraction of the products of the rapidly expanding field of modern biotechnology.

In the decade or so since the first edition, the field of antibiotic research has changed considerably, as have the challenges facing society. In 1983, acquired immunodeficiency syndrome (AIDS) was still in its infancy, and there was little knowledge of the devastation it would cause. Tragic outbreaks of diseases caused by exotic viruses such as Ebola were still only in the minds of science fiction writers. Multiple-antibiotic-resistant *Mycobacterium tuberculosis*, vancomycin-resistant enterococci, *E. coli* O157-H7 and invasive staphylococci were essentially unknown, and the extraordinary promiscuity with which bacteria transfer resistance genes was only whispered in academic circles. Today, we face all these challenges and more. Unfortunately, it is all too likely that we have only scratched the surface and that new challenges to the discovery, production, and use of antibiotics will continue to mount at ever increasing rates.

Thirteen years ago we had only the first glimpses of the utilization of modern industrial biotechnology (i.e., genetic engineering and computerized process control of fermentations) for making new antibiotics or assisting in the overproduction of existing antibiotics. At that time the first antibiotic biosynthesis genes from *Streptomyces* had just been cloned, and expression in heterologous strains and the first fungal antibiotic biosynthesis gene to be cloned, was still a year away from being reported in *Nature*. A decade ago, we could only dream of finding regulatory genes that conferred the overproduction of some antibiotics. Producing novel metabolites via interspecies cloning and cloning genes that conferred specific biochemical modifications on existing structures such as a sterol oxygenase were also far from being realized. In the past 14 years, all these breakthroughs and considerably more have been accomplished.

And so the questions now become: Where has biotechnology of antibiotics gotten us? Where will it lead us into tomorrow?

Modern biotechnology has given us several new products: human insulin, human and bovine growth hormones, and granulocyte colony stimulating factors are just a few examples. Adaptation of genetic engineering and process control has also yielded better methods in the production of traditional products, with new generations of β-lactam antibiotics and enzyme inhibitors, such as pravistatin. In the field of antibiotic production, however, we see only a few examples where genetically engineering and modern biotechnology processes have already been brought into practice. To date, there are no publicly known genetically modified antibiotics or hybrid antibiotics on the market. Similarly, it does not appear that there are any commercial antibiotics currently being overproduced using genetic engineered microorganisms, although this would not necessarily be public knowledge. Does this imply that genetic engineering and sophisticated process control methodologies have little or no future in the antibiotic industry? I believe not. It is the contention of this book that since the first edition was published, the badly needed foundation and data base, from which a new golden era of biotechnology of antibiotics will emanate, has been established. Although the foundation still has some significant cracks and holes, these are being filled, in ever increasing numbers by the industrial and academic research groups who recently have entered the field. This suggests that the maturation of genetic engineering for antibiotic production has begun. This is an essential prerequisite for the eventual and imminent industrial production of genetically engineered antibiotics via biosynthesis pathways.

How will "antibiotic" be defined in this volume? According to Webster, an antibiotic is "a substance produced by a microorganism and able in dilute solution to inhibit or kill another microorganism." Strictly speaking, this definition is still largely accurate. As we face the new millennium, however, it seems that perhaps Webster's definition, introduced by Waksman in 1942, is in need of a practical update. Even the editor of the *Journal of Antibiotics*, Dr. Morisama Yagisawa, has realized the diversity of antibiotics in our modern world, by including in his journal articles covering virtually all areas of bioactive natural products. So, where should the line be drawn between antibiotics and non-antibiotic bioactive metabolites? Certainly, antitumor drugs are antibiotics. They kill not only tumor cells, as well as healthy tissue, but also certain microorganisms. Are cholesterol-lowering agents antibiotics? Again, some of these inhibit or kill microorganisms, but their clinical use has nothing in common with their ability to inhibit the growth of microorganisms. Are β-lactamase inhibitors antibiotics? Their function, presumably in nature and certainly in medicine, is as helper molecules to assist the efficacy of β-lactam antibiotics. Are veterinary growth-promoting natural products antibiotics? Some are known coccidiostats, while the exact function of others is still only marginally understood. Yet, since they function to fatten livestock, they are used in great quantities. Are nisin and related peptides actually antibiotics, or are they just bacteriocins with convenient activities? Are aflatoxins antibiotics? They are microbial secondary metabolites, like most traditional antibiotics, and they kill or inhibit biological entities. Nevertheless, they are not utilized commercially as antibiotics. What about delta-endotoxins of *Bacillus thuringiensis* and *Bacillus sphaericus* antibiotics? Certainly, they kill insects, which are biological entities. They too are produced commercially. In the same light, are algal toxins, *Clostridium botulinum* toxins, and other such proteinaceous toxins antibiotics? Perhaps the definition would be stretched too far to include these. Should immunosuppressive agents be considered? Some exhibit antibiotic activity although it is usually poor; they nevertheless carry out antimetabolic functions. But if immunosuppressants such as cyclosporin and rapamycin are included, why not immunomodulatory proteins such as granulocyte colony–stimulating factors? In this book, the line between antibiotics and other pharmaceutically active natural products has been drawn between those non-protein products that are microbially derived or produced, and those that are derived from plants or animals. While this may appear to be an arbitrary distinction, it does serve the purpose of defining limits. Therefore, while it was very tempting to include a chapter on taxol biosynthesis, its inclusion would have required chapters on vincristine and vinblastine biosynthesis. Moreover, even a single chapter on production of recombinant human protein, tissue plasminogen activator (tPA), for example, would have begged the question of including all of the now thirty or so recombinant proteins on the market. Thus, this book is specific to microbially derived, commercially important bioactive products that are currently available or appear to have a bright future in early 21st-century markets.

Finally, the question of choice must be addressed. Why include two chapters concerning β-lactam antibiotics and another two relating to peptide antibiotics while leaving out many others that are significant to human health but which occupy small niche markets, such as pseudomonic acid (mupirocin). Why include, in some chapters, basic biochemistry and molecular genetics, while in others emphasize industrial scale-up and fermentation processes? Why not include chapters on chemically synthesized antibiotics, or antibiotics such as chloramphenicol, originally produced by Streptomyces fermentations but now chemically synthesized? The answer is that, within the confines of twenty-six chapters, this book endeavors to place itself at the leading edge of the antibiotic biotechnology field, while striking a delicate balance between proven, traditional ("old") technologies and those modern technologies which promise to yield new products and processes as we enter the 21st century. The future of antibiotic production promises to be just such a mixture, with the use of novel biological approaches to solve traditional chemical problems, the development and use of novel screening methods to discover new biological activities, and the application of traditional approaches to genetically engineered microorganisms to overproduce existing or new generations of antibiotics. The contributing authors for this book include several academics, who are often at the leading edge of science and novel concepts but may have never set foot in a production facility; and industrial scientists, who are diverse in their backgrounds and whose areas of expertises range from the genetic engineering of new generations of antibiotics to applying traditional methods to the production of new and unusual molecules.

No book with this scope can be assembled by a single person—particularly one like me, who resides in academia—without the thoughtful assistance and advise of others, particularly those who are associated with industrial antibiotic production. I owe considerable thanks to Dean Taylor for endless hours of fruitful discussion on industrial antibiotic production and potential authors and chapters, and to Arnold Demain for his thoughtful suggestions and gentle reminders to stay close to schedule. I also wish to thank each of the contributors for their considerable efforts and patience with me as I prodded them for updates and new information. I would especially like to thank my wife, Lila, and two sons, Joshua and Justin, for their patience and understanding during the period of this endeavor.

Since entering the field of antibiotic biosynthesis in the early 1980s, I have been inspired by a great number of outstanding scientists. A few have had an enormous influence on my career, whether they know it or not. Thus, it is with great pleasure that I dedicate this book to Heinz Floss and Arnold Demain, colleagues who have taken the time to show me the light and give me much needed encouragement over the past decade, and to David Hopwood, who, through his generosity and kindness, made it possible for me and so many others to delve into the exciting field of streptomycete molecular biology as it unfolded.

William R. Strohl

CONTENTS

Preface   iii

Contributors   ix

PART I   **INTRODUCTION AND APPROACHES FOR IMPROVEMENT IN ANTIBIOTIC PRODUCTION**

1   Industrial Antibiotics: Today and the Future   1
William R. Strohl

2   Molecular Genetic Approaches to Yield Improvement in Actinomycetes   49
Richard H. Baltz

3   Butyrolactone Autoregulators, Inducers of Virginiamycin in *Streptomyces virginiae*: Their Structures, Biosynthesis, Receptor Proteins, and Induction of Virginiamycin Biosythesis   63
Yasuhiro Yamada, Takuya Nihira, and Shohei Sakuda

PART II   **AMINOGLYCOSIDES**

4   Molecular Biology, Biochemistry, and Fermentation of Aminoglycoside Antibiotics   81
Wolfgang Piepersberg

5   Fermentation, Biosynthesis, and Molecular Genetics of Lincomycin   165
Shiau-Ta Chung, Jack J. Manis, Steven J. McWethy, Tom E. Patt, Dennis F. Witz, Holly J. Wolf, and Merle G. Wovcha

PART III   **TEMPLATE-BIOSYNTHESIZED PEPTIDE AND β-LACTAM ANTIBIOTICS**

6   Structure, Function, and Regulation of Genes Encoding Multidomain Peptide Synthetases   187
Peter Zuber and Mohamed A. Marahiel

7   Enzymology of Peptide Synthetases   217
Hans von Döhren and Horst Kleinkauf

8   Comparative Genetics and Molecular Biology of β-Lactam Biosynthesis   241
Ashish S. Paradkar, Susan E. Jensen, and Roy H. Mosher

9   Biosynthesis of Cyclosporins   279
René Traber

10   Echinocandin Antifungal Agents   315
William W. Turner and William L. Current

11   Biochemistry and Genetics of Actinomycin Production   335
George H. Jones and Ullrich Keller

12 Vancomycin and Other Glycopeptides 363
Thalia I. Nicas and Robin D. G. Cooper
13 Thiopeptide Antibiotics 393
Todd M. Smith, Ya-Fen Jiang, and Heinz G. Floss
14 Lipopeptide Antibiotics Produced by *Streptomyces reseosporus*
and *Streptomyces fradiae* 415
Richard H. Baltz

PART IV RIBOSOMALLY SYNTHESIZED PEPTIDE ANTIBIOTICS

15 Nisin and Related Antimicrobial Peptides 437
J. Norman Hansen
16 Cationic Peptides 471
Robert E. W. Hancock and Timothy John Falla

PART V POLYKETIDE ANTIBIOTICS PRODUCED BY TYPE-I MULTIFUNCTIONAL ENZYMES

17 Rapamycin, FK506, and Ascomycin-Related Compounds 497
Kevin A. Reynolds and Arnold L. Demain
18 Rifamycins 521
Giancarlo Lancini and Bruno Cavalleri
19 Polyene Antibiotics 551
José A. Gil and Juan F. Martín

PART VI POLYKETIDE ANTIBIOTICS PRODUCED BY TYPE-II POLYKETIDE SYNTHASE SYSTEMS

20 Anthracyclines 577
*William R. Strohl, Michael L. Dickens, Vineet B. Rajgarhia,
Anton J. Woo, and Nigel D. Priestley*
21 Tetracyclines 659
Iain S. Hunter and Robert A. Hill
22 Antibiotics from Genetically Engineered Microorganisms 683
C. Richard Hutchinson

PART VI PEPTIDYL NUCLEOSIDE ANTIBIOTICS

23 Blasticidin S and Related Peptidyl Nucleoside Antibiotics 703
Steven J. Gould

PART VIII RECOMBINANT BIOCONVERSIONS OF BIOACTIVE MOLECULES

24 New Processes for Production of 7-Aminocephalosporanic Acid
from Cephalosporin 733
Takao Isogai
25 Chemoenzymatic Production of the Antiviral Agent Epivir™ 753
Mahmoud Mahmoudian and Michael J. Dawson
26 Biochemical and Fermentation Technological Approaches to
Production of Pravastatin, a HMG-CoA Reductase Inhibitor 779
Nobofusa Serizawa, Masahiko Hosobuchi, and Hiroji Yoshikawa

Index 807

Contributors

Richard H. Baltz, Ph.D.   Research Advisor, Infectious Disease Research, Lilly Research Laboratories, Eli Lilly and Company, Indianapolis, Indiana

Bruno Cavalleri, Ph.D.   Consultant, Lepetit Research Center, Gerenzano, Italy

Shiau-Ta Chung, Ph.D.   Senior Scientist, Bioprocess Research and Development, Pharmacia and Upjohn, Inc., Kalamazoo, Michigan

Robin D. G. Cooper, D.Sc., Ph.D.   Research Advisor, Infectious Disease Research, Lilly Research Laboratories, Eli Lilly and Company, Indianapolis, Indiana

William L. Current, Ph.D.   Senior Research Scientist, Infectious Disease Research, Lilly Research Laboratories, Eli Lilly and Company, Indianapolis, Indiana

Michael J. Dawson, Ph.D.   Bioprocess Development Group Leader, Bioprocessing Unit, Glaxo Wellcome Research and Development, Stevenage, Herts, England

Arnold L. Demain, B.S., M.S., Ph.D.   Professor of Industrial Microbiology, Department of Biology, Massachusetts Institute of Technology, Cambridge, Massachusetts

Michael L. Dickens, Ph.D.   Department of Microbiology, The Ohio State University, Columbus, Ohio

Timothy John Falla, Ph.D.   Research Fellow, Department of Microbiology, University of Leeds, Leeds, England

Heinz G. Floss, Ph.D.   Professor, Department of Chemistry, University of Washington, Seattle, Washington

José A. Gil, Ph.D.   Associate Professor of Microbiology, Departments of Ecology, Genetics, and Microbiology, University of León, León, Spain

Steven J. Gould, Ph.D.   Professor, Department of Chemistry, Oregon State University, Corvallis, Oregon

Robert E. W. Hancock, Ph.D.   Professor, Departments of Microbiology and Immunology, University of British Columbia, Vancouver, British Columbia, Canada

J. Norman Hansen, Ph.D.   Professor, Departments of Chemistry and Biochemistry, University of Maryland at College Park, College Park, Maryland

Robert A. Hill, Ph.D.   Doctor, Department of Chemistry, University of Glasgow, Glasgow, Scotland

Iain S. Hunter, Ph.D.   Professor, Department of Bioscience and Biotechnology, University of Strathclyde, Glasgow, Scotland

Masahiko Hosobuchi, Ph.D. Assistant Chief Researcher, Biomedical Research Laboratories, Sankyo Company, Ltd., Tokyo, Japan

C. Richard Hutchinson, Ph.D. Professor of Medicinal Chemistry and Bacteriology, School of Pharmacy and Department of Bacteriology, University of Wisconsin, Madison, Wisconsin

Takao Isogai, Ph.D. Research Manager, Fujisawa Pharmaceutical Co., Ltd., Tokodai, Tsukuba, Ibaraki, Japan

Susan E. Jensen, Ph.D. Professor and Chair, Department of Biological Sciences, University of Alberta, Edmonton, Alberta, Canada

Ya-Fen Jiang University of Washington, Seattle, Washington

George H. Jones, Ph.D. Professor, Department of Biology, Emory University, Atlanta, Georgia

Ullrich Keller Technical University Berlin, Berlin, Germany

Horst Kleinkauf, Ph.D. Professor, Department of Biochemistry and Molecular Biology, Technical University Berlin, Berlin, Germany

Giancarlo Lancini, M.D. Consultant in Microbial Chemistry, Lepetit Research Center, Gerenzano, Italy

Mahmoud Mahmoudian, DIC, MSc., Ph.D. Senior Research Biologist, Department of Bioprocessing, Medicines Research Center, Glaxo Wellcome Research and Development, Stevenage, Herts, England

Jack J. Manis, Ph.D. Associate Director, Bioprocess Research Preparations, Pharmacia and Upjohn, Inc., Kalamazoo, Michigan

Mohamed A. Marahiel, Ph.D. Professor, Department of Fachbereich Chemie, Philipps University, Marburg, Germany

Juan F. Martín, Ph.D. Professor, Departments of Ecology, Genetics, and Microbiology, and Institute of Biotechnology, University of León, León, Spain

Steven J. McWethy, Ph.D. Associate Director, Fermentation Production, Pharmacia and Upjohn, Inc., Kalamazoo, Michigan

Roy H. Mosher, Ph.D. Assistant Professor, Department of Biology, University of Illinois at Springfield, Springfield, Illinois

Thalia I. Nicas, Ph.D. Research Scientist, Division of Infectious Diseases, Lilly Research Laboratories, Eli Lilly and Company, Indianapolis, Indiana

Takuya Nihira, Ph.D. Associate Professor, Department of Biotechnology, Osaka University, Osaka, Japan

Ashish S. Paradkar, Ph.D. Post Doctoral Research Associate, Department of Biological Sciences, University of Alberta, Edmonton, Alberta, Canada

Tom E. Patt, Ph.D. Senior Scientist, Bioprocess Research and Development, Pharmacia and Upjohn, Inc., Kalamazoo, Michigan

Wolfgang Piepersberg, Ph.D. Professor, Department of Chemische Mikrobiologie, Bergische Universität GH, Wuppertal, Germany

Nigel D. Priestley, Ph.D. Assistant Professor, College of Pharmacy, The Ohio State University, Columbus, Ohio

Vineet B. Rajgarhia, B.S. Graduate Research Associate, Department of Microbiology, The Ohio State University, Columbus, Ohio

Kevin A. Reynolds, Ph.D. Associate Professor, Department of Pharmaceutical Sciences, School of Pharmacy, University of Maryland at Baltimore, Baltimore, Maryland

Shohei Sakuda, Ph.D. Associate Professor, Department of Applied Biological Chemistry, The University of Tokyo, Tokyo, Japan

Nobufusa Serizawa, Ph.D. Group Director, Biomedical Research Laboratories, Sankyo Company, Ltd., Tokyo, Japan

Todd M. Smith, Ph.D. Department of Biotechnology, University of Washington, Seattle, Washington

William R. Strohl, Ph.D. Professor, Department of Microbiology, The Ohio State University, Columbus, Ohio

René Traber, Ph.D. Senior Scientist, Preclinical Research, Novartis Pharma, Inc., Basel, Switzerland

William W. Turner, M.S. Senior Organic Chemist, Infectious Disease Research, Lilly Research Laboratories, Eli Lilly and Company, Indianapolis, Indiana

Hans von Döhren, M.D. Department of Biochemistry and Molecular Biology, Technical University Berlin, Berlin, Germany

Dennis F. Witz, Ph.D. Senior Research Scientist, Bioprocess Research and Development, Pharmacia and Upjohn, Inc., Kalamazoo, Michigan

Holly J. Wolf, M.S., Ph.D. Director, Department of Bioprocess Research, Pharmacia and Upjohn, Inc., Kalamazoo, Michigan

Anton J. Woo Graduate Research Associate, Department of Microbiology, The Ohio State University, Columbus, Ohio

Merle G. Wovcha, Ph.D. Senior Scientist, Bioprocess Research and Development, Pharmacia and Upjohn, Inc., Kalamazoo, Michigan

Yasuhiro Yamada, Ph.D. Professor, Department of Biotechnology, Osaka University, Osaka, Japan

Hiroji Yoshikawa, Ph.D. Group Director, Biomedical Research Laboratories, Sankyo Company, Ltd., Tokyo, Japan

Peter Zuber, Ph.D. Professor, Department of Biochemistry and Molecular Biology, Louisiana State University Medical Center, Shreveport, Louisiana

1

Industrial Antibiotics: Today and the Future

William R. Strohl

The Ohio State University, Columbus, Ohio

I. CURRENT STATUS OF ANTIBIOTIC DEVELOPMENT

A. What Are Antibiotics?

The concept of "antibiotic" activity was first introduced in 1889 by Paul Vuillemin, who used the term "influences antibiotiques" (antibiotic influences) to describe negative interactions among plants and animals (1). In the 1940s, Waksman coined the term "antibiotic" and described an antibiotic as "a chemical substance derived from microorganisms which has the capacity of inhibiting growth, and even destroying, other microorganisms in dilute solutions" (2). Natural product antibiotics belong to a group of compounds called secondary metabolites, generally characterized by having structures that are unusual compared with those of intermediary metabolites, by being produced at low specific growth rates, and by the fact that they are not essential for growth of the producing organisms in pure culture. Antibiotics are, however, critical to the producing organisms in their natural environment, as they are needed both for survival and competitive advantage (3).

Though Waksman's definition of antibiotics is still true, it is not nearly inclusive enough to describe the vast assortment of antibacterial, antifungal, antiviral, antitumor, and antimetabolic substances known to be produced by microorganisms and macroorganisms today. Part of the reason for this shortcoming is that many pharmacologically active natural products have structures similar to classic bacteriocidal or bacteriostatic agents. Some pharmacologically active compounds, such as cyclosporin and rapamycin, in fact, were originally discovered in antibiotic screening programs. Thus, cyclosporin, a poor antifungal antibiotic but an excellent immunosuppressive agent used to inhibit tissue rejection after organ transplantation, now is typically grouped with other peptide antibiotics. Similarly, tacrolimus (formerly called FK506) and rapamycin, both recently developed immunosuppressive agents, erythromycin, an important bacteriostatic antibiotic, avermectin, a potent antiparasitic agent, and tylosin, a veterinary coccidiostat and growth promotant, all are considered to be members of the macrolide class of "antibiotics." Additionally, there are many chemically synthesized and modified compounds that have been derived biomimetically from natural products, and even more that have been found empirically to possess antibiotic activities.

Table 1 lists some of the antibiological and antimetabolite activities of natural products that might be included within the broader definition of "antibiotics." It is clear that in this modern era of mass screening capabilities and target-based screens, new uses for known compounds, as well as the continued discovery and development of new compounds, will continue to expand.

B. Industrial Antibiotics Market

The world market for anti-infectives has surged from $18 billion in 1994 (4) to $23 billion in 1996 (5), an increase of 28% in just two years. In the United States alone, the 1995 anti-infectives market was greater than $8 billion, with cephalosporins (45%), penicillins (15%), quinolones (11%), tetracyclines (6%), and macrolides (5%) making up the bulk of the sales. Ciprofloxacin, a chemically synthesized fluoroquinone, recently topped all anti-infective drugs with 1993 sales of $1.06 billion.

The antiviral market in 1995 was $1.8 billion and is expected to rise to $3 billion by 1998. The top product in 1995 was acyclovir, with 50% of the market (4). More than 17 million people, however, are infected with HIV, a number that is expected to reach 30 to 40 million by year 2000 (4). With the development of successful new anti-HIV drugs such as 3TC (6) and HIV-proteinase inhibitors (7), it is expected that the antiviral market should increase substantially within the next few years. Similarly, the 1995 world antifungal market, approximately $3 billion, is growing at an astounding rate of 20% annually, driven mostly by the AIDS epidemic, in which opportunistic fungal pathogens cause a large percentage of deaths. Thus, the makeup of the antibiotic market is expected to change dramatically within the next decade.

C. Development of Antibiotics

According to a recent in-depth analysis by Bérdy (8), about 11,900 antibiotics had been discovered through 1994, approximately 6600 (55%) of which were produced by *Streptomyces* spp. The remainder of producing organisms included the filamentous fungi, which produced 2600 (22%), nonactinomycete bacteria, which produced 1400 (12%), and non-*Streptomyces* strains of actinomycetes, which produced 1300 (11%) (8). Of these bioactive natural products, approximately 160 are in clinical use across the world today (8). The Appendix at the end of this chapter lists 252 compounds used clinically and agriculturally in the United States, with selected additions from around the world. Of these compounds, 75 (30%) are natural products, another 75 (30%) are semisynthetic compounds derived from natural products, and the remaining 40% are chemically synthesized compounds. Though this table is not all-inclusive, it does provide a compendium of the most widely used compounds in the United States.

As depicted in Figure 1, the incidence of discovery of new bioactive natural products worldwide was still increasing through 1990 (8), with a projected total of more than 16,000 discovered natural product antibiotics by the year 2000 (Figure 1b). New antibiotics are being discovered at a rate of more than 500 per year, up from 200–300 per year 20 years ago (Figure 1a). Yet, there is the widespread perception in both the scientific literature (9,10) and the popular press (11,12) that the discovery of new natural product antibiotics is on the wane. Figure 2 shows this perception to be largely accurate, at least over the past decade. From 1980 to 1990, more than 4600 new bioactive natural products were discovered worldwide, yet only 3 new natural products and 17 new semisynthetic products reported (either by publication or patent application) since 1980 have been

Table 1 Antibiological Activities of Natural Products in Use, in Development, or of Potential Future Interest

Antibiological activity	Example of natural products
Antibacterial	Streptomycin, tetracycline
Antifungal	Amphotericin B, nystatin
Antiviral	Lamivudine (3TC)
Anthelminthic	Ivermectin
Bacteriostatic cationic peptides	Magainins, defensins, sapecins, bectenecins
Insecticidal	*Bacillus thuringiensis* δ-toxin
Insecticidal	Spinosad
Herbicidal	Phosphinothricin, bialaphos
Anticoccidial	Monensin, nosiheptide
Antitumor	Doxorubicin, mitomycin C
Cytotoxic	Mitoxantrone, mitomycin C
Immunosuppressive	Cyclosporin, rapamycin, tacrolimus
Growth promoters	Monensin
Anticholesterolemic	Lovastatin, pravistatin
Proteinase inhibitors	Aprotinin
Protein kinase inhibitors	Staurosporin
Protein phosphatase inhibitors	Dephostatin
G1- and G2-specific cell cycle inhibitors	Trichostatin A, trapoxin
Matrix metalloproteinase inhibitor	Marimostat
Commercial Fe^{2+} chelator	Desferol (a siderophore)

developed for commercial use in the United States. Moreover, from the early 1960s, when nalidixic acid was developed as the first quinolone antibiotic, to 1996, no new classes of antibiotics have been introduced to the market. In 1993, only 1 new antibiotic was approved by the Food and Drug Administration for use in the United States, none in 1994, and only a few in 1995 and 1996.

Figure 3 indicates the percentage of natural product antibiotics eventually commercialized out of all natural products reported during the same period. Though this percentage is probably not an absolute forecaster, owing to the 7 to 10 years often required for commercialization and clinical testing, it does give a general barometer for commercialization success. From World War II to 1975, approximately 1.6% of all natural product antibiotics reported (either by publication or patent) were commercialized. Since 1975, this number has dropped to about 0.11%. These data suggest that the "Golden Era" of antibiotics, generally recognized as having begun shortly after World War II ended, lasted nearly 30 years. In fact, as shown in Figure 2, 16 natural products first reported in the period of 1971–1975 have since been commercialized. This suggests that since the "Golden Era" of natural products from about the end of World War II to the mid 1970s, fewer and fewer antibiotics have been commercialized from an increasingly larger pool of purified candidate compounds.

Why is this? There are two probable reasons for this. First, traditional methods used to "discover" novel natural products include (a) screening organisms to find ones producing new, structurally and functionally different antibiotics; (b) mutation of microorganisms to produce new activities; (c) fusions of protoplasts of two microorganisms, each

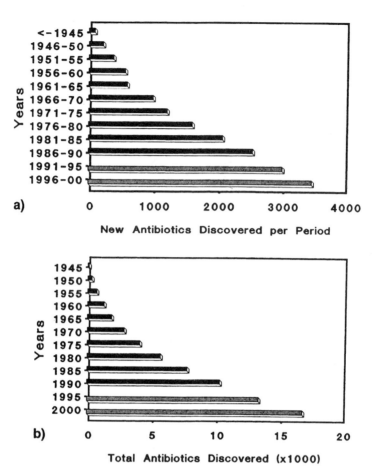

Figure 1 Natural product antibiotics discovered. (a) Number of new natural product antibiotics discovered within each five-year period from 1945. The numbers for the periods 1991–1995 and 1996–2000 (hatched bars) are projected figures. (b) The accumulated totals of natural product antibiotics discovered from 1945 to the year 2000. The numbers for the periods 1991–1995 and 1996–2000 (hatched bars) are projected figures. (Data modified from Ref. 8.)

producing a desired trait, followed by selection for recombinants having combined desired traits; (d) chemical or biochemical modification of a backbone molecule produced by a microorganism; (e) directed biosynthesis by biochemical modification of structures synthesized chemically; and (f) mutasynthesis in which analogs of antibiotics formed by convergent pathways are produced by eliminating the endogenous synthesis of one of the precursors by mutation and replacing the missing building block by exogenously added analogs. Additionally, several important commercial antibiotics, including the carbapenems imipenem and merepenem, have been synthesized chemically, using structures produced in nature as templates for enhanced or more desirable activities.

Past and many current antibiotic screening programs, no matter how sophisticated the screens, have utilized mostly empirical approaches that relied on the principle of serendipity for success. With a large enough sample size, a high enough throughput, and

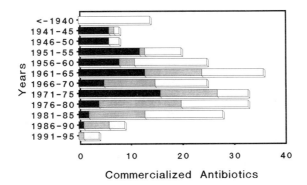

Figure 2 Currently commercialized antibiotics shown in the years in which they were first reported (either by patent application or publication) in five-year blocks from 1945 to 1995. The contributions of natural product antibiotics (solid), semisynthetic antibiotics (shaded), and chemically synthesized antibiotics (hatched) to the totals are indicated. Data are taken from those antibiotics listed in the Appendix and are not necessarily inclusive of all antibiotics commercialized worldwide.

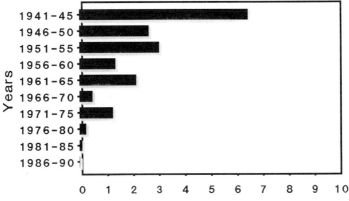

Figure 3 Percentage of natural product antibiotics eventually commercialized out of the total number of natural product antibiotics discovered, given in five-year blocks for the years in which they were first reported (either by patent application or publication).

a broad enough screen base (i.e., number of different activities screened), candidates were always eventually found that could be developed and tested as potential new therapeutic agents. Although these traditional approaches served well and have led to the discovery of most of the current production-scale antibiotics, Figure 3 shows that there has been a diminishing return, most likely due to the rediscovery of known entities. One could only venture a guess at how many times streptomycin and tetracycline have been "rediscovered" in natural products screening programs.

Moreover, existing natural product and chemically synthesized commercial antibacterial antibiotics fall into relatively restricted groups of structures (e.g., β-lactams, aminoglycosides, quinolones, macrolides, glycopeptides) that act on only 15 different bacterial targets (e.g., cell wall assembly, ribosomal protein synthesis, DNA gyrase). In fact, the antibacterial market is dominated by second, third, and fourth generation cephalosporins and penicillins. Successfully commercialized antifungal antibiotics have fallen into the

Table 2 A Partial List of Infectious Agents That Present Serious Problems for Today's Health Care Professionals

Infectious agent/condition	Comments
Bacterial:	
Enterococcus faecium	Most common antibiotic-resistant organism found in long-care facilities; vancomycin-resistant strains increasing; since these organisms are already resistant to most other antibiotics used for their treatment (e.g., aminoglycosides, β-lactams), vancomycin-resistant strains are virtually untreatable with existing antibiotics; as recently as 10 years ago this organism was not predicted as a potentially important pathogen.
Staphylococcus aureus	Methicillin-resistant strains increasing; these strains are currently treatable with vancomycin; the most widely feared possibility is the emergence of vancomycin-resistant staphylococci; also, TSST-1 toxin-producing *S. aureus* strains are the causative agents of toxic shock syndrome, associated with the use of hyperabsorbant tampons.
Acinetobacter baumanni	Newly emergent nosocomial pathogen that can cause sepsis and mortality in infected hospital patients.
Streptococcus pneumoniae	Common pathogen for several diseases is now being found resistant to aminoglycosides, chloramphenicol, ciprofloxacin, tetracycline, and sulfonamides.
Mycobacterium tuberculosis	Rifampin-, isoniazid-, streptomycin-, ethambutol-, and ethionamide-resistant strains have been found that are virtually untreatable with existing antibiotics; cases have increased 28% since the 1980s.
Group A streptococci	Certain strains produce erythrogenic toxins that cause "toxic shock–like" syndrome, a severe form of which can be fatal.
Escherichia coli	Third generation cephalosporin–resistant strains with extended-spectrum β-lactamases are starting to appear.
Escherichia coli O157-H7	New food-borne strain, first isolated in 1982, causes hemorrhagic colitis and other symptoms.
Pseudomonas aeruginosa	Ciprofloxacin-resistant strains of this opportunistic pathogen are beginning to appear.
Legionnella pneumophila	Emergent disease-causing organism discovered in the summer of 1976 at Legionnaires' convention in Philadelphia.
Borrelia burgdorferi	Causative agent of Lyme disease, an emergent infectious disease discovered in the mid 1970s.
Helicobacter pylori	Causative agent for peptic ulcers and stomach cancer; treatable with clarithromycin (acid-stable macrolide) and omeprazole (acid-lowering, cellular proton-pump inhibitor). NIH recently recommended a triple-drug therapy consisting of metronidizole, tetracycline (or alternatively, amoxicillin), and bismuth subsalicylate.
Vibrio cholerae	Reemergence as important infectious agent punctuated by 385,000 cases of cholera in 1994; *Vibrio cholerae* 0139 is a particularly dangerous new variant.
Hemophilis influenzae	One of the organisms causing otitis media, the most common pediatric community-based infection; 20% of all strains are now ampicillin resistant, and more than 50% of strains isolated in Spain are resistant to both chloramphenicol and trimethoprim–sulfamethoxazole.

Table 2 Continued

Infectious agent/condition	Comments
Viral:	
HIV	Promising therapy includes use of combination agents AZT, 3TC, and HIV-1 proteinase inhibitors.
Hantavirus	Rodent-carried virus responsible for deaths in U.S. Southwest; treated with bradykinin antagonist and ribavirin.
Ebola	A filovirus, related to the Marburg virus, that causes hemorrhagic fever. Mortality rate is 50–75%.
Eukaryotic microorganisms:	
Plasmodium falciparum	Several strains of this malaria-causing parasite have become chloroquine resistant.
Candida albicans	Azole-resistant strains are emerging; invasive candidiasis has recently increased 10-fold to become the fourth leading fungal infection in immunocompromised patients.
Invasive pulmonary aspergillosis	Leading cause of death among bone-marrow transplant recipients.
Pneumocystis carinii	Causes a pneumonia that is a leading cause of death in patients with AIDS; this yeastlike organism is naturally resistant to polyene, azole, allylamin, and thiocarbamate antifungal drugs since they all interact with ergosterol present in the membrane of all fungi except *Pneumocystis* spp.
Cryptococcal meningitis	Treated with amphotericin B and flucytosine.
Trichomonas	Metronidazole-resistant strains are emerging.
Cryptosporidium	Water-borne organisms caused an outbreak of diarrhea in Wisconsin in 1994.

same pattern, with most having either polyene- or azole-based structures, and activities directed at cell membrane assembly or integrity.

Virtually every antibiotic discovered or developed over the past 30 years has belonged to the existing classes of antibiotics, that is, variations on known themes for which resistance mechanisms are already entrenched in the environment. Thus, very few antibiotics with substantially different structures or target sites have been discovered to date. There are two significant problems with this trend. First, the law of diminishing returns is more quickly realized with a smaller pool of structure types or sites of activity. Second, acquired or inherited mechanisms conferring resistance to one type of antibiotic often confer resistance to others with similar target sites, activities, or structures. Examples of these include the macrolide–lincosamide–streptogramin (MLS) type of resistance, a broad-based resistance mechanism against many protein-synthesis inhibitory antibiotics (13) and multidrug-resistance exporters (14). Thus, when new, potent antibiotics within the current classes are discovered, their efficacy may already be limited in the clinical setting due to the presence of resistance genes to them.

The conclusions reached from these data argue that instead of continuing the search based only on the discovery of new organisms with antimicrobial activities, future searches need to be directed toward discovery of drugs specifically active against new target sites. This approach, described in more detail in Section IV, is being taken seriously today.

The second likely reason for the dearth of commercialized natural product antibiotics from 1975 to the present is that the U.S. government, pharmaceutical companies, and researchers alike turned their efforts toward the defeat of cancer and heart disease, believing that infectious diseases were under control (15,16).

II.   IMPORTANCE OF CONTINUED DEVELOPMENT OF ANTI-INFECTIVES

A.   Why Do We Need New Antibiotics?

In 1969, the U.S. surgeon general confidently predicted that the war against infectious diseases finally had been won, not only in the United States, but worldwide. That attitude was borne out by government policies in the 1980s, in which funding for infectious disease research was not a high priority (17). During the same period, most of the major pharmaceutical companies decreased research and development on anti-infectives, at least partly because of the absence of economic incentive (16). Thus, in light of this recent history, a valid question that needs to be addressed at this point is why we need to continue to develop new antibiotics with new activities. There are several reasons that we need to develop new antibiotics, preferably with novel structures and activities: (a) new pathogens are evolving at an alarming rate. There are more than 30 new infectious diseases (e.g., AIDS, Ebola, Legionnaires disease, hantavirus, Lyme disease, and the potentially fatal illness caused by food-borne *Escherichia coli* O157:H7; see Table 2) in existence today that were unknown as recently as 20 years ago (18); (b) pathogenic bacteria are acquiring or developing resistance to existing antibiotics and classes of antibiotics in direct correlation with the level of use of those antibiotics to treat them (19). Widespread antibiotic use has resulted in the rapid spread of multidrug-resistant pathogens, and it has become both a local and global health hazard of epidemic proportions; (c) even with the development of remarkable antibiotics that have outstanding biological activities, there are still certain organisms that, in their role as a pathogen, naturally defy even the best antibiotics designed to treat them. Perhaps the best example of this is our current inability to successfully treat *Pseudomonas aeruginosa* infections resulting from cystic fibrosis (20); (d) many potentially important antibiotics have associated toxicities that limit their use. The best example of this is gentamycin and other aminoglycosides, which are limited in effectiveness due to their associated nephrotoxicity and ototoxicity (21). Thus, recent history shows us that not only have we not won the war, but that we face the critical battles ahead to determine if we can win it.

With the statement, "and it is frightening to realize that one single base change in a gene encoding a bacterial β-lactamase can render useless $100 million worth of pharmaceutical research effort" (22), Julian Davies succinctly summed up the problem with development of antibiotic resistance by pathogenic bacteria. The most critical reason for the continued development of new antibiotics is the very expensive and time-consuming race to remain a step ahead of antibiotic-resistance development, which has proceeded at an astonishing rate (23). As it stands today, the development of commercially successful new antibiotics seems not to be keeping pace with the development of resistance to existing agents (24). When the newly emergent antibiotic-resistant strains became prevalent enough to cause widespread concern (over just the past five years or so; 9–12, 16–19, 22–24), there was a marked paucity of new structures and novel activities in the anti-infectives pipeline to take up the fight. Since it requires at least seven years and more than $200 million to get most new drugs approved, this has caused a lag in the number of new antibacterials on the current market that may be able to tackle methicillin- and vancomycin-resistant staphylococci, the ultimate fear of health care professionals. What happens in the way of drug development over the next decade may decide whether we enter a "new era of antibiotics" or a "postantibiotic era," in which the so-called magic bullets would become useless against drug-resistant pathogens (24).

B. Emergence of Antibiotic-Resistant Bacteria

With the emergence of new infectious diseases, as well as the emergence of bacterial strains resistant to existing antibiotics, there is an enormous challenge to pharmaceutical companies, researchers, and governments to develop new methods for treating both existing infectious diseases and those emerging as new health threats.

One of the greatest health threats is the prevalence of untreatable nosocomial infections. Nearly half of all nosocomial infections are caused by *Enterococcus faecium*, *Enterococcus faecalis*, *Streptococcus pneumoniae*, *Staphylococcus aureus*, or *P. aeruginosa* (25). The Centers for Disease Control and Prevention (CDC) estimates that, of the 40 million hospitalizations in the United States each year, 2 million patients contract nosocomial infections, and that as many as 58,000 patients die from them each year (26). According to the CDC, 13,300 U.S. patients died in 1992 of antibiotic-resistant bacterial infections. Additionally, they found that there was a 150% increase in drug-resistant pneumococci between 1987 and 1994 (27), as well as a 20-fold increase in hospital-acquired vancomycin-resistant enterococci (mostly *E. faecium*, but also a fraction of *E. faecalis*) between 1989 and 1993 (0.3% incidence to ca. 8% incidence) (28). Unfortunately, vancomycin-resistant enterococci are nearly untreatable with current antibiotics, with the possible exceptions of the experimental drugs Synercid or teichoplanin, which have been used successfully to treat some cases of vancomycin-resistant enterococci (29). The mortality rate of patients infected with multiple-drug-resistant enterococci is 70%, making this a serious health care problem (29).

C. Antibiotic Resistance: Evolution in Progress

The greatest concern today is that the use of antibiotics results in the development of resistance by pathogens to those antibiotics, a situation coined by Levy in 1992 as *The Antibiotic Paradox* (1). Contrary to popular belief, this is not a new concern. Within four years after the introduction of penicillin during World War II, several strains of penicillin-resistant bacteria were isolated from infected patients (30). As early as 1949, Mary Barber recognized the possibility that drug resistance might be inheritable, rather than attained by simple mutation, when she observed penicillin-resistant staphylococci could lose their resistance (31).

There are several examples of widespread antibiotic use resulting in resistance to the antibiotics used. As Japan was being rebuilt after World War II, sulfonamide-resistant *Shigella* spp. presented a serious health hazard to the population in the form of outbreaks of dysentery. The newly developed antibiotics, streptomycin, tetracycline, and chloramphenicol, were introduced in 1950 to help quell the growing problem. By 1956, however, a strain of *Shigella flexneri* was isolated that was resistant to sulfonamides, streptomycin, tetracycline, and chloramphenicol, and by 1969, 7225 of 10,462 strains tested (69%) were resistant to sulfonamides, streptomycin, tetracycline, and chloramphenicol (32).

Thus, over a period of less than 20 years, nearly 70% of all *Shigella* spp. in Japan became resistant to four antibiotics to which there was minimal resistance prior to their use (32).

In a second example, *E. coli* isolates tested from 1983 through 1990 were universally sensitive to fluoroquinolones (33). From 1991 to 1993, however, 28% of *E. coli* strains tested were resistant to fluoroquinolones. This increase in resistance was directly correlated with the increased use of fluoroquinolones, which were used to treat patients in 1.4% of all cases in 1983–1985, but were used 45% of the time in the period 1991–1993 (33).

It was once thought that microorganisms would never become vancomycin resistant, because the mechanism of action of vancomycin was different from that of other antibiotics (34). Vancomycin has long been the last line of defense against antibiotic-resistant bacteria, particularly methicillin-resistant staphylococci and β-lactam- and aminoglycoside-resistant enterococci. Thus, for several years there was an attitude that if nothing else worked, at least vancomycin would. This illusion was shattered when the discovery of vancomycin-resistant enterococci in England and France was reported in 1987 (35). Now, vancomycin-resistant enterococci are being discovered at an alarming rate, with no new "last line of defense" substitute firmly entrenched on the market (36). Currently, as many as 14% of all patients in some intensive-case units were infected with vancomycin-resistant enterococci (28,36).

Plasmid-encoded TEM- and SHV-type β-lactamases are the most common mechanisms responsible for β-lactam resistance in Gram-negative bacteria (37). These β-lactamases have generally broad substrate specificities for penicillins, as well as some first and second generation cephalosporins, and are responsible for much of the resistance to β-lactams observed in the clinics. It is well documented that as new β-lactams have been developed to resist plasmid-borne β-lactamases, the β-lactamases themselves have evolved (22,37). In an incredible example of directed evolution, TEM- and SHV-type β-lactamases recently have been found containing specific point mutations, all falling in close proximity to the active-site cavity, that confer resistance to third generation cephalosporins and monobactams (37).

Not all clinically significant antibiotic resistance is plasmid- or transposon-mediated. *S. pneumoniae*, the organism with which bacterial transformation was first observed, is the primary causative agent in pneumonia and pediatric otitis media (inner ear infections), and it is also significant in bacterial meningitis and bacteremia. Although *S. pneumoniae* remained penicillin-sensitive for many years, an alarming number of penicillin-resistant *S. pneumoniae* strains have recently been isolated from infected patients, not surprisingly coincident with the use of penicillins to treat these infections (38). These penicillin-resistant *S. pneumoniae* were found not to produce β-lactamases, the common plasmid-borne mechanism for resistance, but instead had developed mutations leading to altered penicillin-binding proteins (PBPs), the target for penicillin activity (38).

S. aureus, a bacterium well adapted to living on human skin, is the major cause of postsurgical and skin infections (39). Unfortunately, this organism is one of the most dangerous bacteria, causing close to 25% mortality among those with severe infections (40). In a demonstration of the Levy's antibiotic paradox, the Oxford strain of *S. aureus*, isolated 50 years ago, was found to be sensitive to virtually every antibiotic tested against it (40). Thus, prior to the use of antibiotics, *S. aureus* contained few, if any, resistance mechanisms. The staphylococci, however, acquired resistance to aminoglycosides very quickly, and by 1992, 32% of *S. aureus* strains tested were found to be resistant to methicillin (the "drug of choice" to treat staphylococcus infections), up from 2% in 1975 (40).

Like pneumococci, methicillin-resistant staphylococci have altered PBPs, giving them a resistance mechanism that cannot be countered easily. Thus, vancomycin has become the drug of last resort to treat methicillin-resistant staphylococci. Ever since E. *faecalis* was shown to transfer vancomycin resistance to S. *aureus* in the laboratory in 1992 (41), one of the greatest fears of health professionals universally has been the emergence of vancomycin-resistant, methicillin-resistant staphylococci (42). Recently, such doubly resistant, virtually untreatable strains have appeared in sporadic cases, confirming the greatest concerns of health care professionals (43). Now the question becomes, will vancomycin-resistant staphylococci emerge faster than the time required to fully develop and test alternatives to vancomycin?

A new mechanism of antibiotic resistance recently was discovered in meropenem-resistant P. *aeruginosa* strains (44). P. *aeruginosa* is an opportunistic pathogen that contributes to nosocomial infections, eye infections, and opportunistic infections of burn patients and those with cystic fibrosis. The mechanism was found to be based on the alteration of outer membrane proteins, causing a reduction in permeability of several antibiotics, including meropenem, through the outer membrane (44). This is a significant finding, since carbapenems (e.g., imipenem) have been considered the antibiotics of choice for the treatment of opportunistic pseudomonads. Moreover, since meropenem has just recently been approved for treatment of bacterial infections, this important finding suggests that antibiotics with completely new structures, activities, and sites of activity may have to be found to combat antibiotic-resistant Gram-negative bacteria in the future.

Finally, antibiotic resistance in Mycobacterium *tuberculosis* is considered to be a major growing problem. Currently, a combination treatment with isoniazid and rifamycin is the method of choice, but many strains of M. *tuberculosis* have recently been found that are resistant to one or both of these antibiotics, and approximately 14% of all tuberculosis cases reported today involve M. *tuberculosis* strains that are resistant to one or more antibiotics (45). The problem facing health care professionals today is that there is no proven effective alternative yet on the market to treat isoniazid- and rifamycin-resistant M. *tuberculosis* (45).

III. ANTIBIOTICS IN THE PIPELINE: A NEW ERA DAWNING TO MEET THE CHALLENGES OF THE TWENTY-FIRST CENTURY

A. A New Era of Antibiotics?

With the recent emergence of new diseases, such as Legionnaires and Lyme diseases, the reemergence of resistant forms of long-known diseases such as tuberculosis, and the emergence of antibiotic-resistant bacteria, a new emphasis has been placed on anti-infective drugs. The contention made here is that this new emphasis, in combination with extraordinary technical advances made in chemistry, biochemistry, molecular biology, and drug formulations over the past few years, will generate a new era of antibiotics, which will be characterized by (a) development of new generations of semisynthetic drugs based on existing structures; (b) revolutionary new therapy regimens developed to deliver drugs more specifically to their intended targets; (c) development of completely new classes of antibacterial, antifungal, and antiviral drugs through combinatorial chemistry and biochemistry approaches, as well as by discovery of novel natural products from exotic sources; (d) more enhanced screening procedures and strategies, including multitudes of

Table 3 Some Promising Antibiotics and Pharmaceutically Active Natural Products Recently Developed or Under Development

Compound	Comments
Synercid	Roche product now in phase III clinical trials; combination of quinupristin (RP57669) and dalfopristin (RP54476), both semisynthetic streptogramins.
HIV proteinase-1 inhibitors	Indinavir, ritonavir, and saquinovir were approved for use in record times (from 42–90 days) in 1995–1996 by the FDA for use in combination therapy against HIV.
3TC and other nucleosides	Approved in 1995 for use in treatment of HIV infections; see Chapter 25.
Echinocandins	Antifungal drugs currently being tested by Eli Lilly; see Chapter 10.
Pneumocandins	Antifungal drugs being tested by Merck.
Polyoxins	Pyrimidine peptide antifungal agents, produced by *Streptomyces cacaoi*, that inhibit cell wall chitin biosynthesis; used to inhibit agriculturally significant fungi.
Spinosyns	Nontoxic bioinsecticides being developed by Eli Lilly from Spinosad, a natural product.
Cationic peptides	Micrologix, Inc., and Magainin Biotech, Inc., are two of the companies developing natural and recombinant cationic peptides for use as enhancers in combination therapy; see Chapter 16.
Lantibiotics	Nisin and other lantibiotics (lanthionin-containing peptides) are being developed by Applied Microbiology, Inc., for use in treatment of peptic ulcer disease, skin infections, periodontal disease, systemic nosocomial infections, and bovine mastitis; see Chapter 15.
Human lactoferrin	Aggenix, Inc., is developing this Fe^{2+}-sequestering glycoprotein as an antibacterial drug.
LY333328	A chloro-biphenyl vancomycin derivative that has considerably higher potency than vancomycin; it is currently undergoing testing by Eli Lilly as a vancomycin alternative; see Chapter 12.
Pirarubicin	A 4′-substituted anthracycline, developed based on the structure of baumycin A; it is considerably less cardiotoxic than doxorubicin while retaining the efficacy; see Chapter 20.
Rapamycin	A macrolide, produced by *Streptomyces hygroscopicus*, under investigation as immunosuppressive agent to combat organ rejection after transplantation; see Chapter 17.
Quinolone antitumor drugs	Quinolones, based on the structure of nalidixic acid, are bacteria DNA gyrase inhibitors; some, however, are also excellent inhibitors of mammalian topoisomerase II, the target of several antitumor drugs, including doxorubicin.
2-Pyridones	Synthesized by transposition of the nitrogen of 4-quinolines; the modifications result in a new series of DNA gyrase inhibitory drugs that have outstanding *in vitro* activities against a broad range of bacteria, including methicillin-resistant staphylococci, vancomycin-resistant enterococci, and ciprofloxacin-resistant bacteria.
Oxazolidinones	Two new oxazolidinones are being tested by Upjohn as potential broad-spectrum antibiotics for use against vancomycin-resistant enterococci and staphylococci.
Glycylglycines	9-Substituted derivatives of tetracyclines for which ribosomal or export-based resistance has not been exhibited. N,N-dimethylglycylamido derivatives of minocycline and 6-demethyl-6-deoxytetracycline are potent, new wide-spectrum antibiotics; see Chapter 21.

Table 3   Continued

Compound	Comments
Everninomycins	Although isolated in the early 1980s, these compounds show strong activity against vancomycin-resistant enterococci and staphylococci; these were originally abandoned as candidates due to some inherent toxicities and the flood of antibiotics on the market in the late 1970s.
PA 1648	Rifampin derivative being developed by PathoGenesis Corp., Seattle, Washington, that has excellent activity against *Mycobacterium tuberculosis* and *Mycobacterium avium-M, intracellulare* complex (MAC), the most common opportunistic bacterial infection of AIDS patients.
Acyclovir-monophosphate	A topical formulation of acyclovir developed by Triangle Pharmaceuticals, Inc., that can be used against herpes labialis.

newly developed target-based screens; and (e) continued and expanded discovery of new pharmacological uses for existing structures and analogs of those structures.

B.   New Antibiotics on the Horizon

As of 1995, there were 79 new, non-AIDS-related anti-infective drugs and vaccines, 28 of which were antibiotics, in development by 49 different U.S. companies (4). Additionally, 103 medicines and vaccines are currently in development for AIDS and AIDS-related opportunistic infections (4). Table 3 lists a few promising anti-infective agents that are currently in clinical testing or that have recently entered the commercial market. A few of these are discussed in more detail in this section.

Is there a new wonder drug out there, coming to the rescue of a world population in need of a cure for vancomycin-resistant Gram-positive bacteria? Possibly, there is. For more than 25 years, pristinamycin has been used in Europe as a drug to combat severe infections caused by both Gram-positive and -negative bacteria, notably without development of resistance against it (46). Pristinamycin is actually a combination of two antibiotics, pristinamycin I_A (a peptidic macrolactone belonging to the streptogramin B group) and pristinamycin II_A (a polyunsaturated macrolactone belonging to the streptogramin A group) (46). Each component alone is bacteriostatic with poor efficacy, but the combination is bacteriocidal with excellent activity against a broad range of bacteria (46). The usefulness of pristinamycin, however, has been limited due to its poor solubility (47). In February 1996, however, Rhône-Poulenc Rhorer introduced Synercid, a new variation on pristinamycin. Synercid (RP59500), which is a mixture of the two water-soluble, semisynthetic streptogramins, quinupristin (RP57669) and dalfopristin (RP54476) (48), is currently in phase III clinical trials worldwide and is currently available in the United States and Europe in an emergency use program. More than 700 patients have recently received Synercid in this program. In one study, 70% of 115 patients with vancomycin-resistant enterococcal infections were successfully treated (i.e., infection cleared) with Synercid (49). Synercid has been found to be bactericidal for most Gram-positive bacteria, but bacteriostatic for *Listeria monocytogenes* (48). In one study, 96% of all staphylococci tested were sensitive to Synercid in vitro (46), suggesting that this drug may become the "vancomycin of the future," that is, a drug of last resort for use against severe bacterial infections. A particularly positive aspect of this combination drug is that it is unaffected by classical rRNA-methylase-conferred MLS resistance mechanisms, the most common resistance mechanisms found in staphylococci (50). Other MLS resistance mechanisms such as acetylation or hydrolysis of streptogramins still affect these compounds, however, so that they are not completely impervious to bacterial resistance mechanisms (50).

As mentioned previously, vancomycin is currently considered the last line of defense against many important Gram-positive pathogenic bacteria, including methicillin-resistant *S. aureus* and antibiotic-resistant *E. faecium*. The increase in vancomycin-resistant strains of both of these organisms has health care professionals extremely worried (42). Eli Lilly has recently been testing an analog of vancomycin currently known as LY333328, a chloro-biphenyl derivative, which is considerably more potent than vancomycin (51). Moreover, LY333328 appears not only to inhibit bacterial growth, but to kill existing bacteria, which may give it a distinct clinical advantage over other existing antibiotics. LY333328, as well as other glycopeptide analogs, has been reported to be very potent against vancomycin-resistant enterococci (52), giving hope for treatment of vancomycin-resistant pathogens.

Meropenem (Merrem, Zeneca Pharmaceuticals; Wilmington, DE) (53) is a new carbopenem antibiotic approved in 1996 for use as a broad-spectrum injectable antibiotic for treatment of intraabdominal infections and for pediatric bacterial meningitis. The only other carbopenem available on the market today is imipenem.

Pharmacia and Upjohn is testing two new drugs in the class of oxazolidones for their ability to treat multiple-drug-resistant strains of *M. tuberculosis* (54). These new antibiotics, obtained from a directed chemical synthesis program, inhibit protein synthesis in a manner different from other protein synthesis–inhibitory antibiotics, have novel structures unrelated to those of other antibiotics, and have a wide spectrum of activity (54). Experiments have shown that, at least in in vitro tests, pathogens do not form resistance against these antibiotics at significant frequencies.

A new aminoglycoside antibiotic, arbekacin, has been developed in Japan for use against methicillin-, gentamycin-, and tobramycin-resistant *S. aureus* strains (55). The incidence of methicillin-resistant *S. aureus* in Japan has risen to nearly 60%, and only vancomycin and the newly developed arbekacin are approved for treatment of these strains. The new aminoglycoside is apparently effective, because the widely distributed resistance mechanism, a bifunctional aminoglycoside phosphotransferase (APH[2″])-6′-acetyltransferase (AAC[6′]), which confers resistance to other aminoglycosides such as gentamycin and tobramycin, is relatively ineffective at modifying the new drug (55). It is probable that within a few years, however, APH(2″)–AAC(6′) will evolve so that it can modify arbekacin.

Another totally new class of drugs being tested as anti-infectives is the cationic peptides (56,57). One example is the development of cationic peptides as "enhancers" that disrupt bacterial membranes by displacing Mg^{2+} (56,57). Magainin Pharmaceuticals, Inc., and Micrologix, Inc., are two companies that are developing cationic peptides, naturally produced antibiotics from tissues as diverse as tongue epithelium and frog skin, as enhancers of normal antibiotic functions. These cationic peptides have marginal anti-infective properties of their own, but when used with other antibiotics, they act synergistically to yield a potent combination (56,57). Just as in the natural environments in which these cationic peptides are produced, it is expected that therapeutic use of these drugs will be best applied as topical antimicrobials or used in "closed spaces" (57).

In some cases, efficacious drugs are available but their synthesis, biosynthesis, or recovery make them extremely expensive and, therefore, less available to needy patients worldwide than desired. The most important discovery made in the anticancer field since doxorubicin has been the finding that paclitaxel (Taxol) has excellent activity against ovarian and breast cancers. Additionally, Taxol and semisynthetic taxanes may be efficacious against a wide range of tumors. Thus far, the greatest impediment to the development of these drugs on a large scale was that they are only found at levels of about 0.01% (w/w) in the bark of several related yew trees, *Taxus brevifolia* (Pacific yew, an endangered species), *Taxus baccata*, *Taxus cuspidata* (Japanese yew), and others (58). Moreover, the chemical synthesis of paclitaxel is very difficult, requiring more than 30 steps. Thus, paclitaxel is currently made semisynthetically from 10-deacetylbaccatin III, produced by the needles of the Himalayan yew (58). Very recently, an important breakthrough was made in the production of paclitaxel in tissue culture. Yukimune et al. (58) discovered that addition of methyl jasmonate to cell cultures of *Taxus* spp. resulted in dramatically increased levels of taxane production. Though their results will not lead immediately to a commercialized process, they are a significant step in the right direction. With this effort and others, we hope to see the commercial production of antitumor taxanes from tissue cultures by the turn of the century.

IV. NEW APPROACHES AND STRATEGIES FOR THE BIOSYNTHESIS OF NEW ANTIBIOTICS AND PHARMACEUTICALLY ACTIVE BIOMOLECULES

A. New Sources of Raw Material for Screening Programs

The questions asked here are (a) Are we doing enough to stay ahead of the ever-increasing pool of antibiotic resistance genes in the environment? and (b) Can we develop antibiotics to which there is no inherent resistance? Based on its mode of action, vancomycin was at one time thought to be an antibiotic to which resistance could not be achieved; yet, we now know that there are specific vancomycin resistance genes in bacterial populations that are becoming rapidly disseminated.

One of the methods used currently is to broaden the source of the screens; hence, companies are now searching for new compounds from samples obtained from tropical rain forests to deserts and oceans. The didemnins, which displayed potent antiviral and antitumor activities, were the first pharmaceuticals obtained from a marine source to be tested in the clinic (59). These, and other marine-derived drugs, have relatively unusual structures that eventually may provide new activities against atypical targets (59).

Some interesting new compounds have been found using expanded sources of raw material, such as myxobacteria, strong antibiotic producers that are just now being mined (60), marine bacteria (59), and bacteria from extreme environments such as hot springs. Even with the expectation that these relatively new sources will yield a new diversity of pharmacologically active agents, however, it is clear that other, new avenues must be found to broaden the chances for development of usable anti-infective agents. Thus, many pharmaceutical companies have retooled their thinking about how to develop new antibiotics.

B. New Uses for Existing Compounds

Most compounds isolated in broad-based screening programs in the past were tested for obvious activities such as an antibacterial, antifungal, and antiviral activities. Over the years, certain compounds originally found to have poor antibiotic activities were later found to have remarkable pharmaceutical activities of other types. Although this typically does not solve the greatest challenge today, namely, the problem of drug-resistant bacteria, it can lead to the discovery of important pharmacologically active drugs for the betterment of society.

The classic example is cyclosporin, a weak antifungal agent produced by *Tolypocladium inflatum* (61), which was later found through the efforts of René Traber to be a useful immunosuppressive agent. This drug was singly responsible for the dramatic increase in the number of successful tissue and organ transplants in recent years. Similarly, FK506 (tacrolimus), rapamycin, and immunomycin, new drugs that may someday replace, or at least share the immunosuppressive market with, cyclosporin, were themselves originally isolated as weak antibiotics.

C. Target-Directed Screens and Rational Drug Design

Traditional screening methods for antibiotics, still in wide use today, were based on the ability of a producing organism, or extract obtained from it, to inhibit the growth of a bacterium, irrespective of the mechanism for its action. In those cases, the mechanism of action was determined later. With the advancement of knowledge and technology, screens can be developed based on a specific activity that can be detected in some automatable manner (62). In the most successful example to date, studies on the life cycle of the human immunodeficiency virus (HIV) demonstrated that the viral-encoded aspartyl proteinase, involved in viral maturation, was required for spread of the virus (7). Thus, target-directed screens for inhibitors specific for the HIV-1 proteinase, that is, target-specific antibiotics (7), have been developed. In 1992, Kuntz (62) described the approaches and requirements for structure-based design. Examples he included as possible targets for inhibition of HIV included HIV-1 proteinase, CD4, gp120, reverse transcriptase, integrase, tat, TAR, and rev (62).

Since most existing antibacterial antibiotics function to inhibit only a few targets, the most obvious approach for the development of completely new classes of anti-infectives is to develop target-specific drugs. Examples of existing bacterial targets as sites for antibacterial activity include dihydropteroate synthase, dihydrofolate synthase, β-lactamases, and aminoglycoside-modifying enzymes (62). Examples of potential sites not already targeted include DNA replication and particularly DNA polymerase III, the cell-division protein FtsZ, antibiotic efflux pumps, leader peptidases responsible for secreting outer membrane proteins, sensor kinase-response regulator two-component systems, and fibronectin-binding mechanisms for those organisms that require binding to fibronectin to confer pathogenicity (63). Desnottes (63) has recently described for each of these potential targets straightforward assays that would allow high-throughput screening methods to be employed. Another possible target in bacteria is phospho-*N*-acetylmuramyl-pentapeptide translocase (translocase I), which catalyzes the first in the cycle of membrane-associated reactions of peptidoglycan biosynthesis (64). Two new antibiotics, liposidomycin B, a potential antimycobacterial natural product, and mureidomycin A, which shows strong antipseudomonad activity, were recently found to inhibit this translocase reaction (64).

Microcide Pharmaceuticals, Inc. (Mountainview, California), which boasts that it is the only company entirely devoted to battling antibiotic-resistant bacterial infections, has developed a method by which they can identify the 5–10% of genes required for the survival of a bacterium, without sequencing the entire genome. They have developed a collaboration with Pfizer to utilize this knowledge in combination with high-throughput screening technology, to develop novel target-based approaches for the discovery of new antibiotics with completely new types of activities (5).

D.   Combinatorial Biochemistry: Hybrid Antibiotics

Hopwood and his colleagues first demonstrated, in 1985, the principle of "hybrid antibiotics," formed by cloning heterologous antibiotic biosynthesis genes from a producing strain into another strain producing a similar compound (65). There are two basic approaches in the application of this principle: (a) cloning of single or multiple genes encoding structural modification (or "decorating") reactions, such as those encoding methyltransferases, hydroxylases, reductases, oxidases, and so forth, to modify basic structures produced by the host organism. This was the approach used by Hopwood et al. (65) in their initial description of hybrid antibiotics; and (b) cloning or mixing and matching of core biosynthetic enzymes, yielding completely new core molecules. This fundamentally novel approach was first employed by Bartel et al. (66), who cloned actinorhodin polyketide synthase (PKS) genes from *Streptomyces coelicolor* into *Streptomyces galilaeus* strains ATCC 31133 and 31671 in efforts to produce new core structures. The principles of recombining type II PKS components, first established by Bartel et al. (66), were placed into practice by Chaitan Khosla, David Hopwood, and their colleagues (67–69), who developed an expression system in which the ever-growing diversity of available type II polyketide biosynthesis gene clusters could be mixed and matched to form completely new combinations of type II polyketide biosynthesis machinery. The results obtained from the mix and match approaches pioneered by Khosla and coworkers have helped to define the roles of components of the type II polyketide biosynthesis clusters. Nevertheless, we are now beginning to appreciate that notions of single protein functionality, such as "chain length factor" and "aromatase," are probably oversimplified. It is beginning to appear that multiple protein components together are responsible for chain length, starter unit selection, and initial folding (70). The combinatorial approach to the development of new aromatic polyketides, reviewed by Hutchinson (71), has resulted in a bevy of new compounds (67–69,71). Nevertheless, many of these new polyketides are not the types of structures on which to base the development of new drugs. A few companies, however, have been developed to take advantage of this approach toward the development of new bioactive compounds.

Another exciting result obtained recently in this area is that domains of modular peptide synthetases were able to be exchanged, resulting in the biosynthesis of novel compounds. This is a very important step, because it suggests that a large number of new peptide-based compounds can be created using libraries of peptide-synthetase modules (72). Similarly, the modules of type I PKSs were recently also recombined in efforts to demonstrate the potential utility of developing recombinant macrolide-type hybrid antibiotics (73).

These "hybrid antibiotic" approaches, at least as practiced thus far, have required intensive molecular work and have resulted in the discovery of relatively few new molecules from much effort and expenditure. Nevertheless, the information from these types of experiments has been used, as mentioned below, to generate an entire library of new recombinant, aromatic polyketides that are being tested for a wide variety of new activities.

E.   Directed Evolution of Enzymes and Pathways

A fundamentally new approach toward the development of better activities and new drugs that has been developed within the past few years is the concept of directed evolution of enzymes and pathways (74–76). The principle of directed evolution is to mimic the natural evolution process, but also to accelerate it in vitro, directing it toward an applied goal, such as an enhanced enzymatic activity, broader or altered substrate specificity, or in the case of application of this principle to pathways, even completely new compounds.

This new concept, first described in by Willem Stemmer in 1994 (74,75), is based on the premise that evolution works more efficiently with blocks of a sequence rather than with point mutations. Thus, rather than evolution based on a series of point mutations, as one would obtain using error-prone polymerase chain reaction (PCR) or other random mutagenesis scanning procedures (76), directed evolution is based on the in vitro shuffling and reassembly of DNA sequences (74,75).

In an exciting new research collaboration between ChromaXome Corporation and Bristol-Meyers Squibb (BMS) (77), the principles of directed evolution have been applied to the development of novel type II polyketide biosynthesis pathways producing aromatic polyketide compounds with enhanced biological activities. DNA from 34 BMS strains, all capable of producing type II polyketides, was isolated and used individually or in pools. Cosmid libraries, containing ca. 40 kbp type II PKS gene clusters and associated genes, were constructed and then digested, mixed and matched randomly, and religated. More than 20 billion protoplasts were transformed with products from 200 ligation reactions, and 10,400 resultant transformants were obtained, 8200 of which were mono-pathway recombinations and 2200 of which were intercluster combinatorial clones (77). Screening revealed 205/8200 (2.5%) type II-PKS-producing clones from the mono-pathway recombinants, 9 of which have been passed on for structure elucidation, and 71/2200 (3.2%) type II-producing clones from the combinatorial pathways, 9 of which are being further tested. Whether this particular set of experiments results in production of new antibiotics is secondary, as the approach has proven the principle, with the result that there was a high probability (ca. 3%) of new structures being obtained (77).

F.   Combinatorial Chemistry

Medicinal chemists have traditionally developed new drugs by modifying natural products handed to them from screening programs (78). The drugs developed using this time-honored approach, however, were typically semisynthetically enhanced versions of existing classes of antibiotics, followed by in vitro and in vivo analysis of their biological activities. In the past few years, however, a completely new approach, or paradigm, has been developed for the search of new bioactive chemicals. In this new approach, termed "combinatorial chemistry," large, random chemical libraries are generated, tested *en masse* using mechanism-based high-throughput screens, and then evaluated further as antibacterials using novel methods and approaches (63).

In present combinatorial chemistry designs, a library of compounds is synthesized quickly on solid support systems or polymers. The library is then released from the support, and the resultant new compounds can be screened for a variety of different activities. As of May 1996, at least 16 new chemical companies were started on the concept of using combinatorial chemistry to search for new pharmacologically active compounds

(79). Some larger pharmaceutical companies, including Abbott, for example, have diminished the role of their traditional natural products screening programs to pursue combinatorial chemistry approaches. Other major pharmaceutical firms are developing collaborations with small, specialized combinatorial chemistry companies to generate large libraries (>100,000) of small-molecule organic compounds that can be screened using high-throughput technology. Many companies are combining different types of novel approaches such as combinatorial chemistry, combinatorial biochemistry, and rational drug design with retooled high-throughput screening methods.

The combinatorial chemistry approach is driven at least in part by the development of automated technology and target-based screens for a wide variety of desired biological activities. Using combinatorial chemistry, a company can synthesize thousands of new compounds per week rather than just hundreds per year. In one example, a company recently produced more compounds (ca. 500,000) in six months using combinatorial chemistry than its medicinal chemists had produced in 50 years using traditional methods (79). When coupled with recently developed automated methods for screening extremely large numbers of compounds (i.e., high-throughput screens), this approach is very attractive to modern pharmaceutical and chemical companies. One drawback to this approach, however, is that it does not take advantage of nature's ability to select for biologically significant functions. Thus, though increasing the numbers game, a substantially greater percentage of the chemicals screened have no chance of possessing biological activities. A modification of the combinatorial chemistry paradigm that addresses this issue is limited- or directed-library combinatorial chemical synthesis, in which several similar structures, perhaps utilizing biomimicry as the starting point, can be generated in a random fashion (80).

It is expected that within a few years, all of the major chemical reactions traditionally run in solutions will be able to be carried out using high-speed, solid-support-based reactions. With this in mind, the ultimate goal of combinatorial chemistry is to marry it with rational drug design, based on knowledge of the three-dimensional, x-ray crystallographic structure of the targets, to generate focused libraries of thousands of similarly structured analogs (79).

V. EPILOG

It is clear from the recent discussion by researchers, physicians, pharmaceutical companies, the film and book industry, and the popular press that society now recognizes the threat posed by newly emerging infectious diseases, reemergent diseases, and drug-resistant pathogenic bacteria. The efforts to tackle these threats are being expanded greatly, and though, in the minds of some pessimists, it may be too little and too late, the effort will eventually result in the discovery of new ways to treat these diseases. The recent payoffs in terms of AIDS treatment, with the development of 3TC and HIV proteinase inhibitors, and the discovery of Synercid are just a few of several emerging success stories. New approaches such as combinatorial chemistry, biochemistry, and directed evolution of genes and pathways, not even imagined a decade ago, promise even faster development of new classes of compounds. In this world of overpopulation and developing health crises, the development of antibiotics to treat infectious diseases remains one of our most critical challenges.

ACKNOWLEDGMENTS

I wish to thank Charles L. DeSanti for reading the manuscript and suggesting modifications. The antibiotics research carried out in my laboratory is supported by the National Science Foundation under grant no. MCB-94-05730.

APPENDIX

Important Antibiotics and Bioactive Natural Products in 1996

Compound or name	Class[a]	Comments
Aclacinomycin A	(NP) Anthracycline antitumor drug	Produced by *Streptomyces galilaeus*; triglycosylated anthracycline antitumor agent used in Japan.
Acyclovir	(C) Nucleoside (guanine) analog	Antiviral drug produced by Glaxo under brand name of Zorivax was tenth most prescribed antibiotic in the United States in 1995; used for treatment of herpes.
Aklomide	(C) Chloronitrobenzamide	Coccidiostat for veterinary use.
Amantadine	(C) Amino-adamantane	Antiviral drug for treatment of influenza A–caused infections.
Amikacin sulfate	(SS) Semisynthetic aminoglycoside antibiotic	Derived from kanamycin A; is modified by only two of the nine resistance modification enzymes known for aminoglycosides; used parenterally for infections caused by Gram-negatives.
Amoxicillin	(SS) Semisynthetic analog of ampicillin	Broad-spectrum, orally administered antibiotic; most widely pharmacy-prescribed antibiotic in the United States in 1995; top producers are Smith-Kline Beecham, Apothecon, and Biocraft.
Amoxicillin/clavulanate	(SS/NP) β-Lactam and β-lactamase inhibitor	Smith-Kline Beecham product, Augmentin, is an oral broad-spectrum antibiotic; claimed 5.6% of the market in 1991 to be the second leading antibiotic worldwide, and was the second most pharmacy-prescribed antibiotic in the United States in 1995.

Compound or name	Class[a]	Comments
Amphotericin B	(NP) Polyene	Broad-spectrum, injectable antimycotic drug; exhibits multiple serious side effects, but is only reliable drug against several deeply invasive fungal infections such as aspergillosis; produced by *Streptomyces nodosus*.
Amphotericin, liposomal	(NP) Liposome-entrapped polyene	Liposome Co. product, Abelcet, has recently been approved for systemic aspergillosis.
Ampicillin	(SS) Semisynthetic β-lactam	6-Amino-penicillin derivative is formulated for oral or parenteral administration.
Ampicillin/sulbactam	(SS/SS) β-Lactam and β-lactamase inhibitor	Roerig product, Unasyn, a combination of an amino-penicillin and an effective β-lactamase inhibitor (both semisynthetic), is an approved injectable, broad-spectrum antibiotic.
Amprolium	(C) Substituted pyrimidine	Coccidiostat for veterinary use; feed additive.
Arbekacin	(SS) Semisynthetic aminoglycoside	Meiji Seika product, Habekacin, is in advanced clinical trials for use against bacteria resistant to other aminoglycoside antibiotics.
Atovaquone	(C) Substituted naphthoquinone	Acute oral treatment of trimethoprim–sulfamethoxazole-resistant *Pneumocystis carinii*–caused pneumonia; used to treat pneumocystis-infected AIDS patients; also antiprotozoal.
Avermectin	(NP) Macrolide	Produced by *Streptomyces avermitilis*; Merck product, Ivermectin, is approved for veterinary use as an antiparasitic; has also been used to treat human onchocerciasis (river blindness).
Azathioprine	(C) Substituted imidazolyl-mercaptopurine	Burroughs Wellcome product, Imuran, was approved in 1994 for use as an immunosuppressant to combat organ rejection in kidney transplants.
Azithromycin	(SS) Semisynthetic erythromycin analog	Pfizer product, Zithromax, is an orally administered "azalide," and subclass of macrolides; active against staphylococci, streptococci, *Moraxella catarrhalis*, and *Haemophilus influenzae*.

Compound or name	Class[a]	Comments
Aztreonam	(C) Broad-spectrum mono-bactam antibiotic	Bristol-Meyers Squibb product, Azactam, is a new, recently approved β-lactamase-stable, broad-spectrum antibiotic, especially active against Gram-negative bacteria; first member of the chemically synthesized monobactams, patterned after monobactam produced by *Chromobacterium violaceum*.
Bacampicillin•HCl	(SS) Semisynthetic β-lactam of penicillin class	Orally administered prodrug of ampicillin with broad spectrum; sensitive to many β-lactamases.
Bacitracin	(NP) Peptide antibiotic complex	Commercial preparation of this topical antibiotic contains 9–22 bacitracin analogs, of which Bacitracin A is the most active; used only in topical applications due to nephrotoxicity; typically used in creams with polymyxin B, or polymyxin B and neomycin sulfate; produced by *Bacillus licheniformis*.
Bambermycins	(NP) Substituted amino-glycosides	Produced by *Streptomyces bambergiensis* and other strains; complex of at least four active components (moenomycins A, B_1, B_2 and C), used in veterinary practice as porcine, avian, and bovine feed additives to promote weight gain.
Bialaphos	(NP) Phosphinoglutamic acid-ala-ala	Produced by *Streptomyces hygroscopicus*; inhibitor of glutamine synthetase; used as nonspecific post-emergent herbicide.
Bleomycin sulfate	(NP) Glycopeptide antitumor antibiotic	Bleomycin A2 is the form used for clinical therapy of some carcinomas and lymphomas; produced by *Streptomyces verticillus*.
Bradykinin antagonist	(NP) Antiviral protein	Cortech product, Bradycor, is a newly approved drug that is used in combination with ribavirin to treat four corners hantavirus infections.
Carbadox	(C) Substituted quinoxaline	Coccidiostat for veterinary use; promotes weight gain.
Carbarsone	(C) Substituted carbamoy-larsinilic acid	Antihistomonad for veterinary use.
Carbenicillin indanyl	(SS) Semisynthetic β-lactam of penicillin class	Prodrug hydrolyzed to carbenicillin; extended spectrum of activity against Gram-negative bacteria.
Carboplatin	(C) Platinum coordinated complex	Used alone or in combination therapy for ovarian cancer.

Compound or name	Class[a]	Comments
Carminomycin	(NP) Anthracycline antitumor drug	Produced by *Actinomadura carminata*; antitumor drug used in Russia for treatment of several cancers.
Cefaclor	(SS) Second generation cephalosporin	In 1991, was top-selling antibiotic for Eli Lilly under the name Ceclor with 6.0% of market; now a generic, with Mylan leading the generic market for this drug in 1995 as ninth most pharmacy-prescribed antibiotic; orally administered drug, widely used for otitis media.
Cefadroxil	(SS) First generation cephalosporin	Orally administered, relatively broad-spectrum antibiotic.
Cefamandole naftate	(SS) Third generation cephalosporin	Broad-spectrum, injectable antibiotic.
Cefazolin sodium	(SS) First generation cephalosporin	Parenterally administered only for serious infections.
Cefepime	(SS) New fourth generation cephalosporin	Bristol-Meyers Squibb product, Maxipime, is a recently approved (1996) broad-spectrum antimicrobial that is active against *Staphylococcus* spp. and *Pseudomonas* spp.; parenterally administered.
Cefixime	(SS) Third generation cephalosporin	Fujisawa product, Cefspan, claimed 1.2% of 1991 world market as nineteenth leading antibiotic; orally administrated, relatively broad spectrum antibiotic.
Cefmetazole sodium	(SS) Second generation cephalosporin	Originally obtained from cephyamycin C, produced by *Streptomyces jumonjinensis*, but now semisynthetically derived from 7-amino cephalosporanic acid; intravenously administered.
Cefonicid sodium	(SS) Second generation cephalosporin	Broad-spectrum, parenterally administered antibiotic; highly resistant to β-lactamases.
Cefoperazone sodium	(SS) Third generation cephalosporin	Broad-spectrum, parenterally administered antibiotic.
Cefotaxime	(SS) Third generation cephalosporin	Claforan, Hoechst brand name, was ninth leading antibiotic worldwide in 1991; very broad spectrum antibiotic; parenteral administration.
Cefotetan, disodium	(SS) Second generation cephalosporin	Zeneca product, Cefotan, is a semisynthetic, broad-spectrum, β-lactamase-resistant cephalosporin approved as an injectable.

Compound or name	Class[a]	Comments
Cefoxitin sodium	(SS) Cepha antibiotic	Broad-spectrum antibiotic derived from cephamycin C produced by *Streptomyces lactamdurans*; β-lactamase-resistant, parenterally administered for severe infections only; Merck brand is Mefoxin.
Cefpodoxime Proxetil	(SS) Third generation cephalosporin	Broad-spectrum, orally absorbed pro-drug ester of active free acid metabolite; Sankyo product, Banan, claimed 1.2% of 1991 worldwide market; highly stable to β-lactamases.
Cefprozil	(SS) Third generation cephalosporin	Broad-spectrum, oral antibiotic.
Ceftazidime	(SS) Third generation cephalosporin	Glaxo brand name, Fortum, gained 2.9% of 1991 market worldwide; used for treatment of *Pseudomonas* infections; broad-spectrum parenteral form resistant to β-lactamases.
Ceftibuten	(SS) Third generation cephalosporin	Schering-Plough product, Cedax, is a new, recently approved (1996) broad-spectrum, orally active antibiotic especially effective for treating infections by Gram-negative bacteria.
Ceftizoxime sodium	(SS) Third generation cephalosporin	Broad-spectrum, highly β-lactamase-resistant parenteral antibiotic.
Ceftriaxone	(SS) Third generation cephalosporin	Roche drug that claimed 5.5% of 1991 antibiotics market; has a long half-life in serum, allowing for once-a-day or twice-a-day administrations; broad-spectrum and parenterally administered.
Cefuroxime	(SS) Second generation cephalosporin	Ceftin (Glaxo) is the orally administered, 1-acetoxy ethyl ester; Zinacef (Glaxo) is the parenterally administered sodium salt; combined drugs ranked fifth with 4.0% of world market in 1991.
Cephalexin	(SS) First generation cephalosporin	Orally administered, relatively narrow spectrum antibiotic; sixth most widely pharmacy-prescribed antibiotic in United States in 1995.
Cephalothin sodium	(SS) First generation cephalosporin	Injectable, used only for serious infections; Lilly product is Keflin.
Cephapirin sodium	(SS) First generation cephalopsorin	Parenterally administered, early cephalosporin.

Compound or name	Class[a]	Comments
Cephradine	(SS) First generation cephalosporin	Orally administered, narrow-range antibiotic used for Group A β-hemolytic streptococci.
Chlorambucil	(C) Mustard-type alkylating agent	Bifunctional alkylating agent used as antineoplastic drug against some lymphomas.
Chloramphenicol	(NP/C) N-Dichloroacyl phenylpropanoid	Broad-spectrum bacteriostat originally discovered as a fermentation product of *Streptomyces venezuelae* but is now synthesized chemically; very inexpensive; still first-line drug against *Salmonella typhi* (causative agent of typhoid fever); reserved for only very serious infections.
Chloroquine	(C) 4-Aminoquinolone	Antimalarial and amebicidal; used for extraintestinal amebiasis.
Chlortetracycline	(NP) Tetracycline	Produced by *Streptomyces aureofaciens*; now used only in ointment form for superficial ocular infections; also used as veterinary feed additive to control bacterial infections and promote weight gain.
Cidofovir	(C) Antiviral	Gilead product, Vistide, was approved in 1996 for treatment of cytomegalovirus retinitis in patients with AIDS.
Cilistatin sodium	(C) Derivatized heptanoic acid	Used in combination therapy with imipenem to inhibit dehydropeptidase-I, the renal enzyme that metabolizes imipenem.
Cinoxacin	(C) Quinolone antibiotic	Orally administered DNA gyrase inhibitor, used primarily for Gram-negatives.
Ciprofloxacin	(C) Fluorinated quinolone antibiotic	DNA gyrase inhibitor; the fourth most pharmacy-prescribed antibiotic in 1995 (4.2% of 1991 world market); Bayer brand, Cipro, a very broad spectrum antibiotic, is produced in oral, parenteral, and ophthalmic forms.
Cisplatin	(C) Heavy metal complex	Antitumor drug used for testicular and ovarian malignancies.
Cladribine	(C) Nucleoside (adenosine) analog	Antitumor drug used for treatment of hairy cell leukemia.

Compound or name	Class[a]	Comments
Clarithromycin	(SS) 6-O-Methylerythromycin	Acid-stable erythromycin analog used in treatment of respiratory tract infections and in treatment of *Helicobacter pylori*; Abbott product, Biaxin, was sixth most pharmacy-prescribed antibiotic in United States in 1995.
Clavulanic acid	(NP) Clavam β-lactam inhibitor	Produced by *Streptomyces clavuligerus*; used in combination therapy with amoxacillin to inhibit β-lactamases produced by pathogens; extends range of the β-lactam.
Clindamycin	(SS) Chlorinated lincomycin analog	Upjohn brand product, Cleocin, claimed 1.3% of 1991 world market as seventeenth leading antibiotic; produced in injectable and oral forms; active against anaerobic bacteria and second-line therapy for methicillin-resistant staphylococci.
Clofazimine	(C) Phenazine derivative	Orally administered antileprosy antibiotic that is bacteriocidal for *Mycobacterium leprae*.
Clopidol	(C) Chlorinated pyridinol	Coccidiostat for veterinary use; promotes weight gain.
Clotrimazole	(C) Oral fluconazole	Schering-Plough product, GyneLotrimin, is used to treat vaginal candidiasis and dermal infections.
Cloxacillin sodium	(SS) β-Lactam of isoxazolyl penicillin series	Chlorinated derivative of oxacillin; highly β-lactamase-resistant; also a veterinary drug used for livestock.
Colistimethate sodium	(NP) Polymyxin E (cyclic peptide antibiotic)	Antibiotic produced by *Bacillus colistinus*; used parenterally for Gram-negative infections, particularly *Pseudomonas aeruginosa*.
Colistin sulfate	(NP) Polymyxin E (cyclic peptide antibiotic)	Topical form used in combination with hydrocortisone, neomycin sulfate, and thonzinium.
Cyclophosphamide	(C) Related to nitrogen mustards	Cytotoxic antitumor drug used in several antitumor combination therapies.
Cycloserine	(NP) Amino acid analog	Produced by *Streptomyces orchidaceus* and chemically synthesized; broad-spectrum, orally administered antibiotic used for antibiotic-resistant *Mycobacterium tuberculosis*; Eli Lilly product is Seromycin.

Compound or name	Class[a]	Comments
Cyclosporin	(NP) Substituted cyclic peptide	Produced by *Tolypocladium inflatum*; Sandoz product, Sandimmune, is used as immunosuppressive agent to combat organ rejection, particularly liver, after transplantation (see Chapter 9).
Cytaribine	(C) Nucleoside analog	Commonly known as ara-C; cytotoxic antitumor drug typically used in combination therapy of acute, nonlymphocitic leukemia.
Dactinomycin	(NP) Actinomycin D (acyl-peptidolactone)	Produced by *Streptomyces parvullus*; antitumor drug used parenterally alone or in combination with other antineoplastic drugs for treatment of a variety of cancers.
Daunorubicin•HCl	(NP) Anthracycline antitumor drug	Produced by *Streptomyces peucetius*, *Streptomyces coeruleorubidus*, and several other streptomycetes; approved for therapy against acute nonlymphocytic leukemia.
Daunorubicin, liposomal	(NP) Liposome-entrapped anthracycline	NeXstar formulation, DaunoXome, was approved recently for treatment of AIDS-related Kaposi's sarcoma
Demeclocycline•HCl	(NP) Chlorinated, demethylated tetracycline analog	Natural analog produced by a mutant of *Streptomyces aureofaciens* is a bacteriostatic agent used as a broad-spectrum antibacterial.
Dicloxacillin sodium	(SS) Dichlorinated β-lactam	Acid-resistant, orally absorbed, broad-spectrum isoxazolyl penicillin highly resistant to β-lactamases.
Didanosine (ddl)	(C) Nucleoside analog	Formerly called dideoxinosine; Bristol-Meyers Squibb product, Videx, is orally administered drug approved for treatment of HIV infections.
Dirithromycin	(SS) Macrolide	Orally administered macrolide approved by the FDA in 1995 for treatment of infections caused by *Streptococcus pneumoniae* (pneumonia) and *Moraxella catarrhalis* (bronchitis), *Mycoplasma pneumoniae*, *Legionella pneumophila*, and *Staphylococcus aureus*; Lilly product, Dynabac, offers advantage for patient compliance as a single-dose-per-day antibiotic.

Compound or name	Class[a]	Comments
Docetaxel	(SS) Semisynthetic taxol	Rhône-Poulenc Rhorer product, Taxotere, was recently approved for treatment of ovarian cancer and is under review for use to treat several other forms of cancer.
Doxorubicin•HCl	(NP) Anthracycline antitumor drug	Produced by mutant of *Streptomyces peucetius*; Pharmacia product, Adriamycin, and generic forms are approved for treatment of a variety of cancers; see Chapter 20.
Doxorubicin, liposomal	(NP) Liposome-entrapped anthracycline	Sequus product, Doxil, was approved recently for treatment of AIDS-related Kaposi's sarcoma.
Doxycycline	(SS) Tetracycline analog	Broad-spectrum bacteriostatic antibiotic derived from oxytetracycline; administered orally or by injection
Efrotomycin	(NP) Natural product antibiotic	Produced by *Streptomyces lactamdurans*; Merck product, Producil, is used as veterinary feed additive to promote porcine weight gain.
Epirubicin	(SS) Anthracycline antitumor drug	4'-*Epi*-doxorubicin produced by chemical modification; approved for treatment of some leukemias.
Erythromycin A	(NP) Macrolide antibiotic	Produced by *Saccharopolyspora erythraea*; available in oral, ophthalmic, or injectable formulations; Tenth leading antibiotic in 1991 with 2.2% of worldwide market; broad-spectrum antibiotic that is drug of choice against *Legionella pneumophila* (Legionnaires disease) and *Mycoplasma* infections.
Ethambutol•HCl	(C) Hydroxymethylpropyl-ethylenediamine	Orally administered tuberculostatic agent used in combination with isoniazid or with isoniazid and streptomycin.
Ethionamide	(C) Substituted nicotinamide	Tuberculostatic agent used in combination therapies.
Etoposide	(SS) Derivative of podophyllotoxin	Commonly known as VP-16; used in combination treatment for small-cell lung and testicular cancer.
Famciclovir	(C) Antiviral cyclic guanine derivative	Prodrug of penciclovir; Smith-Kline Beecham product, Famvir, was approved in 1994 for treatment of Herpes zoster (shingles).
Flomoxef	(SS) Fluorinated oxa-cephalosporin	β-Lactamase-resistant antibiotic; Shionogi brand name, Flumarin, claimed 1.5% of 1991 world market.

Compound or name	Class[a]	Comments
Floxacillin	(SS) Fluorinated derivative of oxacillin	Active against penicillin-resistant staphylococci.
Fluconazole oral	(C) Bis-triazole antifungal antibiotic	First of new class of azoles; available as oral or injectable; Pfizer product, Diflucan, is used to treat vaginal candidiasis; also used to treat cryptococcal meningitis and systemic candidiasis.
Flucytosine	(C) 5-Fluorocytosine	Antifungal agent used for treatment of serious cryptococcal meningitis or candidiasis infections.
Fludarabine phosphate	(C) Fluorinated nucleotide	Analog of vidarabine resistant to deamination; used to treat B-cell chronic lymphocytic leukemia.
Fluorouracil	(C) Fluorinated pyrimidine	Antineoplastic antimetabolite used for treatment of keratoses (topical) and several carcinomas (systemic).
Flurithromycin	(SS) Macrolide	Semisynthetic 8-fluoro-erythromycin; fluoro-group stabilizes the macrolide ring structure; indicated for ear, nose, and throat infections.
Fluvastatin sodium	(C) Hydroxymethylglutaryl-CoA reductase inhibitor	First synthetic HMG-CoA reductase inhibitor; Sandoz product, Lescol, is approved for used in hypercholesterolemia.
Foscarnet sodium	(C) Phosphonoformic acid antiviral agent	Astra USA product, Foscavir, was approved in 1991 for treatment of cytomegalovirus retinitis in patients with AIDS and in treatment of acyclovir-resistant mucocutaneous herpes simplex.
Fosfomycin	(NP) Phosphonic acid	Produced by *Streptomyces* spp.; broad-spectrum antibiotic.
Furazolidone	(C) Nitrofuran	Broad-spectrum antibiotic used for treatment of bacterial or protozoan diarrhea or enteritis; bactericidal.
Fusidic acid	(NP) Steroidal natural product	Produced by *Fusidium coccineum*; active against corynebacteria, coagulase-negative and positive staphylococci, and strict anaerobes.
Ganciclovir sodium	(C) Nucleoside analog	Antiviral oral drug; Syntex product, Cytovene, has been approved for treatment of cytomegalovirus retinitis in patients with AIDS.

Compound or name	Class[a]	Comments
Gemcitabine	(C) Nucleoside analog	Approved in 1996 for treatment of locally advanced and metastatic pancreatic adenocarcinoma; first new pancreatic cancer drug in decades; Eli Lilly product is Gemzac.
Gentamycin sulfate	(NP) Aminoglycoside antibiotic	Produced by *Micromonospora purpurea*; available in injectable, topical, and ophthalmic formulations; very effective antibiotic against Gram-negative bacilli; can be modified by nine different resistance-conferring aminoglycoside phosphotransferases and acetyltransferases.
Goserelin acetate	(C) Synthetic peptide	Zeneca product, Zoladex, is an agonist analog of leutenizing hormone release factor that is approved for treatment of prostate cancer and advanced breast cancer.
Gramicidin	(NP) Peptide antibiotic	Produced by *Bacillus brevis*; used as topical, ophthalmic antibiotic in combination with neomycin and polymyxin B.
Halofuginone HBr	(C) Substituted quinazoline	Coccidiostat for veterinary use; promotes weight gain.
Hygromycin B	(NP) Substitute aminoglycoside	Produced by *Streptomyces hygroscopicus*; veterinary use to control porcine and avian roundworms, nodular worms, and whipworms.
Idarubicin•HCl	(C) Anthracycline antitumor drug	Orally absorbed, chemically synthesized, 4-demethoxydaunorubicin; approved as antileukemic drug.
Idoxuridine	(C) Deoxyiodouridine	Topical ophthalmic antiviral drug.
Ifosfamide	(C) Related to nitrogen mustards	Antitumor drug used in combination therapy as third line against germ cell testicular tumor.
Imipenem	(SS) Carbapenem	Merck product, Primaxin, is a very broad spectrum semisynthetic thienamycin derivative; combined with cilastatin, which prevents renal metabolism by inhibiting dehydropeptidase-1.
Indinavir	(C) HIV-1 protease inhibitor	Merck product, Crixivan, is a newly approved (1996) HIV-1 proteinase inhibitor for use in treatment of AIDS.

Compound or name	Class[a]	Comments
Irinotecan	(C) Antitumor agent	Campo (Rhône-Poulenc Rhorer) and Camptosar (Pharmacia and Upjohn) were approved in 1996 for second-line treatment of colo-rectal cancer (see also topotecan).
Isoniazid	(C) Isonicotinic acid hydrazide	Tuberculostatic agent, available in oral and injectable forms, used in front-line combination therapy with rifampin against *Mycobacterium tuberculosis*.
Itraconazole	(C) Antifungal triazole	Janssen product, Sporanox, has been approved for treatment of histo-plasmosis and blastomycosis.
Josamycin	(NP) Macrolide	Produced by *Streptomyces narbonensis* subsp. *josamyceticus*; 16-membered macrolide ring; used both as human and veterinary product.
Kanamycin sulfate	(NP) Aminocyclitol antibiotic	Produced by *Streptomyces kanamyceticus*; available in oral and injectable formulations; used for short-term treatment of serious infections.
Ketoconazole	(C) Antifungal triazole	Orally active, broad-spectrum antimycotic for systemic and topi-cal treatment of many fungal infections.
Laidlomycin propionate K	(NP) Polyether ionophore	Produced by *Streptomyces* spp., veteri-nary growth promotant.
Lamivudine (3TC)	(SS) Nucleoside analog antiviral drug	Produced using enzymatic and chem-ical reactions (see Chapter 25); Glaxo product, Epivir, was approved in 1995 for use in combi-nation treatment against HIV.
Lasolocid sodium	(NP) Polyether ionophore	Produced by *Streptomyces* spp., veteri-nary use as coccidiostat and growth promotant.
Latamoxef	(SS) Oxycepham	Oxa-substituted, third generation cephalosporin; Eli Lilly product, Moxalactam, has recently been approved as a broad-spectrum, β-lactamase-stable antibiotic; not in wide use in United States due to side effects.

Compound or name	Class[a]	Comments
Lincomycin•HCl	(NP) Lincomycin	Produced by *Streptomyces lincolnensis*; used for treatment in serious infections caused by aerobic Gram-positive pathogens, including streptococci, staphylococci, and pneumococci; also used in veterinary practice as feed additive to promote weight gain.
Lomefloxacin•HCl	(C) Difluoroquinolone	DNA gyrase inhibitor; orally active, very broad spectrum bacteriocidal antibiotic; used for mild infections.
Lomustine	(C) Nitrosourea	DNA- and RNA-alkylating agent used in treatment of Hodgkin's disease and other neoplasias.
Loracarbef	(C) Carbacephem	Synthetic β-lactam of carbacepham class is broad-spectrum antibiotic for oral administration.
Lovastatin	(NP) Hydroxymethylglutaryl-CoA reductase inhibitor	Produced by *Aspergillus terreus*; Merck product, Mevacor, is approved for used in hypercholesterolemia.
Maduramycin ammonium	(NP) Polyether ionophore	Produced by *Nocardia* spp. X-14868; veterinary use as coccidiostat and growth promotant.
Mebendazole	(C) Substituted benzimidazole	Orally absorbed anthelmintic used for treatment of infections caused by pinworm, whipworm, common roundworm, and hookworms.
Mechlorethamine•HCl	(C) Nitrogen mustard	Antineoplastic agent used for treatment of Hodgkin's disease, and some leukemias and sarcomas.
Mefloquine•HCl	(C) Quinoline methanol derivative	Antimalarial agent that works as blood schizonticide.
Meropenem	(C) New carbepenem	Zeneca product, Merrem, is a broad-spectrum intravenous antibiotic approved in 1996 for treatment of complicated intraabdominal infections and pediatric bacterial meningitis.
Methenamine mandelate	(C) Combination of mandelic acid and methenamine	Used for urinary tract infections.
Methicillin	(SS) β-lactam of penicillin class	Standard drug for treatment of *Staphylococcus aureus* infections; available for oral and injectables.
Methotrexate	(C) Antimetabolite	Dihydrofolic acid reductase inhibitor used as antineoplastic drug as well as for treatment of severe psoriasis and adult rheumatoid arthritis.

Compound or name	Class[a]	Comments
Metronidazole	(C) Nitroimidazole	Used in treatment of symptomatic trichomoniasis, acute intestinal amoebiasis, and serious anaerobic infections; used to treat other serious anaerobic infections; Helidac is a combination drug of bismuth subsalicylate, tetracycline, and metronidazole for treatment of *Helicobacter pylori*.
Mezlocillin sodium	(SS) β-Lactam of penicillin class	Broad-spectrum antibiotic for parenteral administration; Mezlin is Miles product.
Miconazole	(C) Substituted azole anti fungal drug	Topical antifungal agent; also used orally or as injectable for treatment of candidiasis and coccidioidomycosis.
Midecamycin	(NP) Marcolide	Produced by *Streptomyces mycarofaciens*; 16-membered macrolide ring.
Milbemectin	(NP) Macrolide	Produced by *Streptomyces hygroscopicus* subsp. *aureolacrimosus*; mixture of milbemycins A_3 and A_4 (3:7 ratio); used in Europe as antiparasitic.
Milbemycins	(NP) Macrolides	Produced by *Streptomyces hygroscopicus* subsp. *aureolacrimosus*; used in Europe as antiparasitic, particularly to treat *Acarocides* (anthelmintic).
Minocycline	(SS) Tetracycline derivative	Orally administered antibiotic used for treatment of tetracycline-resistant staphylococci and diseases caused by rickettsia.
Miocamycin	(SS) Acetylated macrolide	Acetylated ester of midecamycin allows for oral availability.
Mitomycin C	(NP) Antitumor drug	Produced by *Streptomyces caespitosus*; cross-links the complementary strands of DNA with absolute specificity for C-p-G; typically used in combination treatments.
Mitotane (o,p'-DDD)	(C) Chlorinated biphenyl	Adrenal cytotoxic agent used to treat adrenal cortical carcinoma.
Mitoxantrone•HCl	(C) Substituted anthracenedione	Cytotoxic antitumor agent used for treatment of several leukemias.
Monensin sodium	(NP) Polyether ionophore	Produced by *Streptomyces cinnamonensis*; veterinary use as coccidiostat and growth promotant.

Compound or name	Class[a]	Comments
Mupirocin	(NP) Pseudomonic acid A	Produced by *Pseudomonas fluorescens*; Smith-Kline Beecham product, Bactroban Nasal, was approved in 1996 as a topical ointment for treatment of nasal methicillin-resistant *Staphylococcus aureus* infections.
Nafcillin	(SS) β-lactam of penicillin class	Designed as antistaphylococcal drug; used for severe Gram-positive infections.
Naftifine•HCl	(C) Allylamine antifungal agent	Topical antifungal agent that possesses narrow clinical spectrum and poor pharmacokinetics.
Nalidixic acid	(C) DNA gyrase inhibitor	Chemical structure on which fluoroquinolones are based; used for urinary tract infections caused by Gram-negatives; orally administered.
Narasin	(NP) Polyether ionophore	Produced by *Streptomyces aureofaciens*; veterinary use as coccidiostat and growth promotant.
Natamycin	(NP) Tetraene polyene	Produced by *Streptomyces natalensis*; used for ophthalmic treatment against yeasts and fungi.
Neomycin sulfate	(NP) Aminoglycoside antibiotic	Produced by *Streptomyces fradiae*; orally administered bacteriocidal agent used as adjunct to other therapies of bowel problems; also used in combination topical ointment formulation.
Netilmicin	(SS) Aminoglycoside antibiotic	Broad-spectrum semisynthetic aminoglycoside related to sisomicin; formulated as an injectable.
Nevirapine	(C) Antiviral drug	First nonnucleoside reverse transcriptase inhibitor; Boehringer Ingelheim product, Viramune, was approved in 1996 for treatment of AIDS.
Nicarbazine	(C) Pyrimidinol and dinitrocarbanilide	Coccidiostat for veterinary use; promotes weight gain.
Niclosamide	(C) Chloronitrophenyl-chlorsalicylamide	Coccidiostat for veterinary use; promotes weight gain.
Nisin	(NP) Lantibiotic	Produced by *Lactococcus lactis*; food-grade natural antibiotic produced by lactic acid bacteria; see Chapter 15.
Nitrofurantoin	(C) Substituted imidazolidinedione	Orally administered for urinary tract infections.

Compound or name	Class[a]	Comments
Nitrofurazone	(C) Substituted furaldehyde semicarbazone	Topical bacteriocidic agent used in burn cases.
Nitromide	(C) Dintribenzamide	Coccidiostat for veterinary use; promotes weight gain.
Norfloxacin	(C) Fluoroquinolone antibiotic	DNA gyrase inhibitor; Merck product, Noroxin, claimed 1.3% of 1991 world market as sixteenth leading antibiotic; orally administered and very broad spectrum of activity.
Novobiocin sodium	(NP) Coumarin	Produced by *Streptomyces spheroides*; orally administered antibiotic, reserved for only the most severe staphylococcal infections resistant to other treatments.
Nystatin	(NP) Polyene antifungal antibiotic	Produced by *Streptomyces noursei*; broad-spectrum antifungal antibiotic available in topical and oral formulations; used to treat candidiasis; see Chapter 19.
Ofloxacin	(C) Fluorinated carboxyquinolone	Ortho Pharma product, Floxin, is a DNA gyrase inhibitor with very broad spectrum of activity.
Oleandomycin	(NP) Macrolide	Produced by *Streptomyces antibioticus*; antibacterial compound used in feed additives.
Omeprazole	(C) Substituted benzimidazole	Cellular proton-pump inhibitor; Astra/Merck product, Prilosec, has recently been approved for combination therapy with clarithromycin for treatment of *Helicobacter pylori* infections.
Oxacillin sodium	(SS) Isoxazolyl penicillin series	Parenterally administered penicillinase-resistant β-lactam; used for treatment of penicillinase-producing staphylococci.
Oxiconazole nitrate	(C) Azole antifungal agent	Topical agent used for dermal fungal infections.
Oxytetracycline	(NP) Tetracycline	Produced by *Streptomyces rimosus*; bacteriostat with wide spectrum of activity; used for treatment of diseases caused by mycoplasmas and rickettsiae; used to treat acne; also used in veterinary practice as a feed additive to promote weight gain.

Compound or name	Class[a]	Comments
Paclitaxel	(NP) Taxol	Produced by *Taxus* spp. (yew trees); Bristol-Meyers Squibb product, Taxol, was approved in 1994 for treatment of ovarian cancer and breast cancer, and is under investigation for use in treatment of several types of cancer.
Penicillamine	(SS) 3-Mercapto-D-valine	Characteristic product of penicillin degradation; Merck product, Cuprimine, is used for second-line treatment of rheumatoid arthritis.
Penicillin G	(NP) Penicillin	Produced by *Penicillium chrysogenum*; original penicillin, still used for susceptible streptococci, oral anaerobic bacteria, and *Treponema pallidum* (causative agent of syphilis); injectable only, and not effective against most Gram-negative bacteria.
Penicillin V	(SS) Phenoxymethyl analog of penicillin	Apothecon product, Veetids, an acid-stable oral form of penicillin, was seventh most pharmacy-prescribed antibiotic in United States in 1995.
Pentamidine isethionate	(C) Aromatic diamidine	Antiprotozoal agent used especially against *Pneumocystis carinii* caused pneumonia in AIDS patients.
Pentostatin	(NP) Nucleoside analog antineoplastic agent	Produced by *Streptomyces antibioticus*; potent transition state inhibitor of adenosine deaminase; used in treatment of α-interferon-refractive hairy cell leukemia.
Phosphinothricin	(NP) Phosphinoglutamic acid	Produced by *Streptomyces viridochromogenes*; inhibitor of glutamine synthetase; used as nonspecific postemergent herbicide.
Piperacillin sodium	(SS) β-Lactam related to penicillin	Very broad spectrum, parenteral ureidopenicillin that is somewhat sensitive to β-lactamases.
Piperacillin/tazobactam	(SS) β-Lactam and β-lactamase inhibitor	Lederle product, Zosyn, was recently approved as an injectable, very broad spectrum antibiotic; tazobactam is most effective against plasmid-borne β-lactamases.
Plicamycin	(NP) Natural product	Produced by *Streptomyces argillaceus*; also known as mithramycin; antitumor drug used against some testicular tumors.

Compound or name	Class[a]	Comments
Polymyxin B sulfate	(NP) Cyclic peptide antibiotic	Produced by *Bacillus polymyxa*; topical antibiotic used in combination with neomycin and bacitracin; also available for parenteral use against acute infections by *Pseudomonas aeruginosa*.
Polyoxin A	(NP) Nucleoside antibiotic	Produced by *Streptomyces curacaoi* subsp. *asoensis*; specific against phytopathic fungi by inhibiting chitin synthesis; especially used to treat *Alternaria* infections of plants.
Pravastatin	(NP) Hydroxymethylglutanyl-CoA reductase inhibitor	Biochemically synthesized by microbial hydroxylation of mevastatin, a compound produced by *Penicillium citrinum*; Bristol-Meyers Squibb product, Pravachol, is approved for treatment of hypercholesterolemia; see Chapter 26.
Pristinamycin	(NP) Antibiotic mixture	Produced by *Streptomyces pristinaespiralis*; a mixture of streptogramin antibiotics used in Europe; although active against most Gram-positive and -negative bacteria, it has limited use due to lack of solubility; this drug was the basis for development of Synercid.
Pyrantel tartrate	(C) Substituted pyrimidine	Used for veterinary treatment of porcine roundworm and nodular worm infections.
Pyrazinamide	(C) Nicotinamide analog	Orally administered antituberculosis drug; used in combination therapy with rifampin and isoniazid.
Quinine sulfate	(NP) Cinchona alkaloid	Antimalarial; used to treat chloroquine-resistant *Falciparum malaria*.
Quinupristin/dalfopristin	(SS) Streptogramin mixture	Modified from streptogramins produced by *Streptomyces* spp.; Rhône-Poulenc Rhorer drug, Synercid, is currently in advanced trials for treatment of vancomycin-resistant enterococci and methicillin-resistant staphylococci.
Ribavirin	(C) Nucleoside analog	The first synthetic, interferon noninducing, broad-spectrum antiviral nucleoside analog; ICN Pharmaceuticals product, Virazole, is approved for treatment of four corners hantavirus and chronic hepatitis C infections.

Compound or name	Class[a]	Comments
Rifabutin	(SS) Derivative of rifamycin S	Inhibits nucleotide synthesis; orally administered tuberculostatic agent; used against disseminated *Mycobacterium avium* complex in AIDS patients; see Chapter 18.
Rifampin	(SS) Derivative of rifamycin B	Parental compound, rifamycin, is produced by *Streptomyces mediterranei*; orally absorbed, bacteriocidal agent specifically inhibits bacterial RNA polymerase; tuberculostatic; also penetrates white blood cells, so it is effective against intracellular pathogens; see Chapter 18.
Rimantadine	(C) Adamantane derivative	Forest Pharmaceuticals product, Flumadine, has been approved for prophylactic treatment of common flu virus.
Ritonavir	(C) HIV-1 protease inhibitor	Abbott product, Norvir, was approved in 1996 for treatment of HIV.
Robenidine•HCl	(C) Substituted chlorophenyl dihydrazide	Coccidiostat for veterinary use; promotes weight gain.
Rokitamycin	(SS) Esterified macrolide	Propionyl ester of leucomycin A5, produced by *Streptomyces kitasatoensis*; active against *Mycoplasma* spp., and macrolide-resistant strains of *Staphylococcus aureus* and *Streptococcus pyogenes*.
Roxarsone	(C) Nitrophenolarsonic acid	Bacteriostat for veterinary use; promotes weight gain.
Roxithromycin	(SS) Macrolide	9-[O-(2-methoxyethoxy)methyl-oxime] derivative of erythromycin.
Salinomycin	(NP) Polyether ionophore	Produced by *Streptomyces albus*; veterinary use as coccidiostat and growth promotant.
Saquinavir	(C) HIV-1 protease inhibitor	Hoffmann-La Roche product, Invirase, was the first HIV-protease 1 inhibitor approved (1995) for treatment of AIDS; used in combination therapy with AZT and 3TC.
Semduramicin	(SS) Polyether ionophore	Base molecule produced by *Streptomyces* spp.; veterinary use as coccidiostat and growth promotant.
Silver sulfadiazine	(C) Heavy metal substituted sulfa drug	Topical treatment of second and third degree burn wounds; bacteriocidal.

Compound or name	Class[a]	Comments
Simvastatin	(SS) Hydroxymethylglutaryl-CoA reductase inhibitor	Derivative of *Aspergillus terreus* product; Merck product, Zocor, has been approved for treatment of hypercholesterolemia.
Spectinomycin´•HCl	(NP) Aminocyclitol	Produced by *Streptomyces spectabilis*; aminoglycoside-related antibiotic used for treatment of penicillin-resistant *Neisseria gonorrhoeae*; also used in veterinary practice to treat gastroenteritis.
Spiramycin	(NP) Macrolide	Produced by *Streptomyces ambofaciens*; 16-membered macrolide ring; used in France.
Stavudine (d4T)	(C) Nucleoside (thymidine) analog	Bristol-Meyers Squibb product, Zerit, has been approved for treatment of AIDS in patients intolerant to other reverse transcriptase inhibitors.
Streptomycin sulfate	(NP) Aminoglycoside antibiotic	Produced by *Streptomyces griseus*; limited use due to large number of resistant bacteria; used to treat isoniazid-, pyrazinamide-, and rifampin-resistant *Mycobacterium tuberculosis*.
Streptozocin	(NP/C) Glucose analog	Produced by *Streptomyces achromogenes* but synthesized chemically for industry; bacterial and mammalian DNA synthesis inhibitor; used to treat metastatic islet cell carcinoma of pancreas; may also be used in combination therapy for Hodgkin's disease; used experimentally to induce diabetes.
Sulbactam	(SS) Penicillanic acid sulfone	β-Lactamase inhibitor employed in combination therapy with ampicillin.
Sulconazole nitrate	(C) Imidazole derivative	Topical antifungal agent.
Sulfacetamide sodium	(C) Sulfonamide	Used in combination with sulfur as topical acne drug; also used for skin conditions and as secondary antibacterial.
Sulfadiazine	(C) Sulfonamide	Orally administered bacteriostatic agent; used primarily for urinary tract infections.
Sulfadimethoxine	(C) Sulfonamide	Bacteriostat for veterinary use; coccidiostat.

Compound or name	Class[a]	Comments
Sulfamethoxazole	(C) Sulfonamide	Orally administered bacteriostatic agent; used primarily for urinary tract infections; often used in combination therapy with trimethoprim.
Sulfanilamide	(C) Sulfonamide	Topical drug used to treat vulvovaginitis caused by *Candida albicans*.
Sulfanitran	(C) Sulfonamide	Bacteriostat for veterinary use; poultry coccidiostat.
Sulfathiazole	(C) Sulfonamide	Orally administered bacteriostatic agent; used primarily for urinary tract infections.
Sultamicillin	(SS) Double ester of ampicillin and sulbactam	Combination penicillin derivative and β-lactamase inhibitor combined into a single prodrug; Pfizer brand, Unasyn, claimed 1.6% of world market in 1991 as fourteenth leading antibiotic.
Tacrolimus (FK506)	(NP) Macrolide	Produced by *Streptomyces tsukubaensis*; Fujisawa product, Prograf, was approved for use as an immunosuppressant to combat organ rejection in liver transplants.
Taxobactam	(C) β-Lactamase inhibitor	Used in combination therapy with piperacillin to extend range of the β-lactam.
Teichoplanin	(NP) Glycopeptide	Produced by *Actinoplanes teichomyceticus*; similar in structure and activity to vancomycin; limited in use due to associated nephrotoxicity; produced by Lepetit, but still experimental in the United States.
Tenipocide (VM-26)	(SS) Derivative of podophyllotoxin	Phase-specific (late S, early G_2) cytotoxic antitumor drug; inhibits topoisomerase II; used in combination therapy of leukemia and other cancers with other antitumor drugs.
Terbinafine•HCl	(C) Allylamine	Topical antifungal agent; Sandoz product, Lamisil, approved for interdigital tinea infections, has a narrow clinical spectrum and poor pharmacokinetic properties.

Compound or name	Class[a]	Comments
Tetracycline•HCl	(NP) Tetracycline	Produced by *Streptomyces aureofaciens*; bacteriostatic drug available in oral and ophthalmic formulations; used for treatment of several intracellular pathogens and infections caused by *Vibrio* spp.; used in acne treatment.
Thiabendazole	(C) Substituted benzimidazole	Used for treatment of *Ascaris* spp. (roundworm), *Enterobius* spp. (pinworm), hookworm, threadworm, and whipworm, anthelmitic and fungicidal; used in veterinary practice as feed additive.
Thioguanine	(C) Purine analog	Orally administered, antineoplastic drug used in acute nonlymphocytic leukemias and other neoplasms.
Thiotepa	(C) Ethylenimine class	Cytotoxic, alkalating agent used for treatment of adenocarcinomas of breast and ovary.
Tiamulin H-fumarate	(C) Substituted pentacycloocten ester	Antibacterial agent used to treat porcine dysentery caused by *Treponema hyodysenteriae*.
Ticarcillin disodium	(SS) β-Lactam of penicillin class	Broad-spectrum, injectable used primarily for severe infections.
Ticarcillin/clavulanate	(SS/NP) β-Lactam and β-lactamase inhibitor	Smith-Kline Beecham product, Timentin, is approved as an injectable, broad-spectrum antibiotic for use especially in polymicrobial infections.
Tobramycin sulfate	(NP) Aminoglycoside	Produced by *Streptomyces tenebrarius*; parenterally formulated drug used for severe infections; generally effective against Gram-negative bacilli; can be modified by seven different resistance-conferring aminoglycoside phosphotransferases and acetyltransferases.
Tolnaftate	(C) Thiocarbamide antifungal agent	Possesses narrow clinical spectrum and poor pharmacokinetics.
Topotecan	(SS) Semisynthetic analog of camptothecin	Parental compound, camptothecin, is obtained from a Chinese tree, *Camptotheca acuminata*; DNA topoisomerase I inhibitor; Smith-Kline Beecham product, Hycamtin, has been recently approved for treatment of ovarian and colorectal cancers.

Compound or name	Class[a]	Comments
Trimethoprim	(C) Diaminotrimethoxyben-zylpyrimidine	Orally absorbed sulfa-type drug that inhibits dihydrofolate reductase; used for treatment of urinary tract infections caused by Gram-negatives; often used with sulfamethoxazole.
Trimetrexate glucuronate	(C) Diaminoquinazoline	Nonclassical dihydrofolate reductase inhibitor; used to treat pneumonia caused by *Pneumocystis carinii*.
Troleandomycin	(SS) Macrolide antibiotic	Acid-stable acetylated ester of oleandomycin, a product of *Streptomyces antibioticus*; used to treat infections caused by streptococci and pneumococci.
Tylosin phosphate	(NP) Macrolide	Produced by *Streptomyces fradiae*; veterinary use as a feed additive for porcine, avian, and bovine weight gain and improved feed efficiency; often used in combination with other additives; reduces incidence of liver abscesses caused by *Fusobacterium necrophorum*.
Uracil mustard	(C) Nitrogen mustard compound	Orally administered drug used to treat several types of leukemia.
Valacyclovir•HCl	(C) L-Valyl ester prodrug of acyclovir	Glaxo Wellcome drug, Valtrex, was approved in 1995 for treatment of herpes zoster (shingles); this drug is expected to become the successor to acyclovir.
Vancomycin•HCl	(NP) Glycopeptide antibiotic	Produced by *Streptomyces orientalis*; bacteriocidal antibiotic; oral and intravenous formulations; Eli Lilly product, Vancocin, is considered current last line of defense against β-lactam- and aminoglycoside-resistant enterococci and methicillin-resistant staphylococci, among other uses; use is limited by renal toxicity problems at least partly caused by difficulties with purity.
Vidarabene (Ara-A)	(NP) Purine nucleoside antiviral drug	Produced by *Streptomyces antibioticus*; used in ointment for topical treatment of herpes.
Vinblastine sulfate	(NP) Vinca alkaloid	Produced by *Catharanthus roseus* (periwinkle); injectable used to treat a variety of lymphomas, sarcomas, and other neoplasias.

Compound or name	Class[a]	Comments
Vincristine sulfate	(NP) Vinca alkaloid	Produced by *Catharanthus roseus* (periwinkle); injectable used to treat acute leukemia.
Vinorelbine tartrate	(SS) Semisynthetic vinca alkaloid	Vinblastine analog; Burroughs Wellcome product, Navelbine, has been approved for treatment of non-small-cell lung cancer.
Virginiamycin	(NP) Mixture of antibiotics	Produced by *Streptomyces virginiae*; mixture of virginiamycin S_1, a cyclic peptide antibiotic, and virginiamycin M_1, a streptogramin; used as a bovine, porcine, and avian feed additive to promote weight gain and increased feed efficiency.
Zalcitabine (ddC)	(C) Nucleoside analog	Roche product, Hivid, has been approved for treatment of AIDS.
Zidovudine (AZT)	(C) Nucleoside analog	Burroughs Wellcome product, Retrovir, was the first drug approved specifically for treatment of AIDS.

[a] Abbreviations: C, chemically synthesized; NP, natural product; SS, semisynthetic compound.
Sources: Refs. 4 and 81–85.

REFERENCES

1.   Levy SB. The Antibiotic Paradox: How Miracle Drugs Are Destroying the Miracle. New York: Plenum Press, 1992.
2.   Vandamme EJ. Antibiotic search and production: An overview. Vandamme EJ, ed. Biotechnology of Antibiotics. New York: Marcel Dekker, 1984:3–31.
3.   Demain AL. Functions of secondary metabolites. Hershberger CL, Queener SW, Hegeman G, eds. Genetics and Molecular Biology of Industrial Microorganisms. Washington D.C.: American Society for Microbiology, 1989:1–11.
4.   SCRIP's 1995 Yearbook. New York: PharmaBooks Ltd.
5.   Pfeiffer N. New antimicrobial therapies described. Gen Engn News 1996; 16:1,18–19.
6.   Mahmoudian M, Dawson MJ. Chemoenzymatic production of the anti-viral agent Epivir (3TC). Strohl WR, ed. Biotechnology of Antibiotics, 2nd ed. New York: Marcel Dekker, 1997.
7.   Isada CM. Protease inhibitors: Promising new weapons against HIV. Clev Clin J Med 1996; 63:204–208.
8.   Bérdy J. Are actinomycetes exhausted as a source of secondary metabolites? Debabov VG, Dudnik YV, Danilenko VN, eds. Proceedings of the Ninth International Symposium on the Biology of the Actinomycetes. Moscow: All-Russia Scientific Research Institute for Genetics and Selection of Industrial Microorganisms, 1995:13–34.
9.   Neu HC. The crisis in antibiotic resistance. Science 1992; 257:1064–1073.
10. Lappe M. Breakout: The evolving threat of drug-resistant disease. San Francisco: Sierra Club Books, 1995.
11. Lemonick MD. The killers all around: New viruses and drug-resistant bacteria are reversing human victories over infectious disease. Time 1994; September 12:62–69.
12. Begley S. The end of antibiotics. Newsweek 1994; March 28:47–51.
13. Pernodet JL, Fish S, Rouault-Blondelet MH, Cundliffe E. The macrolide-lincosamide-streptogramin B resistance phenotypes characterized by using a specifically deleted, antibiotic-sensitive strain of *Streptomyces lividans*. Antimicrob Agents Chemother 1996; 40:581–585.
14. Lewis K. Multidrug resistance pumps on bacteria: Variations on a theme. Trends Biochem Sci 1994; 19:119–123.
15. Culotta E. Funding crunch hobbles antibiotic resistance research. Science 1994; 264:362–363.
16. Gibbons, A. Exploring new strategies to fight drug-resistant microbes. Science 1992; 257:1036–1038.
17. Lederberg J. Infection emergent. J Am Med Assoc 1996; 275:243–245.
18. The World Health Report, 1996. Geneva: Office of World Health Reporting, World Health Organization.
19. McGowan JE. Antimicrobial resistance in hospital organisms and its relation to antibiotic use. Rev Infect Dis 1983; 5:1033–1048.
20. Wright KC. Cystic fibrosis and the pseudomonads. Brit J Biomed Sci 1996; 53:140–145.
21. Begg EJ, Barclay ML. Aminoglycosides: 50 years on. Brit J Clin Pharmacol 1995; 39:597–603.
22. Davies J. Inactivation of antibiotics and the dissemination of resistance genes. Science 1994; 264:375–382.
23. Cohen ML. Epidemiology of drug resistance: Implications for a post-antimicrobial era. Science 1992; 257:1050–1055.
24. Jernigan DB, Cetron MS, Breiman RF. Minimizing the impact of drug-resistant *Streptococcus pneumoniae* (DRSP): A strategy from the DSRP working group. J Amer Med Assoc 1996; 275:206–209.
25. Brown KS. Pharmaceutical and biotech firms taking on drug-resistant microbes. The Scientist 1996; 10:1,8–9.

26. Wenzel RP. The mortality of hospital-acquired bloodstream infections: Need for a new vital statistic? Int J Epidemiol 1988; 17:225–227.

27. Lederberg J, Shope RE, Oaks SC, eds. Institute of Medicine. Emerging Infections: Microbial Threats to Health in the United States. Washington, D.C.: National Academy of Sciences Press, 1992.

28. Centers for Disease Control and Prevention. Nosocomial enterococci: Resistant to vancomycin—United States, 1989–1993. Morb Mortal Wkly Rep 1993; 42:597–599.

29. Gin AS, Zhanel GG. Vancomycin-resistant enterococci. Ann Pharmacol 1996; 30:615–624.

30. Travis J. Reviving the antibiotic miracle? Science 1994; 264:360–362.

31. Barber M. The incidence of penicillin sensitive variant colonies in penicillinase producing strains of Staphylococcus aureus. J Gen Microbiol 1949; 3:274–279.

32. Falkow S. Infectious Multiple Drug Resistance. London: Pion Ltd., 1975.

33. Murray BE. Can antibiotic resistance be controlled? N Engl J Med 1994; 330:1229–1230.

34. Rowe PM. Preparing for battle against vancomycin resistance. Lancet 1996; 347:252.

35. Uttley AHC, Collins CH, Naidoo J, George RC. Vancomycin-resistant enterococci. Lancet 1988; 1:57–58.

36. Bartlett JG, Froggatt JW III. Antibiotic resistance. Arch Otolaryngol Head Neck Surg 1995; 121:392–396.

37. Collatz E, Labia R, Gutman L. Molecular evolution of ubiquitous β-lactamases towards extended-spectrum enzymes active against newer β-lactam antibiotics. Mol Microbiol 1990; 4:1615–1620.

38. Moreillon P, Wenger A. Antibiotic-resistant pneumococci. Schweiz Mediz Wochensch 1996; 126:255–263.

39. Mayon-White RT, Ducel G, Kereselodze T, Tikomirov E. An international survey of the prevalence of hospital acquired infections. J Hosp Infect 1988; 11(Suppl. A):43–48.

40. Brumfitt W, Hamilton-Miller JMT. The challenge of methicillin-resistant Staphylococcus aureus. Drugs Exp Clin Res 1994; 20:215–224.

41. Noble WC, Virani Z, Cree RGA. Co-transfer of vancomycin and other resistance genes from Enterococcus faecalis NCTC 12201 to Staphylococcus aureus. FEMS Microbiol Lett 1992; 93:195–198.

42. Neu HC. Infection problems for the 1990's: Do we have the answer? Scand J Infect Dis 1993; 91(Suppl):7–13.

43. Christensen KJ, Gubbins PO. Treatment of vancomycin-resistant staphylococcal infections. Ann Pharmacother 1996; 30:288–290.

44. Sumita Y, Fukusawa M. Meropenem resistance in Pseudomonas aeruginosa. Chemother 1996; 42:47–56.

45. Bloom BR, Murray CJL. Tuberculosis: Commentary on a reemergent killer. Science 1992; 257:1055–1064.

46. Barrière JC, Bouanchaud DH, Paris JM, Rolin O, Harris NV, Smith C. Antimicrobial activity against Staphylococcus aureus of semisynthetic injectable streptogramins: RP 59500 and related compounds. J Antimicrob Chemother 1992; 30(Suppl A):1–8.

47. Silver LL, Bostian KA. Discovery and development of new antibiotics: The problem of antibiotic resistance. Antimicrob Agents Chemother 1993; 37:377–383.

48. Nichterlein T, Kretschmar M, Hof H. RP59500, a streptogramin derivative, is effective in murine listeriosis. J Chemother 1996; 8:107–112.

49. Saltus R. Bacterium Enterococcus seen taking hold in hospitals. Boston Globe 1996; February 2.

50. Leclercq R, Nantas L, Soussy C-J, Duval J. Activity of RP59500, a new parenteral semisynthetic streptogramin, against staphylococci with various mechanisms of resistance to macrolide-lincosamide-streptogramin antibiotics. J Antimicrob Chemother 1992; 30(Suppl A):67–75.

51. Nicas TI, Mullem DL, Flokowitsch JE, Preston DA, Snyder NJ, Zweifel MJ, Wilkie SC, Rodriguez MJ, Thompson RC, Cooper RDG. Semisynthetic glycopeptide antibiotics derived from LY264826 active against vancomycin-resistant enterococci. Antimicrob Agents Chemother 1996; 40:2194–2199.

52. Nicas TI, Cooper RDG. Vancomycin and other glycopeptides. Strohl WR, ed. Biotechnology of Antibiotics, 2nd ed. New York: Marcel Dekker, 1997.

53. Shimada J, Kawahara Y. Overview of a new cabapenem, panipenem/betamipron. Drugs Exp Clin Res 1994; 20:241–245.

54. Zurenko GE, Yagi BH, Schaadt, Allison JW, Kilburn JO, Glickman SE, Hutchinson, DK, Barbachyn MR, Brickner SJ. In vitro activities of U-100592 and U-100766, novel oxazolidinone antibacterial agents. Antimicrob Agents Chemother 1996; 40:839–845.

55. Inoue M, Nonoyama M, Okamoto R, Ida T. Antimicrobial activity of arbekacin, a new aminoglycoside antibiotic, against methicillin-resistant *Staphylococcus aureus*. Drugs Exp Clin Res 1994; 30:233–240.

56. Hancock REW, Falla TJ. Cationic peptides. Strohl WR, ed. Biotechnology of Antibiotics, 2nd ed. New York: Marcel Dekker, 1997.

57. Larrick JW, Wright SC. Cationic antimicrobial proteins. Drugs Fut 1996; 21:41–48.

58. Yukimune Y, Tabata H, Higashi Y, Hara Y. Methyl jasmonate–induced overproduction of paclitaxel and baccatin III in *Taxus* cell suspension cultures. Nature Biotechnol 1996; 14:1129–1132.

59. Rinehart KL Jr, Gloer JB, Hughes RG Jr, Renis HE, McGovren, Swynenberg EB, Stringfellow DA, Kuentzel SL, Li LH. 1981. Didemnins: Antiviral and antitumor depsipeptides from caribbean tunicate. Science 1981; 212:933–935.

60. Reichenbach H, Gerth K, Irschik H, Kunze B, Hoefle G. Myxobacteria: A source of new antibiotics. Trends Biotechnol 1988; 6:115–121.

61. Traber R. Biosynthesis of cyclosporins. Strohl WR, ed. Biotechnology of Antibiotics, 2nd ed. New York: Marcel Dekker, 1997.

62. Kuntz ID. Structure-based strategies for drug design and discovery. Science 1992; 257:1078–1082.

63. Desnottes J-F. New targets and strategies for the development of antibacterial agents. Trends Biotechnol 1996; 14:134–140.

64. Brandish PE, Kimura K-I Inukai M, Southgate R, Lonsdale JT, Bugg TDH. Modes of action of tunicamycin, liposidomycin B, and mureidomycin A: Inhibition of phospho-*N*-acetylmuramyl-pentapeptide translocase from *Escherichia coli*. Antimicrob Agents Chemother 1996; 40:1640–1644.

65. Hopwood DA, Malpartida F, Kieser HM, Ikeda H, Duncan J, Fujii I, Rudd BAM, Floss HG, Ōmura S. Production of "hybrid" antibiotics by genetic engineering. Nature 1985; 314:642–644.

66. Bartel PL, Zhu C-b, Lampel JS, Dosch DC, Connors NC, Strohl WR, Beale JM Jr, Floss HG. Biosynthesis of anthraquinones by interspecies cloning of actinorhodin biosynthesis genes in streptomycetes: Clarification of actinorhodin gene functions. J Bacteriol 1990; 172:4816–4826.

67. McDaniel R, Ebert-Khosla S, Hopwood DA, Khosla C. Engineered biosynthesis of novel polyketides. Science 1993; 262:1546–1550.

68. McDaniel R, Ebert-Khosla S, Hopwood DA, Khosla C. Rational design of aromatic polyketide natural products by recombinant assembly of enzymatic units. Nature 1995; 375:549–554.

69. Khosla C, Zawada RJX. Generation of polyketide libraries via combinatorial biosynthesis. Trends Biotechnol 1996; 14:335–341.

70. Rajgarhia VB, Strohl WR. Minimal *Streptomyces* sp. strain C5 daunorubicin polyketide biosynthesis genes required for aklanonic acid biosynthesis. J Bacteriol (1997).

71. Hutchinson CR. Antibiotics from genetically engineered microorganisms. Strohl WR, ed. Biotechnology of Antibiotics, 2nd ed. New York: Marcel Dekker, 1997.

72. Zuber P, Marahiel MA. Structure, function, and regulation of genes encoding multi-domain peptide synthetases. Strohl WR, ed. Biotechnology of Antibiotics, 2nd ed. New York: Marcel Dekker, 1997.

73. Oliynyk M, Brown MJB, Cortés J, Staunton J, Leadlay PF. A hybrid molecular polyketide synthase obtained by domain swapping. Chem Biol 1996; 3:833–839.

74. Stemmer WPC. DNA shuffling by random fragmentation and reassembly: In vitro recombination for molecular evolution. Proc Natl Acad Sci USA 1994; 91:10747–10751.

75. Stemmer WPC. Rapid evolution of a protein in vitro by DNA shuffling. Nature 1994; 370:389–391.

76. Moore JC, Arnold FH. Directed evolution of a para-nitrobenzyl esterase for aqueous-organic solvents. Nature Biotechnol 1996; 14:458–466.

77. Peterson TC. Diverse bioactivities from actinomycete combinatorial biology libraries. Presentation at the Sixth Conference on the Genetics and Molecular Biology of Industrial Microorganisms, Bloomington, Indiana 1996.

78. Petsko GA. For medicinal purposes. Nature 1996; 384(Suppl):7–9.

79. Glaser V. Companies develop novel techniques for maximizing combinatorial library potential. Genetic Engn News 1996; 16:1,19.

80. Hogan JC Jr. Directed combinatorial chemistry. Nature 1996; 384(Suppl 7):17–19.

81. VirSci Corporation (http://www.pharminfo.com/drugdb/dbgn_mnua.html).

82. PDR Generics. Montvale, New Jersey: Medical Economics Data Production Co., 1995.

83. The Merck Index, 12th ed. Whitehouse Station, New Jersey: Merck and Co., 1996.

84. Anonymous. The top 200 drugs, 1996. Amer Druggist 1996; 213:18–27.

85. PharmInfoNet, MCW and FMLH Antibiotic Guide (http://www.intmed.mcw.edu/drug/InfectionRx.html).

2

Molecular Genetic Approaches to Yield Improvement in Actinomycetes

Richard H. Baltz

Lilly Research Laboratories, Eli Lilly and Company, Indianapolis, Indiana

I. INTRODUCTION

Secondary metabolite product yields can be improved by optimizing nutritional and physical components of the fermentation, by genetic modification of the producing organisms, and by iterative combinations of the two processes. This chapter will focus on the genetic modification of the producing organism, with emphasis on the most recent methods that can be applied to this process. Older methods that are still relevant to the process will be briefly discussed and updated when appropriate. Also, the shortcomings of current methods and gaps in information relevant to successful application of some newer procedures will be pointed out.

II. TRADITIONAL METHODS

A. Mutagenesis

A general method of undisputed value to strain improvement is chemical or physical mutagenesis followed by fermentation analysis to identify improved strains. Methods to carry out these procedures have been reviewed (1–3). Of the mutagens analyzed in comparative studies in *Streptomyces fradiae*, N-methyl-N′-nitro-N-nitrosoguanidine (MNNG) was the most potent (1,2), followed by methyl methanesulfonate (MMS), 4-nitroquino-line-1-oxide (NQO), ethyl methanesulfonate (EMS), hydroxylamine (HA), and ultraviolet light (UV). The efficiency of mutagenesis ranged over 1000-fold. MNNG is particularly appealing because of its robustness: it tends to give a plateau of high mutation frequency that is very close to the theoretical optimum level as determined by a Poisson distribution model (1,2).

A potential shortcoming of the Poisson model for determining optimum mutation levels, however, is that it assumes a relatively random distribution of mutations throughout the chromosome. MNNG induces closely linked double mutations near the replication fork in *Escherichia coli* (4,5) and apparently in streptomycetes (6). A study on MNNG-induced mutations in tylosin biosynthetic genes (7), which are now known to be located in a 85 kb region of the *S. fradiae* genome (8,9), indicated that about 5% of the mutants contained two mutations with readily identifiable phenotypes. What was not clear from these studies was whether other silent mutations, potentially deleterious to tylosin production, were present in these strains.

A study by Merson-Davies and Cundliffe (9) has shed new light on this issue. Two of the original *tyl* blocked mutants (7) were analyzed by DNA sequence analysis. The *tylI* mutant gene from strain GS77 contained a single base pair substitution, a GC→AT transition mutation, indicating that this mutant gene contains no silent second-site mutations. Likewise, the *tylB* mutant gene in strain GS50 contains a single GC→AT transition mutation that generates a stop codon. These results suggest that the magnitude of multiple linked mutations induced by MNNG is limited and, thus, may not be a major concern for industrial strain improvement programs. Thus, MNNG may be the mutagen of choice for efficient mutagenesis. The only limitation of MNNG is its specificity for GC base pairs and its high propensity to make GC→AT transition mutations (10), as exemplified in two cases just discussed. Unfortunately, both EMS and NQO also induce mutations in *E. coli* predominantly by the GC→AT transition pathway (10).

It would be very useful to identify other potent chemical mutagens that induce transversion mutations, transition mutations at AT positions, and deletions to complement MNNG, EMS, and NQO in mutagenesis programs.

B.   Genetic Recombination

The potential applications of genetic recombination in industrial streptomycetes have been discussed by Hopwood (11,12), and efficient methods for genetic recombination by protoplast fusion have been available for some time (13–15). In spite of the general availability of protoplast fusion, significant published examples of applications of recombination to strain improvement are lacking. One possibility is that successful applications have been kept as proprietary information. Another possibility is that recombination is not as robust as sequential chemical mutagenesis. Even if recombination is not as robust as random mutagenesis in strain development, it is useful for the construction of recombinants with specific useful traits that cannot be readily generated by mutagenesis. In this regard, it is useful to employ recombination as a complementary method to augment random mutagenesis for strain development.

III.   MOLECULAR GENETIC METHODS

A.   Methods to Overcome Restriction Barriers

Several different methods to introduce plasmid DNA into streptomycete protoplasts have been described (see 16 for references). However, many streptomycetes and other actinomycetes produce restriction endonucleases that can pose serious barriers to protoplast transformation (17–22). Strong restriction can be readily identified by the inability of certain broad host range phages to form plaques on the restricting host (17,18,21,23). Table 1 gives some examples of bacteriophage host ranges on streptomycetes that produce restriction endonucleases, ones that are defective in specific restriction endonucleases, and ones that appear to not express restriction. The producers of the well-characterized restriction endonucleases *Sac*I, *Sac*II, *Sal*I, *Sal*P1, and *Sbo*I showed specific patterns of complete restriction of certain bacteriophages. A mutation that blocked *Sal*I restriction in *Streptomyces albus* G changed the plaque formation pattern from restriction of 8 of 10 bacteriophages to sensitivity to all 10. *S. fradiae* T59235, a tylosin producer, restricted

Table 1   Bacteriophage Plaque Formation on Streptomycetes[a]

Species[a]	Enzyme produced	Plaque formation with the following bacteriophages												
		FP4	FP22	FP43	FP46	FP50	FP54	FP55	FP60	FP61	FP62	VP11	R4	φC31
S. achromogenes	SacI, SacII	–	+	+	+	–		–	+	+	–	–	–	–
S. ambofaciens	—	+	+	+	+	+	+	+	+	+	+	+	+	–
S. albus G	SalI	–	+	–	+	–		–	–	–	–	–	–	
S. albus G	SalI–	+	+	+	+	+		+	+	+	+	+	+	
S. albus P	SalPI (PstI)	+	+	+	+	+		–	+	+	+	+	–	
S. bobilae	SboI	–	+	+	+	+		–	–	–	–	–	–	
S. fradiae T59235	Several	+	+	–	–	+	–	–	+	+	+	+	–	–
S. fradiae PM73	Defective[b]	+	+	+	–	+	+	+	+	+	+	+	–	
S. griseofuscus	—	+	+	+	+	+	+	+	+	+	+	+	+	+
S. lavendulae	SlaI (XhoI)	+	–	–	+	+	–	–	–	+	+	+	+	
S. lipmanii LE32	SliI, SliII[c]	+	+	+	+	+	+	–	+	+	–	–	–	–
S. lipmanii PM87	SliI–, SliII	+	±	+	+	+	+	+	+	+	+	+	–	+
S. phaeochromogenes	SphI	–	+	–	+	+	+	+	+	+	+	+	–	

[a] Data from Cox and Baltz (23); Matsushima et al. (17); Matsushima and Baltz (18); Matsushima and Baltz, unpublished. Bacteriophage lysates were prepared on S. griseofuscus.

[b] Defective in several restriction systems (17).

[c] SliI and SliII have been defined by in vivo restriction and modification of bacteriophages (18). S. lipmanii PM87 is defective in SliI restriction, but not in SliI modification.

7 of 13 bacteriophages. In this case, multiple restriction systems were eliminated by several rounds of mutagenesis and selection for increased transformation frequencies with several different plasmids (17). The relatively nonrestricting derivative PM73 permitted plaque formation by several phages normally restricted by strain T59235. *Streptomyces lipmanii* LE32, which appears to produce two restriction enconucleases, restricted 5 of 10 bacteriophages tested (18). A mutant defective in one of the systems (*Sli*I) fully restricted only 1 of the 10 bacteriophages. Table 1 also shows that *Streptomyces griseofuscus* allowed plaque formation by all 13 bacteriophages tested, and *Streptomyces ambofaciens* permitted plaque formation in 11 of 12 cases. These data suggested that these strains may not express significant levels of restriction.

Table 2 shows some illustrative data on protoplast transformation frequencies in several of these strains. Both *S. ambofaciens* and *S. griseofuscus* were transformed at high frequencies with DNA prepared from heterologous hosts (24,25), confirming that they do not express significant levels of restriction. *S. fradiae* T59235 and *S. lipmanii* LE32, on the other hand, were not readily transformed by DNA prepared from heterologous hosts, but they were transformed efficiently with DNA passaged through homologous hosts. This confirmed that both strains express significant restriction and modification systems that act on plasmid DNA. *S. fradiae* PM73, which contained multiple mutations to eliminate several different restriction systems, was transformed at relatively high efficiencies by plasmids prepared from heterologous and homologous hosts. *S. lipmanii* PM87, a strain defective in one of two *S. lipmanii* restriction systems, allowed an intermediate level of transformation by unmodified plasmid pIJ941. pIJ941 modified for *S. lipmanii* restriction systems transformed *S. lipmanii* LE32 and PM87 at equally high efficiencies. These results support the notion that bacteriophage host range analysis is a good predictor for the expression or lack of expression of significant restriction barriers in streptomycetes.

There are several ways to bypass restriction in streptomycetes. The first is to passage the DNA through a modifying host before attempting to introduce it into the restricting host. This has been shown to work with some small plasmids (24), but it is not a good approach to introduce large plasmids that are effectively restricted in the first host. A second approach is to isolate mutants defective or partially defective in restriction by chemical mutagenesis and selection for improved plasmid transformation (17,18). The obvious

Table 2   Transformation of Streptomycete Protoplasts with Plasmid DNA

Strain	Plasmid	Transformants/μg of DNA[a]		Reference
		Unmodified	Modified	
S. ambofaciens	pIJ702	1×10^5	—	24
	pFJ105	3×10^6	—	24
S. griseofuscus	pHJL193	1.2×10^6	1.2×10^6	25
S. fradiae JS85	pIJ702	$<4.0 \times 10^1$	2.4×10^4	17
	pFJ105	$<4.0 \times 10^1$	1.6×10^4	17
S. fradiae PM73	pIJ702	8.6×10^4	7.5×10^5	17
	pFJ105	4.3×10^4	5.5×10^5	17
S. lipmanii LE32	pIJ941	$<2 \times 10^2$	4×10^4	18
S. lipmanii PM87	pIJ941	2×10^3	5×10^4	18

[a] Unmodified, DNA prepared from heterologous host; modified, DNA prepared from homologous host.

drawbacks of this approach are that it is time consuming, it runs the risk of inadvertant second-site mutations that reduce product yield, and it solves the restriction problem in only a single strain of a single species. A third way to circumvent restriction is to introduce plasmid DNA as a linear concatemer by bacteriophage FP43–mediated transduction (26–30). Presumably, the linear concatemer has a higher probability of forming a modified unrestricted circular plasmid by recombination than a circular monomer does in protoplast transformation. Many species that express potent restriction systems, including several that restrict FP43 itself, are readily transduced by this method (26,27). The transduction method has several advantages: (a) a single transducing lysate can be used to introduce DNA into many different streptomycetes; (b) the physiological stage of cells can be varied to identify conditions to minimize the expression of restriction; (c) in some cases, transducing lysates can be prepared on hosts that modify plasmid DNA for particular restriction systems. The drawback of this method is that its utility is currently limited to self-replicating plasmids derived from pIJ702.

The fourth method is to modify DNA against host restriction in vitro. Matsushima and Baltz (21) have demonstrated that cell-free extracts of *Saccharopolyspora spinosa* can be used to modify plasmid DNA to allow successful protoplast transformation in this highly restricting strain. So far, this method has been limited to a single plasmid. McCue et al. (31) have modified plasmid DNA with a combination of SssI methylase, which methylates CG sequences at the C residue, and AluI methylase, which methylates AGCT sequences at the C residue. The modified plasmids were successfully introduced into *Streptomyces griseus* by protoplast transformation; transformations were not otherwise successful because of the strong restriction barriers.

A fifth method to bypass restriction is to introduce plasmid DNA by conjugation from *E. coli* (22,32,33). In *S. fradiae*, which is highly restricting during protoplast transformation with unmodified plasmid DNA (17,24,29), very high frequencies of exconjugants were obtained (32) by using vectors containing plasmid RK2 *oriT* to drive conjugal transfer from *E. coli* S17-1, a strain that contains plasmid RP4 integrated into the chromosome to provide transfer functions (34,35). In *S. spinosa*, which is highly restricting for bacteriophage plaque formation and protoplast transformation by plasmid DNA (21), very large derivatives of cosmid pOJ436 (32) containing *S. spinosa* DNA were transferred by conjugation from *E. coli* S17-1 and integrated into the *S. spinosa* chromosome at high frequencies (10^{-5} to 10^{-4} per recipient; 33). These striking examples suggest that the single-strand linear concatemers of plasmid DNA can transfer, bypass restriction, form double-strand circular monomers, and integrate by the ϕC31 *att/int* system or by homologous Campbell-like insertions at very high efficiencies. Thus, it appears that conjugation from *E. coli* to actinomycetes may be the method of choice to introduce large plasmids into restricting strains.

A sixth method to bypass apparent restriction is to use a single-strand vector containing a segment of homologous streptomycete DNA to direct homologous recombination into the chromosome (36). This promising method needs further exploration to determine its full utility.

B. Problems Associated with Self-Replicating Plasmids

Many useful self-replicating plasmids have been developed for gene cloning and for construction of recombinant strains (see 16 and references therein). However, a growing body of evidence indicates that the introduction and maintenance of self-replicating

Table 3   Effects of Replicating Plasmid Vectors on Secondary Metabolite Biosynthesis

Strain	Product	Plasmid	Control yield (%)	Reference
Streptomyces spp. 5541	Nemadectins	plJ702	6–9	37
		plJ355	9–10	37
		plJ365	1–13	37
		plJ58	4–6	37
		plJ922	7–16	37
		plJ941	3–7	37
		plJ61	6–8	37
S. acrimycini J12236	Candicidin	plJ699	~30	38
S. fradiae C373.17	Tylosin	plJ702	reduced	39
S. glaucescens	Tetracenomycin	plJ702	~65	40
			~45	
S. toyocaensis	Glycopeptide A47934	plJ702	<20	22

cloning vectors in streptomycetes is generally associated with reductions in secondary metabolite yields.

Table 3 shows several examples of fermentation analyses of streptomycete strains containing freely replicating plasmids. In these cases, the product yields were reduced by varying degrees. The most extensive analysis was carried out in the nemadectin producer, *Streptomyces* spp. 5541. In this case, the strains containing plasmids produced very low yields. When the recombinants were cured of plasmid and refermented, the cured strains produced nemadectin yields equivalent to the original plasmid-free parent strains. This proved that the large reductions in product yield in the recombinants were due to the presence of plasmid DNA. This general phenomenon of inhibition of secondary metabolite production by the presence of self-replicating plasmids may preclude the use of such vectors as a general means to introduce and express cloned DNA to enhance product yield.

C.   Integration of DNA into the Chromosome

An obvious approach to circumvent the problem of replicating plasmid–mediated inhibition of secondary metabolite production is to insert cloned DNA into the chromosome. A number of vectors are now available that are capable of site-specific integration into the chromosome. Table 4 lists some of these along with their salient features.

One approach to chromosomal integration has been to introduce plasmid or bacteriophage integration functions into cloning vectors. Many streptomycete plasmids have the ability to integrate site-specifically into streptomycete genomes (16). Plasmid pSAM2 has been studied in detail, and a number of different cloning vectors have been constructed from this integrating plasmid (41–47). An important unanswered question is whether the integration of pSAM2-based vectors causes negative effects on fermentation yields in highly productive strains. If it does not, then these vectors should be very useful for the construction of recombinant production strains.

A number of vectors have been constructed that use the bacteriophage ϕC31 *att/int* system to direct the insertion of the plasmid into the chromosomal *attB* site (32,48,49). Cosmid pOJ436 (Table 4) was shown to integrate into two different *attB* sites in *S. spin-*

Table 4   Some Integrative Cloning Vectors

Plasmid	Size (kb)	Streptomycete replicon	E. coli replicon	Features[a]	Reference
pPM927	11.6	pSAM2	pBR322	*tsr, stm, spc, ptipA, intp*SAM, *oriT*	41
pKC796	6.7	—	pUC	Am[R], MCS, *int*φC31	42
pOJ436	11.1	—	pUC	Am[R], MCS, *cos, oriT, int*φC31	32
pOJ260	3.5	—	pUC	Am[R], MCS, *oriT*	32

[a]*tsr*, thiostrepton resistance gene; Am[R], apramycin resistance gene; *cos*, λ cohesive end cleavage site; *stm*, streptomycin resistance gene; *spc*, spectinomycin resistance gene; *ptipA*, *tipA* promoter; *intp*SAM, pSAM2 integration function; *int*φC31, φC31 integration function; *oriT*, origin of transfer from RK2; MCS, multiple cloning site.

osa, and integration into at least one of the sites did not cause a reduction in macrolide A83543 production (33). Plasmid pOJ436 and a derivative containing a 35 kb insert of DNA were shown to integrate into a single *attB* site in *Streptomyces toyocaensis*, a glycopeptide antibiotic producer (22). Several of the insertions did not cause significant reductions in glycopeptide A47934 production. These two studies exemplify the utility of cosmid pOJ436 as a method to stably insert DNA into the chromosome without substantially disrupting secondary metabolite production.

A second method to stably insert DNA into the chromosome without disrupting secondary metabolite production is by transposon exchange (50,51). This method relies on the observation that transposons can insert into many different sites in the chromosome, and that a substantial fraction of the insertions, about 50% in the case of the tylosin-producing *S. fradiae* (51), are neutral with respect to secondary metabolite production. The method entails identifying a strain containing a neutral transposon insertion and then using the transposon sequences as regions of homology for double crossovers to insert a gene of interest. This approach has been exemplified by cloning a second copy of the gene encoding a rate-limiting step in tylosin biosynthesis (51; see below).

A third method for the neutral insertion of DNA into the chromosome is to identify a neutral site by transposition or other insertional mutagenesis, to clone the DNA flanking the neutral site, and to use the cloned flanking DNA as regions of homology to insert a gene(s) into the chromosome by homologous double crossovers (52). The advantage of this method is that the recombinants contain cloned genes but no extraneous plasmid or transposon DNA. The advantage of using transposons Tn5096, Tn5099, Tn5099-10, or Tn5100 to identify neutral sites is that they have broad host specificity and contain antibiotic resistance markers that express in actinomycetes and *E. coli* (16,53–58). Thus, DNA flanking the neutral site can be readily cloned in *E. coli*. If this method is used to insert a second copy of a homologous gene, then the recombinant will contain no "foreign" DNA and will have fewer regulatory hurdles to delay the implementation of the strain in production (52). This procedure has been exemplified by the insertion of a second copy of the *tylF* gene into a tylosin production strain of *S. fradiae* (see below).

A fourth method for neutral insertion of DNA is to clone random fragments of chromosomal DNA into a nonreplicating vector (for actinomycetes) that can be introduced into actinomycetes by protoplast transformation or by conjugation from *E. coli*. Recombinants are formed by homologous single crossovers into the chromosome. The disadvantage of this method is that the recombinant contains "foreign" DNA, although the DNA is not self-replicating in actinomycetes. The identification of large segments of chromosomal DNA that can be used for neutral insertion of DNA has been exemplified by studies carried out in *S. spinosa*, a macrolide producing actinomycete (33), using the conjugal vector pOJ436 (Table 4). A technical drawback to this approach is that the insertion of additional copies of homologous genes into such a vector provides two segments of DNA that can participate in homologous recombination into the chromosome. In many cases, the desired recombinants may be readily identified by Southern blot analysis of several different recombinants. This procedure may be impractical if very large DNA segments are to be inserted into the chromosome at a relatively small neutral site. However, this same potential problem exists with the double crossovers using the neutral site insertion procedure.

IV. APPLICATIONS OF MOLECULAR GENETICS TO YIELD IMPROVEMENT

A. Rate-Limiting Steps in Biosynthesis

The concept of improving product yield by increasing the copy number of genes encoding enzymes involved in the rate-limiting steps in secondary metabolite biosynthesis was proposed over a decade ago (59,60), and methods to clone genes involved in antibiotic biosynthesis have been available for some time (61–66). Furthermore, many genes involved in antibiotic biosynthesis have been cloned and analyzed in great detail (16,67). Nonetheless, there are not yet many published examples of using gene cloning to relieve rate limitations (16).

The paucity of examples may be due, in part, to the previously discussed problems of restriction and inhibition of secondary metabolite production by self-replicating cloning vectors. With the chromosome insertion methods and conjugal transfer systems, however, methods are now available to construct recombinant strains with properties suitable for large-scale production. An example is tylosin production in *S. fradiae* (8,60). Highly productive strains of *S. fradiae* accumulate high percentages of macrocin, the immediate precursor of tylosin (68,69). Macrocin lacks the O-methyl group normally present at the 3″ position of the mycinose moiety of tylosin, so that macrocin O-methyltransferase levels may be suboptimal for efficient conversion of macrocin to tylosin in highly productive strains (69). The macrocin O-methyltransferase gene (*tylF*) was cloned (70,71) and initially introduced into a production strain on the replicating plasmid pIJ702 and on the integrating plasmid pKC796 (39). In both cases, the recombinant strains expressed higher levels of macrocin O-methyltransferase and produced higher levels of tylosin, but the presence of either vector caused a decrease in total macrolide yield, reducing the overall potential yield of the process.

However, the neutral insertion of a second *tylF* gene by the transposon exchange and neutral site insertion methods described above have generated stable recombinant strains with substantially improved conversion of macrocin to tylosin, with no reduction in total macrolide products (51,52).

Another laboratory-scale application for yield enhancement has been demonstrated in *Streptomyces clavuligerus* (72). Insertion of a second copy of the *lat* gene into the chromosome caused a two- to fivefold increase in production of β-lactam antibiotics. The *lat* gene encodes lysine ε-aminotransferase, an enzyme involved in the biosynthesis of α-aminoadipic acid, a precursor in penicillin and cephalosporin antibiotic biosynthesis.

These two examples illustrate that both precursor flux, in the case of β-lactam biosynthesis, and antibiotic biosynthetic enzyme levels, in the case of tylosin, can contribute to rate limitations, and that gene cloning and insertion of cloned genes into the chromosome can address either limitation.

B.   Positive and Negative Regulatory Genes

Another appealing molecular genetic approach to yield enhancement is to clone positive regulatory genes and insert them into neutral sites in the chromosome (16), or to disrupt negative regulatory genes. Many global and pathway-specific regulatory genes have been identified in streptomycetes (16,73). Several laboratory-scale examples of enhanced product yield in recombinants have been described (see 16 for a review). A particularly interesting example was the enhancement of spiramycin biosynthesis in S. *ambofaciens* (74). In this case, the positive regulatory gene *srmR* was identified by gene disruption as a mutant defective in multiple steps in spiramycin biosynthesis (75). The *srmR* gene was shown to be a novel transcriptional activator, and the introduction of the cloned *srmR* into a stable S. *ambofaciens* strain on the multicopy vector pHJL401 caused an increase in spiramycin production from 100 to 500 μg/ml. In this case, the introduction of a disrupted *srmR* gene on the same plasmid did not cause an increase or reduction in spiramycin production.

An example of enhancement of antibiotic production by disrupting a global negative regulatory gene has been described by Brian et al. (76). In this case, the *absA* locus of *Streptomyces coelicolor* was first identified by UV-induced mutations that blocked the production of several antibiotics without disrupting differentiation and sporulation (77). The *absA* gene appears to encode a eubacterial two-component sensor kinase involved in a signal transduction process that negatively regulates antibiotic production. Interestingly, the overproduction phenotype was observed only by a gross gene disruption, and not by point mutations. This observation supports the notion that transposition mutagenesis may be a useful adjunct to a comprehensive strain development program (see Section IV.C).

While these and other examples of yield enhancement at the laboratory scale in relatively low producing strains are indeed encouraging, it is not yet known if these approaches will be successful in highly developed production strains in production media. Since improved production yields may be associated with many factors, the early application of manipulating positive and negative regulatory genes in strain development might facilitate the subsequent detection of mutations that influence the flow of precursors into the pathway and enhance the rate of yield improvement.

C.   Other Applications of Transposons

The left end inverted repeat (IR-L) of IS*493*, the progenitor of Tn*5096*, Tn*5099*, Tn*5099-10*, and Tn*5100-4*, contains weak outward reading promoter activity (57). IR-L contains -35 and -10 sequences that conform to consensus prokaryotic promoter sequences. IR-L also contains another potential -35 region that could fuse with a -10 sequence upon insertion. The presence of outward reading promoters and partial promoters has been observed in Gram-negative insertion sequence (IS) elements, and activation of transcription upon transposition has also been observed (78). These observations suggested that transposons derived from IS*493* might be used to activate as well as to disrupt genes. In a recent study in *Streptomyces roseosporus*, it was shown that Tn*5099* insertion mutagenesis could activate the expression of an apparently cryptic pathway for black pigment formation (79). Furthermore, one insertion mutation that enhanced red pigment formation also caused a 60% increase in the lipopeptide antibiotic daptomycin production. It is not known if these mutations are due to the portable promoter in IR-L or to the disruption of negative regulatory elements. However, these questions can be readily addressed, because the DNA flanking the transposition can be cloned directly in *E. coli* selecting for the Am^R marker in Tn*5099*. This general approach is very appealing, since it offers the possibility of assigning the phenotype of yield enhancement to specific genes. The approach can be extended to studying mutations that decrease or abolish antibiotic yield, and it may provide a general method to identify both positive and negative regulatory genes.

V.   SUMMARY

It has taken a concerted effort by many laboratories to advance the molecular genetics of streptomycetes to the relatively elevated position that it enjoys today (16). The practical applications of molecular genetics to yield enhancement have lagged behind somewhat, perhaps for technical reasons described in this chapter. However, many of the technical obstacles have been identified, and potential solutions are now available. The more sophisticated molecular genetic approaches are not likely to supercede the traditional approaches of chemical mutagenesis and recombination; rather, they should be used in a complementary role that will provide a means to learn and exploit knowledge on gene regulation and secondary metabolite biosynthesis to speed the process of strain development.

REFERENCES

1.   Baltz RH. Mutation in *Streptomyces*. Day L, Queener S, eds. The Bacteria, Vol. 9, Antibiotic Producing *Streptomyces*. New York: Academic Press, 1986:61–94.
2.   Baltz RH. Mutagenesis in *Streptomyces* spp. Demain AL, Solomon NA, eds. Manual of Industrial Microbiology and Biotechnology. Washington, D.C.: American Society for Microbiology, 1986:184–190.
3.   Queener SW, Lively DH. Screening and selection for strain improvement. Demain AL, Solomon NA, eds. Manual of Industrial Microbiology and Biotechnology. Washington, D.C.: American Society for Microbiology, 1986:155–169.
4.   Jiménez-Sanchez A, Cerdá-Olmedo E. Mutation and DNA replication in *Escherichia coli* treated with low concentrations of *N*-methyl-*N'*-nitro-*N*-nitrosoguanidine. Mutation Res 1975; 28:337–345.
5.   Cerdá-Olmedo E, Ruiz-Vázquez R. Nitrosoguanidine mutagenesis. Sebek OK, Laskin AI, eds. Genetics of Industrial Microorganisms. Washington, D.C.: American Society for Microbiology, 1979:15–20.
6.   Randazzo R, Sciandrello G, Carere A, Bignami M, Velcich A, Sermonti G. Localized mutagenesis in *Streptomyces coelicolor* A3(2). Mutation Res 1976; 36:291–302.
7.   Baltz RH, Seno ET. Properties of *Streptomyces fradiae* mutants blocked in biosynthesis of the macrolide antibiotic tylosin. Antimicrob Agents Chemother 1981; 20:214–225.
8.   Baltz RH, Seno ET. Genetics of *Streptomyces fradiae* and tylosin biosynthesis. Annu Rev Microbiol 1988; 42:547–574.
9.   Merson-Davies L, Cundliffe E. Analysis of five tylosin biosynthetic genes from the *tylIBA* region of the *Streptomyces fradiae* genome. Mol Microbiol 1994; 13:349–355.
10.   Coulondre C, Miller JH. Genetic studies of the lac repressor IV. Mutagenic specificity in the *lacI* gene of *Escherichia coli*. J Mol Biol 1977; 117:577–606.
11.   Hopwood DA. Genetic recombination and strain improvement. Dev Ind Microbiol 1977; 18:9–21.

12. Hopwood DA. The many faces of recombination. Sebek OK, Laskin AI, eds. Genetics of Industrial Microorganisms. Washington, D.C.: American Society for Microbiology, 1979:1–9.

13. Hopwood DA, Wright HM, Bibb MJ, Cohen SN. Genetic recombination through protoplast fusion in *Streptomyces*. Nature 1977; 268:171–174.

14. Baltz RH. Genetic recombination in *Streptomyces fradiae* by protoplast fusion and cell regeneration. J Gen Microbiol 1978; 107:93–102.

15. Matsushima P, Baltz RH. Protoplast fusion. Demain AL, Solomon NA, eds. Manual of Industrial Microbiology and Biotechnology. Washington, D.C.: American Society for Microbiology, 1986:170–183.

16. Baltz RH. Gene expression in recombinant *Streptomyces*. Smith A, ed. Gene Expression in Recombinant Microorganisms. New York: Marcel Dekker, 1994:309–381.

17. Matsushima P, Cox KL, Baltz RH. Highly transformable mutants of *Streptomyces fradiae* defective in several restriction systems. Mol Gen Genet 1987; 206:393–400.

18. Matsushima P, Baltz RH. *Streptomyces lipmanii* expresses two restriction systems that inhibit plasmid transformation and bacteriophage plaque formation. J Bacteriol 1989; 171:3128–3132.

19. Hu Z, Bao K, Zhou X, Zhou Q, Hopwood DA, Kieser T, Deng Z. Repeated polyketide synthase modules involved in the biosynthesis of a heptaene macrolide by *Streptomyces* sp. FR-008. Mol Microbiol 1994; 14:163–172.

20. Qin Z, Peng K, Zhou X, Liang R, Zhou Q, Chen H, Hopwood DA, Kieser T, Deng Z. Development of a gene cloning systems for *Streptomyces hygroscopicus* subsp. *yengchengensis*, a producer of three useful antifungal compounds, by elimination of three barriers to DNA transfer. J Bacteriol 1994; 176:2090–2095.

21. Matsushima P, Baltz RH. Transformation of *Saccharopolyspora spinosa* protoplasts with plasmid DNA modified *in vitro* to avoid host restriction. Microbiology 1994; 140:139–143.

22. Matsushima P, Baltz RH. A gene cloning system for *Streptomyces toyocaensis*. Microbiology 1996; 142:261–267.

23. Cox KL, Baltz RH. Restriction of bacteriophage plaque formation in *Streptomyces* spp. J Bacteriol 1984; 159:499–504.

24. Matsushima P, Baltz RH. Efficient plasmid transformation of *Streptomyces ambofaciens* and *Streptomyces fradiae* protoplasts. J Bacteriol 1985; 163:180–185.

25. Larson JL, Hershberger CL. Shuttle vectors for cloning recombinant DNA in *Escherichia coli* and *Streptomyces griseofuscus* C581. J Bacteriol 1984; 157:314–317.

26. McHenney MA, Baltz RH. Transduction of plasmid DNA in *Streptomyces* spp. and related genera by bacteriophage FP43. J Bacteriol 1988; 170:2276–2282.

27. McHenney MA, Baltz RH. Transduction of plasmid DNA in macrolide producing streptomycetes. J Antibiot 1989; 42:1725–1727.

28. Hahn DR, McHenney MA, Baltz RH. Properties of the streptomycete temperate bacteriophage FP43. J Bacteriol 1991; 173:3770–3775.

29. Matsushima P, McHenney MA, Baltz RH. Transduction and transformation of plasmid DNA in *Streptomyces fradiae* strains that express different levels of restriction. J Bacteriol 1989; 171:3080–3084.

30. McHenney MA, Baltz RH. Transduction of plasmid DNA containing the *ermE* gene and expression of erythromycin resistance in streptomycetes. J Antibiot 1991; 44:1267–1269.

31. McCue LA, Kwak J, Wang J, Kendrick KE. Analysis of a gene that suppresses the morphological defect of bald mutants of *Streptomyces griseus*. J Bacteriol 1996; 178:2867–2875.

32. Bierman M, Logan R, O'Brien K, Seno ET, Rao RN, Schoner BE. Plasmid cloning vectors for the conjugal transfer of DNA from *Escherichia coli* to *Streptomyces* spp. Gene 1992; 116:43–49.

33. Matsushima P, Broughton MC, Turner JR, Baltz RH. Conjugal transfer of cosmid DNA from *Escherichia coli* to *Saccharopolyspora spinosa*: Effects of chromosomal insertions on macrolide A83543 production. Gene 1994; 146:39–45.

34. Simon R, Priefer V, Pühler A. A broad host range mobilization system for in vivo genetic engineering: Transposon mutagenesis in gram negative bacteria. Bio/technol 1983; 1:784–790.

35. Mazodier P, Petter R, Thompson C. Intergeneric conjugation between *Escherichia coli* and *Streptomyces* species. J Bacteriol 1989; 171:3583–3585.

36. Hillemann D, Pühler A, Wohlleben W. Gene disruption and gene replacement in *Streptomyces* via single stranded DNA transformation of integration vectors. Nucl Acid Res 1991; 19:727–731.

37. Thomas DI, Cove JH, Baumberg S, Jones CA, Rudd BAM. Plasmid effects on secondary metabolite production by a streptomycete synthesizing an anthelminthic macrolide. J Gen Microbiol 1991; 137:2331–2337.

38. Asturias JA, Martín JF, Liras P. Biosynthesis and phosphate control of candicidin by *Streptomyces acrimycini* JI2236: Effect of amplification of the *pabAB* gene. J Ind Microbiol 13; 1994:183–189.

39. Cox KL, Seno ET. Maintenance of cloned biosynthetic genes in *Streptomyces fradiae* on freely-replicating and integrative plasmid vectors. J Cell Biochem 1990; Suppl 14A:93 (abstract).

40. Decker H, Summers RG, Hutchinson CR. Overproduction of the acyl carrier protein component of a type II polyketide synthase stimulates production of tetracenomycin biosynthetic intermediates in *Streptomyces glaucescens*. J Antibiot 1994; 47:54–63.

41. Smokvina T, Mazodier P, Boccard F, Thompson CJ, Guérineau M. Construction of a series of pSAM2-based integrative vectors for use in actinomycetes. Gene 1990; 94:53–59.

42. Kuhstoss S, Richardson MA, Rao RN. Plasmid cloning vectors that integrate site-specifically in *Streptomyces* spp. Gene 1991; 97:143–146.

43. Pernodet J-L, Simonet J-M, Guérineau M. Plasmids in different strains of *Streptomyces ambofaciens*: Free and integrated form of plasmid pSAM2. Mol Gen Genet 1984; 198:35–49.

44. Kuhstoss S, Richardson MA, Rao RN. Site-specific integration in *Streptomyces ambofaciens*: Localization of integration functions in *S. ambofaciens* plasmid pSAM2. J Bacteriol 1989; 171:16–23.

45. Mazodier P, Thompson C, Boccard F. The chromosomal integration site of the *Streptomyces* element pSAM2 overlaps a putative tRNA gene conserved among actinomycetes. Mol Gen Genet 1990; 222:431–434.

46. Smokvina T, Boccard F, Hagège J, Luzzati M, Friedmann A, Pernodet J-L, Guérineau M. Applications of the integrated plasmid pSAM2. Heslet H, Davies J, Florent J, Bobichon L, Durand G, Penasse L, eds. Proceedings of the 6th International Symposium on Genetics of Industrial Microorganisms—GIM90. Strasbourg: Société Francaise de Microbiologíe, 1990:403–412.

47. Boccard F, Smokvina T, Pernodet J-L, Friedmann A, Guérineau M. The integrated conjugative plasmid pSAM2 of *Streptomyces ambofaciens* is related to temperate bacteriophages. EMBO J 1989; 8:973–980.

48. Chater KF. *Streptomyces* phages and their applications to *Streptomyces* genetics. Queener SW, Day LE, eds. Antibiotic-Producing *Streptomyces*. Orlando, Florida: Academic Press, 1986:119–158.

49. Kuhstoss S, Rao RN. Analysis of the integration function of the streptomycete bacteriophage ϕC31. J Mol Biol 1991; 222:897–908.

50. Chung ST, Cross LL. Transposon Tn4556 mediated DNA insertion and site-directed mutagenesis. Heslot H, Davies J, Florent J, Bobichon L, Durand G, Penasse L, eds. Proceedings of the 6th International Symposium on Genetics of Industrial Microorganisms. Strasbourg: Sociéé Francaise de Microbiologie, 1990:207–218.

51. Solenberg P, Cantwell CA, Tietz AJ, Mc Gilvray D, Queener SW, Baltz RH. Transposition mutagenesis in *Streptomyces fradiae*: Identification of a neutral site for the stable insertion of DNA by transposon exchange. Gene 1996; 168:67–72.

52. Baltz RH, McHenney MA, Cantwell CA, Queener SW, Solenberg PJ. Applications of transposition mutagenesis in antibiotic producing streptomycetes. Antonie Leeuwenhoek 1997; 71:179–187.

53. Solenberg PJ, Baltz RH. Transposition of Tn5096 and other IS493 derivatives in Streptomyces griseofuscus. J Bacteriol 1991; 173:1096–1104.

54. McHenney MA, Baltz RH. Transposition of Tn5096 from a temperature-sensitive transducible plasmid in Streptomyces spp. J Bacteriol 1991; 1973:5578–5581.

55. Hahn DR, Solenberg PJ, Baltz RH. Tn5099, a xylE promoter probe transposon for Streptomyces spp. J Bacteriol 1991; 173:5573–5577.

56. Baltz RH, Hahn DR, McHenney MA, Solenberg PJ. Transposition of Tn5096 and related transposons in Streptomyces species. Gene 1992; 115:61–65.

57. Baltz RH, McHenney MA, Solenberg PA. Properties of transposons derived from IS493 and applications in streptomycetes. Baltz RH, Hegeman G, Skatrud PL, eds. Industrial Microorganisms: Basic and Applied Molecular Genetics. Washington, D.C.: American Society for Microbiology, 1993:51–56.

58. Solenberg PJ, Baltz RH. Hypertransposing derivatives of the streptomycete insertion sequence IS493. Gene 1994; 147:47–54.

59. Hopwood DA. Future possibilities for the discovery of new antibiotics by genetic engineering. Salton MRJ, Shockman GD, eds. β-Lactam Antibiotics. New York: Academic Press, 1981:585–598.

60. Baltz RH. Genetics and biochemistry of tylosin production: A model for genetic engineering in antibiotic-producing Streptomyces. Hollaender A, ed. Genetic Engineering of Microorganisms for Chemicals. New York: Plenum Press, 1982:431–444.

61. Hopwood DA, Bibb MJ, Bruton CJ, Chater KF, Feitelson JS, Gil JA. Cloning Streptomyces genes for antibiotic production. Trends Biotechnol 1983; 1:42–48.

62. Martín JF, Gil JA. Cloning and expression of antibiotic production genes. Biotechnol 1984; 2:63–72.

63. Fayerman JT. New developments in gene cloning in antibiotic producing microorganisms. Biotechnol 1986; 4:786–789.

64. Hopwood DA, Kieser T, Lydiate D, Bibb MJ. Streptomyces plasmids: Their biology and use as cloning vectors. Queener SW, Day LE, eds. The Bacteria, Vol. 9, Antibiotic-Producing Streptomyces. New York: Academic Press, 1986:159–229.

65. Hopwood DA, Bibb MJ, Chater KF, Kieser T. Plasmid and phage vectors for gene cloning and analysis in Streptomyces. Method Enzymol 1987; 153:116–166.

66. Rao RN, Richardson MA, Kuhstoss S. Cosmid shuttle vectors for cloning and analysis of Streptomyces DNA. Meth Enzymol 1987; 153:166–198.

67. Seno ET, Baltz RH. Structural organization and regulation of antibiotic biosynthesis and resistance genes in actinomycetes. Shapiro S, ed. Regulation of Secondary Metabolism in Actinomycetes. Boca Raton, Florida: CRC Press, 1989:1–48.

68. Seno ET, Baltz RH. Properties of S-adenosyl-L-methionine: macrocin O-methyltransferase in extracts of Streptomyces fradiae strains which produce normal or elevated levels of tylosin and in mutants blocked in specific O-methylations. Antimicrob Agents Chemother 1981; 20:370–377.

69. Seno ET, Baltz RH. S-adenosyl-L-methionine: macrocin-O-methyltransferase activities in a series of Streptomyces fradiae mutants that produce different levels of the macrolide antibiotic tylosin. Antimicrob Agents Chemother 1982; 21:758–763.

70. Cox KL, Fishman SE, Larson JL, Stanzak R, Reynolds PA, Yeh WK, Van Frank RM, Birmingham VA, Hershberger CL, Seno ET. The use of recombinant DNA techniques to study tylosin biosynthesis and resistance in Streptomyces fradiae. J Nat Prod 1986; 49:971–980.

71. Fishman SE, Cox K, Larson JL, Reynolds PA, Seno ET, Yeh WK, Van Frank R, Hershberger CL. Cloning genes for the biosynthesis of a macrolide antibiotic. Proc Natl Acad Sci USA 1987; 84:8248–8252.

72. Malmberg L-H, Hu W-S, Sherman DH. Precursor flux control through targeted chromosomal insertion of the lysine ε-aminotransferase (*lat*) gene in cephamycin C biosynthesis. J Bacteriol 1993; 175:6916–6924.

73. Champness WC, Chater KF. Regulation and integration of antibiotic production and morphological differentiation in *Streptomyces* spp. Piggot PJ, Moran CP, Jr., Youngman, P., eds. Regulation of Bacterial Differentiation. Washington, D.C.: American Society for Microbiology, 1994:61–93.

74. Geistlich M, Losick R, Turner JR, Rao RN. Characterization of a novel regulatory gene governing the expression of a polyketide synthase gene in *Streptomyces ambofaciens*. Mol Microbiol 1992; 6:2019–2029.

75. Richardson MA, Kuhstoss S, Huber MLB, Ford L, Godfrey O, Turner JR, Rao RN. Cloning of spiramycin biosynthetic genes and their use in constructing *Streptomyces ambofaciens* mutants defective in spiramycin biosynthesis. J Bacteriol 1990; 172:3790–3798.

76. Brian P, Riggle PJ, Santos RA, Champness WC. Global negative regulation of *Streptomyces coelicolor* antibiotic synthesis mediated by an *absA*-encoded putative signal transduction system. J Bacteriol 1996; 178:3221–3231.

77. Adamidis T, Riggle P, Champness WC. Mutations in a new *Streptomyces coelicolor* locus which globally block antibiotic biosynthesis but not sporulation. J Bacteriol 1990; 172:2962–2969.

78. Galas DJ, Chandler M. Bacterial insertion sequences. Berg DE, Howe MM, eds. Mobile DNA. Washington, D.C.: American Society for Microbiology, 1989:109–162.

79. McHenney MA, Baltz RH. Gene transfer and transposition mutagenesis in *Streptomyces roseosporus:* mapping of insertions that influence daptomycin or pigment production. Microbiology 1996; 142:2363–2373.

3

Butyrolactone Autoregulators, Inducers of Virginiamycin in *Streptomyces virginiae:* Their Structures, Biosynthesis, Receptor Proteins, and Induction of Virginiamycin Biosynthesis

Yasuhiro Yamada and Takuya Nihira
Osaka University, Osaka, Japan

Shohei Sakuda
The University of Tokyo, Tokyo, Japan

I.   INTRODUCTION

Virginiamycin has a long history of research on its production, antibacterial activities, mode of action, and biosynthesis, and there are some closely related homologs from different *Streptomyces* species named without any systematic nomenclature. There are, therefore, many synonyms for virginiamycin M_1, such as pristinamycin II_A, streptogramin A, synergistin A, mikamycin A, ostreogrycin A, and vernamycin A; and for virginiamycin M_2, such as pristinamycin II_B and ostreogrycin G. For virginiamycin S, there are three closely related homologs under many names such as pristinamycin I_A, I_B, I_C, streptogramin B, synergistin B_1, mikamycin B, ostreogrycin B, B_2, B_1, and vernamycin B_α, B_β, B_γ. Staphylomycin also was once used as a synonym for virginiamycin M and S.

Streptomyces virginiae mainly produces two types of antibiotics, namely, virginiamycin M and virginiamycin S, as shown in Figure 1 Virginiamycin M has a macrocyclic lactone containing a single amide bond and is a kind of hybrid compound between a macrolide and a deformed cyclic oligopeptide. On the other hand, virginiamycin S is a macrocyclic peptidolactone composed of L-threonine, D-α-aminobutyric acid, L-proline, N-methyl-L-phenylalanine, L-4-oxopipecolic acid, L-phenylglycine, and 3-hydroxypicolinic acid.

The most characteristic feature of this pair of antibiotics is their synergistic effect in the mode of action. The combination of virginiamycin M and S, at the optimum ratio of 3:2, has about a fivefold greater efficacy against *Staphylococcus aureus* compared with that of either used alone (1). The mode of action of virginiamycin, which mainly involves inhibition of protein synthesis at the ribosome, has been reviewed in detail by Cocito (2). Virginiamycin M and S interact with 50S ribosomal subunits, inhibiting elongation processes by preventing the elongation factor (EF) Tu–dependent binding of aminoacyl tRNA to ribosomes and subsequent peptide-bond formation. The plausible target proteins of virginiamycin M on 50S ribosomal subunits were identified. The binding of vir-

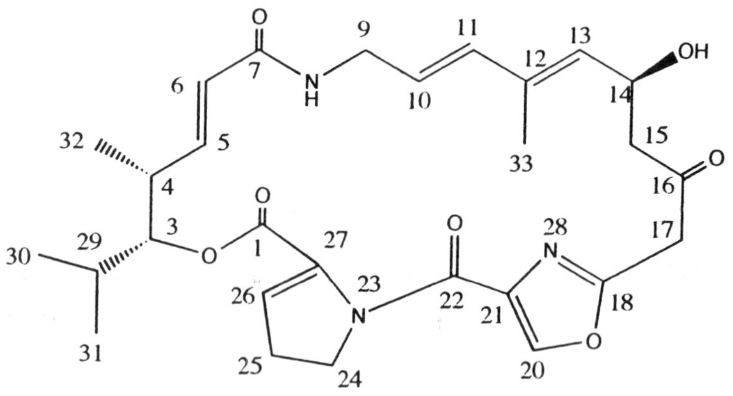

Viginiamycin M₁

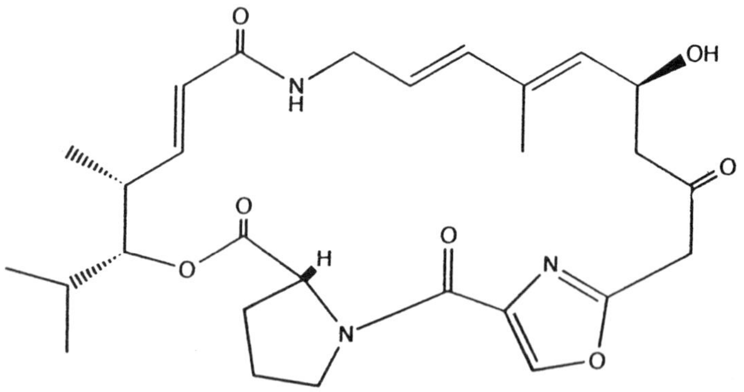

Virginiamycin M₂

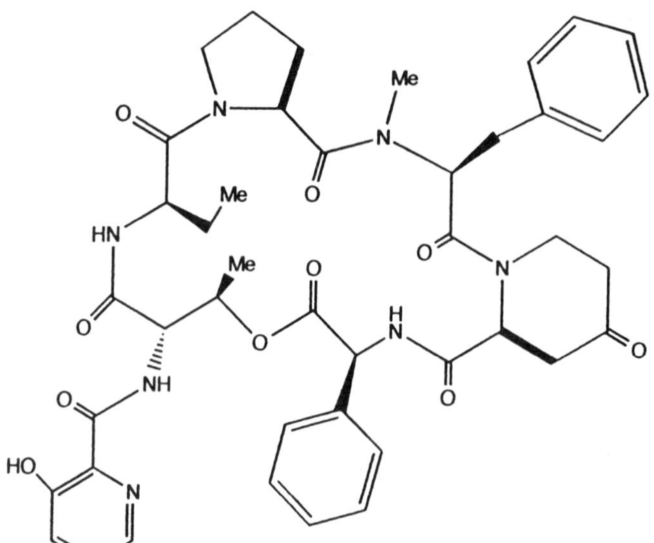

Virginiamycin S

Figure 1   The structures of virginiamycin M and S.

giniamycin M to ribosomes causes a several-fold increase of the affinity of virginiamycin S to this complex; this provides a mechanistic explanation of the synergistic effect (2).

Recently, we have found that an NADPH-dependent reductase in the crude cell extract of *S. virginiae* reduces virginiamycin M to (16R)-16-dihydrovirginiamycin M, with an accompanying decrease to 1/20 of its previous activity. This result suggests the NADPH-dependent reductase in *S. virginiae* seems to play a role of self-resistant pathway in the cells (3).

The historical aspects of the discovery of virginiamycin, the producer strains, and its practical production were described in detail by Biot in the first edition of this book (1). The structure, the chemistry, and especially, the organic synthesis of the virginiamycin groups were well reviewed by Paris et al. of the Rhône–Poulenc group (4). The biosynthesis of virginiamycin M_1, M_2, and S was studied mainly by Kingston and coworkers (5–7) with bio-organic methods. The building blocks and their assembly pattern in virginiamycin molecules M and S are shown in Figures 2 and 3. The genetic basis for virginiamycin biosynthesis is not yet known, and there is no information about a host–vector system that works in *S. virginiae*.

In this chapter, we describe new aspects concerning the induction of virginiamycin production by butyrolactone-type autoregulators. The structures, biosynthesis of butyrolactone autoregulators, and their receptor proteins are also reviewed.

II. THE DISCOVERY OF THE AUTOREGULATOR IN *STREPTOMYCES VIRGINIAE*

At the end of 1960s, Yanagimoto and Terui (8) started studies on the production of virginiamycin using *S. virginiae*. They found some low-molecular-weight compounds from the culture broth of *S. virginiae* that very effectively induce the production of virginiamycin. They named this compound IM (inducing material) and elaborated the assay system to estimate the activity of IM, which is produced at a very low concentration in the culture medium. IM production starts at 12 hr cultivation, and it induces the full production of virginiamycin after 6 hr, at 18 hr of cultivation, as shown in Figure 4. When IM was added to the culture broth at 8 hr, the antibiotics were induced fully at 14 hr of cultivation. Yanagimoto and coworkers partially purified IM, and they predicted that IM has δ- or γ-lactone moiety on the basis of its infrared (IR) spectrum and nuclear magnetic resonance (NMR) signals (9).

In the mid 1980s, we again started the purification of IM, and we purified five closely related compounds (10,11). All of them have a common butanolide skeleton, as shown in Figure 5. These autoregulators were named virginiae butanolide (VB) A, B, C, D, and E. They are produced at about 0.1 μg/ml each in the culture broth of *S. virginiae*, and they induce both virginiamycin M and S at a concentration in the few nanomolar range. The structures of VB were determined by spectroscopy and confirmed by chemical synthesis (10). The structures of known autoregulators isolated from *Streptomyces* are shown in Figure 5.

The first and best-known example of a butyrolactone autoregulator is A-factor from *Streptomyces griseus*, found by Khokhlov and coworkers (12). A-factor induces the production of streptomycin and cytodifferentiation such as aerial mycelium and sporulation in *S. griseus* str⁻ spo⁻ mutants (13). Gräfe's factors, that is, Factor I from *Streptomyces viridochromogenes* (14) and the factors from *Streptomyces bikiniensis* and *Streptomyces cyaneofuscatus* (15), also induce anthracycline antibiotics and cytodifferentiation in *S. griseus*.

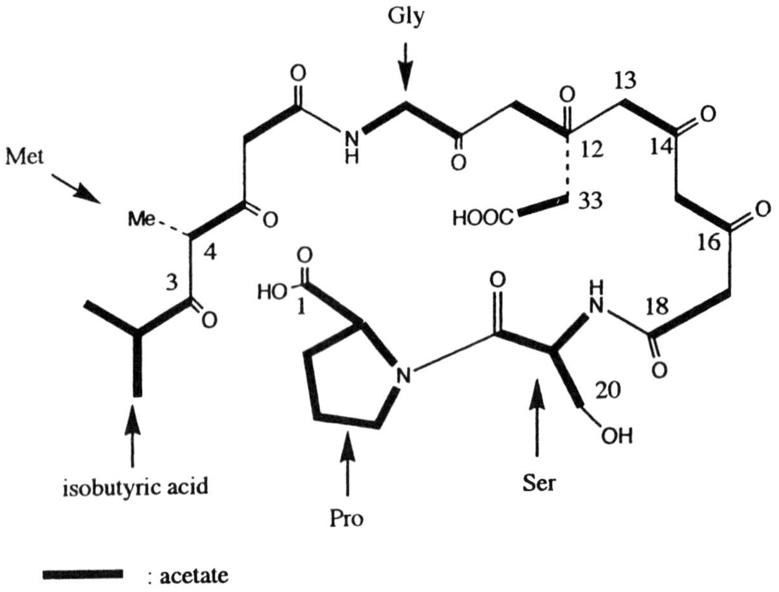

Figure 2   The assembly of building blocks in virginiamycin M.

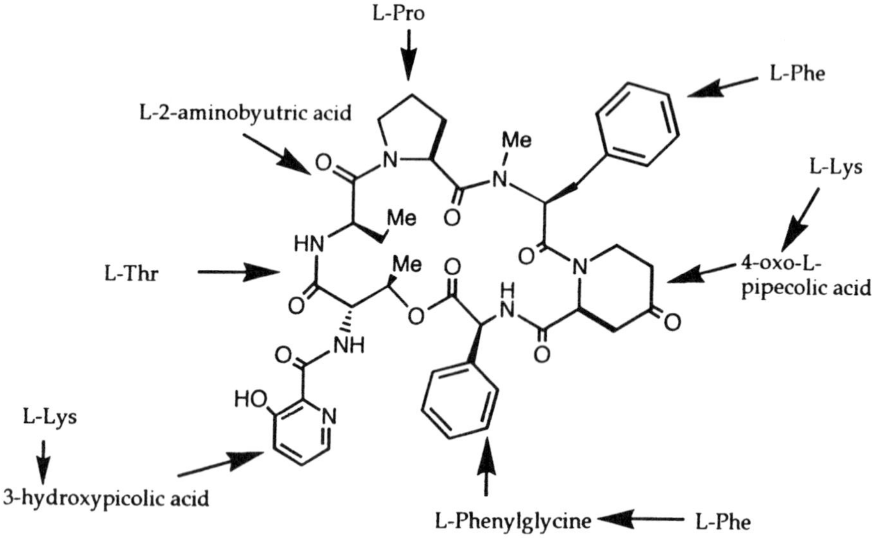

Figure 3   The biosynthesis of virginiamycin S.

Another example is IM-2, the presence of which was originally described in cultures of D-cycloserine producer *Streptomyces* sp. FRI-5 by Yanagimoto (16). IM-2 induces blue pigment production and the shift of produced antibiotics from D-cycloserine to nucleoside antibiotics, such as showdomycin and minimycin (17). We purified IM-2 and determined its structure (18), as shown in Figure 5.

All of these butyrolactone autoregulators have a hydroxymethyl group at C3 and a 1′-hydroxy or 1′-oxo-alkyl substituent at C2. The configuration of the two substituents is

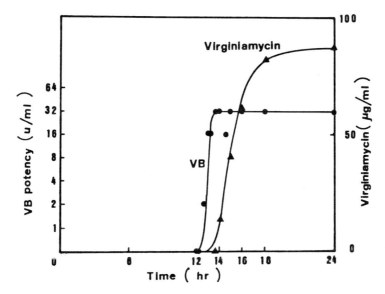

Figure 4   The time course for production of VB (virginiae butanolides) and virginiamycin.

trans (19). The different features among them are the following: (a) the redox state of C6; oxo or hydroxy such as in A-factor and VB, respectively; (b) the orientation of hydroxyl group at C6; α or β in VB and IM-2, respectively; and (c) the length and branching states of alkyl side chains at C2; a good example is IM-2, in which the alkyl side chain is shorter than that of the others, which gives more hydrophilicity to this autoregulator. The *trans* configuration on C2–C3 substituents of all of these autoregulators was established by us (19). The absolute configuration of A-factor and VB A, B, C, and D was determined to be 2R, 3R and 2R, 3R, 6S, respectively, by Mori and coworkers (20–22). That of IM-2 was determined to be 2R, 3R, 6R, by us (23).

All of these autoregulators show activity in the concentration range of a few nanomolars. Combining our surveys (24,25) with the results of Beppu's (13) and Gräfe's groups (26), about 60% of *Streptomyces* species were estimated to produce these butyrolactone autoregulators, although we are not sure about the roles of them in their producers.

III.   THE BIOSYNTHESIS OF VB

The wide distribution of butyrolactone autoregulators and some homologs among industrially useful *Streptomyces* species, as well as their simple but unique structures, attracts our attention to their biosynthetic pathway. The quantity of VB produced by *S. virginiae* is too small for the incorporation experiments using isotope-labeled precursors. During the studies concerning the distribution of VB in *Streptomyces* species, though, we accidentally found one strain of *Streptomyces antibioticus* NF-18 that produces a considerable amount of VB A, a few milligrams per liter, in its culture broth (24). Therefore, we used this strain for the biosynthetic studies of VB. At first, $[1\text{-}^{13}C]\text{-}$ or $[2\text{-}^{13}C]$acetate, $[1\text{-}^{13}C]$isovaleric acid [2], and $[1,3\text{-}^{13}C_2]$glycerol [1] were fed to *S. antibioticus*, and $^{13}C\text{-}$labeled VB A was isolated as the dibenzoate. From the Carbon Magnetic Resonance (CMR) spectra of resulting products, the presumed labeled building blocks were located

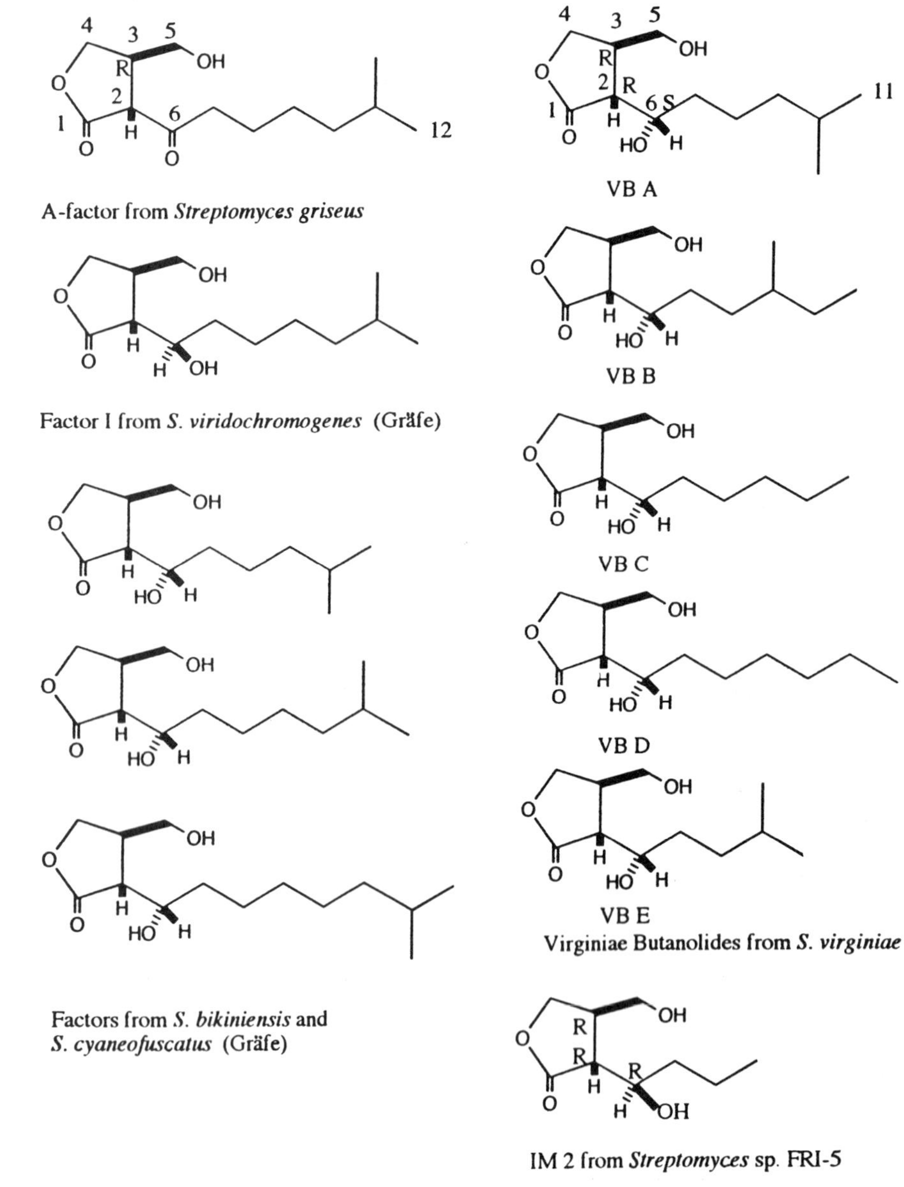

A-factor from *Streptomyces griseus*

Factor I from *S. viridochromogenes* (Gräfe)

Factors from *S. bikiniensis* and
S. cyaneofuscatus (Gräfe)

VB A

VB B

VB C

VB D

VB E
Virginiae Butanolides from *S. virginiae*

IM 2 from *Streptomyces* sp. FRI-5

Figure 5   Butyrolactone autoregulators from *Streptomyces*.

in VB molecule as shown in Figure 6. The incorporation of intact glycerol C_3 unit was confirmed by mass spectral analysis (27).

The postulated key intermediate, 3-oxo-7-methyloctanoate [3], was verified by the incorporation experiment of N-acetyl cysteamine thioester of [2,3-$^{13}C_2$]-3-oxo-7-methyl-octanoate [6] (28). The resulting ^{13}C-labeled VB A dibenzoate clearly showed the retained coupling between C2 and C6 (J = 39.7 Hz), indicating the incorporation of this key intermediate in intact form as shown in Figure 7. The incorporation experiment with [$^2H_5$]glycerol [7] revealed that ^{2}H on C1 and C2 of 7 were stereoselectively deleted dur-

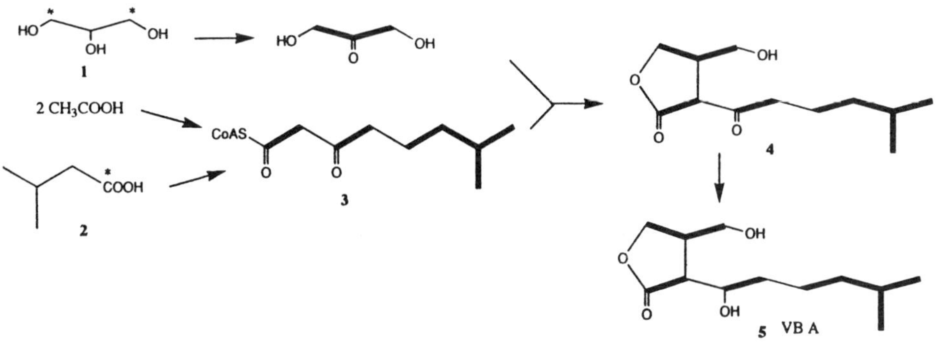

Figure 6   Building blocks of VB A.

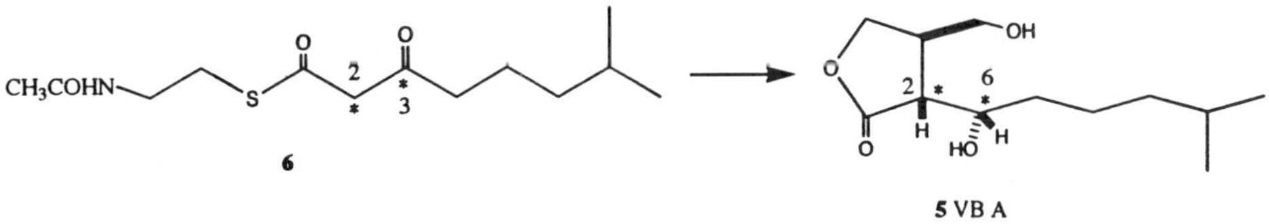

Figure 7   Intact incorporation of $[2,3-^{13}C_2]$-3-oxo-7-methyloctanoate *N*-acetylcysteamine thioester [6] into VB A [5].

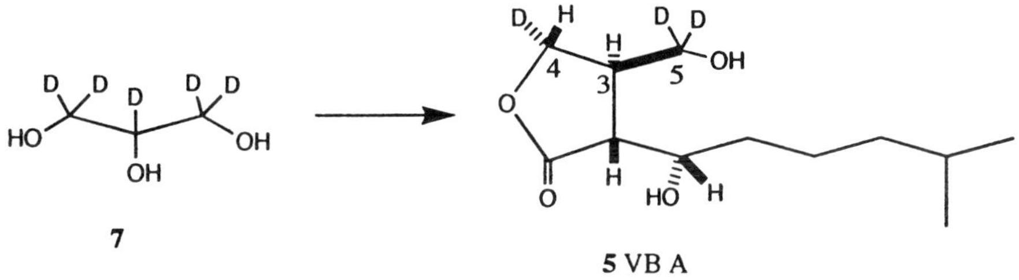

Figure 8   The fate of deuterium on $[^2H_5]$glycerol [7] during the incorporation into VB A [5].

ing the condensation reaction with β-ketoacyl CoA [3], giving mainly $[4-^2H_R, 5-^2H_2]$VB A as shown in Figure 8 (28).

On the basis of these results, the final several steps of VB A were considered as shown in Figure 9. The transesterification between dihydroxyacetone or its phosphate and β-ketoacyl CoA [3] leads to the ester 6 or 9, which undergoes aldol-type condensation to form the butenolide 7 or 10. These very unstable intermediates, which probably can exist only in the enzyme active site, may soon be reduced to 6-dehydro VB A [4] or its phosphate [8]. Then, 6-dehydro VB A [4] is finally reduced to VB A [5] by a hydrogenase. The possible intermediates 6, 7, 8, 9, 4 were chemically synthesized and were used as the substrates for the crude cell-free enzyme system prepared from *S. antibioticus* cells (29). The final product, VB A [5], was converted to the dibenzoate and detected by high-performance liquid chromatography (HPLC). The ester [9] and 6-dehydro VB A [4] were effectively transformed to VB A [5] and the enzymes that catalyze reactions from 9 to 4

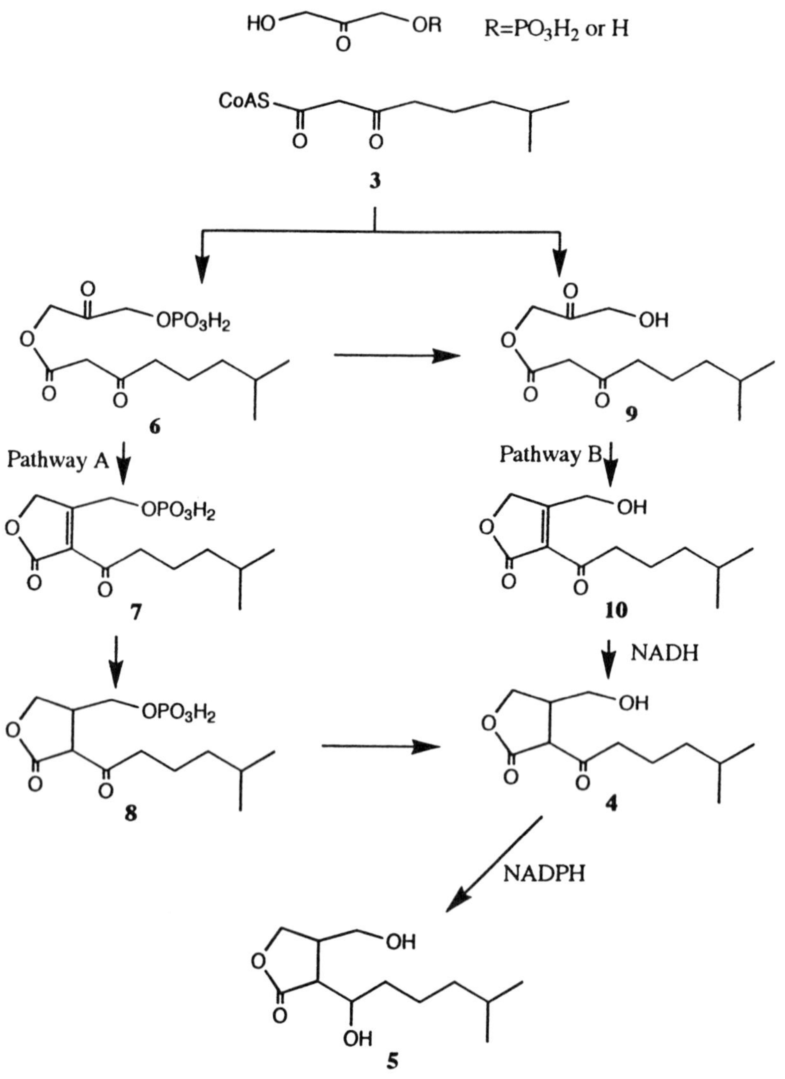

Figure 9 Biosynthetic pathway of VB A involving β-ketoester [9].

and **4** to **5** turned out to be NADH and NADPH dependent, respectively. The phosphorylated compounds such as **6, 7,** and **8** proved to be poor substrates for this crude enzyme system. Therefore, we concluded that pathway B is the most likely for the biosynthesis of VB A, although the paths from **6** to **9** and **8** to **4** were not completely discarded as possibilities (29). Conversion of the ester [9] to VB A [5] in ^2H_2O using the crude enzyme system also supported the result obtained from the experiment shown in Figure 8. C4-H_S was preferably exchanged with ^2H and C2-H, and C3-H also was partially replaced by ^2H.

Taking all these results into consideration, the most plausible mechanism for VB A formation from **9** to **5** are illustrated in Figure 10. After the dehydration of the intramolecular aldol product [11], the double bond delocalized as **12** and the NADH-dependent enzyme delivered the hydride from the *Si* face at C4 or from the *Re* face at C3 (29).

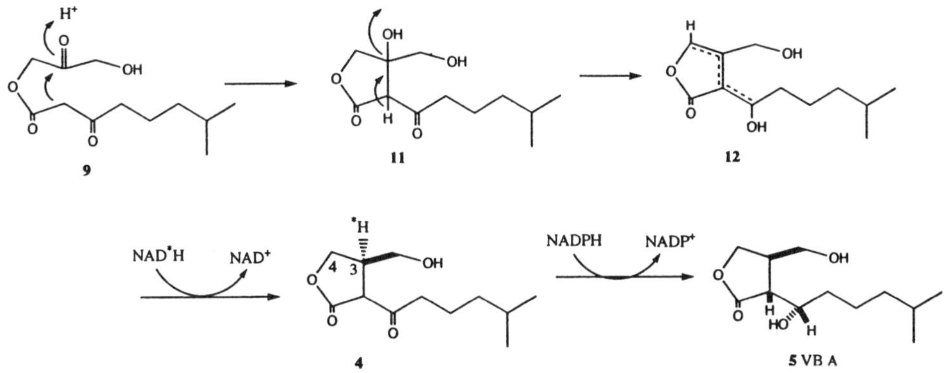

Figure 10 Possible mechanism of VB A formation from the ketoester [9].

The biosyntheses of the other butyrolactone autoregulators in *Streptomyces* species should be basically same as those for VB A in *S. antibioticus*. The minor differences such as the type of starter for the β-ketoacyl CoA, or stereospecificities and equilibrium constants of the final-step hydrogenase or dehydrogenase, cause the three main differences, namely, the length and branching states of C2 alkyl substituents, the redox states at C6, and the configuration of a hydroxyl group at C6.

IV. VIRGINIAE BUTANOLIDE RECEPTOR PROTEIN

From the viewpoint that VBs and related compounds are low-molecular-weight signal substances in actinomycetes corresponding functionally to hormones in plants or vertebrates, they can be considered as *Streptomyces* hormones. If so, *S. virginiae* should have some high-molecular-weight receptor proteins that transmit the signal from the VBs to transcriptional or translational processes in the cells. Based on this hypothesis, we started to search the presumptive VB receptor protein in the cells of *S. virginiae*. To design a suitable ligand for a binding assay, we at first chemically synthesized several VB analogs, and we tested their ability in virginiamycin induction (Figure 11 and Table 1) (30). Structure–activity relationship revealed that almost all parts of the VB molecule are important for its activity, namely, the two hydroxyl groups on C5 and C6, α-orientation of the C6 hydroxyl group, and the chain length of six to eight carbons for C2-alkyl subsituents. Minor deviations from the optimum structure caused drastic decreases in the effectiveness, leaving little freedom in designing a suitable ligand for the binding assay. After several trials, we decided to introduce two ^{3}H atoms to a terminal double bond of a α-hydroxy-ω-heptenyl side chain at C2, resulting in [^{3}H]VB-C$_7$ (**25** in Figure 12), which is a ^{3}H-labeled homolog of VB D and should have a very high affinity toward the receptor. Using this radioactive ligand, we found a binding protein of very high ligand specificity toward VBs in the crude cell-free extract of *S. virginiae* (31,32). The binding protein is present almost exclusively as a soluble cytoplasmic protein, shows dissociation constant (K_d) of several nanomolars, and exists in 30–40 molecules per genome DNA, all of which agreed with the concept of a VB receptor (31).

To characterize the receptor-mediated signal transducing mechanism in triggering physiological differentiation, a large amount of the purified receptor protein will be needed, and we started to purify the VB receptor. At first, we isolated a 36-kDA protein

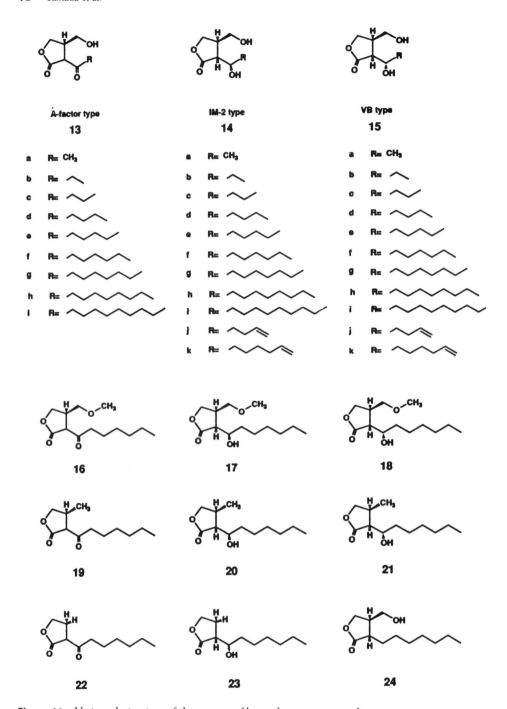

Figure 11   Various derivatives of three types of butyrolactone autoregulators.

Table I   Minimum Effective Concentration of Several VB Analogs in
Virginiamycin Induction

Analogs	A-factor type (μg/ml)	IM-2 type (μg/ml)	VB type (μg/ml)
	13	14	15
a	>100	>100	100
b	10	100	100
c	10	10	10
d	10	1	0.1
e	10	0.1	0.003
f	10	0.01	0.0008
g	10	0.01	0.0008
h	1	0.1	0.1
i	10	1	0.1
j	ND	100	10
k	ND	0.1	0.001
16–18	10	10	1
19–21	1	1	1
22–23	1	1	
24	1		

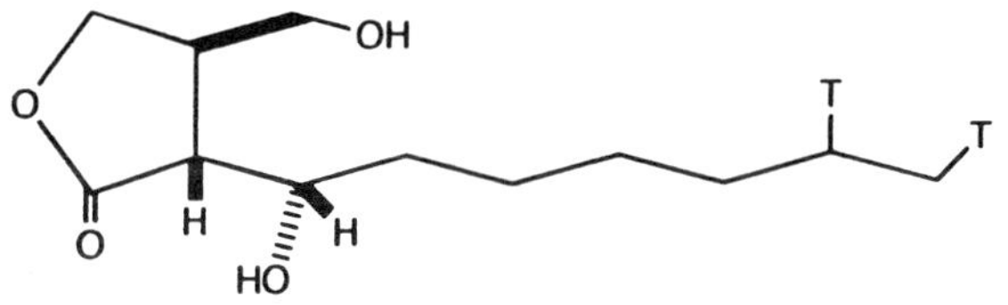

25

Figure 12   Tritium-labeled ligand for binding assay of VB receptor, [^{3}H]VB-C$_7$.

named VbrA that was always present in the active fractions, and the corresponding gene
(*vbrA*) was cloned and sequenced. *vbrA* codes for a protein of 319 amino acids, and C-
terminal two-thirds of the deduced amino-acid sequence showed homology (36%) with
NusG protein of *Escherichia coli* (33). *E. coli nusG* was at first found as an essential host
gene for growth of λ phage, and later it was confirmed to be essential for cell viability as
an antiterminator during the cells transcriptional process. This similarity between VbrA
and an *E. coli* antiterminator protein led us to think that VbrA could be the VB receptor.
However, recombinant VbrA (rVbrA) expressed in *E. coli* by the T7 RNA polymerase
system did not bind VB at all, nor did the immunoprecipitation with anti-rVbrA antibody eliminate VB binding activity from the crude cell-free extract of *S. virginiae* (34).
These findings indicated that VbrA is not a real receptor, and the real one always accompanied VbrA during purification procedure.

Therefore, we again started the purification of the real receptor and obtained a 26-
kDa protein (p26k) after successive purification on anion-exchange, gel filtration,

heparin, and hydrophobic interaction chromatographies. The amino acid sequence of the p26k was partially determined, and degenerate oligonucleotide probes were prepared to clone the corresponding gene by Southern hybridization. The gene thus obtained encodes a protein of 232 amino acids, and its molecular weight was calculated to be 25,001 which agreed well with the value of ca. 26,000 estimated for p26k by sodium dodecyl sulfate–polyacrylamide gel electrophoresis (SDS-PAGE) (34). All the partial amino acid sequences of p26k appeared in the open reading frame (Figure 13). Furthermore, heterologous expression of the gene in *Streptomyces lividans* and *E. coli* gave recombinant p26k possessing very high VB binding activity (Table 2), which confirmed that p26k is exclusively the real VB receptor protein of *S. virginiae*. Therefore, the gene was designated *barA* (butyrolactone autoregulator receptor) (34). Computer search of the databases using the BLAST algorithm revealed that N-terminal sequence of BarA possessed a high level of similarity with several repressors (Figure 14), with local similarity ranging from 55 to 64%. The most homologous region was centered between Val[40] and Lys[61] of BarA, a region that displayed a typical helix-turn-helix DNA binding motif. Therefore, the VB receptor protein (BarA) appears to function as a repressor by binding directly to specific DNA sequences.

Recently, we confirmed the presence of the IM-2-specific binding protein in *Streptomyces* sp. FRI-5, and we purified it to near homogeneity (39). The IM-2-binding protein had a similar molecular weight, of ca. 27,000, to that of BarA. Also, in *S. griseus* IFO 13350, an A-factor-specific binding protein of similar size to BarA also has been found (40,41). Therefore, butanolide receptor proteins in *Streptomyces* species seem to have a molecular weight of 26,000–27,000. To know the possible homology among the genes encoding autoregulator receptor, we have done Southern blot analyses on genomic DNAs from these species as well as from *Streptomyces coelicolor* A3(2) and *S. lividans* TK21 using *barA* as a probe. Unexpectedly, no hybridizing bands were observed even under the mild washing conditions, indicating that there is no general homology among these receptor proteins, although their size and function are supposedly similar (34). The detailed signal transducing mechanism involving these receptor proteins remains as an interesting area of future research. Each of the three known butyrolactone autoregulator receptor proteins, namely, VB receptor, A-factor receptor, and IM-2 receptor, is specific to its own type of autoregulator; the affinity of each toward its own type of autoregulator is at least 100 times higher than that toward different types of autoregulators. These facts suggest that butyrolactone autoregulators might have some ecological roles in many *Streptomyces* species not only to synchronize their life cycle, but also to survive, especially in a nutritionally rich environment.

V. CONCLUSION

We have reviewed the structures, biosyntheses, and receptor proteins of the microbial hormone-like compounds, butyrolactone autoregulators, in *Streptomyces* species, focusing on the virginiae butanolides from *Streptomyces virginiae*. At present, our knowledge in this field is still very poor, but we may suggest that these autoregulators play ecologically important roles for these industrially useful microorganisms. The structures of the butyrolactone autoregulators are unique, but fortunately very simple, and they are quite stable and effective at very low concentrations. Therefore, their chemical synthesis is rather easy for industrial application (10,20,21,23). As for the VBs, at first they were thought

```
                      GGTACCGACCTGTCGGATGGTTTCGGAGGCCAG      33
CAGCGGGTCGTAGCAGCCGTTCACCGGGGTGAAGTAGCTGTGCGCCCTGGGCCACTGCGC      93
CGTCAGGGCGAATCGGTTCTCCGCGGTCCGGCTCCATCCCGTCAGAAACACTTCGGCGAC     153
CGCCGCCCGGTGGACCAGCTCCCGCGGAACCGTGCTGGTCATGGCCGATGCGCGGGCCGG     213
TCGGCCGGTCTGGAACGCCGTTCGCCGGGCCGGGACGGCCACAGGCAGGGTTTCGTTTTC     273
AACCAACACAACAGACATGGAATCCCCCATAGAAACCGATCTCGCGGGAACGGGCGCCTC     333
CCCGTCTCCCCCGCCGATAAGATACATACCAACCGGTTCTTTTGATAGCCGGATGTTGAT     393
CTATCTAGGCTGACTGGCCGGGTCGCCCGACAGCGGCGGATGCATGACAGGAGAAGCCCT     453

ATGGCAGTGCGACACGAACGGGTGGCAGTGCGACAGGAACGGGCCGTCCGCACGCGGCAG     513
 M   A   V   R   H   E   R   V   A   V   R   Q   E   R   A   V   R   T   R   Q
                     N-terminus
GCGATCGTGCGGGCAGCCGCCTCGGTCTTCGACGAGTACGGGTTCGAGGCCGCCACAGTG     573
 A   I   V   R   A   A   A   S   V   F   D   E   Y   G   F   E   A   A   T   V

GCAGAGATCCTCTCGCGGGCCTCGGTCACCAAGGGCGCGATGTACTTCCACTTCGCTTCC     633
 A   E   I   L   S   R   A   S   V   T   K   G   A   M   Y   F   H   F   A   S
                                       fr.24
AAGGAAGAGCTGGCCCGCGGCGTGCTGGCCGAGCAGACCCTGCACGTGGCGGTGCCGGAA     693
 K   E   E   L   A   R   G   V   L   A   E   Q   T   L   H   V   A   V   P   E
         fr.25
TCCGGCTCCAAGGCGCAGGAACTGGTAGACCTCACCATGCTGGTCGCCCACGGCATGCTG     753
 S   G   S   K   A   Q   E   L   V   D   L   T   M   L   V   A   H   G   M   L
                       fr.42
CACGATCCGATCCTGCGGGCGGGCACGCGGCTCGCACTGGACCAGGGGGGCGGTGGACTTC     813
 H   D   P   I   L   R   A   G   T   R   L   A   L   D   Q   G   A   V   D   F

TCCGACGCCAACCCGTTCGGCGAGTGGGGCGACATCTGCGCCCAGCTCCTGGCGGAGGCA     873
 S   D   A   N   P   F   G   E   W   G   D   I   C   A   Q   L   L   A   E   A

CAGGAACGGGGGGAGGTGCTTCCGCACGTGAACCCGAAAAAGACCGGCGACTTCATCGTC     933
 Q   E   R   G   E   V   L   P   H   V   N   P   K   K   T   G   D   F   I   V

GGCTGCTTCACCGGGCTCCAGGCGGTCTCCCGGGTCACCTCCGACCGCCAGGACCTCGGC     993
 G   C   F   T   G   L   Q   A   V   S   R   V   T   S   D   R   Q   D   L   G

CACCGGATCTCGGTGATGTGGAACCACGTGCTGCCCAGCATCGTGCCGGCGTCCATGCTG    1053
 H   R   I   S   V   M   W   N   H   V   L   P   S   I   V   P   A   S   M   L

ACCTGGATCGAAACCGGCGAGGAGCGGATCGGGAAGGTCGCGGCGGCGGCCGAGGCCGCC    1113
 T   W   I   E   T   G   E   E   R   I   G   K   V   A   A   A   A   E   A   A
                                       fr.21
GAGGCTGCGGAGGCCTCCGAGGCCGCCTCCGACGAGTAGGAGCACCGACTTCAGGACATG    1173
 E   A   A   E   A   S   E   A   A   S   D   E   *

CCGGGCACCCAGGGGGTGCCCGGCATGTTTGCTTCCGCCGCCCCACCCGCCCGCGAACGG    1233
GCCGCCGGGCAACGGGGCAGCAAGAACTTCGGCCAAAAACAAGGCAACCGGTCTGGTTTG    1293
ACTTGGCAATCGGGTCTGACGGTTTGTATCGTGATGCCGCAGCGCCGCAACTCGCACCGG    1353
GCGCCCGTTCGGTGTCACGTGCGGGCAGCAGCCGCCTCCCCTCCAGCCGGGGGCTCGGTC    1413
GCCCCTGCGCGCGGCCTTGACCTGCCCGCATCCGAACCACGCCCGCCGGCAGCACACGAG    1473
ACGTTCAGCAAACCGAGCGGTTCGCTTGCCTCAGCCAAACGGTGCACGTCAGGAGTTGCC    1533
TTGACACCCAAACAGGAACGCGCCTTCCGCACCCGCACCCAGCTGGTGCTCTCGGCGGCC    1593
GAGGCCTTCGATCGGCAGGGTTTCGCGACGGCCTCGCTCACCGCCATCAGCAACAGCGCC    1653
GGTGTCAGTAACGGGGCCCTGCACTTCCACTTCGAGAGCAAGGAAGCGCTCGCCGCCGCC    1713
GTCGAAGCGGAGGCGGCCGAGCGGATGCGGACGATCGTCGAC       1755
```

Figure 13 Nucleotide and deduced amino acid sequences of *bar*A encoding the VB receptor protein. Sequences corresponding to the amino acid sequences obtained from the purified protein are underlined. (From Ref. 34.)

Table 2   Functional Expression of the p26k Gene in *Streptomyces lividans* TK21 and in *Escherichia coli*

Host strain	Plasmid	VB binding activity (pmol/100 µl cell extract)	Specific activity (pmol/mg protein)
S. virginiae	—	0.52	0.41
S. lividans TK21	—	0.03	—
S. lividans TK21	pIJ486	0.03	—
S. lividans TK21	pARS701	1.55	1.58
E. coli BL21 (DE3)/pLysS	pET-3d IPTG(–)	0.03	—
E. coli BL21 (DE3)/pLysS	pET-3d IPTG(+)	0.04	—
E. coli BL21 (DE3)/pLysS	pET-p26k IPTG(–)	16.5	15.0
E. coli BL21 (DE3)/pLysS	pET-p26k IPTG(+)	532.2	749.2

```
           1         11        21        31        41        51        61        71

BarA     MAVRHDRVAV RQERAVRTRQ AIVRAAASVF DEYGFEAATV AEILSRASVT KGAMYFHFAS KEELARGVLA EQ
                     **  .  *** .   * . *   * . **   .  *    *     ****   *** .*

TcmR            L  RQRKLRRTRD QLIREALELF LAQGYEHTTV EQIAEAVEVH PRTFFRHFAS KEEVA
                   * .***   .. .  *  *   .. *   *.. .  * * .**  .**.*.**   * .*          .*

EnvR               ALKTRQ ELIETAIAQF AQHGVSKTTL NDIADAANVT RGAIYWHFEN KTQLFNEMWL QQ
                   * ***   *. *  *   .. *   .   **   * **   .**.*.**   * .*

AcrR              KQEAQETRQ HILDVALRLF SQQGVSSTSL GEIAKAAGVT RGAIYWHFKD KSDL
                   * .*.  .. .  ** . *         **  * ** .  ***.** .  ** .*

MtrR               ALKTKE HLMLAALETF YRKGIARTSL NEIAQAAGVT RGALYWHFKN KEDL
                   .  *  * . *  .* . ** **.         **   ** *.**   ** *   . *

ORF188             KD KILGVAKELF IKNGYNATTT GEIVKLSESS KGNLYYHFKT KENLFLEIL
                   *. * .* *   .. * * *   .. * * *            * *

TetR               RE AVIRTALELL NDVGMEGLTT RRLAERLGVQ QPALYWHFKN KRAL
```

Figure 14   Alignment of BarA with several repressors of other origins. Amino acids identical with and similar to those of BarA are indicated by asterisks and dots, respectively. TcmR, a repressor for TcmA involved in tetracenomycin C resistance from *Streptomyces glaucescens* (35); EnvR, a potential repressor for EnvCD involved in septum formation in *E. coli* (GenBank Accession number P31676); AcrR, a potential repressor for AcrAE involved in drug hypersensitivity of *E. coli* (GenBank Accession number P34000); MtrR, a repressor involved in drug efflux system of *Neisseria gonorrhoeae* (36); ORF188, a repressor for an antiseptic resistance gene, qacA, of *Staphylococcus aureus* (37); TetR, a repressor for tetracycline resistance determinant encoded on plasmid pSC101 (38).

only to help earlier production of virginiamycin M and S with similar levels of final yield. Recently, however, we succeeded in enhancing the yield of virginiamycin production by the addition of VB at 8 hr cultivation in an elaborate medium system (42). As for A factor, Beppu et al. (43) found that a mutant of *S. griseus* lacking A-factor receptor produced a higher level of streptomycin than that produced by the wild type. On the basis of these facts, they suggested that A-factor receptor may be a negative regulator of streptomycin production. If this hypothesis is also true for *S. virginae*, the gene disruption of *barA* might enhance virginiamycin production. At present, we know three types of butyrolactone autoregulators, but there is a strong possibility that other autoregulators of unknown types are present in actinomycetes.

The other possible applications of butyrolactone autoregulators are as follows. When the combination of an antibiotics producer and the corresponding autoregulator is revealed, there are possibilities to enhance the yield of antibiotics, to induce production of new antibiotics, and to develop new microbial pesticides for agricultural use or environmental improvement. Smith et al. (44) recently reported that a phytopathogenic bacterium, *Pseudomonas syringae*, produces a signal substance, named syringolide, that has a fused butyrolactone skeleton and is biosynthetically a close relative of the butyrolactone autoregulators of *Streptomyces*. Syringolide is a signal substance for the host plants to prepare against pest invasion, inducing the production of elicitors and phytoallexins. Another well-known group of signal microbial substances is *N*-acyl-homoserine lactone-type autoinducers or autoregulators, which are widely distribute among Gram-negative bacteria (45). As for the induction of antibiotics, *N*-(3-oxohexanoyl)-L-homoserine lactone turned out to be an endogenous inducer of carbapenem antibiotic production in *Erwinia carotovora* (46).

Considering the results described in this chapter, we would like to emphasize the importance of butyrolactone autoregulators as one area of microbial signal substances to be investigated further with regard to its basic science and industrial applications.

REFERENCES

1. Biot AM. Virginiamycin: Properties, biosynthesis, and fermentation. Vandamme EJ, ed. Biotechnology of Industrial Antibiotics, 1st ed. New York and Basel: Marcel Dekker, 1984:695–720.
2. Cocitto C. Antibiotics of the virginiamycin family, inhibitors which contain synergistic components. Microbiol Rev 1979; 43:145–198.
3. Lee C-K, Minami M, Sakuda S, Nihira T, Yamada Y. Stereospecific reduction of virginamycin M1 as the virginiamycin resistance pathway in *Streptomyces virginiae*. Antimicrob Agents Chemother 1996; 40:595–601.
4. Paris JM, Barriere JC, Smith C, Bost PE. The chemistry of pristinamycins. Lukacs G, Ohno M, eds. Recent Progress in the Chemical Synthesis of Antibiotics. Berlin, Heiderberg, New York, London, Paris, Tokyo, Hong Kong, and Barcelona: Springer-Verlag, 1990:183–248.
5. Kingston DGI. The biosynthesis of virginiamycins M_1 and M_2. Petroski RJ, McCormick SP, eds. Secondary-Metabolite Biosynthesis and Metabolism. New York: Plenum Press, 1992:105–117.
6. Reed JW, Kingston DGI. Biosynthesis of antibiotics of the virginiamycin family, 5. The conversion of phenylalanine to phenylglycine in the biosynthesis of virginiamycin S_1. J Nat Prod 1986; 49:626–630.
7. Reed JW, Purvis MB, Kingston DGI, Biot A, Gossele F. Biosynthesis of antibiotics of the virginiamycin family, 7. Stereo- and regiochemical studies on the formation of the 3-hydroxy-picolinic acid and pipecolic acid units. J Org Chem 1989; 54:1161–1165.
8. Yanagimoto M, Terui G. Physiological studies on staphylomycin production: (II) Formation of a substance effective in inducing staphylomycin production. J Ferment Technol 1971; 49:611–618.
9. Yanagimoto M, Yamada Y, Terui G. Extraction and purification of inducing material produced in staphylomycin fermentation. Hakkokogaku 1979; 57:6–14.
10. Yamada Y, Sugamura K, Kondo K, Yanagimoto M, Okada H. The structure of a inducing factors for virginiamycin production in *Streptomyces virginiae*. J Antibiot 1987; 40:496–504.
11. Kondo K, Higuchi Y, Sakuda S, Nihira T, Yamada Y. New virginiae butanolides from *Streptomyces virginae*. J Antibiot 1989; 42:1873–1876.
12. Kleiner EM, Pliner SA, Soifer VS, Onoprienko VV, Balashova TA, Rosynov BV, Khokhlov AS. The structure of A-factor, a bioregulator from *Streptomyces griseus*. Bioorg Khim 1976; 2:1142–1147.

13. Hara O, Beppu T. Mutants blocked in streptomycin production in *Streptomyces griseus*—the role of A-factor. J Antibiot 1982; 35:349–358.

14. Gräfe U, Schade W, Eritt I, Fleck WF, Radics L. A new inducer in anthracycline biosynthesis from *Streptomyces viridochromogenes*. J Antibiot 1982; 35:1722–1723.

15. Gräfe U, Reinhardt G, Schade W, Eritt I, Fleck WF, Radics L. Interspecific inducers of cytodifferentiation and anthracycline biosynthesis from *Streptomyces bikiniensis* and *S. cyaneofuscatus*. Biotechnol Lett 1983; 5:591–596.

16. Yanagimoto M, Enatu T. Regulation of a blue pigment production by γ-nonalactone in *Streptomyces* sp. J Ferment Technol 1983; 61:345–350.

17. Hashimoto K, Nihira T, Sakuda S, Yamada Y. IM-2, a butyrolactone autoregulator, induces production of several nucleoside antibiotics in *Streptomyces* sp. FRI-5. J Ferment Bioeng 1992; 73:449–455.

18. Sato K, Nihira T, Sakuda S, Yanagimoto M, Yamada Y. Isolation and structure of a new butyrolactone autoregulator from *Streptomyces* FRI-5. J Ferment Bioeng 1989; 68:170–173.

19. Sakuda S, Yamada Y. Stereochemistry of butyrolactone autoregulators from *Streptomyces*. Tetrahedron Lett 1991; 32:1817–1820.

20. Mori K, Yamane K. Synthesis of optically active forms of A-factor, the inducer of streptomycin. Tetrahedron 1982; 38:2919–2921.

21. Mori K. Revision of the absolute configuration of A-factor. Tetrahedron 1983; 39:3107–3109.

22. Mori K, Chiba N. Synthesis of optically active virginiae butanolide A, B, C and D and other autoregulators from Streptomycetes. Liebigs Ann Chem 1990; 31–37.

23. Mizuno K, Sakuda S, Nihira T, Yamada Y. Enzymatic resolution of 2-acyl-3-hydroxymethyl-4-butanolide and preparation of optically active IM-2, the autoregulator from *Streptomyces* sp. FRI-5. Tetrahedron 1994; 50:10849–10858.

24. Ohashi H, Zheng YH, Nihira T, Yamada Y. Distribution of virginiae butanolides in antibiotic-producing Actinomycetes, and identification of inducing factor from *Streptomyces antibioticus* as viginiae butanolide A. J Antibiot 1989; 42:1191–1195.

25. Hashimoto K, Nihira T, Yamada Y. Distribution of virginiae butanolides and IM-2 in the genus *Streptomyces*. J Ferment Bioeng 1992; 73:61–65.

26. Eritt I, Gräfe U, Fleck FW. Inducers of both cytodifferentiation and anthracycline biosynthesis of *Streptomyces griseus* and their occurrence in actinomycetes and other microorganisms. Allg Mikrobiol 1984; 24:3–12.

27. Sakuda S, Higashi A, Nihira T, Yamada Y. Biosynthesis of virginiae butanolide A. J Am Chem Soc 1990; 112:898–899.

28. Sakuda S, Higashi A, Tanaka S, Nihira T, Yamada Y. Biosynthesis of virginiae butanolide A, a butyrolactone autoregulator from *Streptomyces*. J Am Chem Soc 1992; 114:663–668.

29. Sakuda S, Tanaka S, Mizuno K, Sukcharoen O, Nihira T, Yamada Y. Biosynthesic studies on virginiae butanolide A, a butyrolactone autoregulator from *Streptomyces*. Part 2. Preparation of possible biosyntheic intermediates and conversion experiments in a cell-free system. J Chem Soc Perkin Trans I 1993; 2309–2315.

30. Nihira T, Shimizu Y, Kim HS, Yamada Y. Structure-activity relationships of virginiae butanolide C, an inducer of virginiamycin production in *Streptomyces virginiae*. J. Antibiot 1988; 41:1828–1837.

31. Kim HS, Nihira T, Tada H, Yanagimoto M, Yamada Y. Identification of binding protein of virginiae butanolide C, an autoregulator in virginiamycin production, from *Streptomyces virginiae*. J Antibiot 1989; 42:769–778.

32. Kim HS, Tada H, Nihira T, Yamada Y. Purification and characterization of virginiae butanolide C-binding protein, a possible pleiotropic signal-transducer in *Streptomyces virginiae*. J Antibiot 1990; 43:692–706.

33. Okamoto S, Nihira T, Kataoka H, Suzuki A, Yamada Y. Purification and molecular cloning of a butyrolactone autoregulator receptor from *Streptomyces virginiae*. J Biol Chem 1992; 267:1093–1098.

34. Okamoto S, Nakamura K, Nihira T, Yamada Y. Virginiae butanolide binding protein from *Streptomyces virginiae*. Evidence that VbrA is not the virginiae butanolide binding protein and reidentification of the true binding protein. J Biol Chem 1995; 270:12319–12326.

35. Guilfoile PG, Hutchinson CR. Sequence and transcriptional analysis of the *Streptomyces glaucescens tcmAR* tetracenomycin C resistance and repressor gene loci. J Bacteriol 1992; 174:3651–3658.

36. Hagman KE, Shafer WM. Transcriptional control of the *mtr* efflux system of *Neisseria gonorrhoeae*. J Bacteriol 1995; 177:4162–4165.

37. Rouch DA, Cram DS, DiBerardino D, Littlejohn TG, Skurray RA. Efflux-mediated antiseptic resistance gene *qacA* from *Staphylococcus aureus*: Common ancestry with tetracycline- and sugar-transport proteins. Mol Microbiol 1990; 4:2051–2062.

38. Unger B, Becker J, Hillen W. Nucleotide sequence of the gene, protein purification and characterization of the pSC101-encoded tetracycline resistance-gene-repressor. Gene 1984; 31:103–108.

39. Ruengjtchatchawalya M, Nihira T, Yamada Y. Purification and characterization of the IM-2 binding protein from *Streptomyces* sp. FRI-5. J Bacteriol 1995; 177:551–557.

40. Miyake K, Horinouchi S, Yoshida M, Chiba N, Mori K, Nogawa N, Morikawa N, Beppu T. Detection and properties of A-factor-binding protein from *Streptomyces griseus*. J Bacteriol 1989; 171:4298–4302.

41. Onaka H, Ando N, Nihira T, Yamada Y, Beppu T, Horinouchi S. Cloning and characterization of the A-factor receptor gene from *Streptomyces griseus*. J Bacteriol 1995; 177:6083–6092.

42. Yang YK, Shimizu H, Shioya S, Suga K, Nihira T, Yamada Y. Optimum autoregulator addition strategy for maximum virginiamycin production in batch culture of *Streptomyces virginiae*. Biotechnol Bioeng 1995; 46:437–442.

43. Miyake K, Kuzuyama T, Horinouchi S, Beppu T. The A-factor-binding protein of *Streptomyces griseus* negatively controls streptomycin production and sporulation. J Bacteriol 1990; 172:3003–3008.

44. Smith MJ, Mazzola EP, Sims JJ, Midland SL, Keen NT, Burton V, Stayton MM. The syringolides: Bacterial C-glycosyl lipids that trigger plant disease resistance. Tetrahedron Lett 1993; 39:223–226.

45. Fuqua WC, Winans S, Greenberg EP. Quorum sensing in bacteria: The LuxR-LuxI family of cell density–responsive transcriptional regulators. J Microbiol 1994; 176:269–275.

46. Bainton NJ, Stead P, Chhabra SR, Bycroft BW, Salmond GPC, Stewart GSAB, Williams P. N-(3-oxohexanoyl)-L-homoserine lactone regulates carbopenem antibiotic production in *Erwinia carotovora*. Biochem J 1992; 288:997–1004.

4

Molecular Biology, Biochemistry, and Fermentation of Aminoglycoside Antibiotics

Wolfgang Piepersberg
Bergische Universität GH, Wuppertal, Germany

I. INTRODUCTION

Aminoglycosides are both indispensable chemotherapeutics and interesting targets of basic research. The most attractive current aspects of aminoglycoside research are (a) the emergent genetic and biochemical data on their biosynthesis and regulation; (b) the molecular mechanisms of resistance development in both producers and clinically relevant pathogens; (c) the molecular aspects of interaction with cellular components in both prokaryotes and man; and (d) new fields of application and new pharmacologically relevant targets such as the successful glycosidase inhibitors. In the future, this research will extend to an analysis of the ecological role of aminoglycosides, their evolutionary significance in nature, and the planned use of their biosynthetic potential in new fields of biotechnological development. The last could include, for example, the modular design of new pathways for related hybrid or totally new products of secondary carbohydrate metabolism as well as the improvement of conventional techniques of fermentation by genetic pathway engineering. Here, we will give an outline of the present state of the art, examples for potential future applications, and some perspectives for unifying view of the basics of the metabolism of secondary (amino) sugars and their derivatives.

This chapter will focus on the pathways for aminoglycoside production and their regulation. In the course of the past 10 to 15 years, the genetics and biochemistry of secondary metabolite production, especially in the bacterial group *Actinomycetales*, has entered a new phase. We can now elucidate in principle the molecular physiology and design of complex biosynthetic pathways for all bioactive natural products of low molecular weight. Here, we report on the current state of knowledge in the field of secondary carbohydrate metabolism, especially that of the aminocyclitol–aminoglycoside antibiotics (ACAGAs). In contrast to the biosynthesis of other chemical groups, such as the polyketides and the nonribosomal peptides, relatively few groups have participated in this pioneering phase of research on this group of natural products. Currently of special interest in ACAGA research are the biochemical pathways themselves: (a) the routes of sugar activation and modification, structural sorting in branched pathways, and the glycosyltransfer reactions, especially of 6-deoxyhexoses; (b) the mechanisms of cyclitol formation, for which two basically different routes are known, and cyclitol modification; (c) the condensation reactions; (d) the flow and sources of intermediate precursor pools into ACAGA molecules; (e) the underlying genetics; and (f) the various levels of regulation, such as general or strain-specific global regulatory networks and the pathway-specific mechanisms of regulation. Examples will be taken mainly from the biosynthetic pathways for streptomycins and fortimicins (astromicins), and 2-deoxystreptamine-(2DOS) and valiol-derived ACAGA pathways. Other important information, such as on the resistance mechanisms in ACAGA producers and new data on the effects of ACAGAs on target sites, will also be reported. The biosynthetic routes for other carbohydrate-derived constituents in extracellular secondary products of bacteria will be compared. Some of the aforementioned topics together with complementary data and aspects have been treated in several reviews in the past 10 years (1–14).

II. NEW GROUPS: DISTRIBUTION AND SCREENING

The detection and description of new natural products clearly belonging to the ACAGA group of secondary metabolites has occurred steadily during the past decade, as is shown in Table 1 (1,12). The most important aminoglycosides are produced by actinomycetes, bacilli, and pseudomonads, with a clear preference for the first group of bacteria (cf. Table 1). The typically encountered toxic side effects of ACAGAs in man, such as oto- and nephrotoxicity (cf. Section VII.A), and the occurrence of widespread resistance determinants in clinical pathogens have diminished the efforts for finding new ACAGAs in most industrial antibiotic screening programs. However, completely different structural subclasses of ACAGAs have been detected when enzyme-specific glycosidase inhibitors, for example, of α-glucosidases, trehalases, and chitinases, have been screened (see Section III for structures). Therefore, several other naturally occurring structural and functional types probably remain to be detected. New techniques and new targets of screening will be used in the future to find new aminoglycosides more directly. Examples of new approaches are to exploit ACAGA-hypersensitive mutants, to use resistance profiles, and genetic screening by use of combinations of pathway-specific gene probes in genomic hybridizations (11,12,16,17).

The pseudomonads making sorbistins (cf. Section III) are not the only Gram-negative unicellular bacteria known to secrete ACAGA-related carbohydrates as diffusible substances. Additional examples include the formation of the hexosamine-based lipo-oligosaccharidic Nod-factors (18) and of N-methyl-*scyllo*-inoamine, as so-called rhizopine (19,20), by rhizobia. However, despite these probably rare cases of diffusible carbohydrates, the Gram-negative organisms produce a wide, variable range of cell-bound and carbohydrate-based extracellular substances that in many instances look like oligomeric secondary metabolites. Examples are the lipopolysaccharides (LPSs) and other heteropolymeric polysaccharides (e.g., the enterobacterial common antigen-ECA). Also, emerging evidence suggests the use of the same gene pool for the production of these polymers and ACAGAs (see Section VII.C).

Glycosidic and/or cyclitol-containing components looking very similar to substructures of ACAGAs, such as glycolipids and other glycoconjugates, also occur in several cellular constituents or extracellular polymers of both archaebacterial and eukaryotic origin. Two examples are the glucosaminyl archaetidyl-*myo*-inositols formed by some methanogenic *Archaea* (21) and the very similar core structure in the oligosaccharidic phosphatidylinositol protein anchors of glycoproteins attached to the outer surface of

Table 1 Chronology of the Detection and Producing Microbial Genera of the Major Aminoglycosides[a]

Aminoglycoside	Year of first description	Producing microbial genera[b]
Streptomycin	1944	S., Strv.
Neomycins	1949	S., Micr.
5'Hydroxystreptomycin	1950	S., Amyc.
Paronomycins (catenulin)	1952	S.
Hygromycin A	1953	S., Coryb.
Kanamycins	1957	S.
Trehalosamines	1957	S.
Hygromycin B	1958	S.
Streptozotocin	1960	S.
Spectinomycin	1961	S.
Bluensomycin (glebomycin)	1962	S.
Gentamicins	1964	Micr.
Kasugamycin	1965	S.
Destomycins	1965	S., Sacch.
Nojirimycin	1966	S.
3-Amino-3-deoxy-D-glucose	1967	Bac.
Apramycin	1968	S., Sacch.
Tobramycin	1968	S.
Sisomicin	1970	Micr.
Ribostamycins	1970	S.
Validamycins	1970	S.
A-396-I	1970	Strv.
Lividomycins	1971	S.
Butirosin	1971	Bac.
Acarbose	1972	Actp.
Myomycin	1973	Noc., Coryb.
SS-56-C	1973	S.
Minosaminomycin	1974	S.
Amylostatins	1974	S., Actp.
Siastatin	1974	S.
Xylostasin	1974	Bac.
Verdamicin	1975	Micr.
Sorbistins	1976	Pseud., Strv.
Seldomycins	1977	S.
LL-BM123α	1977	Noc.
Fortimicins (Astromicins)	1977	Micr.
1-Desoxynojirimycins	1978	S.
Adiposins	1978	S.
Trestatins	1978	S.
Istamycins	1979	S.
Sporaricins	1979	Sacch.
Sannamycin	1979	S.
Dactimicin	1979	Dact.
Oligostatins	1979	S.
Lysinomicin	1981	Micr.
Spenolimycin	1982	S.
Valiolamine	1984	S.
5'-Hydroxy-N-demethyldihydrostreptomycin	1985	S.
1-N-Amidino-1-N-demethyl-2-hydroxy-destomycin	1985	Sacch.
Inosamycins	1985	S.
Neotrehalosadiamine	1986	Bac.
AC4437 (dihydrostreptosylstreptidine)	1986	S.
CV-1	1987	S.
Boholmycin	1988	S.
Ashimycins	1989	S.
Trehazolin	1991	Micr., Amyc.

[a] For references of the first description of ACAGAs before 1980, see ref. 1 and 15; others are cited in texts.

[b] S. = *Streptomyces*; Strv. = *Streptoverticillium*; Micr. = *Micromonospora*; Dact. = *Dactylosporangium*; Amyc. = *Amycolatopsis*; Actp. = *Actinoplanes*; Sacch. = *Saccharopolyspora*; Noc. = *Nocardia*; Coryb. = *Corynebacterium*; Bac. = *Bacillus*; Pseud. = *Pseudomonas*.

eukaryotes, from trypanosomes to mammalian organisms (22). Interestingly, these share the content of nonacetylated glucosamine and the 1-phosphoryl-6-glucosaminyl *myo*-inositol core unit, the biosynthesis of which is currently being studied in the mammalian system (22). These examples could mean that part of the biochemical concept of amino-glycoside biosynthesis is disseminated throughout practically all major groups of organisms, but is used for very different physiological means. The unifying common feature could be their role in the metabolism of extracytoplasmically targeted compounds.

III. STRUCTURAL VERSUS BIOCHEMICAL CLASSES

The definition of aminoglycoside has never been exact nor logical. Until now, the amino-glycosides have mostly been regarded as compounds mainly based on amino-*N*-containing sugars and/or cyclitol derivatives, which are either (pseudo-) oligo- or monosaccharidic in nature. They have been classified according to either their chemical (e.g., structure of aminocyclitol) or their functional classes (e.g., bactericidal versus bacteriostatic translational inhibitors or enzyme inhibitors) (1,15,23–29). The predominant representatives of this group are the (amino)cyclitol–aminoglycosides (ACAGs). However, other amino-sugar-based microbial secondary metabolites, such as monomers and disaccharidic compounds lacking a cyclitol moiety, are also included. Some other groups of secondary metabolites also contain similar carbohydrate components, such as aromatic polyketides, macrolides, glycopeptides, and lincosamides (cf. Ref. 28).

From a biochemical point of view, it would be desirable to group all the secondary metabolites according to "pathway formulas" (similar to E.C. numbers in enzyme nomenclature), that is, according to a neutral, generally applicable system giving equal credit to the major branches of a pathway, especially when the end product is condensed from heterogeneous precursors. In this chapter, we roughly classify the aminoglycoside groups into such a biochemical system by attributing a preliminary pathway formula to each group of closely related end products. The definition of the pathway formulas used here is given in Table 2. A more detailed explanation and a biochemical basis for this system are given in Section V. In its present form, the system represents a simplified and in some cases hypothetical version of the (pseudo-)oligosaccharide biosynthetic pathway. Thus, the coding system employed does not sufficiently distinguish between phases of the pathway before and after condensation reactions of monomeric precursors, and so forth, where we do not know the exact metabolic route. However, the distributions of these fractions of most pathways are practically unknown. Also, for the same reasons the formulas do not pay attention to the modes of activation, types of condensation reactions, and modifications.

A. Streptomycins and Similar Compounds

The streptomycins, historically marking the entrance to aminoglycoside research, are basically composed of a *scyllo*-inositol-derived aminocyclitol (streptidine or bluensidine), a 6-deoxyhexose component (= 6DOH; [dihydro-]streptose or 5′-hydroxystreptose), and an aminohexose derivative (*N*-methyl-L-glucosamine [= NMLGA] or derivatives thereof) (Figure 1). The pathway formula given provisionally is **Ca1(4)–6DOH(2)–HA** (or **–H**). In the past decade, some new members of this family, such as the antibiotics ashimycins (30), AC4437 (31), 6‴-*O*-α-mannopyranosylaminosidostreptomycin (32), and 5′-hydroxy-2″-*N*-demethylstreptomycin (33), have been reported. A short representation of the pathway design for the production of streptomycins is given in Figure 2.

Table 2   Definition of a "Pathway Formula" for the Biosynthesis of ACAGAs

Code	Definition
Ca	Cylitol pathway starting with an inositolphosphate synthaselike mechanism
Ca1	Cylitol pathway starting with D-*myo*-inositol-3-phosphate synthase
Cb	Cylitol pathway starting with a dehydroquinate synthaselike mechanism
Cb1	Cylitol pathway starting with 2-deoxy-*scyllo*-inosose synthase
Cb2	Cylitol pathway starting with valiol synthase
H(A)	(Amino-)hexose pathway[a]
P(A)	(Amino-)pentose pathway[a]
Hep(A)	(Amino-)heptose pathway[a]
Oct(A)	(Amino-)octose pathway[a]
6DOH	(dTDP-)6-Deoxyhexose pathway
[X]	Noncarbohydrate residues

Example:	**HA–(4)Cb1(6)–P(2)–HA**
Meaning:	A 2-deoxyhexitol is glycosylated at positions 4 and 6 by a hexosamine and a pentose that is further 2-glycosylated by a hexosaminyl-unit.

[a] Distinction between nucleosidediphosphate- (NDP-) and phosphate-activated sugar pathways, or the introduction of amino-groups before or after glycosyltransfer, cannot be given at present.

Several other ACAGAs probably are biosynthetically related to streptomycins, as judged from the structure of their cyclitol moieties and other motifs: spectinomycins and the more recently described related spenolimycin (34) (**Ca1(4,5)–6DOH;** Figure 3); kasugamycin and minosaminomycin (**Ca1(4)–6DOH;** Figure 4); compound LL-BM123α (**Ca1(4)–H(4)–HA;** Figure 5); myomycins (**Ca1(4)-HA;** Figure 6); and probably, the new aminoglycoside boholmycin (35) (**HA–(4)Ca1(6)–PA(4)–Hep;** Figure 7). Three further aminoglycosidic components are produced by the LL-BM123α-producing *Nocardia* sp.: the glycocinnamoylspermidines LL-BM123β, LL-BM123γ$_1$, and LL-BM123γ$_2$ (**6DOH(4)–PA(4)–PA;** cf. Figure 5). Though lacking a cyclitol unit, they also resemble the streptomycins or myomycins to some extent because of their strong modification with guanidino-, carbamoyl-, and secondary amino-groups.

B.   2-Deoxystreptamine-Containing Aminoglycosides

Most of the 2-deoxystreptamine (2DOS)-containing aminoglycosides represent a relatively homogeneous biosynthetic group, since they share the common pseudodisaccharidic intermediate paromamine (1,36–38). The most important members of the 2DOS family are the neomycins (**HA–(4)Cb1(5)–P(3)–HA;** Figure 8); the butirosin/-ribostamycins (**HA–(4)Cb1(5)–P;** Figure 9); the kanamycins (**HA–(4)Cb1(6)–HA;** Figure 10); the gentamicins (**HA–(4)Cb1(6)–P** [or **PA**]; Figure 11); and the seldomycins (**HA–(4)Cb1(6)–PA;** Figure 12). Some minor pseudodisaccharidic components are also seen in fermentations of some of the 2DOS groups, such as the biologically active neamine (neomycin A) and seldomycin 2 (Figure 13). These ACAGAs obviously are all rooted in a common basic pathway with paromamine as a common intermediate (Figure 14; cf. Fig. 13). More distantly related groups are the 2DOS-containing, nonparomamine ACAGAs, members of which are the apramycins (**Cb1(4)–OctA(8)–H** [or **HA**]; Figure

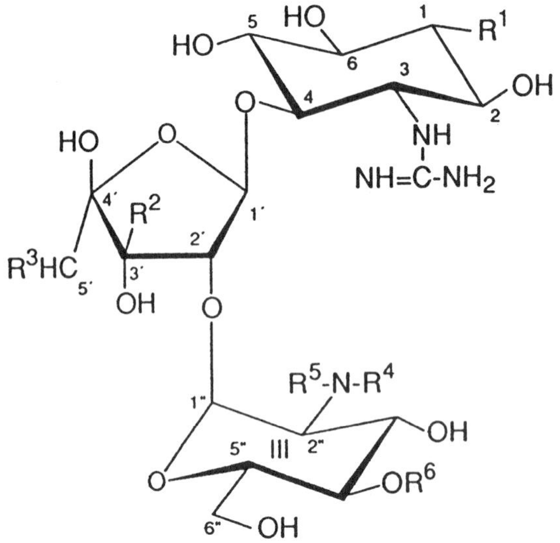

	R^1	R^2	R^3	R^4	R^5	R^6
Streptomycin	$NH\text{-}CNH\text{-}NH_2$	CHO	CH_3	CH_3	H	H
Dihydrostreptomycin	$NH\text{-}CNH\text{-}NH_2$	$CH_2\text{-}OH$	CH_3	CH_3	H	H
5'-Hydroxystreptomycin	$NH\text{-}CNH\text{-}NH_2$	CHO	$CH_2\text{-}OH$	CH_3	H	H
N-Demethylstreptomycin	$NH\text{-}CNH\text{-}NH_2$	CHO	CH_3	H	H	H
Mannosido-Hydroxystreptomycin	$NH\text{-}CNH\text{-}NH_2$	CHO	$CH_2\text{-}OH$	CH_3	H	α-D-mannose (= DM)
Dimannosidostreptomycin	$NH\text{-}CNH\text{-}NH_2$	CHO	CH_3	CH_3	H	α-DM-1,6-α-DM
Bluensomycin	$O\text{-}CO\text{-}NH_2$	$CH_2\text{-}OH$	CH_3	CH_3	H	H
Ashimycin A	$NH\text{-}CNH\text{-}NH_2$	CHO	CH_3	CH_3	H	2'''-carboxy-xylo-furanose (ashimose)
Ashimycin B	$NH\text{-}CNH\text{-}NH_2$	CHO	CH_3	CH_3	$CO\text{-}CH_2\text{-}OH$	α-DM-1,6-α-DM

AC4437 = 5'-Hydroxystreptomycin lacking ring III

Figure 1 Streptomycins and related compounds. The general pathway formula is **Ca1(4)–6DOH(2)–HA** (cf. Table 2).

15) and the hygromycin B/destomycin group (**Cb1(5)–H(2,3)–HepA** or **Ca1(5)–H(2,3)–HepA**; Figure 16). Interestingly, in the latter group there are compounds, such as SS-56-C (cf. Figure 16), that seem to be formed starting from a **Ca1** cyclitol moiety as the aglycone, which could be a strain-specific variation (see also Section III.C). Since this group was extensively studied from the 1950s to the early 1970s, relatively few new members of the 2DOS family of ACAGAs have been described since 1980. Among these are the compounds KA-5685 (4''-deamino-4''-hydroxyapramycin; cf. Figure 15) and 1-N-amidino-1-N-demethyl-2-hydroxy-destomycin (cf. Figure 16), both produced by different strains of *Saccharopolyspora hirsuta* (40,41). Also notable is the fact that the neomycin/ribostamycin-related inosamycins (not shown; cf. Figures 8 and 9) are produced by a strain of *Streptomyces hygroscopicus* (39) on the basis of a monoaminocyclitol, 3-amino-2,3-dideoxy-*scyllo*-inositol, instead of 2DOS as an aglycone.

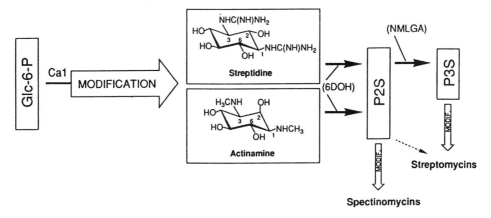

Figure 2   Basic pathway design for the biosynthesis of streptomycins and spectinomycins. Fully modified precursors are condensed to the final products. P2S = pseudodisaccharide; P3S = pseudotrisaccharide; 6DOH = an activated 6-deoxyhexose precursor; NMLGA = NDP-activated N-methyl-L-glucosamine.

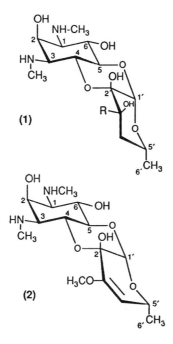

Figure 3   Spectinomycins (**Ca1(4,5)–6DOH**). (1) Spectinomycin (R = OH) and dihydrospectinomycin (R = H); (2) spenolimycin.

C.   Fortimicin (Astromicin)/Istamycin Group

The fortimicin (astromicin)/istamycin group of compounds is a third class of strongly related ACAGAs (**Ca1(6)–Ha** or **Cb1(6)–HA;** Figure 17). The more recently detected fortimicin/istamycin group of aminoglycosides has been intensively studied throughout the 1980s, and several new members or producers have been described: the 2″-N-formimi-

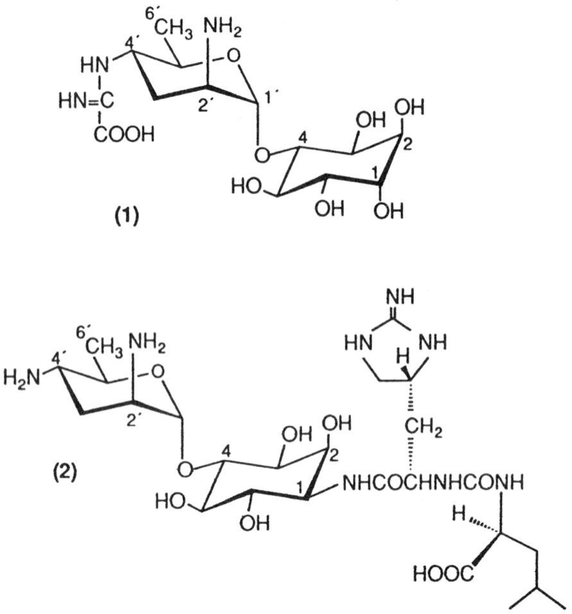

Figure 4   Kasugamycins (**Ca1(4)–6DOH**). (1) Kasugamycin; (2) minosaminomycin.

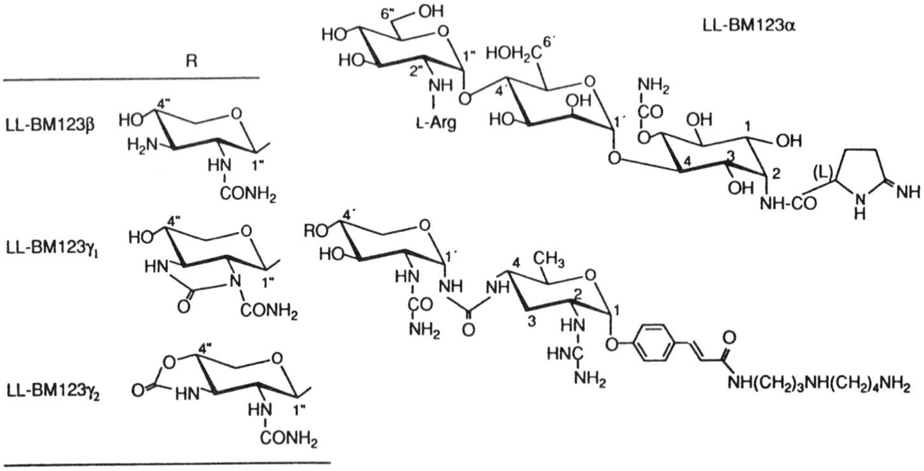

Figure 5   Aminoglycosides of the LL-BM123 complex: LL-BM123α (**Ca1(4)–H(4)–HA**) and the glycocinnamoyl spermidines LL-BM123β, γ₁, and γ₂ (**6DOH(4)–PA(4)–PA**).

doyl derivatives of astromicin (identical with dactimicin) produced by *Micromonospora olivasterospora* (42); derivatives of istamycins A and B produced by *Streptomyces tenjimariensis* (43); and derivatives of sporaricin A produced by *S. hirsuta* (44); or the new variant lysinomicin produced by *Micromonospora pilosospora* (45) (cf. Figure 17). Interestingly, the members of this group produced by *Micromonospora* sp. and *Dactylosporangium* sp. are based on a **Ca1** cyclitol (fortamine), whereas the related compounds produced in

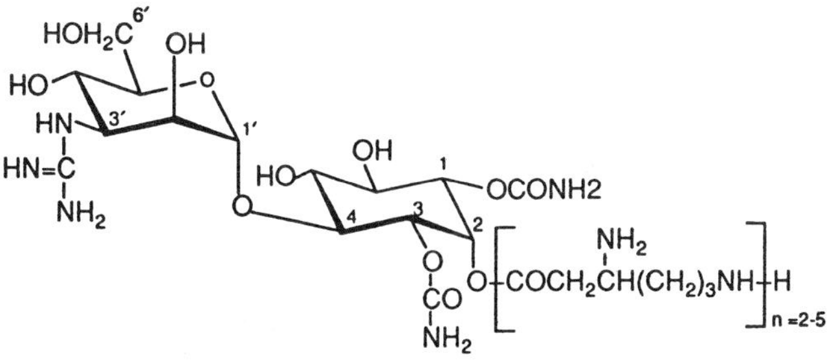

Figure 6 Myomycins (Ca1(4)–HA).

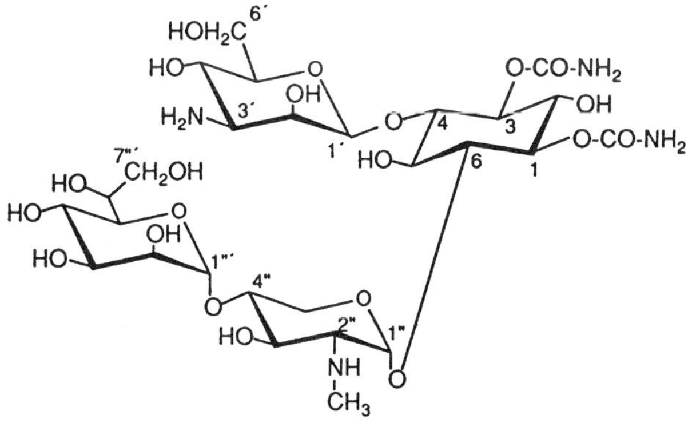

Figure 7 Boholmycin (HA–(4)Ca1(6)–PA(4)–Hep).

Streptomyces sp. (istamycins = ISM; sannamycins) and *Saccharopolyspora* sp. (sporaricins) obviously use a **Cb1**-derived aminocyclitol (2-deoxyfortamine), as outlined in a schematic representation of the pathway design in this class (Figure 18).

D. C$_7$-Aminocyclitol-Aminoglycosides

Another group of ACAGAs containing a C$_7$-cyclitol moiety that is not derived from glucose (see Section V.A) was first described in the early 1970s. This class includes two variably glucosylated aminoglycosides: the validamycins and their nonglucosylated relatives, the validoxylamines (**Cb2(1)–Cb2** for the basic pseudodisaccharide moieties; Figure 19); and the acarbose-related compounds (amylostatins and others) (**Cb2(1)–6DOH** or **Cb2(1)–H** for the basic pseudodisaccharide moieties; Figure 20). Also, a monomeric C$_7$-aminocyclitol, valiolamine, which is assumed to be an intermediate or a side-product of validamycin biosynthesis, has been described more recently as an independent end product of *S. hygroscopicus* subsp. *limoneus* (46). The acarbose-related metabolites of various actinomycetes act as inhibitors of various glycosidases, for example, α-glucosidases and trehalases (26,27). The basic pathway leading to these unusual compounds, despite the use of in vivo labeling studies with stable isotopes (8), has not yet been investigated biochemically.

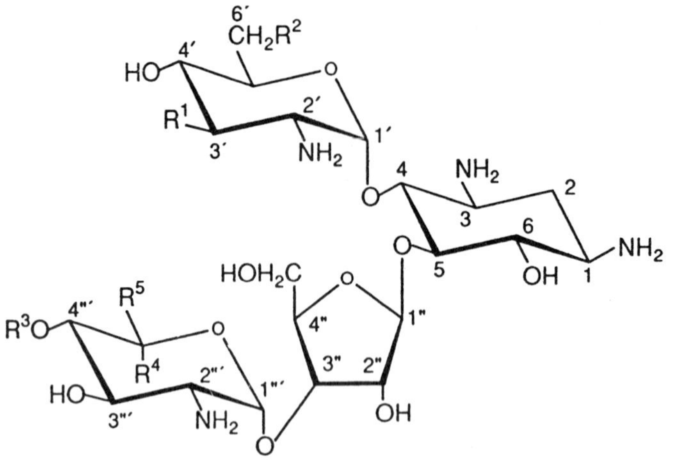

	R^1	R^2	R^3	R^4	R^5
Neomycin B	OH	NH$_2$	H	CH$_2$NH$_2$	H
Neomycin C	OH	NH$_2$	H	H	CH$_2$NH$_2$
Paromomycin I	OH	OH	H	CH$_2$NH$_2$	H
Paromomycin II	OH	OH	H	H	CH$_2$NH$_2$
Mannosylparomomycin	OH	OH	α-D-Man	CH$_2$NH$_2$	H
Lividomycin A	H	OH	α-D-Man	CH$_2$NH$_2$	H
Lividomycin B	H	OH	H	CH$_2$NH$_2$	H

Figure 8 Neomycins and related ACAGAs. The general pathway formula is **HA–(4)Cb1(5)–P(3)–HA.** Neomycin-related compounds, the inosamycins (39), containing 3-amino-2,3-dideoxy-*scyllo*-inositol as cyclitol, also occur as natural products.

E. Other Aminoglycosides

Structurally more distantly related to the aforementioned ACAGA classes, and of even higher uncertainty in their pathway relationships, are a number of old and new aminoglycoside-related secondary metabolites. For instance, the hexitol-containing sorbistins (**Ca1(2)–HA;** Figure 21) are produced, interestingly, in both actinomycetes and Gram-negative bacteria, and their 1,4-diamino-1,4-dideoxysorbitol unit could be formed via ring cleavage of a diaminocyclitol synthesized via the basic **Ca1** pathway. The aminoglycoside hygromycin A (**Ca1(4)–[X]–6DOH;** Figure 22) is of interest, too, since it is produced in the same strain that produces hygromycin B, a **Cb1**-compound (see above). The unusual aminocyclitol moiety of hygromycin A, a *neo*-inosamine-2 in which the 5- and 6-hydroxyls are bridged by a methylene group, however, is presumably also formed via the **Ca1** route.

The monosaccharidic glycosidase inhibitors and antibiotics (**HA;** Figure 23) and several disaccharidic amino-*N*-containing secondary or semisynthetic carbohydrates (**HA(1)–H** or **HA(1)–HA;** Figure 24) lack an (amino-)cyclitol constituent. Some new

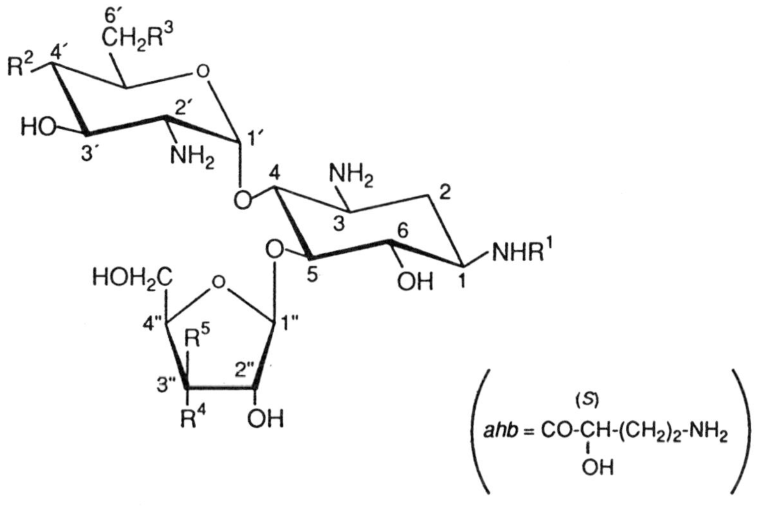

The structure shows a ring system with labeled positions:
6', CH$_2$R^3, R^2, 4', O, 2', R, HO, 3', NH$_2$, 1', O, 4, NH$_2$, 2, 3, 6, NHR^1, O, 5, OH, 1, HOH$_2$C, O, 4", R^5, 1", 3", 2", R^4, OH

$$\left(\ ahb = \underset{\substack{|\\OH}}{CO\text{-}CH}\text{-}(CH_2)_2\text{-}NH_2 \ \right) \quad (S)$$

	R^1	R^2	R^3	R^4	R^5
Butirosin A	ahb	OH	NH$_2$	H	OH
Butirosin B	ahb	OH	NH$_2$	OH	H
Butirosin E$_1$	ahb	OH	OH	H	OH
Butirosin E$_2$	ahb	OH	OH	OH	H
Butirosin C$_1$	ahb	H	NH$_2$	H	OH
Butirosin C$_2$	ahb	H	NH$_2$	OH	H
Ribostamycin	H	OH	NH$_2$	OH	H
Xylostatin	H	OH	NH$_2$	H	OH
LL-BM 408α	H	OH	OH	OH	H

Figure 9 Butirosins and related ACAGAs (HA–(4)Cb1(5)–P).

members of the latter group have been described recently, such as the α,β-glycosidic antibiotic 3,3′-neotrehalosadiamine (cf. Figure 24), which was isolated from a *Bacillus pumilus* via a new screening method for aminoglycoside antibiotics, namely, for its antibacterial activity in an aminoglycoside-hypersensitive strain of *Klebsiella pneumoniae* (47,48). The enzyme inhibitor 1-deoxynojirimycin (DNJ) (cf. Figure 23) was investigated for its biogenesis in a recent study by stable-isotope labeling in *Streptomyces subrutilus* (cf. Section V.B) (49).

Completely new structural classes of ACAGAs have been detected in the past decade with the isolation of the allosamidins (**Ca2?(4)–HA(4)–HA;** Figure 25) and of trehazolin (**Ca1/3?(1,2)–HA;** Figure 26) by screening actinomycete cultures for special groups of glycosidase inhibitors. Allosamidin is the first chitinase inhibitor isolated from streptomycetes (50). Trehazolin (or trehalostatin) is a very specific trehalase inhibitor. It is produced by *Micromonospora* sp. and *Amycolatopsis* sp. (51). The chemical synthesis of trehazolin as well as that of its β-anomer was reported recently (52). In recent studies on the biogenesis of the allosamidins, the direct derivation of the C and N atoms of the allosamizoline moiety from D-glucosamine has been reported (53,54). The C$_6$-aminocyclopentitol moieties in both compounds could either be derived via ring contraction of a

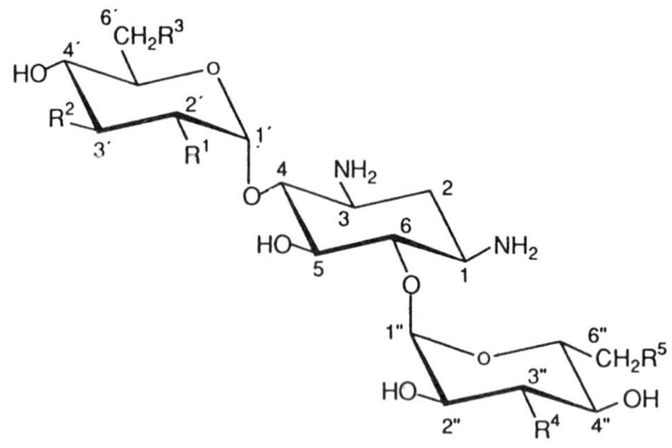

Figure 10 Kanamycins and related ACAGAs (HA–(4)Cb1(6)–HA).

	R^1	R^2	R^3	R^4	R^5
Kanamycin	OH	OH	NH$_2$	NH$_2$	OH
Kanamycin B	NH$_2$	OH	NH$_2$	NH$_2$	OH
Kanamycin C	NH$_2$	OH	OH	NH$_2$	OH
NK-1001	OH	OH	NH$_2$	OH	OH
NK-1012-1	NH$_2$	OH	NH$_2$	OH	OH
Tobramycin	NH$_2$	H	NH$_2$	NH$_2$	OH
Nebramycin 4	NH$_2$	OH	NH$_2$	NH$_2$	OCONH$_2$
Nebramycin 5	NH$_2$	H	NH$_2$	NH$_2$	OCONH$_2$

Ca1-like cyclohexitol or by direct formation via a pentitol(-phosphate) synthase catalyz-ing an unknown new, but Ca1-related, mechanism (called **Ca2** or **Ca3;** cf. the discussion in Section V.A). However, for neither these nor for none of the other natural products mentioned in this section has a biosynthetic study on the enzymatic level been started.

F. Comparison of Basic Pathway Design

The general design of a pathway for the formation of a complex oligomeric secondary metabolite can be subdivided into several phases: (a) activation and (b) modification of the monomeric precursors, (c) oligomerization (condensation of monomers), (d) a second phase of modification of the oligomer, (e) export from the producing cell, and (f) maybe extracellular processing (release) of the active end product from an inactive precursor. These biosynthetic tasks have been quite differently solved in the various producers of ACAGAs. In the formation of streptomycins, most of the modification steps take place at the level of activated monomers (cf. Figure 2; see Section V). In contrast, in the large group of 2DOS-aminoglycosides, although the aminocyclitol is preformed and completely modified, most of the modification of the sugar moieties is transferred to a second phase after condensation of the subunits (cf. Figure 14). Finally, in the fortimicin (astro-micin)/istamycin group, the primary modification of both cyclitol and sugar units takes place after the condensing steps (cf. Figure 18). These differences in pathway design prob-ably have several physiological consequences, such as influences on the product pattern and the regulation of substrate flow, as is outlined in more detail in Sections V.C and VI.

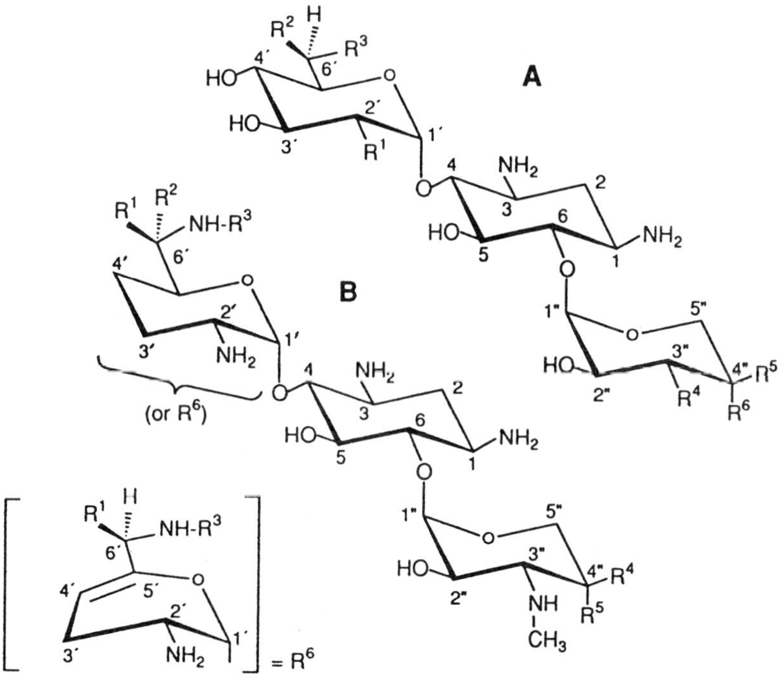

A	R^1	R^2	R^3	R^4	R^5	R^6
Gentamicin A	NH_2	H	OH	$NHCH_3$	OH	H
Gentamicin A_1	NH_2	H	OH	$NHCH_3$	H	OH
Gentamicin A_2	NH_2	H	OH	OH	OH	H
Gentamicin A_3	OH	H	NH_2	$NHCH_3$	H	OH
Gentamicin A_4	NH_2	H	OH	$N(CHO)CH_3$	OH	H
Gentamicin B	OH	H	NH_2	$NHCH_3$	CH_3	OH
Gentamicin B_1	OH	CH_3	NH_2	$NHCH_3$	CH_3	OH
Gentamicin X_2	NH_2	H	OH	$NHCH_3$	CH_3	OH
G-418	NH_2	CH_3	OH	$NHCH_3$	CH_3	OH
JI-20A	NH_2	H	NH_2	$NHCH_3$	CH_3	OH
JI-20B	NH_2	CH_3	NH_2	$NHCH_3$	CH_3	OH

B	R^1	R^2	R^3	R^4	R^5	R^6
Gentamicin C_1	CH_3	H	CH_3	CH_3	OH	-
Gentamicin C_{1a}	H	H	H	CH_3	OH	-
Gentamicin C_2	CH_3	H	H	CH_3	OH	-
Gentamicin C_{2a}	H	CH_3	H	CH_3	OH	-
Gentamicin C_{2-III} [a]	H	H	H	CH_3	OH	-
Sagamicin	H	H	CH_3	CH_3	OH	-
Sisomicin	H	H	H	CH_3	OH	+
Verdamicin	CH_3	H	H	CH_3	OH	+
G-52	H	H	CH_3	CH_3	OH	+
66-40B	H	H	H	OH	H	+
66-40D	H	H	H	H	OH	+

[a] 5'-L-isomer of gentamicin C_{1a}

Figure 11 Gentamicins and related ACAGAs (HA–(4)Cb1(6)–P [or–PA]).

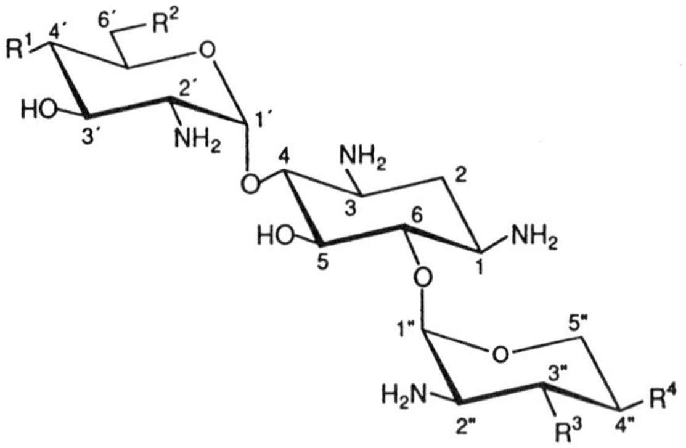

	R¹	R²	R³	R⁴
Seldomycin 1	OH	OH	OH	OH
Seldomycin 3	OH	NH₂	OH	OH
Seldomycin 5	H	NH₂	NH₂	OCH₃

Figure 12 Seldomycins (HA–(4)Cb1(6)–P [or –PA]).

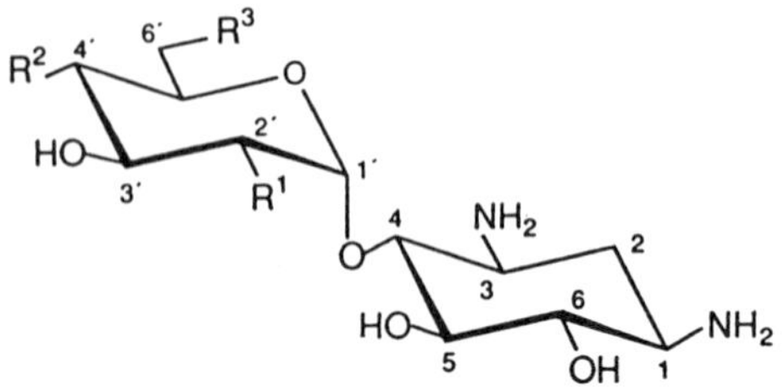

	R¹	R²	R³
Paromamine	NH₂	OH	OH
Neamine	NH₂	OH	NH₂
NK-1003	OH	OH	NH₂
Seldomycin 2	NH₂	H	NH₂

Figure 13 Pseudodisaccharidic 2DOS ACAGAs (Cb1(4)–HA).

G. Semisynthetic Aminoglycosides

Semisynthetic derivatives of chemotherapeutically successful ACAGAs have been obtained in large number by preparative organic chemistry. Interestingly, the only compounds that were chemotherapeutically successful were those into which structural alterations had been introduced that mimicked naturally occurring modifications, thereby resulting in activity against clinically relevant (nosocomial) pathogens with ACAGA-resistance mechanisms. The most important examples are dibekacin (and its derivative

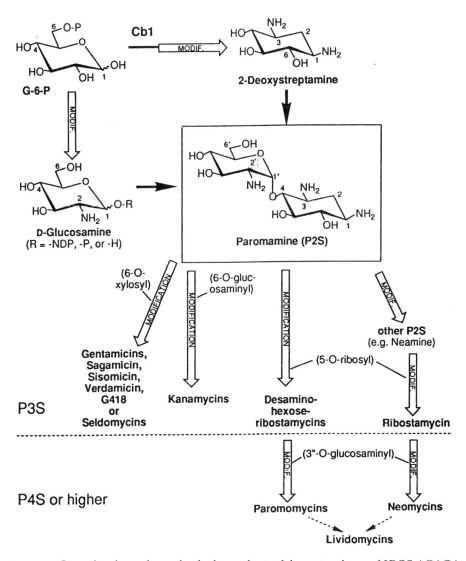

Figure 14 General pathway design for the biosynthesis of the major classes of 2DOS ACAGAs. The central role of the paromamine intermediate is emphasized. The route leading to the seldomycins, whether related to that of the kanamycins or the gentamicins, is unknown. The distribution of modifying phases is indicated with open arrows. P2S, P3S, P4S = pseudodi-, -tri-, or tetrasaccharides, respectively; P = phosphoryl residues.

arbekacin), amikacin, netilmicin, and isepamicin, which are derived from members of the kanamycin and gentamicin groups, respectively (Figure 27). The major alterations leading to potent antibiotics, such as 3,4-dehydroxylation of a hexosamine moiety and introduction of an N^1-α-hydroxy-γ-aminobutyryl residue (= AHB; or its propionyl analog, AHP), also similarly occur in the naturally produced fortimicins (cf. Figure 17) and butirosins (cf. Figure 9), respectively.

Also, some members of the amino-disaccharide family have been prepared semisynthetically, such as the 3-amino-3-deoxy analogs of trehalose and sucrose and their

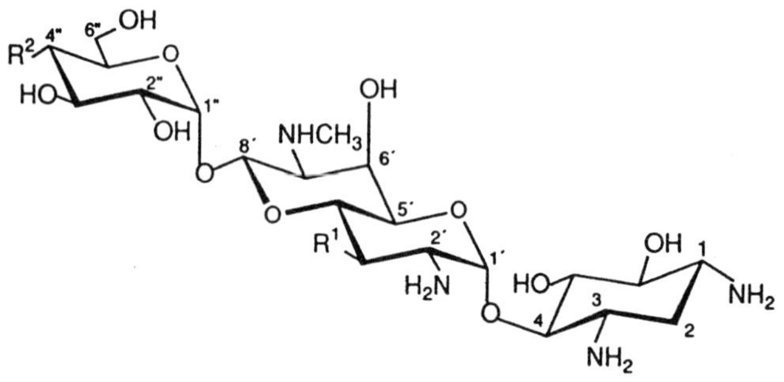

	R¹	R²
Apramycin	H	NH₂
Oxyapramycin	OH	NH₂
Saccharocin (KA-5685)	H	OH

Figure 15 Apramycins and related ACAGAs (Cb1(4)–Oct(8)–H [or –HA]).

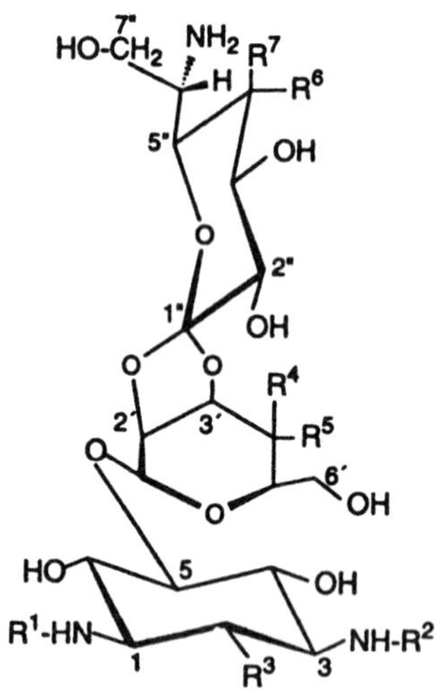

	R¹	R²	R³	R⁴	R⁵	R⁶	R⁷
Hygromycin B	H	CH₃	H	OH	H	OH	H
Destomycin A	CH₃	H	H	OH	H	OH	H
Destomycin B	CH₃	CH₃	H	H	OH	H	OH
Destomycin C	CH₃	CH₃	H	OH	H	OH	H
A-396-I	H	H	H	OH	H	OH	H
A-16316-C	CH₃	CH₃	H	H	OH	OH	H
SS-56-C	H	H	OH	OH	H	OH	H
1-N-Amidino-1-N-demethyl-2-hydroxy-destomycin A	C(NH)NH₂	H	OH	OH	H	OH	H

Figure 16 Destomycins and related ACAGAs (Cb1 [or Ca1](5)–H(2,3)–HepA).

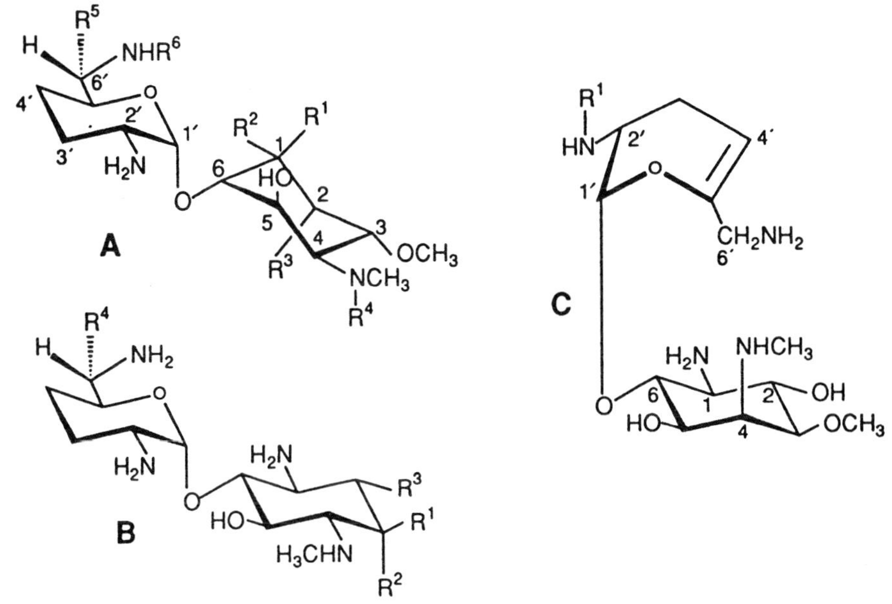

		R^1	R^2	R^3	R^4	R^5	R^6
A	Fortimicin A	NH_2	H	OH	$COCH_2NH_2$	CH_3	H
	Fortimicin B	NH_2	H	OH	H	CH_3	H
	1-*epi*-Fortimicin B	H	NH_2	OH	H	CH_3	H
	Fortimicin C	NH_2	H	OH	$COCH_2NHCONH_2$	CH_3	H
	Fortimicin D	NH_2	H	OH	$COCH_2NH_2$	H	H
	Dactimicin	NH_2	H	OH	$COCH_2NHCH=NH$	CH_3	H
	1-*epi*-Dactimicin	H	NH_2	OH	$COCH_2NHCH=NH$	CH_3	H
	Sporaricin A	H	NH_2	H	$COCH_2NH_2$	CH_3	H
	Sporaricin B	H	NH_2	H	H	CH_3	H
	Istamycin A_0	NH_2	H	H	H	H	CH_3
	Istamycin A	NH_2	H	H	$COCH_2NH_2$	H	CH_3
	(= Sannamycin)						
	Istamycin A_3	NH_2	H	H	$COCH_2NHCH=NH$	H	CH_3
	Istamycin B_0	H	NH_2	H	H	H	CH_3
	Istamycin B	H	NH_2	H	$COCH_2NH_2$	H	CH_3
	Istamycin B_3	H	NH_2	H	$COCH_2NHCH=NH$	H	CH_3
	Istamycin C	NH_2	H	H	$COCH_2NH_2$	H	CH_2CH_3
	Istamycin A_2	NH_2	H	H	$COCH_2NHCONH_2$	H	CH_3
	Fortimicin KH	OCH_3	H	OH	CH_3		
B	Fortimicin KR	H	OCH_3	OH	CH_3		
	Istamycin Y_0	OCH_3	H	H	H		
	Istamycin X_0	H	OCH_3	H	H		
C	Fortimicin KG_3	H					
	Lysinomicin	$COCH_2CHNH_2(CH_2)_3NH_2$					

Figure 17 Fortimicins (astromicins) and related ACAGAs (**Ca1** [or **Cb1**](6)–HA).

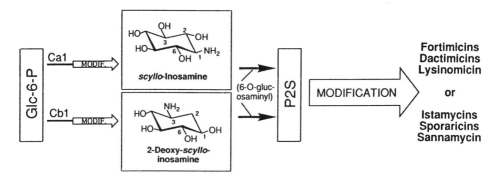

Figure 18 General pathway design for the biosynthesis of the fortimicins and related ACAGAs.

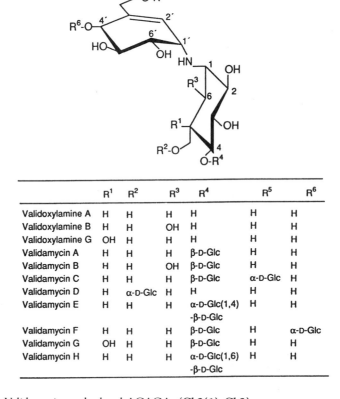

	R¹	R²	R³	R⁴	R⁵	R⁶
Validoxylamine A	H	H	H	H	H	H
Validoxylamine B	H	H	OH	H	H	H
Validoxylamine G	OH	H	H	H	H	H
Validamycin A	H	H	H	β-D-Glc	H	H
Validamycin B	H	H	OH	β-D-Glc	H	H
Validamycin C	H	H	H	β-D-Glc	α-D-Glc	H
Validamycin D	H	α-D-Glc	H	H	H	H
Validamycin E	H	H	H	α-D-Glc(1,4)	H	H
				-β-D-Glc		
Validamycin F	H	H	H	β-D-Glc	H	α-D-Glc
Validamycin G	OH	H	H	β-D-Glc	H	H
Validamycin H	H	H	H	α-D-Glc(1,6)	H	H
				-β-D-Glc		

Figure 19 Validamycins and related ACAGAs (**Cb2(1)–Cb2**).

epimers, T-I, T-II (3-trehalosamine), and T-III or S-I and S-II (3-sucrosamine) (cf. Figure 24) (55), respectively. Except for S-I, these compounds are weak antibiotics; S-I instead is an inhibitor of invertases. These compounds have been obtained by chemoenzymatic synthesis via regioselective oxidation to the 3-ketoforms of trehalose and sucrose by treatment with D-glucoside 3-dehydrogenase from *Flavobacterium saccharophilum*, followed by reductive chemical amination (55).

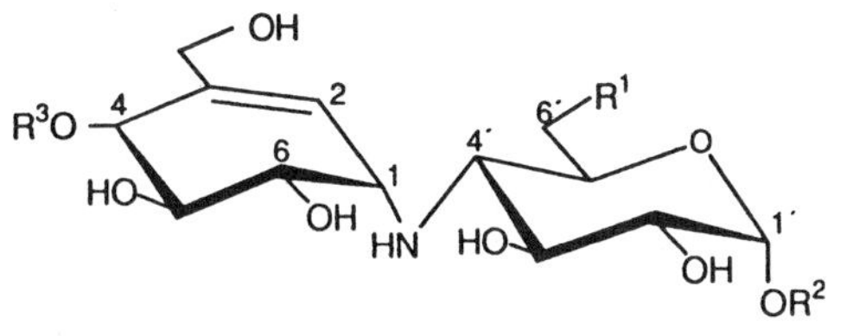

	R^1	R^2	R^3
Amylostatins	H	H, or (α-D-glucopyranosyl)$_n$	H, or (α-D-glucopyranosyl)$_n$
(Acarbose)	H	α-1,4-maltosyl	H
Adiposins	OH	α-1,4-maltosyl	H, or (α-D-glucopyranosyl)$_n$
Trestatins	H	α-1,4-trehalosyl	H, or (core pseudo-trisaccharide)$_n$

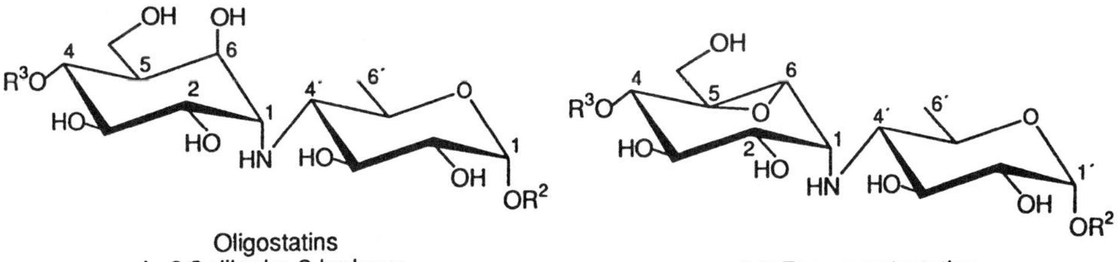

Oligostatins
(= 2,3-dihydro-2-hydroxy-
derivatives of amylostatins)

5,6-Epoxyamylostatins

Figure 20 Amylostatin (acarbose) and related ACAGAs (pathway formula for the core units Cb2(1)–6DOH [or –H]).

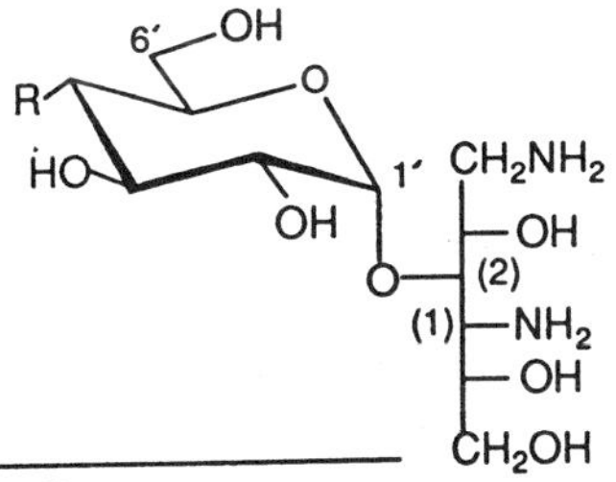

	R
Sorbistin A$_1$	-NH-CO-(CH$_2$)$_2$-CH$_3$
Sorbistin A$_2$	-NH-CO-CH$_2$-CH$_3$
Sorbistin B	-NH-CO-CH$_3$
Sorbistin D	-NH$_2$
Sorbistin C	-OH

Figure 21 Sorbistins (Ca1?(2)–HA). The numbering system is taken from the assumed analogy to streptamine-related aminocyclitols.

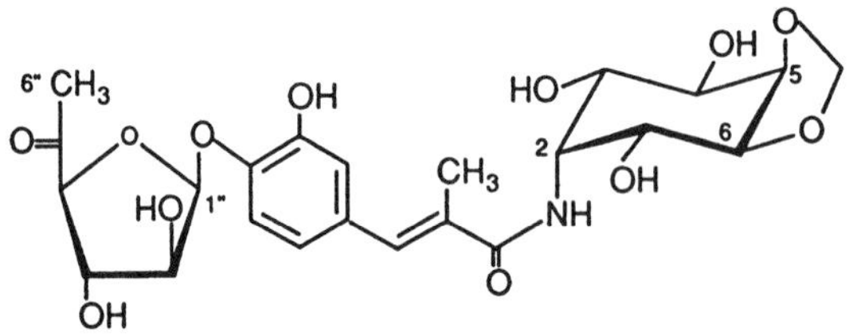

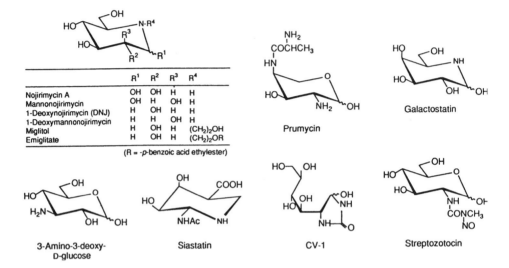

Figure 22 Hygromycin A (Ca1(1)–(X)–6DOH).

Figure 23 Monosaccharidic amino sugar derivatives (**HA**).

IV. GENETICS IN AMINOGLYCOSIDE PRODUCERS

Despite many efforts to understand the molecular genetics of ACAGA-producing actinomycetes and the description of resistance genes (see Section V.C) in nearly all producers of the major chemotherapeuticals in this group, only two systems have been studied in detail thus far, those for streptomycins and fortimicins (astromicins). In the producers of neomycin-like antibiotics, two equivalent but unlinked ACAGA-resistance genes were uniformly found, one of which seemed to be part of the biosynthesis gene cluster (cf. Section IV.C). In none of these strains, however, have the biosynthetic gene clusters clearly been proved to surround one or both of the resistance genes.

A. Genes Involved in the Production of Streptomycins, Bluensomycin, and Spectinomycin

1. Genes Involved in the Production of Streptomycins and Bluensomycin

About 30 genes for the production of (5′-hydroxy-)streptomycin (*str/sts*) and bluensomycin (*blu*) have been cloned and sequenced at least in part, or have been identified by hybridization in various actinomycete strains belonging to the genera *Streptomyces (S.)*, *Streptoverticillium*, and *Amycolatopsis* (Table 3; Figure 28) (4,6,9,10,61,62,64,65; and

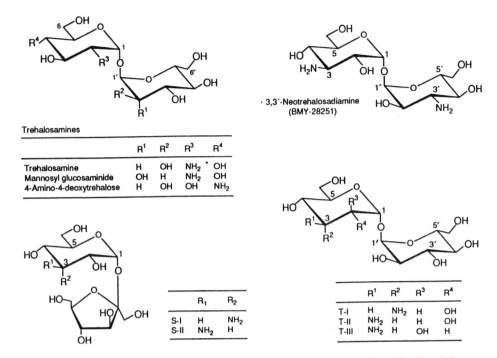

Trehalosamines

	R^1	R^2	R^3	R^4
Trehalosamine	H	OH	NH_2	OH
Mannosyl glucosaminide	OH	H	NH_2	OH
4-Amino-4-deoxytrehalose	H	OH	OH	NH_2

· 3,3'-Neotrehalosadiamine
(BMY-28251)

	R_1	R_2
S-I	H	NH_2
S-II	NH_2	H

	R^1	R^2	R^3	R^4
T-I	H	NH_2	H	OH
T-II	NH_2	H	H	OH
T-III	NH_2	H	OH	H

Figure 24 Aminodisaccharides (**HA(1)–H [or–HA]**). In the compounds of the S and T series, the amino-groups are introduced semisynthetically.

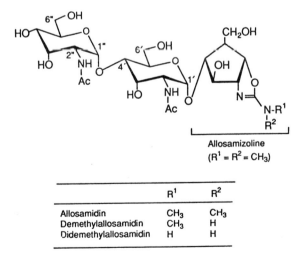

Allosamizoline
($R^1 = R^2 = CH_3$)

	R^1	R^2
Allosamidin	CH_3	CH_3
Demethylallosamidin	CH_3	H
Didemethylallosamidin	H	H

Figure 25 Allosamidins (**Ca2?(4)–HA(4)–HA**).

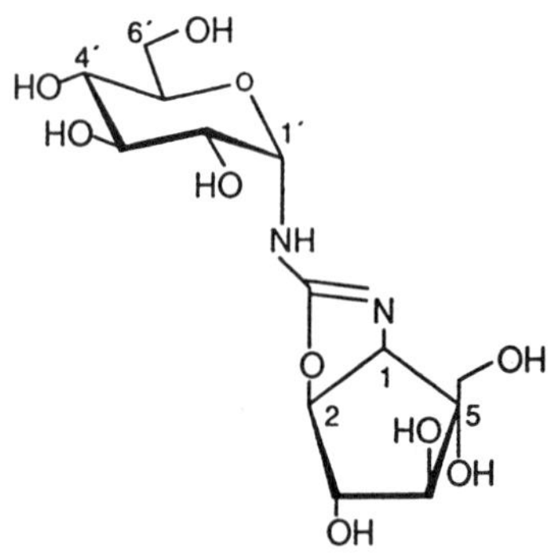

Figure 26 Trehazolin (Ca1/3?(1,2)–HA).

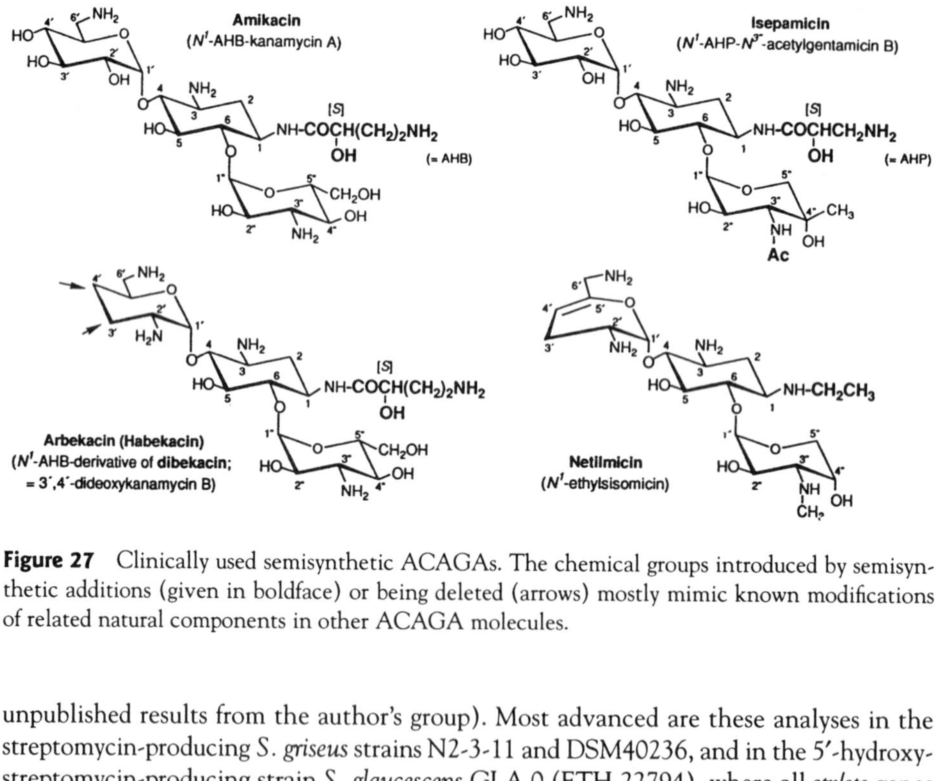

Figure 27 Clinically used semisynthetic ACAGAs. The chemical groups introduced by semisynthetic additions (given in boldface) or being deleted (arrows) mostly mimic known modifications of related natural components in other ACAGA molecules.

unpublished results from the author's group). Most advanced are these analyses in the streptomycin-producing *S. griseus* strains N2-3-11 and DSM40236, and in the 5'-hydroxy-streptomycin-producing strain *S. glaucescens* GLA.0 (ETH 22794), where all *str/sts* genes detected so far are clustered in one region of about 30 to 40 kbp of genomic DNA (cf. Figure 28). The order of genes is functionally mixed, meaning that they are not arranged in subpathway-specific operons. This could reflect the need for a strict coordination of the expression of *str/sts* gene products in order to guarantee a coordinated supply of the activated precursors in the course of streptomycin synthesis. Also, the order and arrangement of individual genes is not the same in both strains, though the majority of the *str/sts* genes identified until now are still organized within the same corresponding operons. The arrangement of these operons also differs considerably in various other producers. Homol-

Table 3 Gene Products and Enzymes Presumed to Be Involved in Streptomycin Production

Gene product[a]	Molecular data[b]		Enzymatic function[c] (preliminary assignment)	Step probably catalyzed[c]	Reference[d]
	MW (kDa)	aa			
Unknown	216 (native)	—	D-myo-inositol-3-phosphate synthetase	1	56
StrO	28	260 (256)	(D-myo-inositol-3-phosphate phosphatase)	2	A, 9
StrI	37	348	(scyllo-inosose dehydrogenase)	3 (or 8)	57
StsC	45	424	scyllo-inosose aminotransferase	4	A, 58
StsE	32	312	(scyllo-inosamine 4-phosphotransferase	5 or 10	58
StrB1	39	347	scyllo-inosamine-4-phosphate amidinotransferase	6 (and 11?)	59
Unknown			(N-amidino-scyllo-inosamine-4-phosphate phosphatase)	(7)	(cf. 60)
StsB	52	490	(N-amidino-scyllo-inosamine dehydrogenase	(8 or 3)	A
StsA	43	410	(3-keto-N-amidino-scyllo-inosamine aminotransferase)	(9 or 21)	A, 9
StrN	36 (35)	320 (316)	(N-amidino-streptamine 6-phosphotransferase)	(10 or 5)	A
StrB2	38 (35)	349 (319)	N-amidino-streptamine-6-phosphate amidinotransferase	11 (or none)	58
StrD	38	355	dTDP-glucose synthase (pyrophosphorylase)	12	58
StrE	36	328	dTDP-glucose 4,6-dehydratase	13	58
StrM	22	200	dTDP-4-keto-6-deoxyglucose 3,5-epimerase	14	58
StrL	32	304	dTDP-4-keto-L-rhamnose reductase (dTDP-L-rhamnose synthase)	15	58
StrH	43	384	(streptidine-6-phosphate dihydrostreptosyltransferase)	(23)	57
StrQ	34	297	CDP-glucose synthase	16	61
StrP	38	358	(NDP-hexose 4-dehydrogenase)	(17 or 20, 18a)	A, 61
StrX	20	182	(NDP-hexose 3,5-epimerase)	(18 or 19a)	62
StrU	46	428	(NDP-hexose oxidoreductase)	(19 or 20, 18a, 20a)	62
StrF	32	281	(NDP-hexose epimerase)	(17a or ?)	57
StrG	23	199	(NDP-hexose epimerase)	(17a or ?)	57
StsG	27	246	(N-methyltransferase)	(22 or 16a)	A
StrS	40	378 (377)	(aminotransferase; unknown function)	(21 or 9)	A, 9
StrT	33		unknown function	?	A
StrY			unknown function	?	61
StrZ			unknown function	?	61
StsD	24	213	unknown function	?	A
StsF	26	236	unknown function	?	A
StrV			(exporter for streptomycin 6-(or 3″-) phosphates)	(25)	A, 62
StrW			(exporter for streptomycin 6-(or 3″-) phosphates)	(25)	A, 62
StrK	46	449 (462)	streptomycin 6-(or 3″-)phosphate phosphatase	27	57
StrA (AphD)	33	307	streptomycin 6-phosphotransferase	28	59
StrR	38 (46)	350 (424)	DNA-binding protein, activator of gene expression		A, 9, 59
AphE	29	272	streptomycin 3″-phosphotransferase	(28a)	63

[a] Cf. Figure 28.

[b] Genetic data from S. griseus N2-3-11 and/or S. glaucescens GLA.0 (from the latter strain given in parentheses if different).

[c] Cf. Figures 29 and 30.

[d] A = Ahlert J, Beyer S, Distler J, Mansouri K, Mayer G, and Piepersberg W, Unpublished data.

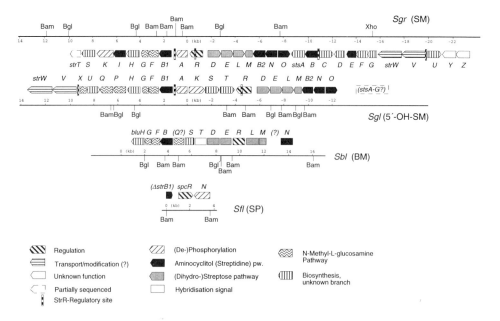

Figure 28   Gene clusters for the production of streptomycins (SM) and the related **Ca**-aminogly-cosides bluensomycin (BM) and spectinomycin (SP). The streptomycete producers investigated most intensively are *S. griseus* (*Sgr*) strains N2-3-11 and DSM40236, *S. glaucescens* (*Sgl*) GLA.0 (ETH 22794), *S. bluensis* (*Sbl*) DSM40564, and *S. flavopersicus* (*Sfl*) NRRL 2820. Restriction maps are given for orientation; the clusters are aligned according to their homologous amidinotransferase [*strB(1)*] genes. Chessboard bars indicate the locations of StrR-binding sites on the DNA.

ogous *str/sts* genes and their gene products in both *S. griseus* and *S. glaucescens* show sequence identity values varying between 58 and 86%. In the corresponding noncoding intercistrons, much less or no significant sequence identity has been found. Thus, the genetic equivalent for the biosynthetic potential of streptomycin formation could be very old in evolutionary terms, being frequently recombined in the actinomycetes.

The enzymatic steps in streptomycin biosynthesis (Figures 29 and 30) that can be postulated from the gene products found by molecular genetics in *S. griseus* and *S. glaucescens* in many cases nicely correspond to those postulated from earlier isotope-labeling, mutant, and enzyme studies (10,23,38,60,66,67). However, some details in the proposed pathway might still have to be revised in the future, although the general outline and phasing of the biochemical route probably will prove to be correct (cf. Figures 2, 29, and 30): (a) formation of the activated precursors, streptidine-6-phosphate, deoxythymidine diphosphate (dTDP)-dihydrostreptose, and NDP-*N*-(methyl)-L-glucosamine; (b) condensation of the precursors to dihydrostreptomycin-6-phosphate; (c) which becomes secreted and probably oxidized while passing the cytoplasmic membrane to give streptomycin-6-phosphate outside the cell; and (d) the liberation of the biologically active streptomycins by a specific phosphatase; (e) After reuptake, streptomycin is rephosphorylated by a streptomycin 6-phosphotransferase, representing the major resistance mechanism (cf. Section V).

The introduction of molecular genetics approaches to the study of streptomycin biosynthesis started with cloning resistance genes in the mid 1980s (reviewed in Refs. 3

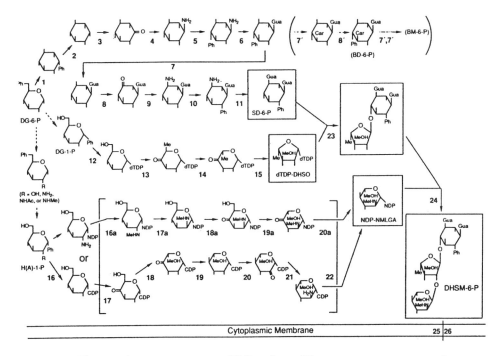

Figure 29 The cytoplasmic streptomycin (SM) pathway. The most important intermediates are boxed. The three activated intermediates principally formed from D-glucose-6-phosphate (DG-6-P) are condensed to dihydro-SM-6-phosphate (DHSM-6-P) in the cytoplasm; this becomes oxidized and dephosphorylated to SM during or after transport through the cytoplsamic membrane (cf. Figure 30). The individual biosynthetic steps are numbered (see text and Table 2). Vertical lines = hydroxyl; Ph = phosphoryl; Gua = guanidyl; Car = carbamoyl; Me = methyl; H(A)-1-P = hexose(amine)-1-phosphate; dTDPG = deoxytymidindiphosphate-glucose; NDP = nucleosidediphosphate [NDP = CDP or UDP]; SD = streptidine; DHSO = dihydrostreptose; NMLGA = N-methyl-L-glucosamine; DHSM = dihydrostreptose.

and 10). These turned out to comprise two genes, *strA (aphD)* and *aphE*, which encode two different streptomycin-phosphotransferases, APH(6) and APH(3″), respectively (63,68–71). Up to the present, only the *strA* gene has been localized within the biosynthesis gene clusters of S. *griseus* and S. *glaucescens* GLA.0. The *aphE* gene, on the other hand, has been shown to occur only in S. *griseus* strains, and it seems not to be part of the *str/sts* cluster (cf. Figure 28). Further streptomycin biosynthetic genes were identified by chromosome walking and genetic complementation of mutants blocked in defined steps (or phases) of the biosynthetic pathway in S. *griseus* (72–74).

Bluensomycin (cf. Figure 1), relative to the other streptomycins, could be formed either via an ancestral precursor pathway for the cyclitol moiety (75), by a parallel development, or even by a degenerated streptidine pathway. Therefore, two producers of bluensomycin, S. *bluensis* DSM40564 and S. *hygroscopicus* subsp. *glebosus* DSM40823, were also incorporated into some comparative analyses of genetic and enzymatic complements (9,75). The order of genes identified by partial sequencing and hybridization studies in S. *bluensis* are given in Figure 28. These studies especially indicated that no second amidino-transferase gene, *strB2*, is present in either bluensomycin producer, though these are found in all streptomycin-producing actinomycetes investigated.

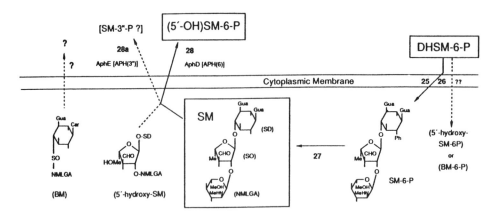

Figure 30 Pathway for the export, oxidation, and release of streptomycin (SM) and SM-resistance mechanisms. For the general numbering and labeling system, see legend to Figure 29. Abbreviations are DHSM-6-P = dihydrostreptomycin-6-phosphate; SM = streptomycin; BM = bluensomycin. The antibiotic, after reuptake into *S. griseus*, becomes rephosphorylated, either at the 6- or 3″-hydroxyls by the resistance enzymes AphD or AphE, respectively.

2. Genes Involved in the Production of Spectinomycins (Actinospectacin)

Spectinomycin and related molecules (Figure 3) are composed of two doubly condensed hexose derivatives, a *myo*-inositol and a 6DOH-derivative (actinospectose, a 4,6-dideoxyhexose), and therefore are **Ca(4,5)–6DOH** compounds, as are, for example, the dihydrostreptosylstreptidine (AC-4437) produced by some streptomycetes (31) or the kasugamycin-related ACAGAs (cf. Figures 1 and 4). Recently, a spectinomycin-resistance-conferring DNA fragment of 3.65 kb was cloned and sequenced from the spectinomycin producer *S. flavopersicus* NRRL2820 (Altenbuchner J and Lyutzkanova D, personal communication). Three of the four reading frames detected showed striking similarity with three genes, *strB1*, *strR*, and *strN*, in the respective clusters of *S. griseus* and *S. glaucescens* (cf. Figure 28). These were preliminarily designated *spcB1*, *spcR*, and *spcN*, respectively. The fourth genetic unit had high similarity with the deleted transposase gene of an IS*112*-element. Therefore, the DNA segment was possibly derived from a rearranged and degenerated gene cluster related to that found in the streptomycin producers. The hypothetical protein product of the *spcB1* gene, if expressed, is doubtless nonfunctional since it is truncated after aa residue no. 90 relative to the *S. griseus* StrB1 protein by a deletion event that probably followed the insertion of an IS*112* element.

Also, the pattern of similarity among the Spc gene products is puzzling (expressed as percent identity): the hypothetical SpcB1 product shows 83.8 and 92.5%, the product of the *strR*-related gene 45.9 and 47.5%, and the product of the *strN*-related gene 29.5 and 29.4% to the StrB1, StrR, and StrN proteins of *S. griseus* and *S. glaucescens*, respectively. It is not yet known whether other production genes for spectinomycin are found adjacent to this cluster. However, this finding strongly supports the hypothesis that an ancestral production gene cluster for streptomycin-like aminoglycosides could have developed into another variant by divergent evolution after degeneration and/or modification. Two or more such clusters may have later recombined with intact *str/sts* gene clusters, thereby creating a new **Ca1–6DOH** pathway yielding simpler but still effective end products, the spectinomycins. The recently described spectinomycin derivative spenolimycin contains a 6DOH moiety with a 3′-O-methyl-group and unsaturated C-3′,4′ bond (cf. Figure 3). These modifications occur also in other streptomycete 6DOH constituents, for example, in sisomicin (cf. Figure 11), fortimicins (cf. Figure 17), and anthracyclines (cf. Chapter 18 in this book). Therefore, the gene cluster in the spenolimycin producer *S. gilvospiralis* could have further recombined with others encoding respective modifications.

B. Genes Involved in the Production of Fortimicins (Astromicins) and Related Aminoglycosides

The genetics of the fortimicin (FTM = astromicin) pathway has been most extensively studied in *Micromonospora olivasterospora* ATCC 21819 (FTM-A producer). Genes for the production of FTM (*fms*) and FTM resistance (*fmr*) all seem to be assembled in a single gene cluster of about 25 to 30 kbp length in this strain (Figure 31 and Table 4) (7,12,76–81,83–86). The *fms* genes have been detected on the basis of self-cloning in mutants blocked in a series of successive steps that had been analyzed earlier and led to the current proposal of the FTM pathway (Figure 32) (87–89). Of the roughly 20 steps of FTM-A biosynthesis, 14 have been identified, mainly by the isolation and analysis of intermediates and their feeding to blocked mutants. The order of identified genes in M. *olivasterospora* is *fms10, 13, 3, 4, 5, 12, 8, 7, 14, 1, 11, (orf2), fmrO, (orf4)*. This DNA segment as a whole only hybridizes to the genomic DNA from *Micromonospora* sp. SF-2089 and *Dactylosporangium matsuzakiense* ATCC 31570 (76). However, the restriction pattern of the hybridizing bands was almost identical only in strain *Micromonospora* sp. SF-2089. In the DNA of the other three producers investigated, *Streptomyces tenjimariensis* ATCC 31603 (istamycins = ISM), *Streptomyces sannanensis* IFO 14239 (sannamycins), and *Saccharopolyspora hirsuta* ATCC 20501 (sporaricins), no hybridization with the 30 kbp fragment from M. *olivasterospora* was observed; but when individual genes for conserved functions were taken as probes, for example, the *fms13* (*sms13*; encoding the N-glycyltransferase) genes, significant hybridization was seen with the DNA from all six producers (80). Thus, it seems likely that all producers of FTM-like aminoglycosides contain highly related gene clusters, originating from a common evolutionary source, with some minor modifications, such as the use of a different gene set for the formation of the (2-deoxy)-*scyllo*-inosose precursor (cf. Figure 18) or the resistance genes (cf. Section

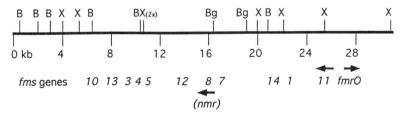

(B = *Bam*HI; Bg = *Bgl*II; X = *Xho*I)

Figure 31   The *fms* gene cluster for fortimicin production in *Micromonospora olivasterospora*. The approximate location of genes complementing mutations in the steps indicated in Figure 32 are given relative to a restriction map (according to Ref. 76). Genes *fms14*, *fms11*, and a fortimicin resistance gene, *fmr*, have been sequenced (77,78).

Table 4 Gene Products and Enzymes Known or Presumed to Be Involved in the Production and Resistance of Fortimicin (FTM)-Group Antibiotics

Gene product[a]	Coding capacity of gene aa[b]	Enzymatic function or step[c] (preliminary assignment)	Remarks[d]	Organism[e]	Reference
Fms1		(D-myo-inositol 2-dehydrogenase)	NAD(P)-dependent?	Mol, Msp, (Dma)	7, 76, 79
Fms2		(scyllo-inosose aminotransferase)	PPL-dependent?	Mol, Msp, (Dma)	7, 76, 79
Fms3		FTM-FU-10 synthesis (D-glucosaminyltransferase)		Mol, Msp, (Dma)	7, 76, 79
Fms4		FTM-AO synthesis		Mol, Msp, (Dma)	7, 76, 79
Fms5		FTM-AO synthesis		Mol, Msp, (Dma)	7, 76, 79
Fms7		FTM-KK1 synthesis		Mol, Msp, (Dma)	7, 76, 79
Fms8		FTM-AP synthesis (FTM-KK1 phosphotransferase)	ATP-dependent, homologous to APH(3')-II	Mol, Msp, (Dma)	7, 76, 79
Fms10		FTM-KH synthesis		Mol, Msp, (Dma)	7, 76, 79
Fms11	(126)	FTM-KR synthesis (FTM-KH epimerase)		Mol, Msp, (Dma)	7, 76, 79
Fms 13 (Sms 13)		FTM-B N-glycyltransferase		Mol, Msp, Dma, Ste, San, Shi	7, 76, 79, 80
Fms14	480	N-formimidoyl FTM-A synthase (oxidase)	FAD, 4-mer	Mol, Msp, (Dma)	7, 76, 77, 79
FmrO (FmrM, FmrD)	293	16S rRNA (G-1405) methyltransferase	SAM-dependent	Mol; Msp, Dma	7, 76, 79, 81
FmrT	211	16S rRNA (A-1408) methyltransferase	SAM-dependent	Ste, (San)	7, 76, 79, 81
KamC	156	16S rRNA (A-1408) methyltransferase	SAM-dependent	Shi	82
Unknown ORF (ORF-2)	99	unknown (upstream fmrO)	(FTM-A synthesis?)	Mol	81
Unknown ORF (ORF-4)	(313)	unknown (downstream fmrO)	(FTM-A synthesis?)	Mol	81
Unknown ORF (ORF-1)	333	(epoxide hydrolase)	(sannamycin synthesis?)	Ste	83
Unknown ORF (ORF-3)	(188)	unknown (downstream fmrT)	(sannamycin synthesis?)	Ste	83

a Cf. Figures 31 and 32.
b In brackets = partial sequence data.
c Cf. Figure 32.
d PPL = pyridoxalphosphate; SAM = S-adenosyl methionine.
e Mol = Micromonospora olivasterospora; MSP = Micromonospora sp. SF-2098; Dma = Dactylosporangium matsuzakiense; San = Streptomyces sannanensis; Ste = S. tenjimariensis; Shi = Saccharopolyspora hirsuta.

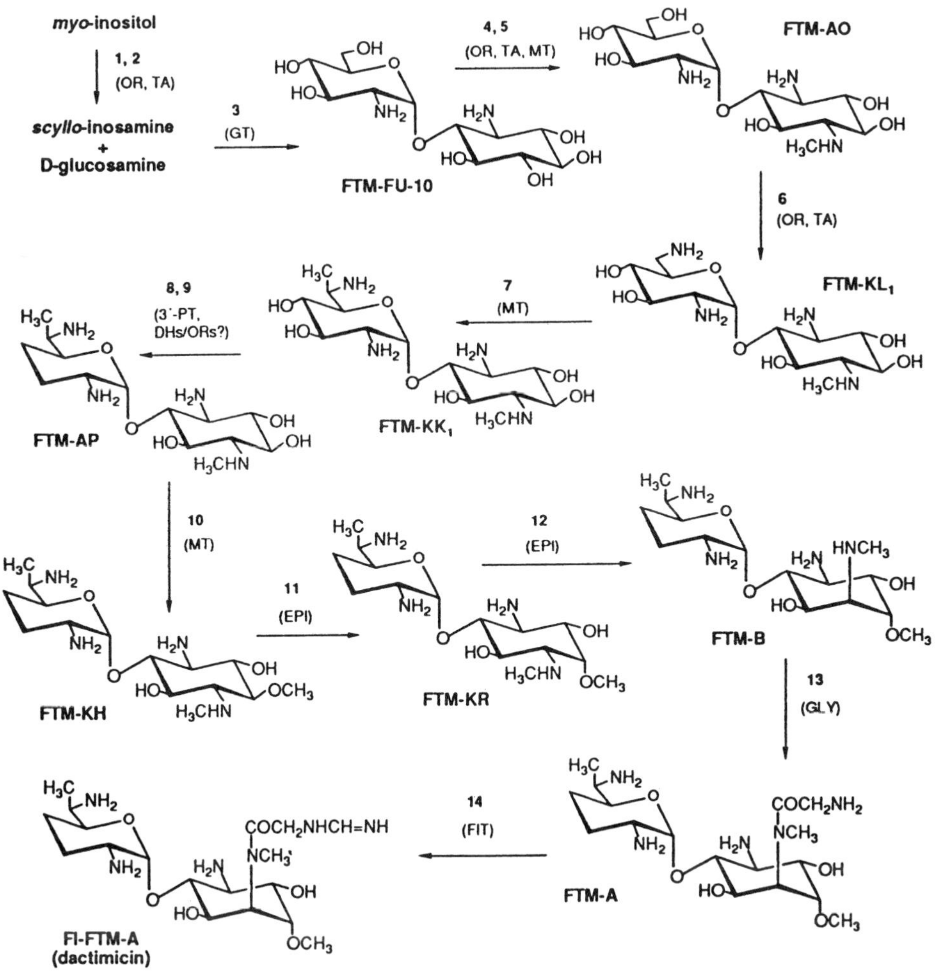

Figure 32 The biosynthetic pathway of fortimicins (FTM = astromicins). The same pathway starting from 2-deoxy-*scyllo*-inosamine appears to be established in the producers of istamycins, sannamycins, and sporaricin. The known intermediates and postulated enzymatic steps are given according to Refs. 7 and 12 (cf. Figure 31 and Table 4). The known or assumed enzymatic conversions involved in the pathway are given: DH = dehydration (dehydroxylation; PMP-dependent) or dehydratation (e.g., enolase); EPI = epimerization; FIT = forimidoyltransfer; GLY = glycyltransfer; GT = glycosyltransfer; MT = methyltransfer; OR = oxidoreduction; PT = phosphotransfer (kinase); TA = transamination.

IV.C). The analysis of blocked mutants and/or conversion studies with ISM intermediates corresponding to the last five intermediates of the FTM pathway (cf. Figure 32) in *S. sannanensis* and *S. tenjimariensis* supported this conclusion (12,42,84,90).

C. Aminoglycoside Resistance Genes in Producers

The analysis of resistance genes in ACAGA-producing actinomycetes and bacilli has provided the most advanced piece of knowledge regarding the genetics of producers

Table 5   Genes and Mechanisms of Self-Resistance in ACAGA Producers

Antibiotic	Producing organism[a]	Resistance gene(s)	Mechanism of resistance[b]	Reference[c]
Streptomycin (SM)	S. griseus	aphD (strA), aphE, [kan]	APH(6), APH(3″), [KM-AAC(3)]	3, 10
5′-OH-SM	S. glaucescens	sph (strA)	APH(6)	3, 10
Neomycin (NM)	S. fradiae	aacC8, aphA-5, aacB (?)	AAC(3), APH(3′), (AAC(2′)?)	3, 91
NM	M. chalcea	aacC9, aphA-5	AAC(3), APH(3′)	3, 91
Paromomycin (PM)	S. rimosus f. paro-momycinus	aacC7, aphA-5	AAC(3), APH(3′)	92, 93
Lividomycin (LM)	S. lividus	aacC, aphA-5	AAC(3), APH(3′)	3, 94
Ribostamycin (RM)	S. ribosidificus	aacC, aphA	AAC(3), APH(3′)	3, 94
Butirosin (BU)	B. circulans	aacC, aphA	AAC(3), APH(3′)	3, 94
Kanamycin (KM)	S. kanamyceticus	aacA, kan	AAC(6′), 16S-MT (G-1405)	3, 94
Hygromycin B (HM-B)	S. hygroscopicus	hyg	APH (7″)	3, 94
HM-B	Sv. eurocidicus	hyg V1, hyg V2	APH (7″), APH(?)	3, 94
Tobramycin (TM) (apramycin; AM)	S. tenebrarius	aacC, aacB, kgmB, kamB [aphD]	AAC(3), TM-AAC(2′), 16S-MT (A-1408), 16S-MT (G-1405), [APH(6)]	3, 94
Gentamicin	M. purpurea		16S-MT (G-1405)	3, 94
Fortimicin (FTM)	M. olivasterospora, M. sp	fmrO (fmrM)	16S-MT(G-1405)	7, 81, 85
Dactimicin	Dact. matsuzakiense	fmrD	16S-MT (G-1405)	7, 85
Istamycin (ISM)	S. tenjimariensis	kamA, (fmrT)	16S-MT (A-1408)	7, 82, 83
Sannamycin	S. sannanensis	fmrS	16S-MT (A-1408)	7, 85
Sporaricin	Sacch. hirsuta	fmrH	16S-MT (A-1408)	7, 85
Spectinomycin (SP)	S. spectabilis	aph, [aac]	APH(?), [AAC(2″)]	12
SP	S. flavopersicus	spcN(?)	APH(?)	A
Kasugamycin (KS)	S. kasugaensis	aac(?), [aacB, aac(?)]	AAC(?), [FTM-AAC(2′), ISM-AAC(2″)]	12

[a] B. = Bacillus; M. = Micromonospora; S. = Streptomyces; Sacch. = Saccharopolyspora; Sv. = Streptoverticillium; Dact. = Dactylosporangium.
[b] AAC = acetyltransferase; APH = phosphotransferase; 16S-MT = 16S rRNA methyltransferase; in [ ] = resistance against other ACAGAs than that produced in the strain.
[c] A = Distler J, Lyutzkanova D, and Altenbuchner J, personal communication.

(Table 5). In all cases studied, at least one resistance gene has been found to be localized in the production gene cluster. Additional ACAGA-resistance genes also might be found in the same strains. Examples are (cf. Table 5) (a) the unlinked *aphD* and *aphE* genes and a cryptic kanamycin resistance gene in *S. griseus* (cf. Table 3 and Figure 28) (82,89,90,95,96); (b) the fortimicin/istamycin resistance determinants in kasugamycin-producing *S. kasugaensis* MB273 (96); (c) a remarkable uniformity is observed in the complement of closely related *aphA* and *aacC* resistance genes in the producers of neomycin-related ACAGAs, namely the neomycin–paromomycin–lividomycin and butirosin–ribostamycin families (cf. Figures 8 and 9). Both genes are required to express full resistance, as is found in the neomycin producer *S. fradiae* (97). This finding is strange, since it was suggested from cloning cosmid libraries from *S. fradiae* ATCC10745, *Micromonospora chalcea* 69-683 (both neomycin producers), and paromomycin-producing *S. rimosus* f. *paromomycinus* that they are not linked physically (91–93,97). Indirect evidence indicates that the *aphA* genes in these producers are linked to the respective production gene clusters and that the AphA enzyme would be required for ACAGA synthesis (98). However, in none of these strains have any biosynthetic genes clearly been proven to exist in the vicinity of either resistance gene, though two putative genes have been identified by DNA sequencing. A reading frame found in a segment of about 4.5 kbp downstream the *aacC8* gene of *S. fradiae* (sequenced from pIJ1) encoded an enzyme belonging to the aspartate aminotransferase family (Pérez-González JA and Piepersberg W, unpublished results; cf. Ref. 97). The speculation remains that two more distantly linked and biosynthetically essential subclusters exist in these strains for which the bridging DNA segment has not yet been detected. In this context, it would be of interest to know whether or not the strain of *S. hygroscopicus* producing the neomycin-related inosamycins also harbors an *aacC* gene, since this should not protect the strain because of the lacking 1-amino group (39). An attractive speculation can be put forward that a rather exceptional genetic situation could be discovered in *S. tenebrarius*, the producer of the nebramycin complex of ACAGAs, which includes the apramycins (cf. Figure 15) and tobramycin (cf. Figure 10). The presence of multiple resistance genes (cf. Table 5) and the strange production profile could indicate that at least two gene clusters, possibly one each for the biosynthesis and resistance for a kanamycin- and a neomycin-related ACAGA, could have been combined in this organism. These could have further evolved to yield a series of new end products, the 12 or more nebramycin factors (1), by recombining with other genes, for example, for an octose pathway.

The difference in the DNA hybridization data for the producers of the two more distant groups of FTM/ISM antibiotics (see Section IV.B) is also reflected by the acquisition of two alternative types of resistance genes (cf. Table 5): (a) *fmrO* (*fmrM*, *fmrD*; from *M. olivasterospora* ATCC 21819, *Micromonospora* sp. SF-2098, and *Dactylosporangium matsuzakiense*, respectively); (b) *fmrT* (*fmrS*, *fmrH*; from *S. tenjimariensis* ATCC 31603, *S. sannanensis* IFO 14239, and *Saccharopolyspora hirsuta* ATCC 20501, respectively). Both of these gene types encode 16S rRNA methyltransferases, but ones that methylate different residues, G-1405 and A-1408, respectively (3,7,78,81,83,85). In each case, the single resistance gene seems to reside in the production gene cluster. However, the resistance genes seem to be differently organized in the gene clusters in the two groups (78).

Resistance-conferring genes for exporter proteins actively transporting antibiotic molecules out of the producer cells have presently been identified only in the gene clusters for nonaminoglycoside antibiotics, such as macrolides, anthracyclines, tetracyclines, and lincosamides (3,10,94; cf. respective chapters in this book). The recent detection of two genes, *strV* and *strW*, conserved in the streptomycin production gene clusters of both *S. glaucescens* and *S. griseus* (cf. Figure 28) and obviously encoding a new type of ABC-transporter (10; S. Beyer, J. Ahlert, and W. Piepersberg, unpublished observations), will lead to discovery of whether or not the ACAGAs have to be actively secreted, too. However, these seem not to confer resistance phenotypes and, therefore, could serve the purpose of transporting inactive final products from the cells only (cf. Section V.E).

Also, ACAGA-resistance determinants can be applied either via selection in the screening programs for new producers of aminoglycoside-related antibiotics (99) or to stimulate aminoglycoside production. For instance, the 6′-acetyltransferase gene (*aacA*) from S. *kanamyceticus* acts to stimulate ACAGA production when cloned on multicopy plasmids into producers of kanamycin or neomycin (100).

V.   BIOGENESIS AND BIOSYNTHETIC PATHWAYS OF AMINOGLYCOSIDE SUBUNITS

In the early phase (until the late 1970s) of pathway analysis, the biochemical origin, or the biogenesis, of the building blocks of the ACAGAs from ordinary metabolites of intermediary metabolism was studied mostly using isotope-labeling analysis (38,66). The only exceptions were presented by the enzymological studies on subpathways for the streptidine (60) and (dihydro-)streptose (67) moieties of streptomycin. Postulates for the biosynthetic pathway for the other groups of ACAGAs could by then be given only from the specific pattern of label in the end products after feeding a variety of precursors. Therefore, the results from more recent biogenesis studies with $1\text{-}^{13}C$- and $6\text{-}^{13}C$-labeled glucose are of special importance, because they suggest that all C_5, C_6, and C_7 units of neomycins and validamycins seem to be formed from intermediates of the pentose phosphate cycle (Figure 33) (8). This probably means that all or most of the fed glucose molecules are generally "equilibrated" by a passage(s) through the pentosephosphate cycle

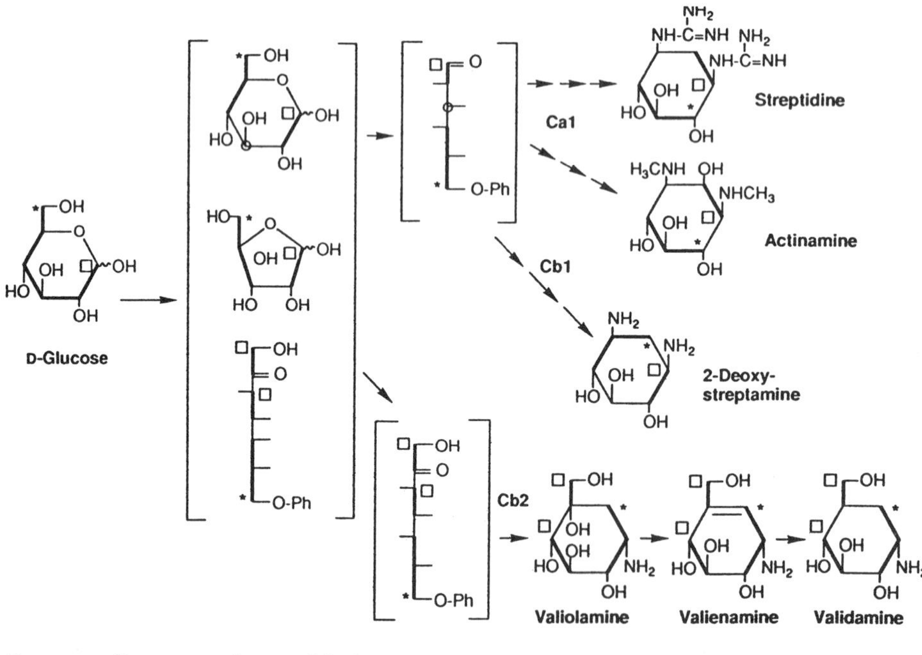

Figure 33   Biogenesis of some of the hexose-, pentose-, and cyclitol-derived components in ACAGAs from $6\text{-}[C^{13}]\text{-}D$-glucose (according to Ref. 8). The labeling patterns in neomycin and validamycin measured by ^{13}C nuclear magnetic resonance (NMR) prove that all units are built up preferentially from C_1 (circled C atoms), C_2, or C_3 units (thick lines) rearranged by transketolase- and transaldolase-catalyzed reactions in passages through the pentosephosphate cycle. The pattern in **Ca1** products is hypothetical. The positions derived from the C6 of D-glucose are marked by a star.

before they become incorporated into secondary carbohydrate components during the production phase. It should be recalled also that this cycle is accessible for hexose molecules on two routes: the decarboxylating hexosemonophosphate shunt, and via intermediates of the upper Embden–Meyerhoff–Parnas pathway, fructose-6-phosphate and glycerolaldehyde-3-phosphate. These data force us to revise some earlier predictions of particular biosynthetic routes for sugar-derived constituents.

A.   (Amino-)Cyclitols

Very different types of cyclitol units, formally derived from cyclohexane and cyclopentane, are found in various groups of secondary metabolites. Besides the ACAGAs these include, for example, pactamycin, the cyclopentanol moiety of which might be formed via *myo*-inositol (**Ca1** mechanism; see below) (8), and several members of the chemical group of secondary nucleosides, such as the antibiotics adenomycin (not shown), aristeromycin, and neplanocin (see below). These sometimes extremely modified derivatives do not allow easy conclusions on their origins before the enzymology of the particular biosynthetic route has been clarified. The two cyclitol forms encountered in the major groups of ACAGAs are either fully hydroxylated/aminated or 2-deoxy forms of C_6-hexitols, mainly derived from the configuration of the diaminocyclitol streptamine, and C_7-hexitols. These are synthesised on two different routes, which we call **Ca** and **Cb** here (cf. Table 2).

   The cyclitol moieties generally may be regarded as aglyca in glycosylation reactions, for example, during the formation of the pseudo-oligosaccharides of the streptomycins (cf. Figure 2), of most 2DOS-containing aminoglycosides (cf. Figure 14), and of the fortimicins and istamycins (cf. Figure 18). Alternatively, they are (co-)substrates in other types of condensation reactions, for example, with another molecule derived from the same pathway or the nonreducing groups of pyranoses (e.g., in the validamycins and amylostatins; cf. Figures 19 and 20). Also, members of a common subfamily of ACAGAs can obviously be synthesized via both alternative aminocyclitol pathways, **Ca1** or **Cb1**. For instance, two of the members of the regularly 2DOS-containing destomycin group have aminocyclitols derived from streptamine. One of these cyclitol moieties even is identical to 1-*N*-amidinostreptamine (see Figure 16) (41), which is an intermediate in the streptomycin pathway (see below). Similarly, beyond the differential formation of a ketoinositol precursor for the fortimicins (**Ca1**) and the istamycins (**Cb1**), the remaining positions of the respective pathways are probably identical (cf. Figures 17 and 32).

I.   The Two Basic Pathways for Cyclitol Formation

The two enzyme mechanisms leading to the formation of (amino-)cyclitols in the major ACAGA classes are provided by the D-*myo*-inositol-3-phosphate synthase (**Ca1**) and 2-deoxy-*scyllo*-inosose synthase (**Cb1**) as shown in Figure 34 (5,8,101,102). The enzyme mechanisms corresponding to that of the 3-dehydroquinate synthase (**Cbn**) seem to be more widespread. Substrates can be D-glucose-6-phosphate, sedoheptulose-7-phosphate or the 5-epimer thereof, or 3-deoxyarabinoheptulosonic acid; or perhaps D-fructose-6-phosphate. The products of **Ca** pathways are cyclitolphosphates, which have to undergo dephosphorylation and further oxidation before a first step of transamination can be passed (cf. Figure 34A). In contrast, the **Cb** route yields 1-keto-2-deoxycyclitols, which can directly be transaminated (cf. Figure 34B).

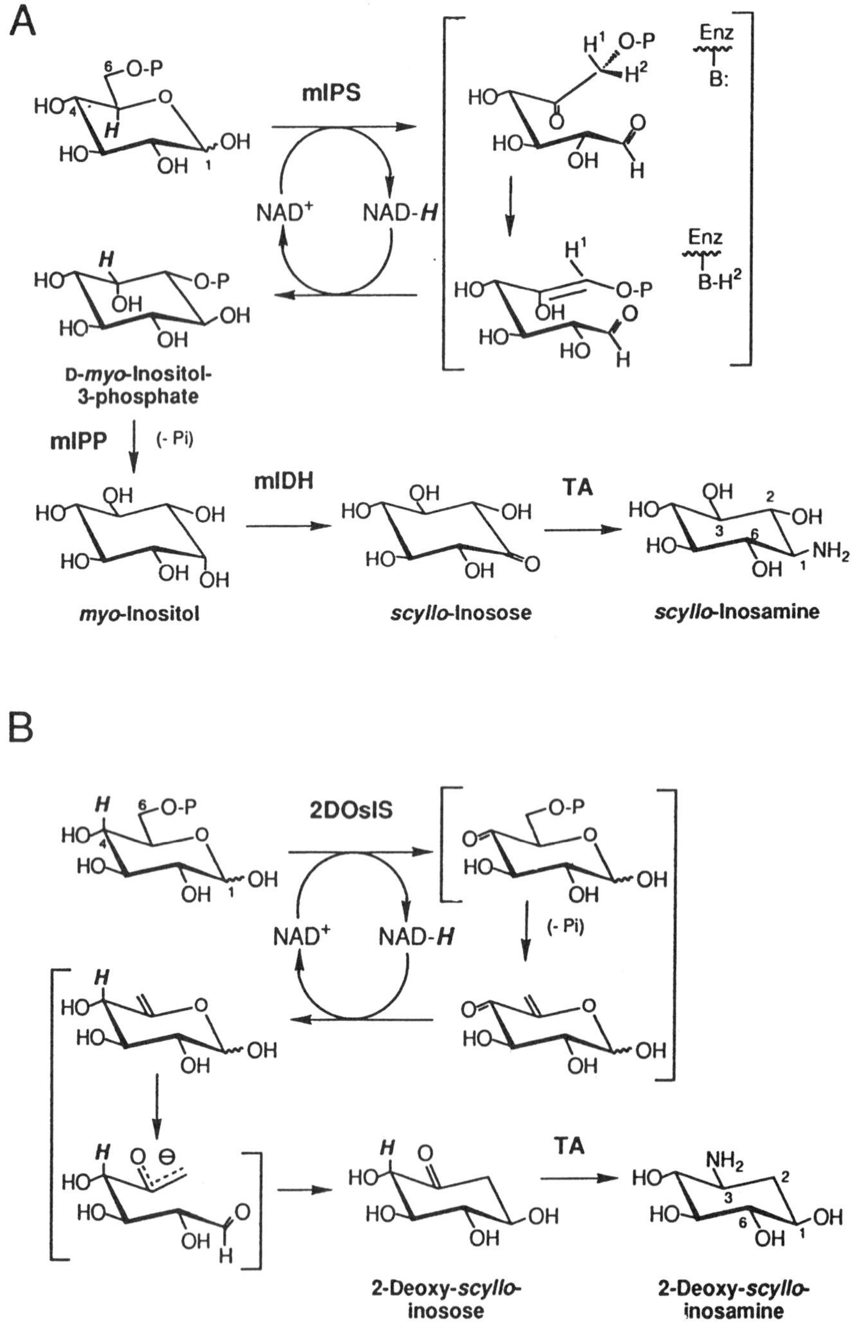

Figure 34   The two general routes to the formation of (amino-)cyclitols. (A) The **Ca1** pathway via D-*myo*-inositol-3-phosphate synthase (mIPS). (B) The **Cb1** pathway via the dehydroquinate synthaselike enzyme 2-deoxy-*scyllo*-inosose synthase (2DOsIS). For the introduction of a first amino-group in the cyclitol in **Ca1**, a dephosphorylation (mIPP), a dehydrogenation (mIDH), and a transamination (TA) step have to follow, whereas in the **Cb1** route transamination is possible directly. For details see Refs. 5, 8, 94, and 99.

The D-myo-Inositol-3-Phosphate Pathway   The first route, designated **Ca1** in this chapter, is via D-*myo*-inositol-3-phosphate, which is synthesized by the NAD$^+$-dependent intramolecular lyase D-*myo*-inositol-3-phosphate synthase (E.C. 5.5.1.4). End products include, for example, the 1,2,3-substituted *myo*-inositol in myomycins (cf. Figure 6), D-*chiro*-inositol (in kasugamycins; cf. Figure 4), D-*myo*-1-deoxy-1-amino-inositol (= D-*myo*-inosamine) (in LL-BM123α; cf. Figure 5), streptidine and bluensidine (cf. Figures 1 and 29), actinamine (in spectinomycins; cf. Figure 3), fortamine (in fortimicins; cf. Figure 17), or streptamine (in SS-56C; cf. Figure 16). The stereochemistry of the reaction (cf. Figure 34A) was studied in the spectinomycin producer (5) and corresponds to that of the mammalian enzyme (103). The enzyme partially purified from strains of *S. griseus* (56) turned out to be quite labile and to have an apparent molecular weight of 216 kDa. It may be more commonly distributed in streptomycetes, since several strains have been found to contain *myo*-inositol in the cell wall fraction, probably as inositides (56,104). However, neither more detailed enzymological data, such as the subunit structure, nor the location and primary structure of its gene have been elucidated for *Streptomyces* spp. The yeast enzyme has been described in more detail and was found to be composed of four 62 kDa subunits, the sequences of which have been determined from the cloned *INO1* gene (105). The reaction catalyzed by the bacterial and the eukaryotic D-*myo*-inositol-3-phosphate synthases follows that of a typical intramolecular aldol condensation (cf. Figure 34A). This involves (a) opening of the pyranose ring and rotation of the C4/C5 bond to place the C6 group in an active position, (b) the reversible oxidation and reduction by NAD$^+$ of the C5 position, (c) the subtraction of the *pro-R*-H atom from C6 and its transfer to the C1 carbonyl, and (d) finally, the use of the β-anomer of D-glucose-6-phosphate as the preferred substrate (5,103). Also, in the sorbistins, a **Ca1** intermediate could be formed first, before ring cleavage and epimerization yield an open-chained 1,4-diamino-1,4-dideoxysorbitol (cf. Figure 21). The derivation of the pentitol moieties in allosamidins (cf. Figure 25) and/or in trehazolin (cf. Figure 26) could also follow **Ca** pathways.

The Dehydroquinate Pathway.   The second general enzymatic mechanism delivering cyclitols, designated **Cb** here, is that of an enzyme family represented by the catalytically NAD$^+$-dependent 3-dehydroquinate synthases acting on open-chained hexose-6- or heptulose-7-phosphates and yielding nonphosphorylated 1-keto-2-deoxy-cyclitols. As end products are found (a) C_6-hexitols, for example, 2-deoxystreptamine (**Ca1**; cf. Figure 34B); (b) C_7-hexitols, for example, valiolamine and its derivatives valienamine and validamine (**Ca2**; cf. Figures 19, 20, and 33); and (c) maybe C_6-pentitols, for example, the cyclitol moieties in aristeromycin and neplanocin (**Ca3**; Figure 35) (8,101, 102,106–109). This mechanism involves first subtracting electrons at C4 of hexosephosphates (C5 of heptulose derivatives); then, elimination of the phosphoester hydroxyl as a leaving group would create a potential for the formation of a carbanion at C6 (C7); finally, after the condensation reaction, the keto-group at C4 (C5) would be reduced to restore the hydroxyl-group (cf. Figure 34B). The mechanism would imply that a 6-deoxy-5-ketoglucose should be a direct intermediate, which was proven by the specific incorporation of this compound, tritium-labeled at C6, specifically into the 2DOS moiety of neomycin (107). The mechanistic equivalence of the ring closure reaction catalyzed by the 2-deoxy-*scyllo*-inosose synthase of the neomycin-producing *S. fradiae* to that exerted by the dehydroquinate synthase on a C_7-sugar acid in the microbial biosynthetic pathway of the aromatic amino acids has been proven (102). For the producers of validamycins, *S. validensis*, and aristeromycin, *S. citricolor*, this same mechanism has only been postulated as yet on the grounds of stable-isotope-labeling studies (8,109). In the

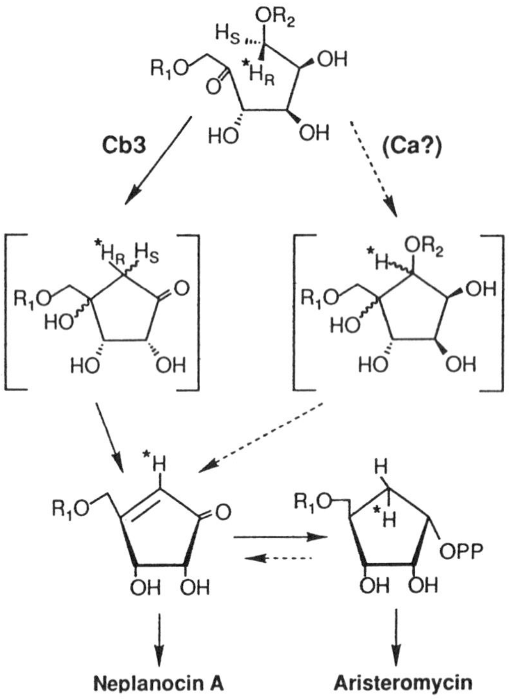

Figure 35   Alternative cyclitol pathways. As an example, the possible biosynthetic routes of the C6-pentitols of aristeromycin and neplanocin A are shown (for details, see text).

latter case, an alternative **Ca**-like mechanism acting on a fructose(-6-phosphate) molecule followed by dehydration and reduction was also discussed (109), which, however, is much less likely (cf. Figure 35). Whether these suggestions also are of relevance for the biogenesis of the pentitol moieties in allosamidins (cf. Figure 25) and/or in trehazolin (cf. Figure 26) is not yet known.

2.   Biosynthesis of Streptidine and Bluensidine

The main difference in the initial intermediates of the **Ca** and **Cb** pathways is that in **Cb** a first transamination step can follow immediately, whereas in **Ca** a phosphatase and an oxidase (dehydrogenase) reaction have to generate a suitable keto intermediate first (cf. Figure 34). The further processing of cyclitol intermediates to aminocyclitols even might at least in part—namely, for the first aminotransfer and further intermediate steps—be very similar, and it might be catalyzed by enzymes related in both structure and substrate specificity. Though these enzymes have not been described for all three major ACAGA classes—the streptomycin-related, 2DOS-containing, and fortimicin-related antibiotics—it can be predicted that at least the first-step cyclitol aminotransferases are probably very similar. This speculation is supported, for example, by the results published by Walker's group on the significant similarity in substrate specificity that the L-glutamine:*scyllo*-inosose aminotransferase (E.C. 2.6.1.50) of S. *griseus* has in common with the L-glutamine:2-deoxy-*scyllo*-inosose aminotransferases in neomycin-producing S. *fradiae*, gentamicin-producing *Micromonospora purpurea,* and spectinomycin-producing *Streptomyces* sp. (60,110,111). However, the incorporation of the second of the 1,3-*cis*-

amino-groups, which stereochemically proceeds in the opposite direction, is interesting for the substrate specificity of the second-step aminotransferases in the biosynthesis of diaminocyclitols.

A biochemical pathway of 11 enzyme-catalyzed steps and remarkable symmetry has been proposed to be involved in the synthesis of streptidine (60,75) (cf. Figure 29). However, the number and identity of the enzymes essential for this route are still matters of debate. By various lines of evidence, SD-6-phosphate is synthesized by two sets of five parallel enzymatic reactions, each basically catalyzed by individual enzymes in streptomycin producers: two cyclitol-phosphate phosphatases, two cyclitol dehydrogenases (oxidizing), two aminotransferases, two phosphotransferases, and two amidinotransferases (cf. Table 3 and Figure 14). The end product of this branch was directly demonstrated to be SD-6-phosphate, which also seems to be the first product made from externally supplied SD in SD⁻ mutants (60,72–74). Also, earlier precursors can become quantitatively incorporated when externally fed into cultures of the wild type or of blocked mutants, such as myo-inositol, scyllo-inosose, scyllo-inosamine, and N-amidino-scyllo-inosamine. The producers of bluensomycin, for example, S. hygroscopicus f. glebosus, seem to lack steps 8 to 11 (cf. Figure 29 and Table 3) (75). In the biosynthesis of bluensidine-6-phosphate, these seem to be replaced by successive carbamoylation and phosphorylation reactions acting on positions 5 and 4 (in the counting system for streptidine) of the N-amidino-scyllo-inosamine precursor, respectively.

Following the formation of D-myo-inositol-3-phosphate, the two initial steps necessary to deliver the ketoinositol intermediate (scyllo-inosose) could be catalyzed by the gene products StrO and StrI encoded by the str/sts gene cluster (cf. Figures 29 and 34A; Table 3). StrO has significant similarity to eukaryotic inositolmonophosphate phosphatases (9), and the StrI protein clearly resembles the myo-inositol-2-dehydrogenase enzyme identified in Bacillus subtilis (112). The StrI and StsB proteins are members of the enzyme family of oxidoreductases (dehydrogenases) with N-terminal dinucleotide-binding folds (57,65). Therefore, StrB is a candidate for the step 8 cyclitol oxidoreductase introducing the 3-keto-group preceding the second transamination step (cf. Figure 29).

Three putative gene products of the str/sts cluster of S. griseus N2-3-11, StrS, StsA, and StsC, distantly resemble known pyridoxal-phosphate (PLP)-dependent aminotransferases (cf. Figure 34 and Table 3) (9–11,65). All three have been expressed in Escherichia coli and assayed for a step 4 transaminase activity. Of these, only StsC protein shows scyllo-inosose aminotransferase activity (E.C. 2.6.1.50); that is, it catalyzes the reversible and PLP-dependent transfer of the α-amino-group of L-glutamine to scyllo-inosose, yielding scyllo-inosamin and α-ketoglutaramate (αKGN; Figure 36) (60,65,110,111). Based on similarities in primary structure, the StsC enzyme, together with the gene products StrS and StsA, are members of a very interesting new class of enzymes (Figures 36A and 37). These include a subfamily of PLP-dependent aminotransferases, the so-called "secondary metabolic aminotransferases" (SMAT), containing a conserved lysine residue that is presumed to serve the binding of PLP via formation of a "Schiffs-base" (cf. Figure 37A). Several other gene products encoded by antibiotic biosynthetic genes and some involved in related or unknown physiological contexts obviously belong to this aminotransferase family, though their enzymatic activities have not yet been proven (11). Besides several putative sugar aminotransferases engaged in the biosynthetic pathways for puromycin, anthracyclines, or macrolides (Table 6) (11,13,120), further examples are (a) the protein MosB of Rhizobium meliloti, which is involved in the metabolism of L-3-O-methyl-scyllo-inosamine (19); (b) the DegT protein of Bacillus stearothermophilus, the expression of which induces increased production of extracellular hydrolases in B. subtilis

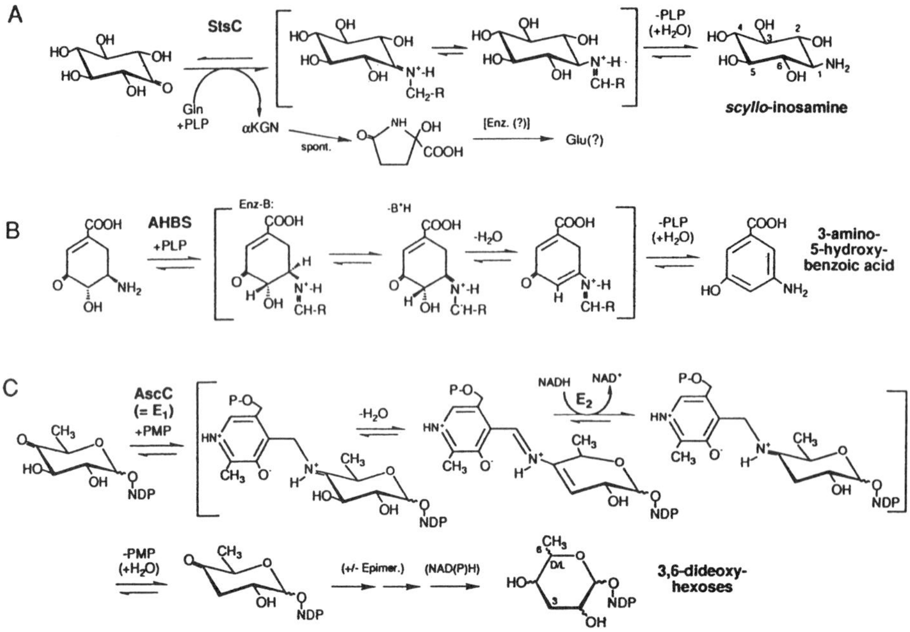

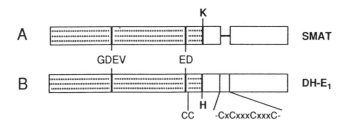

Figure 36 The SMAT (secondary metabolic aminotransferases) family of enzymes: reaction mechanisms. (A) Reaction catalyzed by the pyridoxalphosphate (PLP)-dependent StsC enzyme, an L-glutamine:*scyllo*-inosose aminotransferase. (B) Probable mechanism catalyzed by the StsC-related, PLP-dependent 3-amino-5-hydroxybenzoic acid synthase (AHBS). (C) Mechanism of 3-dehydroxylation in the 3,6-dideoxyhexose pathway of Gram-negative bacteria. E_1 = pyridoxaminephosphate (PMP)-dependent, [2Fe-2S]-containing dehydrase (AscC/RfbH-type); E_3 = NADH-dependent, FAD/[2Fe-2S]-containing reductase (for details, see Ref. 13).

Figure 37 The SMAT family of enzymes: schematic representation of primary structural similarities. (A) The aminotransferase subfamily contains a conserved lysine (K) residue. (B) The dehydrase subfamily (DH-E_1) contains a histidine (H) residue in the same position and several conserved cysteine (C) residues, mostly concentrated in an insert. The N-terminal region of similarity (stippled) and two commonly conserved motifs in both sequences are indicated.

Table 6 Common Enzyme Families in Secondary Carbohydrate Metabolism of Streptomycetes and Gram-Negative Bacteria

Enzyme family[a]	Example Function (postulated)	Gene product	Producing organism/ product[b]	Reference
1. NDP-Hexose synthetases (hexose-1-ph. nucleotidyltransferases)	dTDP-glucose synthase (E.C. 2.7.7.24)	StrD	*S. griseus*, streptomycin (SM)	58
	(dTDP-glucose synthase)	SnoD	*S. nodosus*, amphotericin B	113, A
	dTDP-glucose synthase	TylA1	*S. fradiae*, tylosin	114
	(dTDP-glucose synthase?)	LmbO	*S. lincolnensis*, lincomycin	115
	dTDP-glucose synthase	RfbA	*Salm. enterica* B, LPS O-chain	116
	CDP-glucose synthase (E.C. 2.7.7.33)	StrQ	*S. glaucescens*, 5'-hydroxy-SM	A
	CDP-glucose synthase	RfbF	*Salm. enterica* B, LPS O-chain	116
2. NDP-Hexose 4-(2-) oxidoreductases	dTDP-glucose 4,6-dehydratase (E.C. 4.2.1.46)	StrE	*S. griseus*, SM	58
	(dTDP-glucose 4,6-dehydratase?)	SnoE	*S. nodosus*	113, A
	(dTDP-glucose 4,6-dehydratase?)	TylA2	*S. fradiae*, tylosin	114
	(dTDP-glucose 4,6-dehydratase?)	LmbM	*S. lincolnensis*, lincomycin	115
	dTDP-glucose 4,6-dehydratase	RfbB	*Salm. enterica* B, LPS O-chain	116
	CDP-glucose 4,6-dehydratase	RfbG	*Salm. enterica* B, LPS O-chain	116
	dTDP-L-rhamnose synthase	StrL	*S. griseus*, SM	58, A
	dTDP-L-rhamnose synthase	RfbD	*Salm. enterica* B, LPS O-chain	116
	(NDP-glucose 4-oxidase or epimerase?)	StrP	*S. glaucescens*, 5´hydroxy-SM	11, A
3. NDP-4-Ketohexose isomerases	dTDP-4-keto-6-deoxyglucose 3,5-epimerase (E.C. 5.1.3.13)	StrM	*S. griseus*, SM	58
	dTDP-4-keto-6-deoxyglucose 3,5-epimerase	RfbC	*Salm. enterica* B, LPS O-chain	116
	dTDP-4-keto-6-deoxyglucose isomerase?)	SnoM	*S. nodosus*	113, A
	(NDP-4-ketohexose 3,5-epimerase?)	StrX	*S. glaucescens*, 5'-hydroxy-SM	11, A
4. Ketosugar or ketocyclitol aminotransferases (SMAT)	*scyllo*-inosose 1-AT (E.C. 2.6.1.50)	StsC	*S. griseus*, SM	11, A
	(unknown)	StsA, StrS	*S. griseus*, SM	11, A
	(dTDP-4-keto-6-deoxyglucose 4-AT?)	LmbS	*S. lincolnensis*, lincomycin	115
	(dTDP-3-keto-2-deoxy-L-fucose 3-AT?)	TylB	*S. fradiae*, tylosin	114
	(dTDP-4-keto-6-deoxyglucose 3-dehydrase?)	SnoS	*S. nodosus*	113, A
	(3-amino-5-hydroxybenzoic acid synthase)	RifD	*Amyc. mediterranei*	117
	CDP-4-keto-6-deoxyglucose 3-dehydrase	AscC	*Yers. enterocol.*; LPS O-chain	118, 119

[a] An "enzyme family" is defined as a group of proteins related in both catalytic activity and primary structure; cf. Figures 28 and 46.

[b] *S.* = *Streptomyces*; *Salm.* = *Salmonella*; *Yers.* = *Yersinia*; *Amyc.* = *Amycolatopsis*. LPS = lipopolysaccharide

[c] A = Ahlert J, Beyer S, Verseck S, Distler J, Piepersberg W. Unpublished results.

(121); and (c) the 3-amino-5-hydroxybenzoic acid synthase (AHBS, RifD), a PLP-dependent aromatizing dehydratase, involved in the formation of the aromatic mC_7N units of ansamycins (cf. Figure 36B) (117). A second subfamily is represented by the AscC protein involved in the biosynthesis of the lipopolysaccharide O-chains of *Yersinia enterocolitica* (cf. Figures 36C and 37B; see also Section V.B.1) (13,118,119). Therefore, it seems obvious that one of the genes, *stsA* or *strS*, encodes the N-amindino-*scyllo*-inosamine:L-alanine aminotransferase, the second transaminase necessary for streptidine-6-phosphate formation (cf. Figure 29, step 9; Table 3) (60). The remaining third SMAT enzyme, either of the StrS and StsA proteins, could be involved in the biosynthesis of the hexosamine subunit of streptomycins (cf. Section V.B.3).

The aminocyclitol phosphotransferases catalyzing steps 5 and 10 of the streptidine pathway (cf. Figure 29) could be the gene products StrN and/or StsE (cf. Figure 28 and Table 2). The evidence for this function is still based on protein similarities only (58,65). Both proteins show the typical signature motifs for aminoglycoside phosphotransferases and eukaryotic protein kinases, especially in their probably substrate-binding C-terminal portion (9,63,122,123). Recently, a gene homologous to *strN* was found on a DNA fragment cloned from spectinomycin-producing *S. flavopersicus* that conferred spectinomycin resistance on *S. lividans*. In addition to spectinomycin resistance, phosphorylating activity could be detected in this recombinant *S. lividans* strain (Altenbuchner J, Lyutzkanova D, and Distler J, personal communication). This supports the assumption that *strN* encodes a phosphotransferase. These hypotheses and the exact attribution to a particular phosphorylation step still await experimental verification. The last steps in the two rounds of streptidine formation, the two transamidinations of the cyclitol amino-groups (cf. Figure 29, steps 6 and 11), are characteristic group transfer reactions specific for the particular pathway and are therefore treated further below (see Section V.C).

B.   6-Deoxyhexoses and Other Sugar Components

I.   The General 6-Deoxyhexose Pathway

(6-)Deoxyhexoses (6DOH) can be formed from deoxythymidine diphosphate (dTDP)-glucose, cytidine diphosphate (CDP)-glucose, or guanosine diphosphate (GDP)-mannose in bacteria (10,13,124). In secondary metabolite–producing actinomycetes, D-glucose activated by dTDP seems to be the precursor for most or all 6DOHs that become incorporated into antibiotic-like end products. Catalysis of the first two steps in their pathway is accomplished by the enzymes dTDP-D-glucose synthase (E.C. 2.7.7.24) and dTDP-D-glucose 4,6-dehydratase (E.C. 4.2.1.46), which yield 4-keto-6-deoxyhexose intermediates (Figure 38; cf. Table 6). The 4-keto compounds are used as common key intermediates for branching of the further pathways into the D- and L-series of 6DOH and derivatives. The L-6DOHs are isomerized from the D-configured precursors by use of a 3,5-epimerase (E.C. 5.1.3.13; cf. Figure 38). Frequently, both D- and L-6DOH derivatives are synthesized by this branching route and are specifically incorporated into a particular complex end product, for example, in many macrolides and some angucyclines. In aminoglycosides, 6DOH components are relatively rare, compared with the dominance and variability of modified sugar side chains in other chemical classes of actinomycete secondary metabolites, such as various groups of polyketides and glycopeptides (28). Among the pathway classes of ACAGAs, they are almost exclusively combined with the synthesis of a **Ca1** cyclitol. Therefore, in evolutionary terms, they could form a more closely related subgroup together with the streptomycins even though these have quite different struc-

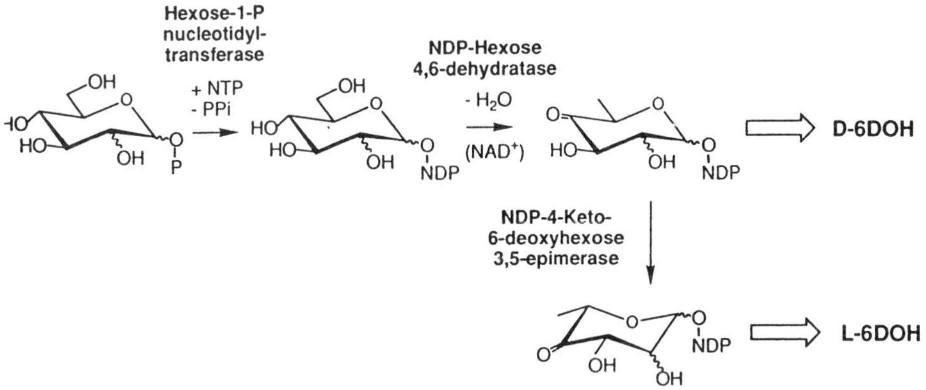

Figure 38 General pathway for the biosynthesis of D- and L-forms of 6-deoxyhexoses (6DOH). Hexose-1-P precursors are either D-glucose-1-P or D-mannose-1-P. P = phosphate; NDP = dTDP, CDP, or GDP.

tures (cf. Figures 1–5) and might be produced via variants of a common ancestral pathway. This view is supported by the detection of a set of genes (*spc* cluster) in a spectinomycin producer that is very similar to *str* gene clusters (cf. Section IV.A; Figure 28).

In the course of the highly flexible 6DOH pathways, several types of further modifications are used. The most important and interesting ones are (a) the deoxygenations (formally: dehydroxylations) at C2, C3, and C4; (b) the transaminations (formally: exchange of hydroxyl- against amino-groups) at C2, C3, and C4; and (c) various forms of isomerization and epimerization steps. Other types of modifications, such as C-, N-, O-, and S-methylations, or transfer reactions for more complex side groups, are also common in the 6DOH pathways. In principle, these sugar-modifying reactions are not restricted to the 6DOH pathways and should act in similar form on other sugar molecules, for example, on other types of NDP-activated precursors or on carbohydrate units already condensed in pseudo-oligosaccharides. Therefore, we here will briefly describe one of these mechanisms, the reductive 3-dehydroxylation, analyzed recently during the studies of the CDP-3,6-deoxyhexose pathway of Gram-negative bacteria (13,116,118,119,125). The enzyme system involved consists of two iron-sulfur proteins, one (called E_1; gene products AscC or RfbH) catalyzing the pyridoxamine-phosphate (PMP)-dependent 3-deoxygenation of the CDP-4-keto-6-deoxy hexose intermediate via an electron transfer mechanism involving formation of radicals and a covalently bound PMP-hexose intermediate (cf. Figure 36C). The electrons for this process are delivered by a second enzyme (E_3), which contains flavine adenine dinucleotide (FAD) besides another [2Fe-2S]-cluster and uses NADH as an electron donor. This type of mechanism could easily play a role in the 3- or 2-deoxygenations of many modified hexose moieties in low-molecular-weight secondary metabolites, as well as in the biosyntheses of several ACAGAs. Examples could be the 3-dehydroxylation reactions on (a) 6DOH sugars of spectinomycins (cf. Figure 3), (b) the purpurosamine moieties of tobramycin and nebramycin factor 5′ (cf. Figure 10), or (c) of many representatives of the gentamicin group (cf. Figure 11B), and (d) of all members of the fortimicin/istamyin group (cf. Figures 17 and 32). Deoxygenations at C2 of pyranoses, as is discussed elsewhere (13), or adjacent to C atoms with bound amino-group could also follow alternative mechanisms.

2.   The L-Dihydrostreptose Pathway

For the streptomycin pathway, Griesbach and collaborators (67) postulated and partially verified, using enzymatic approaches, a route for dTDP-L-dihydrostreptose biosynthesis (steps 12 through 15 in Figure 29) following the basic scheme for L-6DOH formation outlined above (cf. Section V.B.1; Figure 38): starting from D-glucose in form of dTDP-D-glucose, dehydration to dTDP-4-keto-6-deoxyglucose (step 13), epimerization to dTDP-4-keto-L-rhamnose (step 14), and finally, a reduction accompanied by a cleavage and branching of the hexose carbon chain yielding dTDP-L-dihydrostreptose (step 15). The four enzymes catalyzing the synthesis of dTDP-L-dihydrostreptose seem to be encoded by the genes *strD*, *strE*, *strM*, and *strL* (cf. Table 3 and Figure 28) (10,58,59,126).

   An interesting parallel case is manifested in the strong similarity of the StrD, StrE, StrM, and StrL proteins to the products of the respective genes, *rfbA*, *rfbB*, *rfbC*, and *rfbD*, for the biosynthesis of L-rhamnose in salmonellae and other Gram-negative bacteria, underlined by the confirmation of their enzymatic activities in *E. coli* (58,116,126,127). The StrD protein is related to NDP-hexose synthases (hexose-1-phosphate nucleotidyltransferases or pyrophosphorylases; cf. Table 6) (59). Both the StrE and StrL proteins belong to another interesting enzyme family, a subclass of the oxidoreductases with an N-terminal binding site for a dinucleotide coenzyme, the "GalE-family" (Figure 39; cf. Table 6). These act predominantly on the C4, but also on the C2, position of NDP-hexoses and catalyze either dehydrogenation, dehydration, or isomerization (epimerization) reactions. In the latter two cases (e.g., StrE and GalE), tightly bound NAD^+ serves catalytically without measurable accumulation of the reduced form. Others, like the reductases StrL and RfbD, utilize NADPH as the redox coenzyme. Genes similar to all or part of the *strDELM* subcluster are present in many other gene clusters for the production of streptomycete secondary metabolites containing a 6DOH sugar moiety (10,11,13,17). In a screening of streptomycete strains by genomic DNA hybridization, more than 50 of which produced 6DOH-containing secondary metabolites, a majority gave significantly positive signals with at least one of the gene probes derived from *strD*, *strE*, or *strLM* (17). In these experiments, the *strE* gene showed the highest degree of conservation to its counterparts. In each case where the DNA segments hybridizing to these gene probes were analyzed on the molecular level, the respective genes for 6DOH pathways have been proved to occur (113). Thus, this part of the *str* gene cluster appears to be widespread and modularly used among antibiotic-producing streptomycetes and other bacterial groups, and it turned out to be a useful tool in genetic screening approaches.

   Further modifications of dihydrostreptose to streptose or 5′-hydroxystreptose seem to occur on the final condensation products only (cf. Section V.E), rather than during synthesis of the dTDP-activated precursor. The 5′-hydroxy-group in antibiotic produced by *S. glaucescens* is unlikely to stem from the original D-glucose, since then the three enzymes StrE, StrM, and StrL would need to have acquired new substrates and even a new reaction mechanism in the case of the dTDP-D-glucose 4,6-dehydratase.

3.   Hexosamine Pathways

The third moiety of streptomycin, N-methyl-L-glucosamine (NMLGA), is postulated to be formed as a nucleoside diphosphate-activated sugar derived from either D-glucose or D-glucosamine. Nucleosidediphosphate (NDP)-NMLGA synthesis has not yet been studied as intensively as the other branches of the pathway. Earlier biogenesis studies involving isotope labeling suggested that externally administered D-glucosamine is a direct precur-

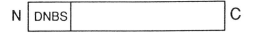

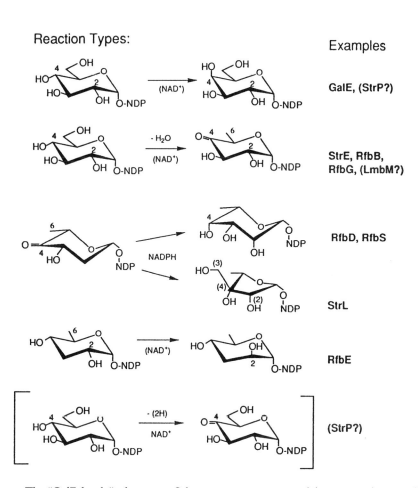

Figure 39   The "GalE family" of enzymes. Schematic representation of the protein chains with an N-terminal dinucleotide binding motif (DNBS). Similarity in protein sequences extends over the full chain length. The family includes 4-epimerases (GalE, StrP?); 4,6-dehydratases (StrE, RfbB, RfbG); reductases (NDP-6DOH synthases; StrL, RfbD, RfbS); 2-epimerases (RfbE); and hypothetical oxidases (dehydrogenases; StrP?).

sor (38,66). Several speculative routes have been postulated including steps for at least three epimerizations, one of which could be divided into separate oxidation and reduction steps at C4 of the hexosamine, followed by N-methylation (38,66,67). Further enzyme-catalyzed conversions would become necessary, such as nucleotidylation, deacetylation of an intermediate, or transamination, if D-glucose or the peptidoglycan precursor uridine diphosphate (UDP)-N-acetyl-glucosamine are substrates (cf. Figure 29).

Thus, the NMLGA branch of the streptomycin pathway remains a puzzle. Not even the direct precursor is known as yet; it could be the 1-phosphates of D-glucose, D-glucosamine, N-acetyl-D-glucosamine, or N-methyl-D-glucosamine. The last is suggested by the finding that a substance identified as UDP-*N*-methyl-D-glucosamine phosphate was accumulated as a transitory metabolite in *S. griseus* before the onset of streptomycin production (127). Also, the additional phosphorylation of UDP-activated hexosamines, which were not accumulated in a mutant obviously blocked in the NMLGA pathway, cannot be explained by the routes postulated so far (128). This situation is reminiscent of the interesting 3'-O-phosphorylation of the purpurosamine moiety in the FTM-KK1 intermediate by the gene product Fms8 of the fortimicin pathway, the function of which is also unknown (76, 79). The Fms8 phosphotransferase was found to be homologous to the APH(3') enzymes encoded by the *nmrA* and *aph* genes of neomycin-producing *Micromonospora* sp. and *S. fradiae*, respectively, and can be replaced by the latter gene products (76,79). However, its involvement in the interesting 3',4'-dehydroxylation remains unclear (cf. Figure 32, steps 8,9). Another unsolved problem is the formation of the *N*-methyl group in NMLGA, which might be introduced at the D-glucosamine level or later in the pathway, even after condensation of the three streptomycin moieties (38,66,67).

The current hypotheses on the NMLGA pathway, as they can be put forward from the genetic and enzymological records, can be summarized as follows: The genes *strPQX* isolated and sequenced from *S. glaucescens*, and *strFG* and *stsG* analyzed from *S. griseus*, appear to be involved in the biosynthesis of NMLGA (57,61,62,65). StrQ was recently shown to have CDP-D-glucose synthase (E.C. 2.7.7.33) activity. This had already been predicted from its similarity in polypeptide sequence to the enterobacterial RfbF proteins (cf. Table 6) (9,116,121,129). Therefore, it could catalyze the hexose-activating step starting the NMLGA pathway (cf. Figure 29, step 16; Beyer S and Piepersberg W, unpublished results). The StrP protein is a member of the GalE family of oxidoreductases (cf. Figure 39), sharing a higher degree of similarity to UDP-glucose 4-epimerases (GalE) than to other members of this group. The StrP enzyme, therefore, could be C4 or C2 oxidorecductase for CDP-activated hexoses (cf. Figure 29, steps 17, 19, or 20) or either a 2-epimerase or a 4-oxidoreductase for alternative NDP-hexose intermediates (cf. Figure 29, steps 17a, 18a, or 20a) of the NMLGA branch (58). The introduction of the amino-group at C2, if being part of a *de novo* hexosamine pathway, could be accomplished with a CDP-2-ketohexose as substrate for an aminotransferase (cf. Figure 29, steps 20 and 21). Candidates for this transaminating enzyme could be either one of the already mentioned gene products, StrS or StsA (cf. Figure 28; Table 3).

The *strFG* genes were mapped in a DNA fragment that complemented a mutant assumed to be blocked in the NMLGA pathway (130). Protein comparisons suggested weak evidence for both StrF and StrG being members of the group of dinucleotide-independent sugar(phosphate) isomerases or epimerases; they might even form a heterodimeric enzyme (57). The gene product StrX is a candidate for a 3,5-epimerase, which is also needed in the biosynthetic route leading to NMLGA (cf. Figure 29, steps 18 or 19a), because of its significant similarity to other NDP-hexose 3,5-epimerases such as StrM (cf. Figure 28 and Table 3) (62). The StsG protein has the three conserved motifs generally found in *S*-adenosylmethionine-dependent methyltransferases (65,131). Therefore, *stsG* could encode the *N*-methyltransferase necessary for streptomycin formation (cf. Figure 16, steps 22 or 16a). Based on these genetic data, the alternative routes for the synthesis of NMLGA are currently favored as working hypotheses; however, to prove one of these several other possibilities, the nature of the precursor molecules and/or the sequence of individual steps will have to be clarified first. The equivalent counterparts of the *strQ*, *strP*, and *strX* genes have as yet not been found in the *str/sts* cluster of *S. griseus*, though earlier hybridization data suggested the localization of distantly related genes at either extreme end of the gene cluster (10). Of the four genes upstream of *strVW* in *S. glaucescens*, only one *strU*, has been found by DNA sequencing distal to *strVW* at the opposite end of the *S. griseus* gene cluster (cf. Figure 28). If *strQ*, *strP*, and *strX* are not found in *S. griseus*, a possible conclusion could also be that the NMLGA pathway could follow in part alternative routes in both strains, that is, in its initial steps. The most important question remaining is whether the amino-nitrogen of NMLGA is introduced via D-glucosamine or via *de novo* synthesis of a 2-aminohexose unit.

In the case of the D-glucosamines as building blocks of 2DOS-containing or fortimicin group ACAGAs, these are obviously incorporated into pseudo-di- or -oligosaccharides as unmodified precursors at the beginning of the respective pathways. However, their status of activation before the glycosyltransfer reaction, for example, nucleotidylation or another type, is unknown. The enzymology creating 3-, 4-, and 6-aminohexoses or 3-aminopentoses in various groups of aminoglycosides seems to be completely different; here, the amino-groups seem to be mostly introduced after oligomer formation. Examples are the 6-amino-groups in the purpurosamines occurring in nearly all 2DOS ACAGAs and fortimicins (cf. Figures 8–12, and 17), the 3-aminoglucose moieties in kanamycins (cf. Figure 10), and the 4-aminoglucose in apramycins (cf. Figure 15). Also, the 2-amino-2-deoxy-D-xylose moieties in the seldomycins are of interest in this context (cf. Figure 14). These could be introduced as a preformed 2-aminopentose in a glycosylation reaction with paromamine as acceptor substrate, analogous to the transfer of a D-xylose unit during the biosynthesis of gentamicins.

As another contrasting example of the biosynthesis of hexosamine-based secondary metabolites, the case of the pseudo-sugar 1-deoxynojirimycin (DNJ; cf. Figure 23) should be mentioned. Recently, the biogenesis of these unusual amino sugars was studied by stable-isotope labeling in *S. subrutilus* (49). As a result, it was postulated that DNJ is the product of a glucose molecule converted, via fructose, 6-oxidation, and reductive 2- or 6-transamination steps, first to mannonojirimycin (Figure 40).

C.   Special Group Transfer Reactions
I.   Amidino- and Carbamoyltransferases

The two *N*-amidinotransferases engaged in the biosynthesis of the streptidine moiety (steps 6 and 11 in Figure 29) seem to be encoded by two closely related genes, *strB1* and *strB2* (cf. Figure 28 and Table 3), present in all streptomycin producers tested (9,10,59,73,74,132,133). Both amidinotransferases of *S. griseus* cloned in *S. lividans* TK23 showed activity in a nonspecific assay that did not differentiate between the first and second transamidination steps (9,59,60,132). Since these enzymes have as yet not been tested individually with their postulated native substrates (see steps 6 and 11 in Figure 29) (60), it remains uncertain whether the assumed functions (StrB1, step 6; StrB2, step 11) are correct (58) or whether StrB1 carries out both steps, as was assumed by others (74). The latter is supported by the puzzling finding that extracts of *S. bluensis* still seemed to contain both enzymatic activities though only the first one is used in the bluensidine pathway (75), and though only the *strB1* gene could be detected by hybridization, cloning, and sequencing in two bluensomycin producers, *S. bluensis* DSM 40564 and *S. hygroscopicus* ssp. *glebosus* DSM 40823 (cf. Figure 28; Ref. 9). The *N*-amidino-*scyllo*-inosamine O-carbamoyltransferase involved in the biosynthesis of bluensomycin (step 7′ in Figure 29) has been described and uses carbamoyl phosphate (not citrulline!) as donor

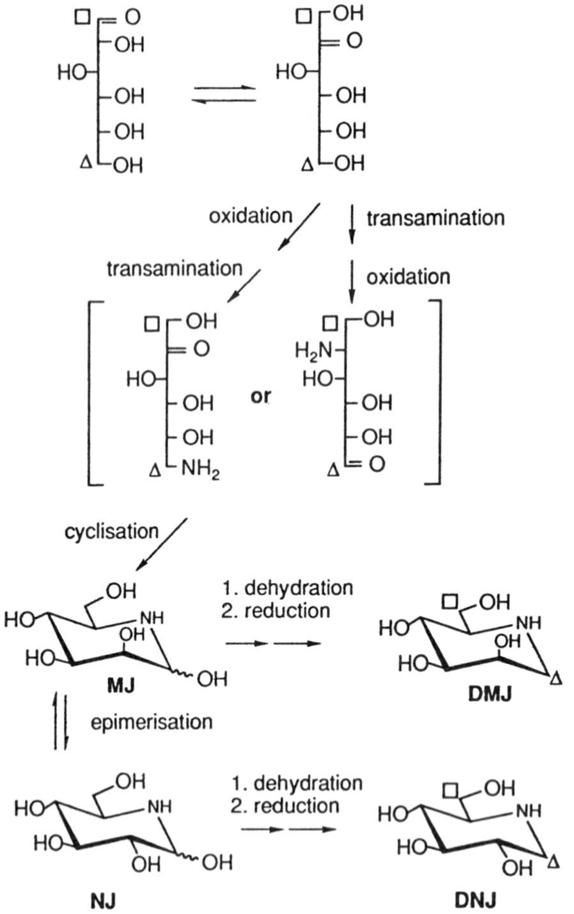

Figure 40   Proposed biogenesis of nojirimycin and related monosaccharide analogs. (D)NJ = (1-deoxy-)nojirimycin; (D)MJ = (1-deoxy-)mannonojirimycin.

cosubstrate (75). Very similar enzymes could be used in the pathways for LL-BM123α (cf. Figure 5), myomycins (cf. Figure 6), and boholmycin (cf. Figure 7). Neither a gene nor a partial protein sequence for a cyclitol O-carbamoyltransferase has been described until now.

2.   Glycyl- and Formimidoyltransferases

Among the biochemically best investigated modifications by side-group extensions of ACAGAs are the two last steps in the common biosynthetic pathway of the fortimicins (FTMs)/istamycins (ISMs), exemplified by the formation of FTM-A (glycyltransfer) and of dactimicin (N-formimidoylation of the glycyl amino-group of FTM-A; cf. Figure 32, steps 13 and 14) (7,12). These are catalyzed by the gene products Fms13 and Fms14, respectively, in M. olivasterospora (cf. Table 3). The genes for these two steps have been cloned, analyzed in part, and found to be present in all producers of FTM/ISM-type aminoglycosides either by hybridization or by activity (77,80). In a blocked mutant of the ISM producer *S. tenjimariensis*, FTM-B was converted into 1-*epi*-FTM-B, dactimicin, and 1-*epi*-dactimicin; *M. olivasterospora* in turn converted ISM-A$_0$ and ISM-B$_0$ into ISM-A3 and ISM-B3, respectively (cf. Figure 17A) (89,90). The mechanism of the glycyltransfer and the putative activation of the glycyl residue (e.g., aminoacyl-adenosine monophosphate [AMP]) have not yet been studied. The N-formimidoyl-group was shown to be also derived from glycine, the C2 group of which was converted via an unusual oxidase mechanism to the formimidoyl-group and probably CO_2 in the presence of molecular oxygen only. This reaction is catalyzed by the FAD-containing Fms14 protein (77).

D. Condensation of Subunits

The major families of ACAGAs are condensed in quite different stages of processing of their subunits (Figure 41; cf. Figures 2, 14, and 18). Oligomerization can be achieved via glycosyltransfer of the NDP-activated and more or less modified monomers (as in the streptomycins), or by use of some other, as yet unknown, ligation reaction(s). Remarkably, this important issue is the least understood in the physiology and biochemistry of formation of (pseudo-)oligosaccharidic natural products in bacteria. For example, the gene products of the *str/sts* and *fms* gene clusters involved in this process have not yet been identified. However, both condensing enzymes for the pseudo-trisaccharide dihydrostreptose-6-phosphate have been detected in cell-free extracts of *S. griseus* (134,135).

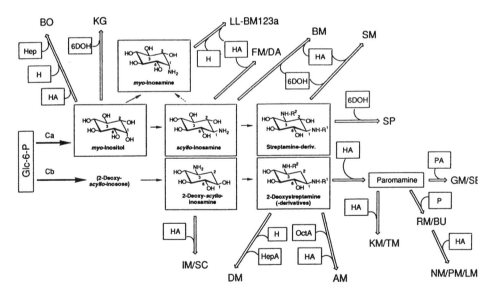

Figure 41   Overview of the pathway design of the major groups of ACAGAs with C$_6$-hexitol units as aglycone. For explanations, see Table 2 and the legends to Figures 2, 14, and 18. AM = apramycins; BM = bluensomycin; BO = boholmycin; DM = destomycins; FM/DA = fortimicins (astromicins) and dactimicin; GM/SE = gentamicins and seldomycins; IM/SC = istamycins and sporaricin; KG = kasugamycins; KM/TM = kanamycins and tobramycin; NM/PM/LM = neomycins, paromomycins, and lividomycins; RM/BU = ribostamycins and butirosins; SM = streptomycins; SP = spectinomycins.

The streptidine-6-phosphate dihydrostreptosyltransferase (E.C. 2.4.2.27) has also been purified, and a homodimeric subunit structure with a molecular weight of 35 kDa for each of the subunits has been determined (134). Weak evidence exists suggesting that this enzyme could be identical with the StrH gene products from S. griseus and S. glaucescens (57,74). For the condensation step in the fortimicin pathway, a mutant and the DNA segment complementing it (gene designation fms3) have been identified (cf. Figures 31 and 32) (7,76,79,86), but neither the gene sequence nor the mechanism catalyzed by the fms3-encoded enzyme have been reported so far. The substrate specificity of the (amino)-cyclitol glycosyltransferases is likely to be very strong. For instance, the N-amidino-scyllo-inosamine-4-phosphate intermediate of the streptidine pathway could be a substrate analog (cf. Figure 30), but it is obviously not used. The inosamycins (cf. Figure 8) are interesting in this respect, since their monoaminocyclitol aglycone indicates that the initial glycosyltransfer reaction toward paromamine could strongly compete for intermediates of the 2DOS pathway in the neomycin–kanamycin–gentamicin group of ACAGAs.

Heterogeneity is observed in the number of saccharidic units in some of the groups of ACAGAs. For example, D-mannosylation at position 4″ of the NMLGA moiety occurs in some streptomycin-producing biovars of S. griseus (29,136). This phenomenon appears to be based on a nonspecific peripheral reaction rather than on an integral step in the biosynthetic pathway, since in the same strains a mannosidohydrolase is formed under carbon catabolite depletion (137). A dimannosylated product also was detected in S. griseus strains (32), as well as products modified at the amino group of the NMLGA subunit; these products of S. griseus FT3-4 were designated ashimycins (30). Also, pseudo-disaccharidic end products of the streptomycin family missing the NMLGA moiety have antibiotic activity and occur as natural end products in fermentations of a Streptomyces sp. strain AC4437 (31). It would be interesting to see whether this strain has an altered pattern of biosynthetic genes, for example, lacking some of the genes for the synthesis of the NMLGA unit or for that of the second glycosyltransferase. Strong variation is also achieved by α- and β-glucosylation in the validamycins. In the amylostatins and trestatins, the transfer of varying numbers of maltose or trehalose residues to the core pseudodisaccharide leads to a large number of variants.

Secondary metabolic glycosyltransferases from actinomycetes involved in the biosynthesis of other carbohydrate-containing antibiotics have not yet been described. However, the detection in both S. lividans and S. antibioticus of a class of macrolide glu-cosyltransferases (MGTs) causing macrolide resistance (138,139) could provide a first clue toward the conclusion that these might be members of one of the glycosyltransferase families that could also be involved in the condensation of some of the ACAGAs. Recently, some genes have been detected in gene clusters for secondary carbohydrate anabolism in streptomycete producers of amphotericin B (SnoT1, SnoT2), erythromycin (EryBV, EryCIII), tylosin (TylY), and daunorubicin (DnrS, DauH) that encode MGT-related proteins and that are mostly associated with gene clusters also encoding 6DOH biosynthetic enzymes (13,113,140–142). Further efforts will also be necessary to analyze the condensation mechanisms for the attachment of the sugar units to the respective cyclitol moieties in the other groups of ACAGAs and to identify their encoding genes. Especially interesting will be the elucidation of condensing mechanisms not following the usual glycosyltransferase mechanisms. These occur, for example, in the Cb2 groups, the validamycins and amylostatins (cf. Figures 19 and 20), or in the formation of some other ACAGA-related compounds, such as the glycocinnamoyl-spermidines containing ureoyl bridges (cf. Figure 5), and in hygromycin A, in which the monoaminocyclitol moiety is bound via an amide bond to the cinnamoic acid–derived spacer constituent (cf. Figure 22).

E.   Secretion by Active Export and Release

In the course of streptomycin production, the final intracellular condensation product, dihydro-streptomycin-6-phosphate, is converted to extracellular streptomycin-6-phosphate by a membrane-associated dehydrogenase (oxidase), probably coupled with active export through the cytoplasmic membrane, since it has been found in the particulate (membrane) fraction and does not require the addition of $NAD(P)^+$ as an electron acceptor (cf. Figures 29 and 30, steps 26 and 27) (143). The oxidase converting dihydrostreptose to streptose has not been purified nor has its electron-accepting cofactor(s) been detected as yet. A candidate gene, strU, found in both S. glaucescens and S. griseus near the putative transporter genes strVW (see below), encodes a protein with significant similarity to dehydrogenases converting alcoholic hydroxyl-groups to aldehyde-groups (cf. Figure 28 and Table 3) (62). However, the properties of the StrU protein, which does not show any indications for a membrane association and carries a typical N-terminal dinucleotide-binding fold, contradict the properties of the oxidase described (143). Therefore, StrU more likely participates in other phases of the pathway, such as the biosynthesis of the NMLGA precursor (cf. Section V.B.3). Also, the 5′-hydroxylase, possibly a cytochrome P_{450} enzyme, necessary for the conversion of the 6DOH (streptose)-containing precursor in the 5′-hydroxystreptomycin producer S. glaucescens, has not been detected as yet. However, a typical cytochrome P_{450} enzyme has not yet been detected among the gene products encoded by the str/sts genes (cf. Table 3).

In the str/sts gene clusters of both S. griseus and S. glaucescens, two tandemly organized genes, strVW, were detected recently that encode proteins of an unusual type of ABC-transporter (cf. Figure 28 and Table 2) (10,62,65). Both proteins show significant but distant similarity, and both contain an N-terminal transmembrane anchor, with each six membrane spanning domains, and a C-terminal ATP-binding domain with the characteristic peptide motifs of ABC-transporters (144). The StrV and StrW proteins could form a membrane-bound pseudo-oligosaccharide export complex. Since streptomycin is secreted in an inactive phosphorylated form (see above), these transmembrane exporters would not result in a resistance phenotype such as the antibiotic-specific ABC-exporters in the producers of anthracyclines, macrolides, and lincosamides (9,115,145,146). Preliminary experiments support this hypothesis, because S. lividans 66 strains carrying a combination of the strA [aphD, APH(6)] and strVW transcription units on plasmids convert added streptomycin to extracellularly accumulated streptomycin-6-phosphate (61). Unfortunately, these constructs turned out to be very unstable; but the phenomenon could not be detected in a strain of S. lividans containing the strA gene alone. Therefore, it will be of interest to investigate if similar transporter genes exist in other aminoglycoside producers, and to determine their substrate profiles.

A different type of membrane-anchored protein was recently identified as the product of the butB gene in Bacillus circulans NRRL B3312 (12,147). The ButB protein is related to the cell-wall-associated S-layer proteins in low-G+C Gram-positive bacteria, and interruption of its gene blocks butirosin production, thus indicating it might also be involved in aminoglycoside export.

In the streptomycin pathway, the final extracellular dephosphorylation step for the release of the biologically active antibiotic is catalyzed by StrK (step 27 in Figure 30)

(57,60). The StrK enzyme was shown to be an extracellular phosphatase specific for strep-tomycin phosphates, with streptomycin-6-phosphate being the preferred substrate. The gene products of the *strK* genes of *S. griseus* and *S. glaucescens* show extensive similarity to alkaline phosphatases, for example, the PhoA protein of *E. coli* (57; Mansouri K and Piepersberg W, unpublished results). The properties of the StrK phosphatase of *S. griseus*, when expressed in *S. lividans*, are in agreement with those reported earlier for the strep-tomycin-phosphate phosphatase (57,60,148).

F.   Aminoglycoside Resistance Mechanisms in Producers

In the past, the investigation of the mechanisms of bacterial resistance against ACAGAs, in both producers and clinically relevant nosocomial pathogens, has con-tributed fundamentally to our understanding of antibiotic resistance phenomena in gen-eral (12,149–151). ACAGA resistance can occur either by mutations, affecting the tar-get site or the uptake, or by specific resistance genes. The identification of the molecular mechanisms of both inactivation of the antibiotic and alteration of the target site by bio-chemical modification in the producers themselves has especially been studied within this group of secondary metabolites (Figure 42; cf. Table 5); again, these were started in pioneering studies with streptomycin (3,94). In fact, the first resistance gene cloned from an antibiotic producer was the gene encoding butirosin-3′-phosphotransferase [APH(3′)-IV] from *B. circulans* (152). Also, the correlation between the phosphorylation of strep-tomycin and its occurence in both a streptomycin producer, *S. griseus* (153,154), and in

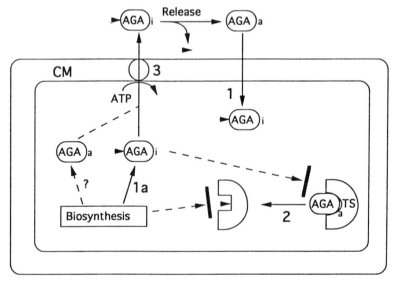

1 Modification
2 Resistant target site (TS)
a, i = Active/inactive secondary metabolite

3 Active export (ATP-driven)
▶ = Modifying group

Figure 42   Schematic representation of some self-protecting resistance mechanisms in producers of ACAGAs. Mechanism 3 (export) is not known to result in a resistance phenotype in the pro-ducers of ACAGAs, but it could be connected with the active transport of modified, inactive prod-ucts out of the cells.

clinical strains of *E. coli* and *Pseudomonas aeruginosa* (155) led, for the first time, to the speculation that transferable antibiotic resistance could in general have evolved from the producers of these natural products (156). Later, ribosomal target-site modification, via specific 16S rRNA methylation, was also identified as a major aminoglycoside resistance mechanism in producers (3,94,157). For the first time, transfer of a gene between Gram-positive and Gram-negative bacteria in nature was demonstrated to occur with an aminoglycoside resistance gene, too; the gene *aphA-3* (kanamycin/neomycin 3′-phosphotransferase) was transferred between enterococci (also streptococci and staphylococci) and *Campylobacter coli* (158). From the producers of aminoglycosides, some of the resistance genes might have spread to other bacteria in earlier evolutionary periods. The mechanisms for the intergeneric transfer of genes are now apparent, and it is interesting to learn that there are related multifactorial systems for intercellular transport of DNA and protein molecules that function specifically between bacteria and unrelated other cell types, such as cells of other bacterial taxa, and plant and animal cells (158–160).

Our knowledge concerning resistance mechanisms in the producers of ACAGAs has accumulated to a greater extent than for any other group of antibiotics. In the producers, three resistance mechanisms have been found: specific phosphorylation and acetylation in various positions of ACAGA molecules, and methylation of 16S rRNA on either A-1408 or G-1405 (cf. Figure 42 and Table 5). Nucleotidylation of ACAGA molecules (aminoglycoside adenylyltransferases [AAD] or nucleotidyltransferases [ANT]), such as encountered with several specificities for all major groups of ACAGAs in many resistant pathogens (149,151), and export resistance do not seem to occur in the producers. However, important questions remained unsolved: for example, what is the contribution of the resistance enzymes to the overall production process, and what is its regulation and their possible interaction with the biosynthetic pathway itself? For the producers of streptomycins, spectinomycin, and fortimicin-group ACAGAs, the relevant results can be summarized in four parts as follows:

First, two resistance enzymes have been detected in the streptomycin-producing strains of *S. griseus* and *S. glaucescens*, encoded by the genes *aphD* [*strA*, *sph*; AphD or APH(6)] and *aphE* [AphE or APH(3″)] (cf. Figures 28 and 30; Table 3) (63,70,71,161–163). The APH(3″) enzyme does not seem to have a counterpart in *S. glaucescens*. The aminoglycoside-resistance mechanisms based on phosphorylation and acetylation were suspected to be derived from biosynthetic enzymes or serve both purposes at the same time, such as the *pac* and *bar* genes encoding puromycin and phosphinothricin acetyltransferases, respectively, (3,60,68,94,122,164,165).

Again, the biosynthetic pathway of streptidine gave the first clues to this speculation, since intermediates in this pathway are successively dephosphorylated and rephosphorylated twice, the last time in the same position (C6 of the aminocyclitol) as is achieved by the resistance enzyme, StrA [APH(6)], in streptomycin producers (cf. Figures 29 and 30) (68). Since this enzyme also has a phosphorylating activity for streptidine and its immediate precursor, *N*-amidinostreptamine (however, at much higher K_M values) (68,70), it was suggested also to be a biosynthetic enzyme. However, as with the APH enzymes, the two gene products StrN and StsE exhibit very similar peptide motifs as are found in the catalytic centers of protein kinases, especially the $HxDx_5Nx_{7-14}UD$ motif (U = hydrophobic residue, e.g., I, V, L), which is probably involved in the transfer of the phosphate group (9,58,166). Therefore, these two proteins are more likely to be the two phosphotransferases involved in the streptidine pathway (see Section V.A). Recently, a spectinomycin resistance gene, encoding a spectinomycin phosphotransferase, was cloned from *S. flavopersicus* NRRL 2820; it showed striking similarity with

StrN of *S. griseus* and *S. glaucescens* (Altenbuchner J, Lyutzkanova D, and Distler J, personal communication). This finding strongly supports the above hypothesis that an ancestral production gene could become a resistance gene by divergent evolution or after degeneration and modification of a preexisting pathway to yield simpler but still effective end products (this could be the case for spectinomycin). Also, the kanamycin-6'-acetyltransferase in *S. kanamyceticus* could, for several reasons, primarily be involved in the acetylation of kanamycin producers (100; see also below).

Second, in *S. griseus* the significance of the AphE [APH(3")] enzyme for resistance or production is still unclear (63,69). It could be either cryptic in the streptomycin-producing strains or, for instance, involved in the occurence of phosphorylated NDP-hexosamines (cf. Section V.B) (128,130). The similarity between the APH(3") enzyme and the APH(3') neomycin-phosphotransferase from *S. fradiae* was used to construct hybrid enzymes (9,123). One of these, which comprised the *N*-terminal half of APH(3") and the C-terminal segment of the APH(3') enzyme, showed neomycin-phosphotransferase activity when expressed in *S. lividans* 66. This supports the postulated correspondence in tertiary structures of aminoglycoside and protein phosphotransferases, especially the localization of the substrate recognition sites in the C-terminal portions (63).

Third, the difference between the two structurally and genetically more distant groups of fortimicin/istamycin-group ACAGAs (see Section IV) is also underlined by the presence of two alternative types of resistance mechanisms: (a) the resistance enzymes FmrO, FmrM, and FmrD are 16S G-1405 rRNA methyltransferases in *M. olivasterospora*, *Micromonospora* sp. SF-2098, and *Dactylosporangium matsuzakiense*, respectively; (b) the FmrT, FmrS, and FmrH gene products are 16S A-1408 rRNA methyltransferases in *S. tenjimariensis*, *S. sannanensis*, and *Saccharopolyspora hirsuta*, respectively (3,7,78,81,83,85). Whether these two types of enzymatic mechanisms have been acquired by chance, for example, after horizontal transfer of part of the production gene clusters devoid of a resistance gene to their current hosts and successive selection for a resistance mechanism, or whether there is a physiological meaning behind this difference is not yet known. Also, it is not known if FTM/ISM producers carry additional resistance mechanisms, such as the modifying 2"- or 2'-*N*-acetyltransferases [AAC(2") or AAC(2')] acting on this group of ACAGAs that have been found in other actinomycetes (see below) (12).

Fourth, resistance to aminoglycosides also occurs as a cryptic or additional phenotypic property in streptomycetes, unrelated to ACAGA production (167). Examples are the cryptic kanamycin-resistance enzyme in *S. griseus* [AAC(3)] or the FTM/ISM-specific 2"- or 2'-*N*-acetyltransferases in the kasugamycin producer *S. kasugaensis* MB273 (96). Also, the ACAGA-resistance profile or individual determinants can be used either as the basis for screening for new producers of ACAGA-like antibiotics (12,99) or to stimulate aminoglycoside production. For instance, the 6'-acetyltransferase gene from *S. kanamyceticus* acts in the latter way when introduced at enhanced gene copy number in kanamycin and neomycin producers (100). This again raises questions about the meaning and effects of two or more different modifying resistance mechanisms for the same class of products, as is observed in all the producers of neomycin/butirosin-related ACAGAs (cf. Table 5).

In conclusion, of the two basic resistance-conferring biochemical phenomena encountered in many other producers of secreted self-toxic natural products, elimination of inhibitory action and export of inhibitor, only the first one seems to be verified in the producers of ACAGAs. In these organisms, suppression of antibiotic action can be achieved either via inactivation of the toxic agent by group transfer or by modification of the target site. Energy-driven exporters nevertheless also might play essential roles in the pathways for ACAGAs, but only to remove the modified and inactive end products from the cells, thus not inducing a resistance phenotype. So, the intracellular antibiotic modification could be directly coupled with export, since the transferred groups could provide part of the substrate recognition properties for the exporter complex. The facilitation of the transport itself could therefore be a second effect, at least for part of the ACAGA phosphoryl- and acetyltransferases, and may explain part of their redundant use (cf. Table 5). A similar effect could be coupled with glucosylation of macrolides by specific UDP-glucose-dependent transferases (MGT) and their export in the oleandomycin producer *S. antibioticus*, causing macrolide resistance (139).

Several implications for the pathway, its physiology, and its evolution could be envisaged if this concept is generally used in the ACAGA-producing bacteria: (a) inactive end products would generally be produced and exported, at least in those cases where ACAGA modification is the major resistance mechanism; (b) ACAGA nucleotidylation is unlikely to occur in the producers, since it would be not economical for the cell; (c) ACAGA modification as a resistance mechanism could have evolved from biosynthetic enzymes; and (d) extracellular hydrolases cleaving off the modifying residues after export should be generally encountered in ACAGA producers. Besides the situation in streptomycin producers, the final possibility could be supported by the existence of both a kanamycin *N*-acetyltransferase and of an *N*-acetylkanamycin amidohydrolase in *S. kanamyceticus* (3,168,169). In conclusion, the resistance by modification could be regarded as a mere self-protection mechanism, enabling the production itself and perhaps facilitated recognition by the export system. The export mechanisms could be of basically different physiological function for all antibiotic-synthesizing bacteria, namely, to transport the compounds out of the cells in order to enable the bioactive end products to reach their natural destinations, namely, targets in other cells.

G.   Diversity and Unifying Themes: A Generalized View

We have seen that there is great diversity in basic pathway design and even in the use of alternative biosynthetic tools and structural elements to reach almost identical biochemical goals (Figure 41). Parts of these pathways seemingly are closely related, whereas others could be although yielding quite distinct end products, such as in the streptomycin–spectinomycin–kasugamycin group. In this case, an ancestral pathway, for example, for streptomycin-related compounds, could have degenerated and been further selected to form several different types of end products. Some ACAGAs are already constructed from a nonaminated cyclitol (e.g., kasugamycins, myomycins, and boholmycin) (cf. Figures 4, 6, and 7), others from monoaminocyclitols (e.g., antibiotic LL-BM123α) (cf. Figure 5) or from diaminocyclitols preformed via a complex branch of the pathway (e.g., streptomycins, spectinomycins, and 2DOS-ACAGAs) (cf. Figures 1 and 8–13). Diaminocyclitols can also be synthesized via later introduction of the second amino-group, as in the fortimicin/istamycin group of ACAGAs. Thus, the sequential distribution of biosynthetic steps that are typical for ACAGA formation over the pathway as a whole can be quite different.

An interesting hypothesis is based on these divergent pathway structures: The design of a pathway together with the specificity of a export system could influence the product pattern. In the producers of the gentamicins, the major modifications occur on the pseudotrisaccharide level; that is, after condensation (cf. Figure 14), a variety of very similar products are made that already could be recognized to some extent by the active exporter. In this manner, a complex mixture of end products could be accumulated in the fermentation medium, the composition of which depends only on the physiological state of the cell, for example, the flux of metabolites through the pathway and the availability of cosubstrates for the modifying enzymes. In contrast, in pathways such as those found in streptomycin biosynthesis, where most of the modification of the subunits is introduced on the monomer level (cf. Figure 2), only a very limited variation of the secreted end product is observed.

The ACAGAs are a class of natural products that appear relatively homogeneous at first glance. However, a considerable diversity in structural elements and a heterogeneity in the currently known design of the biosynthetic pathways are apparent. Nervertheless, ultimately there seem to be several common motifs or individual steps used in the strategies for ACAGA production. A graphic overview summarizing the present postulates on the pathway structures in the producers of the major ACAGA families (cf. Figure 41) reveals several common features:

1. A cyclitol unit is preferably used as an aglycone to form a pseudo-oligosaccharide, maybe because it results in enhanced (bio-)chemical stability and/or specificity in binding to the target site. An alternative view would explain condensations of cyclitols with sugar units by their favorable metabolic coupling, because they are derived from a common precursor pool of carbohydrates centered in the upper glycolytic pathway and the pentosephosphate cycle.

2. Highly conserved enzymes and mechanisms are used in the key modification steps, such as transaminations, transamidinations, other group transfers, and the basic activation and synthesis of glycosidic side chains. Also, here could exist some modification of branching of pathways—different routes might be used to form the same or a very similar end product.

3. Actively exporting systems are postulated to be present in all ACAGA producers and can already now be postulated to play a major role in the specificity of the product patterns.

4. Exporters generally do not seem to confer resistance; this is interpreted as an indication for secretion of inactive modified precursors from which the active component becomes liberated outside the cells by hydrolytic cleavage.

VI.   PHYSIOLOGY AND REGULATION OF AMINOGLYCOSIDE PRODUCTION

The biosyntheses of ACAGAs in sporulating actinomycetes and bacilli, like the production of other secondary metabolites, is probably embedded by strong regulatory links into the cell and differentiation cycle(s) (170). They follow the influences of both external (e.g., nutritional) factors and inherent physiological programs, which are genetically fixed expression patterns of biosynthetic enzymes. Studies with streptomycin-producing S. griseus strains recently led to the proposal of a "decision phase" model for the programming of differentiation and secondary metabolism during early phases of growth in a defined medium (Figure 43) (10,64,171). The phenomenon is also seen in other streptomycetes (172). The decision-making processes are obviously controlled by a complicated, hierarchically organized network of regulatory mechanisms (170,173). These in turn are likely to involve a large variety of global or pathway-specific regulatory proteins, encoded either by genes located in the individual biosynthetic gene clusters or by other, more

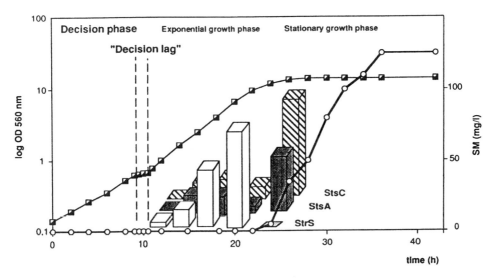

Figure 43 Decision phase model of secondary metabolism and differentiation. The growth, *str/sts* gene expression, and streptomycin (SM) production of *S. griseus* are given as an example. The kinetics of the accumulation of biomass (squares) and of SM (circles) are shown. The columns indicate the relative expression rates of the SMAT enzymes StrS, StsA, and StsC as determined by densidometry of the autoradiographed patterns of proteins from *S. griseus* cells after pulse-labeling with [³⁵S]methionine and separation on two-dimensional protein gels.

pleiotropic, regulatory genes. Also, evidence has been reported that hormonelike autoregulators (e.g., A factor) (14), intracellular signal molecules (e.g., cyclic adenosine monophosphate [cAMP], or guanosine tetraphosphate [ppGpp]), and nutrients (e.g., phosphate, glucose, N sources) control the production of aminoglycosides at the level of gene expression and/or enzyme activity (2,10). However, we are far from having a complete picture of the regulatory cascades acting on any of the ACAGA-producing systems. Some of the more recent results and postulates on the physiology and regulation of streptomycin biosynthesis in *S. griseus* are summarized in Figure 44 (10). The most interesting open questions are, what interrelations exist between primary and secondary carbohydrate metabolism and how the physiological conditions are sensed in order to transfer activating signals to the production gene clusters.

A. Interrelations Between Primary and Secondary Carbohydrate Metabolism

It is known that certain carbon catabolites, the concentration and nature of N source, and phosphate are the major nutritional factors influencing ACAGA production (2,120,174). However, the molecular biology of the involvement of primary metabolic traits in the activation and delivery of precursors has not yet been studied intensively. The dynamics and alterations of precursor pools, as well as the types of nutritional sources and routes used for precursor formation during the production phase in the producers of ACAGAs and other secondary carbohydrates, will have to be determined. Among the main factors to be studied are the fluxes in intermediary C and N metabolism and the origin of the nitrogenous groups in case of the ACAGAs. One of the clues might be given by the finding that there is a strong interaction between the pentosephosphate cycle and

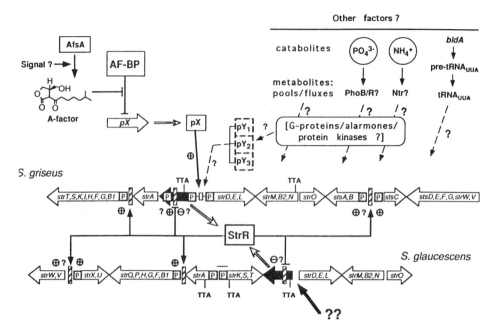

Figure 44 Model for the regulation of streptomycin production in S. *griseus* and S. *glaucescens*. Regulation of the expression of *str/sts* genes by pleiotropic (e.g., A factor) and pathway-specific (e.g., StrR) factors. P = promoters; hatched bars = StrR-binding sites; arrows indicate positive regulatory effects. The *strR* gene of S. *glaucescens* is not regulated by A factor, and it is probably controlled quite differently since the upstream sequences do not show any similarity to those from S. *griseus*. For further explanations, see the text.

the formation of both neomycin and validamycin (8) or the octose moiety of lincomycin (cf. the chapter on lincosamides in this book) (175). Reasons for altered conditions in the primary carbon fluxes could be a changing compartmentation in the filamentous mycelial cells or a difference in the efficiencies of enzymes involved in the conversion of the primary hexosephosphate. Alternatively, the conversion of the major route(s) of intermediary C metabolism for the predominant use in gluconeogenesis could occur during the production phase. Another indication is given by the fact that very few amino acids are usually the preferred sources for nitrogen in the production phases for ACAGAs (2). In the case of S. *griseus*, this is asparagine, though the nitrogenous groups introduced into streptomycin are derived from glutamine, alanine, and arginine (10,64). The regulation of streptomycin production and its growth phase dependence will be discussed in the following section.

B. Regulation of Aminoglycoside Biosynthesis

The physiological changes programmed during the decision phase in S. *griseus*, leading to both differentiation and streptomycin production (cf. Figure 43), depend on the presence of preformed A factor, 2-(6′-methylheptanoyl)-3R-hydroxymethyl-4-butanolide (6,64). However, measurable *de novo* synthesis of A factor occurs later, after the "decision lag" has been passed (10). The significance of other autoregulators, such as factor C (176), for the control of this process is unknown. The hormonelike effect of A factor can be suppressed by high concentrations of L-valine in the medium (171,177). Also, an inhibitor of adenesine diphosphate (ADP)-ribosylation of proteins, 3-aminobenzamide (3-ABA), can suppress sporulation in S. *griseus* 2602 (178). In 3-ABA-resistant mutants of S. *griseus* IFO13189, the production of streptomycin, but not of A factor, is impaired (179). However, 3-ABA does not affect the synthesis of streptomycin in the overproducing strain S. *griseus* N2-3-11 (171). Other physiological changes encountered during the decision lag are (a) increased consumption of amino acids, (b) an increase of intracellular cAMP levels, (c) transient expression of some gene products, and (d) turn-on or shut-off of other genes (6,10,64,171). These effects altogether seem to be an absolute prerequisite for later cell differentiation and streptomycin production. Among the genes switched on are the *str/sts* genes. For example, the A-factor-dependent expression of the aminotransferases StrS, StsA, and StsC occurs 2 to 4 hr after the decision lag, but 10 hr before streptomycin is detectable in the culture medium for the first time (cf. Figure 43). This concept of the induction of secondary metabolism during an early growth phase that is completely separated from the production phase can only be explained when cells concomitantly undergo fundamental changes in their global regulatory networks. Therefore, the existence of signal transduction pathways that might include receptors, transducers, protein kinases, phosphoprotein phosphatases, and second messengers in streptomycetes can easily be imagined. Evidence for the existence in *Streptomyces* of a mixture of typically eubacterial and eukaryote-related phenomena of this type is increasing (170,173,178). Though the direct regulation of the *str* genes and the superimposed regulatory cascades in S. *griseus* are still incompletely understood, a model for the regulation of streptomycin production summarizing the current hypotheses can be proposed (Figure 44).

Repression by glucose and other sugars has been known for a long time for the production of streptomycin, kanamycin, istamycin, and neomycin (2,174). Such repression seems to be caused by the repression of antibiotic biosynthetic enzymes, for example, *N*-acetylkanamycin amidohydrolase (169), rather than by affecting the formation of precursors of secondary metabolites. In *E. coli* and *B. subtilis* (180), carbon catabolite control typically uses the cAMP/cAMP-receptor protein (CAP) system for gene regulation. Although cAMP relieves glucose repression of *N*-acetylkanamycin amidohydrolase in S. *kanamyceticus* (169), direct evidence for the involvement of cAMP in the regulation of ACAGA production is still lacking. The intracellular cAMP concentration falls sharply in the mid to late vegetative growth phase of S. *griseus* S104, before the onset of secondary metabolism (181). Glucose increases cAMP levels in S. *antibioticus* while simultaneously repressing oleandomycin formation (182). There is no evidence that cAMP directly affects streptomycin production in S. *griseus* (171). Instead, the inhibitory action of glucose and related catabolites could be mediated by the glucose kinase. Mutants of S. *coelicolor* lacking this enzyme show normal intracellular levels of cAMP and no glucose-repressed phenotype (183,184). In contrast to these results, glucose-insensitive mutants of S. *kanamyceticus* could be isolated that have wild-type levels of glucose kinase (185).

Again, most of our present knowledge stems from studies on the streptomycin producers (10). Available data and hypotheses on the regulation of the genes for streptomycin production are summarized in the model outlined in Figure 44. Here, we see the different levels and specificities of the regulation of ACAGA biosynthesis. These can be either generally used or strain-specific (e.g., A factor) global regulatory mechanisms that at a lower level guide pathway-specific regulation, such as the StrR-dependent activation of *str/sts* genes in S. *griseus* and S. *glaucescens* (cf. Figure 44) (9,10; Retzlaff L and Distler J, unpublished results).

There is conflicting evidence reported in the literature concerning the influence of the nitrogen source on the production of streptomycin and other aminoglycosides. Nevertheless, ammonium seems to impede synthesis of streptomycin, neomycin, and kanamycin (2), whereas nitrate and some amino acids support the production of ACAGAs, for example, of kanamycin (186) and streptomycin. The stimulation of streptomycin production by alanine, arginine, and/or glutamine can be explained in terms of being direct donors of nitrogenous groups in enzyme-catalyzed steps during streptomycin biosynthesis (cf. Section V). The mechanisms underlying the positive effect of asparagine and proline (2) or the repression of streptomycin synthesis by valine (171,177) in S. griseus are presently not understood at all. These compounds could influence the expression of biosynthetic key enzymes on the genetic level mediated by a NtrB/NtrC-like system or at the physiological level by modulating the activities of primary metabolic enzymes and streptomycin biosynthetic enzymes via metabolites accumulated. Other switches may exert their control by feed-back repression, induction of gluconeogenetic pathways, or metabolic conditions favoring special routes of intermediary metabolism, like the use of the pentosephosphate cycle in the "reverse direction."

The biosynthesis of the classical ACAGAs (e.g., streptomycin, neomycin, kanamycin) is sensitive to a high concentration (>5 mM) of inorganic phosphate (187). The extracellular aminoglycoside-phosphate phosphatase forming the biologically active antibiotic, in the case of streptomycin (cf. Figure 30), from an inactive phosphorylated precursor is inhibited by phosphate. Streptomycin-6-P is accumulated in cultures of S. griseus grown on high concentrations of phosphate or at low pH, due to the inhibition of the streptomycin-6-P phosphatase (StrK) (57). In addition, there is evidence that some secondary metabolic genes are controlled by a PhoB/PhoR-like system, since so-called "Pho boxes" have been detected in phosphate-regulated promoter regions (187,188). Similar structures were also found in the promoter regions of the aphD P2 promoter of S. griseus and the strK (streptomycin-6-P phosphatase) gene of S. glaucescens (64,187).

The possible role of other alarmones, such as guanosine tetra- or pentaphosphates (ppGpp or pppGpp) and the guanosine triphosphate (GTP) pool, in controlling secondary metabolism in streptomycin-producing S. griseus and other antibiotic producers has been studied extensively (189–192). Although relC mutants showed a marked reduction of antibiotic production on complete medium, it was difficult to assess whether the effect on streptomycin production was a direct consequence of the defect in ppGpp formation or an indirect effect of the relC mutation (191). In S. clavuligerus, there is no relationship between the production of ppGpp and that of antibiotics (193). The same observation was made for the streptomycin synthesis in S. griseus on minimal medium, since no significant accumulation of ppGpp could be detected in any growth phase (171).

So-called streptomycete autoregulators have been detected in streptomycin-producing strains of S. griseus (14,176,194,195). These are diffusible low-molecular-weight or proteinaceous substances extractable from the culture fluids and required for the induction of cell differentiation and/or antibiotic production. A factor is essential for streptomycin biosynthesis and differentiation in S. griseus. A factor, which was discovered by Khokhlov and coworkers (194), belongs to a group of chemically similar γ-butyrolactone autoregulators that are synthesized by a variety of Streptomyces spp. (14,196,197). A factor induces streptomycin production and sporulation in A-factor-negative mutants of S. griseus at concentrations as low as 1 nM. The induction by A factor reveals a strict growth phase dependence, namely, in that A factor has to be present during the first hours of growth ("decision phase" model, see below) (10,171). A-factor-induced regulation in S.

griseus depends on an A-factor-binding protein (A-factor receptor protein, ArpA), present in very low amounts (ca. 37 molecules per genome), having a binding constant (K_d) of 0.7 nM, and being encoded by the *arpA* gene (198–200). In two related cases, the virginiae butanolides (VB) of *S. virginiae* (201) and the butanolide autoregulatory factor IM-2 of *Streptomyces* sp. FRI-5 (197), highly specific binding proteins for the individual autoregulators, with similar K_d values, have also been found. All three autoregulator binding proteins have apparent molecular weights of 26 to 27 kDa and in their native states may be dimers (197–200). However, the identity of the butyrolactone receptor proteins with the transcription regulation factor NusG seems not to hold (197,199,202,203), which was claimed previously for the virginiamycin producer *S. virginiae* (201). The butyrolactones are possibly structural and functional analogs to the *N*-acyl homoserine lactones, which act as bacterial communication substances in Gram-negative bacteria (204).

In the proposed model, the A-factor receptor protein acts in the absence of A factor as a repressor for streptomycin biosynthesis and differentiation (cf. Figure 44) (200). In addition A factor stimulates membrane-bound GTPases in *S. griseus* in vivo and in vitro (178). A factor induces the expression of StrR, the activator protein for some of the transcription units in the streptomycin biosynthesis gene cluster (9,59,205). The A-factor-dependent transcription of *strR* seems to be controlled via the A-factor receptor regulating at least one additional A-factor-dependent DNA-binding protein (pX; cf. Figure 44), which binds to an enhancer-like element located upstream of the *strR* promoter (14,196,206). Three additional DNA-binding proteins (pY$_{1-3}$ cf. Figure 44), independent of A-factor induction in *S. griseus*, interact with neighboring sites in the same region upstream of the *strR* gene, suggesting an even more complex regulatory network governing StrR expression (207).

The StrR proteins encoded by the gene clusters for streptomycin biosynthesis of *S. griseus* and *S. glaucescens* have a sequence identity of only 62.8% (10,59,73,74,208). The presence of an activator was first postulated from the phenotype of a mutation and its suppression by complementation with wild-type DNA in *S. griseus* (73,74). Analysis of the mode of action of StrR in *S. griseus* proved that StrR is a DNA-binding protein (9,205). It activates the expression of the *str* genes *strB1*, *stsB* and *stsC*, *strU* and *strV* at the level of transcription by binding to promoter upstream sequences (cf. Figures 28 and 44) (9,62,65,205). These, together with a fourth StrR-binding site identified within the reading frame of the *strR*-gene, are palindromes with the consensus sequence: GTTCGAnnGn(11)CnnCTCAACG (62,65,205). The function of the StrR-binding site within the *strR* gene is still unclear. It could be either negative feed-back regulation of StrR expression, or activation of the promoter P*aph2* located approximately 400 bp downstream of this element (cf. Figure 44). In the *str/sts* gene cluster of *S. glaucescens*, an additional StrR-dependent activation site could also be identified upstream of the divergently oriented genes *strX* and *strV* (cf. Figure 44). Recently, a gene homologous to *strR* was identified on a DNA fragment of *S. flavopersicus* conferring spectinomycin resistance in *S. lividans* (Lyutzkanova D and Altenbuchner J, personal communication). Therefore, it can be speculated that activator proteins homologous to StrR are more widely distributed regulators of biosynthetic genes in producers of ACAGAs. This also supports the suggestion that, especially in those strains using the **Ca1–6DOH** pathway to form streptomycin-related compounds, the biosynthetic capacity could have evolved on the basis of a common ancestral gene cluster.

The global regulatory mechanisms governing both secondary metabolism and differentiation in *Streptomyces* also regulate expression of ACAGA biosynthetic genes. The *bldA* gene coding for a leucine-specific tRNA$_{UUA}$ is one of the candidates for such regulatory switches (cf. Figure 44) (170,173,209–211). *BldA* mutants of *S. griseus* are deficient in aerial mycelium formation and streptomycin production (212). Recently, it was demonstrated that tRNA$_{UUA}$-dependent control could be a key switching process in the onset of differentiation and secondary metabolism (210,211). In *S. griseus, S. glaucescens,* and *S. spectabilis,* the *strR* genes contain a respective TTA triplet in conserved positions in the 5'-section of the respective reading frames (58,59,208; Distler J, Lyutzkanova D, and Altenbuchner J, unpublished results). In the *strN* genes of *S. griseus* and *S. glaucescens,* additional TTA codons were detected. The *strA* (*sph*) gene of *S. glaucescens* also possesses a TTA codon; this, however, is absent from the counterpart of this gene, *strA* (*aphD*), in *S. griseus* (71,163). In *S. coelicolor,* seven different RNA-polymerase sigma factors were identified, and the role of special sigma factors (e.g., WhiG) in controlling differentiation and antibiotic production have been demonstrated (213,214). This could also be the case in controlling the transcription of ACAGA biosynthetic genes, since the similarity of the *str* promoters (*PstrR, Paph,* and *PstrB1*) in *S. griseus* suggests the use of special sigma factors (59).

Several publications report the possible involvement of other factors in the regulation of streptomycin production in *S. griseus* strains (cf. Figure 44): (a) the putative DNA-binding protein ORF1590 necessary for sporulation may also be required for streptomycin production in *S. griseus* (212); (b) ADP-ribosylation of proteins, possibly via influencing membrane-bound G-proteins (GTPases) (178); and (c) C factor, which has been characterized as a cytodifferentiation protein excreted into the medium by *S. griseus* 45H (176). Recently, the demonstration of protein phosphorylation, specifically of protein kinase activities for both L-serine/L-threonine or L-tyrosine residues, in most or all streptomycetes suggests that cascades of protein modification may participate in signal transduction and/or regulatory networks (6,10,172,215–217). Therefore, protein phosphorylation/dephosphorylation also could be involved in the complex regulation of ACAGA synthesis and differentiation in *S. griseus.* Proteins phosphorylated at a tyrosine residue could be detected (215), and specific inhibitors for protein kinases, such as staurosporin, inhibit sporulation (216) and streptomycin production (172) without affecting vegetative growth in strains of this species.

VII.   FUNCTION, ECOLOGY, AND EVOLUTION

It will not be possible to understand the occurrence and evolutionary significance of ACAGAs without gaining fundamental data concerning their ecological function and/or role in the developmental cycle of their producers. Therefore, future basic research will have to concentrate on these aspects in the first case that we are aiming to fully understand the development of the complex biosynthetic pathways for ACAGAs and other secondary carbohydrates. For the purpose of this chapter, we define as "secondary carbohydrate" every product of anabolic (biosynthetic) carbohydrate metabolism beyond glucose and the intermediates of glycolysis and the hexosemonophosphate shunt.

A.   Target-Site Interactions and General Effects on Bacterial and Eukaryotic Cells

Because of the history of ACAGA detection, involving the use of ACAGAs as antibiotic chemotherapeuticals, their molecular effects have been studied exclusively in prokaryotic cells sensitive to ACAGAs and in human cell systems concomitantly coming into contact with these substances, instead of in the ACAGA-producing cells themselves. Nevertheless, the results gained via this indirect route could give clues to the basic meaning of the natural functions of aminoglycosides and their origin. Therefore, the results on the molecular biology of ACAGA action on susceptible cell systems obtained during the past decade will be briefly summarized here.

I. Interactions with Bacterial Cells

The end products of ACAGA pathways are obviously ligands optimized for their target sites; for example, pseudotrisaccharides seem to be the optimal inhibitors of the translational machinery in the 30S subunits of bacterial ribosomes. Where this is not the case, the end products act on alternative targets, such as α-glucosidases or trehalases for the amylostatin-group compounds and trehazolin, or chitinases for the allosamidins. Our knowledge regarding the translational inhibitors is the most advanced, and it is now generally accepted that the antibiotics interact directly with 16S rRNA (see below). Methylation of a single nucleotide out of the about 1600 nucleotides in the 16S rRNA molecules completely suppresses the toxic and pleiotropic effects in the producers of several 2DOS-containing and fortimicin-related ACAGAs (see Section V.F). This finding seems to prove that all the diverse phenomena exerted by these antibacterial compounds depend on the specific interaction with a single target site.

The translational inhibitors among the ACAGAs fall into two functionally different groups: (a) bacteriocidal compounds inducing misreading of the genetic code, for example, the streptomycins, fortimicins, and all 2DOS aminoglycosides (group 1 ACAGAs); and (b) bacteriostatic inhibitors that have no effect on translational accuracy, for example, spectinomycins and kasugamycins (group 2 ACAGAs). Their interaction with the small (30S) subunits of eubacterial ribosomes (eubacterial, mitochondrial, and plastidal ribosomes) is well established (218,219). The group 1 ACAGAs induce mistranslation and rapidly cause loss of all translational activity; group 2 compounds exert a "quasi-relaxed" (Rel$^-$) phenotype similar to the antibiotic chloramphenicol with an uncoupled residual translation of a special group of proteins for a longer period of time (220). Mistranslation is also observed by some aminoglycosides in some, but not all, of the tested genera of the *Archaea* (221). An exception is hygromycin B, which shows functional traits of both groups but does not seem to induce misreading of the genetic code (222). The effects of the group 1 compound streptomycin on the ribosomal elongation cycle in wild-type, streptomycin-resistant or -dependent mutants in RpsL (ribosomal protein S12) of *E. coli* K-12 are still not fully understood. These seem to be associated with the extent of a GTP-hydrolysis idling reaction on cognate EF–Tu ternary complexes and may be interpreted in view of the now-established three ribosomal binding sites for tRNA and the functional interplay between ribosomal subunits in peptidyltransfer and translocation reactions (219,223–225).

The individual binding sites for most of the classical (group 1) ACAGAs on the 16S rRNA are defined by experiments involving cross-linking and protection assays, and site-directed mutagenesis (226–229). The specific interaction of spectinomycin with 16S rRNA bases G-1064 and C-1192 has also been demonstrated recently (230). It is now generally accepted that 16S and 23S rRNAs are ribozymes that are catalytically active constituents of all ribosomes in both decoding and peptidyltransfer (231). The decoding process involves an interaction of a short RNA duplex (paired codon–anticodon) with the P and A sites of the 30S subunits, which is impaired by the mistranslation-inducing

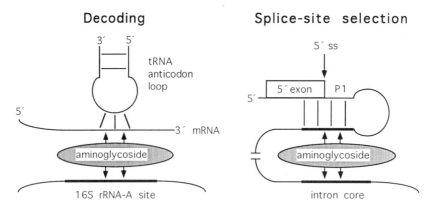

Figure 45   Schematic representation of the interaction of ACAGAs with the ribosomal decoding site on 16S rRNA and the splice site of group I introns (according to Ref. 232).

ACAGAs (Figure 45). Recently, it was also demonstrated that short RNA analogs of the 16S rRNA decoding site specifically interact with both aminoglycosides and the decoding site's RNA ligands, tRNA and mRNA, in the absence of ribosomal proteins (231).

A great surprise was the finding that the self-splicing mechanism of group I introns can be inhibited by certain ACAGAs, especially of the 2DOS family, noncompetitively and with similar selectivity and affinities as the translational process on 16S rRNA in bacteria (232–234). It has been pointed out also that the ACAGA-impaired process of splice site selection by self-splicing group I introns, similar to ribosomal decoding, involves the interaction of three RNA strands (cf. Figure 45) (234). The pseudodisaccharidic ACAGAs lysinomicin (cf. Figure 17) and neamine (cf. Figure 13) competitively inhibit the GTP dependence of the self-splicing reaction in group I introns (235). These findings initiated speculations that aminoglycosides are "molecular fossils" echoing their possible functions as ligands of catalytically active RNAs in a precellular RNA-world (233). An argument in favor of this hypothesis is the finding that all known bactericidal translational inhibitors among the aminoglycosides, though differentially binding, seem to interact with a single common domain in the decoding center of the 16S rRNA of bacterial ribosomes (231).

For many years, the nature of the effects of bactericidal ACAGAs that caused cell death in eubacteria was a matter of debate, and effects other than their direct interaction with the eubacterial ribosome have been suggested to be responsible (25). Besides severe impairment of the initiation and elongation phases of protein synthesis, two phenomena had been observed to be coupled with lethality of ACAGAs. First, the uptake of ACAGAs into both Gram-negative and Gram-positive bacteria shows two-step kinetics, the first phase of which depends on the $\Delta\Omega$ component of the proton motive force or is driven by ATP (236–239). Second, an uptake-mediated disturbance of membrane structure and its associated functions is probably induced by the formation of membrane channels (240,241). Two different models were proposed to explain the pleiotropy of action of ACAGAs: (a) incorporation of misread proteins into the cytoplasmic membrane; and (b) mistranslation of proteins with a short half-life involved in DNA replication and/or cell division, and made at very few copies in a distinct phase of the cell cycle. The first model also would explain the observed drastic increase of aminoglycoside uptake in the second, killing phase. In this phase, the antibiotics are irreversibly accumulated inside the cells in high excess over the number of ribosomes, obviously by electrostatically binding to anionic groups of cytoplasmic macromolecules or by being caged into degradation products of mistranslated proteins (25,241). Also, passage of the ACAGA molecules through the outer membrane of Gram-negative bacteria could be differentially affected by direct interaction of aminoglycosides with porins and/or components of the lipopolysaccharide chains (242).

2. Effects and Target Sites in Eucaryotic Cells

The most important adverse side effects encountered with ACAGAs in human therapy are oto- and nephrotoxicity (243). Therefore, these have been studied extensively for many years. Surprisingly, the emergent biochemical causes of these phenomena seem to be related to the specific interaction of ACAGAs with the mitochondrial 12S rRNA molecules, which are the only representatives of prokaryotic-type rRNAs in mammalian cells. This causality could even be connected to human mitochondrial genetics, since occurence of hypersensitivity toward ACAGAs in patients suffering from ototoxicity was detected after treatment with gentamicin-related 2DOS ACAGAs (244). Hypersensitive persons have been shown to carry an A to G mutation (1555G) in the 12S rRNA. This area of small subunit rRNAs is known to interact with 2DOS ACAGAs and to be involved in the control of codon–anticodon pairing (see above; cf. Figure 45). This defect leads to frequent death of hair cells in the ear. Enhanced production of superoxide by a mistranslated mitochondrial complex I is proposed to be responsible, since about half of the mitochondrial genome is used to encode the proteins of the cytochrome oxidase complex.

Nephrotoxicity is primarily accompanied by membrane damage in the renal tubular cells. The biochemical basis for this effect in man is still not fully understood and could be either caused by an effect on lipid metabolism and structure or by mistranslation of proteins inducing malfunctions of membrane traffic (245). The nephrotoxic effect is also seen in neonates when the mother is treated during gestation (246), and it can be suppressed by polyaspartic acid (247). The possible biochemical effects exerted via impairment of translation (or of group I intron splicing) in the mitochondria of renal cells remain to be demonstrated.

B. Possible Functions for the Producers and Their Ecology

We can only speculate today about the natural functions of these compounds and the identity of their target cells. These, in general terms, could be other cells of the same organism or cells of other organisms, such as competitors (233,248,249). In the first case, we would see hormonelike functions; that is, the target cells would be either nonproducing or otherwise differentiated cell stages within the life cycle of the producer. The functions of ACAGAs in particular are likely to be inhibitory and to be mediated via their specific interactions with 16S rRNAs. But these targets could reside in bacterial competitors, in the mitochondria and/or plastides of eukaryotic cells in the environment, for example, of protozoa or plant roots in soil, or even the aging mycelial cells of the producing actinomycete itself.

A prerequisite for an ecological role of ACAGAs is that they are produced under the natural conditions in the producers' biotope, for example, in soils. Recent investigations with streptomycin producers indicate that they are widespread and that they are enriched in soils under certain conditions of agricultural treatment (250–252). Evidence that streptomycin is really produced in soil also has been presented (253). Therefore, it will be one of the future aims of ACAGA research to study the ecological role of these substances in the biotopes of their producing organisms. It would also be helpful if the driving selective pressure for the transfer of resistance genes from producers to clinical pathogens could still be traced (cf. Section V.F).

C. Evolution of Aminoglycoside Pathways

The majority of the ACAGAs and related compounds treated in this chapter are products of actinomycetes (cf. Table 1). Therefore, the question arises whether or not the evolution of the respective pathways also occured in this lineage of bacterial taxonomy, which is now both physiologically and molecularly defined (254). However, if ACAGAs are ancient natural products, as is suggested by the molecular fossil hypothesis, the evolutionary origins of their biosynthetic pathways also could have preceded the occurence of strictly aerobic bacteria such as the higher actinomycetes (232,248). In that respect, it is interesting to note that many actinomycetes contain inositides in their mixtures of membrane lipids (in contrast to most other bacterial groups; 104). This indicates that **Ca1**-type pathways are also used for more general purposes in ACAGA producers. This is further supported by the recent identification of a new compound, called mycothiol (2-[N-acetylcysteinyl]amido-2-deoxy-a-D-glucopyranosyl-[1→1]-myo-inositol; 255), which is the principal oxygen-protecting thiol in the glutathione-free actinomycetes. This compound could also be regarded as an ACAGA-related structure (**Ca1–HA–[X]**) and an ancient relative of some of their biosynthetic families. When more examples of the gene families involved in these pathways can be compared, the genetic record probably will tell us more about their history (249). Some relationships in protein primary structures already allow reasonable speculations on the derivation of the enzymes for secondary carbohydrate metabolism.

As an example, the emergent similarities in the sets of secondary carbohydrate genes involved in the biosynthesis of antibiotics and in Gram-negative lipopolysaccharide (LPS) O-chains can be considered (11,13,116,125). A comparison shows that two basic mechanisms of the recruitment of necessary biosynthetic enzymes occur: (a) divergent evolution after gene duplication to created new enzymatic function, and (b) horizontal gene transfer to provide flexible means for the selection of new pathway combinations. This can be best shown in a comparison of enzyme proteins with either identical or related functions, with related primary structures, or with both (Figure 46 and Table 6; cf. Sections V.A to V.F). Three examples should illustrate this:

1.   The genes for the functionally identical pairs of dTDP-glucose synthases and dTDP-glucose 4,6-dehydratases in streptomycetes and enterobacteria seem to have been exchanged frequently and freely between unrelated taxa, even though they are organized in common transcription units in each case (cf. Figure 46) (11,116). For instance, in the macrolide producers, the dTDP-glucose synthases (e.g., TylA1) have significantly higher similarities to the respective enzymes (RfbA) encoded by the *rfb* clusters of enterobacteria than to those from other streptomycetes (e.g., StrD); whereas the adjacent gene *tylA2* in the tylosin-producing *S. fradiae* clearly encodes a dTDP-glucose 4,6-dehydratase, which is much more closely related to other counterparts in streptomycetes (e.g., StrE) than to the enterobacterial RfbB proteins. Similar data have been found while comparing the

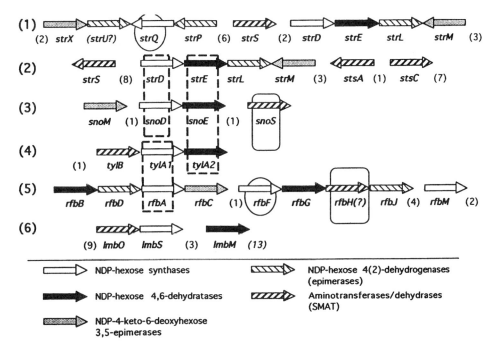

Figure 46 Examples of gene clusters involved in secondary carbohydrate metabolism in antibiotic-producing actinomycetes and in Gram-negative bacteria. Order and orientation of genes in the following gene clusters are compared: *str/sts* cluster of *S. glaucescens* (1) and of *S. griseus* (2), *sno* cluster of amphotericin B–producing *S. nodosus* (3), *tyl* cluster of tylosin-producing *S. fradiae* (4), *rfb* cluster for LPS O-chain biosynthesis from *Salmonella enterica* type B (5), and *lmb/lmr* cluster of lincomycin-producing *S. lincolnensis* (6). Families of structurally and functionally related genes/enzymes are indicated by different shading (see code below; cf. Table 6). The genes framed by a broken line encode functionally identical enzymes that form subfamilies more closely related in primary structures in a taxon-independent manner. Other framed gene pairs are known or believed to encode enzymes with identical or closely related functions.

highly variable gene clusters for LPS O-chain synthesis in different biovars of *Salmonella* and other enterobacteria (13,116). In the latter case, the existence of pairwise-related genes encoding nonidentical functions, namely, the CDP-glucose specific counterparts of RfbA and RfbB, the enzymes RfbF and RfbG, are also found to be encoded by the same transcription unit (cf. Table 6 and Figure 46). Again, in the *str/sts* cluster of *S. glaucescens*, a CDP-glucose synthase is encoded by the *rfbF*-related gene *strQ* (cf. Figures 28 and 29; Table 3).

    2.   Gene duplication clearly was the initial step in the divergent evolution of the aminotransferases of the SMAT family toward the dehydroxylases using pyridoxamine phosphate as a coenzyme and containing an iron-sulfur cluster in addition (cf. Figure 36) (13). The divergence from the related aminotransferases probably arose via mutation of the codon for the conserved lysine residue to a histidine codon, and by insertion of a short DNA sequence with four cysteine codons (cf. Figure 37). However, the sequence distances between the members of the SMAT group of enzymes described until now do not yet allow calculation of an unambiguous tree that more closely relates the

AscC/RfbH-type dehydroxylases to any of the other sequences (for an alignment, see Ref. 11). For instance, the protein similarities between StrS, StsA, and StsC are in the range of 25% sequence identity and, therefore, are too low to suggest gene duplication events as being responsible for their occurence during the evolution of the streptomycin pathway.

3.   An evolutionarily younger example could be found in the enzyme family of amidinotransferases (cf. Table 3), rare enzymes, two of which are encoded by the *strB1* and *strB2* genes in the streptomycin biosynthetic gene clusters (cf. Figures 28 and 29). In contrast, only the *strB1*-equivalent genes, obvious by position and sequence, are present in the respective clusters of bluensomycin producers (cf. Figures 28 and 29) (9,208). Although the region between the genes *strN* and *strM*, which also are adjacent to each other in *S. bluensis,* has not yet been sequenced, a *strB2* gene seems to be lacking based on extensive hybridization studies (cf. Figure 28) (208). An interesting related outgroup enzyme, the glycyl amidinotransferase from rat, has been characterized recently by genetic analysis (256), which allows the calculation of a tree with surprising features (Figure 47). The StrB2-encoding genes in *S. griseus* and *S. glaucescens,* which have been assumed to be derived from the *strB1* genes by gene duplication and rapid divergent evolution in an ancestor of a streptomycin-producing strain (9), seem to be slightly closer to the rat glycyl amidinotransferase. Therefore, the deeper rooting branch point between the StrB2 proteins also could mean that these enzymes are the older ones, and that the close relationships of the StrB1 sequences to each other just reflects their more recent divergence. However, there are several conflicting arguments against both of these hypotheses, such that even an independent invasion of *strB1* and *strB2* genes in the respective production gene clusters could be imagined. Thus, the true evolutionary pathway for the development of these biosynthetic enzymes has to await further clarification based on the discovery of indicative "missing links" in the future.

The conclusion can be drawn that the gene pool from which the biochemical tools for ACAGA production pathways are derived seems to be a highly fluid one, in the sense of being frequently recombined and horizontally disseminated in all prokaryotes, and perhaps in all living organisms. This only can be explained if the gene pool for "secondary carbohydrate" metabolism is subject to continuous selective pressure and if special mechanisms responsible for its mobility have been developed. Specialized transduction or other types of lateral gene transfer have been proposed as responsible for the hot spot–like recombinational activity associated with the *rfb* locus in enterobacteria (116,257). The apparently high mobility of the respective gene pool in streptomycetes could be explained by similar mechanisms in connection, with the strong genomic instabilities associated with the occurence of large (up to 1 Mbp and longer) unstable segments at the ends of linear chromosomes (258–260). The *str/sts* cluster of *S. glaucescens* ETH 22794 was already demonstrated to lie in such an unstable chromosomal region (larger than 1 Mbp) (261).

In summary, the early ACAGA producers obviously followed chaotic trial-and-error approaches in inventing new pathways toward very similar biochemical solutions of probably a common physiological problem. However, they did so by means of a limited number of biochemical tools. Thus, the natural compounds treated in this chapter can be regarded as the results of a directed biochemical evolution. However, the route on which these results were reached obviously was of minor importance and could follow alternative solutions. The easiest explanation for this phenomenon could be that the need for production of ACAGAs and related compounds predated the invention of their now-existing biosynthetic pathways, as is the case for amino acids and nucleotides. Also, the

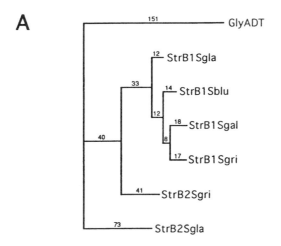

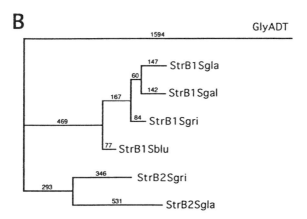

Figure 47   Protein sequence relatedness in streptomycete and mammalian amidinotransferases. Trees have been calculated by the maximum parsimony method (program PAUP 3.1.1) by using the rat L-arginine:glycine amidinotransferase (GlyADT) sequence as an outgroup. (A) Unweighted tree; (B) tree calculated when residues differentially conserved in the StrB1 and StrB2 subfamilies were weighted by a factor of 10. Aligned sequences of aminocyclitol amidinotransferases 1 and 2 (StrB1, 2) were from *S. griseus* (Sgri), *S. glaucescens* (Sgla), *S. galbus* (Sgal), and *S. bluensis* (Sblu).

selective pressure probably was not only aimed to form a particular ligand for a given target site, but also toward a multiplicity of alternative end products with similar, but nonoverlapping, modes of action in taxonomically closely related species or subspecies. This urges the conclusion that the creation of a diversity of ACAGAs was of major selective advantage, for example, to escape specific protection mechanisms or for better distinction in communication processes (see above). In this context, the hypothesis that ACAGAs are "molecular fossils" having had essential functions as ligands or cocatalysts in earlier phases of biochemical evolution, most probably in a primordial RNA world, is still compelling (232). But the selective forces that drove the formation of the recent biosynthetic pathways for ACAGAs must be of quite different and even more individualized (i.e., cell-line-specific) nature, because their specific effects obviously are of value for a limited number of bacterial strains only.

The occurrence of ACAGA-like and highly modified glycosidic or cyclitol-containing products as constituents in many pro- and eukaryotic extracellular polymers, such as cell wall materials (peptidoglycan or pseudomurein), polysaccharides, lipopolysaccharides, glycolipids, and other glycoconjugates, could mean that they have a common evolutionary origin. Maybe, the respective pathways were all developed originally in Gram-negative unicellular bacteria, if these turn out to be the earliest forms of cellular life (cf. Section II) (262,263). The few indications that have been found for the biosynthesis and secretion of carbohydrate-based diffusible substances in Gram-negatives, for example, the sorbistins in pseudomonads (see Section III.E), and the rhizopine *N*-methyl-*scyllo*-inosamine or the Nod-factors from rhizobia (18–20), could mean that these are early oligomeric descendants from originally polysaccharidic substances. The trend to produce low-molecular-weight secondary carbohydrates could have been enforced, for example, (a) with the acquisition of strong developmental cell cycles and differentiation patterns, for example, in the myxobacteria that are also rich in antibiotic production (264); (b) with loss of the outer membrane in the development of the Gram-positive bacterial branch, leading to the differentiating bacilli and actinomycetes; or (c) with the engagement in strong symbiotic or competitive links in association with other cells (e.g., as the rhizobia or the *Frankia* sp.), especially when cells become sessile in particular ecological niches (249). The same general tendency in evolutionary processes could possibly have led also to other metabolites such as secondary peptides, polyketides, nucleosides, alkaloids, and isoprenoids.

VIII. APPLICATION IN BIOTECHNOLOGY

Every biotechnological approach starts with basic research, which in the case of secondary metabolites of the ACAGA class is not as advanced as with many other useful metabolites. Some of the reasons have already been mentioned (see Sections I, II, and IV.G). Our lack of knowledge concerning the biochemistry of the biosynthetic pathways and their regulation exerts a particularly hindering effect and asks for intensified basic research to provide the necessary data for straightforward biotechnological approaches. Various applications of the newly gained data and methodology in biotechnology can be envisaged also in the field of ACAGA development and production, or—in a broader sense—of secondary carbohydrates. These are (a) new rational screening systems, (b) improvement of production strains and fermentation conditions, (c) transfer of production capacities to desired hosts, or (d) hybrid pathway construction by genetic engineering and, ultimately, various levels of further pathway engineering (11).

Genetic screening, for example, by use of pathway-specific gene probes and accompanying the classical biological and biochemical (target-oriented) screening methods, could facilitate and speed the sorting out of wanted and unwanted production capabilities largely without time-consuming isolation and characterization of products. The example of the 6DOH components has already proven very successful (17). The new accessibility of ACAGA structures via new targets of screening, such as the α-glucosidase inhibitors (26,27,265), proved already to be successful with the first substances coming to the market in the treatment of diabetes. Improvement of production yields or saving production costs by more efficient nutrient turnover are further goals that could be sought via rational pathway design. Among the possible strategies, the enhancement of gene doses and/or metabolite fluxes by deregulation or activation are the first and, probably, most efficient ones. Such effects may already be selectable by indirect methods, such as selection for enhanced resistance (266). The transfer of the genetic complement for complete pathways to, and their redesigned regulation in, new host systems for improved production characteristics is an alternative. Because of the placement of ACAGA pathways in complex cell differentiation cycles, this would be especially important when continuous culture techniques should have an advantage in industrial production. Therefore, to learn more about the regulatory mechanisms probably will be a central topic when this kind of pathway engineering is the target in future development.

One of the major goals at present is the biosynthesis of new secondary metabolites by rationally designed hybrid pathways (11,120,267–269). Progress in this field especially has been made with the polyketides, since these are molecules basically made via a process of programmed oligomerization of uniform extender units on a multienzyme complex with well-conserved functional domains or subunits (120,267–269). In contrast, the ACAGA pathways are based on monofunctional enzymes that are products of individual genes and are quite variable in design (see Section V). Also, the biochemistry and chemistry of carbohydrates are complicated, and the intermediates of biosynthetic pathways are mostly quite unstable and inaccessible to synthetic chemistry. Therefore, generally applicable strategies cannot be given as easily, and all possible routes have to be tested separately.

A first target for pathway engineering in the classical antibacterial ACAGAs could be the biological production of the clinically successful semisynthetic derivatives, such as amikacin or the members of the dibekacin/arbekacin family (cf. Figure 27). This approach might be successful, since the chemical modifications were designed in analogy to biochemical modifications naturally occurring in related ACAGA families (see Section III.G). The production in vivo of amikacin by a genetically engineered strain of either the kanamycin A producer S. kanamyceticus or the butirosin producer Bacillus circulans had already been proposed at the beginnings of streptomycete molecular genetics (11,24). The first strategy would imply the transfer of the genes for the biosynthesis and the condensing step of the N^1-α-hydroxy-γ-aminobutyryl unit from B. circulans to a developed strain of S. kanamyceticus. Amikacin was already successfully produced in vivo, though in very low amounts, in a 2DOS-deficient strain of a butirosin producer after feeding kanamycin A (270). Thus, the more complicated transfer of the kanamycin or tobramycin production genes from streptomycetes to B. circulans could also be tried. New bottlenecks in designed pathways like these could become the substrate specificities of the condensing enzymes or of the putative membrane-bound exporters. In our example, the N^1-α-hydroxy-γ-aminobutyryltransferase has to recognize the kanamycin A molecule, and the kanamycin (or butirosin) exporter complex has to accept the hybrid end product as a substrate. Transfer of the genes for the transferases of other types of functional groups, such as the amidino-, carbamoyl-, glycyl-, forimidoyl-, and β-lysyltransferases (cf. Section V.C), among various producers of ACAGAs could also result in interesting new compounds.

The designed mixing of the subpathways for ACAGA subunits could be envisaged as well. For instance, the **Cb** pathways could be exchanged against **Ca** routes, and vice versa. In another line of experimental models, the exchange of the sugar-modifying and -transferring subpathways between producers of related groups of aminoglycosides could be tried, for example, the **PA** pathways between the producers of gentamicins (cf. Figure 11) and seldomycins (cf. Figure 12), or the **6DOH** or **HA** pathways between the producers of streptomycins (cf. Figure 1), spectinomycins (cf. Figure 3), kasugamycins (cf. Figure 4), and boholmycin (cf. Figure 7). Again, the transferases and exporter systems may be limiting in this type of approach. That glycosyltransferases can have adaptable substrate recognition profiles was shown in an elloramycin producer that yielded a glycosylated tetracenomycin after being transformed with the tetracenomycin production genes (271). The genetic and biochemical tools for the production of activated and modified sugar intermediates could be used in the development of biotransformation systems for the in vivo glycosylation of alternative aglycones or for the in vitro enzymatic glycosyltransfer to synthetic aglycones (113).

IX. CONCLUSIONS AND PERSPECTIVE

The group of bacterial secondary metabolites containing amino-nitrogen and (amino-)-cyclitols (ACAGAs) as an aglycone does not represent an isolated metabolic trait of secondary metabolism. Rather, they are one particular class of products of a versatile, ubiquitous secondary carbohydrate metabolism. Our knowledge of the range of natural chemical variants of ACAGAs is probably not complete at present. The investigation of their genetics and of the regulation of the biosynthetic routes is still in its infancy. Accumulating evidence, however, is presented for several common basic features in the productive pathways for ACAGAs and for the use of a common gene pool that can be employed for the modular redesign of these pathways in future. The currently accumulating data from research on these compounds have already influenced the research and development of other carbohydrate-containing groups of low-molecular-weight bioactive molecules, as well as of polysaccharides and glycoconjugates. Also, progress in the field of chemoenzymatic synthesis via providing the biochemical tools, such as enzymes and their substrates (e.g., NDP-activated sugars), is on the horizon. Other fields of application and new structures of ACAGA-related compounds will be accessible by continuing research efforts. It is, therefore, probably not too exaggerated to speculate that the ACAGA group of secondary carbohydrates will also come to be of interest for the development of new pharmaceuticals. Last but not least, emphasis on the importance of these fantastic natural products in basic molecular biological research justifies continuing interest in the biology and evolutionary background of their production.

REFERENCES

1. Umezawa S, Kondo S, Ito Y. Aminoglycoside antibiotics. Rehm H-J, Reed G, eds. Biotechnology, vol. 4. Weinheim: VCH Verlagsgesellschaft, 1986: 309–357.
2. Shapiro S. Regulation of Secondary Metabolism in Actinomycetes. Boca Raton, Florida: CRC Press, 1989.
3. Cundliffe E. How antibiotic-producing organisms avoid suicide. Annu Rev Microbiol 1989; 43:207–233.
4. Mansouri K, Pissowotzki K, Distler J, Mayer G, Heinzel P, Braun C, Ebert A, Piepersberg W. Genetics of streptomycin production. Hershberger CL, Queener SW, Hegeman G, eds. Genetics and Molecular Biology of Industrial Microorganisms. Washington D.C.: American Society for Microbiology, 1989:61–67.
5. Floss HG, Beale JM. Investigation of the biosynthesis of antibiotics. Angew Chem Int Ed 1989; 28:146–177.
6. Distler J, Mansouri K, Mayer G, Stockmann M, Piepersberg W. Streptomycin production and its regulation. Gene 1992; 115:105–111.
7. Hasegawa M. A novel, highly efficient gene-cloning system in Micromonospora applied to the genetic analysis of fortimicin biosynthesis. Gene 1992; 115:85–91.

8. Rinehart KL Jr, Snyder WC, Staley AL, Lau RCM. Biosynthestic studies on antibiotics. Petroski RJ, McCormick SP, eds. Secondary-Metabolite Biosynthesis and Metabolism. New York: Plenum Press, 1992:41–60.

9. Retzlaff L, Mayer G, Beyer S, Ahlert J, Verseck S, Distler J, Piepersberg W. Streptomycin production in Streptomycetes: A progress report. Hegeman GD, Baltz RH, Skatrud PL, eds. Industrial Microorganisms: Basic and Applied Molecular Genetics. Washington D.C.: American Society for Microbiology, 1993:183–194.

10. Piepersberg W. Streptomycin and related aminoglycosides. Vining L, Stuttard C, eds. Biochemistry and Genetics of Antibiotic Biosynthesis. Boston: Butterworth-Heinemann, 1995:531–570.

11. Piepersberg W. Pathway engineering in secondary metabolite-producing actinomycetes. Crit Rev Biotechnol 1994; 14:251–285.

12. Hotta K, Davies J, Yagisawa M. Aminoglycosides and aminocyclitols (other than streptomycin). Vining L, Stuttard C, eds. Biochemistry and Genetics of Antibiotic Biosynthesis Stoneham: Butterworth-Heinemann, 1994:571–595.

13. Liu H-W, Thorson JS. Pathways and mechanisms in the biogenesis of novel deoxysugars by bacteria. Annu Rev Microbiol 1994; 48:223–256.

14. Horinouchi S, Beppu T. A-factor as a microbial hormone that controls cellular differentiation and secondary metabolism in Streptomyces griseus. Mol Microbiol 1994; 12:859–864.

15. Umezawa H, Hooper IR. Aminoglycoside Antibiotics. Berlin: Springer-Verlag, 1982.

16. Numata K, Yamamoto H, Hatori M, Miyaki T, Kawaguchi H. Isolation of an aminoglycoside hypersensitive mutant and its application in screening. J Antibiot 1986; 39:994–1000.

17. Stockmann M, Piepersberg W. Gene probes for the detection of 6-deoxyhexose metabolism in secondary metabolite-producing streptomycetes. FEMS Microbiol Lett 1992; 90:185–190.

18. Denarie J, Cullimore C. Lipo-oligosaccharide nodulation factors: A new class of signaling molecules mediating recognition and morphogenesis. Cell 1993; 74:951–954.

19. Murphy PJ, Heycke N, Banfalvi Z, Tate ME, de Brujin F, Kondorosi A, Tempe J, Schell J. Genes for the catabolism and synthesis of an opine-like compound in Rhizobium meliloti are closely linked and on the Sym plasmid. Proc Natl Acad Sci USA 1987; 84:493–497.

20. Murphy PJ, Trenz SP, Grzemski W, De Bruijn FJ, Schell J. The Rhizobium meliloti rhizopine mos locus is a mosaic structure facilitating its symbiotic regulation. J Bacteriol 1993; 175:5193–5204.

21. Koga Y, Nishihara M, Morii H, Akagawa-Matsushita M. Ether lipids of methanogenic bacteria: Structures, comperative aspects, and biosynthesis. Microbiol Rev 1993; 57:164–182.

22. Englund PT. The structure and biosynthesis of glycosyl phosphatidylinositiol protein anchors. Annu Rev Biochem 1993; 62:112–138.

23. Rinehart KL Jr, Suami T. Aminocyclitol Antibiotics, ACS Symposium Series 125. Washington D.C.: American Chemical Society, 1980.

24. Davies J, Yagisawa M. The aminocyclitol glycosides (aminoglycosides). Vining LC, ed. Biochemistry and Genetic Regulation of Commercially Important Antibiotics. London: Addison-Wesley, 1983:311–354.

25. Davis BD. Mechanism of bactericidal action of aminoglycosides. Microbiol Rev 1987; 51:341–350.

26. Truscheit E, Frommer W, Junge B, Müller L, Schmidt DD, Wingeder W. Chemistry and biochemistry of bacterial alpha-glucosidase inhibitors. Angew Chem Int Ed 1981; 20:744–761.

27. Müller L. Chemistry, biochemistry and therapeutic potential of microbial α-glucosidase inhibitors. Demain AL, Somkuti GA, Hunter-Creva JC, Rossmoore HW, eds. Novel Microbial Products for Medicine and Agriculture. Amsterdam: Elsevier Science Publishers, 1989:109–116.

28. Piepersberg W, Distler J. Aminoglycosides and sugar components in other secondary metabolites. Rehm H-J, Reed G, Pühler A, Stadler P, eds. Biotechnology, 2nd ed., Vol. 7, Products of Secondary Metabolism. Weinheim: VCH, 1997 (in press).

29. Reden J, Dürkheimer W. Aminoglycoside antibiotics. Chemistry, biochemistry, structure-activity relationships. Top Curr Chem 1979; 83:106–170.

30. Tohma S, Kondo H, Yokotsuga J, Iwamoto J, Matsuhashi G, Ito T. Ashimycins A and B, new streptomycin analogues. J Antibiot 1989; 42:1205–1212.

31. Awata M, Muto N, Hayashi M, Yaginuma S. A new aminoglycoside antibiotic, substance AC4437. J Antibiot 1986; 39:724–726.

32. Ikeda Y, Gomi S, Yokose K, Naganawa H, Ikeda T, Manabe M, Hamada M, Kondo S, Umezawa H. A new streptomycin group antibiotic produced by Streptomyces sioyaensis. J Antibiot 1985; 38:1803–1805.

33. Kondo S, Ikeda Y, Ikeda T, Gomi S, Naganawa H, Hamada M, Umezawa H. 5'-Hydroxy-2"-N-demethyldihydrostreptomycin produced by a Streptomyces. J Antibiot 1985; 38:433–435.

34. Karwowski JP, Jackson M, Bobik TA, Prokop JF, Theriault RJ. Spenolimycin, a new spectinomycin-type antibiotic. I. Discovery, taxonomy and fermentation. J Antibiot 1984; 37:1513–1518.

35. Saitoh K, Tsunakawa M, Tomita K, Miaki T, Konishi M, Kawaguchi H. Boholmycin, a new aminoglycoside antibiotic. I. Production, isolation and properties. J Antibiot 1988; 41:855–861.

36. Pearce CJ, Rinehart KL Jr. Biosynthesis of aminocyclitol antibiotics. Corcoran JW, ed. Antibiotics, Vol. 4, Biosynthesis. Berlin: Springer-Verlag, 1981:74–100.

37. Kase H, Odakura Y, Takazawa Y, Kitamura S, Nakayama K. Biosynthesis of sagamicicn and related aminoglycosides. Umezawa H, Demain AL, Hata T, Hutchinson CR, eds. Trends in Antibiotic Research. Genetics, Biosyntheses, Actions, and New Substances. Tokyo: Japan Antibiotics Research Association, 1982:195–212.

38. Okuda T, Ito Y. Biosynthesis and mutasynthesis of aminoglycoside antibiotics. Umezawa H, Hooper IR, eds. Aminoglycoside Antibiotics. Berlin: Springer-Verlag, 1982:111–203.

39. Tsunakawa M, Hanada M, Tsukiura H, Konishi M, Kawaguchi H. Inosamycin, a complex of new aminoglycoside antibiotics. II. Structure determination. J Antibiot 1985; 38:745–751.

40. Kamiya K, Deushi T, Iwasaki A, Watanabe I, Itoh H, Mori T. A new aminoglycoside antibiotic, KA-5685. J Antibiot 1983; 36:738–741.

41. Ikeda Y, Kondo S, Kanai F, Sawa T, Hamada M, Takeuchi T, Umezawa H. A new destomycin-family antibiotic produced by Saccharopolyspora hirsuta. J Antibiot 1985; 38:436–438.

42. Hotta K, Morioka M, Okami Y. Biosynthetic similarity between Streptomyces tenjimariensis and Micromonospora olivasterospora which produce fortimicin-group antibiotics. J Antibiot 1989; 42:745–751.

43. Kondo S, Horiuchi Y, Ikeda D, Gomi S, Hotta K, Okami Y, Umezawa H. 2"-N-Formimidoylistamycin A and B produced by Streptomyces tenjimariensis. J Antibiot 1982; 35:1104–1106.

44. Umezawa H, Gomi S, Yamagishi Y, Obata T, Ikeda T, Hamada M, Kondo S. 2"-N-Formimidoylsporaricin A produced by Saccharopolyspora hirsuta subsp. kobensis. J Antibiot 1987; 40:91–93.

45. Jackson M, Karwowski P, Sinclair AC. Abstracts of the 21st Interscience Conference on Antimicrobial Agents and Chemotherapy. Washington D.C.: American Society for Microbiology, 1981, Abstract 183.

46. Asano N, Kameda Y, Matsui K, Horii S, Fukase H. Validamycin H, a new pseudo-tetrasaccharide antibiotic. J Antibiot 1990; 43:1039–1041.

47. Numata K, Satoh F, Hatori M, Miyaki T, Kawaguchi H. Isolation of 3,3'-neotrehalosadiamine (BMY-28251) from a butirosin-producing organism. J Antibiot 1986; 39:1346–1348.

48. Tsuno T, Ikeda C, Numata K-I, Tomita K, Konishi M, Kawaguchi H. 3,3'-Neotrehalosadiamine (BMY-28251), a new aminosugar antibiotic. J Antibiot 1986; 39:1001–1003.

49. Hardick DJ, Hutchinson DW, Trew SJ, Wellington EMH. Glucose is a precursor of 1-deoxynojirimycin and 1-deoxymannonojirimycin in Streptomyces subrutilus. Tetrahedron 1992; 48:6285–6296.

50. Sakuda S, Isogai A, Matsumoto S, Suzuki A. Search for microbial insect growth regulators. II. Allosamidin, a novel insect chitinase inhibitor. J Antibiot 1987; 40:296–300.

51. Ando O, Satake H, Itoi K, Sato A, Nakajima M, Takahashi S, Haruyama H, Ohkuma Y, Kinoshita T, Enokita R. Trehazolin, a new trehalase inhibitor. J Antibiot 1991; 44:1165–1168.

52. Kobayashi Y, Shiozaki M. Synthesis of trehazolin β-anomer. J Antibiot 1994; 47:243–246.

53. Zhou Z-Y, Sakuda S, Kinoshita M, Yamada Y. Biosynthetic studies of allosamidin. 2. Isolation of didemethylallosamidin, and conversion experiments of ^{14}C-labeled demethylallosamidin, didemethylallosamidin and their related compounds. J Antibiot 1993; 46:1582–1588.

54. Zhou Z-Y, Sakuda S, Yamada Y. Biosynthetic studies on the chitinase inhibitor, allosamidin. Origin of the carbon and nitrogen atoms. J Chem Soc Perkin Trans I 1992; 1992:649–1652.

55. Asano N, Katayama K, Takeuchi M, Furumoto T, Kameda Y, Matsui K. Preparation of 3-amino-3-deoxy derivatives of trehalose and sucrose and their activities. J Antibiot 1989; 42:585–590.

56. Sipos L, Szabo G. Myo-inosotol-1-phosphate synthase in different *Streptomyces griseus* variants. FEMS Microbiol Lett 1989; 65:339–344.

57. Mansouri K, Piepersberg W. Genetics of streptomycin production in *Streptomyces griseus*: Nucleotide sequence of five genes, *strFGHIK*, including a phosphatase gene. Mol Gen Genet 1991; 228:459–469.

58. Pissowotzki K, Mansouri K, Piepersberg W. Genetics of streptomycin production in *Streptomyces griseus*. Molecular structure and putative function of genes *strELMB2N*. Mol Gen Genet 1991; 231:113–123.

59. Distler J, Ebert A, Mansouri K, Pissowotzki K, Stockmann M, Piepersberg W. Gene cluster for streptomycin biosynthesis in *Streptomyces griseus*: Nucleotide sequence of three genes and analysis of transcriptional activity. Nucl Acids Res 1987; 15:8041–8056.

60. Walker JB. Pathways of the guanidinated inositol moieties of streptomycin and bluensomycin. Meth Enzymol 1975; 43:429–470.

61. Beyer S. Molekularbiologische Untersuchungen zur Biosynthese von 5′-Hydroxystreptomycin in *Streptomyces glaucescens* GLA.0. PhD Thesis (Dissertation), Bergische Universitaet GH Wuppertal, 1996.

62. Beyer S, Distler J, Piepersberg W. The *str* gene cluster for the biosynthesis of 5′-hydroxystreptomycin in *Streptomyces glaucescens* GLA.0 (ETH 22794): New operons and evidence for pathway-specific regulation by StrR. Mol Gen Genet 1996; 250:775–784.

63. Heinzel P, Werbitzky O, Distler J, Piepersberg W. A second streptomycin resistance gene from *Streptomyces griseus* codes for streptomycin-3″-phosphotransferase. Relationship between antibiotic and protein kinases. Arch Microbiol 1988; 150:184–192.

64. Distler J, Mayer G, Piepersberg W. Regulation of biosynthesis of streptomycin. Heslot H, Davies J, Florent J, Bobichon L, Durand G, Penasse L, eds. Proceedings of GIM '90, Vol. 1. Paris: Sociécté Française de Microbiologie, 1990:379–392.

65. Ahlert J. Molekularbiologische Untersuchungen zur Biosynthese von Streptomycin in *Streptomyces griseus* N2-3-11: Identifizierung und Expression einer L-Glutamin::*scyllo*- Inosose Aminotransferase. PhD Thesis (Dissertation), Bergische Universitaet GH Wuppertal, 1996.

66. Rinehart KL Jr, Stroshane RM. Biosynthesis of aminocyclitol antibiotics. J Antibiot 1976; 29:319–353.

67. Grisebach H. Biosynthesis of sugar components of antibiotic substances. Adv Carbohydr Chem Biochem 1978; 35:81–126.

68. Walker JB. ATP:streptomycin 6-phosphotransferase. Meth Enzymol 1975; 43:628–632.

69. Walker JB, Walker, MS. ATP:streptomycin 3″-phosphotransferase. Meth Enzymol 1975; 43:632–634.

70. Distler J, Piepersberg W. Cloning and characterization of a gene from *Streptomyces griseus* coding for a streptomycin-phosphorylating activity. FEMS Microbiol Lett 1985; 28:113–117.

71. Distler J, Braun C, Ebert A, Piepersberg W. Gene cluster for streptomycin biosynthesis in *Streptomyces griseus*: Analysis of a central region including the major resistance gene. Mol Gen Genet 1987; 208:204–210.

72. Distler J, Klier K, Piendl W, Werbitzki O, Böck A, Kresze G, Piepersberg W. Streptomycin biosynthesis in *Streptomyces griseus*. I. Characterization of streptomycin-idiotrophic mutants. FEMS Microbiol Lett 1985; 30:145–150.

73. Ohnuki T, Imanaka T, Aiba S. Self-cloning in *Streptomyces griseus* of an *str* gene cluster for streptomycin biosynthesis and streptomycin resistance. J Bacteriol 1985; 164:85–94.

74. Ohnuki T, Imanaka T, Aiba S. Isolation of streptomycin non-producing mutants deficient in biosynthesis of the streptidine moiety or linkage between streptidine-6-phosphate and dihydrostreptose. Antimicrob Agents Chemother 1985; 27:367–374.

75. Walker JB. Possible evolutionary relationships between streptomycin and bluensomycin biosynthetic pathways: Detection of novel inositol kinase and O-carbamoyltransferase activities. J Bacteriol 1990; 172:5844–5851.

76. Dairi T, Ohta T, Hashimoto E, Hasegawa M. Organization and nature of fortimicin A (astromicin) biosynthetic genes studied using a cosmid library of *Micromonospora olivasterospora* DNA. Mol Gen Genet 1992; 236:39–48.

77. Dairi T, Yamaguchi K, Hasegawa M. N-formimidoyl fortimicin A synthase, a unique oxidase involved in fortimicin A biosynthesis: Purification, characterization and gene cloning. Mol Gen Genet 1992; 236:49–59.

78. Ohta T, Dairi T, Hashimoto E, Hasegawa M. Use of a heterologous gene for molecular breeding of actinomycetes producing structurally related antibiotics: Self-defense genes of producers of fortimicin-A (astromicin)-group antibiotics. Actinomycetol 1993; 7:145–155.

79. Dairi T, Ohta T, Hashimoto E, Hasegawa M. Self cloning in *Micromonospora olivasterospora* of *fms* genes for fortimicin A (astromicin) biosynthesis. Mol Gen Genet 1992; 232:270.

80. Ohta T, Hashimoto E, Hasegawa M. Cloning and analysis of a gene (*sms 13*) encoding sannamycin B-glycyltransferase from *Streptomyces sannanensis* and its distribution among actinomycetes. J. Antibiot 1992; 45:1167–1175.

81. Ohta T, Hasegawa M. Analysis of the self-defense gene (*fmrO*) of a fortimicin A (astromicin) producer, *Micomonospora olivasterospora*: Comparison with other aminoglycoside-resistance-encoding genes. Gene 1993; 127:63–69.

82. Holmes DJ, Drocourt D, Tiraby G, Cundliffe E. Cloning of an aminoglycoside-resistance-encoding gene, *kamC*, from *Saccharopolyspora hirsuta*: Comparicon with *kamB* from *Streptomyces tenebrarius*. Gene 1991; 102:19–26.

83. Ohta T, Hasegawa M. Analysis of the nucleotide sequence of *fmrT* encoding the self-defense gene of the istamycin producer, *Streptomyces tenjimariensis* ATCC 31602; comparison with the sequences of *kamB* of *Streptomyces tenebrarius* NCIB 11028 and *kamC* of *Saccharopolyspora hirsuta* CL102. J Antibiot 1993; 46:511–517.

84. Ohta T, Hashimoto E, Hasegawa M. Characterization of sannamycin A–nonproducing mutants of *Streptomyces sannanensis*. J Antibiot 1992; 45:289–291.

85. Ohta T, Dairi T, Hasegawa M. Characterization of two different types of resistance genes among producers of fortimicin-group antibiotics. J Gen Microbiol 1993; 139:591–599.

86. Hasegawa, M. A gene cloning system in *Micromonospora* which revealed the organization of biosynthetic genes of fortimicin A (astromicin). Actinomycetol 1991; 5:126–131.

87. Itoh S, Odakura Y, Kase H, Satho S, Takahashi K, Iida T, Shirahata K, Nakayama K. Biosynthesis of astromicin and related antibiotics. I. Biosynthetic studies by bioconversion experiments. J Antibiot 1984; 37:1664–1669.

88. Odakura Y, Kase H, Itoh S, Satho S, Takasawa S, Takahashi K, Shirahata K, Nakayama K. Biosynthesis of astromicin and related antibiotics. II. Biosynthetic studies with blocked mutants of *Micromonospora olivasteropora*. J Antibiot 1984; 37:1670–1680.

89. Dairi T, Hasegawa M. Common biosynthetic feature of fortimicin-group antibiotics. J Antibiot 1989; 42:934–943.

90. Hotta K, Morioka M, Tohyama H, Okami Y. Biosynthesis of istamycins by *Streptomyces tenjimariensis*. Koyama Y, ed. Trends in Actinomycetology in Japan. Tokyo: Society for Actinomycetes Japan, 1989:61–64.

91. Salauze D, Pérez-González JA, Piepersberg W, Davies J. Characterization of aminoglycoside acetyltransferase-encoding genes of neomycin-producing *Micromonospora chalcea* and *Streptomyces fradiae*. Gene 1991; 101:143–148.

92. Pérez-González JA, Jiménez A. Cloning and expression in *Streptomyces lividans* of a paromomycin phosphotransferase gene from *Streptomyces rimosus* forma *paromomycinus*. Biochem Biophys Res Commun 1984; 125:895–901.

93. López-Cabrera M, Pérez-González JA, Heinzel P, Piepersberg W, Jiménez A. Isolation and nucleotide sequencing of an aminocyclitol acetyltransferase gene from *Streptomyces rimosus* forma *paromomycinus*. J Bacteriol 1989; 171:321–328.

94. Cundliffe E. Self-protection mechanisms in antibiotic producers. Davies J, Chadwick D, Whelan J, Widdows K, eds. Secondary Metabolites: Their Function and Evolution, Ciba Foundation Symp. 171. Chichester: John Wiley and Sons, 1992:199–214.

95. Ishikawa J, Hotta K. Nucleotide sequence and transcriptional start point of the *kan* gene encoding an aminoglycoside 3-*N*-acetyltransferase from *Streptomyces griseus*. Gene 1991; 108:127–132.

96. Hotta K, Ogata T, Mizuno S. Secondary aminoglycoside resistance in aminoglycoside-producing strains of *Streptomyces*. Gene 1992; 115:113–117.

97. Thompson CJ, Kieser T, Ward JM, Hopwood DA. Physical analysis of antibiotic-resistance genes from *Streptomyces*: And their use in vector construction. Gene 1982; 20:51–62.

98. Davies J. A new look at antibiotic resistance. FEMS Microbiol Rev 1986; 39:363–371.

99. Etienne G, Armau E, Dassin M, Tiraby G. A screening method to identify antibiotics of the aminoglycoside family. J Antibiot 1991; 44:1357–1366.

100. Crameri R, Davies JE. Increased production of aminoglycosides associated with amplified antibiotic resistance genes. J Antibiot 1986; 39:128–135.

101. Yamauchi N, Kakinuma K. Confirmation of *in vitro* synthesis of 2-deoxy-*scyllo*-inosose, the earliest intermediate in the biosynthesis of 2-deoxystreptamine, using cell free preparations of *Streptomyces fradiae*. J Antibiot 1992; 45:774–780.

102. Yamauchi N, Kakinuma K. Biochemical studies on 2-deoxy-*scyllo*-inosose, an early intermediate in the biosynthesis of 2-deoxystreptamine. VI. A clue to the similarity of 2-deoxy-*scyllo*-inosose synthase to dehydroquinate synthase. J Antibiot 1993; 46:1916–1918.

103. Wong Y-HH, Sherman WR. Anomeric and other substrate specificity studies with *myo*-inositol-1-P synthase. J Biol Chem 1985; 260:11083–11090.

104. Williams ST, Sharpe ME, Holt JG. Systematic Bacteriology, Vol. 4. Baltimore: Williams and Wilkins, 1989.

105. Paltauf F, Kohlwein SD, Henry SA. Regulation and compartmentalization of lipid synthesis in yeast. Jones EW, Pringle JR, Broach JR, eds. The Molecular and Cellular Biology of the Yeast *Saccharomyces*. Gene Expression. New York: Cold Spring Harbor Laboratory Press, 1992:415–500.

106. Widlanski T, Bender SL, Knowles JR. Dehydroquinate synthase: A sheep in wolf's clothing? J Am Chem Soc 1989 111:2299–2300.

107. Goda SK, Akhtar M. Neomycin biosynthesis: The incorporation of D-6-deoxyglucose derivatives and variously labelled glucose into the 2-deoxystreptamine ring. Postulated involvement of 2-deoxyinosose synthase in the biosynthesis. J Antibiot 1992; 45:984–994.

108. Parry RJ, Bornemann V, Subramanian R. Biosynthesis of the nucleoside antibiotic aristeromycin. J Am Chem Soc 1989; 111:5819–5824.

109. Parry RJ. Investigation of the biosynthesis of aristeromycin. Petroski RJ, McCormick SP, eds. Secondary-Metabolite Biosynthesis and Metabolism. New York: Plenum Press, 1992:89–104.

110. Lucher LA, Chen Y-M, Walker JB. Reactions catalyzed by purified L-glutamine:keto-*scyllo*-inositol aminotransferase, an enzyme required for biosynthesis of aminocyclitol antibiotics. Antimicrob Agents Chemother 1989; 33:452–459.

111. Walker JB. Enzymatic synthesis of aminocyclitol moieties of aminoglycoside antibiotics from inositol by *Streptomyces* spp.: Detection of glutamine-aminocyclitol aminotransferase and

diaminocyclitol aminotransferase activities in a spectinomycin producer. J Bacteriol 1995; 177:818–822.

112. Fujita Y, Shindo K, Miwa Y, Yoshida KI. *Bacillus subtilis* inositol dehydrogenase-encoding gene (*idh*): Sequencing and expression in *Escherichia coli*. Gene 1992; 108:121–125.

113. Piepersberg W, Jimenez A, Cundliffe E, Grabley S, Bräu B, Marquardt R. Glycosyltransferases from streptomycetes as tools in biotransformations. Vassarotti A, ed. BRIDGE Progress Report 1994 (CEC). Brussels: Printeclair, 1995:128–133.

114. Merson-Davies, Cundliffe E. Analysis of five tylosin biosynthetic genes from the *tylIBA* region of the *Streptomyces fradiae* genome. Mol Microbiol 1994; 13:349–355.

115. Peschke U, Schmidt H, Zhang H-Z, Piepersberg W. Molecular characterization of the lincomycin production gene cluster of *Streptomyces lincolnensis* 78-11. Mol Microbiol 1995; 16:1137–1156.

116. Reeves P. Evolution of Salmonella O antigen variation by interspecific gene transfer on a large scale. Trends Genet 1993; 9:17–22.

117. Kim CG, Kirschning A, Bergon P, Ahn Y, Wang JJ, Shibuya M, Floss HG. Formation of 3-amino-5-hydroxy-benzoic acid, the precursor of mC7N units in ansamycin antibiotics, by a new variant of the shikimate pathway. J Am Chem Soc 1992; 114:4941–4943.

118. Thorson JS, Liu H-W. Characterization of the first PMP-dependent iron-sulfur-containing enzyme which is essential for the biosynthesis of 3,6-dideoxyhexoses. J Am Chem Soc 1993; 115:7539–7540.

119. Thorson JS, Liu H-W. Coenzyme B_6 as a redox cofactor: A new role for an old coenzyme? J Am Chem Soc 1993; 115:12177–12178.

120. Vining L, Stuttard C. Biochemistry and Genetics of Antibiotic Biosynthesis. Boston: Butterworth-Heinemann, 1994.

121. Takagi M, Takada H, Imanaka T. Nucleotide sequence and cloning in *Bacillus subtilis* of the *Bacillus stearothermophilus* pleiotropic regulatory gene *degT*. J Bacteriol 1990; 172:411–418.

122. Piepersberg W, Distler J, Heinzel P, Perez-Gonzalez J-A. Antibiotic resistance by modification: Many resistance genes could be derived from cellular control genes in actinomycetes.—A hypothesis. Actinomycetol 1988; 2:83–98.

123. Piepersberg W, Heinzel P, Mansouri K, Mönnighoff U, Pissowotzki K. Evolution of antibiotic resistance and production genes in streptomycetes. Baumberg S, Krügel H, Novack D, eds. Genetics and Product Formation in *Streptomyces*. New York: Plenum Press, 1991:161–170.

124. Gabriel O. Biosynthesis of sugar residues for glycogen, peptidoglycan, lipopolysaccharide, and related systems. Neidhardt FC, ed. *Escherichia coli* and *Salmonella typhimurium:* Cellular and Molecular Biology. Washington DC: American Society for Microbiology, 1987:504–511.

125. Shnaitman CA, Klena JD. Genetics of lipopolysaccharide biosynthesis in enteric bacteria. Micobiol Rev 1993; 57:655–682.

126. Verseck S. Klonierung und Expression von bakteriellen Enzymen der Biosynthese von 6-Desoxyhexose-Derivaten und deren Verwendung zur präparativen Herstellung von dTDP-aktivierten Hexosen. PhD Thesis (Dissertation), Bergische Universitaet GH Wuppertal, 1997.

127. Marumo K, Lindquist L, Verma N, Weintraub A, Reeves P, Lindberg AA. Enzymatic synthesis and isolation of thymidine diphosphate-6-deoxy-D-*xylo*-4-hexulose and thymidine diphosphate-L-rhamnose. Eur J Biochem 1992; 204:539–545.

128. Hirose-Kumagai A, Yagita A, Akamatsu N. UDP-*N*-methyl-D-glucosamine-phosphate. A possible intermediate of N-methyl-L-glucosamine moiety of streptomycin. J Antibiot 1982; 35:1571–1577.

129. Thorson JS, Kelly TM, Liu H-W. Cloning, sequencing, and overexpression in *Escherichia coli* of the α-D-glucose-1-phosphate cytidylyltransferase gene isolated from *Yersinia pseudotuberculosis*. J Bacteriol 1994; 176:1840–1849.

130. Kumada Y, Horinouchi S, Uozumi T, Beppu T. Cloning of a streptomycin-production gene directing synthesis of *N*-methyl-L-glucosamine. Gene 1986; 43:221–224.

131. Kagan RM, Clarke S. Widespread occurence of three sequence motifs in divers S-adenosyl-methionine-dependent methyltransferases suggests a common structure for these enzymes. Arch Biochem Biophy 1994; 310:417–427.

132. Tohyama H, Okami Y, Umezawa H. Nucleotide sequence of the streptomycin phospho-transferase and amidinotransferase of *Streptomyces griseus*. Nucl Acids Res 1987; 15:1819–1834.

133. Mayer G, Vögtli M, Pissowotzki K, Hütter R, Piepersberg W. Colinearity of streptomycin production genes in two species of *Streptomyces*. Evidence for occurence of a second amidino-transferase gene. Mol Gen (Life Sci Adv) 1988; 7:83–87.

134. Kniep B, Grisebach H. Biosynthesis of streptomycin. Purification and properties of a dTDP-L-dihydrostreptose:streptidine-6-phosphate dihydrostreptosyltransferase from *Streptomyces griseus*. Eur J Biochem 1980; 105:139–144.

135. Kniep B, Grisebach H. Biosynthesis of streptomycin. Enzymatic formation of dihydrostrepto-mycin 6-phosphate from dihydrostreptosyl streptidine 6-phosphate. J Antibiot 1980; 33:416–419.

136. Hooper IR. The naturally occurring aminoglycoside antibiotics. Umezawa H, Hooper IR, eds. Aminoglycoside Antibiotics. Berlin: Springer-Verlag, 1982:1–35.

137. Inamine E, Demain AL. Mannosidostreptomycin hydrolase. Meth Enzymol 1975; 43:637–640.

138. Cundliffe E. Glycosylation of macrolide antibiotics in extracts of *Streptomyces lividans*. Antimicrob Agents Chemother 1992; 36:348–352.

139. Vilches C, Hernandez C, Mendez C, Salas JA. Role of glycosylation in biosynthesis of and resistance to oleandomycin in the producer organism, *Streptomyces antibioticus*. J Bacteriol 1992; 174:161–165.

140. Piepersberg W, Stockmann M, Mansouri K, Distler J, Grabley S, Sichel P, Bräu B. German Patent Appl P41 30 967—HOE 91/F 300, 1991.

141. Otten SL, Liu X, Ferguson J, Hutchinson CR. Cloning and characterization of the *Streptomyces peucetius dnr*QS genes encoding a daunosamine biosynthesis enzyme and a glycosyl-transferase involved in daunorubicin biosynthesis. J Bacteriol 1995; 177:6688–6692.

142. Dickens ML, Ye J, Strohl WR. Cloning, sequencing and analysis of aklaviketone reductase from *Streptomyces* sp. strain C5. J Bacteriol 1996; 178:3384–3388.

143. Maier S, Grisebach H. Biosynthesis of streptomycin. Enzymic oxidation of dihydrostrepto-mycin (6-phosphate) to streptomycin (6-phosphate) with a particulate fraction of *Streptomyces griseus*. Biochim Biophys Acta 1979; 586:231–241.

144. Higgins CF. ABC transporters: From microorganisms to man. Annu Rev Cell Biol 1992; 8:67–113.

145. Schoner BE, Geistlich M, Rosteck P, Rao RN, Seno ET, Reynolds P, Cox K, Burgett S, Hershberger C. Sequence similarity between macrolide resistance determinants and ATP-binding transport proteins. Gene 1992; 115:93–96.

146. Fath MJ, Kolter R. ABC transporters: Bacterial exporters. Microbiol Rev 1993; 57:995–1017.

147. Aubert-Pivert E, Davies J. Biosynthesis of butirosin in *Bacillus circulans* NRRL B3312: Iden-tification by sequence analysis and insertional mutagenesis of the *butB* gene involved in antibiotic production. Gene 1994; 147:1–11.

148. Walker JB, Skorvaga M. Streptomycin biosynthesis and metabolism. Phosphate transfer from dihydrostreptomycin 6-phosphate to inosamines, streptamine, and 2-deoxystreptamine. J Biol Chem 1973; 248:2435–2440.

149. Davies J, Smith DI. Plasmid-determined resistance to antimicrobial agents. Annu Rev Microbiol 1978; 32:469–518.

150. Foster TJ. Plasmid-determined resistance to antimicrobial drugs and toxic metal ions in bac-teria. Microbiol Rev 1983; 47:361–409.

151. Shaw KJ, Rather PN, Hare RS, Miller GH. Molecular genetics of aminoglycoside resistance genes and familial relationships of the aminoglycoside-modifying enzymes. Microbiol Rev 1993; 57:138–163.

152. Courvalin P, Weisblum B, Davies J. Aminoglycoside-modifying enzyme of an antibiotic-producing bacterium acts as a determinant of antibiotic resistance in *Escherichia coli*. Proc Natl Acad Sci USA 1977; 74:999–1003.

153. Miller AL, Walker JB. Enzymatic phosphorylation of streptomycin by extracts of streptomycin-producing strains of *Streptomyces*. J Bacteriol 1969; 99:401–405.

154. Nimi O, Ito G, Sueda S, Nomi R. Phosphorylation of streptomycin at C6-OH of streptidine moiety by an intracellular enzyme of *Streptomyces griseus*. Agr Biol Chem 1971; 35:848–855.

155. Umezawa H. Biochemical mechanisms of resistance to aminoglycoside antibiotics. Adv Carbohydr Chem Biochem 1974; 30:183–225.

156. Benveniste R, Davies J. Aminoglycoside antibiotic inactivating enzymes in actinomycetes similar to those present in clinical isolates of antibiotic resistant bacteria. Proc Natl Acad Sci USA 1973; 70:2276–2280.

157. Piendl W, Böck A, Cundliffe E. Involvement of 16S ribosomal RNA in resistance of the aminoglycoside-producers *Streptomyces tenjimariensis*, *Streptomyces tenebrarius*, and *Micromonospora purpurea*. Mol Gen Genet 1984; 197:24–29.

158. Courvalin P. Transfer of antibiotic resistance genes between Gram-positive and Gram-negative bacteria. Antimicrob Agents Chemother 1994; 38:1447–1451.

159. Mazodier P, Davies J. Gene transfer between distantly related bacteria. Annu Rev Genet 1991; 25:147–171.

160. Pohlman RF, Genetti HD, Winans SC. Common ancestry between IncN conjugal transfer genes and macromolecular export systems of plant and animal pathogens. Mol Microbiol 1994; 14:655–668.

161. Distler J, Mansouri K, Piepersberg W. Streptomycin biosynthesis in *Streptomyces griseus*. II. Adjacent genomic location of biosynthetic genes and one of two streptomycin resistance genes. FEMS Microbiol Lett 1985; 30:151–154.

162. Hintermann G, Crameri R, Vögtli M, Hütter R. Streptomycin-sensitivity in *Streptomyces glaucescens* is due to deletions comprising the structural gene coding for a specific phosphotransferase. Mol Gen Genet 1984; 196:513–520.

163. Vögtli M, Hütter R. Characterization of the hydroxystreptomycin phosphotransferase gene (*sph*) of *Streptomyces glaucescens*: Nucleotide sequencing and promoter analysis. Mol Gen Genet 1987; 208:195–203.

164. Vara J, Malpartida F, Hopwood DA, Jiménez A. Cloning and expression of a puromycin *N*-acetyl transferase gene from *Streptomyces alboniger* in *Streptomyces lividans* and *Escherichia coli*. Gene 1985; 33:197–206.

165. Lacalle RA, Tercero JA, Jimenez A. Cloning of the complete biosynthetic gene cluster for an aminonucleoside antibiotic, puromycin, and its regulated expression in heterologous hosts. EMBO J 1992; 11:785–792.

166. Knighton DR, Zeng J, TenEyck LF, Ashford VA, Xuong NH, Taylor SS. Crystal structure of the catalytic subunit of cyclic adenosine monophosphate–dependent protein kinase. Science 1991; 253:407–414.

167. Hotta K, Ishikawa J, Ichihara M, Naganawa H, Mizuno S. Mechanism of increased kanamycin-resistance generated by protoplast regeneration of *Streptomyces griseus*. I. Cloning of a gene segment directing a high level of an aminoglycoside 3-*N*-acetyltransferase activity. J Antibiot 1988; 41:94–103.

168. Demain AL. Carbon source regulation of idiolite biosynthesis in actinomycetes. Shapiro S, ed. Regulation of Secondary Metabolism in Actinomycetes. Boca Raton, Florida: CRC Press, 1989:127–134.

169. Satoh A, Ogawa H, Satomura Y. Regulation of *N*-acetylkanamycin amidohydrolase in the idiophase in kanamycin fermentation. Agric Biol Chem 1976; 40:191–196.

170. Chater KF, Bibb MJ. Regulation of bacterial antibiotic production. Rehm H-J, Reed G, Pühler A, Stadler P, eds. Biotechnology, 2nd ed., Vol. 7, Products of Secondary Metabolism. Weinheim: VCH, 1997 (in press).

171. Neumann T, Distler J, Piepersberg W. Decision phase regulation of streptomycin production in *Streptomyces griseus*. Microbiol 1996;142:1953–1963.

172. Holt TG, Chang C, Laurentwinter C, Murakami T, Garrels JI, Davies JE, Thompson CJ. Global change in gene expression related to antibiotic synthesis in *Streptomyces hygroscopicus*. Mol Microbiol 1992; 6:969–980.

173. Chater KF. Genetics of differentiation in *Streptomyces*. Annu Rev Microbiol 1993; 47:685–713.

174. Vining LC, Doull JL. Catabolite repression of secondary metabolism in actinomycetes. Okami Y, Beppu T, Ogawara H, eds. Biology of Actinomycetes '88. Tokyo: Japan Scientific Societies Press, 1988:406–411.

175. Brahme NM, Gonzalez JE, Mizsak S, Rolls JR, Hessler EJ, Hurley LH. Biosynthesis of the lincomycins. 2. Studies using stable isotopes on the biosynthesis of the methylthiolincosaminide moiety of lincomycin A. J Am Chem Soc 1984; 106:7878–7883.

176. Szeszák F, Vitális S, Békési I, Szabó G. Presence of factor C in *Streptomycetes* and other bacteria. Baumberg S, Krügel H, Novack D, eds. Genetics and Product Formation in *Streptomyces*. New York: Plenum Press, 1991:11–18.

177. Ensign JC. Physiological regulation of sporzlation of *Streptomyces griseus*. Okami Y, Beppu T, Ogawara H, eds. Biology of Actinomycetes '88. Tokyo: Japan Scientific Societies Press, 1988:309–315.

178. Penyige A, Vargha G, Ensign JC, Barabás G. The possible role of ADP ribosylation in physiological regulation of sporulation in *Streptomyces griseus*. Gene 1992; 115:181–185.

179. Ochi K, Penyige A, Barabas G. The possible role of ADP-ribosylation in sporulation and streptomycin production by *Streptomyces griseus*. J Gen Microbiol 1992; 138: 1745–1750.

180. Fisher SH. Glutamine synthesis in *Streptomyces*—a review. Gene 1992; 115:13–17.

181. Ragan CM, Vining LC. Intracellular cyclic adenosine 3′,5′-monophosphate levels and streptomycin production in cultures of *Streptomyces griseus*. Can J Microbiol 1978; 24:1012–1015.

182. Lishnevskaya EB, Kuzina ZA, Asinoovskaya NK, Belousova II, Malkov MA, Ravinskaya AY. Cyclic adenosine-3′,5′-monophosphoric acid in *Streptomyces antibioticus* and its possible role in the regulation of oleandomycin biosynthesis and culture growth. Mikrobiologiya 1986; 55:350.

183. Angell S, Schwarz E, Bibb M. The glucose kinase gene of *Streptomyces coelicolor* A3(2): Its nucleotide sequence, transcriptional analysis and role in glucose repression. Mol Microbiol 1992; 6:2833–2844.

184. Kwakman M, Postma W. Glucose kinase has a regulatory role in carbon catabolite repression in *Streptomyces coelicolor*. J Bacteriol 1994; 176:2694–2698.

185. Flores ME, Ponce E, Rubio M, Huitrón C. Glucose and glycerol repression of α-amylase in *Streptomyces kanamyceticus* and isolation of deregulated mutants. Biotech Lett 1993; 15:595–600.

186. Basak K, Majumdar SK. Utilization of carbon and nitrogen sources by *Streptomyces kanamyceticus* for kanamycin production. Antimicrob Agents Chemother 1973; 4:6–11.

187. Liras P, Asturias JA, Martin JF. Phosphate control sequences involoved in transcriptional regulation of antibiotic biosythesis. TIBTECH 1990; 8:184–189.

188. Martin JF. Molecular mechanisms for the control by phosphate of the biosynthesis of antibiotics and other secondary metabolites. Shapiro S, ed. Regulation of Secondary Metabolism in Actinomycetes. Boca Raton, Florida: CRC Press, 1989:213–237.

189. Ochi K. Metabolic initiation of differentiation and secondary metabolism by *Streptomyces griseus*: Significance of the stringent response (ppGpp) and GTP content in relation to A factor. J Bacteriol 1987; 169:3608–3616.

190. Ochi K. Nucleotide pools and stringent response in regulation of *Streptomyces* differentiation. Okami Y, Beppu T, Ogawara H, eds. Biology of Actinomycetes '88. Tokyo: Japan Scientific Societies Press, 1988:330–337.

191. Ochi K. *Streptomyces griseus*, as an excellent object for studing microbial differentiation. Actinomycetol 1990; 4:23–30.

192. Strauch E, Takano E, Baylis HA, Bibb MJ. The stringent response in *Streptomyces coelicolor* A3(2). Mol Microbiol 1991; 5:289–298.

193. Bascaran V, Sanchez L, Hardisson C, Brana AF. Stringent response and initiation of secondary metabolism in *Streptomyces clavuligerus*. J Gen Microbiol 1991; 137:1625–1634.

194. Khokhlov AS, Tovarova II, Borisova LN, Pliner SA, Shevchenko LA, Kornitskaya EY, Ivkina NS, Rapoport IA. A-factor responsible for the biosynthesis of streptomycin by a mutant strain of *Actinomyces streptomycini*. Doklady Akad Nauk SSSR 1967; 177:232–235.

195. Khokhlov AS. Results and perspectives of actinomycete autoregulators studies. Okami Y, Beppu T, Ogawara H, eds. Biology of Actinomycetes '88. Tokyo: Japan Scientific Societies Press, 1988:338–345.

196. Horinouchi S, Beppu T. Regulation of secondary metabolism and cell differentiation in *Streptomyces*: A-factor as a microbial hormone and the AfsR protein as a component of a two-component regulator system. Gene 1992; 115:167–172.

197. Ruengjitchatchawalya M, Nihira T, Yamada Y. Purification and characterization of the IM-2-binding protein from *Streptomyces* sp. strain FRI-5. J Bacteriol 1995; 177:551–557.

198. Miyake K, Horinouchi S, Yoshida M, Chiba N, Mori K, Nogawa N, Morikawa N, Beppu T. Detection and properties of A-factor-binding protein from *Streptomyces griseus*. J Bacteriol 1989; 171:4298–4302.

199. Onaka H, Ando N, Nihira T, Yamada Y, Beppu T, Horinouchi S. Cloning and characterization of the A-factor receptor gene from *Streptomyces griseus*. J Bacteriol 1995; 177:6083–6092.

200. Miyake K, Kuzuyama T, Horinouchi S, Beppu T. The A-factor-binding protein of *Streptomyces griseus* negatively controls streptomycin production and sporulation. J Bacteriol 1990; 172:3003–3008.

201. Yamada Y, Nihira T, Sakuda S. Biosynthesis and receptor protein of butyrolactone autoregulator of *Streptomyces virginiae*. Actinomycetol 1992; 6:1–8.

202. Miyake K, Onaka H, Horinouchi S, Beppu T. Organization and nucleotide sequence of the *secE–nusG* region of *Streptomyces griseus*. Biochim Biophys Acta 1994; 1217:97–100.

203. Kuberski S, Kasberg T, Distler J. The *nusG* gene of *Streptomyces griseus*: Cloning of the gene and analysis of the A-factor binding properties of the gene product. FEMS Microbiol Lett 1994; 119:33–40.

204. Swift S, Bainton NJ, Winson MK. Gram-negative bacterial communication by *N*-acyl homoserine lactones: A universal language? Trends Microbiol 1994; 2:193–198.

205. Retzlaff L, Distler J. The regulator of streptomycin gene expression, StrR, of *Streptomyces griseus* is a DNA-binding activator protein with multiple recognition sites. Mol Microbiol 1995; 18:151–162.

206. Vujaklija D, Ueda K, Hong S, Beppu T, Horinouchi S. Identification of an A-factor-dependent promotor in the streptomycin biosynthetic gene cluster of *Streptomyces griseus*. Mol Gen Genet 1991; 229:119–128.

207. Vujaklija D, Horinouchi S, Beppu T. Detection of an A-factor-responsive protein that binds to the upstream activation sequence of *strR*, a regulatory gene for streptomycin biosynthesis in *Streptomyces griseus*. J Bacteriol 1993; 175:2652–2661.

208. Mayer G. Molekulare Analyse und Evolution von 5′-Hydroxystreptomycin- und Bluensomycin-Biosynthesegenen aus *Streptomyces glaucescens* GLA0 und *Streptomyces bluensis* ISP 5564. Dissertation, Bergische Universitaet Wuppertal, 1994.

209. Chater KF. Genetic regulation of secondary metabolic pathways in *Streptomyces*. Davies J, Chadwick D, Whelan J, Widdows K, eds. Secondary Metabolites: Their Function and Evolution. Chichester: Wiley and Sons, 1992:144–156.

210. Leskiw BK, Bibb MJ, Chater KF. The use of a rare codon specifically during development. Mol Microbiol 1991; 5:2861–2867.

211. Leskiw BK, Lawlor EJ, Fernandez-Abalos JM, Chater KF. TTA codons in some genes prevent their expression in a class of developmental, antibiotic-negative, *Streptomyces* mutants. Proc Natl Acad Sci USA 1991; 88:2461–2465.

212. McCue LA, Kwak J, Babcock MJ, Kendrick KF. Molecular analysis of sporulation in *Streptomyces griseus*. Gene 1992; 115:173–179.

213. Buttner MJ. RNA polymerase heterogeneity in *Streptomyces coelicolor* A3(2). Mol Microbiol 1989; 3:1653–1659.

214. Champness WC, Chater KF. Regulation and interaction of antibiotic production and morphological differentiation in *Streptomyces* spp. Piggot P, Moran CP Jr, Youngman P, eds. Regulation of Bacterial Differentiation. Washington D.C.: American Society for Microbiology, 1994:61–94.

215. Waters B, Vujaklija D, Gold MR, Davies J. Protein tyrosine phosphorylation in streptomycetes. FEMS Microbiol Lett 1994; 120:187–190.

216. Hong SK, Matsumoto A, Horinouchi S, Beppu T. Effects of protein kinase inhibitors on in vitro protein phosphorylation and cellular differentiation of *Streptomyces griseus*. Mol Gen Genet 1993; 236:347–354.

217. Stowe D, Atkinson T, Mann NH. Protein kinase activities in cell-free extracts of *Streptomyces coelicolor* A3(2). Biochimie 1989; 71:1101–1105.

218. Hill WE, Dahlberg A, Garrett RA, Moore PB, Schlessinger D, Warner JR. The Ribosome: Structure, Function, and Evolution. Washington D.C.: American Society for Microbiology, 1990.

219. Nierhaus KH. The Translational Apparatus. New York: Plenum Press, 1993.

220. Piepersberg W. Aminoglycosid Antibiotika: Wichtige Therapeutika und Objekte der Grundlagenforschung. Forum Mikrobiol 1985; 8/85:153–161.

221. Londei P, Altamura S, Sanz JL, Amils R. Aminoglycoside-induced mistranslation in thermophilic archaebacteria. Mol Gen Genet 1988; 214:48–54.

222. Bakker EP. Aminoglycoside and aminocyclitol antibiotics: Hygromycin B is an atypical bactericidal compound that exerts effects on cells of *Escherichia coli* characteristic for bacteriostatic aminocyclitols. J Gen Microbiol 1992; 138:563–569.

223. Bilgin N, Claesens F, Pahverk H, Ehrenberg M. Kinetic properties of *Escherichia coli* ribosomes with altered forms of S12. J Mol Biol 1992; 224:1011–1027.

224. Moazed D, Noller HF. Interaction of tRNA with 23S rRNA in the ribosomal A, P and E sites. Cell 1989; 57:585–597.

225. Nierhaus KH. Solution of the ribosome riddle: How the ribosome selects the correct aminoacyl-tRNA out of 41 similar contestants. Mol Microbiol 1993; 9:661–669.

226. Moazed D, Noller HF. Interactions of antibiotics with 16S rRNA. Nature 1987; 327:389–394.

227. De Stasio EA, Moazed D, Noller HF, Dahlberg AE. Mutations in 16S ribosomal RNA disrupt antibiotic-RNA interactions. EMBO J 1989; 8:1213–1216.

228. Cundliffe E. Recognition sites for antibiotics within rRNA. Hill WE, Dahlberg A, Garrett RA, Moore PB, Schlessinger D, Warner JR, eds. The Ribosome: Structure, Function, and Evolution. Washington D.C.: American Society for Microbiology, 1990:479–490.

229. Noller HF. On the origin of the ribosome: Coevolution of subdomains of tRNA and rRNA. Gestland RF, Atkins JF, eds. The RNA World. New York: Cold Spring Harbor Laboratory Press, 1993:137–184.

230. Brink MF, Brink G, Verbeet MP, deBoer HA. Spectinomycin interacts specifically with the residues G1064 and C1192 in 16S rRNA, thereby potentially freezing this molecule into an inactive conformation. Nucl Acids Res 1994; 22:325–331.

231. Purohit P, Stern S. Interactions of small RNA with antibiotic and RNA ligands of the 30S subunit. Nature 1994; 370:659–662.

232. Schroeder R, Streicher B, Wank H. Splice-site selection and decoding: Are they related? Science 1993; 260:1443–1444.

233. Davies J, von Ahsen U, Schroeder R. Antibiotics and the RNA world: A role for low-molecular-weight effectors in biochemical evolution. Gestland RF, Atkins JF, eds. The RNA World. New York: Cold Spring Harbor Laboratory Press, 1993:185–204.

234. von Ahsen U, Noller HF. Footprinting the sites of interaction of antibiotics with catalytic group I intron RNA. Science 1993; 260:1500–1503.

235. Rogers J, Davies J. The pseudodisaccharides: A novel class of group I intron splicing inhibitors. Nucl Acids Res 1994; 116:10855–10859.

236. Hancock REW. Aminoglycoside uptake and mode of action with special reference to streptomycin and gentamicin. I. Antagonists and mutants. J Antimicrob Chemother 1981; 8:249–276.

237. Hancock REW. Aminoglycoside uptake and mode of action with special reference to streptomycin and gentamicin. II. Effects of aminoglycosides on cells. J Antimicrob Chemother 1981; 8:429–445.

238. Bryan LE, Kwan S. Roles of ribosomal binding, membrane potential, and electron transport in bacterial uptake of streptomycin and gentamicin. Antimicrob Agents Chemother 1983; 23:835–845.

239. Fraimow HS, Greenman JB, Leviton IM, Dougherty TJ, Miller MH. Tobramycin uptake in *Escherichia coli* is driven by either electrical potential or ATP. J Bacteriol 1991; 173:2800–2808.

240. Davis BD, Chen L, Tai PC. Misread protein creates membrane channels: An essential step in the bactericidal action of aminoglycosides. Proc Natl Acad Sci USA 1986; 83:6164–6168.

241. Busse H-J, Wöstmann K, Bakker EP. The bactericidal action of streptomycin: Membrane permeabilization caused by the insertion of mistranslated proteins into the cytoplasmic membrane of *Escherichia coli* and subsequent caging of the antibiotic inside the cells due to degradation of the proteins. J Gen Microbiol 1992; 138:551–556.

242. Hancock REW, Farmer SW, Li Z, Poole K. Interaction of aminoglycosides with outer membranes and purified lipopolysaccharide and OmpF porin of *Escherichia coli*. Antimicrob Agents Chemother 1991; 35:1309–1314.

243. Pratt WB, Fekety R. The Antimicrobial Drugs. New York: Oxford University Press, 1986.

244. Hutchin, T., Cortopassi, G. Proposed molecular and cellular mechanism for aminoglycoside ototoxicity. Antimicrob Agents Chemother 1994; 38:2517–2520.

245. Kohlhepp SJ, Hou L, Gilbert DN. Pig kidney (LLC-PK1) cell membrane fluidity during exposure to gentamicin or tobramycin. Antimicrob Agents Chemother 1994; 38:2169–2171.

246. Smaoui H. Mallie J-P, Schaeverbeke M, Robert A, Schaeverbeke J. Gentamicin administered during gestation alters glomerular basement membrane development. Antimicrob Agents Chemother 1993; 37:1510–1517.

247. Swan SK, Kohlhepp SJ, Kohnen PW, Gilbert DN, Bennett WM. Long-term protection of polyaspartic acid in experimental gentamicin nephrotoxicity. Antimicrob Agents Chemother 1991; 35:2591–2595.

248. Chadwick D, Whelan J, Widdows K. Secondary Metabolites: Their Function and Evolution, Ciba Foundation Symp. 171. Chichester: John Wiley and Sons, 1992.

249. Piepersberg W. Streptomycetes and corynebacteria. Rehm H-J, Reed G, Pühler A, Stadler P, eds. Biotechnology 2nd ed., Vol. 1. Weinheim: VCH-Verlag, 1993:433–468.

250. Phillips L, Wellington EMH, Rees SB. The distribution of antibiotic resistance patterns within streptomycetes and their use in secondary metabolite screening. J Industr Microbiol 1994; 13:53–62.

251. Phillips L, Wellington EMH, Rees SB, Jun LS, King GP. The distribution of DNA sequences hybridizing with antibiotic production and resistance gene probes within type strains and wild isolates of *Streptomyces* species. J Antibiot 1992; 45:1481–1491.

252. Marsh P, Wellington EMH. Molecular ecology of filamentous actinomycetes in soil. O'Gara F, Dowling DN, Boesten B, eds. Molecular Ecology of Rhizosphere Microorganisms: Biotechnology and the Release of GMOs. Weinheim: VCH, 1994:133–149.

253. Wellington EMH, Marsh P, Toth I, Cresswell N, Huddelston L, Schilhabel MB. The selective effects of antibiotics in soil. Guerrero R, Perdrós-Aló C, eds. Trends in Microbial Ecology. Madrid: Spanish Society for Microbiology, 1993:331–336.

254. Embley TM, Stackebrandt E. The molecular phylogeny and systematics of the actinomycetes. Annu Rev Microbiol 1994; 48:257–289.

255. Newton GL, Arnold K, Price MS, Sherrill C, Delcardayre SB, Aharonowitz Y, Cohem G, Davise J, Fahey RC, Davis C. Distribution of thiols in microorganisms: Mycothiol is a major thiol in most actinomycetes.

256. Guthmiller P, Van Pilsum JF, Boen JR, McGuire DM. Cloning and sequencing of rat kidney L-arginine:glycine amidinotransferase: Studies on the mechanism of regulation by growth hormone and creatine. J Biol Chem 1994; 269:17556–17560.

257. Stevenson G, Neal B, Liu D, Hobbs M, Packer NH, Batley M, Redmond JW, Lindquist L, Reeves P. Structure of the O-antigen of *Escherichia coli* K-12 and the sequence of its *rfb* gene cluster. J Bacteriol 1994; 176:4144–4156.

258. Leblond P, Redenbach M, Cullum J. Physical map of the *Streptomyces lividans* 66 genome and comparison with that of the related strain *Streptomyces coelicolor* A3(2). J Bacteriol 1993; 175:3422–3429.

259. Lin Y-S, Kieser HM, Hopwood DA, Chen CW. The chromosomal DNA of *Streptomyces lividans* 66 is linear. Mol Microbiol 1993; 10:923–933.

260. Altenbuchner J. Hohe genetische Instabilität von Streptomyceten durch chromosomale Deletionen und DNA-Amplifikationen. BioEng 1994; 3/94:33–46.

261. Birch A, Häusler A, Rüttener C, Hütter R. Chromsomal deletion and rearrangement in *Streptomyces glaucescens*. J Bacteriol 1991; 173:3531–3538.

262. Cavalier-Smith T. Kingdom protozoa and its 18 phyla. Microbiol Rev 1993; 57:953–994.

263. Olson GJ, Woese CR, Overbeek R. The winds of (evolutionary) change: Breathing new life into microbiology. J Bacteriol 1994; 176:1–6.

264. Reichenbach H, Höfle G. Production of bioactive secondary metabolites. Dworkin M, Kaiser D, eds. Myxobacteria II. Washington D.C.: American Society for Microbiology, 1993:347–397.

265. Yokose K, Furumai T, Suhara Y, Pirson W. Trestatin: Alpha-amylase inhibitor. Demain AL, Somkuti GA, Hunter-Creva JC, Rossmoore HW, eds. Novel Microbial Products for Medicine and Agriculture. Amsterdam: Elsevier Science Publishers, 1989:117–126.

266. Okami Y. Productivity of aminoglycoside antibiotics with reference to antibiotic resistance of the producer. Kleinkauf H, von Döhren H, Dornauer H, Nesemann G, eds. Regulation of Secondary Metabolite Formation. Weinheim: VCH-Verlag, 1986:333–354.

267. Hopwood DA, Sherman DH, Khosla C, Bibb MJ, Simpson TJ, Fernandez-Moreno MA, Martinez E, Malpartida F. "Hybrid" pathways for the production of secondary metabolites. Heslot H, Davies J, Florent J, Bobichon L, Durand G, Peneasse L, eds. Proceedings of the 6th International Symposium on Genetics of Industrial Microorganisms. Paris: Societe Francaise de Microbiologie, 1990:259–270.

268. Katz L, Donadio S. Polyketide synthesis: Prospects for hybrid antibiotics. Annu Rev Microbiol 1993; 47:875–912.

269. Floss HG, Strohl WR. Genetic engineering of hybrid antibiotics—a progress report. Tetrahedron 1991; 47:6045–6058.

270. Cappelletti LM, Spagnoli R. Biological transformation of kanamycin A to amikacin. J Antibiot 1983; 36:328–329.

271. Decker H, Haag G, Udvarnorki G, Rohr J. Novel genetically engineered tetracenomycins. Angew Chem Int Ed Engl 1995; 34:1107–1110.

5

Fermentation, Biosynthesis, and Molecular Genetics of Lincomycin

Shiau-Ta Chung, Jack J. Manis, Steven J. McWethy, Tom E. Patt, Dennis F. Witz,
Holly J. Wolf, and Merle G. Wovcha
Pharmacia and Upjohn, Inc., Kalamazoo, Michigan

I. INTRODUCTION

Lincomycin was discovered as an antibacterial activity in submerged cultures of *Streptomyces lincolnensis* var. *lincolnensis* (1,2) and identified as the structure shown in Figure 1 (3). This compound was subsequently found to also be produced by certain strains of seven different species of actinomycetes, as listed in Table 1 (4–10). Lincomycin is composed of an amino acid, *trans-N*-methyl-4-*n*-propyl-*L*-proline (commonly referred to as propylhygric acid, or PHA) (11), linked via a peptide bond to a sugar moiety, 6-amino-6,8-dideoxy-1-thio-D-erythro-α-D-galactooctopyranoside (commonly referred to as methylthiolincosamide, or MTL) (12,13). A minor analog, lincomycin B (4′-depropyl-4′-ethyllincomycin), is also normally produced by some strains during the fermentation. Lincomycin and its derivatives (e.g., the more active semisynthetic 7-chloro derivative, clindamycin) are active against most of the common aerobic Gram-positive pathogens including susceptible strains of streptococci, staphylococci, and pneumococci. In addition, clindamycin is effective against certain species of both Gram-negative and Gram-positive anaerobic bacteria (1,14–16). Lincomycin blocks protein synthesis in sensitive strains by preventing binding of aminoacyl-tRNA to the mRNA–ribosome complex in the 50S subunit (17,18). Consistent with this mode of action, one mechanism of resistance to this drug has been shown to be target-site modification involving methylation of adenine residues in 23S RNA (19).

The biosynthesis of lincomycin, its mode of action, and associated resistance mechanisms have been described in several previous reviews (20,21). Since these reports, significant new information has been obtained on the genetics and biochemistry of lincomycin biosynthesis. Most notable in this regard is the isolation, sequencing, and analysis, by Piepersberg and his coworkers (22,23), of a cluster of *S. lincolnensis* genes that may encode the entire lincomycin biosynthetic pathway. This recent information, along with aspects of the lincomycin fermentation process, are the subject of this chapter.

II. FERMENTATION

Lincomycin has been commercially produced by fermentation by The Upjohn Company since the mid 1960s. Mason et al. (1) first reported the production of this antibiotic by a

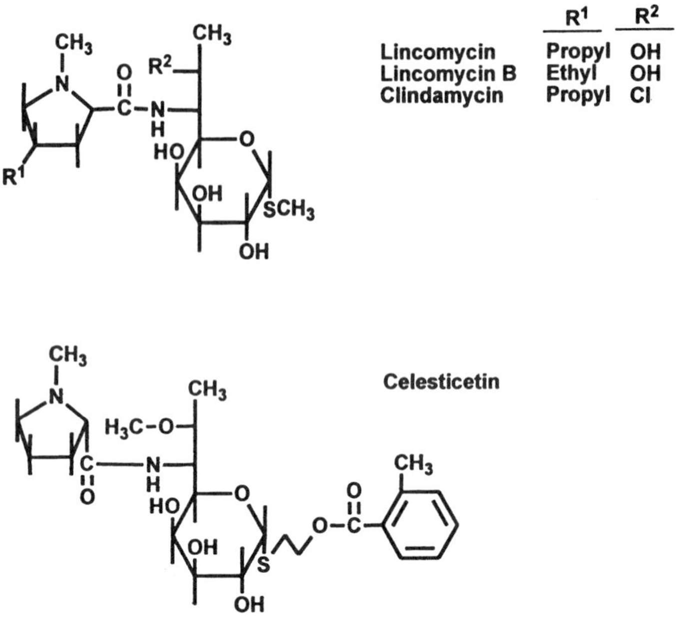

Figure 1   Chemical structures of some lincosamides.

streptomycete, *Streptomyces lincolnensis* var. *lincolnensis*, in 1962. The original composition of matter patent was granted to The Upjohn Company in 1963 (2).

Gonzalez and Miller (21) thoroughly reviewed the fermentation literature on lincomycin in 1985. Recently, a method for determining cell mass via determination of diaminopimelic acid (DAP) concentrations (24) has been applied to profile *S. lincolnensis* growth in seed cultures and fermentations in which complex media containing insoluble materials are used.

A.   Production Cultures, Maintenance, and Storage

Since the review by Gonzalez and Miller (21), only one additional organism has been reported to produce lincomycin. Bibikova et al. (10) reported in 1989 the production of lincomycin by a species of another genus, *Micromonospora halophytica*. This organism was isolated by directed screening on a selective medium containing 50–100 μg/ml of lincomycin. Table 1 summarizes the various actinomyces species that have been reported to produce lincomycin. The *Streptomyces espinosus* culture possesses several interesting characteristics that distinguish it from *S. lincolnensis*: namely, it appears to produce reduced levels of lincomycin B, it is melanin negative, and it produces lincomycin at temperatures of 44 to 48°C (5). Two of the other streptomycete species, *Streptomyces variabilis* and *Streptomyces vellosus*, also appear to be lower lincomycin B producers. The *Streptomyces pseudogriseolus* culture also possesses the melanin-negative phenotype.

Conventional methods of lyophilization and liquid nitrogen freezing have been successfully used in the maintenance and storage of *S. lincolnensis* cultures. Master cell banks composed of spore suspensions may be stored using either of the two methods.

Table 1   Cultures that Produce Lincomycin

Culture	Description	Reference
S. *lincolnensis* var. *lincolnensis*	Original culture	Bergy et al. (2)
S. *espinosus* Dietz, sp. n.	1. Reduced lincomycin B production, melanin negative	1. Argoudelis et al. (4)
	2. Thermophilic	2. Reusser and Argoudelis (5)
S. *pseudogriseolus* chemovar *linmyceticus* Dietz var. nova	Melanin negative	Argoudelis and Coats (6)
S. *variabilis* chemovar *liniabilis* Dietz, var. nova	Lower lincomycin B production	Argoudelis and Coats (7)
Actinomyces roseolus		Kuznetsov et al. (8)
S. *vellosus* Dietz, sp. n.	Lower lincomycin B production	Bergy et al. (9)
Micromonospora halophytica		Bibikova et al. (10)

The master cell bank can be used to inoculate agar slants or a seed medium to generate vegetative growth for liquid nitrogen storage. Either slants or ampoules can be subsequently used as working cultures for inoculation of primary seeds.

B.   Fermentation Process

A typical fermentation sequence employs growing cultures in 1-liter vessels. These may be inoculated with working cultures consisting of either spore suspensions derived from slants or frozen vegetative cultures. Typically, primary seed cultures are incubated until growth occurs; then, they are used to inoculate 2500–7500-liter seed fermenters. After maturation, the seed cultures are transferred to 50,000- to 150,000-liter fermenters at an inoculum level of 1–15% (v/v). Gonzalez and Miller (21) have reported other details for a typical antibiotic fermentation process.

Table A primary seed medium that gives improved performance was developed from that reported previously (21); Yeastolac was replaced with a protein mixture including dried brewer's yeast and yeast extract. Following inoculation, the seed flasks are incubated until seeds reach maturation, as indicated by accumulation of satisfactory levels of biomass. Figure 2 presents average profiles for pH and DAP. A correlation between DAP and dry cell weight was established in a medium with soluble components (data not shown), indicating a ratio of approximately 100 nmol of DAP detected per mg of S. *lincolnensis* dry cell weight. Figure 3 presents typical profiles of pH and DAP for secondary seeds. Maturation of secondary seeds is indicated by a combination of rapid pH decline and accumulation of sufficient quantities of biomass.

Optimal fermentation medium composition and operational specifications are determined from shake-flask, 8-liter, and 250-liter fermentation experiments. Scaled-down versions of production media and conditions are employed in shake-flask fermentations. This provides the capability for evaluation of raw materials, comparison of production strains arising from screening programs, and process diagnosis or troubleshooting efforts. It is important to determine the optimal operating volume when a shake-flask procedure is developed, to ensure that sufficient oxygen transfer is available to support the level of biomass, viscosity, and metabolic rate desired. Fermentation models of laboratory and pilot plant scale have been developed that successfully predict process performance at the production scale. Employing these models, profiles of oxygen uptake rate

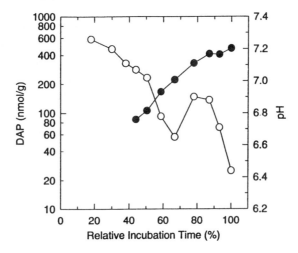

Figure 2   Profiles of diaminopimelic acid (DAP) (●) and pH (○) for S. *lincolnensis* primary seeds. The profiles represent the average of two primary seeds. Approximately 100 nmol DAP represents 1 mg of S. *lincolnensis* cell dry weight.

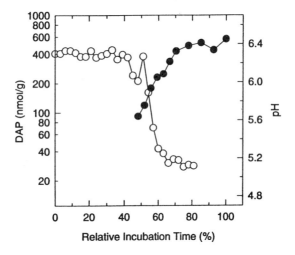

Figure 3   Profiles of DAP (●) and pH (○) for S. *lincolnensis* secondary seeds.

(OUR), dissolved oxygen (DO) concentration, viscosity, and substrate utilization rate are used for successful scale-up of experimental processes from pilot to production settings. Optimization of OUR requires the proper balance between substrate utilization rate, which is greatly influenced by relative solubility and particle size of selected carbon and nitrogen sources, and DO or oxygen availability. Since lincomycin production by S. *lincolnensis* is sensitive to prolonged periods of DO depletion, determination of appropriate agitation rates for particular blade and baffle configurations is important.

Production fermentation media are modifications of the mixtures disclosed by Churchill et al. (25). Figure 4 profiles DAP, colony forming units (CFU), viscosity, and

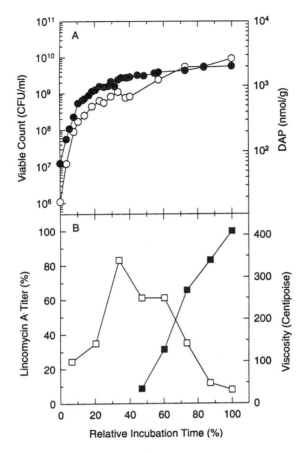

Figure 4   Profiles of DAP (●) and colony forming units (O) (A), and viscosity (□) and relative lincomycin titers (■) (B) from typical *S. lincolnensis* production fermentations. The data presented in each panel were obtained from separate production fermentations.

relative lincomycin titers for typical fermentations. Following a growth phase, indicated by rapid accumulation of DAP and viable cells and increased viscosity values, onset of lincomycin production occurs. A five-fold increase in biomass occurs at the fermentation stage relative to growth in the more stringent seed media. Viscosity values decline as the fermentation progresses, due to fragmentation of mycelia.

C.   Control of Minor Component, Lincomycin B

Lincomycin B (4′-depropyl-4′-ethyllincomycin) was first reported by Argoudelis et al. (26) in 1965 as a minor component in the fermentation by *S. lincolnensis*. Lincomycin B is considered an undesirable side-product since it possesses only approximately 25% (w/w) of the antibacterial activity of lincomycin A (16). It differs from lincomycin A by having one less methylene carbon in the side chain of the propylhygric acid moiety (Figure 1).

Two biochemical approaches were patented for the directed biosynthesis of lincomycin A to give reduced levels of lincomycin B in the fermentation. Visser (27) patented the use of propyl proline addition to lincomycin fermentations as a means to limit lincomycin B formation by *S. lincolnensis*. Propylproline (PPL) is the putative precursor to propylhygric acid in lincomycin A, whereas ethylproline (EPL) is the putative precursor to ethylhygric acid (EHA) of lincomycin B (28). Witz (29) demonstrated the use of L-tyrosine, L-dihydroxyphenylalanine (L-DOPA), and other tyrosine-related compounds for the directed biosynthesis of lincomycin A by *S. lincolnensis*. Witz et al. (28) observed that the addition of L-tyrosine or L-DOPA to fermentation media resulted in the accumulation of PPL and EPL. Although the mechanism by which additions of PPL or L-tyrosine and related compounds result in preferential formation of lincomycin A is not fully understood, the results of these studies suggest that PPL is the preferred substrate over EPL for the enzyme *N*-demethyllincomycin synthetase. This enzyme catalyzes the condensation of MTL with PPL or EPL.

D. Studies of Lincomycin Fermentation in Chemically Defined Media

Fermentation studies performed in chemically defined media have proved useful for determination of the effects of salts, nitrogen, and carbon source on specific rates of lincomycin production by *S. lincolnensis*, and for investigations of culture stability. Formulations of chemically defined media have been reported by Witz et al. (28) and Young et al. (30). Figure 5 shows data consistent with previous reports and profiles the accumulation of biomass (cell dry weight), the pH, the utilization of the carbon sources citrate and glucose, the production of lincomycin, and the specific rate of lincomycin production for a fermentation employing a chemically defined medium. The maximum specific rate of lincomycin production occurs during the latter stages of growth. The specific rate then decreases rapidly during a phase of declining cell mass as carbon sources become depleted.

Phosphate is a physiological regulator of lincomycin production, as observed using defined media employing glucose as the sole source of carbon (30). Maximum specific rates of productivity were detected in the presence of 3 mM phosphate (initial concentration); increased concentrations of phosphate lowered specific rates of productivity, but they substantially increased rates of growth. Lincomycin production is also subject to control by ammonia nitrogen. Ammonium chloride added to a concentration of 25 mM resulted in maximal specific rates of production; as ammonia nitrogen was increased from 40 to 200 mM, a dose-dependent inverse response in productivity was observed (30). Lincomycin production by *S. lincolnensis* was not sensitive to glucose levels of 20–30 g/liter in chemically defined media (30). This is in contrast to the negative effect of glucose on many other antibiotic-producing organisms (31).

E. Lincomycin Assay Methods

Gonzalez and Miller (21) summarized the available biological and chemical assays. Biological diffusion disc plate assay methods were reported by Hanka et al. (32) in 1963 and Neff et al. (33) in 1967. Prescott (34) described a chemical assay for lincomycin in 1966, which was adapted for use with an autoanalyzer. Houtman et al. (35) described a gas–liquid chromatography (GLC) method for the analysis of lincomycin in 1968. More recently, Asmus et al. (36) described a high-performance liquid chromatographic (HPLC) assay method for determination of lincomycin in fermentation broth samples. The chromatographic methods have the advantage over the biological and chemical methods, because both lincomycin A and lincomycin B concentrations can be determined.

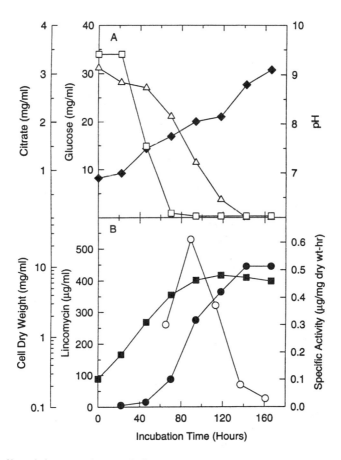

Figure 5 Profiles of glucose utilization (△), citrate utilization (□) and pH (◆) (A), and cell dry weight accumulation (■), lincomycin titers (●) and specific rate of lincomycin productivity (○) (B) by *S. lincolnensis* inoculated into a chemically defined medium. The specific rate of lincomycin production was determined in washed-cell reactions. (From Ref. 16.)

III. LINCOMYCIN BIOSYNTHESIS

As stated above and illustrated in Figure 1, lincomycin A is composed of an amino acid subunit, PHA, and a sugar subunit, MTL. In summary, experiments described below clearly showed that the immediate primary metabolic precursor of PHA is L-tyrosine, with the N-methyl and terminal side-chain methyl groups added in reactions involving transfer from S-adenosylmethionine (28,37,38). The origin of the MTL moiety is less certain, but this seems most likely to involve a nucleotide-activated hexose (23), with the amino group added via a transamination reaction and the S-methyl group added as a single unit (39,40).

A. Biosynthesis of the Amino Acid Moiety

Experiments suggesting the biosynthetic origins of the carbons in the PHA subunit of lincomycin A were carried out by Witz et al. (28). When the producing culture *S. lincolnensis* was fed L-[1-14C]tyrosine, it was found that 14.1% of the label was incorporated into lincomycin A, with all of it going into the carboxyl group of the amino acid moiety. In another experiment in which cells were fed L-[U-^{14}C]tyrosine, essentially all the radioactivity incorporated into lincomycin was again in the amino acid subunit, but the levels were approximately seven times that found when Cl-labeled tyrosine was used. From these results, it was concluded that seven of the nine carbons in the PHA subunit were derived from L-tyrosine. Similar feeding studies using L-[^{15}N]tyrosine demonstrated that the nitrogen of this compound was also efficiently and specifically incorporated into just the PHA portion of lincomycin.

Argoudelis et al. (37) had previously used a combination of radiolabeling and mass spectroscopy to demonstrate that the other two carbons in the PHA subunit, namely, the N-methyl and terminal side-chain methyl groups, originated from the methyl group of methionine.

Information on the pathway by which tyrosine is incorporated into lincomycin came from ^{13}C nuclear magnetic resonance (NMR) studies using deuterated precursors (Rolls JP, unpublished data). In one experiment, it was found that feeding of L-[3',5'-^{2}H]tyrosine resulted in the formation of monodeuterated lincomycin A; the carbon–deuterium bond was at the 5'-position of the PHA subunit. The loss of the 3'-carbon–deuterium bond and the pattern of incorporation observed when radiolabeled L-DOPA was fed to producing cultures were consistent with L-DOPA being an intermediate in the incorporation process. Moreover, a potent tyrosinase activity specific to the lincomycin biosynthetic pathway had been identified and partially characterized in S. lincolnensis (41). As predicted by this pathway, illustrated in Figure 6, incorporation of L-[2',5',6'-^{2}H]DOPA generated trideuterated lincomycin with the label retained at the corresponding positions.

The tyrosinase activity involved in this pathway is clearly distinct from that catalyzing formation of the pigment melanin, because mel deletion mutants have been isolated that retain the capacity to produce significant quantities of lincomycin, for example, LM706 described in Figure 7. Similarly, S. lincolnensis strains in which mel is inactivated by transposon mutagenesis do not make melanin but are unaffected in lincomycin production (Chung ST and Crose LL, unpublished results). This is also consistent with the observation that two other lincomycin producers, S. espinosus and S. pseudogriseolus, lack the mel gene.

More detailed information about the mechanism by which L-DOPA is converted to lincomycins A and B came from studies by Brahme et al. (38). To convert tyrosine via DOPA requires that the aromatic ring be cleaved and, also, that a condensation occurs at the 2'- or 6'-position of tyrosine to form the pyrrolo ring of the PHA or EHA moieties. To study this portion of the lincomycin biosynthetic pathway, they used the labeled compounds L-(3',5'-^{2}H)tyrosine, L-(2',5',6'-^{2}H)DOPA, and L-(6-^{2}H)methionine and a combination of NMR and mass spectral analysis. They were able to rule out parallel biosynthetic pathways leading to PHA via a 3,4-intradiol cleavage of cycloDOPA and to EPL via 2,3-extradiol cleavage of cycloDOPA. These parallel pathways would require a C-methylation step to form both PHA and EHA. The mass spectra analysis of PHA and EHA from the experiment-fed L-(6-^{2}H)methionine was not consistent with the cleavage of cycloDOPA. Only the PHA had the appropriate mass spectra for a C-methylation reaction. The data did support a 2,3-extradiol cleavage of DOPA that leads to PHA via methylation or EHA by protonation (Figure 6).

Similar bioconversions of tyrosine through L-DOPA were reported as the probable pathways leading to the biosynthesis of the C_2- and C_3-proline moieties of the antibiotics

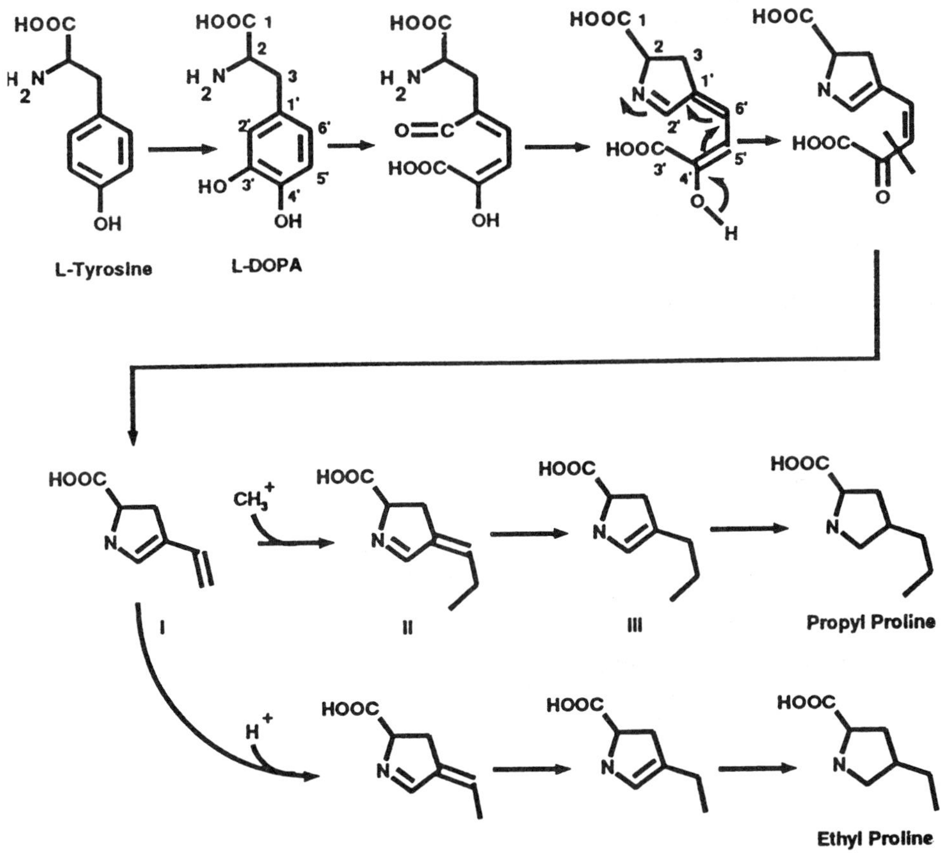

Figure 6   Proposed pathway to PPL and EPL.

anthramycin, tomaymycin, and sibiromycin (42,43). Double-labeling experiments ([^{3}H, ^{14}C]tyrosine) were used in the study to determine the fate of the tyrosine carbon and hydrogen. The data obtained were consistent with a common pathway involving proximal extradiol cleavage of DOPA followed by condensation to form the pyrrolo ring. It appears that lincomycin shares a common biosynthetic pathway from tyrosine.

Further clarification of the final steps in the biosynthesis of PPL from L-tyrosine comes from the studies of Kuo and coworkers (44–46). From a study involving the complementation of *S. lincolnensis* mutants blocked in lincomycin biosynthesis, they discovered that a cofactor was required as a catalytic agent in the biosynthesis of PPL. The cofactor was designed as LCF (lincomycin cosynthetic factor). A structural study involving mass spectroscopy, infrared (IR), ^{13}C NMR, and ^{1}H NMR allowed the assignment of the cofactor structure as 7,8-didemethyl-8-hydroxy-5-deazariboflavin. Interestingly, this cofactor was found earlier to be involved in the biosynthesis of tetracycline in *Streptomyces aureofaciens* (47); when 16 genera of actinomycetes were examined, the cofactor was found in almost every fermentation (45).

The data obtained from the study of the blocked mutant requiring LCF supported the results obtained by Brahme and coworkers (38) to the point of formation of the

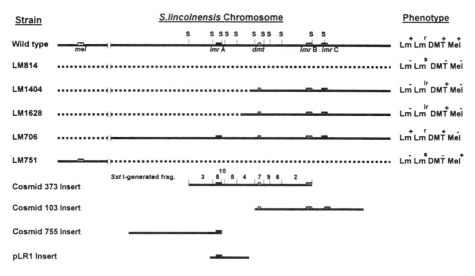

Figure 7 Location and organization of a putative lincomycin biosynthetic gene cluster located close to the *mel* gene on the *S. lincolnensis* chromosome. The segment bounded by *lmrA* and *lmrC* is the 34 kbp region showing strong homology with each of the Lm⁺ *Streptomyces* strains. Cosmids 373, 103, and 755 were isolated from an *SstI*-generated gene bank by homology with *lmrA* and chromosome walking. LM751 and LM814 are LM⁻ mutants in which the entire conserved biosynthetic gene cluster is deleted, and LM814 also lacks the *mel* region. pLRI insert is the 13 kbp *lmrA*-containing fragment obtained by shotgun cloning *BamHI*-digested wild-type chromosome to complement the Lmˢ phenotype of LM814. LM1404 and LM1628 are Lm⁻ mutants containing deletions that terminate within the biosynthetic gene cluster. The exact distance between *mel* and *lmrA* is unknown but exceeds 250 kbp, which is the approximate distance ordered by chromosome walking from each locus. Lmʳ, resistance to lincomycin at concentrations exceeding 1000 μg/ml; Lmˡʳ, low-level lincomycin resistance (MIC ≈ 200 μg/ml in Hickey and Tresner agar); Lmˢ, sensitivity to lincomycin at concentration below 5 μg/ml; MT, N-demethyllincomycin methyltransferase; Mel, melanin; S, *SstI*.

enamine (Figure 6, I). Kuo and coworkers suggest, instead, that an α,β unsaturated imine is formed upon methylation or protonation (Figure 6, II). This modified scheme is consistent with the previously published labeling experiments (40). Knowing that 3-propylidene-Δ^1-pyrroline-5-carboxylic acid (Figure 6, II) accumulates in a mutant lacking a reductase that requires the LCF led Kuo's group to speculate on the remaining biosynthetic steps leading to propylproline. They proposed that the enamine, 3-propyl-Δ^2-pyrroline-5-carboxylic acid (Figure 6, III), is the immediate precursor of propylproline. The modified biosynthetic pathway to PPL then is tyrosine → L-DOPA → → 3-propylidene-Δ^1-pyrroline-5-carboxylic acid → 3-propyl-Δ^2-pyrroline-5-carboxylic acid → PPL.

B.   Biosynthesis of the Sugar Moiety

The MTL amino sugar appears to be structurally unique to lincomycin, but it bears similarity to the amino sugar of celesticetin (Figure 1). The first attempts to elucidate the biosynthetic origins of MTL were the studies reported by Argoudelis et al. (39). They determined that the origin of the S-methyl group of the MTL moiety was derived from

C_1 fragments at the oxidation state of methyl groups. They used a combination of radioactive labeling and mass spectroscopy to determine the origin of the S-methyl group of MTL, as well as the N-methyl and C-methyl groups of the PHA moiety.

Brahme and coworkers (40) approached the study of the origin of the MTL unit of lincomycin by a combination of feeding specifically labeled D-[^{13}C]glucose and identifying the labeled carbon, as well as feeding D-[^{13}C$_6$]glucose and analyzing the ^{13}C–^{13}C spin coupling patterns in MTL and lincomycin. The data suggested that the C_8 carbon skeleton of MTL resulted from the condensation of a pentose unit (C_5) and a C_3 unit. The pentose unit could arise from either the action of the hexose monophosphate shunt on glucose or by condensation of glyceraldehyde-3-phosphate with a C_2 unit from a C_2 donor such as sedoheptulose-7-phosphate. The C_3 unit could be derived from an intact C_3 unit or also result from the combination of a C_2 unit with a C_1 unit (Figure 8, Pathway A).

The terminal steps for converting the resulting C_8 unit to MTL were not determined in the study of Brahme et al. (40). They postulate that an isomerization of the octulose to an octose occurs, followed by dephosphorylation and reduction at the C8 carbon. Then, a transamination of the precursor 6-ketooctose occurs and is followed by a thiomethylation of C1 to complete the synthesis of MTL.

In contrast to the above scheme, analysis of the putative products of a lincomycin biosynthetic gene cluster by Peschke et al. (23) led them to conclude that synthesis of the MTL moiety more likely involves formation of a dTDP-activated hexose (e.g., dTDP-glucose) that is subsequently converted to a dTDP-deoxyamino intermediate followed by glycosylation to form the required C_8 sugar (Figure 8, Pathway B). They suggested that the ^{13}C-labeling pattern obtained by Brahme et al. (40) could support glucose as a starter unit if there is a rapid, efficient equilibrium in the hexosephosphate pool by a hexose monophosphate shunt. This type of rearrangement of labeling was shown by Rinehart et al. (48) to explain labeling patterns in validamycin and neomycin.

Preliminary data have been obtained for the putative transthiomethylation of C1 (Rolls JP and Hessler EJ, unpublished data). The S. lincolnensis culture was fed [^{13}CH$_3$, ^{34}S]-DL-methionine under conditions of lincomycin production. The analysis of the lincomycin showed equal incorporation of ^{13}CH$_3$ from the [^{13}CH$_3$, ^{34}S]-DL-methionine into the C-methyl (the terminal carbon of the PPL side chain), N-methyl, and S-methyl carbons. These results confirmed earlier work that indicated S-adenosyl methionine (SAM) was the source of the methyl groups. The double-labeled methionine experiment was further analyzed to determine whether the group is added to the 6-aminooctose and then subsequently methylated or, alternatively, the S and methyl group are transferred in concert.

The ^{13}CH$_3$ carbon of the thiomethyl group was enriched to a level of 7.8 times the natural abundance as determined by ^{13}C NMR analysis. Mass spectral analysis indicated that the M + 3 (m/e = 211) of the base peak (m/e = 208) in the spectrum was significantly enriched. The enrichment of the M + 3 would be expected if the ^{13}CH$_3$–^{34}S group of methionine is incorporated intact. Further confirmation of an incorporation of ^{13}CH$_3$–^{34}S via transthiomethylation came from an analysis of the cleaved thiomethyl group. The thiomethyl group was analyzed by mass spectroscopy as the dimer of the methanethiol (CH$_3$—S—S—CH$_3$). The base molecular ion of this dimer was m/e = 94, and there was a significant enhancement of the M + 3 molecular ion ($m/2$ = 97). The ratios of M + 2 (incorporation of ^{34}S) to that of M + 3 (incorporation of both the ^{34}S and the ^{13}CH$_3$) for both the MTL (m/e ratio of 210/211) and the methanethiol dimer (m/e ratio of 96/97) were 3.35 and 3.51, respectively. The similarity at these ratios supports the incorporation of the intact ^{13}CH$_3$–^{34}S group.

C. Condensation and N-Methylation

The penultimate step in the biosynthesis of lincomycin is believed to be the formation of the peptide bond between the carboxylic acid analog, PPL, and the amino group of MTL by an adenosine 5'-triphosphate (ATP)-dependent, ribosome-independent N-demethyllincomycin (NDL) synthetase (Figure 8). Evidence supporting such an activity was first provided by Argoudelis et al. (39). They found that when large amounts of MTL are fed to the lincomycin-producing organism, there is an accumulation of NDL well as lincomycin.

The NDL synthetase activity was studied using ^{14}C-labeled propylproline produced via a mutant blocked in both the production of MTL and the final methylation reaction (49). When this mutant is fed MTL, it accumulates NDL. The mutant was fed uniformly labeled [^{14}C]tyrosine and unlabeled MTL to produce [^{14}C]NDL with the majority of the label in the PPL moiety of NDL. The labeled NDL was hydrolyzed under basic conditions to yield [^{14}C]propylproline. The [^{14}C]propylproline was used to study the putative NDL synthetase activity.

The assay protocol for the in vitro study of NDL synthetase was similar to other assays for this type of reaction (50). The reaction mixture contained HEPES buffer (pH 8.0), MgCl$_2$, MTL, ATP, and an ATP-regenerating system of creatine phosphate and creatine kinase. The [^{14}C]propylproline was added, and the reaction was started by the addition of the crude extract from S. lincolnensis grown in chemically defined medium. After a 1 hr incubation at 30°C the [^{14}C]NDL that is formed is separated from the [^{14}C]PPL starting material by either a short resin column of AG1-X2 (OH$^-$ form) or by high-performance liquid chromatography (HPLC).

The NDL synthetase reaction was shown to require ATP, Mg^{2+}, and MTL and to be heat labile. When [^{14}C]propylhygric acid replaced [^{14}C]propylproline in the reaction mixture, there was no incorporation of the label into lincomycin. The pH and temperature optima were determined to be 8.0 and 30°C, respectively. When the crude extract was diluted below a certain critical concentration, the activity diminished dramatically. Enzyme activity was also lost after passing the preparation through a size-exclusion column, but the activity could be recovered by combining specific fractions (51). These studies supported the hypothesis that the nature of the NDL synthetase activity was that of an enzyme complex of readily dissociable, nonidentical subunits. The activity of one of the subunits was identified by a propylproline-dependent ^{32}PP$_i$-ATP exchange assay based on the method used for the tyrocidine synthetase subunit assay (50,52). The peptide antibiotic synthetases of tyrocidine synthetase, edeine synthetase, and gramicidin S synthetase have previously been reported as complexes of readily dissociable, nonidentical subunits (52–54).

The final step in the biosynthesis of lincomycin is the N-methylation of the N-demethyllincomycin formed by condensation of PPL and MTL. An in vitro assay was developed that uses S-[methyl-^{14}C]-adenosyl methionine as a substrate. The labeled lincomycin is separated from the labeled [^{14}C]SAM using basic methylene chloride or HPLC (55). This assay has been used to support shotgun cloning of the methyltransferase gene and to purify the activity to apparent homogeneity (50). Sodium dodecyl sulfate-polyacrylamide gel electrophoretic (SDS-PAGE) analysis of the purified protein indicated a single major band at 29,000 MW. The pI of 5.2 was determined by isoelectric focusing. The pH and temperature optima were determined to be 8.3 and 31°C, respectively. Propylproline, the aglycone moiety of NDL, was not a substrate for the enzyme. The K_m for NDL was determined to be 240 μM, and for SAM 33 μM. S-adenosylhomo-

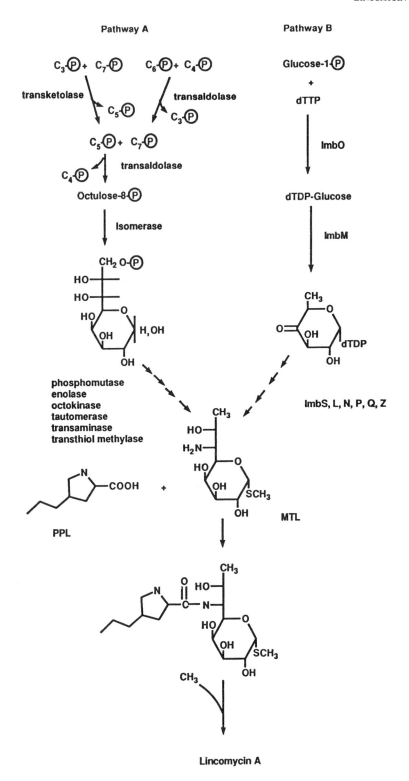

Figure 8   Proposed pathways to MTL and lincomycin.

cysteine, a product of the reaction, was found to be a competitive inhibitor of the reaction. The K_i was determined to be 25 µM (55). These properties of the NDL methyltransferase were similar to properties measured for the S-adenosylmethionine:erythromycin C O-methyltransferase (56) and the S-adenosylmethionine:indolepyruvate 3-methyltransferase (57).

IV. MOLECULAR GENETICS

A. Isolation of a Region of the *S. lincolnensis* Chromosome Coding for Functions Involved in Lincomycin Biosynthesis

With the development of gene cloning techniques for *Streptomyces*, it was soon shown that genes coding for antibiotic biosynthesis were likely to be clustered and closely linked to the corresponding antibiotic resistance determinants (58). That configuration also appeared to exist in *S. lincolnensis*, in that several lincomycin-negative (Lm⁻) mutants isolated from an x-ray-treated cell population were found to also be very sensitive to this drug. Accordingly, shotgun cloning experiments were done in which wild-type *S. lincolnensis* chromosome fragments were used to complement the lincomycin-sensitive (Lmˢ) phenotype of one of these Lm⁻ Lmˢ mutants, LM814. A 13 kbp *Bam*HI fragment was isolated that carries a lincomycin resistance determinant, designated *lmr*A (59). This insert was then used as a probe to identify a cosmid carrying this locus within an *S. lincolnensis* gene bank. Subsequently, the contiguous genomic region around *lmr*A was isolated by chromosome walking.

The extent of the region around *lmr*A involved in lincomycin biosynthesis was inferred from comparative hybridization patterns. As pointed out above, lincomycin is produced by certain strains within seven different species of actinomycetes. Hybridization experiments indicated that the inserts in randomly selected *S. lincolnensis* gene bank cosmids showed little homology under relatively stringent conditions (42°C, 50% formamide) to chromosomal DNA isolated from the other lincomycin producers. In contrast, all but one of the five *Sst*I-generated subfragments of the original 13 kbp *lmr*A-containing insert hybridized strongly to DNA from the Lm⁺ strains, but not to DNA from various Lm⁻ *Streptomyces*, such as *Streptomyces fradiae* and *Streptomyces lividans*. Particularly striking was the finding that the Lm⁺ *S. espinosus* strain BC502 showed strong homology to these fragments, whereas the closely related Lm⁻ *S. espinosus* strain UC5720 did not. These patterns suggested that homology comparisons between Lm⁺ and Lm⁻ strains might indicate the extent of the region near *lmr*A coding for biosynthetic functions. Consistent with that idea, hybridization with subfragments of the ordered gene bank cosmids showed that there was a contiguous highly conserved region in the Lm⁺ strains that was bounded on one end by *lmr*A and extended for about 34 kbp (Figure 7) (60). A similar strategy was employed by Piepersberg and his coworkers (22,23) to identify and isolate this same region from the *S. lincolnensis* production strain 78-11.

B. Analysis of the Conserved Region

The entire conserved region from strain 78-11 was sequenced by Peschke et al. (23) and found to contain 30 open reading frames (Figure 9). The functions encoded for by several of these have been at least partially characterized and are clearly involved in lincomycin production:

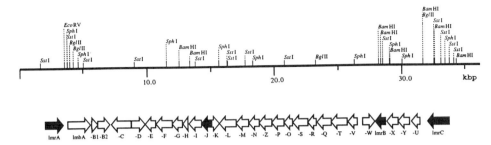

Figure 9   The lincomycin gene cluster. This figure is drawn according to the results of Peschke *et al.* (23). lmb indicates putative biosynthetic genes; lmr indicates genes coding for functions that impart a lincomycin-resistance phenotype; shaded arrows indicate genes encoding characterized functions; white arrows indicate open reading frames of unknown or uncertain function.

1.   **lmrA.**   Subcloning experiments localized *lmr*A on the 2.16 kbp *Sst*I fragment at the leftmost end of the conserved region as depicted in Figure 7 (fragment 8 of cosmid 373) (59). This gene does not confer resistance to the structurally related lincosamide antibiotic celesticetin, nor to macrolides such as erythromycin and tylosin, clearly differentiating it from the macrolide, lincosamide, and streptogramin B-type (MLS) resistance determinants associated with production of those compounds. Surprisingly, *lmr*A also shows little effect against clindamycin, the 7-chloro derivative of lincomycin. Based on its deduced amino acid sequence and a comparison with several known proteins, the *lmr*A gene from *S. lincolnensis* strain 78-11 appears to code for a membrane-integrated protein likely involved in lincomycin export (22).

2.   **lmrB.**   Several observations indicated that there must be at least one other gene in the conserved region, besides *lmr*A, that is involved in specifying resistance to lincomycin. First, hybridization studies showed that two Lm⁻ mutants, LM1628 and LM1404, contained deletions that terminated in the middle of this region and extended leftward, as depicted in Figure 7. Although both mutants lacked *lmr*A, they were still resistant to moderate levels of lincomycin (minimum inhibitory concentration [MIC] ≈ 200 µg/ml in Hickey and Tresner agar versus ≤1 µg/ml for mutants, such as LM814, lacking this entire region). Second, strains in which *lmr*A was inactivated by insertion of the *Streptomyces* transposon Tn4560 (61,62) were also found to be partially resistant to lincomycin (Figure 10). Subsequently, a 2.7 kbp *Sph*I fragment of the conserved region (within fragment 2 of cosmid 373, as indicated in Figure 7) was found by Zhang et al. (22) to contain a gene, designated *lmr*B, which coded for resistance to lincomycin, but again, not to clindamycin, celesticetin, or macrolides. Within the DNA sequence of this fragment, an open reading frame was identified for a protein very similar to several 23S RNA methyltransferases. This indicated that target-site modification was the likely mode of action of the *lmr*B product.

3.   **lmrC.**   More recently, Peschke et al. (23) cloned yet a third subfragment from this cluster that is involved in imparting lincomycin resistance to the producing culture. This gene, designated *lmr*C, flanks the end of the cluster opposite *lmr*A and also codes for a protein with a deduced sequence similar to that of known transport proteins. This is consistent with the properties of strains containing Tn4560 inserted in *lmr*A (mutants III-11 and I-15 in Figure 10) which, whereas only moderately resistant with respect to

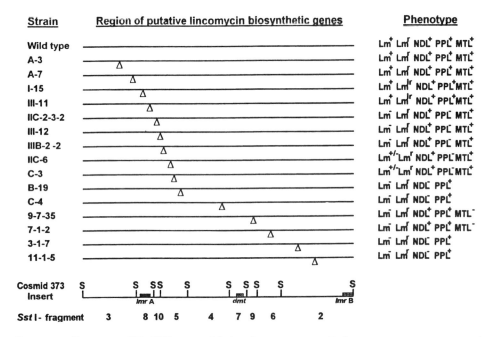

Figure 10 Properties of Tn4560-inserted *S. lincolnensis* mutants. Each mutant contains a copy of Tn4560 (△) at various locations of lincomycin biosynthetic genes. Mutants containing Tn4560 in the SstI-generated fragments 3 and 8 produced lincomycin (Lm⁺), whereas mutants containing it in the fragments 2, 4, 5, 6, 9, and 10 produced no lincomycin (Lm⁻). Lincomycin and *N*-demethyllincomycin (NDL) production were tested by growing the mutants in S-medium and S-medium containing PPL and MTL, respectively. Lm^r, resistance to lincomycin at concentrations exceeding 1000 µg/ml; Lm^{lr}, low-level lincomycin resistance (MIC ≈ 200 µg/ml in Hickey and Tresner agar); S, SstI.

growth on lincomycin-containing agar (MIC ≈ 200 µg/ml), still produced and secreted near-normal levels of lincomycin in liquid fermentations.

    4. **N-demethyllincomycin methyltransferase determinant.**   As described above, the enzyme that converts the penultimate biosynthetic intermediate *N*-demethyl-lincomycin into lincomycin has been identified and purified to homogeneity (50,55). The *N*-terminus of this methyltransferase was sequenced, and the corresponding oligonucleotide prepared (50) and used in hybridization studies to locate that end of the gene on the 2.6 kbp SstI fragment of the conserved region (fragment 7 of cosmid 373). This gene appears to correspond to the open reading frame designated *lmb*J by Peschke et al. (23), all of which is contained within fragment 7. However, subcloned fragment 7 by itself failed to induce methyltransferase activity, indicating that other sequences may also be involved in coding for functional enzyme. In this regard, it is interesting that the apparent molecular weight of the native enzyme was determined by size-exclusion chromatography to be about 300,000, versus 29,000 for the single major band that appeared when this material was subjected to SDS-PAGE (50). These results suggest that the native methyltransferase could be a multimeric complex of similarly sized, but apparently nonidentical, subunits. Possible candidates for an additional subunit gene include the open reading frame designated *lmb*G, which was determined by Peschke et al. (23) to code for

a protein with a molecular weight of approximately 30,000, which also contains a sequence corresponding to the expected SAM-binding site of SAM-dependent methyl-transferases.

Besides these defined determinants, there is evidence that the other, less-characterized, genes in this conserved 34 kbp region may also be lincomycin-specific. For example, insertion of Tn*4560* into many locations within this region blocked lincomycin production (Figure 10) (63,64). Feeding studies with these blocked mutants suggested that genes located in the leftward portion of this region (e.g., in SstI-generated fragments 5 and 10 of cosmid 373) coded for enzymes involved in PPL biosynthesis, whereas insertions in the rightward fragments (e.g., 6 and 9) appeared to disrupt formation of MTL. This is consistent with the locations of functions inferred from analysis of open reading frames in this region (Figure 9) (23). In this analysis, many of the deduced products of the contiguous open reading frames *lmb*A through *lmb*K showed resemblance to enzymes of amino acid metabolism (including *lmb*B1 and *lmb*B2, which were subsequently expressed in *Escherichia coli* and found to code for an uncharacterized L-DOPA-converting activity), whereas the gene products of *lmb*L through *lmb*Q were determined to be most like known sugar-converting enzymes. Thus, genes may be organized by functional pathways within the clustered region. However, insertions at three widely separated sites (mutants B19, C4, 3-1, and 11-1) appeared to block synthesis of *N*-demethyllincomycin from supplied precursors. This suggested that several genes are involved in the synthetase function, which is consistent with purification studies showing that the *N*-demethyllincomycin synthetase is a complex enzyme composed of dissociable, nonidentical subunits.

In comparing the various lincomycin-producing *Streptomyces*, Peschke et al. (23) noted that the order of genes within the conserved segment was the same in each strain, but the segment was apparently located in different genomic regions in these cultures. They suggested that this might reflect transfers of the intact segment via, for example, transposition, conjugation, or transduction and may indicate that all the genes required for lincomycin production are encoded in this segment.

C.   Instability of the *S. lincolnensis* Chromosome at the Region of the Lincomycin Biosynthetic Cluster

There are many reported examples of genetic instabilities in *Streptomyces* that affect a variety of primary and secondary metabolic processes (65). Two chromosomal regions of *S. lincolnensis* that exhibit this characteristic are the lincomycin biosynthetic cluster and the area coding for melanin production. These loci appear to be linked, because at least 5% of the CFU present at the end of normal production fermentations contain deletions encompassing one or both of these regions. As in other *Streptomyces*, the deleted segments in these prototrophic strains can be quite large; chromosome walking experiments have shown that *mel* is greater than 250 kbp from *lmr*A.

Further, several mutants have been found to contain amplified chromosomal sequences. A striking example is LM4344, in which a 23 kbp portion of the lincomycin biosynthetic cluster is highly reiterated (Figure 11) (60). Interestingly, when a DNA fragment containing the junction between these direct repeats was isolated from LM4344 and inserted into the wild-type strain, a high frequency of the resulting transformants were found to also contain amplified chromosomal sequences (66). The reiterations in

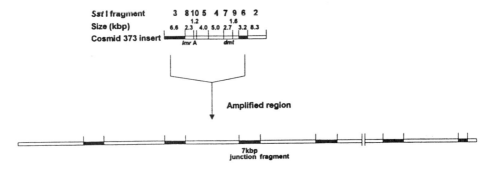

Figure 11   Organization of the amplified chromosomal region in LM4344. Each chromosome is estimated to contain at least 100 copies of the 23 kbp repeated sequence. Chromosome walking experiments showed that there is a large deletion (>150 kbp) extending "leftward" from this region toward the *mel* gene.

these transformants were similar to those found in LM4344, but in some cases they also included vector sequences (Figure 12). Smaller amplified sequences were also frequently generated in *S. lividans* following transformation with this cloned junction fragment. Similarly, it has been shown in other microorganisms that transduction of a segment containing the joint region between copies of a tandemly duplicated region can lead to regeneration of the duplication in the recipient cell (67). The mechanism by which this induced amplification occurs in *S. lincolnensis*, or how it is related to the genetic events that led to LM4344, is unclear. Presumably, first the junction fragment is integrated by a single crossover at the regions of homology, which would generate direct repeats flanking a region similar to that amplified in LM4344. Subsequent recombinational events could result in further amplification of the chromosomal region. However, the level of reiteration seen within the lincomycin biosynthetic cluster in LM4344 is extreme, estimated at more than 100 copies per chromosome, and may involve other unknown elements within this region.

Another striking example of an induced rearrangement in this region of the *S. lincolnensis* chromosome is the finding by Peschke et al. (23) that the entire lincomycin biosynthetic cluster is part of a large duplication of about 500 kbp in the high-titer production strain 78-11, but is present as only a single copy in the wild-type strain NRRL 2936 (which was described as being similar to the parental strain of 78-11). Assuming that this rearrangement occurred during the several mutagenesis and selection steps employed in developing 78-11, it seems likely that gene duplication is at least in part responsible for the enhanced lincomycin productivity of this strain. Clearly, this finding has interesting implications with respect to strategies for culture development in other *Streptomyces*.

ACKNOWLEDGMENT

We thank David P. Brunner for valuable discussions and suggestions, and critical reading of the manuscript.

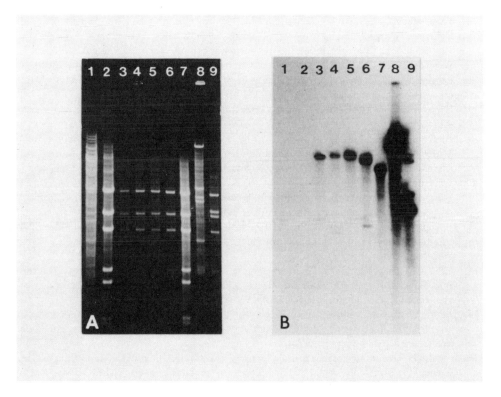

Figure 12 Introduction of the cloned junction fragment into *S. lincolnensis* strains triggers DNA amplifications. *S. lincolnensis* strains LM2 and 1404 (a low-lincomycin-producing mutant derived from LM2), neither of which contains grossly amplified chromosomal sequences such as seen in LM4344, were transformed to thiostrepton resistance (Thio[R]) by pLR1, the plasmid containing the cloned junction fragment. Individual transformants were then passaged serially several times in the absence of Thio, resulting in the loss of free plasmid. Isolates retaining Thio[R] were selected and chromosomal DNA isolated, samples of which were digested with *Sst*I and subjected to electrophoresis on agarose (A). The lanes in this panel are (1) LM2; (2) 4344; (3–6) four independently selected transformants of LM2. All of these transformants contain large amplified regions, most of which are identical or similar to that found in 4344.

The DNA in this gel was then transferred to nitrocellulose and hybridized with ^{32}P-labeled vector (B). Vector DNA appears to be integrated as single (or few) copies in the chromosomes shown in lanes 3–7, but it is part of the regions greatly amplified in the isolates shown in lanes 8 and 9.

REFERENCES

1. Mason DJ, Dietz A, DeBoer C. Lincomycin, a new antibiotic. I. Discovery and biological properties. Sylvester JC, ed. Antimicrobial Agents and Chemotherapy—1962. Ann Arbor, Michigan: American Society for Microbiology, 1963:554–559.
2. Bergy E, Herr RR, Mason DJ. Antibiotic lincolnensin and method of production. 1963; US Patent 3,086,912.
3. Hoeksema H, Bannister B, Birkenmeyer RD, Kagan F, Magerlein BJ, MacKellar FA, Schroeder W, Slomp G, Herr RR. Chemical studies on lincomycin. I. The structure of lincomycin. J Am Chem Soc 1964; 86:4223–4224.

4. Argoudelis AD, Coats JH, Pyke TR. Lincomycin production. 1972; US Patent 3,697,380.
5. Reusser F, Argoudelis AD. Process for preparing lincomycin. 1974; US Patent 3,833,475.
6. Argoudelis AD, Coats JH. Process for producing lincomycin. 1973; US Patent 3,726,766.
7. Argoudelis AD, Coats JH. Process for preparing lincomycin. 1974; US Patent 3,812,014.
8. Kuznetsov VD, Bushueva OA, Bryzgalova LS. Variation of *Actinomyces roseolus*. A lincomycin-producing organism. Antibiotiki 1974; 19:690–693.
9. Bergy ME, Coats JH, Malik VS. Process for preparing lincomycin. 1981; US Patent 4,271,266.
10. Bibikova MV, Singal EM, Ivanitskaia LP, Zhdanovich IuV. Production of lincomycin by *Micromonospora halophytica* culture. Antibiot Khimioter 1989; 34:723–726.
11. Magerlein BJ, Birkenmeyer RD, Herr RR, Kagan F. Lincomycin. V. Amino acid fragment. J Am Chem Soc 1967; 89:2459–2464.
12. Schroeder W, Bannister B, Hoeksema H. Lincomycin. III. The structure and stereochemistry of the carbohydrate moiety. J Am Chem Soc 1967; 89:2448–2453.
13. Slomp G, MacKellar FA. Lincomycin. IV. Nuclear magnetic resonance studies on the structure of lincomycin, its degradation products, and some analogs. J Am Chem Soc 1967; 89:2454–2459.
14. Lewis C, Clapp HW, Grady JE. *In vitro* and *in vivo* evaluation of lincomycin, a new antibiotic. Sylvester JC, ed. Antimicrobial Agents and Chemotherapy—1962. Ann Arbor, Michigan: American Society for Microbiology, 1963:570–582.
15. Mason DJ, Lewis C. Biological activity of the lincomycin related antibiotics. Sylvester JC, ed. Antimicrobial Agents and Chemotherapy—1964. Ann Arbor, Michigan: American Society for Microbiology, 1965:7–12.
16. Grady JE. Recent developments in lincomycin research. Int J Pharmacol 1968; 16:533–538.
17. Chang FN, Sih CJ, Weisblum B. Lincomycin, an inhibitor of aminoacyl SRNA binding to ribosomes. Proc Natl Acad Sci USA 1966; 55:431–438.
18. Cambell JM, Reusser F, Caskey CT. Specificity of lincomycin action on peptidyl transferase activity. Biochem Biophys Res Commun 1979; 90:1032–1037.
19. Skinner R, Cundliffe E, Schmidt FJ. Site of action of a ribosomal RNA-methylase responsible for resistance to erythromycin and other antibiotics. J Biol Chem 1983; 258:12702–12706.
20. Wright JLC. The lincomycin-celesticetin-anthromycin group. Vining LC, ed. Biochemistry and Genetic Regulation of Commercially Important Antibiotics. London: Addison-Wesley, 1983:311–328.
21. Gonzalez JE, Miller TL. Lincomycin. Moo-Young M, ed. Comprehensive Biotechnology. New York: Pergamon Press, 1985:211–223.
22. Zhang HZ, Schmidt H, Piepersberg W. Molecular cloning and characterization of two lincomycin-resistance genes, *lmr*A and *lmr*B, from *Streptomyces lincolnensis* 78-11. Mol Microbiol 1992; 6:2147–2157.
23. Peschke U, Schmidt H, Zhung HZ, Piepersberg W. Molecular characterization of the lincomycin production gene cluster of *Stretomyces lincolnensis* 78-11. Mol Microbiol 1995; 16:1137–1156.
24. Short KA, Campbell CM, Hoogerheide JG, Ceglarek JA. Extraction, quantitation, and use of diaminopimelic acid to measure *Mycobacterium fortuitum* biomass in sterol bioconversions. Abstracts to the 1994 Annual Meeting of the Society for Industrial Microbiology.
25. Churchill BW, Rakow BJ, Bergy ME. Microbiological process for preparing the amino acids *trans*-4-*n*-propyl-L-proline and *trans*-4-ethyl-L-proline. 1973; US Patent 3,753,859.
26. Argoudelis AD, Fox JA, Eble TE. A new lincomycin related antibiotic. Biochemistry 1965; 4:698–703.
27. Visser J. Lincomycin production. 1972; US Patent 3,676,302.
28. Witz DF, Hessler EJ, Miller TL. Bioconversion of tyrosine into the propylhygric acid moiety of lincomycin. Biochemistry 1971; 10:1128–1133.

29. Witz DF. Lincomycin production. 1972; US Patent 3,687,814.

30. Young MD, Kempe LL, Bader FG. Effects of phosphate, glucose, and ammonium on cell growth and lincomycin production by *Streptomyces lincolnensis* in chemically defined media. Biotechnol Bioeng 1985, 27:327–333.

31. Martin JF, Demain AL. Control of antibiotic biosynthesis. Microbiol Rev 1980; 44:230–251.

32. Hanka LJ, Mason DJ, Burch MR, Treick RW. Lincomycin, a new antibiotic. III. Microbiological assay. Sylvester JC, ed. Antimicrobial Agents and Chemotherapy—1962. Ann Arbor Michigan: American Society for Microbiology, 1963:565–569.

33. Neff AW, Barbiers AR, Northam JI. Microbiological methods for assaying lincomycin in animal feed. J Assoc Off Anal Chem 1967; 50:442–446.

34. Prescott GC. Automated assay for the antibiotic lincomycin. J Pharm Sci 1966; 55:423–425.

35. Houtman RL, Kaiser DG, Taraszka AJ. Gas-liquid chromatographic determination of lincomycin. J Pharm Sci 1968; 57:693–695.

36. Asmus PA, Landis JB, Vila CL. Liquid chromatographic determination of lincomycin in fermentation beers. J Chromatogr 1983; 264:241–248.

37. Argoudelis AD, Eble TE, Fox JA, Mason DJ. Studies on the biosynthesis of lincomycin. IV. The origin of methyl groups. Biochemistry 1969; 8:3408–3411.

38. Brahme NM, Gonzalez JE, Rolls JR, Hessler EJ, Mizsak S, Hurley LH. Biosynthesis of the lincomycins. 1. Studies using stable isotopes on the biosynthesis of the propyl- and ethyl-L-hygric acid moieties of lincomycin A and B. J Am Chem Soc 1984; 106:7873–7878.

39. Argoudelis AD, Fox JA, Mason, DJ. Studies on the biosynthesis of lincomycin. II. Antibiotic U-11,973, N-demethyl lincomycin. Biochemistry 1965; 4:710–713.

40. Brahme NM, Gonzalez JE, Mizsak S, Rolls JR, Hessler EJ, Hurley LH. Biosynthesis of the lincomycins. 2. Studies using stable isotopes on the biosynthesis of methylthiolincosaminide moiety of lincomycin A. J Am Chem Soc 1984; 106:7878–7883.

41. Michalik J, Emilianowicz-Czerska W, Switalski L, Raczynska-Bojanowska K. Monophenol monooxygenase and lincomycin biosynthesis in *Streptomyces lincolnensis*. Antimicrob Agents Chemother 1975; 8:526–531.

42. Hurley LH. Elucidation and formulation of novel biosynthetic pathways leading to the pyrrolo[1,4]benzodiazepine antibiotics anthramycin, tomaymycin, and sibiromycin. Acc Chem Res 1980; 13:263–269.

43. Hurley LH, Laswell WL, Ostrander JM, Parry R. Pyrrolo[1,4]benzodiazepine antibiotics. Biosynthetic conversion of tyrosine to the C2- and C3-proline moieties of anthramycin, tomaymycin and sibiromycin. Biochemistry 1979; 18:4230–4237.

44. Coats JH, Li GP, Kuo MS, Yurek DA. Discovery, production, and biological assay of an unusual flavenoid cofactor involved in lincomycin biosynthesis. J Antibiot 1989; 472–474.

45. Kuo MS, Yurek DA, Coats JH, Li GP. Isolation and identification of 7,8-didemethyl-8-hydroxy-5-deazariboflavin, an unusual cosynthetic factor in streptomycetes, from *Streptomyces lincolnensis*. J Antibiot 1989; 42:475–478.

46. Kuo MS, Yurek DA, Coats JH, Chung ST, Li GP. Isolation and identification of 3-propylidiene-Δ^1-pyrroline-5-carboxylic acid, a biosynthetic precursor of lincomycin. J Antibiot 1992; 45:1773–1777.

47. McCormick JRD, Morton GO. Identity of cosynthetic factor 1 of *Streptomyces aureofaciens* and fragment FO from coenzyme F420 of *Methanobacterium* species. J Am Chem Soc 1982; 104:4014–4015.

48. Rinehart KL, Snyder WC, Staley AL, Lau RCM, Biosynthetic studies on antibiotics. Petroski RJ, McCormick SP, eds. Secondary-Metabolite Biosynthesis and Metabolism. New York: Plenum Press, 1992:41–60.

49. Hausknecht EC, Wolf HJ. Preparation and purification of [14C] labeled N-demethyl lincomycin and propylproline from [14C]tyrosine. J Label Compounds Radiopharm 1987; 24:247–253.

50. Hausknecht EC, Horvath BA, Patt TE, Wolf HJ. Characterization of the last two steps of the lincomycin pathway in *S. lincolnensis*. American Society of Pharmacognosy, Ann Arbor, Michigan, 1986, July 27–30.

51. Hausknecht EC, Wolf HJ. Radiometric assay for *N*-demethyllincomycin synthetase. American Society of Microbiology, Annual Meeting, 1986.

52. Lee SG, Lipmann F. Tyrocidine synthetase system. Hash, JH, ed. Methods in Enzymology. Vol. 43. Antibiotics. New York: Academic Press, 1975:585–602.

53. Kyrylo-Borowska Z. Edeine synthetase. Hash, JH, ed. Methods in Enzymology. Vol. 43. Antibiotics. New York: Academic Press, 1975:559–567.

54. Zimmer T-L, Laland SG. Gramicidin S synthetase. Hash, JH, ed. Methods in Enzymology. Vol. 43. Antibiotics. New York: Academic Press, 1975:567–579.

55. Patt TE, Horvath BA. Isolation and characterization of *N*-demethyllincomycin methyltransferase in *Streptomyces lincolnensis*. 13th International Congress of Biochemistry, Amsterdam, The Netherlands, 1985, August 25–30.

56. Corcoran JW. *S*-adenosylmethionine:erythromycin C O-methyltransferase. Hash, JH, ed. Methods in Enzymology. Vol. 43. Antibiotics. New York: Academic Press, 1975:487–498.

57. Speedie MK, Hornemann H, Floss HG. *S*-adenosylmethionine:indolepyruvate 3-methyltransferase. Hash, JH, ed. Methods in Enzymology. Vol. 43. Antibiotics. New York: Academic Press, 1975:498–502.

58. Chater KF, Bruton CJ. Resistance, regulatory and production genes for the antibiotic methylenomycin are clustered. EMBO J 1985; 4:1893–1900.

59. Wovcha MG, Steuerwald DC, Manis JJ. Cloning and characterization of a lincomycin resistance gene from *Streptomyces lincolnensis*. Abstracts of the 5th International Symposium on the Genetics of Industrial Microorganisms. Split, Yugoslavia, September 14–20, 1986; Abstract W4-P4.

60. Patt TE, Manis JJ, Wolf HJ, Wovcha MG. An amplified region of the *Streptomyces lincolnensis* chromosome contains lincomycin resistance and biosynthetic genes. Abstracts of the UCLA Symposia Colloquium on Molecular Genetics of *Streptomyces*. Lake Tahoe, California, March 8–11, 1987.

61. Chung ST. Tn4556, a 6.8 kilobase-pair transposable element of *Streptomyces fradiae*. J Bacteriol 1987; 169:4436–4441.

62. Chung ST. Transposition of Tn4556 in *Streptomyces*. Dev Ind Micrbiol 1988; 29:81–88.

63. Chung ST, Crose LL. Transposon Tn4556-mediated DNA insertion and site-directed mutagenesis. Heslot H, Davies J, Florent J, Bobichon L, Durand G, Peneasse L, eds. Proceedings of the 6th International Symposium on Genetics of Industrial Microorganisms. Strasbourg: Societe Francaise de Microbiologie, 1990:207–218.

64. Chung ST, Crose LL. *Streptomyces* transposon Tn4556 and its applications. Hershberger CL, Queener SW, Hegeman G, eds. Genetics and Molecular Biology of Industrial Microorganisms. Washington, D.C.: American Society for Microbiology, 1989:168–175.

65. Cullum J, Flett F, Piendl W. Genetic instability, deletions, and DNA amplification in *Streptomyces* species. Hershberger CL, Queener SW, Hegeman G, eds. Genetics and Molecular Biology of Industrial Microorganisms. Washington, D.C.: American Society for Microbiology, 1989:127–132.

66. Wovcha MG, Manis JJ, Zwart MA. Isolation of a DNA segment from *Streptomyces lincolnensis* which triggers amplifications when inserted into the chromosomes of *Streptomyces* sp. Abstracts of the 6th International Symposium on the Genetics of Industrial Microorganisms. Strasbourg, France, August 12–18, 1990; Abstract C-16.

67. Anderson RP, Roth JR. Tandem genetic duplication in phage and bacteria. Annu Rev Microbiol 1977; 31:473–505.

6

Structure, Function, and Regulation of Genes Encoding Multidomain Peptide Synthetases

Peter Zuber
Louisiana State University Medical Center, Shreveport, Louisiana

Mohamed A. Marahiel
Philipps University, Marburg, Germany

I. INTRODUCTION

Microorganisms, from a variety of habitats, produce an abundance of low-molecular-weight peptide products that exhibit enormous diversity in chemical structure and bioactivity. These peptide secondary metabolites represent an important class of bacterial and fungal products and have found widespread use in clinical, industrial, and agricultural settings. Many are endowed with antimicrobial activity, whereas others have been exploited as immunomodulators or specific enzyme inhibitors. Some microbial peptides are toxins or virulence determinants produced by plant and animal pathogens, whereas others, while exhibiting little xenotoxic activity, serve as extracellular regulators that mediate intercellular communication between producing organisms.

Some peptides, such as the lantibiotics, are highly stable, multicyclic structures resulting from the proteolytic processing of gene-encoded precursors that have undergone extensive posttranslational modification (1; see Chapter 6 of this book). Many others are not gene-encoded, but are synthesized nonribosomally through a series of reactions catalyzed by large, often multisubunit, enzyme complexes called peptide synthetases (2–6). It is this latter group of peptidelike compounds to which is attributed the remarkable structural diversity of the peptide secondary metabolites. A nonribosomally synthesized peptide can be composed of a linear or cyclic peptide chain and often contains amino acids not found in ribosomally synthesized products. D–Amino acids as well as modified derivatives or precursors of the primary, proteinogenic amino acids are commonly encountered in analyses of peptide antibiotics. Although structurally diverse, most share a common mode of synthesis, the multienzyme thiotemplate mechanism catalyzed by peptide synthetases. In the thiotemplate model, substrate amino acids are first activated to their respective adenylates and are then bound to the active site, or substrate-activating domains of the peptide synthetase, by thioester linkages. The modules are aligned in a sequence that is colinear with the amino acid sequence of the peptide itself. This arrangement of activating domains is called the thiotemplate, since, according to the model, it determines the amino acid sequence of the peptide product. The polypeptide subunits that constitute the peptide synthetase complex are classic examples of multifunctional enzymes, being composed of substrate-activating domains that operate independently of one another, but that also act in concert to catalyze sequential biosynthetic reactions. Not only is the function of the thiotemplate enzyme complex of interest, but the regulation of both the peptide synthetase–catalyzed reactions and the production of the enzyme subunits has recently drawn considerable interest from biochemists and molecular biologists alike.

II. PREVALENCE OF NONRIBOSOMAL PEPTIDE SYNTHESIS

Much of what is known about the thiotemplate mechanism of peptide synthesis is the result of work that focused on the cyclic peptide antibiotics, gramicidin S and tyrocidine (Figure 1), produced by the Gram-positive spore-forming bacterium, *Bacillus brevis* (3,6–12), and studies of the δ-(α-aminoadipyl)-cysteinyl-D-valine (ACV) synthetase, which catalyzes the first step in β-lactam antibiotic synthesis, the formation of the δ-(α-aminoadipyl)-cysteinyl-D-valine tripeptide (13–15). However, other bacteria and many lower eukaryotes that inhabit soil and aquatic environments, including a number of pathogens, produce peptide antibiotics. The large, 18-residue lipodepsipeptide tolaasin (16) is a toxin produced by *Pseudomonas tolaasii*, a mushroom pathogen. Syringomycin (17) and syringotoxin (18) are produced by *Pseudomonas syringae*. The *P. syringae* pv. *phaseolica* produces the peptide phaseolotoxin [N(δ-diaminophosphinyl)–ornithyl–alanyl–homoarginine] (19), most likely by the thiotemplate mechanism (20). Among the eukaryotic plant pathogens, *Cochliobolus carbonum*, a maize fungal pathogen, produces HC-toxin (21,22), and *Fusarium scirpi* produces the n-methyl-depsipeptide, enniatin (23). Iron siderophores, such as enterobactin (24,25) and pyoverdin (26,27), required for virulence by some bacterial pathogens are synthesized by a mechanism closely resembling that of peptide antibiotics. Hepatotoxins such as microcystin (28–31), produced by some freshwater Cyanobacteria are also thought to be produced nonribosomally. The cyclic N-methylated peptide cyclosporin (Figure 1), an immunosuppressive drug, is synthesized by the giant peptide synthetase, cyclosporin synthetase of the fungus *Tolypocladium niveum* (32; see Chapter XX in this book). There is growing evidence that *Streptomyces* utilize nonribosomally synthesized peptides as extracellular regulatory signals and as structural components of aerial mycelia (33,34). Cyclic lipopeptides (35), including antifungal agents and powerful biosurfactants, are produced by species of *Bacillus* (36) and *Arthrobacter* (37). Small lipopeptides synthesized nonribosomally have also been implicated in the establishment of swarming motility and differentiation in *Serratia* (38). Some of the members of the echinocandin class of fungal cell wall synthesis–inhibiting lipopeptides, such as the pneumocandins produced by *Zolarian arboricola* (39), are likely to be synthesized by a thiotemplate mechanism. Having listed these examples, one should keep in mind that the thiotemplate is not the only nonribosomal device for synthesizing peptides. Bacteria produce the cell wall precursor muramyl pentapeptide by a very different mechanism. But even in cell wall biosynthesis, similarities with the enzyme thiotemplate exist, as evidenced by the primary structure homology between the D-alanine-activating enzyme that functions in D-alanyl-lipoteichoic acid synthesis in *Lactobacillus* (40) and the amino acid–activating domains of peptide synthetases.

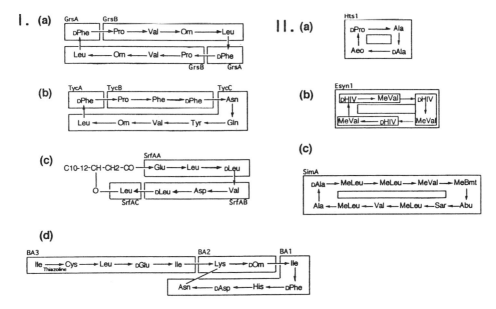

Figure 1 Primary structure of bacterial (I) and fungal (II) peptide antibiotics that are synthesized by the nonribosomal thiotemplate mechanism. (I) (a) gramicidin S, (b) tyrocidine, (c) surfactin, (d) bacitracin; (II) (a) HC-toxin, (b) enniatin A, (c) cyclosporin A. The amino acid sequence of the peptides is shown, as are the names of the enzymes that catalyze synthesis. The order of incorporation is indicated by the arrows, beginning with the amino acid shown below the name of the enzyme subunit.

III. THE THIOTEMPLATE MECHANISM OF PEPTIDE SYNTHESIS

Diagrams of the structures of several peptide antibiotics are shown in Figure 1. Those that are effective bioactive agents are cyclic peptides, as these are inherently more stable than linear peptides. Gramicidin S and tyrocidine are cyclic decapeptides, whereas bacitracin, produced by *Bacillus licheniformis*, is a branched cyclic peptide. Inspection of these three reveals, in addition to the D-form of some substrate amino acids, the presence of other nonprotein amino acids such as ornithine and the thiazoline derivative of isoleucine and cysteine found in bacitracin. The cyclic lipopeptide, surfactin, produced by certain strains of *Bacillus subtilis* contains seven amino acids along with a β-hydroxy fatty acid, which also serves as a member of the cyclic structure. Several lipopeptides such as serrawettin (38) and iturin (35) have similar structures, but the latter possesses a β-amino fatty acid.

Most of the enzymes that catalyze the synthesis of the peptides in Figure 1 have been studied in some detail. A peptide synthetase can be a single multifunctional polypeptide bearing several amino acid–activating domains, each consisting of active-site modules. Such is the case with Hts1 (HC-toxin synthetase) and AcvA [D-(L-α-aminoadipoyl)-L-cysteinyl-D-valine synthetase] (Figure 2). Alternatively, peptide synthetases can be composed of enzyme subunits, each consisting of a subset of the amino acid–activating domains required for complete synthesis, an arrangement most often observed in the thiotemplate enzymes of prokaryotes. Thus, proper subunit interaction may be facilitated by the ordered transcription of subunit genes and the sequential appearance of subunit polypeptides from translating ribosomes. All peptide synthetases of eukaryotes that have

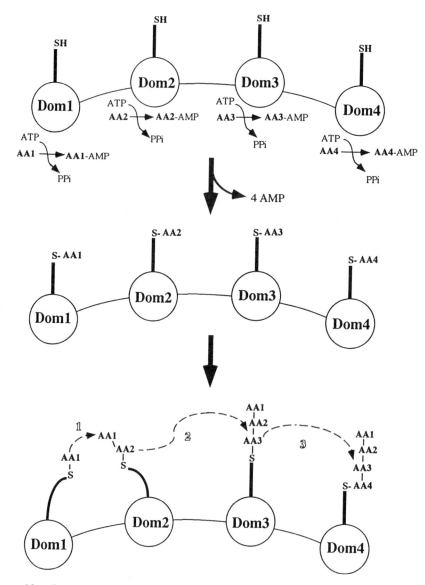

Figure 2 Nonribosomal peptide synthesis catalyzed by a peptide synthetase. Shown at the top is a diagram of the multienzyme thiotemplate consisting of four domains (Dom1, Dom2, Dom3, and Dom4), each bearing a cofactor (vertical bar) with a sulfhydryl-group for substrate amino acid binding. The adenylation reactions catalyzed by each domain for four substrate amino acids (AA1, AA2, AA3, AA4) are indicated. In the middle of the figure is the thiotemplate enzyme bearing the thioester-linked amino acids. At the bottom is the pathway of peptide synthesis charting the movement of the growing peptide chain from one domain to the next (steps 1, 2, and 3).

been examined thus far are composed of single, multifunctional polypeptides, which may be a reflection of the compartmentalization of transcription and translation in eukaryotes as opposed to the two processes being coupled in prokaryotic gene expression.

According to the most recent model of thiotemplate catalyzed peptide synthesis (4,41,42), the enzyme complexes catalyze the activation of the substrate amino acids to form amino acyladenylates at the expense of ATP (adenosine triphosphate) (Figure 2). The activated amino acids are in turn substrates for the formation of the amino acyl–enzyme thioester linkage. The thioester-bound substrates undergo peptide bond formation resulting in the assembly of the peptide product. The original thiotemplate hypothesis (6,11) postulated a central 4'-phosphopantetheine cofactor acting as a swinging arm, transferring the growing peptide chain from one amino acyl–enzyme site to the next, a model that persisted over several decades but was at odds with experiments that examined the accumulated intermediates in peptide synthetase reactions inhibited by the omission of a substrate amino acid, and the phenotype of mutant strains producing gramicidin S synthetase with reduced 4'-phosphopantetheine that were also defective in thioester formation (8,9,43). Instead of a single thioester-linked peptide intermediate accumulating in the mutant, as would be expected in the original thiotemplate model, intermediates of varying length were observed. This apparent contradiction has been resolved with the finding that each amino acid–activating module bears a 4'-phosphopantetheine cofactor site (Figure 2). A new model has emerged postulating the transfer of the growing peptide chain from one domain-linked cofactor to the next. If a mutant were blocked in step 3 of the process diagrammed at the bottom of Figure 2, then the intermediates at module 1, 2, and 3 would accumulate. Synthesis would then be terminated by a cyclization or the simple removal of the linear peptide, which is thought to occur with the aid of a thioesterase that may be a separate protein or an integral part of the synthetase subunit polypeptide. The molecular events associated with initiation of synthesis, transpeptidation, subunit or domain interactions, termination, and cyclization are poorly understood.

IV. ISOLATION OF GENES ENCODING PEPTIDE SYNTHETASES

Several advances in the study of peptide antibiotic biosynthesis have prompted attempts at detailed molecular characterization of peptide synthetases. Investigators have taken advantage of the amino acyladenlylation reaction's reversibility under the appropriate conditions due to its low free energy. An in vitro assay called the ATP-PPi phosphate exchange reaction, involving the use of [^{32}P]pyrophosphate, ATP, the substrate amino acid, and peptide synthetase (44) was developed. Substrate amino acid–dependent incorporation of ^{32}P into ATP can be measured as an indication of the presence of peptide synthetase activity. Using this assay, it has been possible to purify subunits of the enzyme complex and to obtain pure intact peptide synthetase enzyme for catalyzing the synthesis of the entire peptide product in vitro. With the purified subunits, antibodies were raised against peptide synthetase protein and were used for probing expression libraries of *Escherichia coli* to search for recombinant clones bearing peptide synthetase gene DNA (45,46). In an alternative approach, peptide sequencing technology was employed to obtain an amino acid sequence of a peptide fragment of cyclosporin synthetase for the design of an oligonucleotide hybridization probe (32). Clustering of genes encoding the enzymes that catalyze β-lactam synthesis has allowed investigators to isolate the *pcb*AB gene, encoding ACV synthetase of the fungus *Penicillium chrysogenum* (47,48). Cosmid clones overlapping with the isopenicillin synthase gene were found to contain the gene encoding ACV synthetase (49).

A number of fungal and bacterial mutant strains unable to produce peptide antibiotics have been isolated and used to obtain peptide antibiotic biosynthesis gene clusters (49,50), an approach used successfully in the isolation of antibiotic biosynthesis and regulatory genes of various *Streptomyces* species (51–53). The *pcb*AB gene was identified as a cosmid clone that complemented ACV synthetase–deficient mutants of *P. chrysogenum* (54). Transposon insertion mutations that eliminated surfactin production in *B. subtilis* were used to isolate, by chromosome walking, the genes encoding the subunits of surfactin synthetase (50,55).

As expected, the genes encoding the peptide synthetases were found within large transcriptional units (Figure 3). The ACV synthetases are encoded by monocistronic transcription units of near 11 kb, whereas the *srf*A operon encoding the three subunits of surfactin synthetase is 26.2 bp (Figure 3). Cyclosporin synthetase is a massive 1.7 MDa polypeptide encoded by a single open reading frame of 45.8 kb, the largest open reading frame yet identified (32). Nucleotide sequence analysis of peptide synthetase genes and subsequent amino acid sequence prediction have revealed the multidomain organization of the enzymes and enzyme subunits (Figure 3), a finding that came to light during the course of studies on the gramicidin, tyrocidine, and ACV synthetase genes (56–59). Thus, the ACV synthetase of *P. chrysogenum* was found to consist of three, ca. 600 amino acid, domains that are homologous to each other and to those found in the primary struc-

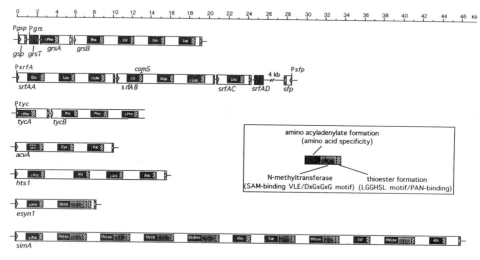

Figure 3 Schematic diagram of the domain organization of peptide synthetases encoded by the bacterial operons *grs*, *srf*A, and *tyc* and the fungal genes *acv*A, *hts*I, *esyn*I, and *sim*Z. Black boxes indicate the amino acid–activating domain adenylation modules, and striped areas show the location of the thioester modules (PAN-binding), located at the C-terminal end of each amino acid–activating domain. Type II domains shown in *esyn*I and *sim*A encode N-methyl peptide synthetases and have in addition an insertion that carries an N-methyltransferase module (SAM-binding). White areas represent the nonconserved spacer regions that separate each amino acid–activating domain. The locations of thioesterase-encoding genes (*grs*T, *srf*AD), *sfp* (and its homolog, *gsp*) and the *comS* gene are shown.

tures of gramicidin S and tyrocidine synthetases. This has become a consistently observed characteristic of peptide synthetase primary structure and corresponds well with the predicted structure of the multidomain thiotemplate as proposed by Lipmann and others (3,6,10).

A recent advance in the identification of peptide synthetase genes is the use of polymerase chain reaction (PCR) technology to amplify a specific sequence from a preparation of genomic DNA (20,60). Using degenerate oligonucleotides corresponding to the sequences encoding the conserved motifs or core sequences that function as sites of ATP binding and thioester formation within the amino acid–activating domain (see below), fragments of genomic DNA were amplified and found to contain sequences of putative peptide synthetase genes. Of course, further analysis is required to determine the exact function of the gene detected in this approach, since a peptide-producing organism may possess a number of peptide synthetase genes/operons, some of which may be cryptic with respect to function or expression (61).

V. ORGANIZATION OF PEPTIDE SYNTHETASES: THE AMINO ACID–ACTIVATING DOMAIN AND IDENTIFICATION OF ADENYLATING AND THIOLESTER MODULES

Early on in the study of peptide synthetase genes, evidence emerged that the enzymes might be composed of semiautonomous domains, when a fragment of the *grs*B gene encoding active Orn-adenylating activity was isolated. But computer-aided database searches performed in a number of laboratories uncovered a large family of acyl-adenylating enzymes that showed homology with the putative amino acid–activating domains of peptide synthetases. Thus, chlorobenzoate:CoA ligases (62), EntE and EntF (24,25) required for enterobactin biosynthesis, fatty acyl:CoA ligases (63), along with peptide synthetase domains (59) all possessed common primary structural motifs at conserved positions within their amino acid sequences. The motifs, thus identified, were proposed to be possible sites for ATP binding, substrate binding, and ATPase activity (59). These can be examined in the alignment of adenylating modules from several peptide synthetases (Figure 4). Shared among the acyl-adenylating enzymes are the five core sequences (Figure 4), including the so-called "signature" sequence core 2 (YSGTTGxP-KGV) (64). Core 2 bears some resemblance to the Walker A box (63) (GxxGxGKT/S) or P loop (65) involved in nucleotide phosphate binding. Core 4 resembles a motif commonly associated with ATPases, and it has been referred to as the ATPase motif (59,66). Some similarity is observed between the sequence around this motif and the Walker B box of nucleotide-binding proteins, both with respect to sequence and position relative to the Walker A box (64).

Protein affinity–labeling experiments supported the assignment of the core sequences 3, 4, and 5 as functioning in ATP interaction. Derivatized ATP analogs that could be cross-linked to the protein were used to identify peptide fragments that could have originated from the ATP-binding domain of tyrocidine synthetase I (TycA) (67,68). The sequence of the purified cross-linked peptide fragments overlapped with the conserved core 3–5 region (Figure 4).

Between core 2 and core 3 is a long stretch of amino acid sequence that contains few blocks of amino acid conservation and is variable in length among the peptide synthetase modules. Cosima et al. (55) have aligned the corresponding sequences from

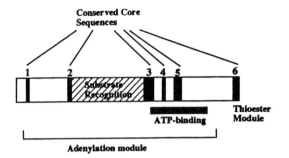

Figure 4   The type I amino acid–activating domain. A schematic diagram of the peptide synthetase amino acid–activating domain I showing the locations of the adenylation and thioester modules along with the sites of the six conserved core sequences. The consensus amino acid sequence of each core sequence is shown. Amino acid positions labeled * are the sites of amino acid substitutions that reduce adenylation activity. The position labeled † is the site of one of the substitutions in a double mutant with reduced adenylating activity. The amino acid position labeled • indicates the site of an amino acid substitution that eliminates thioester activity.

adenylating modules that utilize the same substrate amino acid and found similarities that are not uncovered when several modules of different specificity are compared. These observations prompted them to conclude that the region between core 2 and 3 contained the site of substrate recognition and interaction (Figure 4). Proof of this conclusion awaits biochemical studies.

Initial sequence comparisons failed to identify a possible candidate for thioester formation. A conserved Cys residue somewhere within the vicinity of an adenylating module was predicted to be the thioester site, but no conserved Cys was to be found. A sequence in ACV synthetase similar to the 4′-phosphopantetheine sites of fatty acid and polyketide synthetases suggested the presence of multiple cofactors in peptide synthetases instead of the single cofactor as originally proposed (54). The significance of this observation was not realized, however, until Vater and coworkers isolated a radiolabeled peptide from proteolytically digested GrsB that had been labeled with a [14C]substrate amino acid at its thioester site (12). The peptide corresponded in sequence to the 4′-phosphopantetheine sites identified at the C-terminal end of the amino acid–activating domains of gramicidin S synthetase and ACV synthetase. The sequence (FFxxGG H/D S I/L), referred to as core 6 (Figure 4) (4), is conserved among all of the amino acid–activating domains of peptide synthetases, but it is absent in other acyl-adenylating enzymes. That the cofactor is linked to each amino acid–activating domain has recently been demonstrated (69). The hydroxyl of the conserved Ser is believed to form a phosphodiester linkage with the 4'-phosphopantetheine while the cysteamine- or sulfhydryl-end of the cofactor forms the thioester bond with the carboxyl-group of the substrate amino acid (Figure 5).

To illustrate the modular organization of a peptide synthetase enzyme, the first two domains in a subunit of surfactin synthetase, SrfAB (Figure 3) (55,70), which catalyzes the incorporation of Val, Asp, and D-Leu into the surfactin peptide chain, are depicted in Figure 5. The Val-activating domain AB1 and the Asp-activating domain AB2 each are shown to carry a 4'-phosphopantetheine cofactor with covalently attached substrate amino acid at the thioester module adjacent to the adenylating module. The thioester and adenylation active sites are truly modular in nature. They each can be joined together to form the amino acid–activating domain, or they can be functionally separate active sites. For example, a thioester module is located at a C-terminal proximal position from

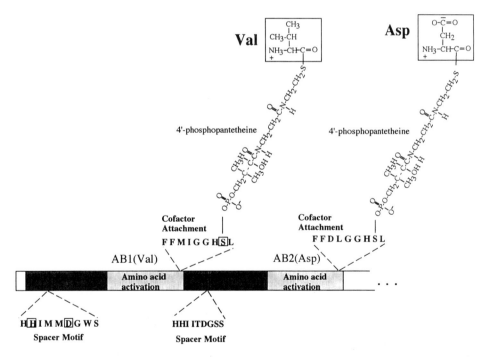

Figure 5 Val- and Asp-activating domains of SrfAB (Surfactin Synthetase 2): A schematic diagram of the first two amino acid–activating domains, AB1 and AB2, of SrfAB, the surfactin synthetase subunit that catalyzes the incorporation of Val, Asp, and D-Leu into the peptide portion of the lipopeptide, surfactin. The darker shaded areas indicate the interdomain regions. The sequences of the spacer motifs are shown. The structure of the 4'-phosphopantetheine cofactor and the amino acid sequence of the 4'-phosphopantetheine attachment site are also shown. The boxed letters indicate the sites of amino acid substitutions that impair peptide synthesis.

the N-methyl-L-valine domain (itself composed of both adenylating and thioester modules) of enniatin synthetase (Figure 2) (23). Here, it is thought to function in the assembly of the depsipeptide nascent chain. Likewise, the adenylating module is often found in enzymes that do not contain a 4′-phosphopantetheine prosthetic group (41,59).

A different type of domain, referred to as the type II domain (Figure 6) (4), which functions in the incorporation of methylated amino acids into a peptide product, is found in the enniatin and cyclosporin synthetases (23,32,71). The type II domain contains a third module bearing a methyltransferase active site positioned between the adenylating and thioester modules. Within this module is a conserved VL E/D xGxGxG motif characteristic of the S-adenosylmethionine (SAM)-dependent methyltransferases. Zocher and coworkers (71) recently examined the binding by photolabeling of radiolabeled SAM to protein fragments of enniatin synthetase produced in *E. coli* by expression of *esynl* gene segments. The valine-adenylating domain and a fragment containing the intact methyltransferase module both were found to bind SAM.

Mutational analysis has been undertaken in several laboratories to understand the significance of the primary structural similarities among amino acid–activating domains. Several Srf⁻ mutant strains of *B. subtilis* bearing deletion, insertion, and missense mutations have been constructed and analyzed for peptide biosynthesis in vivo and for enzyme activity in vitro (72–76). The amino acid–activating domain assignments were made by the analysis of deletion and insertion mutations. The gene/product assignments were determined by analyzing deletion and Tn917 insertion mutants using the ATP-PPi exchange assay. Precise in-frame internal deletions of *srf*AA and *srf*AB were constructed followed by ATP-PPi exchange assays to confirm the colinearity of the amino acid–activating domains with the amino acid sequence of the peptide portion of surfactin (74).

The core 6 sequences encoding the putative thioester modules in the first four domains of surfactin synthetase were subjected to oligonucleotide-mediated, site-directed mutagenesis in order to replace the conserved Ser, thought to be the site of 4′-phosphopantetheine binding, with an Ala (73). Fragments of the mutated DNA, carrying a diagnostic restriction site at the altered sequence, were inserted into integrative plasmids and introduced by genetic transformation into Srf⁺ *B. subtilis* cells. Single crossover recombination resulted in the integration of the mutation-bearing plasmid into the *srf*A genes.

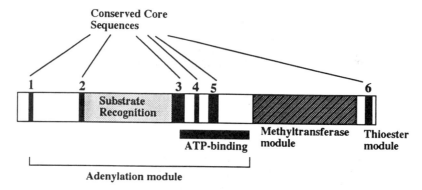

Figure 6 The type II, or N-methyl–amino acid–activating, domain. As in Figure 4, the amino acid–activating domain is shown with adenylating and thioester modules, the ATP-binding region, and the six conserved core sequences. The SAM-dependent N-methyltransferase module is also shown.

Plasmidless segregants were then isolated and were screened for the Ser to Ala mutation by Southern blot analysis of DNA cleaved with the diagnostic restriction enzyme, or by PCR followed by restriction enzyme digestion. Each of the mutations, thus generated and identified, eliminated surfactin production. When analyzed in vitro for both thioester formation and amino acyl-adenylation, it was observed, in the case of the fourth domain catalyzing the activation of Val, that thioester formation was abolished but amino acyl adenylation was unimpaired (76). However, while thioester site mutations in the three domains of srfAA eliminated thioesterification as predicted, adenylation was also impaired (75,76). This suggested that the presence of the cofactor may be required not only for the covalent attachment of the substrate amino acid to the thiotemplate, but also, in some cases, for the proper three-dimensional architecture of individual activating domains.

Another approach to mutationally dissect the amino acid–activating domains of peptide synthetases utilized heterologously expressed peptide synthetase domain DNA. In one study, the tycA gene, of the tyrocidine synthetase operon of B. brevis, encoding the Phe-activating subunit that initiates the synthesis of tyrocidine, was targeted for deletion analysis and in vitro oligonucleotide-mediated mutagenesis (77). The resulting mutant alleles were expressed in E. coli and analyzed for adenylating activity and thioesterification. The analysis of the deletion mutants confirmed the functional significance of the homologous domain found in all peptide synthetases (78). The minimum fragment necessary for amino acid activation was found to correspond closely to the 600-amino-acid homology observed in sequence alignments of peptide synthetase subunits. Mutations in the core 2 (at a conserved Lys) and core 4 (at the conserved Asp) sequences reduced amino acid adenylating activity. In a similar approach, another mutation at a conserved Gly codon within the ATP-binding region of GrsB, which catalyzes the activation of Pro in the gramicidin S biosynthetic pathway, was also found to be required for adenylation (79). Because domains produced in E. coli contain much reduced amounts of 4′-phosphopantetheine cofactor, very little thioester formation was detected when the TycA enzyme was combined with radiolabeled substrate amino acid, but the activity observed depended on the conserved Ser of the thioester site (77). In contrast with the srfAA experiments, the thioester-site Ser codon mutations in tycA and a deletion of the thioester site of GrsA do not cause a significant reduction of adenylating activity of the E. coli–produced enzymes. These experiments lend support to the view of the amino acid–activating domain as consisting of the adenylating and cofactor-bearing thioester modules. However, the analysis of whole synthetase enzymes from bacteria harboring defined mutations is necessary in order to more fully understand the function of the core sequences of the synthetase domains.

VI. ORGANIZATION OF PEPTIDE SYNTHETASES: INTERDOMAIN REGIONS

Between the amino acid–activating domains of peptide synthetases, there is an approximately 500-residue segment that shows fewer regions of amino acid sequence conservation. This interdomain region, or "spacer," contains a conserved motif (the spacer motif, Figure 5) that is found between amino acid–activating domains, but not at the N-terminal region of domains that initiate peptide synthesis (GrsA or TycA) nor at the C-terminus of domains that catalyze the incorporation of the last amino acid of a peptide product (i.e., SrfAC) (70). Between adjacent domains that are situated on different enzyme subunits, such as SrfAA3 and SrfAB1, there are two spacer motifs, in contrast to one motif between domains of a single-subunit polypeptide. The location and distribution of this sequence suggests that it may function somehow in peptide chain elongation. But why it is duplicated between domains of different enzyme subunits is not easily explained. Mutations in the second conserved His and Asp codons of the spacer motif DNA at the N-terminal coding end of *srf*AB eliminate surfactin production but do not affect the level of SrfAB protein (Liu L and Zuber P, unpublished results). To facilitate interdomain interaction was one proposed function of the spacer motif (70).

The region at the C-terminal end of peptide synthetase subunits often functions in the incorporation of a *D*-substrate amino acid (Figure 7A). Recent evidence ascribes the conversion of the L- to the D-configuration to a putative epimerase/racemase active site, a region of conserved amino acid motifs in peptide synthetases that catalyze the incorporation of D-substrates (Figure 7) (70). Deletion of the racemase/epimerase module of GrsA results in the loss of D-Phe formation but does not affect adenylation or thioester formation (78). Unlike an amino acid racemase that bears a pyridoxal phosphate cofactor and catalyzes a one-base mechanism, the epimerases of peptide synthetases are cofactor independent and are thought to catalyze a two-base mechanism of epimerization (83). Several conserved amino acid residues of the epimerase module could be involved in the two-base mechanism (Figure 7B) (70,83). Although the location of the epimerase module is often at the C-terminal end of the peptide synthetase subunit, the first domain of Hts (HC-toxin synthetase) bears an epimerase module that is followed by an extended interdomain region between the first and second amino acid–activating domains (22). Evidently, the epimerase module can function as an internal component of the peptide synthetase subunit provided the proper interdomain context.

Termination of peptide synthesis is believed to involve the activity of the thioesterase active site at the C-terminal end of the subunit that catalyzes the incorporation of the last amino acids into the peptide product. A thioesterase active-site motif GXSXG, found in mammalian fatty acid synthetase thiosterases, is also detected at the C-terminal end of SrfAC (55), GrsB (59), PvnD (27), and ACV synthetases (15).

The interdomain regions can also carry enzyme active-site modules. Enniatin synthetase carries an additional thioester module adjacent to the Val-activating domain (23). In the phytopathogenic pseudomonad that produces coronatine (84), a toxin that causes chlorotic lesions in plants, the enzyme, CmaA, responsible for the incorporation of the precursor coronamic acid, appears to contain an unusual active-site module adjacent to an amino acid–activating domain (85). CmaA is believed to activate isoleucine or alloisoleucine and to catalyze the oxidative cyclization of alloisoleucine to form coronamic acid (2-ethyl-1-aminocyclopropane 1-carboxylic acid). A putative nonheme iron binding region characteristic of enzymes that carry out oxidative cyclization is located on the N-terminal side of the CmaA amino acid–activating domain. The discovery of other active-site modules within or adjacent to the type I amino acid–activating domain extends the number of variations that exist in domain architecture and suggests more ways in which the thiotemplate may be manipulated genetically in the rational design of peptide antibiotics.

VII.   IN VITRO EXAMINATION OF THE THIOTEMPLATE MODEL

Biochemical studies provide evidence for the transfer of the growing peptide chain from one domain to the next in a sequence corresponding to the alignment of substrate-activating domains in the thiotemplate and to the amino acid sequence of the peptide prod-

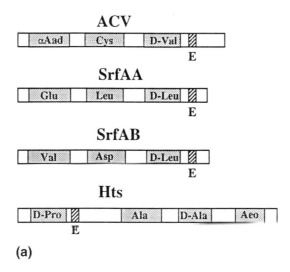

Figure 7 Location and primary structure of epimerase modules. (a) Diagrams showing the organization of the peptide synthetases GrsB, SrfAA, SrfAB, and Hts. The epimerase module is indicated by striped box labeled **E.** (b) Amino acid sequence alignments of epimerase modules from various peptide synthetase subunits. Regions of high conservation are indicated by a white bar below the sequence. Anid ACV epm: *Aspergillus nidulans* ACV synthetase (80); GRS1: gramicidin S synthetase I (57,81); HC syn: HC-toxin synthetase (22); Mle: *Mycobacterium leprae* racemase (NCBI); Nlac ACV: *Nocardia lactamdurans* ACV synthetase (56); Pen ACV: *Penicillium chysogenum* ACV synthetase (47); srfAA: surfactin synthetase I (55,70); srfAB: surfactin synthetase II (55); TycA Rac: Tyrocidine synthetase I (82).

uct (8,9). They also show that epimerization occurs following the synthesis of the peptide, but prior to the peptide's release from the enzyme thiotemplate. Thus, studies of ACMSI and -II (actinomycin synthetase subunits I and II of *Streptomyces chrysomallus* (86), which catalyze the formation of the tripeptide [4-methyl-3-hydroxyanthrinilate (MHA)]–L-Thr–D-Val) provide evidence that the enzyme first catalyzes the formation of the MHA–L-Thr dipeptide followed by the enzyme-bound MHA–L-Thr–Val tripeptide prior to epimerization yielding the MHA–D-Thr–Val product. This was shown by examination of enzyme-bound synthetic intermediates and by measuring hydrogen release resulting from the epimerization reaction. However, recent studies of the ACV synthetase of *Cephalosporium acremonium* suggest a variation on the thiotemplate theme. Shiau and coworkers (87), using the substrates α-aminoadipic acid, the Cys analog O-methyl serine, and L-Valine, observed the formation of dipeptides O-methyl seryl–L-valine and O-methyl seryl–D-valine catalyzed by the ACV synthetase. This finding, and the repeated but unsuccessful attempts to detect the dipeptide intermediate α-aminoadipyl–L-Cys in synthesis using the native substrates, prompted Shiau and colleagues to propose that synthesis of ACV begins with the formation of the enzyme-bound Cys–L-Val dipeptide followed by epimerization to Cys–D-Val and subsequent formation of the final ACV product; a C to N instead of a N to C synthesis (87). However, it was not shown in the experiments using the O-methyl serine substrate that a tripeptide product could be produced from the putative dipeptide intermediate. Additionally, a low yield of dipeptide product was observed in their reactions, which might indicate that the dipeptide was a reaction by-product rather than an intermediate in the synthesis of the ACV tripeptide.

```
Anid ACV epm     51 GSA---SERA YWEGL-LAQT AA--NISALP PVTGTRT-R- ----LARTWS    100
GRS1 rac         51 NSELFLEEAE YWHHL-NYYT DN--VQIKKD YVTMNNK-QK NIRYVGMELT    100
HC syn epm       51 KDIPVDRTVP LIPKIPTADF GYW--GLKHD ENVYGNTVER KI-----PLG     100
MLe rac          51 THPAALDTRS FWIEN-ANKV NLWLADVSLN TDVIQPPGAD DLIRMPCTLS    100
Nlac ACV epm     51 PAE---GERE FWAET-TRDM ES--AELLAQ TEGTTRR-R- ----EEFALT    100
Pen ACV epm      51 ASD---SERN HWNKL-VMET AS--SISALP TSTGSRV-R- ----LSRSLS    100
srfAA epm        51 NSKAFLKEKE YWRQL-EEQA VA--AKLPKD RESGDQR-MK HTKTIEFSLT    100
SrfAB epm        51 QSAHLLQQAE YWSQI-AAEQ VS--P-LPKD CETEQRI-VK DTSSVLCELT    100
TycA Rac c       51 NEADLLSEIP YWESL-ESQA KN--VSLPKD YEVTDCK-QK SVRNMRIRLH    100


Anid ACV epm    101 DDRTVILLNE ASN-QNASIQ DLLLAAVGLA LQQ-VTPGSP SMITLEGHGR    150
GRS1 epm        101 IEETEKLLKN VNKAYRTEIN DILLTALGFA LKE-WADIDK IVINLEGHGR    150
HC syn epm      101 HSITEDLLYK CHDSLHTKTI DVLLAAVLVS FRRSFLDRPV PAVFNEGHGR    150
MLe rac         101 VEQTSEL-DD ARRRFRRSIQ AIVLAALGRT IAQ-TVGDGV VAVELEGEGR    150
Nlac ACV epm    101 APDTRTLLAE SPWAYDTEVN DLLLTATGFA LRS-ITRQAT NHLTVEGHGR    150
Pen ACV epm     101 PEKTASLIQG GIDRQDVSVY DSLLTSVGLA LQH-IAPTGP SMVTIEGHGR    150
srfAA epm       101 AEETEQLTTK VHEAYHTEMN DILLTAFGLA MKE-WTGQDR VSVHLEGHGR    150
SrfAB epm       101 AEDTKHLLTD VHQPYGTEIN DILLSALGLT MKE-WTKGAK IGINLEGHGR    150
TycA Rac c      101 PEETEQLLKH ANQAYQTEIN DLLLAALGLA FAE-WSKLAQ IVIHLEGHGR    150


Anid ACV epm    151 EEIVDPTLDL SRTLGWFTSM YPFEIPPLNV ETLSQGIASL RECLRQVPAR    200
GRS1 epm        151 EEILEQ-MNI ARTVGWFTSQ YPVVLDMQKS DDLSYQIKLM KENLRRIPNK    200
HC syn epm      151 EPGGEDAVDL SRTVGWFTTI SPVYVPEVSP GDILDVVRRV KDYRWATPNN    200
MLe rac         151 S-VLRPDVDV RRTIGWFTNY YPIPLVCVKG QGALAQLDAV HNTLKSIPHY    200
Nlac ACV epm    151 E-LFEGAPDV RDTVGWFTTM HPFAVE-VDP GDLGRSVLAT RANRRRVPHH    200
Pen ACV epm     151 EEV-DQTLDV SRTMGWFTTM YPFEIPRLST ENIVQSVVAV SERFRQVPAR    200
srfAA epm       151 EEIIED-LTI SRTVGWFTSM YPMVLDMKHA DDLGYQLKQM KEDIRHVPNK    200
SrfAB epm       151 EDIIPN-VNI SRTVGWFTAQ YPVVLDISDA DA-SAVIKTV KENLRRIPDK    200
TycA Rac c      151 EDIIEQ-ANV ARTVGWFTSQ YPVLLDLKQT APLSDYIKLT KENMRKIPRK    200


Anid ACV epm    201 GIGFGSL--- -YGYCKHQM- ----PQVTFN YLGQLTSKQS ITDQWALAVG    250
GRS1 epm        201 GIGYEIFKYL TTEYLRPVLP FTLKPEINFN YLGQFDT-DV KTELFT----    250
HC syn epm      201 GFDYFSTKYL TQSGIK-LFE DHLPAEILFN YEGRYQAMES EQTV------    250
MLe rac         201 GIGYGLLRYM -YAPTGRVFS AQRTPDIHFR YVGVVPEPPS VDA-------    250
Nlac ACV epm    201 GIGYGAL--- -FG-GEAPL- ----PAVSFN YLGRLGEGDG QPTE------    250
Pen ACV epm     201 GVGYGTL--- -YGYTQHPL- ----PQVTVN YLGQLARKQS KPKEWVLAVG    250
srfAA epm       201 GVGYGILRYL TAPEHKEDVA FSIQPDVSFN YLGQFDE-MS DAGLFT----    250
SrfAB epm       201 GVGYGILRYF T--ETAETKG FT--PEISFN YLGQFDS-EV KTDFFE----    250
TycA Rac c      201 GIGYDILKHV TLPENRGSLS FRVQPEVTFN YLGQFDA-DM RTELFT----    250
```

(b)

Figure 7 continued.

VIII.   THE DEPSIPEPTIDE SYNTHETASE THIOTEMPLATE

Examination of the enniatin synthetase (23) and comparison with the organization of other peptide synthetases provides insight into the operation of the thiotemplate. Enniatin is a depsipeptide consisting of a six-membered ring composed of alternating D-hydroxy-isovaleric acid (HIV) and N-methyl-L-valine residues. Enniatin synthetase contains two substrate-activating domains that catalyze the formation of the two-residue unit of the six-membered ring, the HIV–(N-Methyl-L-Val) dipeptide. At the carboxy end of the enniatin synthetase protein, there is a third thioester module, which is thought to be a loading site for the assembly of the three dipeptide units. Thus, instead of six individual domains for each of the six enniatin residues, the economical use of genetic information is achieved by the introduction of a third cofactor site for the assembly of presynthesized units. The organization of enniatin synthetase lends support to the new model of the enzyme thiotemplate, the 4'-phosphopantatheine prosthetic group as being not only the site of substrate–enzyme thioester linkage, but also the carrier of the nascent peptide chain.

IX. ENGINEERED BIOSYNTHESIS OF NOVEL PEPTIDE ANTIBIOTICS BY TARGETED DOMAIN REPLACEMENTS

Based on the aforementioned biochemical and structural studies of peptide synthetases of diverse origin, it became clear that these multienzymes are composed of modules that build together the functional units, the amino acid–activating and modifying domains. The implications from these studies revealing the building block arrangement of such multienzymes would be that any peptide could be synthesized by providing a protein template with the appropriate number of amino acid–activating domains that are connected together in the correct order. It had been proposed that one could accomplish this by replacing a domain of peptide synthetase with that of another enzyme, thereby designing a peptide synthetase that could catalyze a product of one's choosing.

Based on the definition of minimal size needed for amino acid activation (77,78), a PCR method was developed for amplification of domain core regions of bacterial and fungal origin (88). The amplified heterologous domains were then used for targeted domain replacements within the srfA operon of B. subtilis. This genetic recombination method was realized in two steps—first, by a specific disruption of the desired domain followed by a gene replacement as summarized in Figure 8. For this approach, an integration vector (pJLA503/5'-3' SRF) for interruption and exchange of the srfAC domain was constructed [88]. The construction was based on an E. coli expression plasmid that contains two DNA fragments (Figure 8, I and III), which were amplified from the srfAC flanking core coding region (Figure 8, 1, II) by PCR. This vector was then used to introduce a selectable marker (cat gene, conferring chloramphenicol resistance) into the srfAC coding region (srfAC::cat) through marker exchange recombination (Figure 8) (88). This was accomplished by selection for CmR and screening for Srf- phenotype. Next, PCR-amplified heterologous amino acid–activating domains were inserted, in frame, between the linkers of the integration vector pJLA/5'-3'-SRF and were used to replace the srfAC::cat-interrupted copy of the srfA operon within the Bacillus chromosome through a second recombination event. This was accomplished by a congression involving selection for a neomycin-resistance gene at an unlinked locus and screening for chloramphenicol sensitivity resulting from the replacement of the cat gene with the peptide synthetase domain construct.

This targeted domain replacement of srfAC was successfully carried out for three bacterial domains of the grs operon activating Phe, Orn, and Leu as well as for the Val- and Cys-activating domains of the fungal acvA gene. Surfactin derivatives produced by the chimeric synthetases were extracted from the cultured broth of different recombinant strains, examined for their hemolytic activity, and analyzed by infrared spectra and mass spectrometry. These studies clearly confirmed the identity of five novel lipopeptides that were produced by the selective domain exchange within the srfA operon. The surfactin isomers were found to carry the desired amino acid residue, as was expected from the corresponding domain replacement.

In general, this approach allows a rational design of peptide antibiotics with defined amino acid sequences through a programmed alteration of peptide synthetase. Therefore,

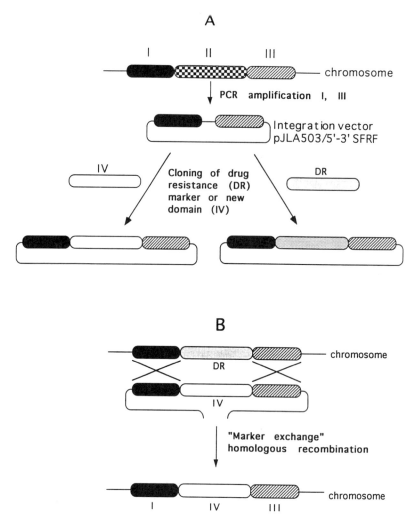

Figure 8 Domain exchange experiment. Marker replacement recombination was carried out to replace the amino acid–activating domain encoded by *Bacillus subtilis srf*AC (surfactin synthetase 3) with those of *Bacillus brevis grs*2 (gramicidin S synthetase 2). (A) DNA sequences of *srf*AC: I and III, which are amplified by PCR, and II, which is to be replaced first by a drug resistance gene (DR) and then by a fragment encoding a heterologous amino acid–activating domain. The amplified sequences I and III are inserted into an *E. coli* plasmid vector unable to replicate in *B. subtilis*. The resulting plasmid is cleaved and ligated with either a fragment encoding a selectable drug resistance gene (DR) or a PCR-amplified sequence encoding an amino acid–activating domain. (B) Transformation with selection for DR results in a deletion of sequence II and replacement with DR DNA. Subsequent congression results in loss of DR and the in-frame insertion of amino acid–activating domain IV. (From Ref. 88.)

these studies may provide new tools for the creation of a diverse class of novel and potentially useful peptide secondary metabolites.

X. SFP AND ITS HOMOLOGS

Most B. subtilis strains, including the strain 168, which is used by many Bacillus geneticists, do not produce the lipopeptide biosurfactant, surfactin. By transforming competent 168 cells with DNA from the surfactin-producing organism B. subtilis ATCC21332, a 168 surfactin producer was obtained (61). The DNA that was transferred to the 168 strain contained the sfp gene, encoding a 226-amino-acid protein of unknown function (89). Sfp appears to be required for the production of peptides that are synthesized by the thiotemplate mechanism. Not only is surfactin production eliminated by deletion of sfp, but the production of an iron siderophore is also reduced. Indeed, sfp mutants grow poorly on medium containing a low Fe concentration (Nakano MM and Zuber P, unpublished results) (90,91). The transcription of srfA and the levels of SrfA subunit proteins are not affected by deletion of sfp. Homologs of Sfp have been found in other bacteria (91,92). An Sfp homolog of B. brevis is encoded by the gsp gene, located upstream from the grs operon but part of a separate transcription unit (90). It has yet to be demonstrated if Gsp is involved in gramicidin production; however, it can complement an sfp mutation with respect to surfactin production and growth on low iron. An sfp homolog required for bacitracin production has been isolated from B. licheniformis by virtue of its ability to promote surfactin production in a nonproducing strain of B. subtilis (Gaidenko T, personal communication). Significant amino acid sequence similarity has been detected between Sfp and EntD (91), which functions in the production of the iron siderophore enterobactin in enteric organisms and is a functional homolog of sfp and sfp[0], a shortened allele of sfp that exists in surfactin nonproducing strains of B. subtilis. An open reading frame (ORF) encoding an Sfp homolog has been discovered in the E. coli genome adjacent to the nik operon, which functions in the uptake of nickel (93). An Sfp homolog has yet to be found in the eukaryotes that are known to produce peptides by the thiotemplate mechanism.

XI. REGULATION OF PEPTIDE ANTIBIOTIC BIOSYNTHESIS

The production of secondary metabolites is normally associated with the bacterium's response to a growth-limiting environment (10,94,95). Depletion of preferred carbon and/or nitrogen sources, along with high cell density or other environmental extremes, will trigger the activation of antibiotic gene expression. This is due to common, global control mechanisms that influence much of what the cell does when it encounters conditions detrimental to normal growth. It has long been known that mutations in spoOA of B. subtilis, an important regulatory gene required for a large part of the bacterium's response to environmental stress, severely impair the production of peptide antibiotics. Suppressors of spoOA that restored production of and resistance to antibiotics were found in abrB, now known to encode a repressor of many stress-induced genes. It is now known that sensing of and response to environmental extremes involve the operation of complex networks of interconnected signal transduction pathways (95–98). The study of the regulation of the srfA operon has uncovered such a regulatory network and illustrates the complexity of the bacterium's response to a changing environment.

A.   The *srf*A Operon: Isolation and Studies of Its Regulation

A genetic approach to the study of antibiotic biosynthesis and its regulation was under-taken that focused on the production of the lipopeptide, surfactin, produced by *B. sub-tilis*. There existed a specific phenotype associated with the production of surfactin: a zone of lysis around colonies of surfactin-producing cells growing on erythrocyte agar plates, resulting from the effect of surfactin's detergent properties (36). Transposon Tn917 insertion mutations that eliminated the zone of lysis (Srf-) uncovered two loci, originally called *srf*A and *srf*B (61,99,100). *srf*B was subsequently found to be a 5 kb deletion adja-cent to the site of Tn917 insertion. The deleted segment contained the so-called early competent genes *com*Q, *com*X, *com*P, and *com*A, the products of which function in the control of competence development. ComX is a peptide pheromone that mediates cell density–dependent control the processing and/or export of which requires ComQ (101). ComX concentration in the medium increases with cell density and triggers the activa-tion of ComP, a membrane protein that is homologous to the histidine protein kinase or the sensor class of two-component regulators found in many prokaryotic organisms (100,102). ComP is believed to undergo autophosphorylation, thereby providing a phos-pho-histidine for ComA, ComP's two-component partner and a member of the response-regulator family of proteins. According to the hypothesis explaining ComP–ComA func-tion (Figure 9), ComA-phosphate becomes a transcriptional activator required for the transcription of the *srf*A operon (103,104).

*srf*A was identified as the site of a Tn917 insertion mutation that eliminated sur-factin production (61). It was also independently identified as *com*L, the site of a Tn917 insertion that impaired competence establishment (105). The method of Youngman and coworkers (106) for creating *lacZ* fusions at the site of Tn917 insertions was employed to create a *srf*A–*lacZ* fusion, expression of which was most active during late stages of the growth curve and required the *com*P and *com*A genes (61,107–109). A strategy of chro-mosome walking from the site of the Tn917 insertion uncovered a large locus, of over 25 kb (50,55). The promoter region was isolated and was found to contain two regions of dyad symmetry immediately upstream of the *srf*A promoter that were required for ComA-dependent transcriptional activation of *srf*A (104,108). Footprint and mutational analy-ses showed that both "ComA boxes" were the sites of ComA-phosphate binding (103), and a mechanism of cooperative interaction between two ComA dimers was proposed (103,104).

Although *com*A is essential for expression of *srf*A, the requirement for *com*P could be bypassed when cells were grown in a medium containing both nutrient broth and glu-cose. This *com*P-independent expression *srf*A was found to require the SpoO phosphore-lay (110), composed of the *spo*OF, *spo*OB, and *spo*OA gene products, all of which are required for sporulation initiation. SpoOF and SpoOA, like ComA, are response-regula-tor proteins of the two-component family. SpoOF is the target of at least two sensors (his-tidine protein kinases) KinA (SpoIIJ) and KinB.

The kinases respond to poorly characterized signals arising from starvation, high cell density, and/or cell division and chromosome replication (110,111). According to the phosphorelay model (110), the kinases autophosphorylate, thereby facilitating the phosphorylation of SpoOF. SpoOF passes the high-energy phosphate to SpoOB, a protein phosphotransferase, which then passes the phosphate on to SpoOA. An additional level of control is exerted by members of the regulatory aspartyl phosphate phosphatase (Rap) family of proteins (112–114). One of these, RapA, has been shown to be a negative reg-ulator of SpoOF by virtue of its ability to catalyze removal of the phosphate from the

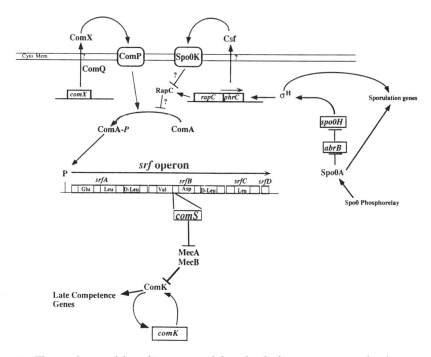

Figure 9 The regulation of the *srf*A operon and the role of *srf*A in competence development. Cell density–dependent control of *srf*A transcription is mediated through ComX, a pheromone that accumulates in late growth cultures. ComX production, processing, and or export requires ComQ. The "sensing" of the pheromone is believed to involve the interaction between the membrane-associated histidine protein kinase ComP and ComX. This activates the phosphorylation of ComA, the positive regulator of *srf*A transcription. Another pathway to *srf*A transcriptional activation involves the extracellular factor CSF (competence-stimulating factor). Its production depends on genes that are required for sporulation initiation, namely, *spo*OH and *spo*OA. SpoOA phosphorylation requires the SpoO phosphorelay (see text) resulting in activated SpoOA, which represses *abr*B. AbrB is a repressor of *spo*OH (encoding the RNA polymerase sigma subunit, s^H) transcription. *spo*OH is required for the production of CSF, suggesting that the j^H form of RNA polymerase initiates transcription at the putative *phr*C gene. The response to CSF requires the SpoOK complex, a peptide permease of the ABC-transporter family. CSF putatively inactivates RapC, a phosphatase negatively controlling ComA. The *srf*A operon encodes the subunits of surfactin synthetase and ComS, a 46-amino-acid peptide that is required for the expression of the late competence genes. The function of *com*S is to activate the transcription of *com*K, which encodes a transcriptional activator of late competence genes. The possible targets of ComS include the *mec*A and *mec*B gene products, which function to inactivate ComK.

conserved aspartyl residue, thereby inactivity SpoOF (113). RapC (112) might play a similar role in the regulation of ComA (Grossman A, personal communication; see below). Rap activity is believed to be regulated in response to high cell density, one of the environmental parameters influencing the cell's decision to undergo sporulation. The *rap* genes reside in operons that also encode small pheromone-like peptides known as Phr's (*p*hosphatase *r*egulators) (112). These are released into the environment, where they increase in concentration as cell density rises. Genetic evidence suggests that the *phr* products serve to downregulate *rap* expression or Rap activity (114). Thus, mutations in *phr*A cause a reduction in sporulation and are suppressed by mutations in *rap*A.

Phosphorylated SpoOA is both a transcriptional activator that stimulates transcription of sporulation genes, and a repressor that acts upon the transcription initiation of *abr*B (115,116), encoding what has been described as a transition state regulator that exerts a negative effect on the transcription of a variety of late growth–induced genes. One of the genes requiring *spo*OA for expression and under the negative control of *abr*B is *spo*OH, which encodes the minor RNA polymerase sigma subunit σ^H (98,117). Recent work of the Grossman laboratory has shown the production of another extracellular peptide factor that activates the transcription of *srf*A, CSF (competence-stimulating factor), which requires the SpoO phosphorelay and SpoOH for production (118). This peptide is encoded by *phr*C (Grossman A, personal communication), which lies in an operon with *rap*C and is believed to be the negative regulator of the RapC aspartyl phosphate phosphatase (119). Utilization of CSF is independent of ComP but requires the SpoOK complex, a peptide transporter of the ABC class (120,121). The function of SpoOK and Csf is the activation of ComA, but how this occurs is not known. Perhaps RapC converts ComA-phosphate to its inactive unphosphorylated form. CSF, in keeping with the proposed function of *phr* products, serves to negatively control RapC. Figure 9 presents a model of the complex regulation affecting *srf*A transcription.

Yet another mode of *srf*A regulation involves the gene *cod*Y, which exerts negative control on certain genes that are activated when the sporulation process is induced (119). CodY is a DNA-binding protein that functions in repressing transcription of genes that are expressed poorly when cells are grown in the presence of exogenous amino acids. Amino acid–dependent *srf*A repression is mediated through *cod*Y, but it is not known if this is a direct or indirect effect.

The surfactin synthetase complex itself is not required for competence development. Deletion analysis indicated that the DNA encoding the fourth amino acid–activating domain, SrfAB1 specifying Val, was required for competence (74). The competence regulatory function of *srf*A has now been ascribed to a small gene located within and out of frame with the *srf*AB gene. This gene, *com*S, encodes a small 46-amino-acid product (122). That translation of the ORF encoded by *com*S is required for competence was shown by suppression of a *com*S amber mutation by a nonsense suppressor tRNA coded for by the *sup*-3 gene (123). The function of *com*S in competence is unknown, but this appears to involve a direct or indirect interaction with the MecB and -A proteins (Medium-independent establishment of competence) (124–126). The *mec* genes are the sites of suppressor mutations that obviate the need for the *com*P, *com*A, and *srf*A system in competence development. MecA and MecB have been shown to function in the inhibition of ComK, which encodes CTF (competence transcription factor), required for the transcription of the late competence genes (81,127,128). ComS could influence MecB and/or MecA activity through DegU (96,97) or SinR (98). Experiments utilizing a synthetic ComS peptide suggest that ComS can form a complex with MecA (Liu L and Zuber P, unpublished results).

DegU is another protein of the response-regulator class that is necessary for competence development and for the production of a number of degradative enzymes that are produced in late growth cultures. Its activity is modulated by the histidine protein kinase encoded by the *deg*S gene, mutations in which inhibit degradative enzyme production but do not effect competence. This observation suggests that the unphosphorylated form of DegU functions in competence development. SinR is a transcriptional regulator that represses certain sporulation genes but is required for competence development. As is the case with comS, null mutations of sinR or degU are suppressed by mecA and mecB mutations (81,126). Thus, degU and sinR, or their products, could be targets of comS activity.

Why is comS situated in its unusual location? The comS amber mutation has no significant effect on surfactin production under the conditions we had tested (123). However, if one views competence as another means by which cells can acquire nutrition by utilizing complex organic polymers (DNA), then there is logic in coregulating the production of a lytic agent (surfactin) with a process designed to import a substance released by cell lysis (the uptake of DNA by competent cells). It is possible that, in addition to its role in competence, comS functions in the autoregulation of srfA. It has been noted that comK somehow exerts a negative effect on srfA expression (81). Thus, comS could function to limit the expression of srfA by releasing comK from Mec-dependent control.

Other control mechanisms could influence srfA expression. As is the case with other peptide synthetase operons, there is a long untranslated region between the transcriptional start site of srfA and the first gene of the operon, srfAA. Recently reported evidence suggests that this sequence and an RNA processing enzyme, Pnp (polynucleotide phosphorylase), function somehow to optimize the translation of srfA mRNA (129).

B. The Regulation of the *grs* and *tyc* Operons

Both the grs and tyc operons (Figure 3) have been isolated from the gramcidin S and tyrocidine producer B. brevis (45,46,57,82,130). Gramicidin S synthetase is composed of two subunits, GrsA and B, encoded by grsA and grsB of the grs operon. GrsA catalyzes the activation of Phe, followed by epimerization to form D-Phe. GrsB contains four domains that catalyze the activation and incorporation of Pro, Val, Orn, and Leu, the Leu-activating domain associated with an epimerase module. Cyclization is achieved by linking two of the resulting D-Phe–Pro–Val–Orn–Leu pentapeptides head to tail. The first gene of the operon, grsT, encodes a product bearing primary structure homology to several thioesterases, but its function is unknown (57). Further upstream and composed of a separate transcription unit is gsp, encoding a homolog of Sfp (89). The tyc operon is composed of three genes that encode the 10 amino acid–activating domains responsible for the incorporation of the substrate amino acids into the tyrocidine decapeptide (82,131).

The promoters of both operons were characterized in hopes of understanding how peptide antibiotic gene transcription is regulated in Bacillus (132,133). Since few procedures have been developed to study gene expression in B. brevis, the expression of the operons was examined in B. subtilis, making use of a phage SPβ-borne lacZ fusion system (134). A transcriptional tycA–lacZ fusion was constructed and used to examine the role of spoO mutations on the tyc operon expression (132). As expected, the expression was observed to increase when cells entered stationary phase of the growth curve, which corresponded with the postexponential increase of tyc mRNA concentration observed in B. brevis. As predicted from earlier studies, tyc–lacZ expression was dramatically reduced in a spoOA mutant, and complete derepression was observed in spoOA and spoOA+ cells when a mutation in abrB (115,135) was present. The expression of tyc–lacZ was constitutive in the abrB mutant, showing that the spoOA–abrB system was primarily responsible for the postexponential induction of tyc. Glucose added to the growth medium causes repression of tyc–lacZ, but this too is relieved by a mutation in abrB.

AbrB is a repressor that binds to DNA in the regulatory region of genes under its control (115). In the case of tycA, DNAase and hydroxyl-radical footprinting studies showed that AbrB recognized a dAT-(deoxyadenylate-thymidylate)rich sequence within the region encoding the long untranslated leader sequence of the *tyc* transcript (136). Protection from hydroxyl-radical cleavage was observed in a string of C residues separated by dAT-rich stretches and aligned on the same face of the DNA helix.

Much less is known about the regulation of *grs*. A *grs–lacZ* fusion was constructed and used to examine *grs* expression in B. *subtilis* (133). As with *tyc*, *grs* expression was activated postexponentially, but later than *tyc* at about 2 hr after the end of exponential growth. Unlike *tyc*, *grs–lacZ* expression required *spo*OH. The promoter sequence of *grs* resembles somewhat promoters that are recognized by the σ^H form of RNA polymerase (137), but the pattern of *grs* expression, occurring 2 hr into stationary phase and well after σ^H-RNA polymerase becomes active, suggests that the interaction of *spo*OH with *grs* may be indirect.

Like so many of the genes that are activated in bacteria by conditions of environmental stress, each of the peptide antibiotic biosynthesis operons described above requires a unique combination of regulatory mechanisms for expression and regulation. *srf*, *tyc*, and *grs* are all influenced by *spo*OA but are regulated by quite different *spo*OA-dependent mechanisms. *srf* is also regulated by an *spo*OA-independent mechanism involving the early *com* genes that govern the cells' response to high cell density.

XII. CONCLUSION: THE FUNDAMENTALS

Much has been learned about the structure of the thiotemplate and the functioning of the substrate-activating domains over the many years since the initial isolation of the peptide synthetases. Yet the most basic aspects of peptide synthesis remain unclear. Our understanding of how the enzyme thiotemplate operates is sketchy at best. It is still not known how transpeptidation occurs or why peptide synthesis initiates at specific domains. It is not known how domain activity is regulated. The details of how epimerization occurs are not known, nor is it known how this reaction affects peptide synthesis. The product of the *sfp* gene and its homologs are thought to function in peptide transport, but evidence for this is not forthcoming. Little is known about the function of the interdomain regions in peptide synthetases. Simple experiments designed to determine how antibiotic biosynthesis gene expression is regulated have uncovered an assortment of links among signal transduction pathways. The imaginative use of molecular genetics and biochemical techniques may yet provide a clearer picture of peptide synthetase function and regulation.

REFERENCES

1. Schnell N, Entian K-D, Schneider U, Gotz F, Zahner H, Kellner R, Jung G. Prepeptide sequence of epidermin, a ribosomally synthesized antibiotic with four sulphide-rings. Nature 1988; 333:276–278.
2. Kleinkauf H, von Döhren H. Nonribosomal biosynthesis of peptide antibiotics. Eur J Biochem 1990; 192:1–15.
3. Kurahashi K. Biosynthesis of peptide antibiotics. Corcoran JW, ed. Antibiotics, Vol. 4. Biosynthesis. Berlin: Springer, 1981:325–352.
4. Stachelhaus T, Marahiel MA. Module structure of genes encoding multifunctional peptide synthetases required for non-ribosomal peptide synthesis. FEMS Lett 1995; 125:3–14.
5. Zuber P. Non-ribosomal peptide synthesis. Curr Opin Cell Biol 1991; 3:1046–1050.

6. Lipmann F. Bacterial production of antibiotic polypeptides by thiol-linked synthesis on protein templates. Adv Microb Phys 1980; 21:227–260.

7. Gevers W, Kleinkauf H, Lipmann F. The activation of amino acids for biosynthesis of gramicidin S. Proc Natl Acad Sci USA 1968; 60:269–276.

8. Gevers W, Kleinkauf H, Lipmann F. Peptidyl transfers in gramicidin S biosynthesis from enzyme-bound thioester intermediates. Proc Natl Acad Sci USA 1969; 63:1335–1342.

9. Kleinkauf H, Roskoski R Jr, Lipmann F. Pantetheine-linked peptide intermediates in gramicidin S and tyrocidine biosynthesis. Proc Natl Acad Sci USA 1971; 68:2069–2072.

10. Katz E, Demain AL. The peptide antibiotics of *Bacillus*: Chemistry, biogenesis and possible functions. Bacteriol Rev 1977; 41:449–474.

11. Lipmann F. On the mechanism of some ATP-linked reactions and certain aspects of protein synthesis. Mc Elroy WDaBG, ed. The Mechanism of Enzyme Action. Baltimore: John Hopkins University Press, 1954:599.

12. Schlumbohm W, Stein T, Ullrich C, Vater J, Krause M, Marahiel MA, Kruft V, Wittmann-Liebold B. An active serine is involved in covalent substrate amino acid binding at each reaction center of gramicidin S synthetase. J Biol Chem 1991; 266:23135–23141.

13. van Liempt H, von Döhren H, Kleinkauf H. δ-(L-α-Aminoadipyl)-L-cysteinyl-D-valine synthetase from *Aspergillus nidulans*. The first enzyme in penicillin biosynthesis is a multifunctional peptide synthetase. J Biol Chem 1989; 264:3680–3684.

14. Zhang J, Demain AL. ACV synthetase. Crit Rev Biotech 1992; 12:245–260.

15. Aharonowitz Y, Bergmeyer J, Cantoral JM, Cohen G, Demain AL, Fink U, Kinghorn J, Kleinkauf H, MacCabe A, Palissa H, Pfeifer E, Schwecke T, van Liempt H, von Döhren H, Wolfe S, Zhang J. δ-(L-α-Aminoadipyl)-L-cysteinyl-D-valine synthetase, the multienzyme integrating the four primary reactions in β-lactam biosynthesis, as a model peptide synthetase. Bio/Technol 1993; 11:807–810.

16. Rainey PB, Brodey CL, Johnstone K. Identification of a gene cluster encoding three high molecular-weight proteins, which is required for synthesis of tolaasin by the mushroom pathogen *Pseudomonas tolaasii*. Mol Microbiol 1993; 8:643–652.

17. Xu GW, Gross DC. Physical and functional analyses of the *syrA* and *syrB* genes involved in syringomycin production by *Pseudomonas syringae* pv. syringae. J Bacteriol 1988; 170:5680–5688.

18. Morgan MD, Chatterjee AK. Genetic organization and regulation of proteins associated with production of syringotoxin by *Pseudomonas syringae* pathovar syringae. J Bacteriol 1988; 170:5689–5697.

19. Moore RE, Niemczura WP, Kwok OCH, Patil SS. Inhibitors of ornithine carbamoyltransferase from *Pseudomonas syringae* pv. phaseolica revised structure of phaseolotoxin. Tetrahedron Lett 1984; 25:3931–3934.

20. Borchert S, Patil SS, Marahiel MA. Identification of putative multifunctional peptide synthetase genes using highly conserved oligonucleotide sequences derived from known synthetases. FEMS Microbiol Lett 1992; 92:175–180.

21. Walton JD. Two enzymes involved in biosynthesis of the host-selective phytotoxin HD-toxin. Proc Natl Acad Sci USA 1987; 84:8444–8447.

22. Scott-Craig JS, Panaccione DG, Pocard J-A, Walton JD. The cyclic peptide synthetase catalyzing HC-toxin production in the filamentous fungus *Cochliobolus carbonum* is encoded by a 15.7-kilobase open-reading frame. J Biol Chem 1992; 267:26044–26049.

23. Haese A, Schubert M, Herrmann M, Zocher R. Molecular characterization of the enniatin synthetase gene encoding a multifunctional enzyme catalysing N-mehtyldepsipeptide formation in *Fusarium scirpi*. Mol Microbiol 1993; 7:905–914.

24. Rusnak F, Sakaitani M, Drueckhammer D, Reichert J, Walsh CT. Biosynthesis of the *Escherichia coli* siderophore enterobactin: Sequence of the *entF* gene, expression and purification of EntF, and analysis of covalent phosphopantetheine. Biochem 1991; 30:2916–2927.

25. Staab JF, Elkins M, Earhart CF. Nucleotide sequence of the *Escherichia coli entE* gene. FEMS Microbiol Lett 1989; 59:15–20.

26. Cox CD, Adams P. Siderophore activity of pyoverdin for *Pseudomonas aeruginosa*. Infect Immun 1985; 5748:130–138.

27. Merriman TR, Merriman ME, Lamont IL. Nucleotide sequence of *pvdD*, a pyoverdine biosynthetic gene from *Pseudomonas aeruginosa*: PvdD has similarity to peptide synthetases. J Bacteriol 1995; 177:252–258.

28. Carmichael WW. The toxins of Cyanobacteria. Sci Am 1994; 270:78–86.

29. Nishiwaki-Matsushima R, Ohta T, Nishiwaki S, Suganuma M, Kohyama K, Ishikawa T, Carmichael WW, Fujiki H. Liver tumor promotion by the cyanobacterial cyclic peptide toxin microcystin-LR. J Cancer Res Clin Oncol 1992; 118:420–424.

30. Sivonen K, Namikoshi M, Evans WR, Carmichael WW, Sun R, Rouhiainen L, Luukkainen R, Rinehart KL. Isolation and characterization of a variety of microcystins from seven strains of the cyanobacterial genus Anabaena. Appl Environ Microbiol 1992; 58:2495–2500.

31. Moore RE. Cyclic peptides and depsipeptides from cyanobacteria: A review. J Ind Microbio 1996; 16:134–143.

32. Weber G, Schorgendorfer K, Schneider-Scherzer E, Leitner E. The peptide synthetase catalyzing cyclosporine production in *Tolypocladium niveum* is encoded by a giant 45.8 kb open reading frame. Cur Genet 1994; 26:120–125.

33. Willey J, Santamaria R, Guijarro J, Geislich M, Losick R. Extracellular complimentation of a developmental mutation implicates a small sporulation protein in aerial mycelium formation by *S. coelicolor*. Cell 1991; 65:641–650.

34. Willey J, Schwedock J, Losick R. Multiple extracellular signals govern the production of a morphogenetic protein involved in aerial mycelium formation by *Streptomyces coelicolor*. Genes Devel 1993; 7:895–903.

35. Vater J. Lipopeptides, an interesting class of microbial secondary metabolites. Schlunegger UP, ed. Biologically Active Molecules. Berlin: Springer-Verlag, 1989:27–38.

36. Arima K, Kainuma A, Tamura G. Surfactin, a crystalline peptidelipid surfactant produced by *Bacillus subtilis*: Isolation, characterization, and its inhibition of fibrin clot formation. Biochem Biophys Res Commun 1968; 31:488–494.

37. Morikawa M, Daido H, Takao T, Murata S, Shimonishi Y, Imanaka T. A new lipopeptide biosurfactant produced by *Arthrobacter sp.* strain MIS38. J Bacteriol 1993; 175:6459–6466.

38. Matsuyama T, Kaneda K, Nakgawa Y, Isa K, Hara-Hotta H, Yano I. A novel extracellular cyclic lipopeptide which promotes flagellum-dependent and -independent spreading growth of *Serratia marcescens*. J Bacteriol 1992; 174:1769–1776.

39. Debono M, Gordee RS. Antibiotics that inhibit fungal cell wall development. Annu Rev Microbiol 1994; 48:471–497.

40. Heaton MP, Neuhaus FC. Biosynthesis of D-alanyl-lipoteichoic acid: Cloning, nucleotide sequence, and expression of the *Lactobacillus casei* gene for the D-alanine-activating enzyme. J Bacteriol 1992; 174:4707–4717.

41. von Döhren H, Pfeifer E, van Liempt H, Lee Y-O, Pavela-Vrancic M, Schwecke T. The nonribosomal system: What we learn from the genes encoding protein templates. Baltz RH, Hegeman GD, Skatrud PL, eds. Industrial Microorganisms: Basic and Applied Molecular Genetics. Washington, D.C.: American Society for Microbiology, 1993:159–167.

42. Zuber P, Nakano MM, Marahiel MA. Peptide Antibiotics. Sonenshein AL Losick R, Hoch JA, eds. *Bacillus subtilis* and Other Gram-Positive Bacteria: Physiology, Biochemistry, and Molecular Biology. Washington, D.C.: American Society for Microbiology, 1993:897–916.

43. Saito Y. Some characteristics of gramicidin S synthetase obtained from mutants of *Bacillus brevis* which could not form D-phenylalanine-L-proline diketopiperazine. Kleinkauf H, von Döhren H, eds. Peptide Antibiotics: Biosynthesis and Functions. Berlin: de Gruyter, 1982:195–207.

44. Lee SG, Roskoski JR, Bauer K, Lipmann F. Purification of the polyenzyme responsible for tyrodicidne synthesis and their dissociation into subunits. Biochem 1973; 12:398–405.

45. Krause M, Marahiel MA, von Döhren H, Kleinkauf H. Molecular cloning of an ornithine-activating fragment of the gramicidin S synthetase 2 gene from *Bacillus brevis* and expression in *Escherichia coli*. J Bacteriol 1985; 162:1120–1125.

46. Marahiel MA, Krause M, Skarpeid H-J. Cloning of the tyrocidine synthetase I gene from *Bacillus brevis* and its expression in *Escherichia coli*. Mol Gen Genet 1985; 201:231–236.

47. Diez B, Gutierrez S, Barredo JL, Solingen P, van der Voort LHM, Martin JF. The cluster of penicillin biosythetic genes. Identification and characterization of the *pcbAB* gene encoding the α-aminoadipyl-cysteine-valine synthetase and linkage to the *pcbC* and *penDE* genes. J Biol Chem 1990; 265:16358–16365.

48. Martin JF, Gutierrez S, Fernandez FJ, Belasco J, Fierro F, Marcos AT, Kosalkova K. Expression of genes and procession of enzymes for the biosynthesis of penicillins and cephalosporins. Antonie van Leeuwenhoek 1994; 65:227–243.

49. Smith DJ, Burnham MKR, Bull JH, Hodgson JE, Ward JM, Browne P, Brown J, Barton B, Earl AJ, Turner G. β-Lactam antibiotic biosynthetic genes have been conserved in clusters in prokaryotes and eukaryotes. EMBO J 1990; 9:741–747.

50. Nakano MM, Magnuson R, Myers A, Curry J, Grossman AD, Zuber P. *srfA* is an operon required for surfactin production, competence development, and efficient sporulation in *Bacillus subtilis*. J Bacteriol 1991; 173:1770–1778.

51. Feitelson JS, Hopwood DA. Cloning of a *Streptomyces* gene for an O-methyltransferase involved in antibiotic biosynthesis. Mol Gen Genet 1983; 190:394–398.

52. Malpartida F, Hopwood DA. Molecular cloning of the whole biosynthetic pathway of a *Streptomyces* antibiotic and its expression in a heterologous host. Nature 1984; 309:462–464.

53. Motamedi H, Hutchinson CR. Cloning and heterologous expression of a gene cluster for the biosynthesis of tetracenomycin C, the anthracycline antitumor antibiotic of *Streptomyces glaucescens*. Proc Natl Acad Sci USA 1987; 84:4445–4449.

54. Gutierrez S, Diez B, Montenegro E, Martin JF. Characterization of the *Cephalosporium acremonium pcbAB* gene encoding a-aminoadipyl-cysteinyl-valine synthetase, a large multidomain peptide synthetase: Linkage to the *pcbC* gene as a cluster of early cephalosporin biosynthetic genes and evidence of multiple functional domains. J Bacteriol 1991; 173:2345–2365.

55. Cosmina P, Rodriguez F, de Ferra F, Grandi G, Perego M, Venema G, van Sinderen D. Sequence and analysis of the genetic locus responsible for surfactin synthesis in *Bacillus subtilis*. Mol Microbiol 1993; 8:821–831.

56. Coque JJR, Martin JF, Calzada JG, Liras P. The cephamycin biosynthetic genes *pcbAB*, encoding a large multidomain peptide synthetase, and *pcbC* of *Nocardia lactamdurans* are clustered together in an organization different from the same genes in *Acremonium chrysogenum* and *Penicillium chrysogenum*. Mol Microbiol 1991; 5:1125–1133.

57. Kratzschmar J, Krause M, Marahiel MA. Gramicidin S biosynthesis operon containing the structural genes *grsA* and *grsB* has an open reading frame encoding a protein homologous to fatty acid thioesterases. J Bacteriol 1989; 171:5422–5429.

58. Smith DJ, Earl AF, Turner G. The multifunctional peptide synthetase performing the first step of penicillin biosynthesis in *Penicillium chrysogenum* is a 421 073 dalton protein similar to *Bacillus brevis* peptide antibiotic synthetases. EMBO J 1990; 9:2743–2750.

59. Turgay K, Krause M, Marahiel MA. Four homologous domains in the primary structure of *grsB* are related to domains in a superfamily of adenylate-forming enzymes. Mol Microbiol 1992; 6:529–546.

60. Turgay K, Marahiel MA. A general approach for identifying and cloning peptide synthetase genes. Peptide Res 1994; 7:238–241.

61. Nakano MM, Marahiel MA, Zuber P. Identification of a genetic locus required for biosynthesis of the lipopeptide antibiotic surfactin in *Bacillus subtilis*. J Bacteriol 1988; 170:5662–5668.

62. Babbitt PC, Kenyon GL, Martin BM, Charest H, Slyvestre M, Scholten JD, Chang H, Liang PH, Dunaway-Mariano D. Ancestry of the 4-chlorobenzoate dehalogenase: Analysis of amino acid sequence identities among families of acyl:adenyl ligases enoyl-CoA hydratases/isomerase and acyl-CoA thioesterases. Biochem 1992; 31:5594–5604.

63. Loyoza E, Hoffmann H, Douglas C, Schulz W, Scheel D, Hahlbrock K. Primary structure and catalytic properties of isoenzymes encoded by the two 4-courmarate:CoA ligase genes in parsley. Eur J Biochem 1988; 176:661–667.

64. Walker JE, Saraste M, Runswick MJ, Gay NJ. Distantly related sequences, in the α- and β-subunit of ATP synthase, myosin, kinases and other ATP-requiring enzymes and common nucleotide binding fold. EMBO J 1982; 1:945–951.

65. Saraste M, Sibbald PR, Wittinghofer A. The P-loop: A common motif in ATP- and GTP-binding proteins. Trends Biochem Sci 1990; 15:430–434.

66. Serrano R, Kielland-Brandt MC, Fink GR. Yeast plasma membrane ATPase is essential for growth and has homology with $(Na^+ + K^+)$, K^+- and Ca^{2+}-Atpases. Nature 1986; 319:689–693.

67. Pavela-Vrancic M, Pfeifer E, von Liempt H, Schafer H-J, von Döhren H, Kleinkauf H. ATP binding in peptide synthetases: Determination of contact sites of the adenine moiety by photoaffinity labeling of tyrocidine synthetase I with 2-azidoadenosine triphosphate. Biochem 1994; 33:6276–6283.

68. Pavela-Vrancic M, Pfeifer E, Schroder W, von Döhren H, Kleinkauf H. Identification of the ATP binding site in tyrocidine synthetase 1 by selective modification with fluorescein 5′-isothiocyanate. J Biol Chem 1994; 269:14,962–14,966.

69. Stein T, Vater J, Krugt V, Wittmann-Liebold B, Franke P, Panico M, McDowell R, Morris HR. Detection of 4′-phosphopantetheine at the thioester binding site for L-valine of gramicidin S synthetase 2. FEBS Lett 1994; 340:39–44.

70. Fuma S, Fujishima Y, Corbell N, D'Souza C, Nakano MM, Zuber P, Yamane K. Nucleotide sequence of 5′ portion of srfA that contains the region required for competence establishment in *Bacillus subtilis*. Nucl Acids Res 1993; 21:93–97.

71. Haese A, Pieper R, von Ostrowski T, Zocher R. Bacterial expression of a catalytically active fragments of the multifunctional enzyme enniatin synthetase. J Mol Biol 1994; 243:116–122.

72. D'Souza C, Nakano MM, Corbell N, Zuber P. Amino-acylation site mutations in amino acid–activating domains of surfactin synthetase: Effects on surfactin production and competence development in *Bacillus subtilis*. J Bacteriol 1993; 175:3502–3510.

73. Galli G, Rodriguez F, Cosmina P, Pratesi C, Nogarotto R, de Ferra F, Grandi G. Characterization of the surfactin synthetase multienzyme complex. Biochim Biophys Acta 1994; 1205:19–28.

74. van Sinderen D, Galli G, Cosmina P, de Ferra F, Withoff S, Venema G, Grandi G. Characterization of the srfA locus of *Bacillus subtilis*: Only the valine-activating domain of srfA is involved in the establishment of genetic competence. Mol Microbiol 1993; 8:833–841.

75. Vollenbroich D, Kluge B, D'Souza C, Zuber P, Vater J. Analysis of a mutant amino acid–activating domain of surfactin synthetase bearing a serine to alanine substitution at the site of carboxylthioester formation. FEBS Lett 1993; 325:220–234.

76. Vollenbroich D, Mehta N, Zuber P, Vater J, Kamp RM. Analysis of surfactin synthetase subunits in srfA mutants of *Bacillus subtilis* OKB105. J Bacteriol 1994; 176:395–400.

77. Gocht M, Marahiel MA. Analysis of core sequences in the D-Phe activating domain of the multifunctional peptide synthetase TycA by site-directed mutagenesis. J Bacteriol 1994; 176:2654–2662.

78. Stachelhaus T, Marahiel MA. Modular structure of peptide synthetases revealed by dissection of the multifunctional enzyme GrsA. J Biol Chem 1996; 270:6183–6189.

79. Tokito K, Hori K, Kurotsu T, Kanda M, Saito Y. Effect of single base substitution at glycine-870 codon of gramicidin S synthetase 2 gene on proline activation. J Biochem 1993; 114:522–527.

80. MacCabe AP, Van Liempt H, Palissa H, Unkles SE, Riach MBR, Pfeifer E, von Döhren H, Kinghorn JR. δ-(L-α-Aminoadipyl)-L-cysteinyl-D-valine synthetase from *Aspergillus nidulans*. J Biol Biochem 1991; 12646–12654.

81. Hahn J, Kong L, Dubnau D. The regulation of competence transcription factor synthesis constitutes a critical control point in the regulation of competence in *Bacillus subtilis*. J Bacteriol 1994; 176:5753–5761.

82. Mittenhuber G, Weckermann R, Marahiel MA. Gene cluster containing the genes for tyrocidine synthetase 1 and 2 from *Bacillus brevis*: Evidence for an operon. J Bacteriol 1989; 171:4881–4887.

83. Stein T, Kluge B, Bater J, Franke P, Otto A, Wittmann-Liebold B. Gramicidin S synthetase I (phenylalanine racemase), a prototype of amino acid racemases containing the cofactor 4'-phosphopantetheine. Biochem 1995; 34:4633–4642.

84. Mitchell RE. Coronatine production by some phytopathogenic pseudomonads. Physiol Plant Pathol 1982; 20:83–89.

85. Ullrich M, Bender CL. The biosynthetic gene cluster for coronamic acid, an ethylcyclopropyl amino acid, contains genes homologous to amino acid–activating enzymes and thioesterases. J Bacteriol 1994; 176:7574–7586.

86. Stindl A, Keller U. Epimerizatoin of the D-valine portion in the biosynthesis of actinomycin D. Biochem 1994; 33:9358–9364.

87. Shiau C-Y, Baldwin JE, Byford MF, Sobey WJ, Schofield CJ. δ-L-(α-Aminoadipoyl)-L-cysteinyl-D-valine synthetase: The order of peptide bond formation and timing of the epimerisation reaction. FEBS Lett 1995; 358:97–100.

88. Stachelhaus T, Schneider, A, Marahiel, MA. Rational design of peptide antibiotics by targeted replacement of bacterial and fungal domains. Science 1995; 269:69–72.

89. Nakano MM, Corbell N, Besson J, Zuber P. Isolation and characterization of *sfp*: A gene required for the production of the lipopeptide biosurfactant, surfactin, in *Bacillus subtilis*. Mol Gen Genet 1992; 232:313–321.

90. Borchert S, Stachelhaus T, Marahiel MA. Induction of surfactin production in *Bacillus subtilis* by *gsp*, a gene located upstream of the gramicidin S operon in *Bacillus brevis*. J Bacteriol 1994; 176:2458–2462.

91. Grossman M, Tuckman TH, Ellestak S, Osborne MS. Isolation and characterization of *Bacillus subtilis* genes involved in siderophore biosynthesis: Relationship between *B. subtilis sfp*^{0} and *Escherichia coli entD* genes. J Bacteriol 1993; 175:6203–6211.

92. Black RA, Wolk CP. Analysis of a Het- mutation in *Anabaena* sp. strain PCC 7128 implicates a secondary metabolite in the regulation of heterocyst spacing. J Bacteriol 1993; 176:2282–2292.

93. Navarro C, Wu LF. Mandrand-Berthelot MA. The *nik* operon of *Escherichia coli* encodes a periplasmic binding-protein-dependent transport system for nickel. Mol Microbiol 1993; 9:1181–1191.

94. Bibb MJ, Andres N, Gamajo HC, Strauch E, Takano E, White J. Stationary-phase production of the antibiotics actinorhodin and undecylprodigiosin in *Streptomyces coelicolor* A3(2) is transcriptionally regulated. Baltz RH, Hegeman GD, Skatrud PL, eds. Industrial Microorganisms: Basic and Applied Molecular Genetics. Washington, D.C.: American Society for Microbiology, 1993:11–24.

95. Chater KF, Brian P, Brown GL, Plaskit KA, Soliveri J, Tan H, Vijgenboom E. Problems and progress in the interactions between morphological and physiological differentiation in *Streptomyces coelicolor*. Baltz RH, Hegeman GD, Skatrud PL, eds. Industrial Microorganisms: Basic and Applied Molecular Genetics. Washington, D.C.: American Society for Microbiology, 1993:151–157.

96. Kunst F, Msadek T, Rapoport G. Signal transduction network controlling degradative enzyme synthesis and competence in *Bacillus subtilis*. Piggot PJ, Moran CP Jr., Youngman P, eds. Reg-

ulation of Bacterial Differentiation. Washington, D.C.: American Society for Microbiology, 1994:1–20.

97. Msadek T, Kunst F, Rapoport G. Two-component regulatory systems. Sonenshein AL, Losick R, Hoch JA eds. *Bacillus subtilis* and Other Gram-Positive Bacteria: Physiology, Biochemistry, and Molecular Biology. Washington D.C.: American Society for Microbiology, 1993:729–746.

98. Smith I. Regulatory proteins that control late-growth development. Sonenshein AL, Losick R, and Hoch JA eds. *Bacillus subtilis* and Other Gram-Positive Bacteria: Physiology, Biochemistry, and Molecular Biology. Washington D.C.: American Society for Microbiology, 1993:785–800.

99. Nakano MM, Zuber P. Cloning and characterization of *srfB*: A regulatory gene involved in surfactin and competence in *Bacillus subtilis*. J Bacteriol 1989; 171:5347–5353.

100. Weinrauch Y, Guillen N, Dubnau DA. Sequence and transcription mapping of *Bacillus subtilis* competence genes *comB* and *comA*, one of which is related to a family of bacterial regulatory determinants. J Bacteriol 1989; 171:5362–5375.

101. Magnuson R, Solomon J, Grossman AD. Biochemical and genetic characterization of a competence pheromone from *Bacillus subtilis*. Cell 1994; 77:207–216.

102. Weinrauch Y, Penchev R, Dubnau E, Smith I, Dubnau D. A *Bacillus subtilis* regulatory gene product for genetic competence and sporulation resembles sensor protein members of the bacterial two-component signal-transduction systems. Genes Devel 1990; 4:860–872.

103. Roggiani M, Dubnau D. ComA, a phosphorylated response regulator protein of *Bacillus subtilis*, binds to the promoter region of *srfA*. J Bacteriol 1993; 175:3182–3187.

104. Nakano MM, Zuber P. Mutational analysis of the regulatory region of the *srfA* operon in *Bacillus subtilis*. J Bacteriol 1993; 175:3188–3191.

105. van Sinderen D, Withof S, Boels H, Venema G. Isolation and characterization of *comL*, a transcription unit involved in competence development of *Bacillus subtilis*. Mol Gen Genet 1990; 224:396–404.

106. Youngman P, Zuber P, Perkins JB, Sandman K, Igo M, Losick R. New ways to study developmental genes in spore-forming bacteria. Science 1985; 218:285–291.

107. Hahn J, Dubnau D. Growth stage signal transduction and the requirements for *srfA* induction in development of competence. J Bacteriol 1991; 173:7275–7282.

108. Nakano MM, Xia L, Zuber P. The transcription initiation region of the *srfA* operon which is controlled by the *comP–comA* signal transduction system in *Bacillus subtilis*. J Bacteriol 1991; 173:5487–5493.

109. Nakano MM, Zuber P. The primary role of *comA* in the establishment of the competent state in *Bacillus subtilis* is to activate the expression of *srfA*. J Bacteriol 1991; 173:7269–7274.

110. Burbulys D, Trach KA, Hoch JA. Initiation of sporulation in *B. subtilis* is controlled by a multicomponent phosphorelay. Cell 1991; 64:545–552.

111. Ireton K, Rudner DZ, Siranosian KJ, Grossman AD. Integration of multiple developmental signals in *Bacillus subtilis* through the SpoOA transcription factor. Genes Devel 1993; 7:283–294.

112. Perego M, Glaser P, Hoch JA. Aspartyl-phosphate phosphatases deactivate the response regulator components of the sporulation signal transduction system in *Bacillus subtilis*. Mol Micobiol 1996; 19:1151–1157.

113. Perego M, Hanstein C, Welsh M, Djavakhishvili T, Glaser P, Hoch JA. Multiple protein-aspartate phosphatases provide a mechanism for the integration of diverse signals in the control of development in *B. subtilis*. Cell 1994; 79:1847–1855.

114. Perego M, Hoch JA. Cell-cell communication regulates the effects of protein aspartate phosphatases on the phosphorelay controlling development in *Bacillus subtilis*. Proc Natl Acad Sci USA 1996; 93:1549–1553.

115. Strauch MA, Spiegelman GB, Perego M, Johnson WC, Burbulys D, Hoch JA. The transition state transcription regulator AbrB of *Bacillus subtilis* is a DNA binding protein. EMBO J 1989; 8:1615–1621.

116. Strauch MA, Webb V, Speigelman B, Hoch J. The SpoOA protein of *Bacillus subtilis* is a repressor of the *abrB* gene. Proc Natl Acad Sci USA 1990; 87:1801–1805.

117. Carter HL III, Moran CP. New RNA polymerase sigma factor under *spoO* control in *Bacillus subtilis*. Proc Natl Acad Sci USA 1986; 83:9438–9442.

118. Solomon JM, Magnuson R, Srivastava A, Grossman AD. Convergent sensing pathways mediate response to two extracellular competence factors in *Bacillus subtilis*. Genes Devel 1995; 9:547–558.

119. Slack FJ, Serror P, Joyce E, Sonenshein AL. A gene required for nutritional repression of the *Bacillus subtilis* dipeptide permease operon. Mol Microbiol 1995; 15:689–702.

120. Perego M, Higgins CF, Pearce SR, Gallagher MP, Hoch JA. The oligopeptide transport system of *Bacillus subtilis* plays a role in the initiation of sporulation. Mol Microbiol 1991; 5:173–185.

121. Rudner DZ, Ledeaux JR, Ireton K, Grossman AD. The spoOK locus of *Bacillus subtilis* is homologous to the oligopeptide permease locus and is required for sporulation and competence. J Bacteriol 1991; 173:1388–1398.

122. D'Souza C, Nakano MM, Zuber P. Identification of *comS*, a gene of the *srfA* operon that regulates the establishment of genetic competence in *Bacillus subtilis*. Proc Natl Acad Sci USA 1994; 91:9397–9401.

123. D'Souza C, Nakano MM, Frisby DL, Zuber P. Translation of the open reading frame encoded by *comS*, a gene of the *srf* operon, is necessary for the development of genetic competence but not surfactin biosynthesis in *Bacillus subtilis*. J Bacteriol 1995; 177:4144–4148.

124. Dubnau K, Roggianni M. Growth medium–independent genetic competence mutants of *Bacillus subtilis*. J Bacteriol 1990; 172:4048–4055.

125. Kong L, Siranosian KJ, Grossman AD, Dubnau D. Sequence and properties of *mecA*: A negative regulator of genetic competence in *Bacillus subtilis*. Mol Microbiol 1993; 9:365–373.

126. Msadek T, Kunst F, Rapoport G. MecB of *Bacillus subtilis* is a pleiotropic regulator of the ClpC ATPase family, contolling competence gene expression and survival at high temperature. Proc Natl Acad Sci USA 1994; 91:5788–5792.

127. van Sinderen D, Venema G. *comK* acts as an autoregulatory control switch in the signal transduction route to competence in *Bacillus subtilis*. J Bacteriol 1994; 176:5762–5770.

128. Kong L, Dubnau D. Regulation of competence-specific gene expression by Mec-mediated protein-protein interaction in *Bacillus subtilis*. Proc Natl Acad Sci USA 1994; 91:5793–5797.

129. Luttinger A, Hahn J, Dubnau D. Polynucleotide phosphorylase is necessary for competence development in *Bacillus subtilis*. Mol Microbiol 1996; 19:343–356.

130. Hori K, Yamamoto Y, Minetoki T, Kurotsu T, Kanda M, Miura S, Okamura K, Furujama J, Saito Y. Molecular cloning and nucleotide sequence of the gramicidin S synthetase I gene. J Biochem 1989; 106:639–645.

131. Weckermann R, Furba§ R, Marahiel MA. Complete nucleotide sequence of *tycA* gene coding the tyrocidine synthetase 1 from *Bacillus brevis*. Nucl Acids Res 1988; 16:11841.

132. Marahiel MA, Zuber P, Czekay G, Losick R. Identification of the promoter for a peptide antibiotic gene from *Bacillus brevis* and studies on its regulation in *Bacillus subtilis*. J Bacteriol 1987; 169:2215–2222.

133. Marahiel MA, Nakano MM, Zuber P. Regulation of peptide antibiotic production in *Bacillus*. Mol Microbiol 1993; 7:631–636.

134. Zuber P, Losick R. Role of AbrB in the SpoOA- and SpoOB-dependent utilization of a sporulation promoter in *Bacillus subtilis*. J Bacteriol 1987; 169:2223–2230.

135. Perego M, Spiegelman GB, Hoch JA. Structure of the gene for the transition state regulator *abrB*: Regulator synthesis is controlled by the SpoOA sporulation gene in *Bacillus subtilis*. Mol Microbiol 1988; 2:689–699.

136. Furbaß R, Gocht M, Zuber P, Marahiel MA. Interaction of the AbrB, a transcriptional regulator from *Bacillus subtilis*, with the promoters of the transition state–activated genes *tycA* and *spoVG*. Mol Gen Genet 1991; 225:347–354.

137. Moran CP Jr. RNA polymerase and transcription factors. Sonenshein AL, Losick R, Hoch JA, eds. *Bacillus subtilis* and Other Gram-Positive Bacteria: Physiology, Biochemistry, and Molecular Biology. Washington D.C.: American Society for Microbiology, 1993:653–667.

138. MacCabe AP, Van Liempt H, Palissa H, Unkles SE, Riach MBR, Pfeifer E, von Döhren H, Kin ghorn JR. δ-(L-α–Aminoadipyl)-L-cysteinyl-D-valine synthetase from *Aspergillus nidulans*. J Biol Chem 1991; 266:1246–12654.

7
Enzymology of Peptide Synthetases

Hans von Döhren and Horst Kleinkauf
Technical University Berlin, Berlin, Germany

I. INTRODUCTION

Peptides, especially cyclic peptides, have gained increasing attention as potential drugs regularly detected by target- and mechanism-based screens. This is well reflected by the variety of chapters in this volume treating peptide antibiotics, such as β-lactams (1,2), the classical *Bacillus* peptides gramicidin, tyrocidine, and surfactin (3), and lipopeptides like daptomycin (4), cyclosporins (5), thiopeptides (6), vancomycin (7), echinocandins (8), lantibiotics (9), and virginiamycin (10). In addition, peptide bonds are contained in some macrolides (rapamycin, FK-506) (11) and aminoglycosides (lincomycin, butirosine) (12). The enzymology of precursor activation and peptide bond formation is similar in all these systems, except for lantibiotics employing multienzymes rather than directly converting mRNA transcripts via the ribosomal system (13). The unique structures of peptides offer distinct, useful measures of variation by residual exchanges or the introduction of modified precursor amino acids. These are especially relevant in the case of cyclic structures originating from enzymatic systems. However, the understanding of the architecture of their enzyme templates is still incomplete. The current state of the art thus permits the variation of identified genes (14), whereas the defined construction of any desired peptide structure is subject of continuing research.

In this chapter, we summarize the research on the enzymology of bioactive peptides; structures and regulation of multidomain peptide synthetase genes are treated separately by Zuber and Marahiel (3).

II. THE NONRIBOSOMAL SYSTEMS OF PEPTIDE SYNTHESIS

From biosynthetic studies conducted in the peptide field, three groups of basic pathways have emerged (15): the ribosomal system, the stepwise condensing enzyme systems, and the polyenzyme systems referred to as nonribosomal systems. These can be described from the similarities of the gene structures involved, the similarities of certain motifs contained in their functional elements, or the basic chemistry of amino acid activation and condensation reactions. Peptide structures generally provide clues to their biosynthetic origins, from amino acid constituents, additional constituents, and structural features. All peptides originate from linear structures (16).

A. Systems Modifying Ribosomally Made Precursors

Peptides encoded by mRNA are restricted to the 20 protein amino acids and selenocysteine. The occurrence of a single nonprotein residue already implies an enzymatic origin. In the last years, however, an increasing number of peptide modifications have been identified, including the in-chain epimerization of single residues (17–19), dehydration and thioether cross-links (20–22), and cyclizations including side-chain carboxyl-groups (23–25). A new type of reaction extending the linear template function is the splicing of proteins (26–28). Enzyme studies for the respective modifications are just beginning.

So far, it remains fairly easy to identify nonprotein amino acid residues originating from the set of protein amino acids. Any non–amino acid constituent and structurally unusual amino acids will point directly to an enzymatic origin.

B. Scope of Peptide Structures

Enzymatically formed peptides contain a number of structural elements not present in ribosomally formed peptides (16). In addition to α-carboxyl-α-amino(imino)-group linkages, these structures may contain carboxyl-groups located in 2-,3-,4-, or 5-position, 2-amino-groups, not only peptide but ester bonds, and linkages to compounds like carboxylic acids or amines. The list of possible posttranslational modifications exceeds the respective list for ribosomal peptides. Most prominent are the various modes of cyclization.

C. Amino Acid–Adding Systems

Amino acid–adding systems will not be considered in detail in this chapter. These enzyme systems are quite well characterized and comprise sets of interacting enzymes catalyzing the addition of single amino acids. The best-studied examples are the biosynthesis of glutathion (29), the 4′-phosphopantetheine moiety of coenzyme A (30), and the murein part of bacterial cell walls (31). Many of the respective enzymes in various organisms have been characterized, some have been crystallized (32–34), and quite a few gene sequences have been obtained. Most of the enzymes catalyze carboxyl-group activation by cleavage of the terminal phosphate of adenosine-5′-triphosphate (ATP), producing adenosine-5′-diphosphate (ADP) and phosphate. The bacterial cell-wall-forming systems, in particular, are of prime importance in the evaluation of antibacterial compounds.

In addition, several amino acid–adding systems have become known in the aminoacylation of viral RNAs (35), proteins (36), muropeptides (37), and polymers, such as teichoic acids (38). Whereas the first three systems employ specific aminoacyl-tRNAs, the last system structurally resembles acyl–coenzyme A synthetases, and it transfers an activated D-Ala to an acyl carrier protein transporter (39). Peptide bond formation occurs in all of these systems by separate transferases.

A special case of stepwise amino acid addition is repeated condensation to arrive at polymer structures. Such systems functioning in analogy to, for example, polyhydroxybutyrate-forming enzymes produce, for example, poly-D-glutamic acids (40,41), and they presumably are related to the polyenzyme type of peptide synthetases. These enzymes, condensing 3-carboxyl-groups, produce a size-defined polymer of about 10^6 Da. Other systems may produce poly-Lys chains of much smaller size, 25 residues (42). Even branched peptide-forming systems have been reported (43). None of these systems has been characterized in detail.

D. Polyenzyme Systems

Polyenzyme systems have received great interest for a variety of reasons. In the early stages of genetic information analysis, peptide-forming polyenzymes were an alternative to the ribosomal pathway (44). Their presence seemed to point to a remnant of early evolution (45). For the most part, genetic analysis has now established these enzyme systems as one of the complex devices evolved to accomplish efficiently the synthesis of complex metabolites in the cellular environment (46). It becomes evident that genetic elements referred to as modules encode distinct biosynthetic functions; these modules are arranged so that sequential processes, sometimes of more than 40 reactions, proceed in an ordered manner in the required cellular compartment(s). This holds not only for peptides, but also for polyketides, compounds of mixed origin, and presumably for most metabolites.

Polyenzymes can be recognized at the gene level by repeated modules encoding defined motifs for amino acid activation, aminoacylation, or peptide bond formation. The number of repeats corresponds to the number of residues in the peptide (13). At the protein level, polyenzymes can be recognized by their outstanding sizes, related to the 3 kb size of a single module, which corresponds to a set of domains of about 120 kDa required for the incorporation of one residue into a peptide. Up to now, cyclosporin synthetase at 1.7 MDa is the largest synthetase known, encoded by a 45.6 kb gene with no introns (47). This polyenzyme catalyzes the formation of a cyclo-undecapeptide in a sequence of 40 reactions (48). Current studies in the enzymology of peptide synthetases are compiled in Table 1.

III. ORGANIZATION OF PEPTIDE-SYNTHESIZING POLYENZYME SYSTEMS

With the isolation and sequencing of genes of the peptide synthetase forming the tripeptide β-lactam precursor δ-(L-α-aminoadipyl)-L-cysteinyl-D-valine (ACV), the biosynthetic link of peptide antibiotics became obvious (49,50). Bacterial and fungal systems possess a similar modular organization and highly conserved motifs. These details are discussed at the gene level by Zuber and Marahiel (3). The functional characterization of peptide synthetases will be discussed below.

A. Structure–Function Analysis

Structure–function analysis of peptide synthetases includes classical enzyme studies with no link to structural data. These have been carried out with enzyme kinetics, substrate analogs, inhibition studies, and the isolation of intermediates and products. Engineering approaches have employed mostly fragment expression and site-directed mutagenesis. In addition, first experiments with chimeric structures have been performed.

I. Amino Acid Activation

Amino Acid Selection.   Substrate selection involves recognition, formation of adenylate, and selection in an aminoacyl transfer reaction (Figure 1). It thus formally resembles protein biosynthesis, although there are no correction functions comparable to tRNA- and elongation-factor-mediated deacylation. The view of reduced specificity and thus relaxed product composition, however, should be corrected with the notion that

Table I Current State of Research on Peptide Synthetases

Peptide	Organism	Structural type[a]	Gene cloned	Enzymology
Linear				
Carnosine	*rat*	P-2	−	+
Bacilysin	*Bacillus subtilis*	P-2-M	(+)	(+)
ACV		P-3	+	+
	Aspergillus nidulans		+	+
	Penicillium chrysogenum		+	(+)
	Acremonium chrysogenum		+	+
	Streptomyces clavuligerus		+	+
	Nocardia lactamgenus		+	−
	Lysobacter sp.		+	
Ergotpeptides	*Claviceps purpurea*	R-P-3-M	−	+
Bialaphos	*Streptomyces hygroscopicus*	P-3	+	−
Leupeptin	*Streptomyces exfoliatus*	R-P-3	−	+
Edeine	*Bacillus brevis Vm4*	P-5-M	−	+
Anguibactin	*Vibrio anguillarum*	R-P-2-M	+	−
Yersiniabactin	*Yersinia enterocolitica*	R-P-2-M	+	−
Phaseolotoxin	*Pseudomononas syringae* pv. *ph.*	P-4-M	(+)	−
Victorin	*Cochliobolus victoriae*	R-P-5-M	(+)	−
Ardacin	*Kibdelosporangium aridum*	P-7-M	(+)	−
Pyoverdin	*Pseudomonas aeruginosa*	R-P-8-M	+	−
Linear gramicidin	*Bacillus brevis*	P-15-M	−	+
Alamethicin	*Trichoderma viride*	P-19-M	−	+
Cyclopeptides				
Cyclopeptin	*Penicillium cyclopium*	C-2	−	+
Enterochelin	*Escherichia coli*	P-C-E-3	+	+
HC-toxin	*Cochliobolus carbonum*	C-4	+	+
Chlamydocin	*Diheterospora chlamydosporia*	C-4	(+)	−
Cyl-2	*Cylindrocladium macrosporum*	C-4	(+)	−
Tentoxin	*Alternaria alternata*	C-4	−	+
Ferrichrome	*Aspergillus quadricinctus*	C-6	−	+
	Ustilago maydis		+	−
Echinocandin	*Aspergillus nidulans*	R-C-6	−	(+)
Microcystin	*Microcystis aeruginosa*	C-7	(+)	(+)
A-90	*Anabaena A-90*	C-7	(+)	−
Iturin	*Bacillus subtilis*	C-8	(+)	−
Gramicidin S	*Bacillus brevis ATCC 9999*	C-(P-5)$_2$	+	+
Tyrocidine	*Bacillus brevis ATCC 8185*	C-10	+	+
Cyclosporin	*Tolypocladium niveum*	C-11	+	+
Mycobacillin	*Bacillus subtilis*	C-13	−	+
Lactones				
Actinomycin	*Streptomyces clavuligerus*	R-(L-5)$_2$	−	+
Destruxin	*Metarhizium anisopliae*	L-6	+	(+)
Etamycin	*Streptomyces griseus*	R-L-7	−	(+)
Surfactin	*Bacillus subtilis*	L-8	+	+
Quinomycin	*Streptomyces echinatus*	(R-P-4)$_2$	−	+
R106	*Aureobasidium pullulans*	L-9	−	(+)
Syringomycin	*Pseudomonas syringae*	R-L-9	(+)	−

Table 1   Current State of Research on Peptide Synthetases (Continued)

Peptide	Organism	Structural type[a]	Gene cloned	Enzymology
Linear				
Syringostatin	*Pseudomonas syringae*	R-L-9	(+)	–
SDZ 90-215	*Septoria* sp.	L-10	–	+
SDZ 214-103	*Cylindrotrichum oligosporum*	L-11	(+)	+
Branched polypeptides				
Victorin	*Cochliobolus victoriae*	R-P-5-C-3	(+)	
Polymyxin	*Bacillus polymyxa*	R-P-10-C-7	–	+
Bacitracin	*Bacillus licheniformis*	R-P-12-C-7	(+)	+
Nosiheptide	*Streptomyces actuosus*	R-P-13-C-10-M	–	+
Thiostrepton	*Streptomyces laurentii*	R-P-17-C-10-M	–	+
Branched peptidolactones				
Lysobactin	*Lysobacter* sp.	P-11-L-9	(+)	+
A21798C	*Streptomyces roseosporus*	R-P-13-L-10	(+)	+
A54145	*Streptomyces fradiae*	R-P-13-L-10	–	+
CDA	*Streptomyces coelicolor*	R-P-12-L-11	(+)	–
Tolaasin	*Pseudomonas tolaasi*	R-P-18-L-5	(+)	–
Depsipeptides				
Enniatin	*Fusarium oxysporum, F. scirpi*	D-6	+	+
Beauvericin	*Beauveria bassiana*	D-6	–	+
Related systems				
D-Ala addition to lipoteichoic acid	*Lactobacillus casei*	ester	+	+
Saframycin Mx1	*Myxococcus xanthus*	quinone peptide	+	–
Coronatin	*Pseudomonas syringae*	acyl amino acid	+	(+)
FK506 (immunomycin)	*Streptomyces tsukubaensis*	macrolide	+	(+)
Rapamycin	*Streptomyces*	macrolide	+	(+)

[a] The abbreviations used are P peptide, C cyclopeptide, L lactone, D depsipeptide, E ester, R acyl, M modified. The structural types are defined by the number of amino-, imino-, or hydroxy acids in the precursor chain. The ring sizes of cyclic structures are indicated in the number following C, L, D, or E, defining the type of ring closure.
For references, see Refs. 13 and 49–52.

certain residues in peptides are quite rigorously restricted, which might be related to their functional role. This is obvious by inspection of peptide families. The classical example is gramicidin S, which had been considered as a single product for a long time, until Nozaki and Muramatsu (51) and Thibault et al. (52) demonstrated a set of substitutional variants in the commercial extract (Figure 2a). Replacement of ornithine by lysine had also been demonstrated by feeding studies (53). In contrast, the related tyrocidine has been known as a mixture of analogs with exchanges in the positions of aromatic amino acids for a long time (Figure 2b). It is obvious here, as in the coproduced linear gramicidin (Figure 2c), that there are various degrees of discrimination of substrates. In vitro examination of enzyme systems revealed the acceptance of a variety of natural and synthetic analogs, but at the same time a second step of discrimination became apparent. Some

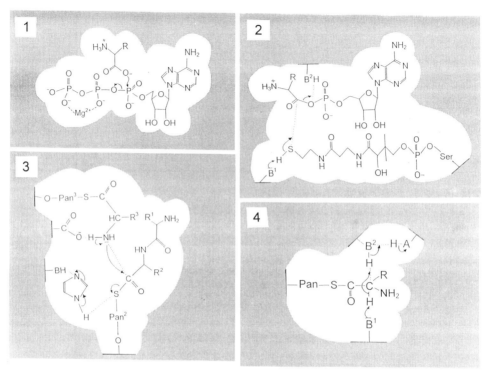

Figure 1   Schematic views of reactions involved in peptide biosynthesis. (1) Adenylate formation involving nucleophilic attack of the carboxyl-group at the α-phosphate of the MgATP^{2-}-complex with release of MgPP$_i^{2-}$; (2) aminoacylation of the pantetheine cofactor by formation of the thiolate anion, attack of the mixed anhydride, and release of AMP; (3) tentative view of the peptide bond formation by nucleophilic attack of the aminoacyl-nitrogen at the preceding thioester-carboxyl, involving deprotonation–protonation; (4) epimerization of an aminoacyl-thioester, a reaction differing from those catalyzed by the well-characterized amino acid racemases. (Altered from Ref. 13.)

compounds are substrates in the adenylate formation reaction but are not incorporated into the peptide. Examples are phenylserine in case of gramicidin S (54) and glutamate in case of the penicillin tripeptide precursor ACV (55). Substrate recognition could partially be determined by cytoplasmic concentrations of precursors, but also shifted by compartmentation of enzymes. A study of several strains of *Fusarium* producing different families of enniatins has revealed variable substrate profiles of the respective synthetases (56). Discrimination of substrates may be more or less pronounced. Whereas in gramicidin S formation substituted prolines are accepted as substrates, in the echinocandin-type acylhexapeptide producers *Aspergillus nidulans* and *Zalerion arboricola*, hydroxy-proline is discriminated over Pro (57). In contrast, in the production of neoviridogrisein, the direct precursor D-hydroxy-Pro may be exchanged to the nonhydroxylated analog by feeding of Pro (58).

Substrate selection is thus subject to controls at (a) the recognition level, (b) formation of the adenylate, (c) stability of the adenylate, (d) transfer of the acyl residue to the cofactor (aminoacylation or acylation), (e) stability of this acyl intermediate, (f) proper functioning of the acyl intermediate in peptide (or ester) bond formation, and (g) stability of the respective peptidyl intermediates in the biosynthetic cycle. The control of the recognition level is contained in the protein structure of the adenylate domain. Alignments searching for conserved regions should identify the common nucleotide-binding sites and adenylate-forming active sites (see below). Unconserved regions would help to assign substrate specificity. The suspected C–D stretch has been shown by Cosmina et al. (59) to align for substrate groups. If all members of the adenylate family are compared, this stretch identifies enzymes according to their substrates in well-established cases like acetyl-, long-chain acyl-, and 4-coumaroyl-CoA synthetases, luciferases, and several peptide synthetase domains (von Döhren H, unpublished data).

Nucleotide Binding.   As schematically depicted in Figure 1, adenylate formation proceeds from a divalent metal-ion complex of ATP. In case of the gramicidin S system, only Mg^{2+}, Mn^{2+}, and Ca^{2+} were accepted from a collection of cations (60). The nucleotide specificity has been investigated in both the gramicidin S system and ACV synthetase (55,60). 2'-deoxy-adenosine-5'-triphosphate (2'-dATP) and guanosine-5'-triphosphate (GTP) are, for example, less efficiently used substrates. Studies with nucleotide analogs and substituted ATPs indicate a binding preference for the anti conformation, since preferred syn conformers with substitutions in the 8-position are not accepted as substrates in several systems (60). Substrate profiles found for peptide synthetases differ from those of aminoacyl-tRNA synthetases, indicating their structural dissimilarity, which has been confirmed by sequence analysis of the respective genes (13). Similarity searches conducted on nucleotide-binding enzymes, including adenylate-forming synthetases, have led to no obvious results. Thus, the adenosine-5'-monophosphate (AMP)-forming tyrocidine synthetase/insect luciferase family appears to be a unique collection of adenylate-forming enzymes, which is readily identified by its signature sequence SGTTGxPKG (13,61). A collection of other key motifs described is shown in Table 2.

Structure–Function Studies.   Studies on the alteration of single amino acid residues have yet to assign functions to side chains. Yoshitaka Saito and colleagues have, by sequencing of defective gramicidin S synthetase 2 multienzyme genes, identified four Gly conversions to either Glu or Asp, leading to inactivation of adenylate formation in the respective domains: the first Gly in the signature SGTTG, a conserved Gly between the C- and D-motifs, and two Gly within the D-motif (YGxFE) and G-motif (KxRGxRIExGEIE) (62,63). Investigating conserved Lys residues expected to function in ionic attachment of the triphosphate moiety of ATP, Gocht and Marahiel (64) demonstrated a drastic reduction of adenylate formation upon changing the PKG in the signature sequence to PTG. Less reduction has been observed with PRG (90%, retention of charge and size) (64) and PQG (60%, retention of size) in the valine domain of surfactin synthetase 2 (65). Change of the H-motif NGK to NGQ in the same domain reduced the activity by 94% (65). A domain carrying changes in both the C- and H-motifs was inactive. Affinity-labeling studies were performed with both 2-azido-ATP and the versatile nucleotide mimic fluorescein 5'-isothiocyanate (FITC) (66,67). Surprisingly the distant motifs G and H were tagged. This was unexpected, since in the N-methyl amino acid–forming systems of enniatin synthetase and cyclosporin synthetase, N-methyl-transferase domains have been found inserted between the G- and H-motifs, dividing the adenylate domain into the segments A1 and A2 (Figure 3). Are the late motifs H and I involved in adenylate formation? The answer cannot yet be unambiguously given, since a truncated A to G segment of tyrocidine synthetase 1 proved to be inactive (Dieckmann R and von Döhren H, unpublished result). The recently described substrate-free crystal

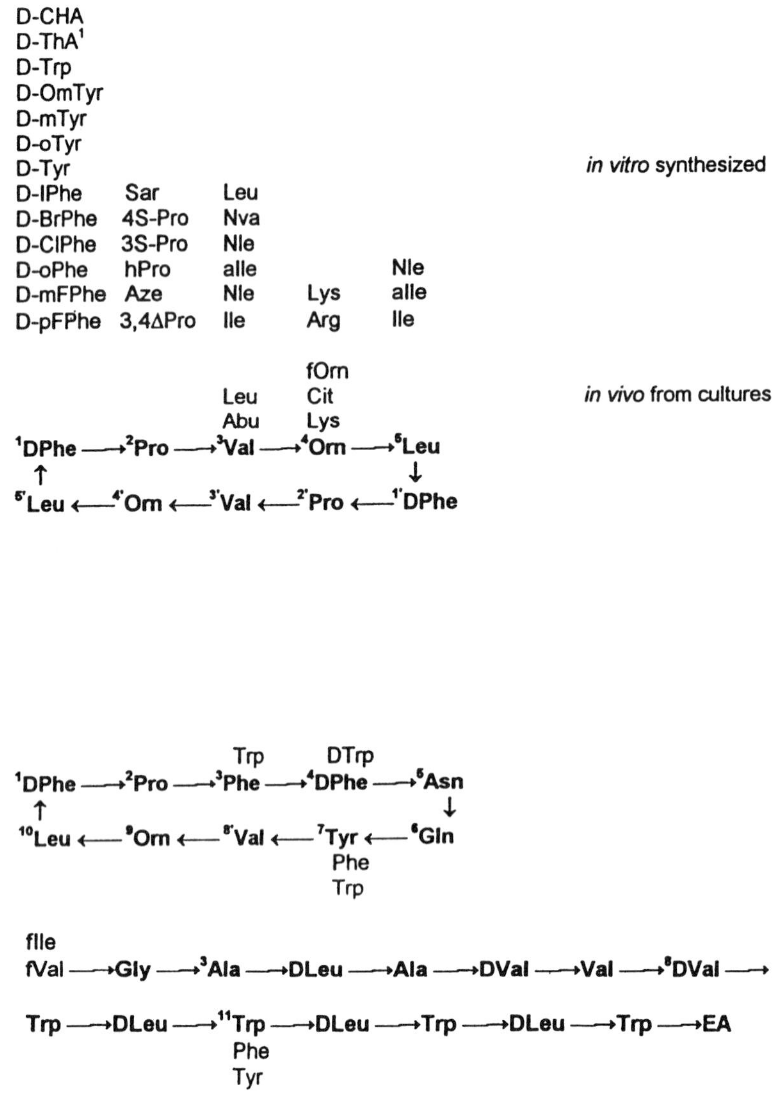

```
D-CHA
D-ThA¹
D-Trp
D-OmTyr
D-mTyr
D-oTyr
D-Tyr                                                    in vitro synthesized
D-IPhe     Sar     Leu
D-BrPhe    4S-Pro  Nva
D-ClPhe    3S-Pro  Nle
D-oPhe     hPro    alle            Nle
D-mFPhe    Aze     Nle     Lys     alle
D-pFPhe    3,4ΔPro Ile     Arg     Ile


                                fOrn
                   Leu          Cit                       in vivo from cultures
                   Abu          Lys
  ¹DPhe ──→²Pro ──→³Val ──→⁴Orn ──→⁵Leu
    ↑                                  ↓
  ⁵ʹLeu ←──⁴ʹOrn ←──³ʹVal ←──²ʹPro ←──¹ʹDPhe
```

```
                   Trp     DTrp
  ¹DPhe ──→²Pro ──→³Phe ──→⁴DPhe ──→⁵Asn
    ↑                                   ↓
  ¹⁰Leu ←── ⁹Orn ←── ⁸Val ←── ⁷Tyr ←── ⁶Gln
                             Phe
                             Trp


  fIle
  fVal ──→Gly ──→³Ala ──→DLeu ──→Ala ──→DVal ──→Val ──→⁹DVal ──→

  Trp ──→DLeu ──→¹¹Trp ──→DLeu ──→Trp ──→DLeu ──→Trp ──→EA
               Phe
               Tyr
```

Figure 2 Peptide analogs formed by *in vivo* and *in vitro* biosynthesis. (a) Analogs of gramicidin S isolated from cultures or obtained by *in vitro* enzymatic synthesis. Note that due to the symmetry of the compound, in principle both mono- and disubstituted anologs may be found. (b) Analogs of tyrocidine isolated from cultures. Note the similar specificities of positions 3 and 4, the restriction to Phe in position 1, and Tyr acceptance only in position 7. (c) Analogs of linear gramicidin isolated from cultures. Note that only Trp in position 11 is variable, and only Val in position 1.

structure of firefly luciferase indicates the involvement of at least part of the H-motif in the adenylate-forming reaction (68).

The C-terminal boundary of the adenylate domain has been deduced from limited proteolysis and sequence alignments (69), which have identified also similarities of structural organization of the adjacent pantetheine-attaching region (motif J) with various acyl carrier proteins.

Table 2   Consensus Sequences of Motifs

Adenylate domains

A:	LTxxELxxxAxxLxR
B:	AVxxAxAxYVxIDxxYPxER
C:	YTSGTTGxPKG
D:	IIxxYGxT
E:	GELxIxGxxVAR
F:	RLYRTGDL
G:	IEYLGRxDxQVKIRxxRIELGEIE
H:	LxxYMVP
I:	LTxxGKLxRKAL

Acyl carrier domains

J:	LGGxSIxAI

Elongation (1)/epimerization (2) domains

K	(B1): YPSVxxQxRMYIL,	(B2): LxPIQxWF
L	(B1): LIxRHExL,	(B2): LxxxHD
M	(B1): DMHHIIxDGxSxxI	(B2): HHxxVDxVSWxIL
N	(B1): LSKxGQxDIIxGTPxAGR	(B2): VxxEGHGRE
O	(B1): IxGMFVNTxLALR,	(B2): TVGWFTxxxPxxL
P:		(B2): PxxGxGy
Q:		(B2): VxFNYLG

N-methyltransferases

M1:	GxDFxxWTSMYDG
M2:	LEIGTGTGMVLFNLxxxxGL
M3:	VxNSVAQYFP
M4:	ExxEDExLxxPAFF
M5:	HVExxPKxMxxxNELSxYRYxAV
M6:	GxxVExSxARQxGxLD

The various enzymes of this adenylate-forming family catalyze a set of reactions, including (a) phosphoryl-group-mediated cleavage of adenylates with substrate release, and (b) aminoacylation of CoA- or protein-bound pantetheine. The first set of reactions includes the substrate-dependent isotope exchange reaction

$$E + RCOOH + MATP^{2-} \rightarrow E\{RCO\text{-}AMP\} + MPP_i^{2-} \quad (1)$$

as well as the formation of various nucleotide polyphosphates by adenylation of polyphosphates or triphosphates (70–73):

$$E + MATP^{2-} \rightarrow E\{AMP\} + MPP_i^{2-} \quad (2)$$

$$E\{RCO\text{-}AMP\} + P_n \rightarrow E + AP_{n+1} + RCOOH \quad (3)$$

$$E + MATP^{2-} + P_n \rightarrow E + AP_{n+1} + MPP_i^{2-} \quad (4)$$

$$E\{RCO\text{-}AMP\} + NTP \rightarrow E + Ap_4N + RCOOH \quad (5)$$

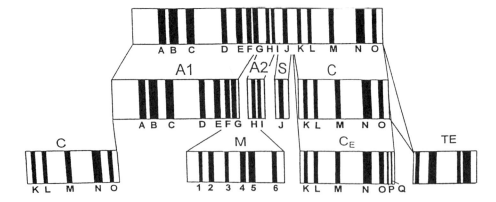

Figure 3 Peptide synthetase modules. A peptide synthetase module (top) can be dissected into submodules catalyzing adenylate formation (A1 and A2), an acyl carrier module (S), and a condensing module (C); condensing modules with epimerizing function have two additional motifs (C$_E$). N-methyltransferase modules (M) are inserted between A1 and A2. For terminating reactions, a thioesterase module (TE) may be added.

The physiological functions of these reactions are not understood, but compounds like A$_2$P$_4$ or A$_2$P$_5$ have been implicated in signaling pathways (73,74), originally termed alarmones (75). Acyl-CoA synthetases and insect luciferases show different preferences for polyphosphate substrates, whereas no data have been reported for peptide synthetases.

2.   Aminoacyl- and Peptidyl-Transport

Aminoacylation has initially been ascribed to cysteinyl side chains (15), until peptide synthetase sequencing work first completed on the ACV synthetase from *Penicillium chrysogenum* revealed the absence of conserved cysteine residues. With a considerable effort Vater and coworkers have verified the attachment of 4′-phosphopantetheine at the J-motif in the gramicidin S system (76–79). Acylation or aminoacylation of the pantetheine cysteamine thiol is another similarity to acyl-CoA synthetases and luciferases:

$$E^{1-1} \{RCO\text{-}AMP\} + E^{1-2}\text{-pan-SH} \longrightarrow E^{1-1} + AMP + RCO\text{-}S\text{-pan-}E^{1-2} \quad (6)$$

$$E\{RCO\text{-}AMP\} + CoASH \longrightarrow E + AMP + RCO\text{-}SCoA \quad (7)$$

The notations E^{1-1} and E^{1-2} indicate the subsites 1 and 2 in the direct neighborhood of the site 1 of a multifunctional protein.

From the pH dependence of the reaction, the formation of a thiolate anion can be concluded (80, Figure 1). Both types of synthetases can be expected to have binding sites for 4′-phosphopantetheine and, presumably, CoA. The possible transfer of acyl or aminoacyl residues to acyl carrier proteins (ACPs) has not been investigated. However, Heaton and Neuhaus (38) have uncovered a unique mode of D-Ala attachment to teichoic acids, consisting of a D-Ala adenylate-forming enzyme, a D-Ala carrier protein, and a respective transferase. Both ACP from *Escherichia coli* and *Streptomyces erythreae* also accepted the aminoacyl residue.

Do these results rule out the participation of cysteine residues in the catalytic cycle of peptide synthetases? Occasionally, conserved Cys residues are found within groups of adenylate domains or carrier protein domains. Gocht and Marahiel have studied the E-motif Cys-364 of tyrocidine synthetase 1. Alteration to Ser increased the aminoacylation level, whereas adenylate formation was essentially unchanged; no effect has been found on the epimerization reaction catalyzed by this single-unit peptide synthetase (66). Involvement of Cys in the epimerization reaction had been postulated by Kanda and coworkers (81), but functional groups related to this modification are thought to be located in the elongation domain. How can the improvement of aminoacylation be understood? This reaction represents the charging of the cysteamine thiol and is conventionally measured by a filter binding assay. Thioester-attached aminoacyl residues can be detached by performic acid. This type of assay is mainly limited by hydrolytic instability of the aminoacyl thioesters. Half-lives of these have been estimated (82,83), and they vary considerably, depending on their structure. An increase of charging could thus be related to an improved rate of aminoacylation, and decreased rate of hydrolytic deacylation, but also to a charging of noncatalytic side chains. Nonspecific charging of nonthiol side chains has been observed with proteins like BSA or lysozyme in adenylate formation assays. Attachment is presumably by peptide bond formation (Pfeifer E and von Döhren H, unpublished data). Substitutions of the conserved J-motif serines to alanines in the surfactin system and the gramicidin S system have demonstrated the complete loss of the aminoacylation reaction, and indicate the requirement of posttranslational modification for thioester formation (85,86).

Aminoacylation assays have revealed that overexpressed peptide synthetases are only incompletely posttranslationally modified by pantetheine. Tyrocidine synthetase 1 expressed in E. coli contains about 1.5% holo-enzyme (80). The reduced cofactor content leads to decreased activities in aminoacylation and epimerization reactions, which require the cofactor (64,80,84). Some evidence has been obtained that apo-enzymes may slightly differ from holo-enzymes with respect to catalytic properties (80). Addition of 4′-phosphopantetheine is thought to be catalyzed by a holo-enzyme synthase utilizing CoA:

$$\text{apo-peptide synthetase} + \text{CoA} \xrightarrow{\text{holo-enzyme synthase}} \text{holo-peptide synthetase} + 3',5'\text{-ADP} \quad (8)$$

The reaction has been studied in some detail in the modification of ACP in E. coli (87), rat liver (88,89), and spinach chloroplasts (90,91), and recently the ACP-holo-enzyme synthase from E. coli has been characterized and identified as the dpj gene (92). However, this synthase failed to modify expressed tyrocidine synthetase 1 (Pfeifer E and Lambalot R, unpublished results). A holo-peptide synthetase synthase has been detected in extracts of the tyrocidine producer Bacillus brevis ATCC 8185 and the enniatin-producing Fusarium scirpi (Pfeifer E, unpublished results).

For more than two decades, the rotating cofactor model originally proposed by Laland et al. and Lipmann et al. has been associated with peptide synthetases, although it did not explain all experimental data (15). So in vitro systems with incomplete substrate amino acid supply accumulate all possible intermediate peptides. This result could hardly be explained with the presence of a single 4′-phosphopantetheine. In addition, Saito and coworkers (93) had obtained pantetheine-free mutant multienzymes in the gramicidin S system, impaired in epimerization and aminoacylation functions. The absence of conserved cysteines and the presence of multiple pantetheine attachment consensus sequences obtained from numerous gene sequence data definitely support a multiple-carrier model. For the gramicidin S system, Vater and coworkers have succeeded in demonstrating the presence of the cofactor at all five predicted sites, utilizing a negative replacement labeling technique with mass spectrometric detection of the modified peptides (77–79).

The transport of intermediates thus involves the simultaneous binding, presumably at the elongation domain, of two acylated 4'-phosphopantetheine moieties, and their positional arrangement to permit peptide bond formation. In analogy with the ribosomal system, binding sites resembling the A- and P-sites could be envisioned. However, the repertoire of peptide synthetases exceeds the ribosomal aminoacyl/peptidyl system considerably (Table 3).

Whereas generally the ribosomal A-site requires a free amino-group and L-configuration, the enzymatic A-site analog also may direct *N*-substituted aminoacyl-groups and D-configurated groups including hydroxy acids. A respective model is shown in Figure 4.

3. Epimerization

It has long been thought that epimerization would occur at the thioester stage of the activated amino acid. This had been concluded from the studies on gramicidin S and tyroci-

Table 3   Types of Elongation Reactions in the Nonribosomal System

A-site	P-site	System
Aminoacyl	D-Aminoacyl	Gramicidin S, tyrocidin initiation
		Intermolecular transfer
Aminoacyl	Acyl	Surfactin initiation, ACV initiation
Aminoacyl	Formyl-aminoacyl	Gramicidin initiation
Aminoacyl	Peptidyl	General elongation
D-Aminoacyl	Peptidyl	General elongation
Aminoacyl	D-Peptidyl	Elongation, intermolecular transfer
N-Methyl-aminoacyl	D-Aminoacyl	Cylosporin initiation

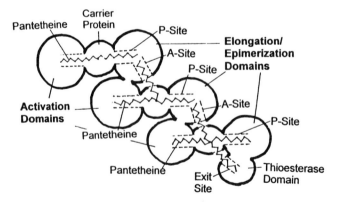

Figure 4   Scheme of elongation in the nonribosomal system, employing the terminology of the ribosomal system. The aminoacyl residue is attached as thioester to its tRNA analog cofactor 4'-phosphopantetheine. This residue swings to its respective A-site on the elongation domain. The respective peptidyl residue, equally thioester-bound to its 4'phosphopantetheine carrier, swings to a respective P-site, and condensation is catalyzed by a peptidyltransferase center, transferring the peptidyl residue onto the aminoacyl residue with peptide bond formation. The free cofactor is now aminoacylated to function in its respective A-site, whereas the elongated peptide docks to the following P-site. In contrast to the ribosome, each step has its own petidyltransferase center on the elongation domain, and A- and P-sites may vary in their selection properties (see Table 3).

dine biosynthesis (15). Analysis of the configuration of the thioester-bound amino acids yielded L,D-mixtures with the D-configuration dominating. Surprisingly, in both actinomycin (94) and ACV synthetases (95–97) enzyme-bound valine showed exclusively L-configuration. Stindl and Keller (94) have shown that the dipeptide intermediate of actinomycin is enzyme attached as a racemate, indicating that epimerization occurs at the dipeptide stage. In ACV synthesis, the tripeptide is released so fast that no intermediate can be trapped. The stereospecificity of the peptide-releasing thioesterase has been changed by mutation of an active serine residue (96,97). In that case, the LLL-tripeptide can be detected by in vitro synthesis. Release should be catalyzed by hydrolysis of the thioester intermediate. When amino acid analogs Glu or OMe-Ser have been used, the dipeptides Cys-D-Val and OMe-Ser-D,L-Val have been formed in low yields (98,99). The data seem to indicate that the first peptide bond has not been formed, and that the release of the dipeptide is catalyzed by the thioesterase. It has also been suggested that the "first" peptide bond is formed only in the second step. Clarification must come from the analysis of intermediate thioesters.

In conclusion, the available data suggest that epimerization occurs at the peptidyl stage, and only in the special case of initiation is it conferred to the aminoacyl stage. Analysis of sequence data of elongation modules involved in the addition of D–amino acids from L-isomers revealed altered motifs K, L, M, N, and O, and the additional motifs P and Q, absent in elongation modules directly incorporating L– or D–amino acids (80) (Figure 3). From amino acid sequence alignments, de Crécy–Lagard et al. (100) have suggested that a 350-amino-acid domain comprising the motifs L–O either catalyzes epimerization or condensation reactions. The striking similarity of the M-motif with key motifs of chloramphenicol acetyltransferases and dihydrolipoamide acyltransferases has been pointed out. This analysis missed the additional motifs P and Q, and it restricted the domains to a single function. This seems to correlate well with the occurence of D–amino acid residues in interdomain peptidyl transfer positions in prokaryotic systems. There are, however, various examples of intradomain peptidyl transfers of thioesters with anchored D–amino acid residues, for example, in the linear gramicidin and bacitracin systems, as well as in the eukaryotic HC-toxin synthetase. The latter example indeed shows a unique bifunctional elongation domain with two M-motifs, but additional sequence data will have to verify the coupled epimerization/condensation functions.

4. N-Methylation

N-Methylation was first studied in the case of enniatin synthetase (101). The intermediate N-methyl-valine was detected, indicating that the reaction took place at the aminoacyl thioester stage. The reaction required S-adenosylmethionine, and it was inhibited by methyltransferase inhibitors like sinefungin (102). The methyltransferase was located by affinity labeling and specific immunodetection procedures (103). Sequencing of the enniatin synthetase gene revealed that the transferase module was inserted in the adenylate module, separating it into two submodules (A1 and A2, Figure 3) (104). Structure analysis of the related firefly luciferase identified these two submodules as N- and C-terminal fragments (68). Sequencing of the cyclosporin synthetase gene provided seven additional N-methyltransferase modules (47), and alignments provide five highly conserved motifs for identification (13), including the methyltransferase-specific sequence. N-methylation is not restricted to eukaryotes; several prokaryotic N-methylated peptides also are under investigation, including actinomycin and daptomycin (105,106).

5.   Acylation

N-Acylations largely resemble the condensation of various starter acyl-groups in polyketide formation. The respective acyl-CoA derivative, presumably derived from a pathway-integrated fatty acid or polyketide synthase, is transferred to the first amino group of a thioester-bound aminoacyl residue, requiring the action of an acyltransferase. Such acyltransferases have been partially purified from the polymyxin (107) and surfactin biosynthetic systems (108,109). So far, sequence data is missing, but presumably similarity to known transferases from the polyketide field can be expected.

Acylation by aromatic carboxylic acids proceeds by direct activation and transfer. A well-studied example seemed to be the enterobactin-forming system in *E. coli*. Initiation seemed to require the interaction of a dihydroxybenzoate-activating enzyme (EntE) with a serine-activating multienzyme (EntF) (110). Walsh and colleagues (111,112), could show that entE resembles an adenylate-forming module, similar to acyl-CoA synthetases, and entF a peptide synthetase, consisting of elongation domain, adenylation domain, and acyl carrier protein domain. The synthetases were sequenced and overexpressed, but apparently the lack of pantothenylation hindered the expected initiation.

Keller and coworkers succeeded in the preparation of several aromatic carboxylic acid–activating starter enzymes involved in the biosynthesis of actinomycin (4-methyl-3-hydroxyanthranilic acid) (105,113,114), triostin (quinoxaline-2-carboxylic acid) (105,115), and mikamycin (3-hydroxypicolinic acid) (105,116). More recently, related enzymes have been identified in the Actinomycetes that form the thiopeptides nosiheptide and thiostrepton (117,118), and in the pristinamycin biosynthetic system (de Crécy-Lagard V, personal communication). Whether direct acylation of the pantetheine-attached starter amino acid occurs, or an additional transferase function is required, has not been settled.

B.   System Identification and Analysis

Metabolite-producing enzyme systems are embedded into a complex cellular context. Besides genes for the actual bond making in the metabolite basic structure, essential additional functions include (a) regulation of biosynthetic genes, (b) precursor biosynthesis, (c) transport of precursors and product, and (d) intrinsic resistance against or export of the metabolite. In none of the systems under study has the complete set of genes been evaluated. The progress, however, is obvious if the data from nonpeptide metabolites are compared.

The regulation of the respective biosynthetic pathways should be connected with external and internal inducer signals. Such signals could be related to stress conditions, such as depletion of any nutrient source or metal ions such as Fe^{3+}, or the presence of oxygen. The ecological view of external signals of competing organisms has so far been neglected, but some data have been obtained in invasive processes, like plant infection by strains of *Pseudomonas*. Here, evidence for the induction of peptide biosynthesis by plant substances has been obtained (119,120). Likewise, cell isolates from the plant pathogenic fungus *Botrytis cinerea* may induce the production of antifungal peptaibols of the trichorzianine type together with chitobiohydrolase, endochitinase, and β-1,3-glucanase in *Trichoderma harzianum* (121).

1.   Prediction of Organization

The organization of peptide biosynthetic systems is primarily approached from the amino acid composition of the product. From the protein side, large multifunctional enzymes are identified as peptide synthetases by immunoassays, and functionally characterized by amino acid substrate selection. Alternatively, the organization of gene structures will be inspected for correlation with the structure predicted from the presumed pathway. Finally, gene structures and enzyme structures have to be matched to verify the assumptions.

Recent examples of these approaches include ACV synthetases (122,123), surfactin synthetases (59,109,124,125), HC-toxin synthetase (126), cyclosporin synthetase (5,47), and enniatin synthetase (103). The difficult part is to provide meaningful amino acid sequence data from the very large proteins, generally to be derived from peptide fragments.

The prediction of organization will follow the current state of knowledge, deriving several rules. These include the following:

1. The number of adenylate modules should correspond to the number of residues in the peptide. In case of repetitive structures, modules may be reused, as, for example, in case of enniatin formation.
2. The N-terminal starting amino acid is obvious in linear structures, still obvious in acylated cyclopeptides or peptidolactones, but not generally predictable in cyclopeptides.
3. Prokaryotic systems analyzed so far vary considerably in their extent of integration. Systems ranging from one to six modules have been characterized, and substantial evidence for even larger multienzymes exists, for example, in the cases of lysobactin (127,128) and syringopeptins (Zocher R, personal communication). The only completely integrated system in prokaryotes found so far is the ACV synthetase, which is also speculated to be transferred by genetic exchange (1).
4. The known eukaryotic systems are fully integrated, ranging from 2 to 11 modules.
5. Each adenylate module (50–60 kDa) is associated with an acyl acarrier module (10 kDa) and an elongation/epimerization module (40–50 kDa). It is still not settled if module positions have to be conserved. Thus, whereas generally the sequence adenylate (A)–acyl carrier (C)–elongation (E) is found, cyclosporin synthetase starts with an elongation domain, followed by 11 sets of A–C–E modules. Generally, an elongation module in the N-terminal position of a multienzyme indicates catalysis of an acyl, amino acyl, or peptidyl transfer.
6. Acylation of peptides by aliphatic or aromatic carboxylic acids is followed by different routes. The respective carboxylic acids are supplied by linked polyketide synthases, either of the fatty acid or various polyketide synthase types, and introduced as either CoA esters or activated directly as adenylates. Several such activating systems have been characterized (see Section III.A.5). To initiate peptide synthesis with CoA esters, respective transferases are required;
7. N-Methylation requires an additional methyltransferase module, which in the eukaryotic systems identified to date is inserted in the adenylate domain.

These rules permit a rough prediction of the information content required for a peptide synthetase system. Shortcomings are still the lack of information concerning various modification reactions including hydroxylation, oxidation, O-methylation, and formation of thiazolidine and oxazoline rings from cysteine and serine side chains. Also, side-chain glycosylation and inter–side chain linking by ether or C–C bonds, as, for example, in the vancomycin type of glycopeptides, have not yet been studied.

2. Relations to Other Biosynthetic Systems

Several metabolites that have been identified contain both peptide bonds and polyketide features. Lipophilic amino acids like Bmt [(4R)-4-[(E)-2-butenyl]-4-methyl-L-threonine] or aromatic amino-acids like phenylglycine are manufactured by associated enzyme systems. Whereas their activation proceeds by adenylate formation and enzyme aminoacylation, acylation of starter amino acids and initiation of polyketide synthesis both proceed from CoA esters, and they require transferase functions. In both peptide- and polyketide-forming systems, intermediates remain attached at an acyl carrier domain via 4′-phosphopantetheine (129). Additional similarities may be unraveled in the near future, when oxygenation/hydroxylation modules of peptide synthetases are evaluated, and possible extensions of aminoacyl or peptidyl intermediates by, for example, malonyl-CoA will be investigated. Such reactions have been implied in the biosynthesis of bleomycin (130) and echinocandin (57). In addition, glycosyltransferases operating in various modifications may belong to similar enzyme classes.

The arrangement of various biosynthetic modules to facilitate a multistep process is obviously not restricted to certain classes of compounds. However, the adaptation of each module to its specific function in a given system is still an open issue.

C. Manipulation of Systems

I. In Vivo and In Vitro Synthesis of Peptide Analogs

To change the composition of peptides or peptide families, the supply of direct precursors is convenient. Certain positions may show a less restricted substrate selection and permit the in vivo synthesis of new compounds by culture feeding. Available examples have been reviewed recently (131). Most extensively studied has been the cyclosporin system, both in vivo and in vitro (48). Cyclosporin synthetase can be prepared conveniently from production strains, thus permitting the facile preparation of peptide analogs (Figure 5). Likewise, the peptidolactone analog SDZ 104-125 synthetase has been studied for analog production (132).

Attempts to direct biosynthesis may sometimes lead to surprises, as in the case of D-threonine, which was introduced into the cyclosporin system to replace the initiating D-alanine. From in vitro studies it soon became evident that the D-alanine activation site did accept D-alanine, D-serine, and related derivatives, but not D-threonine (132). Culture feeding led to N-methyl-4isoleucyl-cyclosporin (133). Presumably, the D-threonine is metabolized to L-allo-threonine by a nonspecific alanine racemase and, not being a substrate for cyclosporin synthetase, may enter the isoleucine pathway. Alternatively, as is known from the the bacterium Serratia marcescens, a specific D-threonine dehydratase may be induced and directly convert D-threonine to L-isoleucine. Site 4 of cyclosporin synthetase, which activates leucine, differs from the other leucine-activating sites in its low level of discrimination between leucine and isoleucine. The initial ratio of these is 5:1 in the employed medium, and the postulated shift in this ratio leads to a cyclosporin analog devoid of immunosuppressive activity, retaining affinity to cyclophilin, but the complex no longer binds to calcineurin. Physiological effects for the producer have not been followed, but interestingly the analog has potential anti-HIV1 activity.

Together with the data on gramicidin S (134) and enniatins (135), the following conclusions can be drawn:

1. The positional exchange by feeding is largely determined by the respective substrate selection properties of the specific site.

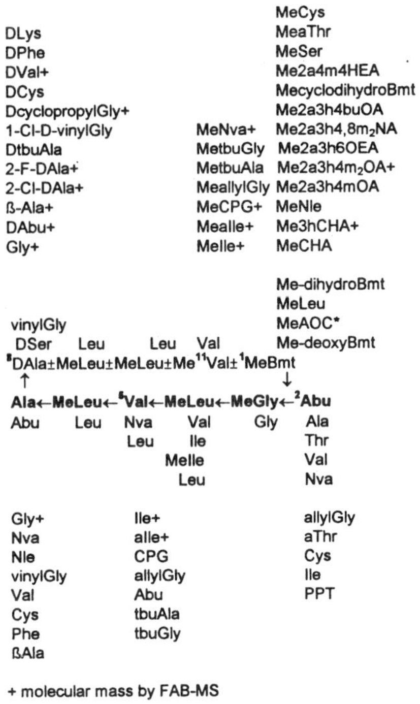

```
                                      MeCys
DLys                                  MeaThr
DPhe                                  MeSer
DVal+                                 Me2a4m4HEA
DCys                                  MecyclodihydroBmt
DcyclopropylGly+                      Me2a3h4buOA
1-Cl-D-vinylGly        MeNva+         Me2a3h4,8m₂NA
DtbuAla                MetbuGly        Me2a3h6OEA
2-F-DAla+              MetbuAla        Me2a3h4m₂OA+
2-Cl-DAla+             MeallylGly      Me2a3h4mOA
ß-Ala+                 MeCPG+          MeNle
DAbu+                  MeaIle+         Me3hCHA+
Gly+                   MeIle+          MeCHA

                                      Me-dihydroBmt
                                      MeLeu•
vinylGly                              MeAOC*
  DSer    Leu    Leu   Val            Me-deoxyBmt
ᵇDAla±MeLeu±MeLeu±Meᵃ¹¹Val±ᶦMeBmt
   ↑                        ↓
Ala←MeLeu←⁵Val←MeLeu←MeGly←²Abu
Abu    Leu   Nva   Val   Gly   Ala
             Leu   Ile         Thr
                   MeIle       Val
                   Leu         Nva

Gly+       Ile+       allylGly
Nva        aIle+      aThr
Nle        CPG        Cys
vinylGly   allylGly   Ile
Val        Abu        PPT
Cys        tbuAla
Phe        tbuGly
ßAla
```

+ molecular mass by FAB-MS

Figure 5 Cyclosporins synthesized *in vitro*. Changed positions are indicated, and generally single replacements have been reported, except for substitutions at positions 5 and 11 showing double replacement, or even tripüle replacement for 2, 5 and 11 in case of e.g. Nva or allyl-glycine. Compounds directly placed at the cyclosporin A-structure have also been isolated from fermentations, and were available as reference compounds. All other compounds have been described by chromatographic evidence or additional mass spectra (+). Abbreviations used are: Abu–aminobutyrate, allylGly–allyl–glycine, 2a3h4buOH–2-amino-3-hydroxy–4-butyloctanoic acid, 2a3h4, 8m₂NA–2-amino-3-hydroxy-4, 8-dimethylnonanoic acid, 2a3h6OEA–2-amino-3-hydroxyoct-6-enoic acid, 2a3h4m₂OA-2-amino-3hydroxy4,4-dimethylocanoic acid, 2a4mHEA–2-amino-4-methylhex-4-enoic acid, AOC–aminooctanoic acid, CHA–cyclohexyl-alanine, 2-Cl-DAla–2-chloro-D-alanine, CPG–cyclopropyl-glycine, cyclopropylGly–cyclopropyl-glycine, D–D-configuration, 2-F-DAla–2-fluoro-D-alanine, 3hCHA–3-hydroxy-cyclohexyl-alanine, Me–N-methyl-, Nle–norleucine, PPT–phosphinothricine, tbuAla–t-butyl-alanine, tbuGly–t-butyl-glycine. (Reprinted with permission from (48); for details see (132)).

2. Precursors may be subject to modification and thus lead also to unexpected new products.

3. Poor substrates will reduce the product yield according to their rate of incorporation. If more than one position is exchanged, the respective rates of product formation are roughly additive.

4. Likewise, in the synthesis of unmethylated analogs of *N*-methyl-peptides, rates decrease dramatically to about 10% for each unmethylated residue. Thus, de-dimethyl or de-trimethyl compounds are rarely observed.

5. Certain analogs may exert inhibitory properties on the peptide synthetase, which could be related to product inhibition, or (not investigated) in vivo to more complex mechanisms of product inhibition involving regulatory components of targets of resistance.

2. Engineering of Systems

To introduce defined positional exchanges known from gene sequence alterations in ribosomal peptide formation, somewhat more complex approaches are required. Since the active-site architecture of amino acid–activating modules is not known in detail, the present approach considers the exchange of complete modules. Thus, Stachelhaus et al. (14) have replaced the terminal adenylate and acyl carrier modules of surfactin synthetase 3 by respective sets of modules from either a *Bacillus* system (gramicidin S) or a fungal ACV synthetase. The procedure involving double crossover has been described in detail in the respective chapter (3). Other strategies of direct selection procedures in gene replacement approaches have been designed for Streptomycetes (136) or have been employed in engineering of ACV synthetase from *Aspergillus nidulans* (137,138). So, respective variations of peptide synthetase structures are and will be the subject of investigation, as the production of surfactin analogs has demonstrated (14). Open questions remaining are (a) the actual performance of newly constructed systems, and (b) their improvement in case of poor performance. The fragment replacement indeed seems to mimic natural processes of gene recruitment into multienzyme structures, which, however, is presumably connected to yet unidentified natural selection processes.

IV. CONCLUSIONS

Studies on nonribosomal peptide formation by multienzymes have demonstrated the modular organization of these systems. As in the case of polyketide formation, the linear arrangements of modules determine their sequential operation. Their various modes of integration, however, are still not understood. It is evident that substrate-activating sites introducing amino and imino acids as well as hydroxy acids have different specificities. Thus, variations in the structures of side chains are easily accomplished, and these exceed the variability of polyketide systems in this respect. Work is in progress to make use of such systems for structure–function studies in the analysis of natural products and in the biosynthesis of new products. Future efforts will be directed to linking system variations to various selection processes.

REFERENCES

1. Demain AL. Comparative biochemistry and fermentation of β-lactam biosynthesis. Strohl W, ed. Biotechnology of Antibiotics, 2nd ed. New York: Marcel Dekker, 1997.
2. Jensen SE, Paradkar AS, Mosher RH. Comparative genetics of β-lactam antibiotic production. Strohl W, ed. Biotechnology of Antibiotics, 2nd ed. New York: Marcel Dekker, 1996.
3. Marahiel MA, Zuber P. Structure, function and regulation of genes encoding multi-domain peptide synthetases. Strohl W, ed. Biotechnology of Antibiotics, 2nd ed. New York: Marcel Dekker, 1997.
4. Baltz RH. Daptomycin and A54145. Strohl W, ed. Biotechnology of Antibiotics, 2nd ed. New York: Marcel Dekker, 1997.
5. Traber R. Biosynthesis of cyclosporins. Strohl W, ed. Biotechnology of Antibiotics, 2nd ed. New York: Marcel Dekker, 1997.
6. Floss HG. Thiopeptide antibiotics. Strohl W, ed. Biotechnology of Antibiotics, 2nd ed. New York: Marcel Dekker, 1997.

7. Nicas T, Cooper R. Vancomycin and other glycopeptides. Strohl W, ed. Biotechnology of Antibiotics, 2nd ed. New York: Marcel Dekker, 1997.

8. Current W, Turner W. Echinocandins—cyclic peptide antifungal drugs for the future. Strohl W, ed. Biotechnology of Industrial Antibiotics, 2nd ed. New York: Marcel Dekker, 1996.

9. Hansen JN. Nisin and related lantibiotics. Strohl W, ed. Biotechnology of Antibiotics, 2nd ed. New York: Marcel Dekker, 1997.

10. Yamada Y. Butyrolactone autoregulators and their role in virginiamycin biosynthesis. Strohl W, ed. Biotechnology of Antibiotics, 2nd ed. New York: Marcel Dekker, 1997.

11. Jeong BC, Demain AL. Rapamycin, FK-506 and immunomycin-related immunosuppressants. Strohl W, ed. Biotechnology of Antibiotics, 2nd ed. New York: Marcel Dekker, 1997.

12. Chung ST, Lincomycin/clindamycin. Strohl W, ed. Biotechnology of Antibiotics, 2nd ed. New York: Marcel Dekker, 1997.

13. Kleinkauf H, von Döhren H. A nonribosomal system of peptide biosynthesis. Eur J Biochem 1996; 236:335–351.

14. Stachelhaus T, Schneider A, Marahiel MA. Rational design of peptide antibiotics by targeted replacement of bacterial and fungal domains. Science 1995; 269:69–72.

15. Kleinkauf H, von Döhren H. Nonribosomal biosynthesis of peptide antibiotics. Eur J Biochem 1990; 192:1–15.

16. von Döhren H. Complilation of peptide structures: A biogenetic approach. Kleinkauf H., von Döhren H, eds. Biochemistry of Peptide Antibiotics. Berlin: de Gruyter 1980, 411–507.

17. Kreil G. Conversion of L- to D-amino acids: A posttranslational reaction. Science 1994; 266:996–997.

18. Heck SD, Siok CJ, Krapcho KJ, Kelbaugh PR, Thadeio PF, Welch MJ, Williams RD, Ganong AH, Kelly ME, Lanzetti AJ, Gray WR, Phillips D, Parks TN, Jackson H, Ahlijanian MK, Saccomano NA, Volkmann RA. Functional consequences of posttranslational isomerization of Ser[46] in a calcium channel toxin. Science 1994; 266:1065–1068.

19. Mor A, Amiche M, Nicolas P. Enter a new post-translational modification: D–Amino acids in gene-encoded peptides. Trends Biochem Sci 1992; 17:481–485.

20. Gasson MJ. Lantibiotics. Vining LC, Stuttard C, eds. Genetics and Biochemistry of Antibiotic Production. Boston: Butterworth-Heinemann 1995, 283–306.

21. Sahl H-G, Jack RW, Bierbaum G. Biosynthesis and biological activities of lantibiotics with unique post-translational modifications. Eur J Biochem 1995; 230:827–853.

22. Jack RW, Sahl H-G. Unique peptide modifications involved in the biosynthesis of lantibiotics. Trends Biotechnol 1995; 13:269–278.

23. Fréchet D, Giutton JD, Herman F, Faucher D, Helynck G, Monegier du Sorbier B, Ridoux JP, James-Sarcouf E, Vuilhorgne M. Solution structure of RP 71955, a new 21 amino acid tricyclic peptide active against HIV-1 virus. Biochem 1994; 33:42–50.

24. Potterat O, Stephan H, Metzger JW, Gnau V, Zähner H, Jung G. Aborycin—a tricyclic-21-peptide antibiotic isolated from *Streptomyces griseoflavus*. Liebigs Ann 1994; 1994:741–743.

25. Martínez-Bueno M, Maqueda M, Gálvez A, Samyn B, van Beeumen J, Coyette J, Valdivia E. The cyclic structure of the enterococcal peptide antibiotic AS-48. J Bacteriol 1994; 176:6334–6339.

26. Cooper AA, Stevens TH. Protein splicing: Self-splicing of genetically mobile elements at the protein level. Trends Biochem Sci 1995; 20:351–356.

27. Kane PM, Yamashiro CT, Wolczyk DF, Neff N, Goebl M, Stevens TH. Protein splicing converts the yeast TFP1 gene product to the 69-kD subunit of the vacuolar H(+)-adenosine triphosphatase. Science 1990; 250:651–657.

28. Hirata R, Ohsumk Y, Nakano A, Kawasaki H, Suzuki K, Anraku Y. Molecular structure of a gene, VMA1, encoding the catalytic subunit of H(+)-translocating adenosine triphosphatase from vacuolar membranes of *Saccharomyces cerevisiae*. J Biol Chem 1990; 265:6726–6733.

29. Meister A. Glutathione metabolism. Meth Enzymol 1995; 251:3–7.

30. Shimizu S, Tani Y, Ogata K. Synthesis of coenzyme A and its biosynthetic intermediates by microbial processes. Meth Enzymol 1979; 62:236–245.

31. Bugg TDH, Walsh CT. Intracellular steps of bacterial cell wall peptidoglycan biosynthesis. Enzymology, antibiotics and antibiotic resistance. Nat Prod Rep 1992; 6:199–215.

32. Fan C, Moews PC, Shi Y, Walsh CT, Knox JR. A common fold for peptide synthetases cleaving ATP to ADP: Glutathione synthetase and D-alanine:D-alanine ligase of *Escherichia coli*. Proc Natl Acad Sci USA 1995; 92:1172–1176.

33. Fan C, Moews PC, Walsh C. Vancomycin resistance: Structure of D-alanine:D-alanine ligase at 2.3 Å resolution. Science 1994; 266:439–443.

34. Benson TE, Filman DJ, Walsh CT, Hogle JM. An enzyme-substrate complex involved in bacterial cell wall biosynthesis. Nature Struct Biol 1995; 8:644–653.

35. Giegé R, Puglisi JD, Florentz C. tRNA structure and aminoacylation efficiency. Progr Nucl Acid Res 1993; 45:129–206.

36. Soffer RL. Aminoacyl-tRNA transferases. Adv Enzymol 1974; 40:91–139.

37. Kamiryo T, Matsuhashi M. The biosynthesis of the cross-linking peptides in the cell wall peptidoglycan of *Staphylococcus aureus*. J Biol Chem 1972; 247:6305–6311.

38. Heaton, MP, Neuhaus, FC. Role of the D-alanyl carrier protein in the biosynthesis of D-alanyl-lipoteichoic acid. J Bacteriol 1994; 176:681–690.

39. Perego M, Glaser P, Minutello A, Strauch MA, Leopold K, Fischer W. Incorporation of D-alanine into lipoteichoic acid and wall teichoic acid in *Bacillus subtilis*—identification of genes and regulation. J Biol Chem 1994; 270:15598–15606.

40. Cromwick AM, Gross RA. Investigation by NMR of metabolic routes to bacterial gamma-poly(glutamic acid) using C-13-labeled citrate and glutamate as media carbon sources. Can J Microbiol 1995; 41:902–909.

41. Birrer GA, Cromwick AM, Gross RA. Gamma-Poly(glutamic acid) formation by *Bacillus licheniformis* 9945a: Physiological and biochemical studies. Int J Biol 1994; 16:265–275.

42. Shoji S, Sakai H. Poly-L-lysine produced by Streptomycetes. III. Chemical studies. Agric Biol Chem 1981; 45:2503–2508.

43. Simon RD. The biosynthesis of multi-L-arginyl-poly(L-aspartic acid) in the filamentous bacterium *Anabaena cylindrica*. Biochim Biophys Acta 1976; 422:407–418.

44. von Döhren H, Kleinkauf H. Research on nonribosomal systems: Biosynthesis of peptide antibiotics. Kleinkauf H, von Döhren H, Jaenicke L, eds. The Roots of Modern Biochemistry: Fritz Lipmann's Squiggle and Its Consequences. Berlin: Walter de Gruyter 1988:355–367.

45. Lipmann F. Search for remnants of early evolution in present-day metabolism. Biosystems 1975; 6:234–238.

46. Kleinkauf H, von Döhren H. The nonribosomal peptide biosynthetic system—on the origins of structural diversity of peptides, cyclopeptides and related compounds. Antonie van Leeuwenhoek 1994; 67:229–242.

47. Weber G, Schorgendörfer K, Schneider-Scherzer E, Leitner E. The peptide synthetase catalyzing cyclosporine production in *Tolypocladium niveum* is endoded by a giant 45.8-kilobase open reading frame. Curr Genet 1994; 26:120–125.

48. Kleinkauf H, von Döhren H. Biosynthesis of cyclosporins and related peptides. Anke T, ed. Fungal Biotechnology. Chapman and Hall, Weinheim 1997.

49. Smith DJ, Burnham MKR, Bull JH, Hodgson JE, Ward JM, Browne P, Brown J, Barton B, Earl AJ, Turner G. β-Lactam biosynthetic genes have been conserved in clusters in prokaryotes and eukaryotes. EMBO J 1990; 9:741–747.

50. Kleinkauf H, van Liempt H, Palissa H, von Döhren H. Biosynthese von Peptiden: Ein nichtribosomales System. Naturwissenschaften 1992; 79:153–162.

51. Nozaki S, Muramatsu I. Natural homologs of gramicidin S. J Antibiot 1987; 37:689–690.

52. Thibault P, Faubert D, Karunanithy S, Boyd RK, Holmes CFB. Isolation, mass spectrometric characterization, and protein phosphatase inhibition properties of cyclic peptide analogs of gramicidin S from *Bacillus brevis* (Nagano strain). Biol Mass Spectrom 1992; 21:367–379.

53. Haring V. Diploma thesis, TU Berlin 1983.
54. Kleinkauf H, von Döhren H. A survey of enzymatic biosynthesis of peptide antibiotics. Trends in Antibiotic Research. Japan Antibiotics Res. Ass. 1982:220–232.
55. Baldwin JE, Shiau C-Y, Byford MF, Schofield CJ. Substrate specificity of L-δ-(α-aminoadipoyl)-L-cysteinyl-D-valine synthetase from *Cephalosporium acremonium*: Demonstration of the structure of several unnatural tripeptide products. Biochem J 1994; 301:367–372.
56. Pieper R, Kleinkauf H, Zocher R. Enniatin synthetases from different Fusaria exhibiting distinct amino acid specificities. J Antibiot 1992; 45:1273–1277.
57. Adefarati AA, Giacobbe RA, Hensens OD, Tkacz JS. Biosynthesis of L-671,329, an echinocandin-type antibiotic produced by *Zalerion arboricola*: Origins of some of the unusual amino acids and the dimethylmyristic acid side chain. J Am Chem Soc 1991; 113:3542–3545.
58. Okumura Y. Biosysthesis of viridogrisein. Kleinkauf H, von Döhren H, eds. Biochemistry of Peptide Antibiotics. Berlin: de Gruyter, 1990:365–378.
59. Cosmina P, Rodriguez F, de Ferra F, Grandi G, Perego M, Venema G, van Sinderen D. Sequence and analysis of the genetic locus responsible for surfactin synthesis in *Bacillus subtilis*. Mol Microbiol 1993; 8:821–831.
60. Pavela-Vrancic M, Pfeifer E, Freist W, von Döhren H. Nucleotide binding by multienzyme peptide synthetases. Eur J Biochem 1994; 220:535–542.
61. Toh H. N-terminal halves of gramicidin S synthetase 1, and tyrocidine synthetase 1 as novel members of the firefly luciferase family. Protein Sequ Data Anal 1990; 3:517–521.
62. Saito M, Hori K, Kurotsu T, Kanda M, Saito Y. Three conserved glycine residues in valine activation of gramicidin S synthetase 2 from *Bacillus brevis*. J Biochem 1994; 117:276–282.
63. Tokita K, Hori K, Kurotsu T, Kanda M, Saito Y. Effect of single base substitutions at glycine-870 codon of gramicidin S synthetase 2 gene on proline activation. J Biochem 1993; 114:522–527.
64. Gocht M, Marahiel MA. Analysis of core sequences in the D-Phe activating domain of the multifunctional peptide synthetase TycA by site directed mutagenesis. J Bacteriol 1994; 176:2654–2662.
65. Hamoen LW, Eshuis H, Jongbloed J, Venema G, van Sinderen D. A small gene, designated *ComS*, located within the coding region of the fourth amino acid–activation domain of *srfA*, is required for competence development in *Bacillus subtilis*. Mol Microbiol 1995; 15:55–63.
66. Pavela-Vrancic M, Pfeifer E, van Liempt H, Schäfer H-J, von Döhren H, Kleinkauf H. ATP binding in peptide synthetases: Determination of contact sites of the adenine moiety by photoaffinity labeling of tyrocidine synthetase 1 with 2-azidoadenosine triphosphate. Biochem 1994; 33:6276–6283.
67. Pavela-Vrancic M, Pfeifer E, Schröder W, von Döhren H, Kleinkauf H. Identification of the fluorescein 5′-isothiocyanate binding site in tyrocidine synthetase 1. J Biol Chem 1994; 269:14962–14966.
68. Conti E, Franks NP, Brick P. Crystal structure of firefly luciferase throws light on a superfamily of adenylate forming enzymes. Structure 1996; 4:287–298.
69. Dieckmann R, Lee Y-O, van Liempt H, von Döhren H, Kleinkauf H. Expression of an active adenylate-forming domain of peptide synthetases corresponding to acyl-CoA-synthetases. FEBS Lett 1995; 357:212–216.
70. Garrido S, Zaera E, Torrecilla A, Sillero A, Sillero MAG. Labeled adenosine(5′)tetraphospho(5′)adenosine (Ap(4)A) and adenosine(5′)tetraphospho(5′)nucleoside (Ap(4)N). Synthesis with firefly luciferase. J Biochem Biophys Meth 1995; 30:191–198.
71. Guranowski A, Sillero MAG, Sillero A. Adenosine 5′-tetraphosphate and adenosine 5′-pentaphosphate are synthesized by yeast acetyl coenzyme A synthetase. J Bacteriol 1994; 176:2986–2990.
72. Ortiz B, Sillero A, Sillero MAG. Specific synthesis of adenosine(5′)tetraphospho(5′)nucleoside and adenosine(5′)oligophospho(5′)adenosine (n > 4) catalyzed by firefly luciferase. Eur J Biochem 1993; 212:263–270.

73. Sillero MAG, Guranowski A, Sillero A. Synthesis of dinucleotide polyphosphates catalyzed by firefly luciferase. Eur J Biochem 1991; 202:507–513.

74. Lee PC, Bochner BR, Ames BN. ApppppA, heat shock stress, and cell oxidation. Proc Natl Acad Sci USA 1983; 80:7496–7500.

75. Stephens JC, Artz SW, Ames BN. Guanosine 5'-diphosphate 3'-diphosphate (ppGpp): Positive effector for histidine operon transcription and general signal for amino acid deficiency. Proc Natl Acad Sci USA 1975; 72:4389–4393.

76. Schlumbohm W, Stein T, Ullrich C, Vater J, Krause M, Marahiel MA, Kruft V, Wittmann-Liebold B. An active site serine is involved in covalent substrate amino acid binding at each reaction center of gramicidin S synthetase. J Biol Chem 1991; 266:23135–23141.

77. Stein T, Vater J, Kruft V, Wittmann-Liebold B, Franke P, Panico M, Dowell RM, Morris HR. Detection of 4'-phosphopantetheine at the thioester binding site for L-valine of gramicidin S synthetase 2. FEBS Lett 1994; 340:39–44.

78. Stein T, Kluge B, Vater J, Franke P, Otto A, Wittmann-Liebold B. Gramicidin S synthetase 1 (phenylalanine racemase), a prototype of amino acid racemases containing the cofactor 4'-phosphopantetheine. Biochem 1995; 34:4633–4642.

79. Stein T, Vater J. Amino acid activation and polymerization at modular multienzymes in nonribosomal peptide biosynthesis. Amino Acids 1996; 10:201–227.

80. Pfeifer E, Pavela-Vrancic M, von Döhren H, Kleinkauf H. Characterization of tyrocidine synthetase 1 (TY1): Requirement of post-translational modification for peptide biosynthesis. Biochem 1995; 34:7450–7459.

81. Kanda M, Hori K, Kurotsu T, Miura S, Yamada Y, Saito Y. Sulfhydryl groups related to the catalytic activity of gramicidin S synthetase 1 of *Bacillus brevis*. J Biochem 1981, 90:765–771.

82. Gadow A, Vater J, Schlumbohm W, Palacz Z, Salnikow J, Kleinkauf H. Gramicidin S synthetase: Stability of reactive thioester intermediates and formation of 3-amino-2-piperazine-dione. Eur J Biochem 1983, 132:229–234.

83. Schlumbohm W. Thesis, TU Berlin, 1990.

84. Hori K, Yamamoto Y, Minetoki T, Kurotsu T, Kanda M, Miura S, Okamura K, Furuyama J, Saito Y. Molecular cloning and nucleotide sequence of the gramicidin S synthetase 1 gene. J Biochem 1989; 106:639–645.

85. Vollenbroich D, Kluge B, D'Souza C, Zuber P, Vater J. Analysis of mutant amino acid–activating domain of surfactin synthetase bearing a serine-to-alanine substitution at the site of carboxylthioester formation. FEBS Lett 1993; 325:220–224.

86. Vollenbroich D, Mehta N, Zuber P, Vater J, Kamp RM. Analysis of surfactin synthetase subunits in Srfa mutants of Bacills subtilis Ole B 105. J Bacteriol 1994; 176:395–400.

87. Alberts AW, Vagelos PR. Acyl carrier protein. VIII. Studies of acyl carrier protein and coenzyme A in *Escherichia coli* pantothenate or β-alanine auxotrophs. J Biol Chem 1966; 241:5201–5204.

88. Tweto J, Liberati M, Larabee AR. Protein turnover and 4'-phosphopantetheine exchange in rat liver fatty acid synthetase. J Biol Chem 1971; 246:2468–2471.

89. Sohby C. Regulation of fatty acid synthetase activity. J Biol Chem 1979; 254:8561–8566.

90. Elhussein SA, Miernyk JA, Ohlrogge JB. Plant holo-(acyl carrier protein) synthase. Biochem J 1988; 252:39–45.

91. Fernandez MD, Lamppa GK. Acyl carrier protein import into chloroplasts. J Biol Chem 1991; 266:7220–7226.

92. Lambalot RH, Walsh CT. Cloning, overproduction, and characterization of the *Escherichia coli* holo-acyl carrier protein synthase. J Biol Chem 1995; 270:24658–24661.

93. Hori K, Kanda M, Kurotsu T, Miura S, Yamada Y, Saito Y. Absence of pantothenic acid in gramicidin S synthetase 2 obtained from some mutants of *Bacillus brevis*. J Biochem 1981; 90:439–447.

94. Stindl A, Keller U. Epimerization of the D-valine portion in the biosynthesis of actinomycin D. Biochem 1994; 33:9358–9364.

95. Schwecke T, Aharonowitz Y, Palissa H, von Döhren H, Kleinkauf H, van Liempt H. Enzymatic characterisation of the multifunctional enzyme δ-(L-α-aminoadipyl)-L-cysteinyl-D-valine synthetase from *Streptomyces clavuligerus*. Eur J Biochem 1992; 205:687–694.

96. Kallow W. Thesis, TU Berlin, 1996.

97. Kallow W, von Döhren H, Kennedy J, Turner G. Abstracts of the Third European Conference of Fungal Genetics. Münster, 1996:159.

98. Shiau C-Y, Baldwin JE, Byford MF, Schofield CJ. δ-L-(α-Aminoadipoyl)-L-cysteinyl-D-valine synthetase: Isolation of L-cysteinyl-D-valine, a shunt product, and implications for the order of peptide bond formation. FEBS Lett 1995; 375:303–306.

99. Shiau C-Y, Baldwin JE, Byford MF, Sobey WJ, Schofield CJ. δ-L-(α-Aminoadipoyl)-L-cysteinyl-D-valine synthetase: The order of peptide bond formation and the timing of the epimerization reaction. FEBS Lett 1995; 358:97–100.

100. de Crécy-Lagard V, Marliére P, Saurin W. Multienzymatic non ribosomal peptide biosynthesis: Identification of the functional domains catalysing peptide elongation and epimerization. C R Acad Sci Paris 1995; 318:927–936.

101. Billich A, Zocher R. N-methyltransferase function of the multifunctional enzyme enniatin synthetase. Biochem 1987; 26:8417–8423.

102. Billich A, Zocher R. Biosynthesis of N-methylated peptides. Kleinkauf H, von Döhren H, eds. Biochemistry of Peptide Antibiotics. Berlin: de Gruyter 1990, 57–80.

103. Pieper R, Haese A, Schröder W, Zocher R. Arrangement of catalytic sites in the multifunctional enzyme enniatin synthetase. Eur J Biochem 1995; 230:119–126.

104. Haese A, Schubert M, Herrmann M, Zocher R. Molecular characterization of the enniatin synthetase gene encoding a multifunctional enzyme catalysing N-methyl-depsipeptide formation in *Fusarium scirpi*. Mol Microbiol 1993; 7:905–914.

105. Keller U. Peptidolactones. Vining LC, Stuttard C, eds. Genetics and Biochemistry of Antibiotic Production, Boston: Butterworth-Heinemann 1995, 173–196.

106. Weßels P. Thesis, TU Berlin, 1995.

107. Komura S, Kurahashi K. Biosynthesis of polymyxin E by a cell-free enzyme system. IV. Acylation of enzyme bound L-2,4-diaminobutyric acid. J Biochem 1985; 97:1409–1417.

108. Menkhaus M. Thesis, TU Berlin, 1994.

109. Menkhaus M, Ullrich C, Kluge B, Vater J, Vollenbroich D, Kamp RM. Structural and functional organization of the surfactin biosynthetic multienzyme system. J Biol Chem 1993; 268:7678–7684.

110. Greenwood KT, Luke RKJ. Studies on the enzymatic synthesis of enterochelin in *Escherichia coli* K-12, *Salmonelle typhimurium* and *Klebsielle pneumoniae*. Physical association of enterochelin synthetase components in vitro. Biochim Biophys Acta 1980; 614:185–195.

111. Rusnack F, Sakaitani M, Drueckhammer D, Reichert J, Walsh CT. Biosynthesis of the *Escherichia coli* siderophore enterobactin—sequence of the *entF*-gene, expression and purification of EntF, and analysis of covalent phosphopantetheine. Biochem 1991; 30:2916–2927.

112. Reichert J, Sakaitani M, Walsh CT. Characterization of EntF as a serine-activating enzyme. Protein Sci 1992; 1:549–555.

113. Keller U, Kleinkauf H, Zocher R. 4-Methyl-3-hydroxy-anthranilic acid activating enzyme from actinomycin producing *Streptomyces chrysomallus*. Biochem 1984; 23:1479–1484.

114. Keller U, Schlumbohm W. Purification and characterization of actinomycin synthetase I, a 4-methyl-3-hydroxy-anthraniilic acid-AMP ligase from *Streptomyces chrysomallus*. J Biol Chem 1992, 267:11745–11752.

115. Schlumbohm W, Keller U. Chromophore activating enzyme involved in the biosynthesis of the mikamycin B antibiotic etamycin from *Streptomyces griseovirides*. J Biol Chem 1990; 265:2156–2161.

116. Glund K, Schlumbohm W, Bapat M, Keller U. Biosynthesis of quinoxaline antibiotics: Purification and characterization of the quinoxaline-2-carboxylic acid activating enzyme from *Streptomyces triostinus*. Biochem 1990; 29:3522–3527.

117. Smith TD, Priestley ND, Knaggs AR, Nguyen T, Floss HG. 3,4-Dimethylindole-2-carboxylate and 4-(1-hydroxyethyl)quinoline-2-carboxylate activating enzymes from the nosiheptide and thiostrepton producers, *Streptomyces actuosus* and *Streptomyces laurentii*. Chem Commun 1993; 1612–1614.

118. Strohl WR, Floss HG. Thiopeptides. Vining LC, Stuttard C, eds. Genetics and Biochemistry of Antibiotic Production. Boston: Butterworth-Heinemann 1995, 223–238.

119. Mazzola M, White FF. A mutation in the indole-3-acetic acid biosynthesis and syringomycin production. J Bacteriol 1994; 176:1374–1382.

120. Mo YY, Geibel M, Bansall RF, Gross DC. Analysis of sweet cherry (*Prunus avium* L) leaves for plant signal molecules that activate the *syrB* gene required for synthesis of the phytotoxin, syringomycin, by *Pseudomonas syringae* pv syringae. Plant Physiol 1995; 107:603–612.

121. Schirmbock M, Lorito M, Wang YL, Hayes CK, Avisan-Atac I, Scala F, Harman GE, Kubicek CP. Parallel formation and synergism of hydrolytic enzymes and peptaibol antibiotics, molecular mechanisms involved in the antagonistic action of *Trichoderma harzianum* against phytopathogenic fungi. Appl Environm Microbiol 1994; 60:4364–4370.

122. MacCabe AP, van Liempt H, Palissa H, Unkles SE, Riach MBR, Pfeifer E, von Döhren H, Kinghorn JR. δ-L-(α-Aminoadipoyl)-L-cysteinyl-D-valine synthetase from *Aspergillus nidulans*: Molecular characterization of the *acvA* gene encoding the first enzyme of the penicillin biosynthetic pathway. J Biol Chem 1991; 266:12646–12654.

123. Baldwin JE, Bird JU, Field RA, O'Callaghan NM, Schofield CJ, Willis AC. Isolation and partial characterization of ACV synthetase from *Cephalosporium acremonium* and *Streptomyces clavuligerus*. Evidence for the presence of phosphopantothenate in ACV synthetase. J Antibiot 1991; 44:241–248.

124. Ullrich C, Kluge B, Palacz Z, Vater J. Cell-free biosynthesis of surfactin, a cyclic lipopeptide produced by *Bacillus subtilis*. Biochem 1991; 30:6503–6508.

125. Galli G, Rodriguez F, Cosmina P, Pratesi C, Nogarotto R, de Ferra F, Grandi G. Characterization of the surfactin synthetase multienzyme complex. Biochim Biophys Acta 1994; 1205:19–28.

126. Scott-Craig JS, Panaccione DG, Pacard JA, Walton JD. The cyclic peptide synthetase catalysing HC toxin production in the filamentous fungus *Cochliobolus carbonum* is encoded by a 15.7 kilobase open reading frame. J Biol Chem 1992; 267:26044–26049.

127. Kopiez H. Thesis, TU Berlin, 1994.

128. Lück-Klatte B. Thesis, TU Berlin, 1994.

129. Kleinkauf H, von Döhren H. Links between polyketide and peptide forming enzyme systems. J Antibiot 1995; 48:563–567.

130. Takita T. Chemistry of bleomycin. Umezawa H, Takita T, Shiba T, eds. Bioactive Peptides Produced by Microorganisms. Halsted Press Kodansha Tokyo 1978:35–70.

131. Thiericke R, Rohr R. Biological variation of microbial metabolites by precursor-directed biosynthesis. Nat Prod Rep 1993; 10:263–289.

132. Lawen A, Traber R. Substrate specificities of cyclosporin synthetase and peptolide SDZ 214-103 synthetase. J Biol Chem 1993; 268:20452–20465.

133. Traber R, Kobel H, Loosli H-R, Senn H, Rosenwirth B, Lawen A. [Melle⁴]cyclosporin, a novel natural cyclosporin with anti-HIV activity: Structural elucidation, biosynthesis and biological properties. Antiviral Chem Chemother 1994; 5:331–339.

134. Kleinkauf H, von Döhren H. Cell-free biosynthesis of peptide antibiotics. Vezina C, Singh K, eds. Advances in Biotechnology, Vol. 3. Oxford: Pergamon Press, 1981:83–88.

135. Madry N, Zocher R, Kleinkauf H. Selective synthesis of depsipeptides by the immobilized multienzyme enniatin synthetase. Eur J Appl Microbiol Biotechnol 1983; 17:75–79.

136. Baltz RH, Hosted TJ. Molecular genetic methods for improving secondary metabolite production in actinomycetes. Trends Biotechnol 1996; 14:245–250.

137. Kennedy J. Thesis, University of Sheffield, 1995.

138. Kennedy J, Turner G. Abstracts of the Third Euruopean Conference on Fungal Genetics. Münster, 1996:160.

8

Comparative Genetics and Molecular Biology of β-Lactam Biosynthesis

Ashish S. Paradkar and Susan E. Jensen
University of Alberta, Edmonton, Alberta, Canada

Roy H. Mosher
University of Illinois at Springfield, Springfield, Illinois

I. INTRODUCTION

β-Lactam antibiotics have enjoyed a long history of use as chemotherapeutic agents, and even today, they account for more than 50% of all antibiotics prescribed worldwide. By targeting bacterial cell wall biosynthesis, they combine the desirable properties of low toxicity and very effective bactericidal activity. The widespread use of compounds such as penicillin G and ampicillin is also attributable to their cost-effectiveness as treatments for life-threatening diseases. The low cost of these agents is, in turn, a direct result of the tremendous increases in fermentation yields that have been achieved through years of strain improvement, fermentation optimization, and refinement of downstream processing. This chapter will not attempt to document the yield improvements that have occurred through these traditional means over the 50 years that β-lactam compounds have been in clinical use, as these subjects have been covered elsewhere (1,2). Nor will it examine the detailed biochemical and biophysical data that are beginning to explain the unique mechanisms of action of the various biosynthetic enzymes involved in the production of β-lactam compounds (3,4). Rather, it will focus on the current state of knowledge of the genetics and molecular biology of β-lactam antibiotic biosynthesis, building on similar reviews that have been published (5–7). In particular, emphasis will be placed on comparisons between the various producing species, both prokaryotic and eukaryotic.

II. GENES IN PENICILLIN/CEPHALOSPORIN BIOSYNTHESIS

The biosynthesis of the penicillin/cephalosporin group of antibiotics involves a common pathway, with certain core activities conserved among all producer microorganisms that have been examined so far. These producer species include a number of filamentous fungi, most notably members of the genera *Penicillium*, *Cephalosporium*, and *Aspergillus*, a number of actinomycetes including *Streptomyces* and *Nocardia* spp., and examples of other bacterial species such as *Flavobacterium* and *Lysobacter* spp. In every case, the pathway begins with the condensation of the three precursor amino acids, L-α-aminoadipate, L-cysteine, and L-valine, to form a tripeptide intermediate, δ-L-(α-aminoadipyl)-L-cysteinyl-D-valine (ACV). ACV is then converted to isopenicillin N, which is subsequently modified to give a variety of end products such as hydrophobic penicillins, cephalosporins, and cephamycins (Figure 1). Since cephamycins are just modified forms of cephalosporins, and arise from the same basic pathway, the term cephalosporin will be used throughout this chapter to include both cephalosporin and cephamycin compounds.

A. α-Aminoadipic Acid: A Common Precursor, but Different Biosynthetic Origins

A notable difference exists between fungal and bacterial β-lactam producer species with regard to the formation of α-aminoadipate, one of the three precursor amino acids of all penicillins and cephalosporins (Figure 2). This difference results from the separate pathways for lysine metabolism found in eukaryotes and prokaryotes. In eukaryotes, including fungal β-lactam-producing species, lysine is biosynthesized via a pathway in which α-aminoadipate occurs as an intermediate (8), and it can be drawn off for penicillin/cephalosporin biosynthesis (9). On the other hand, in prokaryotes, lysine is biosynthesized via a different route without the involvement of α-aminoadipate (10,11), and therefore, the prokaryotic β-lactam-producing species have evolved a different strategy to make α-aminoadipate. In *Streptomyces* spp. and *Nocardia lactamdurans*, α-aminoadipate is formed by the catabolism of lysine in a two-step process (12,13). In the first step, lysine is converted to 1-piperidine-6-carboxylate, catalyzed by the enzyme lysine ε-aminotransferase (LAT). Since LAT is present only in penicillin/cephalosporin-producing actinomycetes but is absent in nonproducers, and since the gene encoding this enzyme (*lat*) is clustered with other penicillin/cephalosporin biosynthetic genes in both *Streptomyces clavuligerus* (14,15) and *N. lactamdurans* (16), LAT is considered to be a part of the penicillin/cephalosporin biosynthetic pathway (Figure 2). In the second step, 1-piperidine-6-carboxylate is converted to α-aminoadipate by the putative enzyme piperidine-6-carboxylate dehydrogenase. Despite the recognition that such an enzyme activity must be involved, no data are available to document the presence of this activity. Similarly, although a number of penicillin/cephalosporin gene clusters from prokaryotic producer species have been partially or fully sequenced, no candidate genes that could encode a piperidine-6-carboxylate dehydrogenase have been discovered.

In fungi, although α-aminoadipate is available from the lysine biosynthetic pathway, it could also be obtained from a lysine catabolic pathway, similar to that found in the actinomycetes, and be channeled into penicillin biosynthesis. In keeping with this possibility, a lysine auxotroph of *Penicillium chrysogenum* with a block before α-aminoadipate formation was found to produce penicillin in a lysine-supplemented medium, and it showed LAT activity (17). Therefore, in fungi, in addition to the lysine biosynthetic pathway, lysine catabolism may also provide α-aminoadipate for penicillin biosynthesis; however, the relative contribution of each pathway is unclear.

B. Common Early Genes

The first two steps of the common penicillin/cephalosporin biosynthetic pathway bring about the condensation of the three precursor amino acids, α-aminoadipate, cysteine, and valine, to form the tripeptide ACV, and the subsequent cyclization of ACV to form

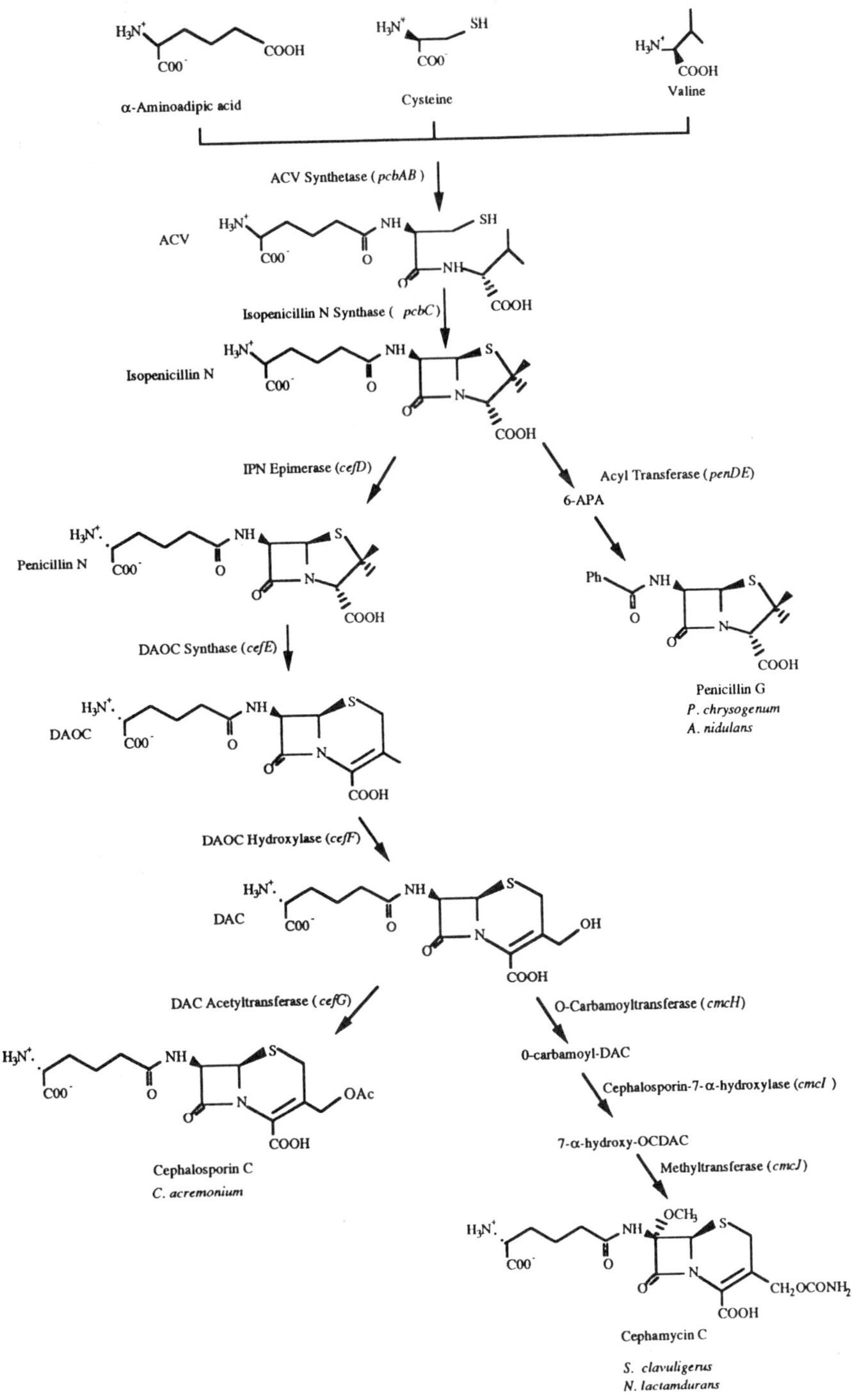

Figure 1   The common pathway for biosynthesis of penicillins, cephalosporins, and cephamycins in bacteria and fungi. Abbreviations: ACV, δ-(L-α-aminoadipyl)-L-cysteinyl-D-valine; IPN, isopenicillin N; 6-APA; 6-aminopenicillanic acid; DAC, deacetylcephalosporin C; DAOC, deacetoxycephalosporin C; OCDAC, o-carbamoyl-deacetoxycephalosporin C. The genes are indicated in parentheses.

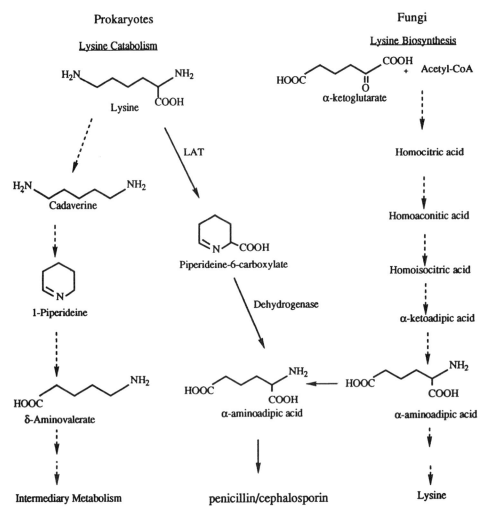

Figure 2   Lysine metabolism and its relationship to α-aminoadipic acid production in bacteria and fungi. Abbreviation: LAT, lysine ε-aminotransferase.

isopenicillin N, the first β-lactam intermediate in the pathway. These reactions are catalyzed by ACV synthetase and isopenicillin N synthase, respectively, and are invariably present in all prokaryotic and fungal producer species.

1.   ACV Synthetase (pcbAB)

The formation of ACV is mediated by a single, large (approximately 420 kDa) polypeptide, ACV synthetase (ACVS). The gene *pcb*AB, which encodes ACVS, has been completely sequenced from three separate fungal species, *P. chrysogenum* (18,19) *Cephalosporium acremonium* (20), and *Aspergillus nidulans* (21), and from one actinomycete, *N. lactamdurans* (22). Partial sequence information, including the 5′- and 3′-ends of the *pcb*AB gene, is also available from *S. clavuligerus* (15,23,24). The deduced amino acid sequences of all *pcb*AB genes studied to date share extensive sequence homology and show the presence of three repeated domains (25) (Figure 3). These three domains align

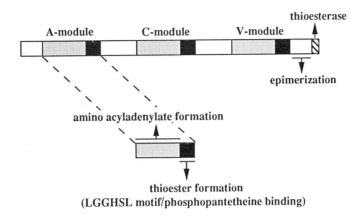

Figure 3   The modular organization of the ACVS polypeptide. Abbreviations: A, α-aminoadipate domain; C, cysteine domain; V, valine domain.

well with each other, and they also align with similar domains present in the gramicidin synthetase I and tyrocidine synthetase I subunits of the multi-subunit peptide synthetase complexes of *Bacillus brevis* (26,27). Therefore, ACV synthesis is thought to occur via a nonribosomal protein thiotemplate mechanism similar to that employed by peptide antibiotic synthetases in *Bacillus* (28). This mechanism typically involves a series of reactions in which the substrate amino acids are first activated as aminoacyl adenylates and then covalently bound to the thiol groups of phosphopantetheine cofactors by thioester linkages. Subsequently, the amino acids are linked to each other sequentially by transpeptidation, during which the phosphopantetheine cofactors transfer the activated amino acid or growing peptide chain from one active site to the next. By analogy with the *Bacillus* peptide synthetases, the three repeated domains are thought to represent modules containing the active sites for the adenosine 5′-triphosphate (ATP)-mediated activation of α-aminoadipate, L-cysteine, and L-valine, in that order (Figure 3). The valine domain also contains an additional region, responsible for the epimerization of L-valine to D-valine. As observed with other peptide synthetases, each domain shows a highly conserved phosphopantetheine binding motif toward the carboxy-terminal end, and this motif includes a conserved serine residue associated with phosphopantetheine binding. A fourth domain, found toward the carboxy-terminal end of the ACVS polypeptide, resembles the thioesterase protein of the gramicidin synthetase complex, and also thioesterases of fatty acid synthetases. This fourth domain may therefore be involved in the release of the final peptide product from the enzyme active site. Thus, ACVS is mechanistically very similar to other peptide synthetases from *Bacillus*. However, unlike the multi-subunit organization of these *Bacillus* peptide synthetases, all of the enzyme functions involved in ACVS activity, namely, activation, epimerization, and polymerization, are contained within different domains of one large polypeptide. In this respect, ACVS more closely resembles fungal peptide synthetases such as cyclosporin synthetase (29), and the smaller size of ACVS (420 compared with 1400 kDa) makes it an attractive system in which to study this single multifunctional polypeptide type of nonribosomal peptide synthesis.

2.   Isopenicillin N Synthase (pcbC)

The tripeptide ACV is cyclized to form isopenicillin N, the first β-lactam-containing intermediate in the pathway, by isopenicillin N synthase (IPNS). The gene encoding

IPNS, *pcb*C, has been cloned and sequenced from a variety of bacterial and fungal sources (22,30–35). As with *pcb*AB, *pcb*C sequences from different sources show extensive similarity at both the nucleotide and deduced amino acid sequence level. However, identification of residues important for catalysis has not been possible because the similarities between the deduced protein sequences from the different *pcb*C genes extend throughout the entire protein, and the sequences show little similarity to any other known proteins. IPNS activity requires molecular oxygen and iron, and it is stimulated by the presence of ascorbate. Since this activity is almost completely inhibited in presence of chemical reagents that modify cysteine residues covalently (3), much attention was focused initially on the presence and function of the different cysteine residues. All fungal IPNS proteins that have been examined so far, namely, from *C. acremonium* (36), *P. chrysogenum* (37,38), and *A. nidulans* (39) contain two cysteine residues at positions 106 and 255 (with respect to the *C. acremonium* sequence; Figure 4). However, replacement of Cys-106 by a serine residue in the *C. acremonium* IPNS by site-directed mutagenesis of the *pcb*C gene resulted in the loss of 97% of the activity, whereas a similar replacement at the 255 position decreased activity by only 50% (40). Since neither replacement completely abolished activity, both Cys residues were concluded to be important, but not essential for activity, and since the replacement at Cys-106 caused a greater detrimental effect, Cys-106 was more important than Cys-255. The importance of Cys-106 was again exemplified by the conservation of this residue in all prokaryotic IPNS enzymes, along with a stretch of eight amino acids around Cys-106 that are either identical or highly conserved in all prokaryotic and fungal IPNS enzymes (Figure 4) (30). Cys-255 is also highly conserved among all IPNS enzymes examined so far, with the exception of *N. lactamdurans*, which contains the Cys-106 but has an Ala-255 residue in place of Cys-255 (22). Replacement of Cys-106 and Cys-255 by serine residues in the *S. clavuligerus* IPNS led to decreases in activity of 96 and 47%, respectively, similar to that seen with *C. acremonium* IPNS, again suggesting the relative importance of Cys-106 over Cys-255 (41).

It was originally thought that Cys-106 might be involved in substrate binding, whereas Cys-255 could be important for stabilization of the protein (42). However, spectroscopic analyses of wild-type and mutant forms of *C. acremonium* IPNS in the presence of ACV, iron, and nitrous oxide, an oxygen analog, suggested that the cysteine residues of the enzyme do not interact covalently with the cysteine group of ACV, nor do they coordinate with the iron; rather, they facilitate the binding of ACV to the active site of the enzyme (43,44). Recently, a model has been proposed for the active site of IPNS in which it is suggested that a reactive iron atom coordinates with six ligands in an octahedral symmetry (45). In this model, four of these endogenous ligands are provided by three histidine residues and one aspartate residue, and the remaining two exogenous ligands are provided by ACV and oxygen (45). The energy from these interactions is subsequently used to remove four protons from ACV and form the β-lactam and thiozolidine rings, resulting in the formation of isopenicillin N. More recently, the crystal structure of the Mn^{2+}-IPNS from *A. nidulans* has been elucidated (46), which has revealed that the four endogenous ligands involved in binding the metal ion are His-214, Asp-216, His-270, and Gln-330 (Figure 5). Indeed, both His-214 and His-270 are highly conserved in all IPNS enzymes (Figure 4), and site-directed mutagenesis of both histidine residues, individually, resulted in a total loss of the enzyme activity in *C. acremonium* (47). Since mutagenesis of other well-conserved histidine residues had a less detrimental effect on the enzyme activity, the involvement of only two histidine ligands, His-214 and His-270, in the iron-containing active site seems more likely than the three histidine residues pro-

```
1                                                      50
MGS..VSKAN VPKIDVSP.L FGDDQAAKMR VAQQIDAASR DTGFFYAVNH    A. nidulans
MAS..TPKAN VPKIDVSP.L FGDNMEEKMK VARAIDAASR DTGFFYAVNH    P. chrysogenum
MGSVPVPVAN VPRIDVSP.L FGDDKEKKLE IAARIDRACR DTGFFYAVNH    C. acremonium
....MRNHAD VPVIDISG.L SGNDMDVKKD IAARIDRACR GSGFFYAANH    Flavobacterium sp.
....MRNHAD VPVIDISG.L SGNDMDVKKD IAARIDRACR GSGFFYAANH    L. lactamgenus
.MPVLMPSAH VPTIDISP.L FGTDAAAKKR VAEEIHGACR GSGFFYATNH    S. clavuligerus
.MPILMPSAE VPTIDISP.L SGDDAKAKQR VAQEINKAAR GSGFFYASNH    S. jumonjinensis
..MKMPSAE  VPTIDVSP.L SGGDAQEKVR VGQEINKACR GSGFFYAANH    N. lactamdurans
.MPIPMLPAH VPTIDISP.L SGGDADDKKR VAQEINKACR ESGFFYASHH    S. griseus
.MPVLMPSAD VPTIDISP.L FGTDPDAKAH VARQINEACR GSGFFYASHH    S. lipmanii
.MPVLMPSAD VPTIDISPQL FGTDPTPRRT SRGRSTRPAR GSGFFYASHH    S. cattleya
```

```
51            *                                        100
GINVQRLSQK TKEFHMSITP EEKWDLAIRA YNKEHQDQVR AGYYLSIPGK
GVDVKRLSNK TREFHSITTD EEKWDLAIRA YNKEHQDQIR AGYYLSIPEK
GVDLPWLSRE TNKFHMSITD EEKWQLAIRA YNKEHESOIR AGYYLPIPGK
GVDLAALQKF TTDWHMAMSA EEKWELAIRA YNPAN.PRNR NGYYMAVEGK
GVDLAALQKF TTDWHMAMSP EEKWELAIRA YNPAN.PRNR NGYYMAVEGK
GVDVQQLQDV VNEFHGAMTD QEKHDLAIHA YNPDN.PHVR NGYYKAVPGR
GVDVQLLQDV VNEFHRNMSD QEKHDLAIHA YNKDN.PHVR NGYYKAIKGK
GVDVQRLQDV VNEFHRTMSP QEKYDLAIHA YNKNN.SHVR NGYYMAIEGK
GIDVRRLQDV VNEFHRTMTD EEKYDLAIHA YNKNN.PRTR NGYYMAVKGK
GIDVLLKDV  VNEFHRTMTD QEKHDLAIHA YNENN.SHVR NGYYMARPGR
GIDVRRLQTW SNES.TTMTD QRSTTWRSTR YNENN.SHVR NGYYMARPGR
```

```
101  *                                                 150
KAVESFCYLN PNFTPDHPRI QAKTPTHEVN VWPDETKHPG FQDFAEQYYW
KAVESFCYLN PNFKPDHPLI QSKTPTHEVN VWPDEKEQYW FREFAEQYYW
KANESFCYLN PSFSPDHPRI KEPTPMHEVN IWPDEAKHPG FRAFAEKYYW
KANESFCYLN PSFDADHATI KAGLPSHEVN IWPDEARHPG MRRFYEAYFS
KAVESFCYLN PSFDADHATI KAGLPSHEVN IWPDEARHPG MRRFYEAYFS
KAVESFCYLN PDFGEDHPMI AAGTPMHEVN LWPDEERHPR FRPFCEGYYR
KAVESFCYLN PSFSDDHPMI KSETPMHEVN LWPDEEKHPR FRPFCEEYYW
KAVESFCYLN PSFSEDHPEI KAGTPMHEVN SWPDEEKHPS FRPFCEEYYR
KAVESWCYLN PSFSEDHPQI RSGTPMHEGN IWPDEKRHQR FRPFCEQYYR
KTVESWCYLN PSFGEDHPMI KAGTPMHEVN VWPDERHPD FRSFGEQYYR
ETVESWCYLN PSFGEDHPMM KAGTPMHEVN VWPDEERHPD FGSFGEQYHR
```

```
151  *                                                 200
DVFGLSSA.L LKRGYALALGK EENFFARHFK PDDTLASVVL .IRYPYLDPY
DVFGLSSA.L LRGYALALGK EEDFFSRHFK KEDALSSVVL .IRYPYLNPI
DVFGLSSA.V LRGYALALGK DEDFFTHRSR RDTTLSSSVVL .IRYPYLDPY
DVFDVAAV.I LRGFAIALGR EESFFERHFS MDDTLSAVSL .IRYPFLENY
DVFDVAAV.I LRGFAIALGR EESFFERHFS MDDTLSAVSL .IRYPFLENY
QMLKLSTV.1 MRGLALALGR PEHFFDAALA EQDSLSSVSL .IRYPFLEEY
QLLRLSTV.I MRGYALALGR REDFFDEALA EADTLSSVSL .IRYPYLEEY
TMHRLSKV.L MRGFALALGK DERFFPEALK EADTLSSVSL .IHYPYLEDY
DVFSLSKV.L MRGFALALGK PEDFFDASLS LADTLSAVTL .IRYPYLEDY
EVFRLSKVFL LRGFALALGK PEEFFENEVT EEDTLSCRSL MIRYPYLDPY
EVSASRRCC. .CGASRWRRQ AGESSSNEVT EEDTLSAVSM .IRYPYLDPY
```

```
201  #          #                                      250
PEAAIKTAAD GTKLSFEWHE DVSLITVLYQ SNVQNLQVET AAGYQDIEAD
PPAAIKTADD GTKLSFEWHE DVSLITVLYQ SDVANLQVEM PQGYLDIEAD
PEPAIKTADD GEKLSFEHHQ DVSLITVLYQ SDVQNLQVKT PQGWQDIQAD
P..PLKLGPD GEKLSFEHHQ DVSLITVLYQ TAIPNLQVET AEGYLDIPVS
P..PLKLGPD GQLLSFEDHL DVSMITVLFQ TQVQNLQVET VDGWRDIPTS
P..PVKTGPD GTKLSFEDHL DVSMITVLFQ TQVQNLQVET VDGWQDIPRS
P..PVKTGPD GEKLSFEDHF DVSMITVLYQ TEVQNLQVET VDGWRDLPTS
P..PVKTGPD GTKLSFEDHL DVSMITVLFQ TEVQNLQVET ADGWDLPTS
P..PVKTGPD GTKLSFEDHL DVSMITVLFQ TEVQNLQVET VDGWQSLPTS
PEAAIKTGPD GTRLSFEDHL DVSMITVLFQ TEVQNLQVET VDGWQSLPTS
PEAAIKTGPD GTRLSFEDHL DVSMITVLSK TEVQNLQVET VDGWQSLPTS
```

```
251     *                      *                       300
DTGYLINCGS YMAHLTNNYY KAPIHRVKWV NAERQSLPFF VNLGYDSVID
DNAYLVNCGS YMAHITNNYY PAPIHRVKWV NEERQSLPFF VNLGFNDTVQ
DTGFLINCGS YMAHITDDYY PAPIHRVKWV NEERQSLPFF VNLGWEDTIQ
DEHFLVNCGT YMAHITNGY  PAPVHRVKYI NAERLSIPFF ANLSHASAID
DEHFLVNCGT YMAHITNGY  PAPVHRVKYI NAERLSIPFF ANLSHASAID
ENDFLVNCGT YMAHVTNDYF PAPNHRVKFV NAERLSLPFF LNGHEAVIE
DEDFLVNCGT YMGHITHDYF PAPNHRVKFI NAERLSLPFF LNAGNSVIE
DTDFLVNAGT YLGHLTNDYF PSPLHRVKFV NAERLSLPFF FHAGQHTLIE
GENFLINCGT YMGYLTNDYF PAPNHRVKFI NAERLSLPFF LHAGHTTVME
GENFLINCGT YLGYLTNDYF PAPNHRVKYV NAERLSLPFF LHAGQNSVMK
GENFLINCGT YLGYLTNDYF PAPNHRVKYV NAERLSLPFF LHAGQNSVMK
```

```
301        #                            341
PFDPREP... .NGKSDREP  LSYGVDYLQNG LVSLINKNGQ T
PWDPSKE... .DGKTDQRP  ISYGVDYLQNG LVSLINKNGQ T
PWDPATAKDG AKDAAKDKPA ISYGEYLOGG  LRGLLINKNGQ T
PFAP.PP... YAPAGNPT   VSYGDYLQHG  LLDLIRANGQ T
PFAP.PP... YAPARGNPT  VSYGDYLQHG  LLDLIRANGQ T
PFVPEGA... SEEVR.NEA  LSYGDYLQHG  LRALIVKNGQ T
PFVPEGA... AGTVK.NPT  TSYGEYLQHG  LRALIVKNGQ T
PFFPDGA... PEGKQGNEA  VRYGDYLNHG  LHSLIVKNGQ T
PFSPEDT... RG.KELNPP  VRYGDYLQQA  SNALIAKNGQ T
PFHPEDT... .GDRKLNPA  VTYGEYLQEG  FHALIAKNVQ T
PFTRRT.... .GDRKLNPA  VTYGEYLQBG  FTR...... T
```

Figure 4 A multiple alignment of the derived IPNS amino acid sequences from 11 β-lactam-producing microorganisms. This alignment was constructed using PILEUP and PRETTY programs from the Wisconsin Package Version 8.1 (Genetics Computer Group, Madison, Wisconsin). The GenBank or SWISSPROT accession number for each of the sequences is as follows: *Aspergillus nidulans* (M21882); *Penicillium chrysogenum* (P08703); *Cephalosporium acremonium* (P05189); *Flavobacter acremonium* (P05189); *Flavobacterium sp.* (P16020); *Lysobacter lactamgenus* (X56660); *Streptomyces clavuligerus* (P10621); *Streptomyces jumonjinensis* (P18286); *Nocardia lactamdurans* (P27744); *Streptomyces lipmanii* (M22081); *Streptomyces cattleya* (D78166); *Streptomyces griseus* (X54609). Please note that because gaps have been introduced into the alignment at various places, the numbering of amino acid residues in the figure differs from that used in the body of the chapter, where the numbering conforms to that used for the *C. acremonium* IPNS. Proposed active-site metal-binding amino acids have been marked with a #; other residues that may be found in the active site have been marked with a *.

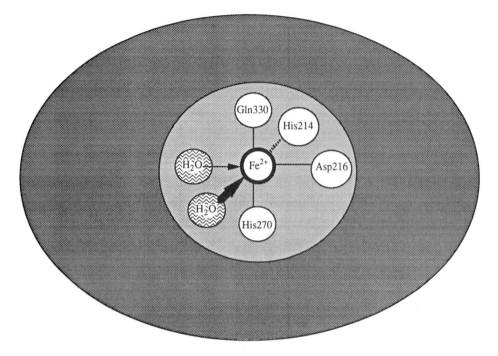

Figure 5   A schematic diagram of the *A. nidulans* IPNS active-site structure, adapted from that proposed by Roach et al. (46), depicting the amino acid residues involved in the coordination of divalent iron.

posed earlier. Similarly, Gln-330 is also conserved in all IPNS enzymes except that of *N. lactamdurans*, where Asn-330 is present instead (Figure 4).

Another residue of demonstrated importance for catalysis is Pro-285, since a change to leucine in a *C. acremonium* spontaneous mutant resulted in a total loss of activity (48). Moreover, this residue is invariably present in all of the prokaryotic and fungal genes (Figure 4). However, the precise role of this proline residue in the IPNS reaction is not clear at present.

C.   Late Genes in the Biosynthesis of Hydrophobic Penicillins

Isopenicillin N can be considered a branch point intermediate in the penicillin/cephalosporin pathway, and its conversion to a variety of hydrophobic penicillins, for example, penicillin G, represents the final step in the penicillin-forming branch of the pathway. This reaction is found only in penicillin-producing fungi such as *P. chrysogenum* and *A. nidulans*, and it is absent in cephalosporin-producing fungi and prokaryotes (3). It is still unclear whether the conversion involves a one- or a two-step process. Either the α-aminoadipate moiety of isopenicillin N is exchanged in a single step with one of a variety of substituted acetic acid derivatives that are present intracellularly as CoA derivatives, or alternatively, the α-aminoadipate moiety is first removed by an amidohydrolase to form 6-aminopenicillanic acid (6-APA) followed by reaction with a CoA derivative to form the corresponding penicillin (49). The enzyme catalyzing this reaction, acyl-CoA-isopenicillin acyltransferase (ACT), exists as a heterodimer consisting of two subunits of 29 and 11 kDa (50,51). ACT is a multifunctional enzyme that contains acyl-CoA-isopenicillin N acyltransferase (IAT), acyl-CoA:6-APA acyltransferase (AAT), and isopenicillin N amidohydrolase and penicillin amidase activities. Both of the subunits are derived from a 40 kDa preprotein by a posttranslational processing mechanism and are encoded by a single gene, *penDE*, which has been cloned and sequenced from two fungal β-lactam producers (51–53). The genes from both *P. chrysogenum* and *A. nidulans* show a high degree of similarity, and unlike the other early pathway genes, both contain three introns at the same relative positions. The significance of these introns will be discussed later. The sequences encoding the 11 kDa subunit precede those that encode the 29 kDa subunit, with the processing site present between Gly-102 and Cys-103 (54,55). It is likely that the processing involves an autocatalytic mechanism, since the 29 kDa protein was detected in an in vitro transcription/translation system using the entire cloned *penDE* gene (56). Expression of the *penDE* gene and its various derivatives in an *Escherichia coli* expression system has suggested that formation of an active ACT requires a cooperative interaction between the two polypeptides during their synthesis and folding. AAT activity was observed only when the two polypeptides were synthesized either from an intact *penDE* gene, or from the separately cloned *penD and penE* regions encoding the 11 and 29 kDa subunits coexpressed from two different plasmids (56). Activity was not observed in expression systems encoding the individual subunits, nor was activity recovered upon mixing of these extracts. Therefore, the subunit interaction is necessary for the proper synthesis of ACT and its enzyme activity.

Cloning and sequencing of *penDE* genes from various nonproducing mutants of *P. chrysogenum* that lacked IAT activity identified two point mutations in the region corresponding to the 29 kDa subunit (57). The Gly-150 → Val mutation is located in a region that is highly conserved in both *P. chrysogenum* and *A. nidulans* genes, whereas the Glu-258 → Lys mutation was in a less conserved region. Notably, since these mutants also lacked amidohydrolase activity, the residues Gly-150 and Glu-258 have been implicated as part of an active site that is shared by other enzyme activities associated with ACT. Recently, a sequence of amino acids in the ACT protein from *P. chrysogenum* and *A. nidulans* was identified that shows a weak similarity to sequences in other pathway enzymes, including deacetoxycephalosporin C synthase (DAOCS) and deacetylcephalosporin C synthase (DACS) from *S. clavuligerus*, DAOCS/DACS from *C. acremonium*, and IPNS from *S. clavuligerus*, *Streptomyces lipmanii*, *C. acremonium*, and *Flavobacterium* sp. (58). In all of the aforementioned enzymes, the residues Ser-227, Gln-234, and Asn-239 (relative to the *P. chrysogenum* ACT protein) are highly conserved. Because all of these enzymes bind β-lactam ring-containing substrates, these conserved residues may be necessary for substrate recognition. Site-directed mutagenesis of Ser-227 to Ala abolished IAT and AAT activities and also the processing of the 40 kDa proenzyme, suggesting a role for Ser-227 in substrate binding and processing (58). Similarly, mutation of Ser-309 to Ala abolished both IAT and AAT activities but not processing, thus implicating Ser-309 in the catalytic mechanism.

D.   Common Genes in the Cephalosporin Pathway

Channeling of the branch point intermediate isopenicillin N into the cephalosporin pathway requires several enzymatic activities that are found only in cephalosporin-producing fungi (e.g., *C. acremonium*) and prokaryotes (e.g., *Streptomyces*, *N. lactamdurans*, *Lysobacter lactamgenes*, and *Flavobacterium* spp.) but are absent in the penicillin-producing fungi.

1. Isopenicillin N Epimerase (cefD)

In the first reaction that commits an organism to cephalosporin formation, isopenicillin N is epimerized to penicillin N. The epimerization is carried out by isopenicillin N epimerase, encoded by *cef*D gene. Although isopenicillin N epimerase activity has been demonstrated in *C. acremonium* (59), the extreme lability of the fungal enzyme has precluded further purification of the enzyme and cloning of the corresponding gene. However, the prokaryotic counterpart of this enzyme shows greater stability and has been purified from *S. clavuligerus* (60,61) and *N. lactamdurans* (62), and the corresponding genes have been cloned, sequenced, and expressed in *E. coli* and *Streptomyces lividans*, respectively (63,64). The purified enzyme contains one molecule of pyridoxal-5'-phosphate per molecule of the enzyme, a cofactor commonly associated with epimerase/racemase activities. A consensus pyridoxal-phosphate-binding sequence SXHKXL has been identified in the genes from both organisms (64). The sequence is part of an identical stretch of 21 amino acids and may be important for catalysis. Recently, the *cef*D gene has also been identified in *L. lactamgenes* and expressed in *E. coli* (35).

2. DAOCS–DACS (cefE–cefF)

The next reaction in the pathway is an important step in cephalosporin biosynthesis since it involves the expansion of the five-membered thiazolidine ring of penicillin N into the six-membered dihydrothiazine ring, characteristic of all cephalosporins. The ring-expanding reaction is catalyzed by deacetoxycephalosporin C synthase (DAOCS), encoded by *cef*E, and results in the formation of deacetoxycephalosporin C (DAOC, Figure 1). Subsequent hydroxylation of deacetoxycephalosporin C by the enzyme deacetyl-cephalosporin C synthase (DACS), encoded by *cef*F, gives deacetylcephalosporin C (DAC). Both enzyme activities were demonstrable in *C. acremonium*; however, the activities could not be separated from each other by a variety of purification schemes (65,66). Furthermore, the identical substrate requirements of both enzymes, which include molecular oxygen, iron, and α-ketoglutarate, led to the proposal that both DAOCS and DACS were encoded by a single bifunctional protein. The cloning of the corresponding gene, and its expression in *E. coli*, confirmed that, in *C. acremonium*, DAOCS and DACS activities reside on a single polypeptide encoded by *cef*EF (67). In contrast, both DAOCS and DACS activities were clearly separable from each other in *S. clavuligerus*, although the purified DAOCS showed a weak DACS activity and DACS exhibited a low DAOCS activity (68). Moreover, the *S. clavuligerus* genes encoding these activities, *cef*E and *cef*F, have been cloned and mapped close to, but separate from, each other (69,70). Thus, the presence of two separate enzymes in *S. clavuligerus*, versus a single bifunctional enzyme in *C. acremonium*, is a major point of difference in the cephalosporin pathways present in the prokaryotic and the eukaryotic organisms. Separate genes for *cef*E and *cef*F have also been identified in *N. lactamdurans* (71), and the same situation is suspected for *L. lactamgenes*, where *cef*E showed DAOCS activity when expressed in *E. coli* but lacked detectable DACS activity (35). The prokaryotic *cef*E and *cef*F genes are very similar to one another and to the fungal *cef*EF gene, although the latter has an extension of 20 codons at the 3'-end of the gene (7).

The deduced protein sequences of *cef*E, *cef*F, and *cef*EF genes from both sources show a weak but significant similarity to IPNS, possibly a reflection of the fact that all of these enzymes require molecular oxygen and iron for activity (67). Interestingly, the strongest similarity to the IPNS sequence is present around Cys-106, a residue known to

be important for IPNS activity. This similarity suggests that *cef*EF sequences corresponding to those around Cys-106 in IPNS could also be important for DAOCS/DACS activity, even though Cys-106 is no longer believed to be directly involved in substrate binding in the IPNS reaction.

E. Late Genes in Cephalosporin C Biosynthesis

DAC is the branch point intermediate where the cephamycin and cephalosporin pathways diverge (Figure 1). In the last step of the cephalosporin biosynthetic pathway, which
is seen in some actinomycetes but most notably in the fungus C. *acremonium*, DAC is
acetylated to form cephalosporin C in a reaction catalyzed by DAC acetyltransferase
(DACAT). DACAT is encoded by *cef*G, which has been cloned and sequenced from C.
acremonium (72). The gene has two introns and shows high similarity to other eukaryotic
acetyltransferases, notably homoserine-o-acetyltransferases involved in methionine
biosynthesis. Among prokaryotes, although S. *clavuligerus* and S. *lipmanii* are known to
produce 7-α-methoxycephalosporin C (73), there have been no reports of a DACAT
enzyme, nor has the corresponding gene been located in these organisms.

As another option, DAC can be converted to cephabacins in L. *lactamgenes*.
Cephabacins are cephalosporins that contain a 7-formylamino substituent and an
oligopeptide side chain at the C3 position of the molecule, and because of this structure
they possess remarkable stability against β-lactamases (74). However, there is no further
information about the late enzymes or genes involved in the conversion of DAC to
cephabacins.

F. Late Genes in Cephamycin C Biosynthesis

The production of cephamycins has been observed only in actinomycetes, and not in
fungi. Actinomycetes, including S. *clavuligerus*, N. *lactamdurans*, and *Streptomyces cattleya*, have the ability to convert DAC to cephamycin C via several "late" steps of the
pathway (Figure 1). These reactions include o-carbamoylation at C3 of DAC, followed
by hydroxylation and methylation at C7. The carbamoylation is carried out by carbamoyltransferase (OCT), which requires ATP, Mn^{2+}, and Mg^{2+}, as well as carbamoyl
phosphate, and has been partially characterized from both S. *clavuligerus* (75) and N. *lactamdurans* (76). The gene encoding OCT, *cmc*H, has been identified within the
cephamycin biosynthetic gene clusters of S. *clavuligerus* and N. *lactamdurans* (76).

The hydroxylation at C7 is mediated by the enzyme cephalosporin 7-α-hydroxylase,
which has been purified from S. *clavuligerus* (77) and partially characterized from N. *lactamdurans* (78). The corresponding *cmc*I genes have been identified from both organisms
and expressed in S. *lividans* (78,79). The subsequent methylation at C7 is catalyzed by a
methyltransferase, and the gene *cmc*J encoding this activity has been identified in the N.
lactamdurans gene cluster (78). Although some *Streptomyces* spp. also produce cephamycins
A and B (80), which differ from cephamycin C in the nature of the substituent groups at
C3, the reactions involved in their biosynthesis have not been investigated.

G. Other Accessory Genes

Since penicillins and cephalosporins are antibiotics that inhibit biosynthesis and assembly of the peptidoglycan-containing cell walls present in prokaryotes (81), it is imperative for the prokaryotic penicillin/cephalosporin producers to possess a mechanism for

self-protection. In prokaryotes, genes encoding self-resistance functions are typically clustered together with the biosynthetic genes involved in formation of any particular antibiotic (82). On the other hand, since eukaryotic cell walls do not contain peptidoglycan, fungal penicillin/cephalosporin producers may be naturally resistant to these antibiotics and not need a resistance gene. It has been noted previously that most species of *Streptomyces*, including both penicillin/cephalosporin producers and nonproducers, are intrinsically resistant to moderate to high levels of penicillin (83). Both β-lactamases (84) and atypical penicillin-binding protein (PBP) profiles have been detected in some nonproducing species (85,86), which may explain their tolerance to β-lactam antibiotics. The existence of similar resistance mechanisms in at least some penicillin/cephalosporin-producing species is also evident from the recent identification of the genes *cmc*PBP and *cmc*Bla, encoding a PBP and a β-lactamase, respectively, within the gene cluster of *N. lactamdurans* (87). The deduced protein sequence of these genes shows significant similarity to corresponding penicillin-interacting proteins from the nonproducing *Streptomyces* species. Similarly, a β-lactamase gene has been recently identified in the cephalosporin cluster of *L. lactamgenes* (35). In *S. clavuligerus*, PBPs with very low affinities for β-lactams have been detected (86), but attempts to detect a β-lactamase activity have yet to be successful. However, the lack of detection of a β-lactamase activity must be viewed with caution, because this organism produces two kinds of β-lactamase inhibitors, clavulanic acid (88) and β-lactamase inhibitor protein (BLIP) (89), which might preclude detection of such an activity. The counterparts of the *N. lactamdurans* *cmc*PBP and *cmc*Bla genes have not yet been identified in *S. clavuligerus*. Nonetheless, a gene, *pcb*R, has been found immediately downstream of the *pcb*C gene in *S. clavuligerus*, which encodes a putative protein showing no similarity to the protein encoded by *cmc*PBP of *N. lactamdurans*; instead, it shows a significant similarity to the members of the high-molecular-weight class B PBPs from other bacteria. The highest similarity observed is to the low-affinity PBPs, PBP3r and PBP5, from *Enterococcus hirae* (90; Paradkar AS, Aidoo KA, and Jensen SE, unpublished observations). The 58 kDa PcbR protein showed in vitro penicillin-binding activity in the presence of high penicillin concentrations, whereas gene disruption of *pcb*R was only possible in an antibiotic nonproducing strain of *S. clavuligerus* and resulted in penicillin sensitivity (Paradkar AS, Aidoo KA, and Jensen SE, unpublished observations). These results have suggested that *pcb*R encodes a low-affinity PBP responsible at least in part for the self-resistance mechanism associated with penicillin/cephalosporin production in *S. clavuligerus*.

Besides resistance genes, antibiotic biosynthetic gene clusters may also contain genes encoding transport/export proteins that ensure proper secretion of the antibiotic molecule (91). In *N. lactamdurans*, a gene, *cmc*T, has been identified in the penicillin/cephalosporin gene cluster that encodes a potential transmembrane protein possibly involved in export of the antibiotics (87).

III. MOLECULAR ARCHITECTURE AND EVOLUTION OF PENICILLIN/CEPHALOSPORIN BIOSYNTHETIC GENES

Classical genetic mapping and molecular cloning studies have revealed that antibiotic biosynthesis and resistance genes are invariably clustered on the chromosomes of *Streptomyces* and other actinomycetes (92,93). In keeping with this general rule, the penicillin/cephalosporin biosynthetic genes from all bacterial species studied to date have

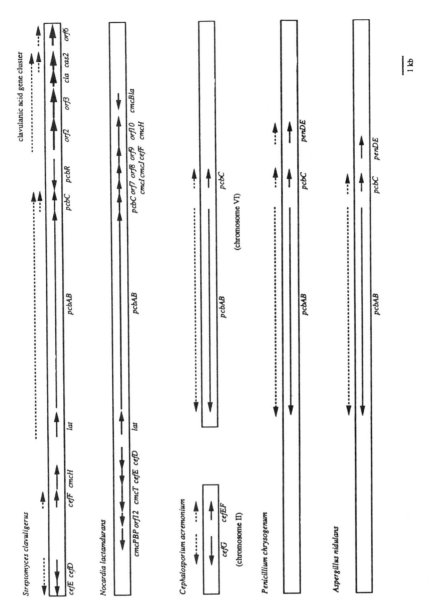

Figure 6   Molecular arrangement of penicillin/cephalosporin biosynthetic genes in bacteria and fungi. The solid arrows represent genes and the dashed arrows represent transcripts. Please refer to the text for gene designations.

been found to be organized into clusters (5) (Figure 6). It was somewhat surprising, however, to find that the penicillin/cephalosporin biosynthetic genes from fungal producer species were also tightly clustered, even though the fungal genes are expressed as individual, monocistronic transcripts (Figure 6). Since the fungal and bacterial penicillin/cephalosporin biosynthetic genes share extensive sequence similarities as well as a conspicuous similarity in organization, a common evolutionary pathway, involving one or more horizontal transfers of production genes between penicillin/cephalosporin-producing actinomycetes and the eukaryotic ancestors of present-day fungal penicillin/cephalosporin producers, has been proposed (5,7).

A. Prokaryotic Gene Arrangement

Among the prokaryotic producers, the gene clusters from S. *clavuligerus* and N. *lactamdurans* have been most extensively characterized. The arrangement of the three early genes as a closely spaced group is conserved in both of the actinomycetes. The genes *lat*, *pcb*AB, and *pcb*C all lie in the same transcriptional orientation, and they are sequentially arranged on the chromosome in the same order as the first steps of the cephamycin C biosynthetic pathway (15,16). In S. *clavuligerus*, the intergenic region between *lat* and *pcb*AB is 152 bp (15) and that between *pcb*AB and *pcb*C is 31 bp (23), whereas in N. *lactamdurans*, the genes are even more tightly linked, with only 64 bp present between *lat* and *pcb*AB (16) and no intergenic region between *pcb*AB and *pcb*C (22). This close spacing of the early genes was suggestive of an operon-like structure, perhaps facilitating coordinate expression. Indeed, in S. *clavuligerus* transcriptional analysis has indicated that these genes are transcribed as a large polycistronic *lat*–*pcb*AB–*pcb*C transcript originating from upstream of *lat* and terminating immediately downstream of *pcb*C (94).

Although a long polycistronic transcript could provide a means to ensure coordinate synthesis of the first three enzymes of the pathway, transcriptional and sequence analyses suggest that the *pcb*C gene within the operon can also be transcribed and regulated independently. S1 nuclease analysis of the region upstream of *pcb*C has shown that, besides the polycistronic transcript, *pcb*C is also expressed from its own specific promoter, which is embedded within the *pcb*AB coding sequences, to give an approximately 1.2 kb monocistronic transcript (34,94,95). Similar monocistronic transcripts have been detected in a cephamycin-producing *Streptomyces griseus* strain (34); however, the significance of this transcript in IPNS synthesis is unclear, since no conditions have been discovered in which production of the small transcript is enhanced or repressed relative to the long transcript.

There is no evidence for the presence of a transcription start site within the *lat*–*pcb*AB intergenic region (94). On the other hand, it has been reported that sequences within *lat* (extending from –192 to –522 bp relative to the *pcb*AB start codon) possess promoter activity when tested in a high-copy-number promoter probe plasmid (24). However, S1 nuclease protection analysis of S. *clavuligerus* RNA failed to detect any transcription start sites originating within this region; instead, it pointed to the presence of a transcript that spanned this entire region. Therefore, it seems very likely that *lat* and *pcb*AB are coexpressed together with *pcb*C.

It is also worth noting that a terminator-like sequence is present immediately downstream from *lat* in the intergenic region between *lat* and *pcb*AB (15), which could allow selective expression of *lat* by dissociating its transcription from that of the downstream genes in the operon. However, S1 nuclease (94) and promoter probe analyses (24) indicated no evidence of termination of the *lat* transcript at this terminator, and they suggested rather that *lat* transcription proceeds into the downstream genes. An antitermination mechanism, which would allow transcription to proceed through the terminator when antibiotic production conditions are favorable, has been postulated (24). However, such a mechanism could not be ubiquitous, since the N. *lactamdurans lat*–*pcb*AB intergenic region does not show the presence of terminator-like sequences (16).

The midpathway genes, cefD and cefE, which together direct the conversion of isopenicillin N to deacetoxycephalosporin C, form another tightly linked group that is conserved in all of the prokaryotic clusters. In S. clavuligerus, the cefD and cefE genes, with an 81 bp intergenic region present between them, are located approximately 7 kb upstream of lat, and both are expressed on a large (>10 kb), divergent (with respect to lat) transcript (15,63,96). The large transcript extends considerably past the cefE gene and, therefore, must encode other, as yet unidentified genes that lie outside of the known cephamycin gene cluster. Likewise, in N. lactamdurans, the cefD and cefE genes are located upstream of, but much closer to, lat than in S. clavuligerus (0.7 vs. 7 kb) (64,87). Also, these genes do not have any intergenic region present between them; instead, they appear to be translationally coupled (64). Available data suggest that in the gene clusters of other Streptomyces spp. and Flavobacterium sp., cefD and cefE are also located upstream from lat (97).

The midpathway gene cefF, which is involved in the conversion of deacetoxy-cephalosporin C to deacetylcephalosporin C, and cmcH, the late gene involved in the conversion of DAC to O-carbamoyl-DAC, are clustered and oriented in the same direction, in both S. clavuligerus and N. lactamdurans. However, the location of the cefF–cmcH cluster relative to the lat–pcbAB–pcbC cluster is not well conserved in the two actinomycetes. In S. clavuligerus, the cefF–cmcH cluster is located about halfway between cefD and lat, oriented in the opposite direction relative to cefD, and possibly expressed on its own transcript (15,70,76). However, in N. lactamdurans, the cefF–cmcH cluster has been located downstream of pcbC together with other late genes, namely, cmcI and cmcJ, which direct the final steps in the conversion of O-carbamoyl-DAC to cephamycin C (64,78,87,98). These genes, cmcI–cmcJ–cefF–cmcH, appear to form a third closely spaced group in N. lactamdurans and may be coordinately expressed (see Figure 6). The presumptive counterparts for cmcI and cmcJ in S. clavuligerus have yet to be located and identified. Instead, at the corresponding location (i.e., downstream of pcbC) in S. clavuligerus, a cluster of genes, involved in the biosynthesis of clavulanic acid, has been located (90,99).

The differences in gene organization between the penicillin/cephalosporin biosynthetic gene clusters of S. clavuligerus and N. lactamdurans may result from differences in the genes surrounding the clusters, and they may or may not affect expression of the genes. In other antibiotic-producing actinomycetes, in particular the aromatic polyketide producers, some differences can be observed in the order and expression of homologous genes within apparently closely related biosynthetic clusters, especially when comparing across species boundaries (100,101). Perhaps even more significantly, the streptomycin biosynthetic gene clusters of S. griseus and Streptomyces glaucescens show many similarities, but they also show distinct differences in the organization and expression of clearly homologous genes (102). Presumably, the variance observed between the S. clavuligerus and N. lactamdurans clusters reflects differences in growth requirements and time since species divergence, as well as the need to coordinate gene expression with other, perhaps diverse, global regulatory mechanisms.

B. Fungal Gene Arrangement

In the fungal producers, the penicillin/cephalosporin biosynthetic genes are also arranged in clusters, although the precise chromosome on which they are located varies from species to species (103). Strikingly, the genes are not as closely spaced as in the prokaryotes, and intergenic regions as large as 800–900 bp are common. This greater spacing may be necessary to accommodate the more complex features of the eukaryotic transcription machinery; or since fungal genes are not expressed as multicistronic transcripts, it may simply reflect the absence of any pressure to keep intergenic distances short. The fungal and prokaryotic arrangements of penicillin/cephalosporin biosynthetic genes are also similar in that *pcb*AB and *pcb*C are found adjacent to one another, but they differ in transcriptional organization. The *pcb*AB and *pcb*C genes are divergently transcribed in fungi, as opposed to the operon-like transcriptional arrangement seen in the prokaryotes. The intergenic region between the two genes presumably contains promoters that cause divergent transcription of the *pcb*AB and *pcb*C genes to give approximately 11 and 1.2 kb transcripts, respectively (19–21,104,105). The large *pcb*AB transcript in fungal producers is more stable than its prokaryotic counterpart, but this is likely just due to the presence of more stabilizing features on eukaryotic mRNAs in general. Large *pcb*AB transcripts have been detected in all three fungal producer species.

In penicillin producers such as *P. chrysogenum* and *A. nidulans*, the *pen*DE gene, which encodes the last enzyme of the penicillin pathway, is located downstream from the *pcb*C gene and is oriented in the same direction (19,52,106,107) (Figure 3). The *pcb*C–*pen*DE intergenic region in *P. chrysogenum* is 1.5 kb (19,51,107), compared with 0.8 kb in *A. nidulans* (51), and in *P. chrysogenum*, the *pen*DE gene is transcribed over 1.15 kb (52,107).

In the cephalosporin C producer, *C. acremonium*, the *pcb*AB and *pcb*C genes for the early steps of the pathway are grouped together on chromosome VI, whereas the *cef*EF and *cef*G genes for the late steps of the pathway are located on chromosome II (108). The location of the putative *cef*D gene in the *C. acremonium* genome is at present unknown. Like the early genes, the *cef*G and *cef*EF genes, although grouped together, are oppositely oriented and expressed from divergent promoters contained within the 938 bp intergenic region (72,109). The *cef*G and *cef*EF genes are transcribed over 1.4 and 1.2 kb, respectively (72).

C.   Origin and Evolution

The conserved clustering of penicillin/cephalosporin biosynthetic genes in both the prokaryotes and eukaryotes has suggested, at least for the early pathway genes, a bacterial genesis. From an evolutionary perspective, there are two major branch point metabolites in the penicillin/cephalosporin biosynthetic pathway: (a) isopenicillin N, which can be either converted to the hydrophobic penicillins or epimerized to penicillin N and shunted toward cephalosporin biosynthesis; and (b) deacetylcephalosporin C, which can be either transacetylated to form cephalosporin C or shunted toward cephamycin C production. Both isopenicillin N and deacetylcephalosporin C, therefore, represent important evolutionary landmarks with respect to the proposed transfer of penicillin/cephalosporin biosynthetic genes between prokaryotes and eukaryotes.

A comparison of IPNS-encoding genes from a diverse group of Gram-positive bacterial and fungal β-lactam producers suggested that all *pcb*C genes, whether fungal or bacterial, are descended from a common ancestral gene that existed approximately 370 million years ago. This was a pivotal discovery because previous studies had shown that fungi and bacteria diverged almost 2 billion years ago. A horizontal transfer of genes, well after the proposed split of eukaryotes from prokaryotes, was thus postulated. The recent sequence-similarity studies that also included the IPNS genes from the two Gram-negative β-lactam producers, *Flavobacterium* sp. and *L. lactamgenes*, have suggested that the proposed horizontal transfer between the bacteria and fungi may have occurred before the divergence of Gram-negative and Gram-positive bacteria about 1–1.5 billion years ago. Because there is a possibility that the rate of evolutionary change in IPNS genes is not constant between organisms, the absolute validity of either of these proposals cannot yet be substantiated (Figure 7) (5,35,98,110,111). Furthermore, the overall direction of transfer is uncertain.

A number of factors weighed in favor of a prokaryote to fungus transfer: (a) An analysis of the percent G+C content of a number of fungal IPNS genes showed that they possess an uneven distribution of nucleotides, leading to a biased codon usage more typical of that used by the high-percentage G+C genomes of actinomycetes than of other fungal genes (5,112); (b) The arrangement of biosynthetic genes in clusters is a common feature of prokaryotic chromosomes but is less common in fungi (67); (c) The β-lactam biosynthetic genes are scattered into subclusters on different chromosomes within the C. *acremonium* genome, whereas they are all tightly clustered on the chromosomes of actinomycete producers. It seems more likely that the genes were clustered in their original host and then dispersed when introduced into a new host rather than vice versa (111); (d) The greater complexity and variety of β-lactam structures produced by bacteria is consistent with a longer evolutionary history for β-lactam biosynthesis in prokaryotes (5,98); and (e) The central pathway genes common to all penicillin/cephalosporin producers lack introns, whereas genes encoding uniquely fungal enzyme activities contain introns (98).

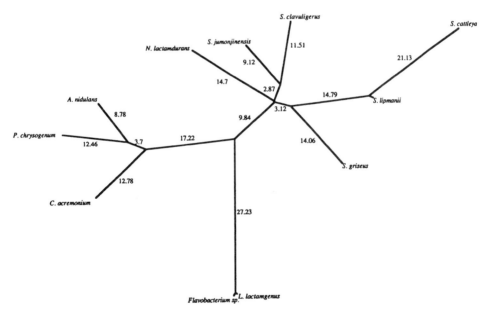

Figure 7 A phylogenetic tree depicting the evolutionary relatedness of the derived IPNS amino acid sequences from 11 β-lactam-producing microorganisms. The unrooted tree was constructed using the DISTANCES and GROWTREE programs from the Wisconsin Package Version 8.1 (Genetics Computer Group, Madison, Wisconsin 53711) and the DRAWTREE program (Felsenstein J. 1993. PHYLIP [Phylogeny Inference Package] Version 3.5c). The Jukes–Cantor distance correction method was used to compensate for multiple substitutions, and evolutionary distances were estimated using a neighbor-joining method. The branch lengths are proportional to the number of nonsynonymous substitutions per 100 amino acids.

Furthermore, if gene transfer did take place between bacteria and fungi, it may have occurred on more than one occasion (113). Two hypotheses for horizontal gene transfer have been suggested: (a) the evolutionary distance hypothesis, and (b) the topological hypothesis. Briefly, the first proposal argues that a single transfer of penicillin/cephalosporin biosynthetic genes occurred approximately 40 million years before the divergence of *Cephalosporium*, *Penicillium*, and *Aspergillus* species from their common ancestor. The second hypothesis suggests that at least two horizontal transfers took place, such that all the genes required for penicillin/cephalosporin biosynthesis were transferred to an ancestor of *Cephalosporium*, whereas those for just penicillin production were transferred to a common ancestor of *Penicillium* and *Aspergillus* species. Arguments concerning both hypotheses are ongoing, and the issues have yet to be conclusively resolved.

In *C. acremonium*, DAOCS and DACS activities are encoded by one gene, *cef*EF. Initially, it was assumed that *cef*EF arose via gene fusion, following the horizontal transfer of the *cef*E and *cef*F genes from a bacterial cephalosporin producer (67). However, sequence analysis has shown that the derived amino acid sequences of both *cef*E and *cef*F from *S. clavuligerus* align with that of *cef*EF across their entire sequences. This finding is more consistent with the theory that *cef*EF, encoding a bifunctional DAOCS/DACS activity, evolved initially in a prokaryotic ancestor and subsequently diverged via gene duplication into separate *cef*E and *cef*F genes. This proposal was subsequently supported by the discovery that highly purified *S. clavuligerus* DAOCS showed low but detectable levels of DACS activity, and purified DACS showed weak but measurable DAOCS activity (5,70,114). Therefore, the *cef*EF gene likely evolved in a prokaryotic host and was subsequently transferred to a fungal host before the gene duplication and divergence of *cef*EF into separate *cef*E and *cef*F genes occurred in prokaryotes. In keeping with this theory, the *cef*EF gene of *C. acremonium* would encode an enzyme similar to the putative primordial prokaryotic DAOCS/DACS.

As mentioned previously, none of the fungal genes involved in the early and midpathway steps possessed intervening sequences (introns) (98). In contrast, both the *pen*DE and *cef*G genes, directing the last steps of penicillin and cephalosporin biosynthesis, respectively, possessed multiple introns (51,72,98). Introns are an almost exclusive trait of eukaryotic genomes; this suggests that the early and midpathway genes (*pcb*AB, *pcb*C, and *cef*EF) are of bacterial origin, whereas the late pathway genes are of a more recent and fungal origin. Supporting this, sequence analysis has shown that the derived amino acid sequence of *cef*G is highly similar to that of yeast homoserine acetyltransferases (72,109).

It is likely, therefore, that penicillin/cephalosporin biosynthetic genes were at some point transferred from prokaryote to eukaryote, but evidence for the exact mechanism by which this process occurred is lacking. Recent studies have shown that under the appropriate conditions, plasmid DNA can be conjugated from *E. coli* to the yeast *Saccharomyces cerevisiae*, thus providing an example of genetic exchange between prokaryote and eukaryote (113). Since both actinomycetes and fungi exist naturally in the soil environment, and many have filamentous stages in their life cycles, it might well be expected that they come into frequent and close contact with each other. Because neither is motile, cell–cell interaction could take place for extended periods of time, perhaps long enough for conjugation or natural transformation processes to occur. Since actinomycetes, especially the *Streptomyces*, undergo a complex differentiation process during which the substrate mycelium is lysed and cell contents are released into the surrounding environment, the possibility of soil fungi encountering substantial quantities of bacterial DNA would also seem realistic. The exact mechanism by which exogenous prokaryotic genetic material could be incorporated, maintained, and expressed in the foreign genomes is unclear, although processes involving illegitimate recombination and favored by natural selection might be suspected.

IV. REGULATION OF PENICILLIN/CEPHALOSPORIN BIOSYNTHESIS

Early evidence that antibiotic production is subject to complex regulation came from the observation that production is typically dissociated from cell growth. This evidence of regulation was further substantiated by growth medium optimization studies aimed at achieving higher yields. Such studies yielded a wealth of data that suggested that the timing and extent of antibiotic production are dictated by nutrient availability and other environmental factors (115). Although the situation varies from one organism to another, in general, production is inhibited by high levels of easily metabolizable carbon, nitrogen, and phosphate sources. In both fungal and prokaryotic producers, some of these effects are due to transcriptional regulation of the genes encoding the key pathway enzymes, although the details of the regulatory features of these pathways are only beginning to be elucidated.

In *S. clavuligerus*, studies on the transcriptional regulation of some genes of the penicillin/cephalosporin pathway have identified transcription start points and putative promoter sequences (Table 1). The transcription start site of the long polycistronic *lat–pcb*AB–*pcb*C transcript has been identified as a T residue 88 bp upstream from *lat*, whereas that of the short *pcb*C monocistronic transcript has been identified as a C residue 92 bp upstream from *pcb*C (94,95). The transcription start point of the other polycistronic transcript expressed from the *cef*D–*cef*E cluster has been mapped to an A residue 130 bp upstream from *cef*D (63). The –10 and –35 promoter sequences of *cef*D/*cef*E show some similarity to both *E. coli* (116) and *Streptomyces* (117) consensus promoter sequences. Interestingly, the –10 region of *lat* and *pcb*C are identical but show little similarity to the *E. coli* or *Streptomyces* consensus sequences, which is in agreement with the general promoter heterogeneity seen in this genus. The *lat* –35 region has high similarity to corresponding sequences from the *cef*D/*cef*E promoter, whereas those of *pcb*C showed some

Table I Comparison of Promoters from the Penicillin/Cephalosporin Cluster of *Streptomyces clavuligerus*

Promoter	Sequence	Transcription start site, distance from the initiation codon
E. coli consensus[a]	T T G A C a–17bp–T A t A a T	
Streptomyces consensus[a]	T T G A C r–18bp–T A g r r T	
lat	T G G A A G–17bp–G T G G G T	T, 88 bp
*pcb*C	T G C A C G–18bp–G T G G G T	C, 92 bp
*cef*D/*cef*E	T T G A A G–18bp–C A G A A T	A, 130 bp

[a] Uppercase letters show nucleotides that are highly conserved, lowercase letters show nucleotides that are significantly conserved; r, purine (a or g).

similarity to other genes involved in secondary metabolism (94). Both the long *lat–pcb*AB–*pcb*C and the short *pcb*C transcripts show temporal regulation, which suggests that the temporal expression of both *lat* and *pcb*C is regulated at transcriptional level. Since the time course of appearance and the amount of the monocistronic *pcb*C transcript synthesized are very similar to those of the long polycistronic transcript, the identical –10 regions of their promoters may be involved in bringing about some type of coordinate regulation (94).

Among fungal producers, the transcription start sites for the divergently expressed *pcb*AB (21) and *pcb*C (118) genes have been identified in *A. nidulans*. The putative promoter sequences and other upstream sequences of the two genes are quite different, although it could be expected that if both genes were coordinately expressed they would share some common features. The *pcb*C promoter sequences, which have also been identified in *P. chrysogenum* (37) and *C. acremonium* (104), show common eukaryotic core promoter motifs like the TATA and CAAT sequences. In contrast, the *pcb*AB promoter sequences, which have been identified in *A. nidulans* (21), do not show any such motif. The *A. nidulans pcb*AB–*pcb*C intergenic region contains a 53 bp sequence of dyad symmetry present equidistant from both genes (21); however, its involvement in the expression of these genes is presently not clear. Recently, multiple transcription start sites were detected within 100 nucleotides of the start codon for the *pen*DE gene of *A. nidulans* (119). However, since no TATA motifs were detected within 200 nucleotides of the transcription start site, other cis-acting sequences are thought to be involved in transcription initiation.

The *pcb*C transcripts appear preferentially during the late stages of the growth cycle in *C. acremonium* and *A. nidulans*, suggesting a temporal mode of expression occurring at the transcriptional level (104,120). In *A. nidulans*, where transcription of *pcb*C is most well studied, the 872 bp *pcb*AB–*pcb*C intergenic region was analyzed in both orientations for promoter activity using the *lacZ* reporter gene system. Though temporal expression was the same for both genes, the *pcb*C promoter also showed a separate mode of regulation, carbon catabolite repression (CCR) (121). Repressing amounts of glucose in the medium not only decreased penicillin production, it also significantly repressed the expression of the *pcb*C, but not the *pcb*AB, gene fusion (121). In a separate study, the levels of *pcb*C transcripts were several times as high in the presence of nonrepressible as compared with repressible carbon sources (122). Therefore, the CCR of penicillin production is mediated through the transcriptional control of at least one pathway gene, *pcb*C. Since mutations in *cre*A, a gene mediating CCR of primary metabolic genes in fungi, did not significantly derepress *pcb*C expression, another *cre*A-independent mechanism of CCR is implicated in the regulation of *pcb*C expression (122). Although details of this mechanism are unclear, sequences between –1334 to –966 (relative to the *pcb*C start codon), which are located within the *pcb*AB coding region, are implicated in CCR. When the region upstream of *pcb*C was sequentially deleted from the 5′-end and the deletions tested for promoter activity by a *lacZ* gene fusion technique, a deletion that encompassed these sequences gave derepressed levels of *lacZ* activity in the presence of a repressing carbon source (118). Nonetheless, the mechanism of CCR may be complex, since other sequences still further upstream from –1334 and sequences within the *pcb*AB–*pcb*C intergenic region also seem to be involved in modulating the *lacZ* activity (118). It has been shown that the expression of the *pcb*C gene also appears to be under the control of a pH regulatory system (123). External alkaline pH bypasses CCR, resulting in derepression of the *pcb*C transcript in the presence of repressing carbon sources.

However, since an acidic pH does not prevent carbon derepression of *pcb*C, it seems that CCR and pH regulation are mechanistically different, but they may act in concert at alkaline pH (123). It has now been shown that at alkaline pH the *pcb*C transcription is positively regulated by PacC, a transcription factor that contains three putative Cys_2His_2 zinc fingers, which are characteristically present in some eukaryotic transcription factors, and that is encoded by the *pac*C gene (124). A region of PacC protein including the zinc finger sequences was overexpressed in *E. coli* and was shown to be able to bind in vitro at several places upstream from the *pcb*C gene in a sequence-specific manner. A consensus sequence, GCCAA(G)G, has been derived from the sequence comparisons of the PacC-binding sites (124).

The fungal β-lactam genes also show regulatory mechanisms that are unique to the organism. A case in point is the repression of *pcb*C and *pcb*AB expression by nitrogen, which is observed in *P. chrysogenum* but not *A. nidulans*. The nitrogen repression of *pcb*C and *pcb*AB is thought to be mediated by NRE, the global nitrogen regulatory protein, which also regulates a variety of genes involved in nitrogen metabolism (125). The NRE protein contains a single zinc finger motif, and the domain containing this motif binds specifically to many sites within the intergenic promoter region of the *pcb*C and *pcb*AB genes. The binding sites contain a motif, GATA, which is also the binding site for a variety of eukaryotic transcription factors belonging to the GATA protein family (125). Interestingly, the intergenic region of *P. chrysogenum* contains six GATA sequences as opposed to only one GATA sequence present in *A. nidulans*, which does not show nitrogen regulation, suggesting the importance of GATA sequences in this type of regulation.

There is some evidence to indicate that there are still more types of regulatory mechanisms that control the expression of *pcb*C and *pcb*AB genes. Using gene fusion technology, several trans-acting regulatory mutations have been identified that negatively affect the expression of the reporter gene placed under the control of *pcb*C or *pcb*AB promoter regions (126,127). However, since the analysis of the genes corresponding to these mutations has not been described yet, details of the regulatory mechanisms associated with these mutations is not clear at present. Similar gene fusion experiments have revealed a motif GGCCAATC in the *pcb*C–*pcb*AB intergenic region, which when deleted led to a positive effect on *pcb*C expression but a negative effect on *pcb*AB expression in *A. nidulans* (128). This suggests that the sequence containing this motif could bind to either one dual-function transcription factor, or a group of proteins, which could then positively regulate *pcb*C and negatively regulate *pcb*AB. This motif is also conserved in *P. chrysogenum* and *C. acremonium* *pcb*C–*pcb*AB intergenic regions, leading to the idea that the mechanism involved may be conserved in these organisms. Thus, the β-lactam biosynthetic genes in fungi seem to be under the control of a complex regulatory network involving a variety of cis- and trans-acting elements.

Antibiotic biosynthetic gene clusters often contain specific regulatory genes, encoding transcriptional activators or repressors that act to regulate the biosynthetic genes in a coordinate manner in order to achieve optimal levels of antibiotic production (91). A mechanism for coordinate regulation is particularly necessary in the fungal systems, where all pathway genes are independently transcribed. In prokaryotes, the coordinate expression of genes is partly achieved by the operon arrangement of the genes within the cluster. However, the coordinate expression of these groups of genes would still require a common regulatory mechanism. Many observations suggest the presence of such a mechanism in fungal as well as prokaryotic producers, although the details of it are presently obscure.

In the fungus *C. acremonium*, methionine stimulates antibiotic production, which results from a coordinate increase in the levels of transcripts encoded by *pcb*AB, *pcb*C, *cef*EF, and to some extent, *cef*G (105). Sequences like CANNTG, which recognize many eukaryotic regulatory factors, are present in the upstream regions of all four genes, and they may be involved in coordinate regulation of transcription of these genes. Furthermore, pleiotropic mutants of *P. chrysogenum* have been isolated and characterized, and these show reduced amounts of all biosynthetic enzymes and produce low levels of penicillin (129). These mutants could be defective in a regulatory gene involved in coordinate expression of all biosynthetic genes.

In *S. clavuligerus*, *lat* promoter activity, as determined by measuring *xylE*-encoded catechol-2,3-dioxygenase activity in a *xylE* reporter gene fusion system, was more than 2500 times as high when the construct was present at high copy number in the native host, than when present in a heterologous, penicillin/cephalosporin nonproducing host (94). Therefore, a host-specific transcriptional factor acting specifically on the *lat* promoter/upstream region must be present in *S. clavuligerus* to explain such high transcriptional activity. Moreover, as in *P. chrysogenum*, pleiotropic antibiotic-blocked mutants of *S. clavuligerus* have been isolated that show no IPNS, ACVS, LAT, or DAOCS activity, products of two different operons within the cluster (Jensen SE, unpublished observations). These pleiotropic mutants could also be explained by the presence of a host-specific transcriptional factor regulating penicillin/cephalosporin biosynthetic genes.

V. GENETICS OF CLAVULANIC ACID BIOSYNTHESIS

A totally separate biosynthetic scheme is entailed in the formation of another group of β-lactam compounds, known as the clavams. These compounds differ from the penicillin/cephalosporin group of β-lactams in having oxygen in place of sulfur in the second ring of the bicyclic nucleus, which is referred to as an oxazolidine ring (3) (Figure 4). The production of clavams is a property that is shared by many actinomycetes, including penicillin/cephalosporin producers, for example, *S. clavuligerus*, *S. lipmanii*, *Streptomyces jumonjinensis*, and *Streptomyces katsuharamanus* (99), as well as a nonproducing species, *Streptomyces antibioticus* (130,131); however, this property has not yet been reported in fungi. Clavulanic acid is a clavam well known for its potent β-lactamase inhibitory activity, which makes it valuable as a chemotherapeutic agent when used in combination with conventional penicillins and cephalosporins for the treatment of infections by β-lactamase-producing organisms. The remarkable efficacy of Augmentin, a commercial combination drug composed of amoxycillin and clavulanic acid, resulted in this one product taking 5.6% of the market share for all antibacterials in 1991, with world sales estimated at $850 million. The β-lactamase inhibitory activity of clavulanic acid is related to its specific ring stereochemistry, which is opposite to that found in all other clavams (132). Clavams other than clavulanic acid all have similar nuclear structures, but their biological activities range from antibacterial to antifungal in nature, and none have β-lactamase inhibitory activity.

Biochemical experiments have demonstrated that the pathway for clavulanic acid biosynthesis begins with the condensation of the amino acid arginine with a three-carbon glycolytic intermediate (133,134) (Figure 8). Because one of the components in this reaction is not an amino acid, an ACVS-like peptide synthetase may not be present, and the condensation may involve a different reaction mechanism. The early steps of the pathway, which at present are not fully understood, lead to the formation of the interme-

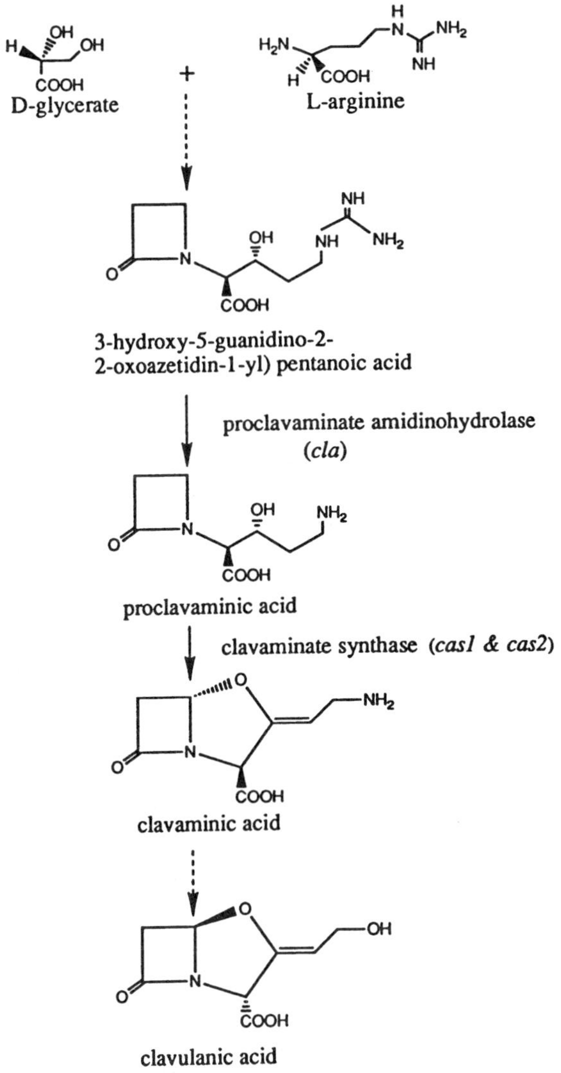

Figure 8 The pathway for biosynthesis of clavulanic acid. Genes are indicated in parentheses.

diate 5-guanidino-(2-oxoazetidin-1-yl)pentanoic acid, which is subsequently converted to 3-hydroxy-5-guanidino-2-(2-oxoazetidin-1-yl)pentanoic acid (135,136). The next intermediate in the pathway is proclavaminic acid, which is converted to clavaminic acid and finally to clavulanic acid (137,138). Radiolabeling of precursors and feeding experiments suggest that pathways for clavulanic acid and the other clavams have a common origin, and that they share intermediates at least up to the level of proclavaminic acid or even beyond (139,140).

The best-studied enzyme in the pathway is clavaminate synthase (CAS), which is involved in the conversion of proclavaminic acid to clavaminic acid (see Figure 8). CAS oxidatively catalyzes the formation of the oxazolidine ring, which is characteristic of all clavams, including clavulanic acid. Initially, CAS activity was studied in the clavulanic acid producer, *S. clavuligerus* (141,142), but recently CAS activity has also been detected in *S. antibioticus*, purified (143,144), and correlated with the production of clavams other than clavulanic acid. Therefore, CAS may be considered a key enzyme in the formation of all clavams in general. Interestingly, CAS is an α-ketoglutarate-dependent oxygenase that requires molecular oxygen and iron for activity, a property it shares with DAOCS/DACS enzymes of penicillin/cephalosporin pathway (141,142). However, cloning of the corresponding genes and comparison of their deduced amino acid sequences revealed no significant relationship between these two dioxygenases, which belong to a larger class of α-ketoglutarate-dependent oxygenases (145). In *S. clavuligerus*, CAS activity is associated with two separate proteins, CAS1 and CAS2, which are encoded by two very similar but separate genes, *cas1* and *cas2* (145). Proclavaminate amidinohydrolase (PAH), encoded by *cla*, is another enzyme in the pathway that has been characterized (136). This enzyme catalyzes the removal of amidino group from 3-hydroxy-5-guanidino-2-oxoazetidinyl pentanoic acid to give proclavaminic acid (see Figure 8).

In *S. clavuligerus*, the genes encoding clavulanic acid biosynthetic enzymes have been located immediately downstream from the penicillin/cephalosporin gene cluster (99,146,147) (Figure 6). A 12 kb DNA fragment from *S. clavuligerus*, which is located immediately downstream from *pcbC* and conferred upon *S. lividans* the ability to produce a clavulanic acid–like activity, has been sequenced completely (90,148). The genes *cas2* and *cla* have been located on this fragment grouped with two other upstream unidentified genes in an operon-like arrangement. Transcriptional analysis indicates that all four genes are expressed together to form a 5.3 kb polycistronic transcript; however, *cas2*, which is located at the distal end of the operon, is also expressed as a 1.2 kb monocistronic transcript (149). Sequence analysis of DNA fragments that complemented different mutants blocked in clavulanic acid production has identified other pathway genes present immediately downstream from *cas2* (150). Similarly, gene disruption analysis has indicated genes present downstream from *cas2* are also essential for clavulanic acid biosynthesis (Paradkar AS, Aidoo KA, and Jensen SE, unpublished observations); however, their precise role in the pathway is not fully understood at present.

The gene *cas1*, encoding the CAS1 isoenzyme, has been found to be separated from *cas2* by at least 20 kb of DNA (145). Supporting this, *cas1* is not present on the 12 kb DNA fragment carrying *cas2* and other clavulanic acid pathway genes, and therefore its location relative to *cas2* is unknown (148). Gene disruption of *cas2* resulted in a strain that was blocked in clavulanic acid biosynthesis when grown in a defined production medium, but the strain did make clavulanic acid when grown in a soy-based fermentation medium, although at levels 60% of the wild type. This leaky phenotype of the *cas2*-disrupted strain in soy medium, but not in the defined medium, correlated well with the presence of *cas1* transcripts in soy but not defined medium. Therefore, despite its unknown location, *cas1* can be recruited for clavulanic acid biosynthesis. Since *cas2* transcripts were detected in both media, it follows that *cas1* and *cas2* show significant differences in their nutritional regulation, but they both contribute to clavulanic acid production (149).

Available data suggest that the clavulanic acid biosynthetic genes in *S. jumonjinensis* and *S. katsuharamanus* are also located immediately downstream from the penicillin/cephalosporin gene cluster (99). The clustering of genes encoding biosynthetic enzymes for production of a β-lactamase inhibitor together with those encoding biosynthetic enzymes for production of β-lactam antibiotics, even though both types of compounds entail totally different biosynthetic schemes, is very intriguing. Perhaps the close juxtaposition of the gene clusters reflects a common regulatory mechanism that would allow coregulation of production of the antibiotics and the inhibitor. Coordinated production would confer upon the producing host a selective advantage, not only over the β-lactam-susceptible microorganisms in nature, but also over those that develop resistance by acquiring the ability to produce β-lactamases.

VI. APPLICATIONS OF MOLECULAR GENETICS IN BIOTECHNOLOGY

Strain improvement of β-lactam-producing microorganisms is an ongoing process that has been under way for the past 40 years. Standard or classical techniques, such as screening for new soil isolates, mutagenesis and screening for high producers, and the selection of high producers by growth on metabolic inhibitors, have resulted in the isolation of *Penicillium* strains that produce up to 50,000 times the amount of penicillin produced by Fleming's original isolate in 1928 (109,151). Nevertheless, in recent years, the efficacy of these empirical and somewhat random methods of strain improvement has declined significantly, leading to smaller and smaller incremental increases in production levels with each round of selection (109,152).

The advent of molecular techniques for manipulating the genetic material of filamentous fungi combined with the elucidation of the major enzymatic steps in the β-lactam biosynthetic pathway have resulted in the isolation, cloning, and expression of many of the genes that direct β-lactam production (153). These accomplishments have resulted in a growing number of attempts to directly modify existing pathways and, in some instances, create novel pathways for β-lactam biosynthesis (152–155).

Detailed kinetic studies, as well as a growing appreciation of the regulatory mechanisms governing secondary metabolism, have allowed the identification of rate-limiting reactions that create putative bottlenecks in β-lactam production pathways (156). Molecular genetic approaches to strain improvement, therefore, seek to alleviate such problems by directly targeting enzymes that may catalyze rate-limiting reactions and/or by creating entirely novel biosynthetic pathways, one enzyme at a time. One ultimate, long-term goal of such studies is the cell-free synthesis of β-lactam antibiotics, whereby the complete control of the biosynthetic pathway, its components, and its output is possible (157).

Perhaps the best-documented and most successful application of molecular genetics to strain improvement was the alleviation of one of the bottlenecks in the cephalosporin C pathway in C. *acremonium*. (153,158) A high-level producing strain of C. *acremonium* was found to accumulate penicillin N in its culture broth. This strongly suggested that a metabolic bottleneck was occurring due to a rate-limiting DAOCS/DACS reaction. To test this proposal, additional copies of the previously cloned C. *acremonium* cefEF gene were introduced into the fungus. Approximately 25% of the transformants showed up to 50% improvement in cephalosporin C production, although this increment dropped to 15% when a high-producing clone was scaled up to production level. It was concluded, however, that even a 15% increase in production was significant, given the already high level of production by the parental strain. As might be predicted, the recombinant strain no longer accumulated penicillin N, and Southern blot analysis revealed that the hyperproducing strain possessed one extra copy of the cefEF gene that had integrated heterologously at a location in the genome different from that of the native gene.

Recently, the cefG gene, encoding DAC acetyltransferase, was cloned from a wild-type strain of C. *acremonium* and was located just upstream of the cefEF gene (109). When cefG was reintroduced into a DAC acetyltransferase mutant of C. *acremonium*, a gene dosage effect was observed; transformants showed a direct correlation between the number of copies of *cef*G integrated into the mutant genome and the level of cephalosporin C produced. This effect was also observed when the *cef*G gene was reintroduced into the wild-type strain, strongly suggesting that DAC acetyltransferase was rate-limiting in this strain. Moreover, it was noted that the *cef*EF-encoding DNA fragment, used by Skatrud et al. (158) to enhance cephalosporin C production in *C. acremonium*, also contained the closely linked *cef*G gene. This may call into question whether it was the *cef*EF gene or *cef*G that caused the improved production in that study. If the production strain used by Skatrud et al. (158) was in fact rate-limiting for DAC acetyltransferase rather than DAOCS/DACS, then the penicillin N that accumulated in that strain might have resulted from feed-back inhibition of DAOCS/DACS by DAC. The introduction of a fragment containing the *cef*EF and *cef*G genes, therefore, would have resolved the rate-limiting reaction as well as the feed-back loop. However, it is also well known that industrial production strains from different lineages have very different biosynthetic capabilities, and so it is quite possible that DAOCS/DACS was the actual rate-limiting step in the strain used by Skatrud et al. (158).

In a similar study aimed at improving penicillin production by *P. chrysogenum*, a 5.1 kb *Sal*I fragment, carrying the closely linked *pcb*C and *pen*DE genes of *P. chrysogenum*, was used to transform a production strain of the fungus. A number of transformants that produced 18 to 40% more penicillin V than the parental strain were isolated. The variability among the transformants was thought to be due to differences in the location of plasmid integration and to differences in the number of integrated copies (159,160). Previous attempts to improve penicillin production by reintroduction of the *pcb*C gene alone were unsuccessful. This failure was attributed to the preexistence of multiple copies of the *pcb*C gene in many of the high-producing industrial strains of *P. chrysogenum*, and it suggested that the *pen*DE gene that was responsible for the improvement in production (155).

Molecular genetics has also been used to design new biosynthetic pathways. The current process for producing 7-aminodeacetoxycephalosporanic acid (7-ADCA), a precursor for a number of clinically important cephalosporins (e.g., cephalexin, cephradine, and cefadroxil), involves a four-step chemical ring expansion of penicillin G and a final enzymatic deacylation (161). The chemical reactions involved require large quantities of expensive, environmentally unfriendly solvents. An enzymatic or fermentative process producing large amounts of DAOC, which could be enzymatically deacylated to 7-ADCA, would be far more cost-effective and environmentally sound (153).

Production strains of *C. acremonium* accumulate only small amounts of DAOC; most of the intermediate is rapidly hydroxylated to DAC by the bifunctional DAOCS/DACS. Attempts to disable the DACS portion of the enzyme genetically without losing the DAOCS function were unsuccessful (161). Therefore, *cef*E and *cef*D genes from *S. clavuligerus* and *S. lipmanii*, respectively, were introduced into a high-titer penicillin-producing strain of *P. chrysogenum*. Stable transformants were isolated that produced low but detectable levels of DAOC as well as slightly lowered levels of penicillin V. It was suggested that optimization of DAOC production by the recombinant strain would require disabling the *pen*DE gene and perhaps increasing the gene dosage of *cef*D and *cef*E; however, targeted gene disruption in production strains possessing multiple copies of the *pen*DE gene could prove difficult (161,162).

Another approach to producing 7-ADCA centered on the high-level expression of the *S. clavuligerus cef*E gene in *P. chrysogenum*. This was accomplished by removing the prokaryotic promoter and transcriptional terminator regions from the *S. clavuligerus cef*E gene and replacing them with the analogous regions from the *P. chrysogenum pcb*C gene. The overexpressed DAOCS, however, was unable to ring-expand the penicillin G formed by the *P. chrysogenum* host. Ultimately, it is hoped that site-directed mutagenesis, guided by x-ray crystallographic analysis, will lead to a DAOCS enzyme with an altered substrate specificity, allowing the enzymatic ring expansion of either penicillin G or V in vivo (163,164).

Pathway bioengineering has also been successfully applied to the fermentative production of 7-aminocephalosporanic acid (7-ACA). Until recently, 7-ACA, a precursor for a number of clinically important cephems such as cephaloglycine and cephalothin, was produced via an inefficient and expensive chemical deacylation of highly purified cephalosporin C (165). However, by introducing hybrid genes for D–amino acid oxidase from *Fusarium solani* and cephalosporin acylase from *Pseudomonas diminuta* into *C. acremonium*, a recombinant strain was isolated that produced low but industrially promising amounts of 7-ACA by fermentation.

A novel fermentative process for the production of both 7-ADCA and 7-ACA has been recently developed. It was found that if a high-titer penicillin-producing strain of *P. chrysogenum* was fed adipate, significant levels of adipyl-6-aminopenicillanic acid (adipyl-6-APA) accumulated in culture broths (167). Recombinant plasmids, carrying hybrid *cef*E (from *S. clavuligerus*), and *cef*EF + *cef*G (from *C. acremonium*) genes, were each introduced into the *P. chrysogenum* host. Transformants carrying the hybrid *cef*E gene produced almost equivalent amounts of adipyl-6-APA and adipyl-7-ADCA when grown in adipate-supplemented medium. Likewise, transformants carrying the hybrid *cef*EF and *cef*G genes produced adipyl-6-APA, adipyl-7-ADCA, adipyl-7-ADAC (adipyl-7-aminodeacetylcephalosporanic acid), and adipyl-7-ACA. Transformants carrying just the *cef*EF gene produced all of the above except for 7-ACA (167). The overall results strongly suggested that both the *S. clavuligerus* DAOCS and the *C. acremonium* DAOCS/DACS enzymes were capable of ring-expanding adipyl-6-APA. The same transformants, however, were unable to ring-expand penicillin V when fed phenoxyacetic acid. Interestingly, these results contrasted sharply with those obtained by others who found that cell-free extracts of *S. clavuligerus* containing DAOCS activity were unable to ring-expand adipyl-6-APA (168).

Purified adipyl-7-ADCA and adipyl-7-ACA from culture broths could be readily deacylated by a *Pseudomonas*-derived glutaryl amidase to produce, respectively, 7-ADCA and 7-ACA. Interestingly, production levels of adipyl-7-ADCA and adipyl-7-ACA by the recombinant strains were substantially enhanced by applying classical methods of strain improvement to the transformants. The production levels of 7-ACA and 7-ADCA by these strains strongly suggested the possibility for commercial development (167).

VII.   FUTURE PROSPECTS

The application of molecular genetics to strain improvement in the β-lactam-producing species has just begun. To date, it has allowed us to manipulate only a few of the parameters controlling secondary metabolism and has resulted in very modest gains in production efficiency. Future uses of molecular techniques will most likely revolve around identifying the transcriptional and regulatory mechanisms that limit or restrict the expression of native or foreign genes in producing strains. Furthermore, a growing knowledge of the biochemical and biophysical properties of the biosynthetic enzymes will ultimately permit their manipulation at the molecular level guided by x-ray-crystallographic analysis of active-site structures; this may in turn allow the synthesis of a wider range of bioactive precursors and metabolites.

These optimistic projections are based solely on a consideration of the scientific merits of the application of recombinant DNA technology to the production of antibiotics. However, they do not take into account the impact of several sociological factors that may make the future less promising. For example, the genetically manipulated industrial strain of *C. acremonium*, improved by the introduction of an additional copy of *cef*EF, was developed right up to the point of introduction into the fermentation plant, but it still has not been used for industrial production of cephalosporin C. The reasons can be traced to factors such as persistent uncertainty about the acceptance by consumers of products resulting from recombinant technology, but also to strategic decisions by pharmaceutical companies to purchase antibiotic starting materials from offshore fermentation facilities rather than produce them in-house. Finally, the current trend seen in some pharmaceutical companies to turn away from antibiotics as preferred targets for new drug development may further limit the application of molecular genetics to antibiotic production. This disturbing trend is partly due to the difficult economic realities involved in trying to achieve a reasonable rate of return on the development of a new antibiotic, where the expense of bringing the product to market may not be recovered before the appearance of antibiotic resistance reduces the marketability of the product. We are left in the unfortunate situation that, at the very time that the rapid spread of antibiotic-resistant organisms makes the need for new classes of antibiotics most pressing, the economic costs of discovering and developing these new antibiotics is discouraging such research. Perhaps as the problem of antibiotic resistance becomes even more acute, research into the development of new antibiotics will, of necessity, come back into favor, and the full force of molecular genetics will be brought to bear on the problem.

REFERENCES

1.   Corbett K. The history of antibiotic production. From "bedpans" to fermenters. The Biochemist 1990; 12:8–13.
2.   Veenstra AE, Niekus HGD. Penicillin production at Royal Gist-Brocades. Kleinkauf H, von Döhren H, eds. Fifty Years of Penicillin Application: History and Trends. Prague: Public Ltd., 1994:47–53.
3.   Baldwin JE, Schofield C. The biosynthesis of β-lactams. Page MI, ed. The Chemistry of β-Lactams. London: Blackie Academic and Professional, 1992:1–78.
4.   Baldwin J. Studies on the synthesis of penicillin—isopenicillin N synthase (IPNS). Kleinkauf H, von Döhren H, eds. Fifty Years of Penicillin Application: History and Trends. Prague: Public Ltd., 1994:151–169.
5.   Aharonowitz Y, Cohen G, Martin JF. Penicillin and cephalosporin biosynthetic genes: Structure, organization, regulation and evolution. Annu Rev Microbiol 1992; 46:461–496.
6.   Martin JF, Coque JJR, Gutierrez S, Barredo JL, Diez B, Montenegro E, Calzada JG, Liras P. Clusters of genes involved in penicillin and cephalosporin biosynthesis. Kleinkauf H, von Döhren H, eds. Fifty Years of Penicillin Application: History and Trends. Prague: Public Ltd., 1994:97–114.
7.   Jensen SE, Demain AL. Beta-Lactams. Vining LC, Stuttard C, eds. Genetics and Biochemistry of Antibiotic Biosynthesis. Stoneham, Massachusettes: Butterworth-Heinemann, 1994:239–268.

8. Bhattarcharjee JK. α-Aminoadipate pathway for the biosynthesis of lysine in lower eukaryotes. Crit Rev Microbiol 1985; 12:131–151.

9. Luengo JM, Revilla G, Lopez MJ, Villanueva JR, Martin JF. Inhibition and repression of homocitrate synthase by lysine in *Penicillium chrysogenum*. J Bacteriol 1980; 144:869–876.

10. Umbarger H. Amino acid biosynthesis and its regulation. Annu Rev Biochem 1978; 47:533–606.

11. Vining LC, Shapiro S, Madduri K, Stuttard C Biosynthesis and control of β-lactam antibiotics: The early steps in the "classical" tripeptide pathway. Biotech Adv 1990; 8:159–183.

12. Kern BA, Hendlin D, Inamine E. L-Lysine ε-aminotransferase involved in cephamycin C synthesis in *Streptomyces lactamdurans*. Antimicrob Agents Chemother 1980; 17:676–685.

13. Madduri K, Stuttard C, Vining LC. Lysine catabolism in *Streptomyces* spp. is primarily through cadaverine: β-Lactam producers also make α-aminoadipate. J Bacteriol 1989; 171:299–302.

14. Madduri K, Stuttard C, Vining LC. Cloning and location of a gene governing lysine ε-aminotransferase, an enzyme initiating β-lactam biosynthesis in *Streptomyces* spp. J Bacteriol 1991; 173:985–988.

15. Tobin MB, Kovacevic S, Madduri K, Hoskins JA, Skatrud PL, Vining LC, Stuttard C, Miller JR. Localization of lysine ε-amino-transferase (lat) and δ-(L-α-aminoadipyl)-L-cysteinyl-D-valine (ACV) synthetase (pcbAB) genes from *Streptomyces clavuligerus* and production of lysine ε-aminotransferase activity in *Escherichia coli*. J Bacteriol 1991; 173:6223–6229.

16. Coque JJR, Liras P, Laiz L, Martin JF. A gene encoding lysine 6-aminotransferase, which forms the β-lactam precursor α-aminoadipic acid, is located in the cluster of cephamycin biosynthetic genes in *Nocardia lactamdurans*. J Bacteriol 1991; 173:6258–6264.

17. Esmahan C, Alvarez E, Montenegro E, Martin JF. Catabolism of lysine in *Penicillium* leads to formation of 2-aminoadipic acid, a precursor of penicillin biosynthesis. Appl Environ Microbiol 1994; 60:1705–1710.

18. Smith DJ, Earl AJ, Turner G. The multifunctional peptide synthetase performing the first step in penicillin biosynthesis in *Penicillium chrysogenum* is a 421,037 dalton protein similar to *Bacillus brevis* peptide antibiotic synthetase. EMBO J 1990; 9:2743–2750.

19. Diez B, Gutierrez S, Barredo JL, van Soligen P, van der Voort LHM, Martin JF. The cluster of penicillin biosynthetic genes: Identification and characterization of the pcbAB gene encoding the (α-aminoadipyl)-L-cysteinyl-D-valine synthetase and linkage to the pcbC and penDE genes. J Biol Chem 1990; 265:16358–16365.

20. Gutierrez S, Diez B, Montenegro E, Martin JF. Characterization of the *Cephalosporium acremonium* pcbAB gene encoding α-aminoadipylcysteinyl-valine synthetase, a large multidomain peptide synthetase: Linkage to the pcbC gene as a cluster of early cephalosporin-biosynthetic genes and evidence of multiple functional domains. J Bacteriol 1991; 173:2354–2365.

21. MacCabe AP, van Liempt H, Palissa H, Unkles S, Riach MBR, Pfeifer E, von Döhren H, Kinghorn JR. δ-(L-α-Aminoadipyl)-L-cysteinyl-D-valine synthetase from *Aspergillus nidulans*: Molecular characterization of the acvA gene encoding the first enzyme of the penicillin biosynthetic pathway. J Biol Chem 1991; 266:12646–12654.

22. Coque JJR, Martin JF, Calzada FG, Liras P. The cephamycin biosynthetic genes pcbAB, encoding a large multidomain peptide synthetase, and pcbB of *Nocardia lactamdurans* are clustered together in organization different from the same genes in *Acremonium chrysogenum* and *Penicillium chrysogenum*. Mol Microbiol 1991; 5:1125–1133.

23. Doran JL, Leskiw BK, Petrich AK, Westlake DWS, Jensen SE. Production of *Streptomyces clavuligerus* isopenicillin N synthase in *Escherichia coli* using two-cistron expression systems. J Indust Microbiol 1990; 5:197–206.

24. Yu H, Serpe E, Romero J, Coque JJ, Maeda K, Oelgeschlager M, Hintermann G, Liras P, Martin JF, Demain AL, Piret J. Possible involvement of the lysine ε-aminotransferase gene (lat) in the expression of the genes encoding ACV synthetase (pcbAB) and isopenicillin N synthetase (pcbC) in *Streptomyces clavuligerus*. Microbiol 1994; 140:3367–3377.

25. Aharonowitz Y, Bergmeyer J, Cantoral JM, Cohen G, Demain AL, Fink U, Kinghorn J, Kleinkauf H, MacCabe A, Palissa H, Pfeifer E, Schwecke T, van Liempt H, von Döhren H, Wofe S, Zhang J. δ-(L-α-aminoadipyl)-L-cysteinyl-D-valine synthetase, the multienzyme integrating four primary reactions in β-lactam biosynthesis, as a model peptide synthetase. Bio/Technol 1993; 11:807–810.

26. Krause M, Marahiel MA. Organization of the biosynthesis genes for the peptide antibiotic gramicidin S. J Bacteriol 1988; 170:4669–4674.

27. Mittenhuber G, Weckermann R, Marahiel MA. Gene cluster containing the genes for tyrocidine synthetase 1 and 2 from *Bacillus brevis*: Evidence for an operon. J Bacteriol 1989; 171:4881–4887.

28. Kleinkauf H, von Döhren H. Biosynthesis of peptide antibiotics. Annu Rev Microbiol 1987; 41:259–289.

29. Dittman J, Wenger RM, Kleinkauf H, Lawen A. Mechanism of cyclosporin A biosynthesis. Evidence for synthesis via a single linear undecapeptide precursor. J Biol Chem 1994; 269:2841–2846.

30. Cohen G, Shiffman D, Mevarech M, Aharonowitz Y. Microbial isopenicillin N synthase genes: Structure, function, diversity and evolution. Trends Biotechnol 1990; 8:105–111.

31. Leskiw BK, Aharonowitz Y, Mevarech M, Wolfe S, Vining LC, Westlake DWS, Jensen SE. Cloning and nucleotide sequence determination of the isopenicillin N synthetase gene from *Streptomyces clavuligerus*. Gene 1988; 62:187–196.

32. Shiffman D, Cohen G, Aharonowitz Y, Palissa H, von Döhren H, Kleinkauf H, Mevarech M. Nucleotide sequence of the isopenicillin N synthase gene (pcbC) of the Gram negative *Flavobacterium* sp. SC 12,154. Nucl Acids Res 1990; 18:660.

33. Shiffman D, Mevarech M, Jensen SE, Cohen G, Aharonowitz Y. Cloning and comparative sequence analysis of the gene coding for isopenicillin N synthase in *Streptomyces*. Mol Gen Genet 1988; 214:562–569.

34. Garcia-Dominguez M, Liras P, Martin JF. Cloning and characterization of the isopenicillin N synthase gene of *Streptomyces griseus* NRRL 3851 and studies of expression and complementation of the cephamycin pathway in *Streptomyces clavuligerus*. Antimicrob Agents Chemother 1991; 35:44–52.

35. Kimura H, Izawa M, Sumino Y. Molecular analysis of the gene cluster involved in cephalosporin biosynthesis from *Lysobacter lactamgenes* YK90. Appl Microbiol Biotechnol 1996; 44:589–596.

36. Samson SM, Belagaje R, Blankenship DT, Chapman JL, Perry D, Skatrud PL, VanFrank RM, Abraham EP, Baldwin JE, Queener SW, Ingolia TD. Isolation, sequence determination and expression in *Escherichia coli* of the isopenicillin N synthetase gene from *Cephalosporium acremonium*. Nature 1985; 318:191–194.

37. Barredo JL, Cantoral JM, Alvarez E, Diez B, Martin JF. Cloning, sequence analysis and transcriptional study of the isopenicillin N synthase of *Penicillium chrysogenum* AS-P-78. Mol Gen Genet 1989; 216:91–98.

38. Carr LG, Skatrud PL, Scheetz ME, Queener SW, Ingolia TD. Cloning and expression of the isopenicillin N synthetase gene from *Penicillium chrysogenum*. Gene 1986; 48:257–266.

39. Ramon D, Carramolino L, Patino C, Sanchez F, Peñalva MA. Cloning and characterization of the isopenicillin N synthetase gene mediating the formation of the β-lactam ring in *Aspergillus nidulans*. Gene 1987; 57:171–181.

40. Samson SM, Chapman JL, Belagaje R, Queener SW, Ingolia TD. Analysis of the role of cysteine residues in isopenicillin N synthetase activity by site-directed mutagenesis. Proc Natl Acad Sci USA 1987; 84:5705–5709.

41. Durairaj M, Leskiw BK, Jensen SE. Genetic and biochemical analysis of the cysteinyl residues of isopenicillin N synthase from *Streptomyces clavuligerus*. Can J Microbiol 1996 42:870–875.

42. Kriauciunas A, Frolik CA, Hassell TC, Skatrud PL, Johnson MG, Holbrook NL, Chen VJ. The functional role of cysteines in isopenicillin N synthase. J Biol Chem 1991; 266:11779–11788.

43. Chen VJ, Orville AM, Harpel MR, Frolik CA, Surerus KK, Munck E, Lipscomb JD. Spectroscopic studies of isopenicillin N synthase. J Biol Chem 1989; 264:21677–21681.

44. Orville AM, Chen VJ, Kriauciunas A, Harpel MR, Fox BG, Munck E, Lipscomb JD. Thiolate ligation of the active site Fe^{2+} of isopenicillin N synthase derives from substrate rather than endogenous cysteine: Spectroscopic studies of site specific Cys → Ser mutated enzymes. Biochem 1992; 31:4602–4612.

45. Scott RA, Wang S, Eidness MK, Kriauciunas A, Frolik CA, Chen VJ. X-ray absorption spectroscopic studies of the high-spin iron (II) active site of isopenicillin N synthase: Evidence for Fe-S interaction in the enzyme-substrate complex. Biochem 1992; 31:4596–4601.

46. Roach PL, Clifton IJ, Fulop V, Harlos K, Barton GJ, Hajdu J, Andersson I, Schofield CJ, Baldwin JE. Crystal structure of isopenicillin N synthase is the first from a new structural family of enzymes. Nature 1995; 375:700–704.

47. Tan DSH, Tiow-Suan S. Functional analysis of conserved histidine residues in *Cephalosporium acremonium* isopenicillin N synthase by site-directed mutagenesis. J Biol Chem 1996; 271:889–894.

48. Ramsden M, McQuade BA, Saunders K, Turner MK, Harford S. Characterization of a loss-of-function in the isopenicillin N synthetase gene of *Acremonium chrysogenum*. Gene 1989; 85:267–273.

49. Queener SW, Neuss N. The biosynthesis of β-lactam antibiotics. Moran EB, Morgan M, eds. The Chemistry and Biology of β-Lactam Antibiotics, Vol. 3. London: Academic Press, 1982:1–81.

50. Whiteman PA, Abraham EP, Baldwin JE, Fleming MD, Schofield CJ, Sutherland JD, Willis AC. Acyl-coenzyme A:6-aminopenicillanic acid acyltransferase from *Penicillium chrysogenum* and *Aspergillus nidulans*. FEBS Lett 1990; 262:342–344.

51. Tobin MB, Fleming MD, Skatrud PL, Miller JR. Molecular characterization of the acyl-coenzyme A:isopenicillin N acyltransferase gene (penDE) from *Penicillium chrysogenum* and *Aspergillus nidulans* and activity of recombinant enzyme in *Escherichia coli*. J Bacteriol 1990; 172:5908–5914.

52. Barredo JL, van Soligen P, Diez B, Alvarez E, Cantoral JM, Kattevilder A, Smaal EB, Groenen MAM, Veenstra AE, Martin JF. Cloning and characterization of acyl-CoA:6-APA acyltransferase gene of *Penicillium chrysogenum*. Gene 1989; 83:291–300.

53. Montenegro E, Barredo JL, Gutierrez S, Diez B, Alvarez E, Martin JF. Cloning, characterization of the acyl-CoA:6-amino penicillanic acid acyltransferase gene of *Aspergillus nidulans* and linkage to the isopenicillin N synthase gene. Mol Gen Genet 1990; 221:322–330.

54. Aplin RT, Baldwin JE, Cole SCJ, Sutherland JD, Tobin MB. On the production of α,β-heterodimeric acyl-coenzyme A:isopenicillin N acyltransferase of *Penicillin chrysogenum*: Studies using a recombinant source. FEBS Lett 1993; 319:166–170.

55. Tobin MB, Cole SC, Miller JR, Baldwin JE, Sutherland JD. Amino acid substitutions in the cleavage site of acyl coenzyme A: isopenicillin N acyl transferase from *Penicillium chrysogenum*. Gene 1995; 162:29–35.

56. Tobin MB, Baldwin JE, Cole SCJ, Miller JR, Skatrud PL, Sutherland JD. The requirement for subunit interaction in the production of *Penicillium chrysogenum* acyl-coenzyme A:isopenicillin N acyltransferase in *Escherichia coli*. Gene 1993; 132:199–206.

57. Fernandez FJ, Gutierrez S, Velasco J, Montenegro E, Marcos AT, Martin JF. Molecular characterization of three loss-of-function mutations in the isopenicillin N–acyltransferase gene (penDE) of *Penicillium chrysogenum*. J Bacteriol 1994; 176:4941–4948.

58. Tobin MB, Cole SCJ, Kovacevic S, Miller JR, Baldwin JE, Sutherland JD. Acyl-coenzyme A:isopenicillin N acyltransferase from *Penicillium chrysogenum*: Effect of amino acid substitutions at Ser^{227}, Ser^{230} and Ser^{309} on proenzyme cleavage and activity. FEMS Microbiol Lett 1994; 121:39–46.

59. Jayatilake S, Huddleston JA, Abraham EP. Conversion of isopenicillin N into penicillin N in cell-free extracts of *Cephalosporium acremonium*. Biochem J 1981; 194:645–647.

60. Jensen SE, Westlake DWS, Wolfe S. Partial purification and characterization of isopenicillin N epimerase activity from *Streptomyces clavuligerus*. Can J Microbiol 1983; 29:1526–1531.

61. Usui S, Yu CA. Purification and properties of isopenicillin N epimerase from *Streptomyces clavuligerus*. Biochim Biophys Acta 1989; 999:78–85.

62. Laiz L, Liras P, Castro JM, Martin JF. Purification and characterization of the isopenicillin N epimerase from *Nocordia lactamdurans*. J Gen Microbiol 1990; 136:663–671.

63. Kovacevic S, Tobin MB, Miller JR. The β-lactam biosynthesis genes for isopenicillin N epimerase and deacetoxycephalosporin C synthetase are expressed from a single transcript in *Streptomyces clavuligerus*. J Bacteriol 1990; 172:3952–3958.

64. Coque JJ, Martin JF, Liras P. Characterization and expression in *Streptomyces lividans* of cefD and cefF genes from *Nocordia lactamdurans*: The organization of the cephamycin gene cluster differs from that in *Streptomyces clavuligerus*. Mol Gen Genet 1993; 236:453–458.

65. Scheidegger A, Kuenzi MT, Nuesch J. Partial purification and catalytic properties of a bifunctional enzyme in the biosynthetic pathway of β-lactams in *Cephalosporium acremonium*. J Antibiot 1984; 37:522–531.

66. Dotzlaf JE, Yeh WK. Copurification and characterization of deacetoxycephalosporin C synthetase/hydroxylase from *Cephalosporium acremonium*. J Bacteriol 1987; 169:1611–618.

67. Samson SM, Dotzlaf JE, Slisz ML, Becker GW, van Frank RM, Veal LE, Yeh W, Miller JR, Queener SW, Ingolia TD. Cloning and expression of the fungal expandase/hydroxylase gene involved in cephalosporin biosynthesis. Bio/Technol 1987; 5:1207–1216.

68. Jensen SE, Westlake DWS, Wolfe S. Deacetoxycephalosporin C synthetase and deacetoxycephalosporin C hydroxylase are two separate enzymes in *Streptomyces clavuligerus*. J Antibiot 1985; 38:263–265.

69. Kovacevic S, Weigel BJ, Tobin MB, Ingolia TD, Miller JR. Cloning, characterization, and expression in *Escherichia coli* of the *Streptomyces clavuligerus* gene encoding deacetoxycephalosporin C synthetase. J Bacteriol 1989; 171:754–756.

70. Kovacevic S, Miller JR. Cloning and sequencing of the β-lactam hydroxylase gene (cefF) from *Streptomyces clavuligerus*: Gene duplication may have led to separate hydroxylase and expandase activities in the actinomycetes. J Bacteriol 1991; 173:398–400.

71. Coque JJR, Enguita FJ, Cardoza RE, Martin JF. Characterization of the cefF gene of *Nocardia lacamdurans* encoding a 3′-methylcephem hydroxylase different from the 7-cephem hydroxylase. Appl Microbiol Biotechnol 1996; 44:605–609.

72. Gutierrez S, Velasco J, Fernandez FJ, Martin JF. The cefG gene of *Cephalosporium acremonium* is linked to the cefEF gene and encodes a deacetylcephalosporin C acetyltransferase closely related to homoserine O-acetyltransferase. J Bacteriol 1992; 174:3056–3064.

73. O'Sullivan J, Abraham EP. The conversion of cephalosporins to 7-α-methoxycephalosporins by cell-free extracts of *Streptomyces clavuligerus*. Biochem J 1980; 186:613–616.

74. Nozaki Y, Okonogi K, Katayama N, Ono H, Harada S, Kondo M, Okazaki H. Cephabacins, new cephem antibiotics of bacterial origin. 4. Antibacterial activities, stability to β-lactamases and mode of action. J Antibiot (Tokyo) 1984; 37:1528–1535.

75. Brewer SJ, Taylor PM, Turner MK. An adenosine triphosphate-dependent carbamoyl-phosphate-3-hydroxymethylcephem-O-carbamoyltransferase from *Streptomyces clavuligerus*. Biochem J 1980; 185:555–564.

76. Coque JJR, Llarena FJP, Enguita FJ, De La Fuente JL, Martin JF, Liras P. Characterization of the cmcH genes of *Nocardia lactamdurans* and *Streptomyces clavuligerus* encoding a functional 3′-hydroxymethyl cephem O-carbamoyltransferase for cephamycin biosynthesis. Gene 1995; 162:21–27.

77. Xiao X, Wolfe S, Demain AL. Purification and characterization of cephalosporin 7-α-hydroxylase from *Streptomyces clavuligerus*. Biochem J 1991; 280:471–474.

78. Coque JJR, Enguita FJ, Martin JF, Liras P. A two-protein component 7-α-cephem-methoxylase encoded by two genes of the cephamycin C cluster converts cephalosporin C to 7-methoxycephalosporin C. J Bacteriol 1995; 177:2230–2235.

79. Xiao X, Hintermann G, Hausler A, Barker PJ, Foor F, Demain AL, Piret J. Cloning of a *Streptomyces clavuligerus* DNA fragment encoding the cephalosporin 7-α-hydroxylase and its expression in *Streptomyces lividans*. Antimicrob Agents Chemother 1993; 37:84–88.

80. Gordon EM, Sykes RB. Cephamycin antibiotics. Morin RB, Gorman M, eds. Chemistry and Biology of β-Lactam Antibiotics. New York: Academic Press, 1982:199–364.

81. Frere JM, Nguyen-Disteche M, Coyette J, Joris B. Mode of action: Interaction with the penicillin binding proteins. Page MI, ed. The Chemistry of β-Lactams. Glasgow: Blackie Academic and Professional, Chapman and Hall, 1992:148–197.

82. Cundliffe E. How antibiotic-producing organisms avoid suicide. Annu Rev Microbiol 1989; 43:207–234.

83. Ogawara H. Antibiotic resistance in pathogenic and producing bacteria with special reference to β-lactam antibiotics. Microbiol Rev 1981; 45:591–619.

84. Forsman M, Haggstrom B, Lindgren L, Jaurin B. Molecular analysis of β-lactamases from four species of *Streptomyces*: Comparison of amino acid sequences with those of other β-lactamases. J Gen Microbiol 1990; 136:589–598.

85. Nakazawa H, Horikawa S, Ogawara H. Penicillin-binding proteins in *Streptomyces* strains. J Antibiot 1981; 34:1070–1072.

86. Horikawa S, Nakazawa H, Ogawara H. Penicillin-binding proteins in *Streptomyces cacaoi* and *Streptomyces clavuligerus*. J Antibiot 1980; 33:1362–1368.

87. Coque JJR, Liras P, Martin JF. Genes for a β-lactamase, a penicillin-binding protein and a transmembrane protein are clustered with the cephamycin biosynthetic genes in *Nocardia lactamdurans*. EMBO J 1993; 12:631–639.

88. Reading C, Cole M. Clavulanic acid: A beta-lactamase-inhibiting beta-lactam from *Streptomyces clavuligerus*. Antimicrob Agents Chemother 1977; 11:852–857.

89. Doran JL, Leskiw BL, Aippersbach S, Jensen SE. Isolation and characterization of a β-lactamase inhibitory protein from *Streptomyces clavuligerus* and cloning and analysis of the corresponding gene. J Bacteriol 1990; 172:4909–4918.

90. Jensen SE, Alexander DC, Paradkar AS, Aidoo KA. Extending the β-lactam biosynthetic gene cluster in *Streptomyces clavuligerus*. Baltz RH, Hegeman GD, Skatrud PL, eds. Industrial Microorganisms: Basic and Applied Molecular Genetics. Washington, D.C.: American Society for Microbiology, 1993:169–176.

91. Martin JF, Liras P. Organization and expression of genes involved in the biosynthesis of antibiotics and other secondary metabolites. Annu Rev Microbiol 1989; 43:173–206.

92. Chater KF. The improving prospects for yield increase by genetic engineering in antibiotic-producing streptomycetes. Bio/Technol 1990; 8:115–121.

93. Martin JF. Clusters of genes for the biosynthesis of antibiotics: Regulatory genes and overproduction of pharmaceuticals. J Ind Microbiol 1992; 9:73–90.

94. Petrich AK, Leskiw BK, Paradkar AS, Jensen SE. Transcriptional mapping of the genes encoding the early enzymes of the cephamycin biosynthetic pathway of *Streptomyces clavuligerus*. Gene 1994; 142:41–48.

95. Petrich AK, Wu X, Roy KL, Jensen SE. Transcriptional analysis of the isopenicillin N synthase–encoding gene of *Streptomyces clavuligerus*. Gene 1992; 111:77–84.

96. Kovacevic S, Tobin MB, Miller JR. Linkage of β-lactam biosynthetic genes in *Streptomyces clavuligerus*: Cloning and transcriptional studies. Kleinkauf H, von Döhren H, eds. Fifty Years of Penicillin Application: History and Trends. Prague: Public Ltd., 1994:132–134.

97. Smith DJ, Burnham MKR, Bull JH, Hodgson JE, Ward JM, Brown P, Brown J, Barton B, Earl AJ, Turner G. β-Lactam antibiotic biosynthetic genes have been conserved in clusters in procaryotes and eucaryotes. EMBO J 1990; 9:741–747.

98. Queener SW. Molecular biology of penicillin and cephalosporin biosynthesis. Antimicrob Agents Chemother 1990; 34:943–948.

99. Ward JM, Hodgson JE. The biosynthetic genes for clavulanic acid and cephamycin production occur as a "super cluster" in three *Streptomyces*. FEMS Microbiol Lett 1993; 110:239–242.

100. Hutchinson CR. Anthracyclines. Vining LC, Stuttard C. eds. Genetics and Biochemistry of Antibiotic Production. Toronto: Butterworth-Heinemann, 1995:331–357.

101. Han L, Yang K, Ramalingam E, Mosher RH, Vining LC. Cloning and characterization of polyketide synthase genes for jadomycin B biosynthesis in *Streptomyces venezuelae* ISP5230. Microbiology 1994; 140:3379–3389.

102. Piepersberg W. Streptomycin and related aminoglycosides. Vining LC, Stuttard C, eds. Genetics and Biochemistry of Antibiotic Production. Toronto: Butterworth-Heinemann, 1995:531–570.

103. Fierro F, Gutiérrez S, Díez B, Martín JF. Resolution of four large chromosomes in penicillin-producing fungi: The penicillin gene cluster is located on chromosome II (9.6 Mb) in *Penicillium notatum* and chromosome I (10.4 Mb) in *Penicillium chrysogenum*. Mol Gen Genet 1993; 241:573–578.

104. Smith AW, Ramsden M, Dobson MJ, Harford S, Peberdy JF. Regulation of isopenicillin N synthetase (IPNS) gene expression in *Acremonium chrysogenum*. Bio/Technol 1990; 8:237–240.

105. Velasco J, Gutierrez S, Fernandez FJ, Marcos AT, Arenos C, Martin JF. Exogenous methionine increases levels of mRNAs transcribed from pcbAB, pcbC and cefEF genes, encoding enzymes of the cephalosporin biosynthetic pathway in *Acremonium chrysogenum*. J Bacteriol 1994; 176:985–991.

106. MacCabe AP, Riach MBR, Unkles SE, Kinghorn JR. The *Aspergillus nidulans* npeA locus consists of three contiguous genes required for penicillin biosynthesis. EMBO J 1989; 9:279–287.

107. Diez B, Barredo JL, Alvarez E, Cantoral JM, van Solingen P, Van der Voort LMH, Martin JF. Two genes involved in penicillin biosynthesis are linked in a 5.1 kb SalI fragment in the genome of *Penicillium chrysogenum*. Mol Genet Genet 1989; 218:572–576.

108. Skatrud PL, Queener SW. An electrophoretic molecular karyotype for an industrial strain of *Cephalosporium acremonium*. Gene 1989; 78:331–338.

109. Mathison L, Soliday C, Stepan T, Aldrich T, Rambosek J. Cloning, characterization, and use in strain improvement of the *Cephalosporium acremonium* gene cefG encoding acetyltransferase. Curr Genet 1993; 23:33–41.

110. Weigel BJ, Burgett SG, Chen VJ, Skatrud PL, Frolik CA, Queener SW, Ingolia TD. Cloning and expression in *Escherichia coli* of isopenicillin N synthetase genes from *Streptomyces lipmanii* and *Aspergillus nidulans*. J Bacteriol 1988; 170:3817–3826.

111. Miller JR, Ingolia TD. Cloning and characterization of beta-lactam biosynthetic genes. Mol Microbiol 1989; 3:689–695.

112. Peñalva MA, Moya A, Dopaza J, Ramon D. Sequences of isopenicillin N synthetase genes suggest horizontal gene transfer from prokaryotes to eukaryotes. Proc R Soc London Ser 1990; 241:164–169.

113. Peñalva MA, Espeso E, Orejas M, Gomez-Pardo E. Evolution and control of gene expression of the *Aspergillus nidulans* isopenicillin N synthase gene. Kleinkauf H, von Döhren H, eds. Fifty Years of Penicillin Application: History and Trends. Prague: Public Ltd., 1994:224–230.

114. Skatrud PL, Tobin MB, Miller JR, Kovacevic S, Hoskins J, Queener SW, Ingolia TD. Evidence for horizontal transfer in the evolution of the beta-lactam biosynthetic pathway. Kleinkauf H, von Döhren H, eds. Fifty Years of Penicillin Application: History and Trends. Prague: Public Ltd., 1994:231–232.

115. Demain AL, Aharonowitz Y, Martin JF. Metabolic control of secondary biosynthetic pathways. Vining LC, ed. Biochemistry and Genetic Regulation of Commercially Important Antibiotics. Reading, Massachusetts: Addison-Wesley, 1983:49–72.

116. Hawley DK, McClure WR. Compilation and analysis of *Escherichia coli* promoter DNA sequences. Nucl Acids Res 1983; 11:2237–2255.

117. Strohl W. Compilation and analysis of DNA sequences associated with apparent strepto-mycete promoters. Nucl Acids Res 1992; 20:961–974.

118. Perez-Esteban B, Orejas M, Gomez-Pardo E, Peñalva MA. Molecular characterization of a fungal secondary metabolism promoter: Transcription of the *Aspergillus nidulans* isopenicillin N synthetase gene is modulated by upstream negative elements. Mol Microbiol 1993; 9:881–895.

119. Litzka O, Bergh KT, Brakhage AA. Analysis of the regulation of the *Aspergillus nidulans* penicillin biosynthesis gene aat (penDE), which encodes acyl coenzyme A:6-aminopenicil-lanic acid acyltransferase. Mol Gen Genet 1995; 249:557–569.

120. Peñalva MA, Vian A, Patino C, Perez-Aranda A, Ramon D. Molecular biology of penicillin production in *Aspergillus nidulans*. Hershberger CL, Queener SW, Hegeman G, eds. Genetics and Molecular Biology of Industrial Microorganisms. Washington, D.C.: American Society for Microbiology, 1989:256–261.

121. Brakhage AA, Browne P, Turner G. Regulation of *Aspergillus nidulans* penicillin biosynthesis and penicillin biosynthesis genes acvA and ipnA by glucose. J Bacteriol 1992; 174:3789–3799.

122. Espeso EA, Peñalva MA. Carbon catabolite repression can account for the temporal pattern of expression of a penicillin biosynthetic gene in *Aspergillus nidulans*. Mol Microbiol 1992; 6:1457–1465.

123. Espeso EA, Tilburn J, Arst HN Jr, Peñalva MA. pH regulation is a major determinant in expression of a fungal penicillin biosynthetic gene. EMBO J 1993; 12:3947–3956.

124. Tilburn J, Sarkar S, Widdick DA, Espeso EA, Orejas M, Mungroo J, Peñalva MA, Arst HN. The *Aspergillus* PacC zinc finger transcription factor mediates regulation of both acid- and alkaline-expressed genes by ambient pH. EMBO J 1995; 14:779–790.

125. Haas H, Marzluf GA. NRE, the major nitrogen regulatory protein of *Penicillium chrysogenum*, binds specifically to elements in the intergenic promoter regions of nitrate assimilation and penicillin biosynthetic gene clusters. Curr Genet 1995; 28:177–183.

126. Perez-Esteban B, Gomez-Pardo E, Peñalva MA. A lacZ reporter fusion method for the genetic analysis of regulatory mutations in pathways of fungal secondary metabolism and its applications to the *Aspergillus nidulans* penicillin pathway. J Bacteriol 1995; 177:6069–6076.

127. Brakhage AA, Den Brulle JV. Use of reporter genes to identify recessive trans-acting muta-tions specifically involved in the regulation of *Aspergillus nidulans* penicillin biosynthesis genes. J Bacteriol 1995; 177:2781–2788.

128. Bergh KT, Litzka O, Brakhage AA. Identification of a major cis-acting DNA element con-trolling the bidirectionally transcribed penicillin biosynthesis genes acvA (pcbAB) and ipnA (pcbC) of *Aspergillus nidulans*. J Bacteriol 1996; 178:3908–3916.

129. Cantoral JM, Gutierrez S, Fierro F, Gil-Espinosa S, van Liempt, Martin JF. Biochemical char-acterization and molecular genetics of nine mutants of *Penicillium chrysogenum* impaired in penicillin biosynthesis. J Biol Chem 1993; 268:737–744.

130. Wanning M, Zahner H, Krone B, Zeeck A. Ein neues antifungisches β-lactam antibioticum der clavam-reihe. Tetrahedron Lett 1981; 22:2539–2540.

131. Rohl F, Rabenhorst J, Zahner H. Biological properties and mode of action of clavams. Arch Microbiol 1987; 147:315–320.

132. Muller JC, Toome V, Pruess DL, Blount JF, Weigele M. Ro 22-5417, a new clavam antibiotic from *Streptomyces clavuligerus*. III. Absolute stereochemistry. J Antibiot 1983; 36:217–225.

133. Valentine BP, Bailey CR, Doherty A, Morris J, Elson SW, Baggaley KH, Nicholson NH. Evi-dence that arginine is a later metabolic intermediate than ornithine in the biosynthesis of clavulanic acid by *Streptomyces clavuligerus*. J Chem Soc Chem Commun 1993:1210–1211.

134. Townsend CA, Ho MF. Biosynthesis of clavulanic acid: Origin of the C3 unit. J Am Chem Soc 1985; 107:1066–1068.

135. Elson SW, Baggaley KH, Fulston M, Nicholson NH, Tyler JW, Edwards J, Holms H, Hamil-ton I, Mousdale DM. Two novel arginine derivatives from a mutant of *Streptomyces clavuligerus*. J Chem Soc Chem Commun 1993:1211–1212.

136. Elson SW, Baggaley KH, Davison M, Fulston M, Nicholson NH, Risbridger GD, Tyler JW. The identification of three new biosynthetic intermediates and one further biosynthetic enzyme in the clavulanic acid pathway. J Chem Soc Chem Commun 1993:1212–1214.

137. Baldwin JE, Adlington RM, Bryans JS, Bringhen O, Coates JB, Crouch NP, Lloyd MD, Schofield CJ, Elson SW, Baggaley KH, Cassels R, Nicholson N. Isolation of dihydro-clavaminic acid, an intermediate in the biosynthesis of clavulanic acid. Tetrahedron 1991; 47:4089–4100.

138. Townsend CA, Krol WJ. The role of molecular oxygen in clavulanic acid biosynthesis: Evidence for a bacterial oxidative deamination. J Chem Soc Chem Commun 1988:1234–1236.

139. Iwata-Reuyl D, Townsend CA. Common origin of clavulanic acid and other clavam metabolites in *Streptomyces*. J Am Chem Soc 1992; 114:2762–2763.

140. Janc JW, Egan LA, Townsend CA. Emerging evidence for a shared biosynthetic pathway among clavulanic acid and the structurally diverse clavam metabolites. Bioorg Med Chem Lett 1993; 3:2313–2316.

141. Elson SW, Baggaley KH, Gillett J, Holland S, Nicholson NH, Sime JT, Woroniecki SR. Isolation of two novel intracellular β-lactams and a novel dioxygenase cyclising enzyme from *Streptomyces clavuligerus*. J Chem Soc Chem Commun 1987:1736–1738.

142. Salowe SP, Marsh EN, Townsend CA. Purification and characterization of clavaminate synthase from *Streptomyces clavuligerus*: An unusual oxidative enzyme in natural product biosynthesis. Biochem 1990; 29:6499–6508.

143. Baldwin JE, Fujishma Y, Goh KC, Schofield CJ. Enzymes of valclavam biosynthesis. Tetrahedron Lett 1994; 35:2783–2786.

144. Janc JW, Egan LA, Townsend CA. Purification and characterization of clavaminate synthase from *Streptomyces antibioticus*. J Biol Chem 1995; 270:5399–5404.

145. Marsh EN, Chang MDT, Townsend CA. Two isozymes of clavaminate synthase central to clavulanic acid formation: Cloning and sequencing of both genes from *Streptomyces clavuligerus*. Biochem 1992; 31:12648–12657.

146. Bailey CR, Butler MJ, Normansell MJ, Rowlands ID, Winstanley DJ. Cloning a *Streptomyces clavuligerus* genetic locus involved in clavulanic acid biosynthesis. Bio/Technol 1985; 2:808–811.

147. Aidoo KA, Wong A, Alexander DC, Rittamer RA, Jensen SE. Cloning, sequencing and disruption of a gene from *Streptomyces clavuligerus* involved in clavulanic acid biosynthesis. Gene 1994; 147:41–46.

148. Aidoo KA, Paradkar AS, Alexander DC, Jensen SE. Use of recombinant DNA techniques to study the production of β-lactam compounds in *Streptomyces clavuligerus*. Gullo VP, Hunter-Cevera JC, Cooper R, Johnson RK, eds. Developments in Industrial Microbiology, Vol. 33. Fredricksburg, Virginia: Society of Industrial Microbiology, 1993:219–236.

149. Paradkar AS, Jensen SE. Functional analysis of the gene encoding the clavaminate synthase 2 isoenzyme involved in clavulanic acid biosynthesis in *Streptomyces clavuligerus*. J Bacteriol 1995; 177:1307–1314.

150. Hodgson JE, Fosberry AP, Rawlinson NS, Ross HNM, Neal RJ, Arnell JC, Earl AJ, Lawlor EJ. Clavulanic acid biosynthesis in *Streptomyces clavuligerus*: Gene cloning and characterization. Gene 1995; 166:49–55.

151. Elander RP, Chiang SJ. Genetics and antibiotic process improvement: From classical genetics to genetic engineering. Prokop A, Bajpai RK, Ho CS, eds. Recombinant DNA Technology and Applications. Toronto: McGraw-Hill, 1991:153–170.

152. Skatrud PL, Hoskins J, Wood JS, Tobin MB, Miller JR, Kovacevic S, Cantwell CA, Queener SW. Genetic manipulation of the β-lactam antibiotic biosynthetic pathway. Leatham GF, ed. Frontiers in Industrial Mycology. New York: Chapman and Hall, 1992:40–53.

153. Skatrud PL. Genetic engineering of β-lactam antibiotic biosynthetic pathways in filamentous fungi. TIBTECH 1992; 10:324–329.

154. Yeh WK, Queener SW. Potential industrial use of cephalosporin biosynthetic enzymes and genes: An overview. Ann NY Acad Sci 1990; 613:128–141.

155. Vichitsoonthonkul T, Chu YW, Sodhi HS, Saunders G. β-Lactam antibiotics produced by genetically engineered filamentous fungi. Murooka Y, Imanaka T, eds. Recombinant Microbes for Industrial and Agricultural Applications. New York: Marcel Dekker, 1994:119–135.

156. Malmberg L-H, Sherman DH, Hu W-S. Analysis of rate-limiting reactions in cephalosporin biosynthesis. Ann NY Acad Sci 1992; 665:16–26.

157. Wolfe S, Demain AL, Jensen SE, Westlake DWS. Enzymatic approach to synthesis of unnatural beta-lactams. Science 1984; 226:1386–1392.

158. Skatrud PL, Tietz AJ, Ingolia TD, Cantwell CA, Fisher DL, Chapman JL, Queener SW. Use of recombinant DNA to improve production of cephalosporin C by Cephalosporium acremonium. Bio/Technol 1989; 7:477–485.

159. Veenstra AE, van Solingen P, Huininga-Muurling H, Koekman BP, Groenen MAM, Smaal EB, Kattevilder A, Alvarez E, Barredo JL, Martín JF. Cloning of penicillin biosynthetic genes. Hershberger CL, Queener SW, Hegeman G, eds. Genetics and Molecular Biology of Industrial Microorganisms. Washington, D.C.: American Society for Microbiology, 1989:262–269.

160. Veenstra AE, Bovenberg RAL, van Solingen P, Müller WH, van der Voort LHM. The acyl-transferase of Penicillium chrysogenum: Characterization of the enzyme and use of its gene in strain improvement. Kleinkauf H, von Döhren H, eds. Fifty Years of Penicillin Application: History and Trends. Prague: Public Ltd., 1994:188–198.

161. Beckmann R, Cantwell C, Whiteman P, Queener SW, Abraham EP. Production of deacetoxycephalosporin C by transformants of Penicillium chrysogenum: Antibiotic biosynthetic pathway engineering. Baltz RH, Hegeman GD, Skatrud PL, eds. Industrial Microorganisms: Basic and Applied Molecular Genetics. Washington, D.C.: American Society for Microbiology, 1993:177–182.

162. Cantwell C, Beckmann R, Whiteman P, Queener SW, Abraham EP. Isolation of deacetoxycephalosporin C from fermentation broths of Penicillium chrysogenum transformants: Construction of a new fungal biosynthetic pathway. Proc R Soc Lond B 1992; 248:283–289.

163. Cantwell CA, Beckmann RJ, Dotzlaf JE, Fisher DL, Skatrud PL, Yeh W-K, Queener, SW. Cloning and expression of a hybrid Streptomyces clavuligerus cefE gene in Penicillium chrysogenum. Curr Genet 1990; 17:213–221.

164. Queener SW, Beckmann RJ, Cantwell CA, Hodges RL, Fisher DL, Dotzlaf JE, Yeh W-K, McGilvray D, Greaney M, Rosteck P. Improved expression of a hybrid Streptomyces clavuligerus cefE gene in Penicillium chrysogenum. Ann NY Acad Sci 1994; 721:178–193.

165. Matsumoto K. Bioconversion of penicillins and cephalosporins with biocatalysts. Kleinkauf H, von Döhren H, eds. Fifty Years of Penicillin Application: History and Trends. Prague: Public Ltd., 1994:276–286.

166. Isogai T, Fukagawa M, Aramori I, Iwami M, Kojo H, Ono T, Ueda Y, Kohsaka M, Imanaka H. Construction of a 7-aminocephalosporanic acid (7ACA) biosynthetic operon and direct production of 7ACA in Acremonium chrysogenum. Bio/Technol 1991; 9:188–191.

167. Crawford L, Stepan AM, McAda PC, Rambosek JA, Conder MJ, Vinci VA, Reeves CD. Production of cephalosporin intermediates by feeding adipic acid to recombinant Penicillium chrysogenum strains expressing ring expansion activity. Bio/Technol 1995; 13:58–62.

168. Maeda K, Luengo JM, Ferrero O, Wolfe S, Lebedev MY, Fang A, Demain AL. The substrate specificity of deacetoxycephalosporin C synthase ("expandase") of Streptomyces clavuligerus is extremely narrow. Enz Microbiol Technol 1995, 17:231–234.

9
Biosynthesis of Cyclosporins

René Traber

Novartis Pharma, Inc., Basel, Switzerland

I. INTRODUCTION

Cyclosporins, produced as secondary metabolites by various fungi imperfecti and a few ascomycetes, represent a class of neutral cyclic peptides that are composed of 11 aliphatic hydrophobic amino acids. Cyclosporins exert remarkable biological effects such as antifungal, antiparasitic, anti-inflammatory, and immunosuppressive activities (1).

Cyclosporin A (CyA), the main metabolite (Figure 1), specifically suppresses T-lymphocyte proliferation without affecting other immunological functions (3) and has proven to be the first selective immunosuppressive drug (4). It is in clinical use successfully worldwide under the trade name Sandimmun/Neoral to prevent allograft rejection in organ and bone marrow transplantations (5). Further indications for CyA include the treatment of various diseases originated by autoimmune disorders. The efficacy and the clinical benefit of CyA have been demonstrated for patients affected in the diseases rheumatoid arthritis, severe generalized chronic psoriasis, idiopathic nephrotic syndrome (hypoalbuminemia), and autoimmune uveitis (Behçet's disease); positive effects have also been described in cases of insulin-dependent diabetes mellitus (6,7). In some patients, especially when CyA is administrated in higher doses, renal dysfunction has been observed (8), but this side effect can be significantly reduced by careful drug monitoring (9).

In addition, CyA plays an important role as an investigational drug both in the field of multidrug resistance in cancer chemotherapy by restoring sensitivity of tumor cells to antineoplastic agents (10), and also against the human immune deficiency (HIV) virus by selectively inhibiting HIV-1 replication (11–13).

In the last few years, CyA has had—and will continue to have—a great impact on basic research in understanding the biochemical events in T-cell activation and signal transduction. At the cellular level, CyA shows a high affinity to its receptor, the cytosolic protein cyclophilin (14,15). The cyclophilins reveal peptidyl-prolyl cis–trans isomerase activity catalyzing the cis–trans isomerization of peptide bonds involving prolyl residues (16). The effector domain of the cyclosporin–cyclophilin complex binds to the serine–threonine phosphatase calcineurin. Comprehensive reviews on the molecular mechanism of immunosuppressive agents (17) and on the specific interaction of CyA and analogs with cyclophilins (18) have been recently published.

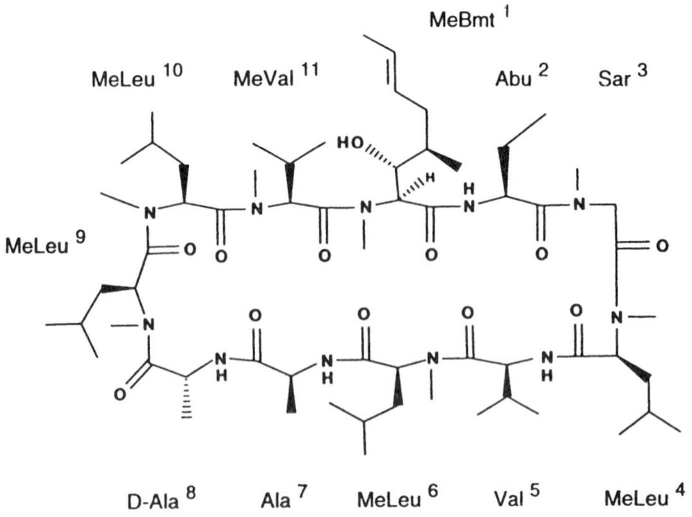

Figure 1   Structure of cyclosporin A. Abu, L-2-aminobutyric acid; Bmt, (4*R*)-4-[(*E*)-2-butenyl]-4-methyl-L-threonine (= (2*S*, 3*R*, 4*R*, 6*E*)-2-amino-3-hydroxy-4-methyloct-6-enoic acid); Me, *N*-methyl; Sar, sarcosine. The numbering system of amino acids corresponds to the sequence in the Edman degradation (2).

In the search for new CyA analogs with improved therapeutic properties, a broad variety of new cyclosporins has been prepared by chemical derivatization and total synthesis (for a review, see Ref. 19) as well as by fermentation using selected precursors and by in vitro biosynthesis. In the last decade, deep insight in the biosynthesis of cyclosporins has been gained. This knowledge will be extensively reviewed in this chapter.

II.   TAXONOMY OF CYCLOSPORIN-PRODUCING ORGANISMS

In the course of a microbiological screening program, in the early 1970s CyA and the minor metabolites CyB and CyC were isolated from cultures of two fungi imperfecti identified as *Cylindrocarpon lucidum* Booth NRRL 5760 and *Tolypocladium inflatum* Gams (originally classified as *Trichoderma polysporum* (Link ex Pers.) Rifai) NRRL 8044 (20). The two strains were obtained from soil samples collected in Wisconsin and in the Hardanger Vidda (Norway), respectively. Since its original description (21), the genus *Tolypocladium* has been revised and extended, and the particular CyA-producing strain NRRL 8044 was reclassified to *Tolypocladium niveum* (Rostrup) Bissett (22). However, this neotypification has later been considered to be inappropriate (23); in the literature both names are used, but the majority of authors adhere to *T. inflatum*. Further confusion in nomenclature was introduced by von Arx (24), who proposed to merge the genus *Tolypocladium* with the genus *Beauveria* and, subsequently, to assign the cyclosporin-producing organism to *Beauveria nivea*. This reclassification, though taken over by the American Type Culture Collection (25), has hardly been followed by the scientific community. It has been proposed to retain the name *T. inflatum* W. Gams for the fungal strain NRRL 8044 that produces CyA (26).

Various different fungal taxa producing CyA and its congeners will be extensively discussed in Section VII; also, new cyclosporin analogs described from other fungal sources will be mentioned there.

III. FERMENTATION AND ISOLATION OF NATURAL CYCLOSPORINS

The fungal strain *T. inflatum* NRRL 8044 grows best on a medium composed of malt extract, yeast extract, and agar within the temperature range 6 to 33°C; the optimal temperature is about 24°C. After a cultivation time of 12 to 14 days, cyclosporin production is reached (20). *C. lucidum* NRRL 5760, which produces only in static surface culture, is less suitable. For production of CyA, selected mutants obtained from the original strain of *T. inflatum* by treatment with ultraviolet (UV) light or *N*-methyl-*N'*-nitro-*N*-nitrosoguanidine are used under aerated submerged culture conditions. In large-scale fermentation tanks, a medium containing glucose as carbon source and casein-pepton as nitrogen source, supplemented with trace elements (ions of Zn, Mn, Mo, Cu, Fe) and vitamins (thiamine, biotin, pyridoxine), is recommended (27). The production of CyA is monitored by high-performance liquid chromatography (HPLC) and, after a fermentation time of 14 days on average, an optimal concentration is attained (20). The crude cyclosporins are extracted with an organic solvent, preferably ethyl acetate, and the complex mixture is separated by applying systematic chromatographical methods such as Sephadex gel filtration, and silica gel and reversed-phase medium- and high-pressure chomatography. First, the quantitatively dominating CyA and CyC were isolated in pure form (2), followed by the congeners B, D, and E (28). From large-scale fermentations, by further processing of minor fractions and mother liquors, more than 25 individual natural cyclosporins presently have been isolated from *T. inflatum*, some of them occuring only in trace amounts (29). In several cases, the yields could be significantly improved by adding specific amino acids to the culture medium (see Section VI.A).

Independently from us at Sandoz Laboratories, Agathos and Lee (30) studied the influence of amino acids on the production of CyA by *T. inflatum* and found an enhancing effect of externally supplied L-valine in a chemically defined medium, raising the final CyA titer to 710 mg/liter, compared with only 130 mg/liter without L-valine supplementation. Furthermore, Agathos and Chun report that immobilization of *T. inflatum* spores into porous celite beads results in an up to threefold higher cyclosporin formation than for the free cell culture (31).

IV. STRUCTURAL VARIATIONS IN NATURAL CYCLOSPORINS

Characteristic structural features of natural cyclosporins include a unique unsaturated β-hydroxy-α-amino acid with a C_9 skeleton, (2S, 3R, 4R, 6E)-3-hydroxy-4-methyl-2-methylamino-oct-6-enoic acid, the *N*-methylation of several of the 11 amino acids, and the presence of D-alanine in the molecule. The individual cyclosporins differ from each other by variation of one or two amino acid constituents. The most frequent diversity occurs in position 2, which can be occupied by L-2-aminobutyric acid (CyA), L-alanine (CyB), L-threonine (CyC), L-valine (CyD), or L-norvaline (CyG). *N*-Demethyl analogs are encountered in positions 1, 6, 9, 10, and 11. Modifications at position 5 are illustrated by L-norvaline in CyM and L-leucine in Cy26 instead of L-valine. In position 7, a second

L-2-aminobutyric acid can substitute for L-alanine (CyV). N-Methyl-L-leucine in position 4 may be replaced by N-methyl-L-isoleucine (Cy29) or by L-valine in CyQ and CyS. Regarding possible biosynthetic pathways, variations at position 1 are of special interest: CyF and CyK contain deoxy-MeBmt, whereas N-methyl-L-2-amino-octanoic acid is found in CyZ. Both building units probably stem from a common precursor of the genuine amino acid (4R)-4-[(E)-2-butenyl]-4-methyl-L-threonine (Bmt). A full exchange of this characteristic structural unit by N-methyl-L-leucine is observed in CyO. At present, positions 3 and 8 containing sarcosine and D-alanine, respectively, are the only conserved building units.

CyH (32), which contains N-methyl-D-valine at position 11 instead of the natural L-epimer, is not a product of direct biosynthesis (see Section VI.E). In our current understanding of CyH formation, during the extraction of CyA with acidic alcoholic solution, a small portion isomerizes to form iso-CyA (2) which then can convert into CyH or back into CyA.

The structures of cyclosporins A–Z and 26–30 are indicated in Table 1.

V.   BIOSYNTHESIS OF CYCLOSPORIN A PRECURSORS

CyA contains three nonproteinogenic amino acids: D-alanine in position 8, L-2-aminobutyric acid in position 2, and in position 1, the unusual amino acid Bmt, which, until today, has been described in the literature uniquely as a building element of cyclosporins (29) and the related peptolide SDZ 214-103 and its congeners (33).

A.   Biosynthesis of the Amino Acid Bmt

In 1983, in a first series of experiments using isotope-labeled precursors, Kobel et al. (34) showed that ^{13}C-labeled acetate is incorporated in vivo into Bmt in a polyketide-like manner. The C-methyl in position 4 of the carbon chain as well as the seven N-methyl-groups originate from the S-methyl of methionine. Incorporation studies with doubly labeled [*methyl*-(^{13}CD$_3$)]methionine suggested that the C-methyl-transfer to the ketide chain of Bmt proceeds in the form of an intact CD$_3$ unit. These findings later were well confirmed by feeding experiments using selectively labeled [^{13}C]glucose (35).

Based on these results, Offenzeller et al. (36) proposed a concept for the biosynthesis of Bmt (Figure 2), involving two phases: (a) a basic assembly process comprising head-to-tail coupling of four acetate units, the respective reduction and dehydration steps, and most probably, the methylation reaction; and (b) a subsequent transformation process introducing the amino function. Alternative possibilities are conceivable, but the basic assembly process has to result in either compound A, 3(R)-hydroxy-4(R)-methyl-6(E)-octenoic acid, or in compound B, 4(R)-methyl-(E, E)-2,6-octadienoic. To distinguish between these principal routes, in vivo incorporation of [1-^{13}C, ^{18}O$_2$]acetate into Bmt was studied. Retention of ^{18}O, evidenced by a significant upfield shift of the ^{13}C nuclear magnetic resonance (NMR) signal of C3, strongly favored structure A as an intermediate. In parallel, an in vitro enzymatic system was established by purifying crude extracts from *T. inflatum*; it enabled identification of 3(R)-hydroxy-4(R)-methyl-6(E)-octenoic acid (compound A) as an in vitro product of Bmt polyketide synthase (36). Depending on the degree of purity of the enriched enzyme fraction, two additional methylated in vitro products were detected and characterized as 4(R)-methyl-(E, E)-2,6-octadienoic

Table 1 Chemical Structures of Cyclosporins A to Z and 26 to 30

Metabolite	Amino acid composition[a]										
	1	2	3	4	5	6	7	8	9	10	11
CyA	MeBmt	Abu	Sar	MeLeu	Val	MeLeu	Ala	D-Ala	MeLeu	MeLeu	MeVal
CyB	MeBmt	Ala	Sar	MeLeu	Val	MeLeu	Ala	D-Ala	MeLeut	MeLeu	MeVal
CyC	MeBmt	Thr	Sar	MeLeu	Val	MeLeu	Ala	D-Ala	MeLeu	MeLeu	MeVal
CyD	MeBmt	Val	Sar	MeLeu	Val	MeLeu	Ala	D-Ala	MeLeu	MeLeu	MeVal
CyE	MeBmt	Abu	Sar	MeLeu	Val	MeLeu	Ala	D-Ala	MeLeu	MeLeu	Val
CyF	Deoxy-MeBmt	Abu	Sar	MeLeu	Val	MeLeu	Ala	D-Ala	MeLeu	MeLeu	MeVal
CyG	MeBmt	Nva	Sar	MeLeu	Val	MeLeu	Ala	D-Ala	MeLeu	MeLeu	MeVal
CyH	MeBmt	Abu	Sar	MeLeu	Val	MeLeu	Ala	D-Ala	MeLeu	MeLeu	D-MeVal
CyI	MeBmt	Val	Sar	MeLeu	Val	MeLeu	Ala	D-Ala	MeLeu	Leu	MeVal
CyK	Deoxy-MeBmt	Val	Sar	MeLeu	Val	MeLeu	Ala	D-Ala	MeLeu	MeLeu	MeVal
CyL	Bmt	Abu	Sar	MeLeu	Val	MeLeu	Ala	D-Ala	MeLeu	MeLeu	MeVal
CyM	MeBmt	Nva	Sar	MeLeu	Nva	MeLeu	Ala	D-Ala	MeLeu	MeLeu	MeVal
CyN	MeBmt	Nva	Sar	MeLeu	Val	MeLeu	Ala	D-Ala	MeLeu	Leu	MeVal
CyO	MeLeu	Nva	Sar	MeLeu	Val	MeLeu	Ala	D-Ala	MeLeu	MeLeu	MeVal
CyP	Bmt	Thr	Sar	MeLeu	Val	MeLeu	Ala	D-Ala	MeLeu	MeLeu	MeVal
CyQ	MeBmt	Abu	Sar	Val	Val	MeLeu	Ala	D-Ala	MeLeu	MeLeu	MeVal
CyR	MeBmt	Abu	Sar	MeLeu	Val	Leu(?)	Ala	D-Ala	MeLeu	Leu(?)	MeVal
CyS	MeBmt	Thr	Sar	Val	Val	MeLeu	Ala	D-Ala	MeLeu	MeLeu	MeVal
CyT	MeBmt	Abu	Sar	MeLeu	Val	Leu	Ala	D-Ala	MeLeu	Leu	MeVal
CyU	MeBmt	Abu	Sar	MeLeu	Val	MeLeu	Ala	D-Ala	MeLeu	MeLeu	MeVal
CyV	MeBmt	Abu	Sar	MeLeu	Val	MeLeu	Abu	D-Ala	MeLeu	MeLeu	MeVal
CyW	MeBmt	Thr	Sar	MeLeu	Val	MeLeu	Ala	D-Ala	MeLeu	MeLeu	Val
CyX	MeBmt	Nva	Sar	MeLeu	Val	MeLeu	Ala	D-Ala	Leu	MeLeu	MeVal
CyY	MeBmt	Nva	Sar	MeLeu	Val	Leu	Ala	D-Ala	MeLeu	MeLeu	MeVal
CyZ	MeAoa	Abu	Sar	MeLeu	Val	MeLeu	Ala	D-Ala	MeLeu	MeLeu	MeVal
Cy26	MeBmt	Nva	Sar	MeLeu	Leu	MeLeu	Ala	D-Ala	MeLeu	MeLeu	MeVal
Cy27	Bmt	Val	Sar	MeLeu	Val	MeLeu	Ala	D-Ala	MeLeu	MeLeu	MeVal
Cy28	MeLeu	Abu	Sar	MeLeu	Val	MeLeu	Ala	D-Ala	MeLeu	MeLeu	MeVal
Cy29	MeBmt	Abu	Sar	MeIle	Val	MeLeu	Ala	D-Ala	MeLeu	MeLeu	MeVal
Cy30	MeLeu	Val	Sar	MeLeu	Val	MeLeu	Ala	D-Ala	MeLeu	MeLeu	MeVal

[a] Bmt = (2S, 3R, 4R, 6E)-2-amino-3-hydroxy-4-methyloct-6-enoic acid = (4R)-4-[(E)-2-butenyl]-4-methyl-L-threonine; Abu = L-2-aminobutyric acid; Aoa = L-2-aminooctanoic acid; Nva = L-norvaline; Me = N-methyl.

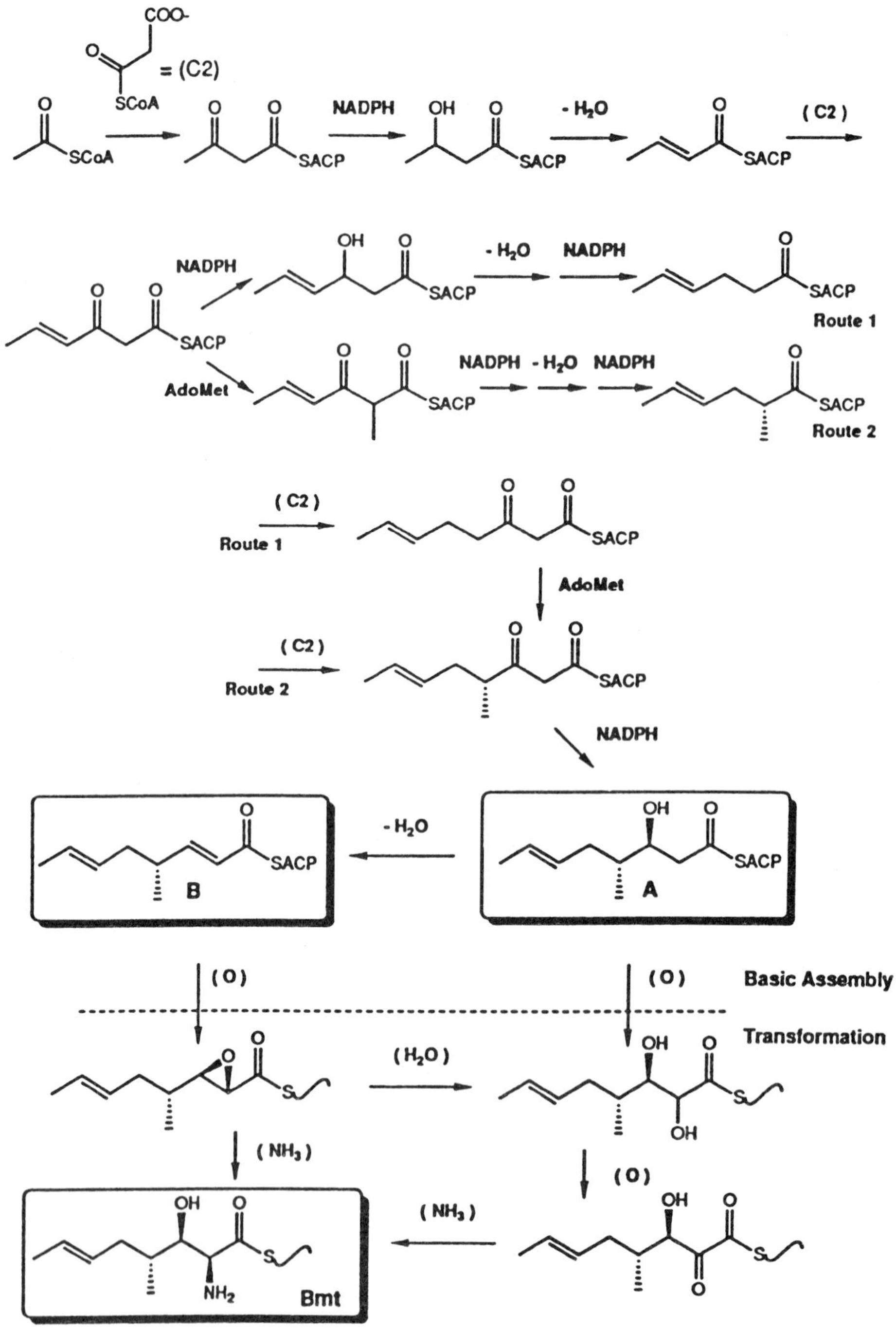

Figure 2 Possible routes of the biosynthetic pathway of Bmt. Polyketide biosynthesis is assumed to take place in an enzyme-bound form (ACP = acyl carrier protein). The product compound A is released from the Bmt synthase as a coenzyme A thioester, suggesting that subsequent transformation to Bmt takes place upon this activated intermediate. (From Ref. 36, with permission.)

and 4(R)-methyl-6(E)-octenoic acid by liquid chromatography–mass spectrometry analysis. They represent most likely artifacts produced by unknown enzymes, since the preservation of the ^{18}O from [1-^{13}C, $^{18}O_2$]acetate excludes a biosynthetic pathway via compound B. With progressive purification of Bmt polyketide synthase, these two substances are formed in decreasing amounts. The optimal activity of the enzyme lies around pH 7 and at 35°C.

The question remains, by which route is the C-methyl-group attached to the carbon chain following the proposed biosynthetic scheme (Figure 2)? Using the enzymatic in vitro system for Bmt polyketide synthase, it was possible—for the first time in polyketide biosynthesis—to elucidate the exact stage by unambiguously identifying 3-oxo-4(E)-hexenoic acid as the key intermediate for C-methylation (37).

These findings have been corroborated by in vivo feeding experiments with the fungus using deuterium-labeled acetate as precursor (37). CyA samples isolated from fermentations supplemented with either [1-^{13}C, $^2H_3$]- or [2-^{13}C, $^2H_3$]acetate were analyzed by ^{13}C and ^2H NMR techniques. The NMR measurements, showing an incorporation rate of about 20-fold over natural abundance, revealed for the terminal methyl-group (C8) of Bmt a deuterium distribution CD_3:CHD_2:CH_2D:CH_3 of 14:65:12:9. At the olefinic double bond (C6), about 11% deuterium is retained, whereas in position C4 deuterium is completely lost. Also, at C2, in the course of the transformation process to introduce the amino function, deuterium is eliminated, as expected. The above results are well in accordance with the conclusions drawn from studies using the in vitro assay for Bmt polyketide synthase and thus provide further evidence for route no. 2 as the biosynthetic pathway.

Furthermore, in vitro experiments demonstrated the successful substitution of the starter unit acetyl-CoA by intermediates of the first elongation cycle such as acetoacetyl-CoA and crotonyl-CoA; butyryl-CoA leads, besides other products, to the saturated 3-hydroxy-4-methyl-octanoic acid.

Interestingly, the Bmt backbone 3(R)-hydroxy-4(R)-methyl-6(E)-octenoic acid is not released from the enzyme as a free carboxylic acid, but as a coenzyme A thioester. Thus, we suggested (36) that the subsequent transformation to Bmt takes place on this activated intermediate. Currently, experimental studies are ongoing to investigate in detail these reaction steps.

B. Biosynthesis of the Other Constituent Amino Acids of Cyclosporin A

Of the nonproteinogenic amino acids L-2-aminobutyric acid and D-alanine, the latter is derived from L-alanine by a specific fungal racemase recently described (38). This enzyme catalyzes the reversible racemization of alanine, showing a maximal reaction velocity at pH 8.8 and 42°C for the L to D direction, and requires pyridoxal phosphate as the exclusive cofactor. Molecular mass determinations of the denatured enzyme by sodium dodecyl sulfate (SDS)–polyacrylamide gel electrophoresis (PAGE) gave a value of 37 kDa, whereas gel filtration calibration studies yielded a value between 120 and 150 kDa, indicating an oligomeric native structure.

To gain insight into the primary metabolism and the origin of L-2-aminobutyric acid, an overproducing strain of *T. inflatum* was grown on minimal medium containing either [1-^{13}C]-, [2-^{13}C]-, [3-^{13}C]-, or [6-^{13}C]glucose as the only carbon source (35). From NMR analysis of the four differently ^{13}C-labeled CyA samples, as exemplified in Figure 3 for [1-^{13}C]- and [6-^{13}C]glucose, it was concluded that L-2-aminobutyric acid originates

CsA: [1-¹³C]Glc and [6-¹³C]Glc

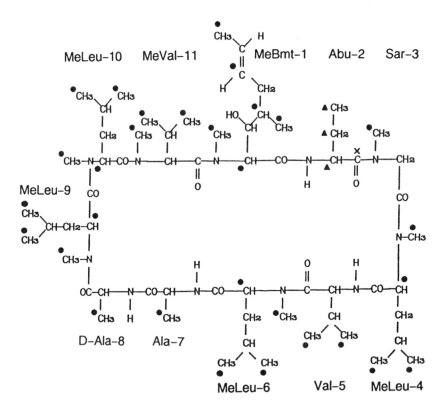

Figure 3   ¹³C incorporation into Cyclosporin A by growth of *T. inflatum* on a 1:1 mixture of [1-¹³C]glucose or [6-¹³C]glucose and unlabeled glucose as sole carbon source. The symbols depict ¹³C enrichment as follows. Growth on [1-¹³C]glucose: (●) 13–15%; (▲) 6–8%; (×) 2–4%; no symbol, natural abundance. Growth on [6-¹³C]glucose: (●) 20–25%; (▲) 11–13%; (×) 4–6%; no symbol, natural abundance. (Reproduced from Ref. 35.)

mainly from oxaloacetate via acetyl-coenzyme A and the Krebs cycle; minor biosynthetic routes, however, such as the citramalate pathway were also seen to contribute. The ¹³C-labeling pattern also clearly revealed that the other constituent amino acids of cyclosporin are synthesized by classical biochemical pathways (Figure 4).

The ¹³C enrichment in cyclosporin is significantly lower by growth on [1-¹³C]glucose than by growth on [6-¹³C]glucose. This difference arises because C1 of glucose is lost by decarboxylation when glucose is fed through the pentosephosphate pathway. The relative flux through the pentosephosphate pathway versus glycolysis was estimated as 40%.

According to the preliminary studies of Kobel et al. (34), the *N*-methyl-groups originate from the methyl of methionine, which in turn stems from Cβ of serine. Thus,

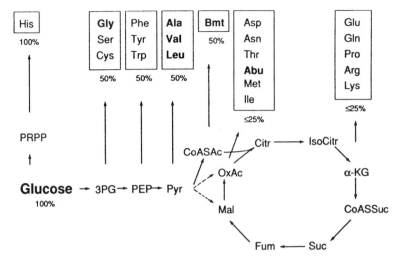

Figure 4 Biosynthesis of constituent amino acids of cyclosporin A from glucose with expected maximum label incorporation at a given position when grown on 100% selectively enriched [^{13}C]glucose. Key intermediates of glycolysis and the Krebs cycle are depicted in abbreviated form. Flux of carbon atoms through the pentosephosphate pathway is neglected. The amino acids occurring in cyclosporin A are shown in bold type; for abbreviations, refer to Figure 1. CoASSuc, succinyl-coenzyme A; Citr, citrate; IsoCitr, isocitrate; α-KG, α-ketoglutarate; Fum, fumarate; Mal, malate; OxAc, oxaloacetate; Pyr, pyruvate; Suc, succinate; PEP, phospho*enol*pyruvate; PG, 3-phosphoglycerate; PRPP, phosphoribosylpyrophosphate. (Reproduced from Ref. 35.)

the seven *N*-methyl carbons carried labels when CyA was produced from [1-^{13}C]glucose and [6-^{13}C]glucose.

VI. BIOSYNTHESIS OF CYCLOSPORINS

A nonribosomal biosynthetic pathway is clearly indicated for CyA, considering its cyclic structure, the partial *N*-methylation of the 11 peptide bonds, the uncommon building units Bmt, L-2-aminobutyric acid, and D-alanine, and the plethora of isolated congeners. Nonribosomal biosynthesis directed by multienzyme thiotemplates have been reported for other small peptides of microbial origin, such as gramicidin S and enniatin (for a review, see Ref. 39).

A. Precursor-Directed Biosynthesis of Cyclosporins

A strong influence on the biosynthesis of peptide metabolites exerted by exogenously supplied amino acid precursors has been observed earlier both in prokaryotes and eukaryotes (40). In the cyclosporin series, addition of specific amino acids in excess to the fermentation medium effects a shift in the ratio of the various cyclosporins produced, especially by influencing position 2. For example, addition of DL-2-aminobutyric acid suppresses the biosynthesis of the minor congeners, with CyA becoming almost the exclusive metabolite. CyG, usually found only in trace amounts, can be produced in high percentage by external supply of L-norvaline (27).

Incorporation of foreign amino acids into various positions can also be attained, as illustrated by the formation of [L-Allylgly²]CyA when DL-α-allylglycine is fed as precursor. Exogenously supplied L-3-cyclohexylalanine results in a predominant production of [MeCyclohexylala¹]CyA (replacement of MeBmt). It is noteworthy that DL-threo-3-cyclohexylserine, a closer mimetic to Bmt, was not incorporated into cyclosporins by the organism; only the usual pattern of cyclosporins A, B, and C was observed.

D-Alanine in position 8 can be successfully substituted for by D-serine to give the corresponding analogs [D-Ser⁸]CyA, [D-Ser⁸]CyB, [D-Ser⁸]CyC, [D-Ser⁸]CyD, and [D-Ser⁸]CyG (41). Also, the monohalogenated 3-fluoro-, 2-deutero-3-fluoro-, and 3-chloro-D-alanines are substrates for competitive in vivo incorporation leading to [3-fluoro-D-Ala⁸]CyA (42), [2-deutero-3-fluoro-D-Ala⁸]CyA (43), and [3-chloro-D-Ala⁸]CyA, respectively. Because the latter amino acids, especially 2-deutero-3-fluoro-D-alanine, act as potent inhibitors of alanine racemase (44), the conversion of L-alanine to D-alanine is blocked, and therefore, the biosynthesis of "normal" CyA is suppressed.

The variability of position 8 by feeding other D–amino acids to the fungus was found to be rather low; for example, supplying D-2-aminobutyric acid or D-norvaline results in an increase of CyA and CyG formation, respectively, via epimerization of the precursor, presumably by the Ala-racemase. Attempts to prepare the [D-Thr⁸]CyA analog by feeding D-threonine to the culture medium did not lead to the desired compound, but, surprisingly, to a novel member of the cyclosporin family, namely, [MeIle⁴]CyA (designated Cy29; Table 1), which turned out to be a very potent anti-HIV-1 agent in vitro (13,45). The role of D-threonine supplementation in inducing [MeIle⁴]CyA formation is not clear. It is feasible that D-threonine is epimerized to L-allo-threonine by the nonspecific alanine racemase present in *T. inflatum*. L-Allo-threonine, after being transformed by L-threonine dehydratase, which has been described as being nonspecific in regard to the stereochemistry of the β-position (46), may enter the biosynthetic pathway to L-isoleucine. The rapid racemization of D-threonine would overcome, in this model, the known strong inhibition of L-threonine dehydratase by D-threonine (47). Alternatively, the presence or induction of a specific D-threonine dehydratase in the fungus *T. inflatum*, as has been observed in the bacterium *Serratia marcescens* (48), is also conceivable. In this model, D-threonine would be directly converted to L-isoleucine.

In summary, the incorporation of constitutional and foreign amino acids is a further characteristic indication for a nonribosomal biosynthetic pathway for cyclosporins. However, exchange of amino acid constituents is limited; many substrates tried were not incorporated or acted to suppress in vivo cyclosporin biosynthesis (e.g., DL-3-aminobutyric acid or S-ethyl-L-methionine).

B. Cyclosporin Synthetase

In 1990, Lawen and Zocher (49) described the purification and characterization of the enzyme cyclosporin synthetase, isolated from the mycelium of the strain *T. inflatum* NRRL 8044 (S 7939/45). This enzyme synthesizes cyclosporin A by a thiotemplate mechanism starting from the precursor amino acids in their unmethylated form, utilizing adenosine triphosphate (ATP)/Mg²⁺, and with S-adenosyl-L-methionine as methyl donor. The first attempts (50) to establish the cell-free synthesis of cyclosporin A were not successful, but they led to a partially enriched enzyme that could synthesize the diketopiperazine *cyclo*-(D-Ala–MeLeu), which represents a partial sequence of cyclosporin A. Later investigations (51) showed that the aforementioned diketopiperazine was also detected in the mycelium of a cyclosporin nonproducing strain (mutant YP 582), whereas the mycelium of the producing strain 7939/45 did not contain this compound. Interestingly, in the cyclosporin-blocked mutant, the amino acid Bmt is released in free form the culture medium (52).

I. *Molecular Mass of Cyclosporin Synthetase*

Measurements of the molecular mass of the native cyclosporin synthetase were originally performed by ultracentrifugation in glycerol gradients and by SDS–polyacrylamide gel electrophoresis using enniatin synthetase (250 kDa) (53), linear gramicidin synthetase 2 (350 kDa) (54), and tyrocidine synthetase 3 (450 kDa) (55) as standards. The extrapolation of molecular masses of the calibration proteins resulted in a molecular mass of at least 650–800 kDa for cyclosporin synthetase (49). In spite of this high value, it was not possible to dissociate the enzyme into subunits using urea or detergents like SDS, nor β-mercaptoethanol; cyclosporin synthetase behaves as a single polypeptide chain and appears not to be glycosylated.

It later became evident that the molecular mass of cyclosporin synthetase was drastically underestimated. For δ-(L-α-aminoadipyl)-L-cysteinyl-D-valine (ACV) synthetase, the first enzyme in the penicillin biosynthesis, the molecular mass could be calculated from the nucleotide sequence of the open reading frame (56,57) to be in the range of 420–425 kDa, instead of 230 kDa as determined from SDS-PAGE. Based on a molecular weight of 420 kDa for ACV synthetase as a reference, the estimate for the molecular mass of cyclosporin synthetase was corrected up to about 1.5 MDa (Figure 5). To overcome the basic difficulty in determining very high molecular masses of proteins with the SDS-PAGE method due to the lack of appropriate standards, cesium chloride density gradient centrifugation was used as an alternative approach. Only minute protein concentrations such as 10–50 nM are required, due to the extremely sensitive fluorescence detection system of the analytical ultracentrifuge (Figure 6). This method yielded for cyclosporin synthetase an average molecular mass of 1.4 MDa with a maximum error of ±160 kDa (58).

Recently, the cyclosporin synthetase gene has been cloned and sequenced; it contains a giant 45.8 kb open reading frame, which codes for a peptide of 15,281 amino acids with a calculated M_r of 1,689,243 (60). This value is in good agreement with the result of 1.5 MDa obtained from SDS–polyacrylamide gel analyses as well as the slightly underestimated value of the CsCl density gradient centrifugation experiments. Moreover, the knowledge of the gene confirms the findings (49) that cyclosporin synthetase consists of a single polypeptide chain.

From all data available so far on peptide and depsipeptide synthetases, it appears that enzymes of bacterial origin such as gramicidin S synthetase, tyrocidine synthetase, or actinomycin synthetase (all reviewed in Ref. 61) have subunit structure, whereas fungal enzymes such as SDZ 214-103 synthetase (62) (see Section VI.C), SDZ 90-215 synthetase (63), and cyclosporin synthetase consist of single polypeptide chains. Cyclosporin synthetase represents the most complex one. Like type I polyketide synthases, these enzymes are designated "multifunctional polypeptides"; the bacterial enzymes, on the other hand, are called "multienzyme complexes," analogous to type II polyketide synthases (64).

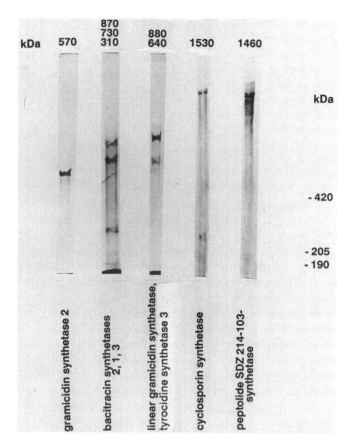

Figure 5   Molecular mass estimation of peptide synthetases in one 3% SDS-PAGE. The molecular masses of the reference proteins recombinant tyrocidine synthetase 2 (190 kDa), myosin (205 kDa), and ACV synthetase (420 kD) are indicated. Extrapolation results in molecular masses of 570 kDa for gramicidin synthetase 2 (lane 1), 310, 730, and 870 kDa for bacitracin synthetases 2, 1, and 3 (lane 2), 640 and 880 kDa for linear gramicidin synthetase 2 and tyrocidine synthetase 3 (lane 3), 1530 kDa for cyclosporin synthetase (lane 4), and 1460 kDa for peptolide SDZ 214-103 synthetase (lane 5). (From Ref. 58, with permission.)

2.   Mechanism of Cyclosporin A Biosynthesis

As already outlined in the first publication on the characterization of cyclosporin synthetase (49), this multifunctional enzyme follows a thiotemplate mechanism. This mechanism, elucidated by the group of Lipmann (65), closely resembles the biosynthesis of fatty acids. In a first step, cyclosporin synthetase activates all constituent amino acids of cyclosporin A in their unmethylated form as aminoacyl adenylates by reaction with ATP (measured by amino acid–dependent ATP–pyrophosphate exchange (49), or directly proved by the use of adenylates as substrates for cyclosporin A biosynthesis (66)); this step also occurs in the ribosomal mechanism. The second step in the nonribosomal mechanism consists of a transesterification of the enzyme-bound activated amino acids onto reactive thiol groups of the enzyme. Thus, cyclosporin synthetase can be radiolabeled by covalent binding of ^{14}C-labeled substrates (e.g., valine and leucine), ATP, and Mg^{2+}. Fur-

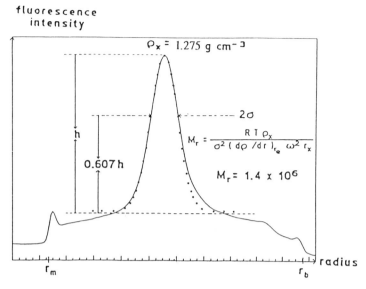

Figure 6 Molecular mass estimation of cyclosporin synthetase by density gradient centrifugation. Cyclosporin synthetase purified by glycerol gradient ultracentrifugation (49) has been labeled with 4'-([(iodoacetyl)amino]methyl)fluorescein; 8.8 μg of this enzyme preparation (end concentration 25 μg/ml) was analyzed by CsCl density gradient centrifugation at 40,000 rpm in an analytical ultracentrifuge equipped with a fluorescence detection system. The profile shows the distribution of fluorescence intensity monitored after 9 hr. Circles designate the best fit to the Gaussian distribution equation $f(r) = (1/\sigma\sqrt{2\pi}) \exp [-(r-r_x)^2/2\sigma^2]$. r_m represents the meniscus, r_b the bottom of the measuring cell, r_x the radial position of the protein band, and σ the bandwidth. (From Ref. 59, with permission.)

thermore, specific SH-blocking agents like iodoacetamide or 2,2'-dithiopyridine inhibited cyclosporin biosynthesis; this effect could be reversed by 1,4-dithioerythritol (66).

Cyclosporin synthetase accepts only the unmethylated precursor amino acids of cyclosporins. N-Methylation takes place at the stage when the thioesters are bound to the enzyme; N-methyl-transfer activity is an integral part of cyclosporin synthetase, and S-adenosyl-L-methionine acts as the methyl-group donor. These findings are supported by photoaffinity-labeling experiments using ^{14}C-labeled S-adenosyl-L-methionine as well as by the observations that N-methylated amino acids can be split off the protein by performic acid oxidation (49). Biosynthesis of an unmethylated cyclosporin has not been observed; the reason may be that at position 3 a N-methylated amino acid (sarcosine) is needed, which greatly facilitates the formation of a β-turn, as conformational studies have shown (67). Here, experiments using cyclosporin synthetase isolated from a mutant strain (YP 582) are of interest. This mutant enzyme no longer synthesizes CyA, but it yields as major product the diketopiperazine cyclo-(D-Ala–MeLeu). When S-adenosyl-L-methionine is omitted from the incubation mixture, the unmethylated diketopiperazine cyclo-(D-Ala–Leu) is consequently obtained, though its formation is about 20 times slower than that of corresponding methylated product (51).

Regarding the elongation steps to build up the amino acid sequence, the thiotemplate mechanism as proposed by Lipmann (65) suggests a central 4'-phosphopantetheine arm that acts as a carrier of the growing peptide chain. Taking in account a length of 20

Å for the 4′-phosphopantetheine molecule, it is able to reach up to six of the active centers of an enzyme (68). Therefore, cyclosporin synthetase would have to be equipped with at least two 4′-phosphopantetheine molecules catalyzing the synthesis of at least two linear precursor peptide chains. Although it was shown that cyclosporin synthetase contains more than one 4′-phosphopantetheine molecule, it was not possible to determine the exact stoichiometry of 4′-phosphopantetheine bound to cyclosporin synthetase (49).

To gain insight into the chain elongation process during cyclosporin biosynthesis, experiments were performed to isolate linear precursor peptides. Using cyclosporin synthetase from the strain *T. inflatum* 7939/45 and short incubation times, four linear precursor peptides were identified after thioester breakage, namely the di-, tri-, and tetrapeptides H–D-Ala–MeLeu–OH, H–D-Ala–MeLeu–MeLeu–OH, and H–D-Ala–MeLeu–MeLeu–MeVal–OH, respectively, and the nonapeptide H–D-Ala–MeLeu–MeLeu–MeVal–MeBmt–Abu–Sar–MeLeu–Val–OH (69). The four intermediate peptides represent partial sequences of CyA, all starting with D-Ala as the N-terminal amino acid. These results indicate that the biosynthesis of cyclosporin A proceeds by a stepwise elongation via a single linear precursor peptide starting with D-Ala (66). Notably, the linear undecapeptide H–D-Ala–MeLeu–MeLeu–MeVal–MeBmt–Abu–Sar–MeLeu–Val–MeLeu–Ala–OH could not be detected, suggesting that the cyclization reaction, the last step in cyclosporin biosynthesis, is rather fast.

In summary, cyclosporin synthetase, the most complex multifunctional enzyme known so far, catalyzes at least 40 reaction steps: 11 aminoadenylation reactions, 11 transthiolation reactions, 7 N-methylation reactions, 10 elongation reactions, and the final cyclization reaction (Figure 7). In a modified thiotemplate mechanism that has been proposed (70), each active site carries its own 4′-phosphopantetheine residue, and therefore, a central 4′-phosphopantetheine arm limited in its geometry is not required (Figure 8).

This model is in accordance with the results from gradient sedimentation experiments in the analytical ultracentrifuge, which indicate an oblate overall shape of the enzyme. It was calculated that the oblate ellipsoid looks like a discus of 330 Å in diameter and 46 Å in thickness (58). Revision of the calculations for a molecular mass of 1.69 MDa gave slightly corrected values of 322 Å in diameter and 54 Å in thickness (Schmidt B, personal communication).

The sequence of the open reading frame of the cyclosporin synthetase gene shows 11 homologous modules (60), which are supposed to be responsible for the activation of the 11 constitutive amino acids of CyA. Two types of domains are found, those with and those without putative N-methyltransferase activity. The polypeptide sequence belonging to a 45 kDa fragment of cyclosporin synthetase is recognized to have N-methyltransferase activity (60) and to be very similar to a corresponding sequence present in enniatin synthetase (72); all seven of these cyclosporin synthetase partial sequences are highly conserved. The order of domains of the two types corresponds with the order of N-methylated and nonmethylated amino acids in CyA.

A 130 kDa cyclosporin synthetase fragment obtained by proteolytic digestion could be characterized by its capacity to activate L-alanine (60). This permits, according to its position in the deduced amino acid sequence (N-terminus at position 13,601), assignment of the eleventh domain to L-alanine activation. This amino acid is known as the last to be added to the growing peptide chain (59).

The C-terminal end of domain 11 is not the C-terminus of cyclosporin synthetase, but approximately 500 amino acids of nondomain sequence follow. As the biosynthesis of

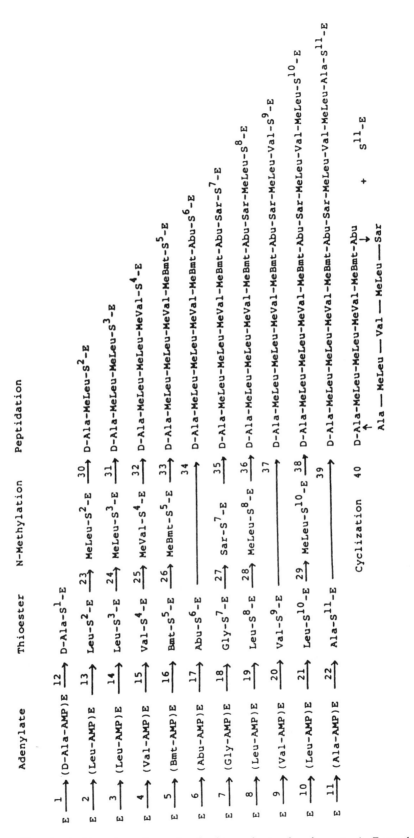

Figure 7 Hypothetical reaction scheme for the biosynthesis of cyclosporin A. E stands for cyclosporin synthetase; S^n, superscript numbers refer to active sites according to the elongation sequence; numbers above arrows indicate partial reaction steps.

A.

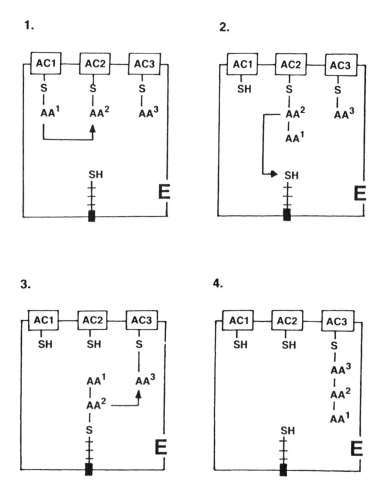

Figure 8a "Thiotemplate" mechanism (A) and "modified thiotemplate" mechanism (B) for peptide biosynthesis. (A) Activated amino acids (AA1, AA2, AA3, ...) are bound to thiol groups cysteine residues at the corresponding active centers (AC1, AC2, AC3, ...). A central 4′-phosphopantetheine arm (‡SH) acts as carrier to build up the peptide chain via transthiolation reactions. E stands for enzyme. (B) Each active center carries its own 4′-phosphopantetheine residue (‡SH) at which the corresponding activated amino acid is bound and transported to each next active center for elongation of the peptide chain (1, 2, 4). The 4′-phosphopantetheine arms themselves are bound covalently over specific serine residues (denoted O) to the enzyme. In this model (3), a central 4′-phosphopantetheine arm is not needed (?). (Adapted from Ref. 71.)

cyclosporins includes ring closure as the final step, it is speculated (60) that the above peptide sequence, which shows no significant homology to domains 1 to 11, harbors this function. The dimensions of cyclosporin synthetase deduced from the CsCl gradient centrifugation measurements imply a ring structure for the 11 domains, each domain folded on the other.

In this context, recent experiments to study the denaturation of the multifunctional polypeptide cyclosporin synthetase have to be mentioned (73). They show that at

B.

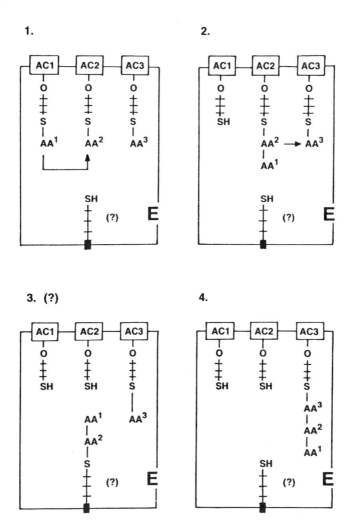

Figure 8b

least two stages of reversible enzyme denaturation with urea are passed. With increasing concentrations of urea (up to 0.8 M), cyclosporin A biosynthesis becomes inhibited and finally stops; only the diketopiperazine *cyclo*-(D-Ala–MeLeu), representing the first two amino acids of the growing peptide chain of CyA, is still detectable. At higher urea concentrations, the enzyme preparation becomes totally inactive. Formation of *cyclo*-(D-Ala–MeLeu) is interpreted as an unfolding of some of the other nine enzyme domains while the two amino acid–activating domains 8 and 9 are still functional.

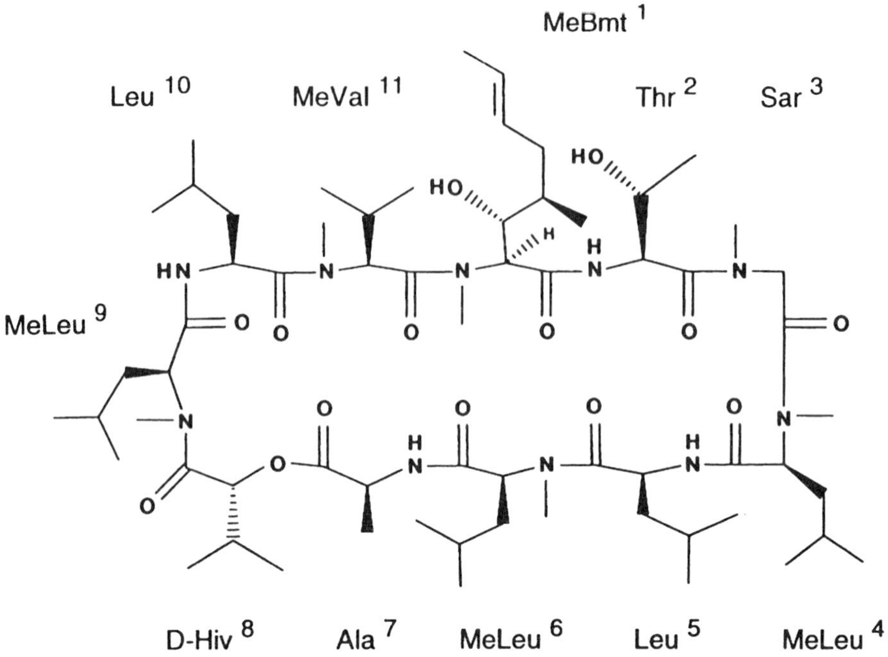

Figure 9   Structure of peptolide SDZ 214-103; D-Hiv, D-2-hydroxyisovaleric acid.

C.   Peptolide SDZ 214-103 Synthetase

In the search for new immunosuppressants, in 1988, the novel cyclosporin-related peptolide SDZ 214-103 (=[Thr^2, Leu^5, D-Hiv^8, Leu^{10}]cyclosporin) was discovered at Sandoz Ltd. (33). SDZ 214-103 (Figure 9) is produced by the fungus *Cylindrotrichum oligospermum* (Corda) Bonorden and exerts similar biological activities as CyA. The main structural difference lies in the presence of D-2-hydroxyisovaleric acid at position 8 instead of D-alanine, resulting in an ester bond. From crude extracts of the mycelium of the producing strain, we were able to prepare an enzyme fraction capable of synthesizing in vitro the peptolide when the constitutive amino acids Bmt, Gly, Thr, Val, Leu, and the hydroxy acid D-Hiv, ATP, and S-adenosyl-L-methionine are incubated (62) (Figure 10). Peptolide SDZ 214-103 synthetase does not synthesize cyclosporin, nor does cyclosporin synthetase synthesize the peptolide.

Peptolide synthetase elutes from sizing columns in the same volume as cyclosporin synthetase. Using SDS-PAGE analysis, a molecular mass only slightly lower than that of cyclosporin synthetase is determined (74) (Figure 5). Peptolide synthetase appears to be one multienzyme polypeptide and is also not glycosylated. It cross-reacts with antibodies directed specifically against cyclosporin synthetase. Although both enzymes are similar in many characteristics, they are clearly distinct in their specificities in regard to the various positions of the cyclosporin and peptolide rings (see Section VI.E).

Peptolide synthetase follows, as has been determined so far, the same principal biosynthetic mechanism as cyclosporin synthetase and catalyzes at least 39 partial reac-

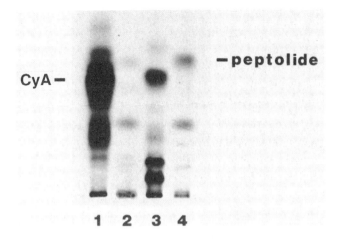

Figure 10   Thin-layer chromatographic (TLC) separation of *in vitro* synthesized cyclosporin A and peptolide SDZ 214-103. Cyclosporin synthetase (lanes 1 and 3) or peptolide synthetase (lanes 2 and 4) were incubated with all constituent amino acids for cyclosporin A (lanes 1 and 2) or for the peptolide (lanes 2 and 4), the necessary cosubstrates, and S-adenosyl-L-[*methyl*-14C]methionine as radiolabel. The ethyl acetate–extractable reaction products were separated on silica gel plates with water-saturated ethyl acetate as mobile phase. The positions of reference samples of CyA and the peptolide are indicated. (From Ref. 62, with permission.)

tion steps: 11 aminoadenylation reactions, 11 transthiolation reactions, 6 N-methylation reactions, and the final cyclization step. The experimental data available suggest that the D-hydroxy acid in position 8 is the starting point of the biosynthesis.

D.   Natural Peptolide SDZ 214-103 Minor Metabolites

Compared with the plethora of natural cyclosporins isolated from large-scale fermentations of *T. inflatum*, only a very limited series of peptolide SDZ 214-103 minor components are produced by the fungus *C. oligospermum* (33) (Table 2). Interestingly, natural variations do not occur in position 2 as in cyclosporins, but in position 5, leading to [Val5]- and [Ile5]SDZ 214-103. As a novel feature, hydroxylation at the terminal methyl-group of MeBmt is encountered in the natural compound [8'-Hydroxy-MeBmt1]SDZ 214-103, whereas neither the deoxy- nor the N-demethyl-MeBmt analog are observed; a replacement of MeBmt by a mimetic such as MeLeu (as in CyO) is also not found. N-Demethylated congeners appear in position 3, for the first time ([Gly3]SDZ 214-103), and in position 4 ([Leu4]SDZ 214-103), but so far not in the other MeLeu units (positions 6 and 9) or in the MeVal position 11.

The few modifications observed within the group of SDZ 214-103 metabolites reflect the distinctly higher substrate specificity of peptolide synthetase compared with that of cyclosporin synthetase, as will be discussed in Section VI.E.

Table 2 Chemical Structures of Natural SDZ 214-103 Minor Metabolites

Metabolite	Amino (hydroxy) acid composition										
	1	2	3	4	5	6	7	8	9	10	11
SDZ 214-103	MeBmt	Thr	Sar	MeLeu	Leu	MeLeu	Ala	D-Hiv	MeLeu	Leu	MeVal
[Gly³]-214-103	MeBmt	Thr	**Gly**	MeLeu	Leu	MeLeu	Ala	D-Hiv	MeLeu	Leu	MeVal
[Leu⁴]-214-103	MeBmt	Thr	Sar	**Leu**	Leu	MeLeu	Ala	D-Hiv	MeLeu	Leu	MeVal
[Val⁵]-214-103	MeBmt	Thr	Sar	MeLeu	**Val**	MeLeu	Ala	D-Hiv	MeLeu	Leu	MeVal
[Ile⁵]-214-103	MeBmt	Thr	Sar	MeLeu	**Ile**	MeLeu	Ala	D-Hiv	MeLeu	Leu	MeVal
[8′-OH-MeBmt¹]-214-103	**8′-OH-MeBmt**	Thr	Sar	MeLeu	Leu	MeLeu	Ala	D-Hiv	MeLeu	Leu	MeVal

E. *In Vitro* Synthesis of Cyclosporin A and Peptolide SDZ 214-103 Analogs

Using an enzyme preparation isolated from an improved strain of *T. inflatum* (7939/45), Lawen et al. (75) established a reproducible method for the in vitro biosynthesis of cyclosporins in microgram quantities. In addition to CyA and its known natural congeners, a large series of new cyclosporins not accessible by fermentation became available (76,77). Also, a broad variety of new peptolide SDZ 214-103 analogs were prepared using the peptolide in vitro system (76). For stability reasons, both enzymes were incubated at suboptimal temperature (6°C) with the necessary amino acids (hydroxy acid) together with ATP, MgCl$_2$, and S-adenosyl-L-methionine for 7 days. The cyclopeptides were extracted with ethyl acetate and purified by preparative HPLC. If sufficient material was obtained, fast atom bombardment mass spectra (FAB-MS) were recorded for structural proof, and/or immunosuppressive activity, characteristic for this class of compounds, was measured (76) (Tables 3 and 4).

1. Position 1

The substrate specificities for all of the 11 amino (hydroxy) acid sites, as far as experimentally accessible, have been investigated in detail (76). Of special interest is position 1, as in most natural cyclosporins and in all peptolides it carries the unique structural element Bmt, which is crucial for high immunosuppressive activity (78). The naturally occuring deoxy analogs (CyF and CyK), and CyZ, which contains N-methyl-L-2-aminooctanoic acid instead of MeBmt, indicates that neither the 3-hydroxy-group nor the double bond is essential for substrate recognition by cyclosporin synthetase. These findings are supported by the successful incorporation of L-2-amino-3-hydroxy-4-methyloctanoic acid (dihydro-Bmt), L-3-cyclohexylalanine, and L-3-hydroxy-3-cyclohexylalanine, the last two mimetics of deoxy-Bmt and Bmt, respectively. The steric requirements for the 4-methyl-group in Bmt seem to be minimal: L-2-amino-3-hydroxy-4,4-dimethyloctanoicacid(4-methyl-dihydro-Bmt), L-2-amino-3-hydroxy-4-butyloctanoic acid, and L-2-amino-3-hydroxy-oct-6-enoic acid (4-demethyl-Bmt) are all recognized as substrates. The length of the alkyl side chain, as far as tested, may range from three carbon atoms (Leu) to seven (L-2-amino-3-hydroxy-4,8-dimethylnonanoic acid); L-norleucine and L-2-amino-4-methylhex-4-enoic acid, each containing a four-carbon chain, seem to be incorporated, too. On the other hand, threonine, with a two-carbon chain, is not an effective substrate for that position, and serine may be incorporated to a low extent. Interestingly, the hydrolysis artifact *cyclo*-(dihydro-Bmt) (29) is accepted by the enzyme. Aromatic amino acids such as L-phenylalanine and L-tyrosine are not substrates for position 1; tyrosine totally inhibits cyclosporin biosynthesis. Charged amino acids, for example, phosphinotricin (2-amino-4-(hydroxymethylphosphinyl)butanoic acid), are not incorporated.

For peptolide SDZ 214-103 synthetase, we expected to observe a similar substrate specificity as in the case of cyclosporin synthetase, especially for position 1. Surprisingly, however, the enzymes differ much in their substrate recognition. In general, cyclosporin synthetase accepts a much broader pattern of amino acids at more sites than does peptolide SDZ 214-103 synthetase. To illustrate, in position 1, peptolide synthetase recognizes only the saturated Bmt, L-2-amino-3-hydroxy-4-methyloctanoic acid (dihydro-Bmt), whereas, unlike with cyclosporin synthetase, L-2-amino-3-hydroxy-4,4-dimethyloctanoic acid (4-methyl-dihydro-Bmt), L-2-amino-3-hydroxy-oct-6-enoic acid (devoid of 4-methyl moiety), and enlarged alkyl-groups (*n*-butyl) are not accepted. This means that the stereochemistry of the 4-methyl-group is probably critical for sub-

Table 3   Incorporation Studies with Various Amino Acids into Cyclosporin A[a]

Precursor	New substance detected	Cochromatography with reference[b]	TLC R_f value[c]	HPLC α-value[d]	New cyclosporin isolated[e]	FAB-MS value (M + H[+])	Immunosuppressive activity
Position 1							
L-2-Amino-3-hydroxy-4-methyloctanoic acid	+	+	0.40	12.18	−		
L-2-Amino-3-hydroxy-4,4-dimethyl-octanoic acid	+	+	0.43	13.74	+	1217	n.d.[f]
L-3-Cyclohexylalanine	+	+	0.48	19.79	−		
Leu	+	+	0.43	11.04	−		
L-2-Aminooctanoic acid	+	+	0.55	24.58	−		
3-Hydroxy-3-cyclo-hexyl-L-alanine	+	n.a.[g]	0.37	12.01	+	1203	+
L-2-Amino-3-hydroxy-oct-6-enoic acid	+	+	0.40	9.00	−		
L-2-Amino-3-hydroxy-4,8-dimethyl-nonanoic acid	+	+	0.37	27.73	−		
L-2-Amino-3-hydroxy-4-butyloctanoic acid	+	n.a.	0.40	21.86	−		
cyclo-(dihydro-Bmt)	+	+	0.47	10.82	−		
L-Norleucine	+	n.a.	0.42	n.d.	−		
L-2-Amino-4-methyl-hex-4-enoic acid	+	n.a.	0.36	13.82	−		
Ser	+	+	0.10	4.10	−		
allo-Thr	+	n.a.	0.22	4.50	−		
Cys	+	n.a.	0.21	5.36	−		
Position 2							
Ala	+	+	0.26	7.48	−		
Val	+	+	0.45	14.22	−		
Thr	+	+	0.17	6.37	−		
Nva	+	+	0.41	12.96	−		
L-Allylglycine	+	+	0.48	10.14	−		
allo-Thr	+	+	0.26	7.06	−		
Ile	+	+	0.40	n.d.	−		
Cys	+	+	0.48	n.d.	−		
Positions 4,6,9, and 10							
Val[h]	+	+	0.19	4.84	−		
L-2-Amino-4-methyl-hex-4-enoic acid	+	n.a.	0.36	n.d.	−		
L-Norvaline	+	n.a.	0.27	n.d.	−		
L-Norleucine	+	n.a.	0.30	n.d.	−		
L-tert-Butylalanine	+	n.a.	0.47	n.d.	−		
Positions 5 and 11							
L-Norvaline	+	n.a.	0.38	10.20	+	1202.7	+
allo-Ile	+	n.a.	0.55	15.77	+	1230.9	+
Ile	+	n.a.	0.50	8.40	+	1230	n.d.

Table 3   (*Continued*)

Precursor	New sub-stance detected	Cochroma-tography with reference[b]	TLC R_f-value[c]	HPLC α-value[d]	New cyclosporin isolated[e]	FAB-MS value (M + H[+])	Immunosup-pressive activity
Leu	+	n.a.	0.45	n.d.	−		
L-Cyclopropylglycine	+	n.a.	0.51	12.87	+	n.d.	+
Abu	+	n.a.	0.12	n.d.	−		
L-Allylglycine	+	n.a.	0.63	n.d.	−		
L-*tert*-Butylalanine	+	n.a.	0.48	n.d.	−		
Position 7							
Gly	+	n.a.	0.23	7.96	+	1188	+
Abu	+	+	0.48	11.97	+	1216	+
L-Norvaline	+	n.a.	0.60	14.57	+	n.d.	+
L-Norleucine	+	n.a.	0.32	n.d.	−		
L-Vinylglycine	+	n.a.	0.51	n.d.	−		
Val	+	n.a.	0.33	n.d.	−		
Cys	+	n.a.	0.47	n.d.	−		
Phe	+	n.a.	0.32	n.d.	−		
Position 8							
D-Abu	+	n.a.	0.43	13.09	+	1216	+
D-Ser	+	+	0.26	5.45	−		
Gly	+	+	0.21	7.58	+	1188	+
3-Fluoro-D-alanine	+	+	0.46	9.84	+	1220	+
3-Chloro-D-alanine	+	+	0.49	11.73	+	n.d.	+
D-Vinylglycine	+	n.a.	0.45	12.11	+	1214	+
D-Cyclopropylglycine	+	n.a.	0.48	15.20	+	n.d.	+
D-Cys	+	+	0.40	12.06	−		
D-Phe	+	+	0.63	35.49	+	n.d.	+
D-Val[i]	+	−	0.33	11.68	+	1216	+
D-*tert*-Butylalanine	+	n.a.	0.34	n.d.	−		
D-Lys	+	+	0.32[j]	5.43	−		
1-Chloro-D-vinyl-glycine	+	n.a.	0.45[k]	n.d.	−		

[a] For each position studied, three assays were performed: one with all constitutive amino acids of CyA (control), a second without the original amino acid of the respective position, and a third with the new amino acid.

[b] Cochromatography in thin-layer chromatography (TLC) and in high-performance liquid chromatography (HPLC).

[c] TLC system: silical gel 60 high-performance TLC plates, water-saturated EtOAc, 2 × 10 cm.

[d] HPLC system: LiChrospher 100 RP-$_{18}$ column (5 μm, 125 × 4 mm; Merck Darmstadt) at 75°C; mobile phase: acetonitrile–water–ortho phosphoric acid (630:370:0.1 by vol); detection 210 nm. The α-factor is defined as relative retention time $[(t_{R,1} - t_0)/(t_{R,2} - t_0)] \times 10$, where $t_{R,1}$ and $t_{R,2}$ are the corresponding retention times, and t_0 is the dead retention time. CyA is taken as reference compound (α = 10.00).

[e] Isolation of unlabeled cyclosporins by preparative HPLC was performed as described in (74).

[f] n.d., not done.

[g] n.a., reference not available.

[h] Only the incorporation of the unmethylated valine in position 4 was observed (74).

[i] The data obtained argue strongly against the synthesis of [D-Val[8]] CyA; nevertheless, they indicate incorporation of D-Val into position 8. We prefer the interpretation that [Gly[7], D-Val[8]] CyA is made by the enzyme because of steric hindrance of the valine in position 8.

[j] For separation of this basic cyclosporin, another solvent had to be used: CHCl$_3$:MeOH:AcOH = 80:20:2 (R_f for CyA = 0.86).

[k] Since the preparation of 1-chloro-D-vinylglycine contains some 20% of D-vinylglycine, [D-vinylglycine[8]] CyA is made by the enzyme.

Table 4   Incorporation Studies with Various Amino and Hydroxy Acids into Peptolide SDZ 214-103[a]

Precursor	New substance detected	Cochromatography with reference[b]	TLC R_f value[c]	HPLC α-value[d]	New peptolide isolated[e]	FAB-MS value (M + H[+])	Immunosuppressive activity
Position 1							
L-2-Amino-3-hydroxy-4-methyloctanoic acid	+	+	0.43	23.4	–		
L-3-Cyclohexylalanine	+	n.a.[f]	0.57	35.0	+	n.d.[g]	+
Leu	+	n.a.	0.48	23.0	+	n.d.	+
3-Hydroxy-3-cyclohexyl-L-alanine	+	n.a.	0.38	n.d.	–		
cyclo-(dihydro-Bmt)	+	n.a.	0.76	31.3	+	n.d.	+
Position 2							
L-3-Hydroxynorvaline	+	n.a.	0.55	23.5	+	1261	+
Abu	+	n.a.	0.65	26.4	+	n.d.	+
L-Norvaline	+	n.a.	0.68	32.2	+	n.d.	+
L-Norleucine	+	n.a.	0.70	37.6	+	n.d.	+
Ala	+	n.a.	0.45	n.d.	–		
Val	+	n.a.	0.67	n.d.	–		
L-tert-Butylalanine	+	n.a.	0.51	n.d.	–		
Positions 4,5,6,9, and 10							
Leu[h]	+	+	0.39	n.d.	–		
L-Norleucine	+	n.a.	0.42	n.d.	–		
Val	+	n.a.	0.37	n.d.	–		
Val[i]	no						
Ile[j]	+	+	0.39	n.d.	–		
(3-Trimethylsilyl)-L-alanine	+	n.a.	0.48	n.d	–		
L-2-Amino-4-methyl-hex-4-enoic acid	+	n.a.	0.43	n.d	–		
Position 11							
Abu	+	n.a.	0.53	12.7	+	1234	+
allo-Ile	+	n.a.	0.51	23.4	+	1261	+
Leu	+	n.a.	0.56	22.2	+	n.d.	+
L-Cycloproylglycine	+	n.a.	0.44	33.4	+	n.d.	+
L-Vinylglycine	+	n.a.	0.51	25.8	+	n.d.	+
L-Allylglycine	+	n.a.	0.47	29.6	+	n.d.	+
L-tert-Butylalanine	+	n.a.	0.50	30.2	+	n.d.	+
L-Norvaline	+	n.a.	0.50	n.d	–		
Position 7							
Abu	+	n.a.	0.43	22.9	+	1261	+
L-Vinylglycine	+	n.a.	0.47	31.7	+	n.d.	+
L-Norvaline	+	n.a.	0.67	28.1	+	n.d.	+
Cys[k]	+	n.a.	0.49	32.1	+	n.d.	+

Table 4 (*Continued*)

Precursor	New substance detected	Cochromatography with reference[b]	TLC R_f-value[c]	HPLC α-value[d]	New peptolide isolated[e]	FAB-MS value (M + H+)	Immunosuppressive activity
Position 8							
D-Lactic acid	+	n.a.	0.37	10.5	+	1219	+
D-2-Hydroxybutyric acid	+	n.a.	0.41	15.1	+	1233	+
D-2-Hydroxy-*n*-valeric acid	+	n.a.	0.42	18.5	+	1247	+
D-Hiv	+	n.a.	0.42	19.0	+	n.d.	+
D-2-Hydroxy-3-methyl-valeric acid	+	n.a.	0.42	23.6	+	1261	+
D-Hydroxyisocaproic acid	+	n.a.	0.43	23.9	+	1261	+

[a]For each position, three assays were performed: one with all constitutive amino acids of SDZ 214-103 and D-Hiv (control), a second without the corresponding building unit, and a third with the new amino or hydroxy acid.

[b]Cochromatography in thin-layer chromatography (TLC) and in high-performance liquid chromatography (HPLC).

[c]TLC system: silical gel 60 high-performance TLC plates, water-saturated EtOAc, 2 × 10 cm.

[d]HPLC system: LiChrospher 100 RP-$_{18}$ column (5 μm, 125 × 4 mm; Merck) at 75°C; mobile phase: acetonitrile–water–orthophosphoric acid (630:370:0.1 by vol); detection 210 nm. The α-factor is defined as relative retention time $[(t_{R,1} - t_0)/(t_{R,2} - t_0)] \times 10$, where $t_{R,1}$ and $t_{R,2}$ are the corresponding retention times, and t_0 is the dead retention time. CyA is taken as reference compound ($\alpha = 10.00$).

[e]Isolation of unlabeled peptolides by preparative HPLC was performed as described in (74).

[f]n.a., reference not available.

[g]n.d., not done.

[h]Only the incorporation of the unmethylated leucine in position 4 was observed.

[i]Addition of Val to the SDZ 214-103 synthesis incubation mixture did not yield the formation of the natural compound [Val5]SDZ 214-103.

[j]Only the incorporation of the unmethylated isoleucine in position 5 was observed.

[k]Amounts of the synthesized new peptolide were too low to yield an FAB mass spectrum. Without this, we were not able to decide from our data whether this substance is [Cys7]SDZ 214-103 or not.

strate recognition. On the other hand, as with cyclosporin synthetase, the 3-hydroxy function is not essential; incorporation of both L-3-cyclohexylalanine and L-3-hydroxy-3-cyclohexylalanine is effective. A chain length exceeding eight carbon atoms, as in L-2-amino-3-hydroxy-4,8-dimethylnonanoic acid, is not tolerated. As in the case of cyclosporin synthetase, addition of L-tyrosine to the incubation mixture inhibits peptolide SDZ 214-103 biosynthesis.

2. Position 2

Among the natural cyclosporins, the greatest variability is observed at position 2 (Abu, Ala, Thr, Val, Nva); for the peptolide SDZ 214-103, no natural modifications at this site are known. Using the in vitro system for biosynthesis of cyclosporins, a few examples of further amino acids could be added: L-cysteine and L-allo-threonine are incorporated, but neither serine and 3-hydroxy-norvaline nor homoserine are incorporated. Halogen atoms at C3 prevent the incorporation of the corresponding amino acids, and a double bond at C4 is tolerated (L-allylglycine), but not at C3 (L-vinylglycine). The length of the side chain may vary from one C atom (Ala) up to three (L-norvaline), but an elongated chain as in L-norleucine is not accepted. Steric hindrance is also an important factor: L-leucine, L-isoleucine, L-cyclopropylglycine, and L-*tert*-butylglycine do not serve as substrates for cyclosporin synthetase.

In peptolide SDZ 214-103 and its natural congeners, position 2 is occupied solely by L-threonine, a unit also found in the natural CyC. Other building blocks known for position 2, such as Ala, Abu, Val, and Nva, are only incorporated to a minor extent into SDZ 214-103 analogs, if at all. These findings explain our earlier negative in vivo feeding experiments. On the other hand, the elongated threonine, L-3-hydroxynorvaline, is well incorporated by peptolide synthetase (but not by cyclosporin synthetase). However, in contrast to the successful in vitro incorporation, attempts to prepare the new analog [3-HydroxyNva²]SDZ 214-103 by precursor-directed biosynthesis using the fungus failed.

L-Allylglycine, which is a good substrate for cyclosporin synthetase, is not tolerated by peptolide synthetase; L-norleucine, with an *n*-butyl chain at Cα, is a substrate for the enzyme but is not accepted by cyclosporin synthetase. Halogen-substituted amino acids, such as 3-fluoro- and 3-chloro-L-alanine, do not serve as substrates, nor does L-cysteine or L-ornithine. Interestingly, the 3-hydroxy-group is only accepted in its original stereochemistry; the epimeric L-allo-threonine, which is a substrate of cyclosporin synthetase, is not incorporated.

3.   *Position 3*

Position 3, occupied by sarcosine (= *N*-methylglycine), is the most conserved site. Apart from glycine, only D-alanine was found to be recognized. Other D–amino acids, for example, D-proline and DL-cyclopropylglycine, which are capable of stabilizing the β-turn in the cyclosporin molecule, are not accepted by either enzyme.

4.   *Positions 4, (5), 6, 9, and 10*

Studies focusing exclusively on one particular position of the four *N*-methyl-L-leucines (positions 4, 6, 9, and 10) are not possible because the assay system only provides information about amino acids than can or cannot exchange all of them. In the cyclosporin series, there are two exceptions due to the availability of natural reference compounds, namely in position 4: (a) CyQ and CyS, in which valine substitutes for leucine; and (b) the isoleucine analog [MeIle⁴]CyA. After addition of isoleucine to the CyA incubation mixture to allow the enzyme to incorporate *N*-methylleucines in positions 6, 9, and 10 simultaneously, [MeIle⁴]CyA is formed as major product, indicating that cyclosporin synthetase exhibits a very high affinity for isoleucine only at position 4 (45). It seems that all leucines in cyclosporin can only be replaced by the unbranched hydrophobic amino acids L-norvaline and L-norleucine. Thus, the observed overall substrate specificity for positions 4, 6, 9, and 10 is possibly much higher than for each individual site under consideration.

In the peptolide SDZ 214-103, leucine occupies the five positions 4, 5, 6, 9, and 10; at three of them (positions 4, 6, and 9), Leu is *N*-methylated. Therefore, the characterization of substrate specificities of specific leucine sites is even more difficult than that discussed for cyclosporins. Evidently, L-valine and L-norleucine appear to be accepted for all leucines in peptolide SDZ 214-103. From large-scale fermentations, the isoleucine-5 analog has been isolated as natural minor metabolite (Hofmann H, unpublished results).

5.   Position(s) (5 and) 11

The valine-containing positions 5 and 11 (cyclosporin synthetase) and 11 (peptolide SDZ 214-103 synthetase) exhibit a moderate substrate specificity. One of the β-methyl-groups of the valines may be exchanged for either a hydrogen (Abu) or an ethyl-group (allo-Ile) or one methyl-group for a hydrogen atom and the other for an ethyl-group (L-norvaline). It is remarkable that L-isoleucine is a substrate only for cyclosporin synthetase, indicating that the stereochemistry of Cβ is discriminating for position 11 of peptolide synthetase. The unsaturated analog of L-norvaline, L-allylglycine, is accepted by both enzymes to a minor degree. O-Methyl-L-threonine, a mimic of L-valine or L-isoleucine, is not incorporated (similar to O-methylaspartic acid instead of Leu). Furthermore, the α-branched 2-aminoisobutyric acid cannot replace either Abu at position 2 nor valine at positions 5 and 11; it acts, not unexpectedly, as a strong inhibitor of in vitro cyclosporin biosynthesis (76).

As discussed for the leucine sites, only the sum of the specificities of positions 5 and 11 is determined in the case of cyclosporin synthetase. Since in peptolide SDZ 214-103 position 11 is the single one containing a valine moiety, it is easier to study. At position 11 both enzymes resemble each other the most, but the general rule that peptolide synthetase exerts the higher substrate specificity is also valid for this site.

6.   Position 7

The last position in the biosynthetic pathway appears to have a very high substrate specificity. In vivo, the only modification encountered so far is the substitution for L-alanine by L-2-aminobutyric acid, yielding the natural CyV. The latter is formed in vitro as the main reaction product besides [Gly7]CyA when Ala is omitted in the incubation mixture. Some further evidence has been found for the incorporation of L-norvaline and L-vinylglycine (to a small extent). Many substituents that are good substrates of position 8 in the D-configuration (3-fluoro-alanine, 3-chloro-alanine, cyclopropylglycine, and serine) do not serve at all as substrates for position 7. An even higher substrate specificity of this site is exerted, once again, by peptolide SDZ 214-103 synthetase.

7.   Position 8

Position 8 is the only position containing a D–amino acid in cyclosporin, and it is the starting position of the biosynthetic process (66). For recognition by cyclosporin synthetase, all substrates for that position must be present in the D-configuration, except glycine. Slight modification of the alkyl chain in D-Ala is allowed: D-Abu, D-vinylglycine, D-cyclopropylglycine, and probably D-valine are substrates for position 8, but longer or more bulky (e.g., D-norvaline, D-isoleucine, DL-*tert*-butylglycine) side chains are not tolerated. The successful in vitro synthesis of the new cyclosporin analog [D-Abu8]CyA is an illustrative example (Figure 11a). In vivo experiments with feeding of D-Abu to the fungus do not lead to the formation of the envisaged compound; rather, CyA production is stimulated, probably due to the epimerization of D-Abu into the L-form by the nonspecific alanine racemase. In the case of [D-Abu8]CyA, sufficient material could be prepared by enzymatic synthesis; thus, the structure was confirmed by FAB-MS show-

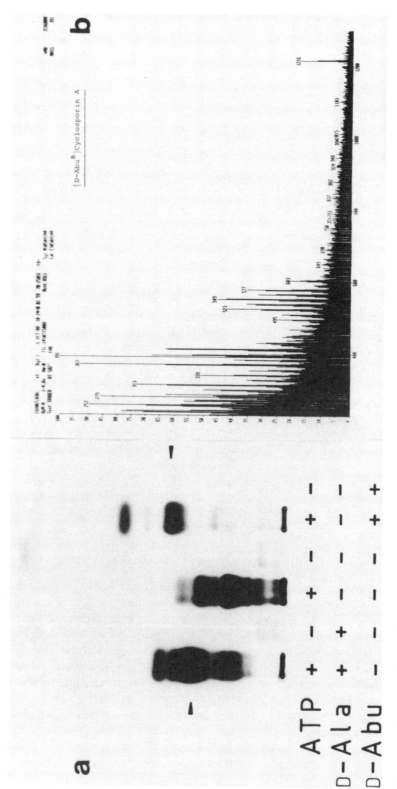

Figure 11 *In vitro* synthesis of [D-Abu8]cyclosporin A. (a) When all constitutive amino acids of CyA are incubated together with ATP, Mg^{2+}, S-adenosyl-L-[^{14}C-*methyl*]-methionine, and the enzyme fraction, the main reaction product is CyA (left arrow). If D-Ala is exchanged for D-Abu, the new product [D-Abu8]CyA is synthesized (right arrow). The thin-layer chromatographic (TLC) separation of ethyl acetate–extractable reaction products is shown as autoradiogram. (b) Fast atom bombardment mass spectrum of [D-Abu8]CyA, showing the correct molecular ion peak (1216(M + H)$^+$). (From Ref. 59, with permission.)

Table 5   Immunosuppressive Activity of *In Vitro* Synthesized Cyclosporin A and Peptolide
SDZ 214-103 Analogs

Cyclopeptide	Biosynthesis	Activity[a]
Cyclosporin A (Sandimmun)	Natural	+++
Cyclosporin A	Enzymatic	+++
[Me-3-hydroxy-cyclohexylalanine^1]CyA	Enzymatic	++
[Nva^{2,5}, MeNva^{11}]CyA	Enzymatic	++
[Nva^5, MeNva1^{11}]CyA	Enzymatic	++(+)
[aIle^5, aMeIle^{11}]Cya	Enzymatic	++
[aIle^{5,11}]Cya	Enzymatic	+
[Cyclopropylglycine^5, MeCyclopropylglycine^{11}]CyA	Enzymatic	++(+)
[Gly^7]CyA	Enzymatic	++
[β-Ala^7]CyA	Enzymatic	++
[Gly^{7,8}]CyA	Enzymatic	++
[Abu^7, D-Abu^8]CyA	Enzymatic	++
[Gly^8]CyA	Enzymatic	++(+)
[β-fluoro-D-Ala^8]CyA	Enzymatic	++
[β-chloro-D-Ala^8]CyA	Enzymatic	++
[D-Abu^8]CyA	Enzymatic	++
[D-Cyclopropylglycine^8]CyA	Enzymatic	++(+)
[D-Vinylglycine^8]CyA	Enzymatic	++(+)
[D-Phe^8]CyA	Enzymatic	+
[β-Ala^8]CyA	Enzymatic	++
SDZ 214-103	Natural	+++
SDZ 214-103	Enzymatic	+++
[MeCyclohexylalanine^1]SDZ 214-103	Enzymatic	++
[3-Hydroxynva^2]SDZ 214-103	Enzymatic	+++
[Abu^7]SDZ 214-103	Enzymatic	++(+)
[D-Lactic acid^8]SDZ 214-103	Enzymatic	+++
[D-2-Hydroxybutyric acid^8]SDZ 214-103	Enzymatic	+++
[D-2-Hydroxy-n-valeric acid^8]SDZ 214-103	Enzymatic	+++
[D-2-Hydroxy-3-methylvaleric acid^8]SDZ 214-103	Enzymatic	++(+)
[D-2-Hydroxyisocaproic acid^8]SDZ 214-103	Enzymatic	++
[MeAbu^{11}]SDZ 214-103	Enzymatic	++(+)
[MeLeu^{11}]SDZ 214-103	Enzymatic	++
[aMeIle^{11}]SDZ 214-103	Enzymatic	++(+)

[a]+++ = strong immunosuppressive activity; ++ = moderate activity; + = weak activity.

ing the correct molecular ion peak at m/z 1216 (Figure 11b), the immunosuppressive activity in vitro was measured to about a factor of 5 lower than the activity of CyA (Table 5).

If D-alanine is missing in the incubation mixture, glycine takes its position, and [Gly^8]cyclosporin is formed in high yield. Also, the combined replacement of D-Ala (position 8) and L-Ala (position 7) can be achieved by omitting both D-Ala and L-Ala or by substituting for them with D,L-Abu; [Gly^{7,8}]CyA and [Abu^7, D-Abu^8]CyA, respectively, are obtained.

Regarding the substitution of D-alanine by D-valine, in vitro synthesis of [D-Val⁸]CyA per se is not achieved as indicated by the FAB-MS (*m/z* 1216 instead of the expected value of 1230). To interpret the difference in 14 mass units, we propose that, as a result of the branched side chain of valine, the enzyme selects for the neighboring position 7 a "smaller" amino acid leading to the formation [Gly⁷, D-Val⁸]CyA. On the other hand, the incorporation of D-cyclopropylglycine as a close, but sterically less demanding, analog of D-valine yields, although in small amounts, [D-cyclopropylglycine⁸]CyA. The β-position of D-Ala may carry a hydroxyl- (D-Ser), a sulfhydryl- (D-Cys), or a halogeno-function (3-fluoro-D-Ala, 3-chloro-D-Ala), but the double- and triple-substituted amino acids 3,3-difluoro-D-Ala and 3,3,3-trifluoro-D-Ala are no longer substrates of cyclosporin synthetase. An elongated side chain in the polar precursors, exemplified by 3-chloro-D-vinylglycine or both D-Thr and D-allo-Thr, is not tolerated. Interestingly, the aromatic amino acid D-phenylalanine serves as a minor substrate for the enzyme.

D-Hydroxy acids, like D-2-hydroxyisovaleric acid, the corresponding building unit of peptolide SDZ 214-103, and D-lactic acid, the isosteric compound to D-Ala, are not incorporated into position 8 by cyclosporin synthetase (62). Thus, cyclosporin synthetase is not capable of introducing an ester linkage between positions 7 and 8, as does peptolide SDZ 214-103 synthetase.

Peptolide SDZ 214-103 synthetase recognizes, as far as been analyzed, D-2-hydroxy acids carrying various alkyl chains at the α-carbon, ranging from methyl (D-lactic acid) to butyl (D-2-hydroxycaproic acid). Methyl branches at C3 (D-hydroxyisovaleric acid, D-2-hydroxy-3-methylvaleric acid) and C4 (D-2-hydroxy-4-methylvaleric acid = D-2-hydroxyisocaproic acid) are accepted as well. On the other hand, the α-branched D-2-hydroxyisobutyric acid is not a substrate. For position 8, several differences in the substrate specificities of the enzymes become evident. D-Ala is the building block of all natural cyclosporins, and the isosteric D-lactic acid is a good substrate of peptolide synthetase. While glycine can replace D-Ala in cyclosporins, its isoster, glycolic acid, is not incorporated by peptolide synthetase. Whereas both enzymes efficiently incorporate the corresponding precursors with an ethyl side chain (D-Abu or D-2-hydroxybutyric acid), the propyl-group is accepted only by peptolide synthetase (D-2-hydroxy-*n*-valeric acid) but not as D-norvaline in the case of cyclosporin synthetase. The isoster of the natural D-2-hydroxyisovaleric acid unit in the peptolide, the amino acid D-valine, is incorporated into cyclosporins as discussed above, but D-leucine, the isoster of D-2-hydroxy-4-methylvaleric acid, is not accepted. Polar substituents in the hydroxy acids are a limitation, too; the D-serine isoster D-glyceric acid is not accepted as a substrate.

Whereas D-phenylalanine serves as a substrate for cyclosporin synthetase, the isoster D-phenyllactic acid is not incorporated into the peptolide.

Peptides are not substrates of cyclosporin synthetase as has been described for gramicidin S synthetase 2 (79). Neither the dipeptide D-Ala–MeLeu nor the nonapeptide D-Ala–MeLeu–MeLeu–MeVal–MeBmt–Abu–Sar–MeLeu–Val is incorporated into CyA in vitro. Remarkably, though, cyclosporin synthetase is capable of introducing a β-alanine into position 7 or 8 instead of the α-alanines present in CyA, leading to the formation of a 34-membered ring instead of the "normal" 33-membered ring (77). To our knowledge, enzymatic synthesis of such ring-enlarged cyclopeptides has not been described in the literature before. Both [β-Ala⁷]CyA and [β-Ala⁸]CyA show moderate immunosuppressive activity (Table 5). Peptolide SDZ 214-103 synthetase, on the other hand, did not incorporate either β-Ala in position 7 or a D-β-hydroxy acid in position 8.

VII. CYCLOSPORIN A AND NOVEL CYCLOSPORINS FROM DIVERSE FUNGAL TAXA

In addition to the original cyclosporin-producing fungi. *T. inflatum* and *C. lucidum*, in the last decade a series of microorganisms belonging to various fungal taxa were discovered that produce CyA (and CyB, CyC), usually in low titers (1 to 10 mg/liter). Within this group, a *Trichoderma viride* strain (80) and various strains of *Fusarium* (81–83) and *Neocosmospora* (81,84), besides a complex group of hyphomycetes, for example, *Tolypocladium* sp., *Acremonium*, *Beauveria*, and *Chaunopycnis* (for a review, see Ref. 85). We presume that the natural, nonmutated cyclosporin A–producing strains coproduce the known congeners, mainly CyB and CyC, by merit of a common multienzyme polypeptide as characterized in detail from *T. inflatum*.

Different patterns of cyclosporin biosynthesis in fungi have begun to emerge. As a first example, the peptolide SDZ 214-103 (=[Thr^2, Leu^5, D-Hiv^8, Leu^{10}]cyclosporin) was obtained from cultures of *C. oligospermum* (Corda) Bonorden (33). This fungus was isolated from leaf litter collected in the Swiss Jura. Also, the fungus *Stachybotrys chartarum* has been reported to produce the new compound FR901459 = [Thr^2, Leu^5, Leu^{10}]CyA, but none of the other known cyclosporins (86). Two further examples were discovered in our laboratories, namely, the production of the novel [Thr^2, Leu^5, Ala^{10}]CyA by a strain identified as *Acremonium luzulae* (Fuckel) W. Gams, and of [Thr^2, Ile^5]CyA by a strain classified as a *Leptostroma* anamorph of *Hypoderma eucalyptii* Cooke and Harkn. (87). The usual pattern of known cyclosporins is not found in either organism. The two compounds represent hitherto unique members of the cyclosporin family: in [Thr^2, Leu^5, Ala^{10}]CyA, the *N*-methylleucine unit at position 10 is exchanged against alanine; and in [Thr^2, Ile^5]CyA, for the first time, isoleucine occurs in position 5 of the peptide ring. Recently, [Leu^4]CyA, representing a new structural variation, and [MeLeu^1]CyA, identical with our minor component Cy28 from *T. inflatum*, were isolated from the mycelium of surface-cultivated *Tolypocladium terricola* (88). Interestingly, [MeLeu^4]CyA has also become available as *N*-demethylation product of CyA by microbial biotransformation with *Actinoplanes* sp. ATCC 53771 (89).

The antifungal antibiotic ramihyphin A from *Fusarium solani*, described several years ago, turned out to be identical with CyA (90).

VIII. OUTLOOK

The mechanism of cyclosporin biosynthesis is now widely understood, as key enzymes Bmt synthase, alanine racemase, and cyclosporin synthetase are necessary to build up the cyclic undecapeptide. Still more experimental work has to be performed on the biosynthesis of the peptolide SDZ 214-103 to fully characterize the enzymes and the pathways involved.

The in vitro systems established for the synthesis of CyA and the peptolide SDZ 214-103, as well as the detailed knowledge of the biosynthesis of the amino acid Bmt, will, furthermore, enable access to new cyclosporin and peptolide analogs with an enhanced or altered spectrum of biological effects, for example, exerting anti-HIV activity.

Screening of a broad variety of microorganisms over the last decade has revealed diverse fungal taxa producing CyA and its congeners; even some cyclosporins that contain novel structural modifications have been detected in this way. Surely, that list will be further enlarged in the near future.

The manipulation of the giant cyclosporin synthetase gene by DNA-mediated transformation represents the first step toward gene engineering. By exchanging parts of the gene coding for amino acid–specific domains, mutated genes will be gained with the aim of directing the synthesis of new cyclosporins or of cyclosporins that at present are only obtained as minor products in the normal biosynthesis.

ACKNOWLEDGMENT

I express great appreciation to my colleague Alfons Lawen (Monash University, Clayton, Victoria, Australia; formerly at Technical University, Berlin) for his valuable comments regarding this chapter.

REFERENCES

1. von Wartburg A, Traber R. Cyclosporins, fungal metabolites with immunosuppressive activities. Ellis GP, West GB, eds. Progress in Medicinal Chemistry, Vol. 25. Amsterdam: Elsevier Science Publishers 1988:1–33.
2. Rüegger A, Kuhn M, Lichti H, Loosli HR, Huguenin R, Quiquerez C, von Wartburg A. Cyclosporin A, ein immunsuppressiv wirksamer Peptidmetabolit aus *Trichoderma polysporum* (Link ex Pers.) Rifai. Helv Chim Acta 1976; 59:1075–1092.
3. Borel JF, Feurer C, Gubler HU, Stähelin H. Biological effects of cyclosporin A: A new anti-lymphocytic agent. Agents Actions 1976; 6:468–475.
4. Borel JF. Editorial: Ciclosporin and its future. Prog Allergy 1986; 38:9–18.
5. Borel JF. Pharmacology of cyclosporine (Sandimmune). IV. Pharmacological properties *in vivo*. Pharmacol Rev 1989; 41:259–371.
6. Feutren G, von Graffenried B. Cyclosporin A: Pharmacology and therapeutic use in autoimmune diseases. Rugstad HE, Endresen L, Forre O, eds. Immunopharmacology in Autoimmune Diseases and Transplantation. New York: Plenum Press, 1992:159–173.
7. Borel JF, Feutren G, Baumann G, Hiestand PC. Cyclosporin and some new immunosuppressive drugs in the treatment of autoimmune diseases. Lydyard PM, Brostoff J, eds. Autoimmune Disease. Oxford: Blackwell Science, 1994:169–217.
8. Mason J. Pathophysiology and toxicology of Cyclosporine in humans and animals. Pharmacol Rev 1989; 41:423–434.
9. Quesniaux VFJ. Pharmacology of cyclosporine (Sandimmune): Immunochemistry and monitoring. Pharmacol Rev 1989; 41:249–258.
10. Gavériaux C, Boesch D, Boelsterli JJ, Bollinger P, Eberle MK, Hiestand P, Payne T, Traber R, Wenger R, Loor F. Overcoming multidrug resistance in Chinese hamster ovary cells *in vitro* by cyclosporin A (Sandimmune) and non-immunosuppressive derivatives. Br J Cancer 1989; 60:867–871.
11. Andrieu JM, Even P, Venet A, Tourani JM, Stern M, Lowenstein W, Audroin C, Eme D, Masson D, Sors H, Israel-Biet D, Beldjord K. Effects of cyclosporin on T-cell subsets in human immunodeficiency virus disease. Clin Immunol Immunopathol 1988; 47:181–198.
12. Karpas A, Lowdell M, Jacobson SK, Hill F. Inhibition of human immunodeficiency virus and growth of infected T cells by the immunosuppressive drugs cyclosporin A and FK 506. Proc Natl Acad Sci USA 1992; 89:8351–8355.

13. Rosenwirth B, Billich A, Datema R, Donatsch P, Hammerschmid F, Harrison R, Hiestand P, Jaksche H, Mayer P, Peichl P, Quesniaux V, Schatz F, Schuurman HJ, Traber R, Wenger R, Wolff B, Zenke G, Zurini M. Inhibition of HIV-1 replication by SDZ NIM 811, a non-immunosuppressive cyclosporin A analog. Antimicrob Agents Chemother 1994; 38:1763–1772.

14. Handschumacher RE, Harding MW, Rice J, Drugge RJ, Speicher DW. Cyclophilin: A specific cytosolic binding protein for cyclosporin A. Science 1984; 226:544–547.

15. Weber C, Wider G, von Freyberg B, Traber R, Braun W, Widmer H, Wüthrich K. The NMR structure of cyclosporin A bound to cyclophilin in aqueous solution. Biochem 1991; 30:6563–6574.

16. Fischer G, Wittmann-Liebold B, Lang K, Kiefhaber T, Schmid FX. Cyclophilin and peptidyl-prolyl *cis-trans* isomerase are probably identical proteins. Nature 1989; 337:476–478.

17. Baumann G. Molecular mechanism of immunosuppressive agents. Transplant Proc 1992; 24 (Suppl 2):4–7.

18. Lawen A. Biosynthesis and mechanism of action of cyclosporins. Ellis GP, Luscombe DK, eds. Progress in Medicinal Chemistry, Vol. 33. Amsterdam: Elsevier Science Publishers, 1996:53–97.

19. Fliri HG, Wenger R. Cyclosporine: Synthetic studies, structure-activity relationships, biosynthesis and mode of action. Kleinkauf H, von Döhren H, eds. Biochemistry of Peptide Antibiotics. Berlin, New York: Walter de Gruyter, 1990:245–287.

20. Dreyfuss M, Härri E, Hofmann H, Kobel H, Pache W, Tscherter H. Cyclosporin A and C, new metabolites from *Trichoderma polysporum*. Eur J Appl Microbiol 1976; 3:125–133.

21. Gams W. *Tolypocladium*, eine Hyphomycetengattung mit geschwollenen Phialiden. Persoonia 1971; 6:185–191.

22. Bissett J. Notes on *Tolypocladium* and related genera. Can J Bot 1983; 61:1311–1329.

23. Cannon PF. International Commission on the Taxonomy of Fungi (ICTF): Name changes in fungi of microbiological, industrial and medical importance. Part 2. Microbiol Sci 1986; 3:285–287.

24. von Arx JA. *Tolypocladium*, a synonym of *Beauveria*. Mycotaxon 1986; 25:153–158.

25. Catalogue of Filamentous Fungi. Jong SC, Edwards MJ, eds. Rockeville: American Type Culture Collection (ATCC) 18th ed. 1991:75.

26. Dreyfuss MM, Gams W. Proposal to reject *Pachybasium niveum* Rostrup in order to retain the name *Tolypocladium inflatum* W. Gams for the fungus that produces cyclosporin. Taxon 1994; 34:660–661.

27. Kobel H, Traber R. Directed biosynthesis of cyclosporins. Eur J Appl Microbiol Biotechnol 1982; 14:237–240.

28. Traber R, Kuhn M, Loosli HR, Pache W, von Wartburg A. Neue Cyclopeptide aus *Trichoderma polysporum*: die Cyclosporine B, D and E. Helv Chim Acta 1977; 60:1568–1578.

29. Traber R, Hofmann H, Loosli HR, Ponelle M, von Wartburg A. Neue Cyclosporine aus *Tolypocladium inflatum*. Die Cyclosporine K–Z. Helv Chim Acta 1987; 70:13–36.

30. Lee J, Agathos SN. Dynamics of L-valine in relation to the production of cyclosporin A by *Tolypocladium inflatum*. Appl Microbiol Biotechnol 1991; 34:513–517.

31. Chun GT, Agathos SN. Immobilization of *Tolypocladium inflatum* spores into porous celite beads for cyclosporine production. J Biotechnol 1989; 9:237–254.

32. Traber R, Loosli HR, Hofmann H, Kuhn M, von Wartburg A. Isolierung und Strukturermittlung der neuen Cyclosporine E, F, G, H und I. Helv Chim Acta 1982; 65:1655–1677.

33. Dreyfuss MM, Schreier MH, Tscherter H, Wenger R (Sandoz Ltd.). Cyclosporin peptolides, their preparation by fermentation or chemical synthesis, and their use as pharmaceuticals. European Patent Application 0 296 123 A2; June 15, 1988. [Chem Abstr 1989; 111:152146a.]

34. Kobel H, Loosli HR, Voges R. Contribution to knowledge of the biosynthesis of cyclosporin A. Experientia 1983; 39:873–876.

35. Senn H, Weber C, Kobel H, Traber R. Selective ^{13}C-labelling of cyclosporin A. Eur J Biochem 1991; 199:653–658.

36. Offenzeller M, Su Z, Santer G, Moser H, Traber R, Memmert K, Schneider-Scherzer E. Biosynthesis of the unusual amino acid (4R)-4-[(E)-2-butenyl]-4-methyl-L-threonine of cyclosporin A. Identification of 3(R)-hydroxy-4(R)-methyl-6(E)-octenoic acid as a key intermediate by enzymatic *in vitro* synthesis and by *in vivo* labeling techniques. J Biol Chem 1993; 268:26127–26134.

37. Offenzeller M, Santer G, Totschnig K, Su Z, Moser H, Traber R, Schneider-Scherzer E. Biosynthesis of the unusual amino acid (4R)-4-[(E)-2-butenyl]-4-methyl-L-threonine of cyclosporin A: Enzymatic details of the polyketide pathway. Biochem 1996; 35:8401–8412.

38. Hoffmann K, Schneider-Scherzer E, Kleinkauf H, Zocher R. Purification and characterization of eucaryotic alanine racemase acting as key enzyme in cyclosporin biosynthesis. J Biol Chem 1994; 269:12710–12714.

39. Kleinkauf H, von Döhren H. Nonribosomal biosynthesis of peptide antibiotics. Eur J Biochem 1990; 192:1–15.

40. Katz E, Demain AL. The peptide antibiotics of Bacillus: Chemistry, biogenesis and possible functions. Bacteriol Rev 1977; 41:449–474.

41. Traber R, Hofmann H, Kobel H. Cyclosporins: New analogues by precursor directed biosynthesis. J Antibiot 1989; 42:591–597.

42. Patchett AA, White RF, Goegelman RT. A new cyclosporin derivative with modified "8-amino acid." U.K. Patent Application BG 2 206 119 A; June 20, 1988.

43. Hensens OD, White RF, Goegelman RT, Inamine ES, Patchett AA. The preparation of [2-deutero-3-fluoro-D-Ala[8]]cyclosporin A by directed biosynthesis. J Antibiot 1992; 45:133–135.

44. Wang E, Walsh C. Suicide substrates for the alanine racemase of *Escherichia coli* B. Biochem 1978; 17:1313–1321.

45. Traber R, Kobel H, Loosli HR, Senn H, Rosenwirth B, Lawen A. [MeIle[4]]Cyclosporin, a novel natural cyclosporin with anti-HIV activity: Structural elucidation, biosynthesis and biological properties. Antivir Chem Chemother 1994; 5:331–339.

46. Davies L. Functional and stereochemical specificity at the β carbon atom of substrates in threonine dehydratase-catalyzed α,β elimination reactions. J Biol Chem 1979; 254:4126–4131.

47. Faleev NG, Martinkova NS, Sadovnikova MS, Saporovskaya MB, Belikov VM. The L- and D-threonine dehydratases accompanying L-tyrosine phenol-lyase: Selective decomposition of D-threonine in racemic mixture. Enz Microb Technol 1982; 4:164–168.

48. Crout DHG, Gregorio MVM, Müller US, Komatsubara S, Kisumi M, Chibata O. Stereochemistry of the conversions of L-threonine and D-threonine into 2-oxobutanoate by the L-threonine and D-threonine dehydratases of *Serratia marcescens*. Eur J Biochem 1980; 106:97–105.

49. Lawen A, Zocher R. Cyclosporin synthetase: The most complex peptide synthesizing multienzyme polypeptide so far described. J Biol Chem 1990; 265:11355–11360.

50. Zocher R, Nihira T, Paul E, Madry N, Peeters H, Kleinkauf H, Keller U. Biosynthesis of cyclosporin A: Partial purification and properties of a multifunctional enzyme from *Tolypocladium inflatum*. Biochemistry 1986; 25:550–553.

51. Dittmann J, Lawen A, Zocher R, Kleinkauf H. Isolation and partial characterization of cyclosporin synthetase from a cyclosporin non-producing mutant of *Beauveria nivea*. Biol Chem Hoppe-Seyler 1990; 371:829–834.

52. Sanglier JJ, Traber R, Buck RH, Hofmann H, Kobel H. Isolation of (4R)-4-[(E)-2-butenyl]-4-methyl-L-threonine, the characteristic structural element of cyclosporins, from a blocked mutant of *Tolypocladium inflatum*. J Antibiot 1990; 43:707–714.

53. Zocher R, Keller U, Kleinkauf H. Enniatin synthetase, a novel type of multifunctional enzyme catalyzing depsipeptide synthesis in *Fusarium oxysporum*. Biochemistry 1982; 21:43–48.

54.   Akers HA, Lee SG, Lipmann F. Identification of two enzymes responsible for the synthesis of the initial portion of linear gramicidin. Biochem 1977; 16:5722–5729.

55.   Lee SG, Roskoski Jr R, Bauer K, Lipmann F. Purification of the polyenzymes responsible for tyrocidine synthesis and their dissociation into subunits. Biochem 1973; 12:398–405.

56.   Smith DJ, Earl AJ, Turner G. The multifunctional peptide synthetase performing the first step of penicillin biosynthesis in *Penicillium chrysogenum* is a 421 073 dalton protein similar to *Bacillus brevis* peptide antibiotic synthetases. EMBO J 1990; 9:2743–2750.

57.   Díez B, Gutiérrez S, Barredo JL, van Solingen P, van der Voort LH, Martin JF. The cluster of penicillin biosynthetic genes: Identification and characterization of the *pcb*AB gene encoding the α-aminoadipyl-cysteinyl-valine synthetase and linkage of the *pcb*C and *pen*DE genes. J Biol Chem 1990; 265:16358–16365.

58.   Schmidt B, Riesner D, Lawen A, Kleinkauf H. Cyclosporin synthetase is a 1.4 MDa multienzyme polypeptide. Re-evaluation of the molecular mass of various peptide synthetases. FEBS Lett 1992; 307:355–360.

59.   Lawen A, Dittmann J, Schmidt B, Riesner D, Kleinkauf H. Enzymatic biosynthesis of cyclosporin A and analogues. Biochimie 1992; 74:511–516.

60.   Weber G, Schörgendorfer K, Schneider-Scherzer E, Leitner E. The peptide synthetase catalyzing cyclosporine production in *Tolypocladium niveum* is encoded by a giant 45.8-kilobase open reading frame. Curr Genet 1994; 26:120–125.

61.   Merrick WC. Mechanism and regulation of eukaryotic protein synthesis. Microbiol Rev 1992; 56:291–315.

62.   Lawen A, Traber R, Geyl D. *In vitro* biosynthesis of [Thr^2,Leu^5,D-Hiv^8,Leu^{10}]cyclosporin, a cyclosporin-related peptolide with immunosuppressive activity by a multienzyme polypeptide. J Biol Chem 1991; 266:15567–15570.

63.   Lee C, Lawen A. *In vitro* biosynthesis of peptolide SDZ 90-215 by a 1.2 MDa multienzyme polypeptide. Biochem Mol Biol Int 1993; 31:797–805.

64.   Nomenclature for multienzymes—recommendations 1989 of the Nomenclature Committee of the International Union of Biochemistry (NC-IUB). Eur J Biochem 1989; 185:485–486.

65.   Lipmann F. Attempts to map a process evolution of peptide biosynthesis. Science 1971; 173:875–884.

66.   Dittmann J, Wenger RM, Kleinkauf H, Lawen A. Mechanism of cyclosporin A biosynthesis: Evidence for synthesis via a single linear undecapeptide precursor. J Biol Chem 1994; 269:2841–2846.

67.   Loosli HR, Kessler H, Oschkinat H, Weber HP, Petcher TJ, Widmer A. Peptide conformations: The conformation of cyclosporin A in the crystal and in solution. Helv Chim Acta 1985; 68:682–702.

68.   Kleinkauf H, von Döhren H. Biosynthesis of peptide antibiotics. Annu Rev Microbiol 1987; 41:259–289.

69.   Kleinkauf H, Dittmann J, Lawen A. Cell-free biosynthesis of cyclosporin A and analogues. Biomed Biochim Acta 1991; 50:S219–S224.

70.   Schlumbohm W, Stein T, Ullrich C, Vater J, Krause M, Marahiel MA, Kruft V, Wittmann-Liebold B. An active serine is involved in covalent substrate amino acid binding at each reaction center of gramicidin S synthetase. J Biol Chem 1991; 266:23135–23141.

71.   Dittmann J. Untersuchungen zum Mechanismus der *in vitro* Biosynthese von Cyclosporin A. Ph.D. Thesis, Technical University of Berlin, 1992.

72.   Haese A, Schubert M, Herrmann M, Zocher R. Molecular characterization of the enniatin synthetase gene encoding a multifunctional enzyme catalyzing N-methyldepsipeptide formation in *Fusarium scirpi*. Mol Microbiol 1993; 7:905–914.

73.   Dittmann J, Vaillant F, Kleinkauf H, Lawen A. Reversible denaturation of cyclosporin synthetase by urea. FEBS Lett 1996; 380:157–160.

74.   Lawen A, Traber R, Geyl D. *In vitro* biosynthesis of [Thr^2,Leu^5,D-Hiv^8,Leu^{10}]cyclosporin, a cyclosporin-related immunosuppressive peptolide. Biomed Biochim Acta 1991; 50:S260–S263.

75. Lawen A, Traber R, Geyl D, Zocher R, Kleinkauf H. Cell-free biosynthesis of new cyclosporins. J Antibiot 1989; 42:1283–1289.

76. Lawen A, Traber R. Substrate specificities of cyclosporin synthetase and peptolide SDZ 214-103 synthetase. Comparison of the substrate specificities of the related multifunctional polypeptides. J Biol Chem 1993; 268:20452–20465.

77. Lawen A, Traber R, Reuille R, Ponelle M. *In vitro* biosynthesis of ring-extended cyclosporins. Biochem J 1994; 300:395–399.

78. von Wartburg A, Traber R. Chemistry of the natural cyclosporin metabolites. Prog Allergy 1986; 38:28–45.

79. von Dungen A, Vater J, Kleinkauf H. Biosynthesis of gramicidin S with the aid of dipeptides by gramicidin S synthetase. Eur J Biochem 1976; 66:623–626.

80. Gauze GF, Terekhova LP, Maximova TS, Brazhnikova MG, Federova GF, Borisova VN. Screening of new antibiotics of cyclosporin group. Antibiotiki 1983; 28:243–245.

81. Dreyfuss MM. Neue Erkenntnisse aus einem pharmakologischen Pilz-Screening. Sydowia 1986; 39:22–36.

82. Hong L, Tang X, Miao C, Wang Y. Cyclosporin produced by *Fusarium solani* sp. no. 4–11. Isolation, separation, purification, and identification. Kangshengsu 1984; 9:5–15.

83. Sawai K, Okuno T, Terada Y, Harada Y, Sawamura K, Sasaki H, Takao S. Isolation and properties of two antifungal substances from *Fusarium solani*. Agric Biol Chem 1981; 45:1223–1228.

84. Nakajima H, Hamasaki T, Tanaka K, Kimura Y, Udagawa S, Horie Y. Production of cyclosporin by fungi belonging to the genus *Neocosmospora*. Agric Biol Chem 1989; 53:2291–2292.

85. Dreyfuss MM, Chapela IH. Potential of fungi in the discovery of novel, low-molecular weight pharmaceuticals. Gullo VP, ed. The Discovery of Natural Products with Therapeutic Potential. Boston: Butterworth-Heinemann, 1994:49–80.

86. Sakamoto K, Tsujii E, Miyauchi M, Nakanishi T, Yamashita M, Shigematsu N, Tada T, Izumi S, Okuhara M. FR901459, a novel immunosuppressant isolated from *Stachybotrys chartarum* no. 19392. J Antibiot 1993; 46:1788–1798.

87. Traber R, Dreyfuss MM. Occurence of cyclosporins and cyclosporin-like peptolides in fungi. J Ind Microbiol 1996 (in press).

88. Jegorov A, Matha V, Sedmera P, Havliček V, Stuchlik J, Seidel P, Šimek P. Cyclosporins from *Tolypocladium terricola*. Phytochem 1995; 38:403–407.

89. Kuhnt M, Bitsch F, France J, Hofmann H, Sanglier JJ, Traber R. Microbial biotransformation of cyclosporin A. J Antibiot 1996; 49:781–787.

90. Proska B, Uhrín D, Kovácik V, Voticky Z, Betina V. Identity of the antibiotic ramihyphin A and cyclosporin A. Folia Microbiol 1991; 36:141–143.

10
Echinocandin Antifungal Agents

William W. Turner and William L. Current

Lilly Research Laboratories, Eli Lilly and Company, Indianapolis, Indiana

I. INTRODUCTION

Fungal infections range from superficial conditions of the skin (e.g., ringworm and athlete's foot) and nails (onychomycoses) to disseminated life-threatening diseases. During the past decade, the incidence of life-threatening fungal infections has increased dramatically (1). Major factors responsible for this dramatic rise include increased use of broad-spectrum antibiotics, marked increases in the numbers of immunocompromised persons (e.g., AIDS, cancer, and transplant patients), more aggressive medical procedures with increased use of invasive techniques and prosthetic devices, and an aging patient population.

Pathogenic fungi responsible for life-threatening infections in the immunocompromised host include *Candida* spp., *Aspergillus* spp., *Pneumocystis carinii*, *Cryptococcus neoformans*, and *Histoplasma capsulatum*. Present therapeutic options for the treatment of such fungal infections are limited to compounds in two classes, the polyenes and the azoles. Amphotericin B, a polyene antifungal agent, has broad-spectrum activity; however, its utility is limited by nephrotoxicity. This compound may be used alone or in combination with 5-fluorocytosine. Newer azoles, such as fluconazole, are fungistatic agents that are relatively safe and free of side effects; however, resistance is emerging. Just five years after its introduction, an alarming proportion of *Candida* spp. isolated from AIDS patients are resistant to fluconazole (2).

Because only a limited number of agents are available for the treatment of life-threatening fungal infections and because resistance may further limit the utility of the newer azoles, there is an urgent need for new antifungal agents with different modes of action. Among drug discovery targets being investigated to address this urgent need, those in the fungal cell wall appear to be promising. This chapter briefly reviews the composition of the fungal cell wall, presents glucan synthesis as a target for antifungal drug discovery, and considers the potential utility of the echinocandin class of antifungal agents.

II. FUNGAL CELL WALL COMPOSITION AND STRUCTURE

Much of our limited knowledge of the chemical composition and structure of the fungal cell wall comes from studies of the yeasts *Saccharomyces cerevisiae* (3–7) and *Candida albi-*

cans (8–10). The cell wall represents 15–25% of the dry weight of yeast (7) and, therefore, represents an important investment by the cell. Historically, the fungal cell wall was regarded by many as a rigid, inert exoskeleton providing structural support to the plasma membrane and cytoplasm. We now know that this cellular organelle has many vital functions, including regulation of cell shape; physical protection and osmotic stabilization of the protoplast; support for a number of enzymes; prevention of passage of certain large molecules; mediation of adherence and agglutination; and protection from cell lysis by other microorganisms and by host phagocytes.

The fungal cell wall is composed primarily of carbohydrate, some of which is covalently linked to protein (5). Glucan polymers of (1,3)- and (1,6)-β-linked D-glucose residues and α-mannan (highly glycosylated, secreted mannoproteins) each make up approximately 50% of the dry weight of the yeast cell wall. Chitin, linear chains of (1,4)-β-linked N-acetyl-D-glucosamine, makes up approximately 2% of the dry weight of the cell walls obtained from stationary phase yeast. β-Glucans have been divided into three fractions: alkali-soluble (1,3)-β-D-glucans with 10% (1,6)-β-branches; alkali-insoluble (1,3)-β-D-glucans with rare (1,6)-β-branches; and highly branched (1,6)-β-D-glucan containing 20% (1,3)-β-branches (11–13). The (1,3)-β-D-glucans are believed to contain approximately 1500 glucose residues, whereas the smaller (1,6)-β-D-glucans contain 150–200. The alkali-soluble and -insoluble (1,3)-β-D-glucan fractions are now regarded as one, varying only in the extent of cross-linking with chitin (14,15).

III. ANTIFUNGAL AGENTS THAT AFFECT FUNGAL CELL WALL BIOSYNTHESIS AND/OR FUNCTION

Within the potential complexity of the carbohydrate structures of the fungal cell wall are a number of molecular targets that provide opportunities for antifungal drug discovery. Ideally, molecular targets unique to fungi and essential for viability represent the best candidates. Mannans do not appear to be unique, because similar O- and N-glycosylated proteins are found in all eukaryotes. However, the benanomycins and pradimicins are an interesting group of antifungal agents that form Ca+-dependent, insoluble complexes with yeast mannans, resulting in subsequent alterations of plasma membrane permeability. Major cell wall targets unique to fungi for which potentially useful antifungal compounds have been identified are the enzymes involved in chitin synthesis and glucan synthesis. Polyoxins and nikkomycins, analogs of uridine 5'-diphosphate-N-acetyl-D-glucosamine (the natural substrate), are competitive inhibitors of chitin synthases. Compounds of the echinocandin lipopeptide family and the papulacandin glycolipid family are noncompetitive inhibitors of (1,3)-β-D-glucan synthase. A review of these cell wall active agents has been published (16).

IV. THE ECHINOCANDIN ANTIFUNGAL AGENTS

The name echinocandin was originally applied to a small family of cyclic lipopeptide antifungal natural products having the same cyclic peptide nucleus (the echinocandin nucleus) but different fatty acid side chains. Cyclic lipopeptide antifungal agents referred to as the echinocandins are now represented by more than 20 isolated natural products belonging to six different families (Figure 1) and a large number of semisynthetic analogs

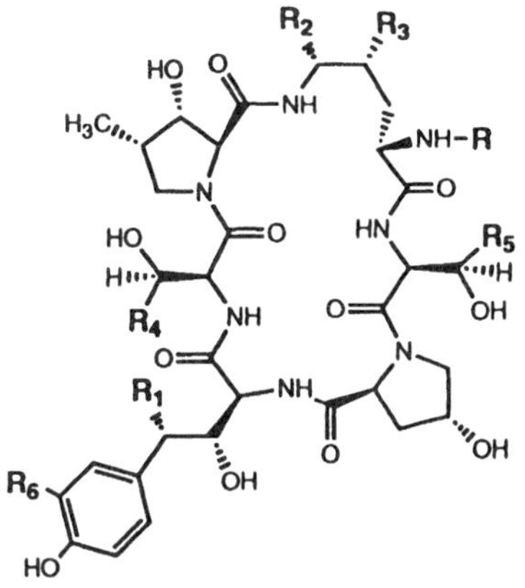

Echinocandin Lipopeptide Family	R	R_1	R_2	R_3	R_4	R_5	R_6
Echinocandin B	Linoleoyl	OH	OH	OH	CH_3	CH_3	H
C	Linoleoyl	H	OH	OH	CH_3	CH_3	H
D	Linoleoyl	H	H	H	CH_3	CH_3	H
Aculeacin Aγ	Palmitoyl	OH	OH	OH	CH_3	CH_3	H
Mulundocandin	12-Methylmyristoyl	OH	OH	OH	H	H	H
Sporiofungin A	10,12-Dimethylmyristoyl	OH	OH	OH	CH_2CONH_2	H	H
Pneumocandin A_0	10,12-Dimethylmyristoyl	OH	OH	OH	CH_2CONH_2	CH_3	H
WF11899A	Palmitoyl	OH	OH	OH	CH_2CONH_2	CH_3	OSO_3H

Figure 1   Representatives of the six naturally occurring families of echinocandin lipopeptide antifungal agents.

derived from several of the naturally occurring compounds. In this chapter we have expanded the use of the name echinocandin to refer to this entire class of cyclic lipopeptide antifungal agents along with the smaller family that was originally isolated. All of these agents are inhibitors of glucan synthesis. The driving force for the synthetic efforts within several families of this class has been the combination of potent antifungal activity and perceived low level of toxicity of some of these compounds. Early observations of the activity of the echinocandins implied that, although they were fungicidal, their spectrum was narrow and limited to *Candida* spp. With more study and with the discovery of more potent semisynthetic analogs, the spectrum has been expanded to include other pathogenic fungi, such as *Aspergillus* spp. and *P. carinii*. These improvements have increased the probability that a clinically successful compound will be identified from the echinocandin class in the near future.

A.   Mode of Action of Echinocandin Antifungal Agents

Antifungal agents of the echinocandin class (both natural products and semisynthetic analogs) that have been studied to date are inhibitors of fungal wall biosynthesis. They are noncompetitive inhibitors of (1,3)-β-D-glucan synthase, an enzyme (enzyme complex) that forms glucan polymers that make up a major portion of the cell wall of many pathogenic fungi (17–20). A schematic representation of fungal cell wall glucan synthesis and its inhibition by echinocandin agents is shown in Figure 2. Polymers of (1,3)-β-D-glucan are produced by an enzyme complex composed of at least two subunits (21). One subunit is in the plasma membrane (or endoplasmic reticulum?) and is thought to be the catalytic component because it is protected from heat denaturation by the substrate, UDP-glucose. A second subunit binds guanosine 5′-triphosphate and associates with and activates the catalytic component. The activating component can be separated from the membrane-bound complex with salt and detergent. Another possible function within the glucan synthase complex is transport of the polymer out of the cell. It is not known if a separate subunit is responsible for export of the (1,3)-β-D-glucan polymer. Once outside the cell, the glucan polymer becomes cross-linked with other glucan polymers and with chitin, by enzymes such as the glucosyltransferase encoded by the *BGL2* gene (22).

B. The Naturally Occurring Echinocandins

Echinocandin B (ECB) was the first factor isolated and was identified as the major component in the echinocandin family of compounds produced by *Aspergillus nidulans* or *Aspergillus rugulosis*. Investigators at Ciba-Geigy (23), Sandoz (24), and Eli Lilly independently discovered this agent at about the same time, with the earliest publication appearing in 1974. Structures of various natural product members of the echinocandin class, representing six echinocandin families, are shown in Figure 1.

All natural product members of the echinocandin class have a cyclic hexapeptide ring with a fatty acid side chain attached to the α-amino-group of the ornithine. All members contain an unusual, hydroxyl-substituted, homotyrosine residue, two substi-

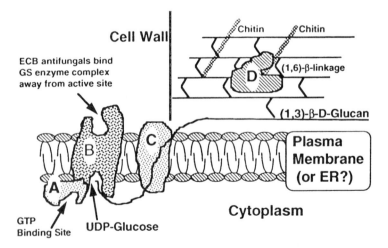

Figure 2   Diagrammatic representation of fungal cell wall (1,3)-β-D-glucan synthesis. The glucan synthase complex is composed of at least two components: A, a subunit that binds GTP and activates the catalytic subunit (B), which polymerizes UDP-glucose into (1,3)-β-D-glucan polymers. Another functional component (C) of the complex is responsible for transport of the glucan polymer out of the cell. Extracellular enzymes, such as glucosyltransferases (D) form glucan–glucan and glucan–chitin cross-links.

tuted prolines, and a hydroxyl-substituted ornithine cyclized at the δ-amino-group. The most common variation among the echinocandins is the degree of hydroxylation of the amino acids.

An echinocandin is grouped into one of six families of antifungal agents by the type of fatty acid side chain and substitution patterns of the amino acids. Family differences also include two residues of the peptide nucleus that are some combination of threonine, serine, or 3-hydroxyglutamine. When R_2 (Figure 1) is a hydroxyl, the molecule contains a very unusual hemiaminal functionality, which greatly increases its instability under high pH conditions.

Isolation of the aculeacin family from *Aspergillus aculeatus* by the chemists at Toyo Jozo revealed a group of compounds with a cyclic peptide nucleus similar to that of the echinocandins described above, but with side chains other than linoleic acid (25). Mulundocandin (26), isolated at Hoechst from *Aspergillus sydowi*, has serines replacing the two threonines in the ring and has a 12-methylmyristoyl side chain.

Two closely related families of compounds are the sporiofungins (27) from *Cryptosporiopsis* sp., isolated at Sandoz, and the pneumocandins (28) isolated from *Zalerion arboricola* by researchers at Merck. Members of these two families have a 3-hydroxyglutamine replacing one of the threonines of the ring. At Fujisawa, compounds were isolated from *Coleophoma empetri* and given the designation WF11899 (29). Compounds in this latter family have a 3-hydroxyglutamine residue and also a water-solubilizing sulfate residue on the homotyrosine phenyl ring. These are the only naturally occurring water-soluble echinocandins reported at the time of this writing.

C. Semisynthetic Echinocandins

Of the six naturally occurring echinocandin families, only the original echinocandins and the pneumocandins have been subjected to extensive structure–activity studies by synthetic alteration. Structure–activity work based on WF11899 has been conducted by scientists at Fujisawa, but only limited data was found in the patent literature at the time of this writing (30,31). The remainder of this section describes the structure–activity studies of the echinocandin and pneumocandin derivatives.

1. Echinocandin Derivatives

Discovery of Orally Active Echinocandins.   Echinocandin B is a potent anticandidal agent but was never used clinically because of toxicity, primarily associated with hemolysis. Early studies with the echinocandins demonstrated that both the antifungal potency and the hemolytic properties of these compounds were altered by changes in the fatty acid side chain. Hydrogenolysis of the two double bonds in the linoleic side chain of ECB gave a tetrahydro derivative, which was more potent against *C. albicans* but was even more hemolytic. Discovery of a practical way to remove enzymatically the natural side chain then provided an avenue for large-scale structure–activity studies of the side chain of ECB. Investigators at Eli Lilly were able to use a deacylase found in the fermentation broth of *Actinoplanes utahensis* to cleave the linoleic side chain from ECB to give the deacylated cyclic peptide (ECBnuc) (32). Without the side chain, ECBnuc did not inhibit the enzyme and had no whole cell activity. Activity was restored to various degrees by reacylation with synthetic side chains. Structure–activity studies demonstrated that both antifungal activity and hemolytic potential increased as the length of nonbranched alkyl side chains increased. Structurally, a phenyl-group was incorporated into the side chain

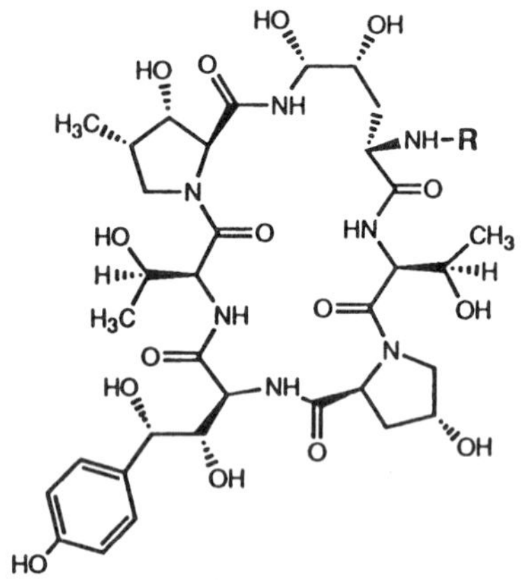

Compound	R	MIC (μg/ml)	ED₅₀ (mg/kg) ip	oral
Echinocandin B (ECB)	Linoleoyl	0.625	28.0	>100
Cilofungin	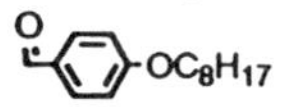 (structure) -OC₈H₁₇	0.156	7.6	>100
LY225489	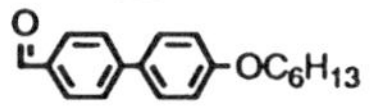 (structure) -OC₆H₁₃	0.039	1.1	NT
LY280949	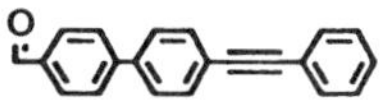 (structure)	0.039	0.6	18.8
LY303366	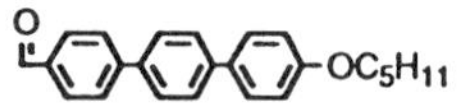 (structure) -OC₅H₁₁	0.010	0.3	7.8

Figure 3 Structure and anti-*Candida* activity of echinocandin B and selected semisynthetic analogs. MIC, minimal inhibitory concentrations against *C. albicans* A26 (ATCC62342) determined by a microbroth dilution assay; ED50, calculated dose for 50% survival of mice with a lethal infection of *C. albicans* A26 (ATCC62342).

and the length of the alkyl portion of the side chain was adjusted to produce an analog, LY121019 (cilofungin), that was not hemolytic and that retained the antifungal activity of ECB (Figure 3). LY121019 had potent anti–*C. albicans* activity in vitro and was effective in a murine model of disseminated candidiasis (Figure 3). Cilofungin was the first compound of this class to enter clinical evaluation, and initial results of the treatment of *Candida* esophagitis (33) and disseminated candidiasis (34) were promising. Unfortunately, nephrotoxicity, attributed to polyethylene glycol, in the IV formulation and failure to identify a clinically acceptable substitute to solubilize cilofungin resulted in discontinuation of clinical evaluation (35).

Continuation of structure–activity studies led to incorporating additional aromatic rings into the side chain, substitutions that resulted in antifungal activity that was more potent than that of cilofungin (Figure 3). For example, a biphenyl analog with a C6 alkyl tail (LY225489) had a four-fold improvement in potency against *C. albicans* in vitro and an eight-fold improvement in efficacy, when administered parenterally, in a murine model of *C. albicans* infection. Adding a phenylethynyl-group to the biphenyl gave a very unusual, totally rigid side chain analog (LY280949) with antifungal activity and efficacy in animal models similar to that of LY225489. Unexpectedly, LY280949 was the first echinocandin compound to exhibit oral efficacy in an animal model of fungal infection (Figure 3).

Structure modifications aimed at optimizing this activity led to a group of compounds with an oral ED_{50} below 10 mg/kg. From this group of compounds, it was determined that a linearly rigid section of the side chain is crucial for this desired property. Also, addition of a flexible alkyl section maximized antifungal potency, perhaps by a crucial adjustment of the lipophilicity of this region of the molecule. One member of this group, LY303366, the side chain of which has a rigid terphenyl head and a flexible C5 tail, was chosen as a next generation clinical candidate (Figure 3).

In Vitro Activity of LY303366.   LY303366 has potent in vitro activity against all *Candida* spp. studied to date (Table 1). Compared with cilofungin, LY303366 was far more potent and had a broader spectrum of activity.

With the widespread use of fluconazole, there have been increasing reports of resistance by *Candida* spp. Resistance may be due either to the acquisition of an inherently resistant species of *Candida* or to the development of resistance by a previously susceptible strain of *C. albicans* (2). LY303366 is active against *Candida* spp. that are inherently resistant to fluconazole, such as *Candida glabrata* and *Candida krusei* (Table 1), and isolates of *C. albicans* that are resistant to azole antifungal agents (Table 2). This lack of cross resistance should be anticipated, since the mode of action of LY303366, inhibition of cell wall biosynthesis, is different from that of the azoles, which inhibit ergosterol biosynthesis.

LY303366 was more potent than amphotericin B against >100 isolates of *C. albicans* in an agar dilution assay using Sabaroud's medium and in a broth microdilution assay (36) using antibiotic medium 3 (AB3) or RPMI 1640 medium (Table 3). The susceptibility of *C. albicans* isolates to LY303366 was similar in the agar dilution assay and microbroth dilution assay using RPMI 1640 medium (36). LY303366 was more potent when tested in the microbroth dilution assay using AB3 (Table 3).

One feature of the newer analogs of the echinocandin class of antifungal agents is their rapid fungicidal activity. For *C. albicans* and other *Candida* spp., the minimal inhibitory concentration (MIC) and the minimal fungicidal concentration (MFC) of LY303366 are similar, rarely differing by more than a single twofold dilution.

Table 1   Geometric Mean Minimal Inhibitory Concentrations[a] of LY303366, Cilofungin, and Amphotericin B Against Four (*Candida parapsilosis*) or Five (Other *Candida* spp.) Clinical Isolates

Antifungal agent	*Candida albicans*	*Candida parapsilosis*	*Candida glabrata*	*Candida krusei*	*Candida tropicalis*
LY303366	0.01	0.26	0.01	0.02	0.02
Cilofungin	0.25	>20	2.87	1.32	0.87
Amphotericin B	0.03	0.05	0.05	0.08	0.06

[a] Minimal inhibitory concentrations (MIC, mg/ml) were determined by a broth microdilution method adapted from the tentative reference method (document M27-T) recommended by the Committee on Antifungal Susceptibility Testing (36). Antibiotic medium 3 was used rather than RPMI 1640 medium. The MIC is defined as the lowest concentration of compound that completely inhibited growth when tested with LY303366, cilofungin, or amphotericin B.

Table 2   Minimal Inhibitory Concentrations[a] of Antifungal Agents Against Clinical Isolates of
Candida albicans that Are Susceptible or Resistant to Azole Antifungal Agents

Antifungal agent	C. albicans CA4[b]	C. albicans CA3[b]	C. albicans ATCC62342[b]	C. albicans A26[c]
LY303366	0.01	0.02	0.01	0.01
Cilofungin	5.0	5.0	20.0	0.63
Amphotericin B	0.08	0.31	0.16	0.63
Fluconazole	>80	>80	>80	0.16
Miconazole	5.0	80	10	0.04
SCH 39304	>80	>80	>80	0.04

[a] Minimal inhibitory concentrations (MIC, µg/ml) were determined by a broth microdilution method adapted
from the tentative reference method (document M27-T) recommended by the Committee on Antifungal
Susceptibility Testing (36) using RPMI-1640 plus MOPS buffer medium. The MIC is defined as the lowest concentration of compound that completely inhibited growth when tested with LY303366 or amphotericin B.
However, the MIC for an azole such as fluconazole represented the lowest concentration of compound that
inhibited growth by ≥80% compared with untreated controls.
[b] Clinical isolate resistant to fluconazole.
[c] Clinical isolate susceptible to fluconazole (ATCC62342).

Our studies of the activity of LY303366 against *C. albicans* clearly demonstrate that
this compound and related ECB analogs are fungicidal and that they act rapidly in vitro
(Tables 4 and 5). A 5 min pulse of LY303366 at the MIC (0.01 µg/ml) killed >90% of C.
albicans growing in YPD medium at 30°C (37,38). LY303366 is more potent and acts
more rapidly than cilofungin and amphotericin B. All three of these compounds are considered fungicidal (Table 6). The fungistatic property of fluconazole was evident when
compared with the fungicidal compounds LY303366, cilofungin, and amphotericin B
(Table 6). Rapid fungicidal activity may prove useful in the treatment of life-threatening
fungal infections in the immunocompromised host.

LY303366 is active against *Aspergillus fumigatus* in vitro; however, this activity is
not exhibited by traditional MIC or MFC endpoints. There are two distinct break points
that one can observe in microbroth dilution assays. The first break point (cilofungin, 0.25
µg/ml; LY303366, 0.12 µg/ml) is an abrupt change from confluent growth as a hyphal mat
to the growth of small discrete microcolonies with altered morphological features, including thick, highly branched hyphae with swollen ends. The second break point (cilofungin, 25 µg/ml; LY303366, 3.1 µg/ml) occurs at a higher concentration and is the transition from the presence of small numbers of microcolonies to no visible colonies. We
believe that the first break point, the minimal effective concentration (MEC), more
closely correlates with activity in animal models (see below) than does the second break
point.

Efficacy of LY303366 in Animal Models of Fungal Infection.   The potent in vitro
activity of LY303366 against *C. albicans* translated into good efficacy in stringent models
of disseminated candidiasis (Table 7) (39,40). LY303366 was active in a murine model
of disseminated candidiasis when administered intraperitoneally or orally. In this model
of disseminated candidiasis, LY303366 was more effective on a mg/kg basis than cilofungin or amphotericin B when given intraperitoneally to mice that were immunosuppressed
by x-irradiation.

Table 3 Minimal Inhibitory Concentrations of LY303366 and Amphotericin B that Inhibited 50% (MIC$_{50}$) and 90% (MIC$_{90}$) of 107 Clinical Isolates of C. *albicans* Tested by an Agar Dilution Assay[a] or by Broth Microdilution Assays Using RPMI 1640 Medium (RPMI) or Antibiotic Medium 3 (AB3)[b]

Antimicrobial agent (number of isolates tested)	Range	MIC$_{50}$	MIC$_{90}$
Agar dilution assay$_a$			
LY303366 (107)	0.002 to 0.625	0.039	0.156
Amphotericin B	0.312 to >20	1.25	5.0
Broth microdilution—AB3[b]			
LY303366 (115)	0.001 to 1.25	0.001	0.02
Amphotericin B (112)	0.20 to 0.625	0.02	0.78
Broth microdilution—RPMI[b]			
LY303366 (113)	0.001 to 1.25	0.02	0.156
Amphotericin B (114)	0.078 to 1.25	0.156	0.625

[a] MICs (µg/ml) were determined by a twofold serial agar dilution method in Sabouraud's dextrose agar (Difco Laboratories, Detroit, Michigan). LY303366 was dissolved in 100% methanol, diluted to the appropriate concentration in 50% methanol, and then tested at the desired concentration in agar containing 5% (v/v) methanol. Cultures of C. *albicans* were grown on Sabouraud's dextrose agar slants at 35°C overnight. Cultures were suspended in sterile saline and adjusted to a final concentration of 5×10^6 conidia/ml in sterile broth. A portion (about 2.0 µl) of the dilution was inoculated with an inoculation apparatus (Cathra dispenser, MCT Medical Browne Systems Cathra Systems, St. Paul, Minnesota). The final inoculum size was approximately 10^4 colony forming units (CFU) per spot. Each plate was inoculated with 37 spots. Plates were incubated for 48 hr at 35°C. MICs are defined as the lowest concentration at which no growth was visible.

[b] MICs were determined by a broth microdilution method adapted from the tentative reference method (document M27-T) recommended by the Committee on Antifungal Susceptibility Testing (36). Antibiotic medium 3 or RPMI-1640 plus MOPS buffer medium was used. The MIC is defined as the lowest concentration of compound that completely inhibited growth when tested with LY303366 or amphotericin B.

In a murine model of organ recovery, LY303366 significantly reduced the number of fluconazole-resistant C. *albicans* in the kidneys of animals treated orally for 4 days with twice the ED$_{50}$. Similar treatment with fluconazole did not reduce the number of C. *albicans* recovered from the kidneys (Figure 4). In the same animal model, LY303366 also significantly reduced the number of fluconazole-nonsusceptible C. *krusei* in the kidneys of animals treated orally for 4 days with twice the ED$_{50}$. Similar treatment with fluconazole did not reduce the number of C. *krusei* recovered from the kidneys (data not shown).

In a murine model of organ recovery, LY303366 significantly reduced the number of A. *fumigatus* recovered from the kidneys and was as effective as amphotericin B on a mg/kg basis when both were administered intraperitoneally (Figure 5). In the model used to obtain the data shown in Figure 5, it is not certain if the compounds used exhibited activity against germinating conidia or if they were effective against hyphae within the tissues. To be effective in this stringent model, even the high levels of amphotericin B (10 mg/kg) must be given within 1 hr after inoculation of A. *fumigatus* spores, before hyphae are established in tissues. We then developed a DBA/2 mouse model to ensure

Table 4 Rapid Killing of C. *albicans* A26 (ATCC62342) by LY303366 (LY) Confirmed by Standard Microbiological Plate Counts[a]

Study no.	Mean plate count (CFU/ml × 1000)				Percent reduction in colony forming units[a]	
	Control at 5 min	LY at 5 min	Control at 3 hr	LY at 3 hr	LY at 5 min	LY at 3 hr
1[b]	940	30	940	42	97.0	96.0
2	2100	19	1100	32	99.1	97.1
3	630	3.5	580	5.8	99.5	99.0

[a] Approximately 1×10^6 C. *albicans* per ml were either pulsed for 5 min in YPD broth containing LY303366 (0.01 µg/ml), then washed in YPD and resuspended in fresh YPD without LY303366 for 3 hr at 30°C (LY at 5 min), or were incubated continuously in LY303366 for 3 hr (LY at 3 hr) and then washed in YPD. After the approximate 3 hr incubation period, 50 µl of the cultures (containing approximately 50,000 cells) and 50 µl of 10-fold serial dilutions (1- to 10,000-fold) from LY303366-treated and nontreated controls were plated in duplicate on YPD agar, and colony forming units (CFU) were determined after 48 hr of growth at 30°C (plate counts). Percent reductions represent the number of CFU in control cultures minus the number of CFU in corresponding LY303366-treated cultures
[b] Data from study 1 are also reported in Table 5.

Table 5 Flow Cytometry and Standard Plate Count Assay[a] Demonstrating that >90% of the Cells in a Growing C. *albicans* A26 (ATCC62342) Culture Were Killed by a 5 Min Pulse of LY303366 at 0.01 µg/ml in YPD Broth

Test compound	Percent PI positive		Mean plate count (CFU × 10,000)	
	5 min pulse	3 hr incubation	5 min pulse	3 hr incubation
LY303366	95	96	15	21
None (control)	not done	5	not done	469

[a] Flow cytometry assays (37,38) utilize propidium iodide (PI) as a viability probe. Approximately 1×10^6 C. *albicans* per ml were either pulsed for 5 min in YPD broth containing LY303366 (0.01 mg/ml), then washed in YPD and resuspended in fresh YPD without LY303366 for 3 hr at 30°C (5-min pulse), or were incubated continuously in LY303366 for 3 hr (3 hr incubation) and then washed in YPD. After the approximate 3 hr incubation period, 50 ml of the YPD containing cells (approximately 50,000 cells) and 50 ml of 10-fold serial dilutions (1- to 10,000-fold) were plated in duplicate on YPD agar and CFU were determined after 48 hr of growth at 30°C (plate counts). One milliliter aliquots were also incubated in PI for 15 min and then examined with flow cytometry to determine the percentage of fluorescent cells (percent PI positive).

that compounds were treating established infections, ones in which hyphae were present in tissues. In the DBA/2 model, mice were given dexamethasone (4.6 mg/liter in drinking water, beginning 4 days before inoculation of A. *fumigatus* and continuing throughout the study) and test compounds were first administered 24 hr after inoculation of spores, at which time long, branched hyphae were demonstrated in numerous organs. In the DBA/2 murine model of disseminated aspergillosis, LY303366 had an ED_{50} of less than 3 mg/kg when administered intraperitoneally once daily for 9 days (Figure 6). Because of its toxicity in this model, amphotericin B at 10 mg/kg could not be used. A lower dose of ampho-

Table 6 Comparison of Rapid Killing of C. *albicans* A26 (ATCC62342) by LY303366, Cilofungin, Amphotericin B, and Fluconazole[a]

Compound	Concentration[b] (mg/ml)	Exposure time	Percent PI positive[c]	Percent reduction in CFU
LY303366	0.01 (1 × MIC)	5 min pulse	95	96
Cilofungin	0.63 (1 × MIC)	3 hr	>90	>90
Amphotericin B	0.20 (2 × MIC)	5 min pulse	<10	67
Fluconazole	4.00 (>10 MIC)	90 min	<10	0

[a] Concentrations of all compounds listed are mg/ml in YPD broth. Flow cytometry assays and standard plate counts were performed as described in the footnote to Table 5.
[b] Parenthetical quantities are the multiples of the minimum inhibitory concentrations present.
[c] With respect to flow cytometry assay utilizing propidium iodide as a viability probe, as described in the footnote to Table 5.

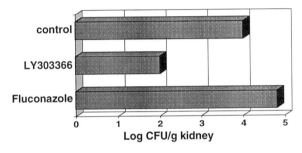

Figure 4 Renal recovery of C. *albicans* CA4 (fluconazole-resistant clinical isolate). Mice were challenged intravenously with 2×10^5 cells and treated orally twice daily for 4 days with $2 \times ED_{50}$. (From Ref. 39.)

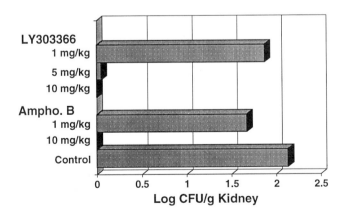

Figure 5 Renal recovery of A. *fumigatus* WM-1. Mice were challenged intravenously with 1×10^5 conidia and then treated intraperitoneally twice daily for 4 days with LY303366 or with amphotericin at 0, 4, 24, and 48 hr after inoculation of conidia. The levels of amphotericin used are approximately the same (1 mg/kg) or 10 times (10 mg/kg) the dose used in humans.

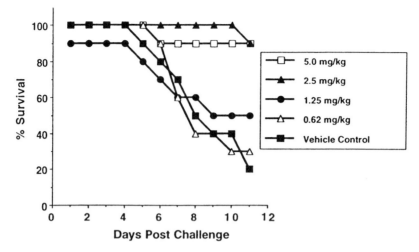

Figure 6   Survival of dexamethasone-immunosuppressed DBA/2 mice following once daily IP treatments with LY303366 administered for 8 days, beginning 24 hours after IV inoculation of 100 conidia of *A. fumigatus* WM-1.

tericin B (1 mg/kg intraperitoneally on days 1, 3, 5, and 7) was used, but survival was only 20%.

In a *P. carinii* model, LY303366 reduced the number of cysts in the lungs of heavily infected, immunosuppressed rats by more than 99% when administered orally at 5 mg/kg once daily for 4 days (Figure 7). Prophylactic oral administration of 1 mg/kg twice daily for 4 weeks resulted in >90% reduction in all life-cycle forms (data not shown). Thus, it appears that cysts of *P. carinii* are disrupted by LY303366. Details of the animal model have been published (41).

Pharmacokinetic Properties of LY303366.   Preliminary studies in rats and dogs suggested that the pharmacokinetic properties of LY303366 differ markedly from those of

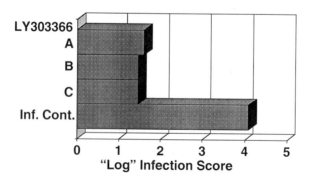

Figure 7   Mean infection scores of *P. carinii* cysts in homogenates of lung tissues in our four-day cyst reduction model (41). Immunosuppressed rats were allowed to develop heavy *P. carinii* infections, they were treated with LY303366 for up to 4 days, and the numbers of cysts in the lungs were counted microscopically. Treatment groups were: A, animals receiving a single 10 mg/kg IV dose 4 days prior to necropsy; B, animals receiving a single 5 mg/kg IV dose 4 days prior and daily 5 mg/kg oral doses on days 1–4 prior to necropsy; C, animals receiving daily oral doses on days 1–4 prior to necropsy. Infected control (Inf. cont.) animals received no therapy for *P. carinii* pneumonia.

cilofungin (42). Some of the most important differences between LY303366 and cilofungin as they relate to the treatment of fungal infections are stated below. LY303366 was absorbed orally, whereas cilofungin was not. LY303366 had a half-life in rats of 18 to 26 hr, whereas cilofungin had a half-life of approximately 40 min. The amount of compound that penetrated into tissues was higher for LY303366 than for cilofungin. In rats, the concentration of [^{14}C]LY303366 was higher in target organs of fungal infection (e.g., liver, spleen, kidney, lungs) than in the plasma. LY303366 may enter the central nervous system, whereas cilofungin appears to be excluded from this compartment. Higher than plasma counts of radioactivity appeared in the brains of rats following administration of [^{14}C]LY303366. Higher than MIC concentrations of LY303366 were found in the plasma of both rats and dogs for many hours following a single oral dose. Data shown graphically in Figure 8 demonstrate this feature in dogs.

2. Pneumocandin Derivatives

Development of a Water-Soluble Pneumocandin. The first member of the pneumocandin class to be isolated was pneumocandin A_0 (Figures 1 and 9), a compound that is less hemolytic than other members of the naturally occurring echinocandins (43). The anti-*Candida* activity of pneumocandin A_0 (L-671,329), as determined by in vitro broth dilution assays and by a murine kidney clearance assay, is comparable with that of cilofungin (Table 8). Of the pneumocandin natural products, pneumocandin B_0 (Figure 9) appears to be the most potent glucan synthase inhibitor; however, its in vitro and in vivo antifungal activity is comparable with that of pneumocandin A_0 (Table 8) (44). Pneumocandin B_0 differs from pneumocandin A_0 only in the absence of a methyl on one of the proline rings. Since both compounds have low water solubility and are difficult to formulate for IV administration, scientists at Merck embarked on a study to find a water-soluble prodrug. This research produced the compound L-693,989, a phosphate monoester at the phenolic hydroxyl of the homotyrosine residue of pneumocandin B_0 (45). As shown in Table 8, the water-soluble L-693,989 was as effective as its parent in a murine model of candidiasis. This compound is a prodrug, since the phosphate ester is cleaved in the presence of tissue phosphatases to give the active parent compound pneumocandin

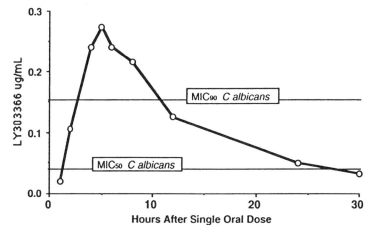

Figure 8 Mean plasma concentrations of LY303366 after administration of a single 10 mg/kg oral dose to beagle dogs (n = 3). The MIC$_{90}$ and MIC$_{50}$ of >100 clinical isolates of C. *albicans* as determined by our most stringent *in vitro* assay (Table 3) are shown.

Table 7   *In Vivo* antifungal Efficacies (ED$_{50}$) of LY303366, Cilofungin, Amphotericin B, Fluconazole, and Itraconazole in a Mouse Survival Model of Disseminated *C. albicans* Infection[a]

Antifungal compound	Route (no. of mice)	Dose range (mg/kg)	Total no. of doses	Timing of doses	ED$_{50}$ (mg/kg)
LY303366	IP (8)	10–0.039	4	0, 4, 24, 48 hr	0.3
LY303366	PO (10)	12.5–1.56	8	2 × day for 4 days	7.8
Cilofungin	IP (8)	40–5	3	0, 4, 24, 48 hr	7.6
Cilofungin	PO (8)	50–12.5	8	2 × day for 4 days	>50
Amphotericin B	IP (8)	12.5–0.78	3	0, 4, 24 hr	4.0
Fluconazole	PO (8)	1.0–0.062	8	2 × day for 4 days	0.3
Itraconazole	PO (8)	50–3.12	8	2 × day for 4 days	15.5

[a] ED$_{50}$s were estimated on the basis of survival at 7 days after challenge by using the analysis method of Reed and Muench (1938, J Hyg. 27:493–497)). ICR mice were immunosuppressed by sublethal x-irradiation and 24 hr later were inoculated IV with 2×10^6 *C. albicans* A26 (ATCC62342) per mouse. Mice treated IP were given four doses beginning within 15 min after inoculation of *C. albicans*. Mice treated orally (PO) were given two doses per day, the first dose beginning within 30 min after inoculation of *C. albicans*.

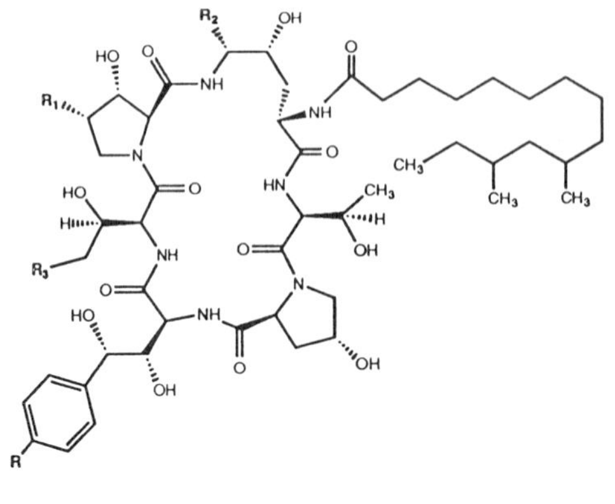

Compound	R	R$_1$	R$_2$	R$_3$
Pneumocandin A$_0$	OH	CH$_3$	OH	CONH$_2$
Pneumocandin B$_0$	OH	H	OH	CONH$_2$
L-693,989	OPO(OH)$_2$	H	OH	CONH$_2$
L-705,589	OH	H	OCH$_2$CH$_2$NH$_2$	CONH$_2$
L-731,373	OH	H	OH	CH$_2$NH$_2$
L-733,560	OH	H	OCH$_2$CH$_2$NH$_2$	CH$_2$NH$_2$

Figure 9   Structures of naturally occurring and selected semisynthetic analogs of compounds in the pneumocandin family of echinocandins.

Table 8 Comparison of the Aqueous Solubilities, Potency of Glucan Synthase Inhibition (IC_{50}), Minimal Concentration of Each Compound that Is Fungicidal to 90% of *C. albicans* Isolates Tested (MFC_{90}), and Minimum Effective Doses that Clear 99% of the *C. albicans* from the Kidneys of Infected Mice of Two Naturally Occuring and a Synthetic Prodrug Pneumocandin, L-693,989

Test compound	Solubility (mg/ml)	Glucan synthase IC_{50}[a] (μM)	*C. albicans* MFC_{90}[b] ($\mu g/ml$)	Kidney clearance assay[c] (MED_{99} mg/kg)
Pneumocandin A_0 (l-671,329)	<0.1	0.20	0.50	2.5
Pneumocandin B_0 (L-688,786)	<0.1	0.07	0.25	3
L-693,989	>42	>10	2	3
Cilofungin	not done	1.0	0.5	3

[a] Concentration at which 50% of the measurable polymerization of UDP-glucose into (1,3)-β-D-glucan is inhibited. The *in vitro* assay was performed as described previously (43).

[b] MFC_{90}, the minimal concentration that kills 90% of all of the *C. albicans* isolates tested (43).

[c] Minimum concentration of compound, administered intraperitoneally twice daily for 4 days, that resulted in a 99% reduction (compared with nontreated controls) in colony forming units of *C. albicans* recovered from the kidneys of infected mice on day 7 (TOKA assay, 43).

B_0. Unlike the parent compound, the phosphate prodrug (L-693,989) has minimal glucan synthase inhibition and in vitro anti-*Candida* activities.

Pneumocandins with Increased Antifungal Potency. Continued synthetic work has led to much more active compounds containing cationic amino solubilizing groups (46). The newest compounds were modified at one or both of two sites on the cyclic peptide portion of the molecule (Figure 9). With pneumocandin B_0 as the parent, conversion of the hemiaminal site to a β-aminoethyl ether gives L-705,589. Conversion of the β-hydroxyglutamine of pneumocandin B_0 to a β-hydroxyornithine gives L-731,373. Both of these modifications are combined in L-733,560. As can be seen in Table 9, L-731,373 and L-733,560 were more potent in vitro than L-705,589 against several species of *Candida*; however, L-733,560 was clearly the most effective of the three compounds in a mouse candidiasis survival model (47,48). It was also the most potent of the three in a murine model of *C. albicans* organ clearance. The minimal fungicidal concentrations of L-733,560 against *Candida* spp. appear to be comparable with those of amphotericin B, and both compounds, when administered parenterally, were highly effective in a survival model of murine candidiasis (Table 9). However, when L-733,560 was given orally, an ED_{50} of >50.0 mg/kg was reported for the survival assay.

These pneumocandins were also effective as parenteral agents in a mouse disseminated *A. fumigatus* model. L-733,560 and L-705,589 had ED_{90}s of 0.48 and 0.12 mg/kg, respectively, in a 28-day survival study in which the control, amphotericin B, had an ED_{90} of 0.36 mg/kg. L-731,373 was much less active, with an ED_{90} of >20.0 mg/kg. This interesting result shows the value of the aminoethyl ether moiety in enhancing the *Aspergillus* activity. As with cilofungin and LY303366, the pneumocandins do not appear to have potent activity against *A. fumigatus* by classic in vitro broth dilution methods but dramatically affect cell morphology at low concentrations.

Table 9   Enzyme Inhibition (IC_{50}) Minimum Fungicidal Concentrations that Inhibited 90% of Fungal Growth (MFC_{90}) of Species of *Candida*, and Effective Dose Allowing 50% Survival (ED_{50}) of *C. albicans*–Infected Mice of Three Cationic Pneumocandins.

Test compound	Glucan synthase IC_{50}[a]	MFC_{90}[b](μg/ml)					C. albicans ED_{50}[c]
		C. albicans	C. parapsilosis	C. glabrata	C. krusei	C. tropicalis	
L-705,589	11	0.5	4	2	8	0.5	0.84
L-731,373	10	≤0.06	1	0.25	0.25	≤0.06	0.62
L-733,560	1	0.5	0.5	0.5	0.5	0.25	0.15
AMB	NA	1	1	0.5	1	0.5	0.3

[a] Concentration (nM) at which 50% of the measurable polymerization of UDP-glucose into $(1,3)$-β-D-glucan is inhibited. The *in vitro* assay was performed as described previously (43).
[b] MFC_{90}, the minimal concentration that kills 90% of all *C. albicans* isolates tested (47).
[c] Minimum concentration of compound, administered intraperitoneally twice daily for 4 days, that resulted in 50% survival (compared with nontreated controls) of mice infected with *C. albicans* (48).

All three cationic pneumocandins were very active against *P. carinii* in an immunosuppressed-rat model (49). When given intraperitoneally, L-733,560, L-705,589, and L-731,373 had ED_{90}s for cyst clearance of 0.01, 0.03, and 0.03 mg/kg, respectively. When dosed orally, these values were 2.2, 5.0, and 4.0 mg/kg. This good level of oral efficacy against *P. carinii* contrasts with the poor oral efficacy in the murine candidiasis models. L-733,560 was also quite effective prophylactically, with the ED_{90} for daily oral treatment at 2.2 mg/kg. Daily oral treatment of 6.25 mg/kg completely prevented the proliferation of both *P. carinii* cysts and trophozoites (47).

Pharmacokinetic Properties of Pneumocandins.   Pharmacokinetic studies demonstrated that the plasma half-lives of the semisynthetic derivatives administered intravenously have been extended when compared with that of pneumocandin B_0 (50). In mice, the half-life of pneumocandin B_0 was 0.99 hr, whereas those of L-705,589, L-731,373, and L-733,560 were 7.95, 2.73, and 5.95 hr, respectively. In Rhesus monkeys, the pattern is the same, with reported half lives of 0.73, 12.0, 4.68, and 11.8 hr for pneumocandin B_0, L-705,589, L-731,373, and L-733,560, respectively.

V.   CONCLUSIONS

During the past decade, the number of patients with life-threatening fungal infections has increased dramatically. Present therapeutic options available for the treatment of such infections are limited to amphotericin B and several azoles. Toxicity of amphotericin B limits its utility, and development of resistance to azoles may threaten the long-range utility of this class of antifungal agents. Therefore, there is a need for new antifungal agents having a mode of action different from those of the antifungal drugs presently available. Ideally, a new antifungal agent should be potent, broad-spectrum, fungicidal, and safe and effective when administered orally and parenterally. The search for such an agent has led several groups to study one of the fungal-specific targets in the cell wall—

glucan synthesis. Compounds of the echinocandin class are known inhibitors of (1,3)-β-D-glucan synthase, a fungal-specific enzyme that polymerizes UDP-glucose into the (1,3)-β-D-glucan polymers that make up the major carbohydrate scaffolding of the fungal cell wall. New semisynthetic echinocandin analogs such as LY303366 are markedly improved compared with cilofungin with respect to potency, rapidity of cidal activity, spectrum of cidal activity, efficacy (oral and parenteral) in animal models of fungal infection, and pharmacokinetic properties. Compared with cilofungin, the semisynthetic pneumocandin analog L-733,560 is much more potent and is more effective as a parenteral agent for the treatment of fungal infections in laboratory animals. These documented improvements provide encouragement that LY303366, L-733,560, or a related echinocandin antifungal agent has the potential of becoming a useful drug for the treatment of life-threatening fungal infections caused by important opportunistic pathogens such as *Candida* spp., *Aspergillus* spp., and *Pneumocystis carinii*.

REFERENCES

1. Georgopapadakou NH, Tkacz JS. The fungal cell wall as a drug target. Trends Microbiol 1995; 3:98–104.
2. Rex JH, Rinaldi MG, Pfaller MA. Resistance of *Candida* species to fluconazole. Antimicrob Agents Chemother 1995; 39:1–8.
3. Ballou CE. Isolation, characterization, and properties of *Saccharomyces cerevisiae mnn* mutants with non-conditional protein glycosylation defects. Meth Enzymol 1990; 185:440–470.
4. Cabib E, Roberts R. Synthesis of the yeast cell wall and its regulation. Annu Rev Biochem 1982; 51:763–793.
5. Fleet GH. Cell walls. Rose AH, Harrison JS, eds. The Yeasts, Vol. 4, 2nd ed. London: Academic Press, 1991:199–277.
6. Klis FM. Review: Cell wall assembly in yeast. Yeast 1994; 10:851–869.
7. Stratford M. Another brick in the wall? Recent developments concerning the yeast cell envelope. Yeast 1994; 10:1741–1752.
8. Reiss E. Molecular organization of the fungal cell wall. Reiss E, ed. Molecular Immunology of Mycotic and Actinomycotic Infections. New York: Elsevier, 1986:5–25.
9. Ruis-Herrera J. Fungal Cell Wall: Structure, Synthesis, and Assembly. Boca Raton, Florida: CRC Press, 1991:1–248.
10. Shepherd MG. Cell envelope of *Candida albicans*. CRC Crit Rev Microbiol 1987; 15:7–25.
11. Manners DJ, Masson AJ, Patterson JC. The structure of a β-1,3-D-glucan from yeast cell walls. Biochem J 1973; 135:19–30.
12. Manners DJ, Masson AJ, Patterson JC, Bjorndal H, Lindberg H. The structure of a β-1,6-D-glucan from yeast cell walls. Biochem J 1973; 135:31–36.
13. Fleet GH, Manners DJ. Isolation and composition of an alkali-soluble glucan from the cell wall of *Saccharomyces cerevisiae*. J Gen Microbiol 1976; 94:180–192.
14. Brown JL, Kossaczka Z, Jiang B, Bussy H. A mutational analysis of killer toxin resistance in *Saccharomyces cerevisiae* identifies new genes involved in (1,6) β glucan synthesis. Genetics 1993; 133:837–849.
15. Hong Z, Mann P, Brown NH, Tran LE, Shaw KJ, Hare RS, DiDomenico B. Cloning and characterization of KNR4, a yeast gene involved in (1,3)-β-glucan synthesis. Mol Cell Biol 1994; 14:1017–1025.
16. Debono M, Gordee RS. Antibiotics that inhibit fungal cell wall development. Annu Rev Microbiol 1994; 48:471–497.
17. Tang J, Parr TR Jr. W-1 solubilization and kinetics of inhibition by cilofungin of *Candida albicans* (1,3)-β-D-glucan synthase. Antimicrob Agents Chemother 1991; 35:99–103.

18. Gordee RS, Debono M, Parr TR Jr. The fungal cell wall—a target for lipopeptide antifungal agents. Fernandes PB, ed. New Approaches for Antifungal Drugs. Boston: Birkhauser Press, 1992:46–63.

19. Tang J, Parr TR Jr, Turner W, Debono M, LaGrandeur L, Burkhardt F, Rodriguez M, Zweifel M, Nissan J, Clingerman K. LY303366: A noncompetitive inhibitor of (1,3)-β-D-glucan synthase from *Candida albicans* and *Aspergillus fumigatus*. Thirty-third Interscience Conference on Antimicrobial Agents and Chemotherapy, New Orleans, October 17–20, 1993: Abstract 367.

20. Beaulieu D, Tang J, Yan SB, Vessels JM, Radding JA, Parr TR Jr. Characterization and cilofungin inhibition of solubilized *Aspergillus fumigatus* (1,3)-β-D-glucan synthase. Antimicrob Agents Chemother 1994; 38:937–944.

21. Kang MS, Cabib E. Regulation of fungal cell wall growth: A guanine nucleotide-binding, proteinaceous component required for activity of (1,3)-β-D-glucan synthase. Proc Natl Acad Sci USA 1986; 83:5808–5812.

22. Goldman RC, Sullivan PA, Zakula D, Capobianco JO. Kinetics of β-1,3 glucan interaction at the donor and acceptor sites of the fungal glucosyltransferase encoded by the *BGL2* gene. Eur J Biochem 1995; 227:372–378.

23. Benz F, Knusel F, Nuesch J, Treichler H, Voser W, Nyfeler R, Keller-Schierlein W. Stoffwechselprodukte von Microorganismen. Echinocandin B, ein neuartiges Polypeptid-Antibioticum aus *Aspergillus nidulans* var. *echinulatus*: Isolierung und Bausteine. Helv Chim Acta 1974; 57:2459–2477.

24. Keller-Juslen C, Kuhn M, Loosli H-R, Pechter TJ, Weber HP, Wartburg A. Struktur des Cyclopeptid-Antibiotikums SL 7810 (= echinocandin B). Tetrahedron Lett 1976; 17: 4147–4150.

25. Mizuno K, Yagi A, Satoi S, Takada M, Hayashi M, Asano K, Matsuda T. Studies on aculeacin. I. Isolation and characterization of aculeacin A. J Antibiot 1977; 30:297–302.

26. Roy K, Mukhopadhyay T, Reddy GCS, Desikan KR, Ganguli BN. Mulundocandin, a new lipopeptide antibiotic. I. Taxonomy, fermentation, isolation and characterization. J Antibiot 1986; 40:275–280.

27. Pache W, Dreyfuss M, Traber R, Tscherter H. Sporiofungins, new antifungal antibiotics of the cyclopeptide group. Proceedings of the Thirteenth International Congress of Chemotherapy, Vienna, Austria 1983: PS 4.8/3, Part 115, Abstract 10.

28. Schwartz RE, Giacobbe RA, Bland JA, Monaghan RL. L-671,329, a new antifungal agent I. Fermentation and isolation. J Antibiot 1989; 42:163–167.

29. Iwamoto T, Akihiko F, Sakamoto K, Tsurumi Y, Shigematsu N, Yamashita M, Hashimoto S, Okuhara M, Kohsaka M. WF11899A, B and C, novel antifungal lipopeptides I. Taxonomy, fermentation, isolation and physico-chemical properties. J Antibiot 1994; 47:1084–1091.

30. Toshiro I, Akihiko F, Kumiko N, Yasuhisa T, Nobuharu S, Chiyoshi K, Motohiro H, Masakuni O, Kazuo S, Hihji K, Hidenori O. Cyclic polypeptide with antibiotic activity, process for its preparation and pure culture of a Coelomycetes strain. European Patent Application 0,462,531 A2; 1991.

31. Ohki H, Tomishima M, Yamada A, Takasugi H. Cyclic antimicrobial peptides and preparation thereof. European Patent Application 0,644,199 A1; 1995.

32. Boeck LD, Fukuda DS, Abbott BJ, Debono M. Deacylation of echinocandin B by *Actinoplanes utahensis*. J Antibiot 1989; 42:382–388.

33. Copley-Merriman CR, Ransburg NJ, Crane LR, Kerkering TM, Pappas PG, Pottage JC, Hyslop DL. Cilofungin treatment of *Candida* esophagitis: Preliminary phase II results. Thirtieth Interscience Conference on Antimicrobial Agents and Chemotherapy, Atlanta, GA, 1990: Abstract 581.

34. Copley-Merriman CR, Gallis H, Graybill JR, Doebbeling BN, Hyslop DL. Cilofungin treatment of disseminated candidiasis: Preliminary phase II results. Thirtieth Interscience Conference on Antimicrobial Agents and Chemotherapy, Atlanta, GA, 1990: Abstract 582.

35. Doebbeling BN, Fine BD, Pfaller MA, Sheetz CT, Stokes JB, Wenzel RP. Acute tubular necrosis (ATN) and anion-gap acidosis during therapy with cilofungin (LY121019) in polyethylene glycol (PEG). Thirtieth Interscience Conference on Antimicrobial Agents and Chemotherapy, Atlanta, GA, 1990: Abstract 583.

36. Galgiani JN, Bartlett MS, Espinel-Ingroff A, Fromtling RA, Pfaller M, Rinaldi MG. Reference Method for Broth Dilution Antifungal Susceptibility Testing of Yeasts: Proposed Standard. NCCLS Document M27-T, Vol. 15, No. 10. Villanova, Pennsylvania: NCCLS, 1995.

37. Petersen BH, Green L, Steimel L, Hyslop D, Current WL. Use of flow cytometry for determination of minimal exposure time for effective antifungal activity of LY303366 and other antifungal compounds. Thirty-third Interscience Conference on Antimicrobial Agents and Chemotherapy, New Orleans, October 17–20, 1993: Abstract 362.

38. Green L, Petersen BH, Steimel L, Haeber P, Current W. Rapid determination of antifungal activity by flow cytometry. J Clin Microbiol 1994; 32:1088–1091.

39. Zeckner D, Butler T, Boylan C, Boyll B, Lin Y, Raab P, Schmidtke J, Current W. LY303366, activity in a murine systemic candidiasis model. Thirty-third Interscience Conference on Antimicrobial Agents and Chemotherapy, New Orleans, October 17–20, 1993: abstract 365.

40. Zeckner D, Butler T, Boylan C, Boyll B, Lin Y, Raab P, Schmidtke J, Current W. LY303366, activity against systemic aspergillosis and histoplasmosis in murine models. Thirty-third Interscience Conference on Antimicrobial Agents and Chemotherapy, New Orleans, October 17–20, 1993: Abstract 364.

41. Boylan CJ, Current WL. Improved rat model of Pneumocystis carinii pneumonia; induced laboratory infections in Pneumocystis-free animals. Infect Immun 1992; 60:1589–1597.

42. Zornes L, Stratford R, Novilla M, Turner D, Boylan C, Boyll B, Butler T, Lin Y, Zeckner D, Turner W, Current W. Single dose IV bolus and oral administration pharmacokinetics of LY303366, a new lipopeptide antifungal agent related to echinocandin B, in female Lewis rats and beagle dogs. Thirty-third Interscience Conference on Antimicrobial Agents and Chemotherapy, New Orleans, October 17–20, 1993: Abstract 370.

43. Bartizal K, Abruzzo G, Trainor C, Krupa D, Nollstadt K, Schmatz D, Schwartz R, Hammond M, Balkovec J, Vanmiddlesworth F. In vitro antifungal activities and in vivo efficacies of 1,3-β-D-glucan synthesis inhibitors L-671,329, L-646,991, tetrahydroechinocandin B, and L-687,781, a papulacandin. Antimicrob Agents Chemother 1992; 36:1648–1657.

44. Schmatz DM, Abruzzo G, Powles MA, McFadden DC, Balkovec JM, Black RM, Nollstadt K, Bartizal K. Pneumocandins from Zalerion arboricola IV. Biological evaluation of natural and semisynthetic pneumocandins for activity against Pneumocystis carinii and Candida species. J Antibiot 1992; 45:1886–1891.

45. Balkovec JM, Black RM, Hammond ML, Heck JV, Zambias RA, Abruzzo G, Bartizal K, Kropp H, Trainor C, Schwartz RE, McFadden DC, Nollstadt KH, Pittarelli LA, Powles MA, Schmatz DM. Synthesis, stability, and biological evaluation of water-soluble prodrugs of a new echinocandin lipopeptide. Discovery of a potential clinical agent for the treatment of systemic candidiasis and Pneumocystis carinii pneumonia (PCP). J Med Chem 1992; 35:194–198.

46. Bouffard FA, Zambias RA, Dropinski JF, Balkovec JM, Hammond ML, Abruzzo GK, Bartizal KF, Marrinan JA, Kurtz MB, McFadden DC, Nollstadt KH, Powles MA, Schmatz DM. Synthesis and antifungal activity of novel cationic pneumocandin B_0 derivatives. J Med Chem 1994; 37:222–225.

47. Bartizal K, Scott T, Abruzzo GK, Gill CJ, Gill CJ, Pacholok C, Lynch L, Kropp H. In vitro evaluation of the pneumocandin antifungal agent L-733560, a new water-soluble hybrid of L-705589 and L-731373. Antimicrob Agents Chemother 1995; 39:1070–1076.

48. Abruzzo GK, Flattery AM, Gill CJ, Kong L, Smith JG, Krupa D, Pikounis VB, Kropp H, Bartizal K. Evaluation of water-soluble pneumocandin analogs L-733560, L-705589, and L-731373 with mouse models of disseminated aspergillosis, candidiasis, and cryptococcosis. Antimicrob Agents Chemother 1995; 39:1077–1081.

49. Schmatz DM, Powles MA, McFadden D, Nollstadt K, Bouffard FA, Dropinski JF, Liberatio P, Andersen J. New semisynthetic pneumocandins with improved efficacies against *Pneumocystis carinii* in the rat. Antimicrob Agents Chemother 1995; 39:1320–1323.
50. Hajdu R, Thompson R, White K, Stark-Murphy B, Kropp H. Comparative pharmacokinetics of three water-soluble analogues of the lipopeptide antifungal compound L-688,786 in mice and rhesus monkeys. Thirty-third Interscience Conference on Antimicrobial Agents and Chemotherapy, New Orleans, October 17–20, 1993: Abstract 357.

11

Biochemistry and Genetics of Actinomycin Production

George H. Jones
Emory University, Atlanta, Georgia

Ullrich Keller
Technical University Berlin, Germany

I. INTRODUCTION

Actinomycins are acylpeptide lactones produced by a large number of *Streptomyces* strains. They consist of two pentapeptide lactone rings, which are attached via their amino-groups to the two carboxy-groups of actinocin, a phenoxazinone dicarboxylic acid. Besides the unique acyl residue, actinocin, actinomycins contain unusual amino acids such as *D*- and *N*-methyl amino acids and have both peptide and ester bonds in their chains (See Figure 1 for the structure of actinomycin D.) This indicates that the biosynthesis system of this class of compounds is one of the most complex among microbial peptide synthesis systems. Both bi- and monocyclic acylpeptide lactones exert a wide spectrum of biological activities, which makes the study of their genetics and biochemistry important for understanding the basis of their formation, and for enabling the engineering of new compounds that might be accessible by future manipulation of genes involved in acylpeptide lactone formation.

Although a cell-free system capable of supporting the complete synthesis of actinomycin (acm) has not yet been developed, much information on the enzymology of acm biosynthesis has been developed. In addition, some of the factors involved in the regulation of acm production have also been identified. This chapter will summarize early and recent studies on the chemistry, production, biosynthesis, and genetics of the actinomycins.

II. CHEMISTRY AND PRODUCTION OF ACTINOMYCIN

Table 1 (adapted from ref. 1) lists a number of acm-producing streptomycetes and the acm complexes they produce. Structures of actinomycins have been reviewed previously (2–4) and will not be discussed in detail here. There are many different actinomycins that arise by substitutions in several positions of their pentapeptide lactone rings with

Table I   Actinomycin-Producing Streptomycetes and the
acm Complexes They Produce

Name of organism	Actinomycin complex
Streptomyces antibioticus	A
Streptomyces flavus	C
Streptomyces flaveolus	A
Streptomyces parvus	A
Streptomyces chrysomallus	C
Streptomyces flavus	X
Streptomyces flavus	I
Streptomyces flavus-parvus	X
Streptomyces parvulus	D
Streptomyces michiganensis	X
Streptomyces fradiae	Z
Streptomyces melanochromogenes	K
Streptomyces aureofaciens	P_2

Adapted from Ref. 1.

homologous amino and imino acids. These substitutions typically occur in the positions occupied by D-valine, proline, or sarcosine in the structure shown in Figure 1. The positions occupied by N-methylvaline and threonine (Figure 1) are generally invariant.

An actinomycin-producing organism, when cultured without the addition of amino acids (the normal conditions for fermentation), will usually produce a number of acm forms simultaneously. For example, *Streptomyces chrysomallus* produces a mixture of actinomycins C1, C2, and C3, which vary at the D-valine position of the pentapeptide chain (5). *Streptomyces antibioticus*, on the other hand, produces a number of actinomycins that differ at the proline position in the pentapeptide chain (6,7). Growth of producing organisms in the presence of particular amino acids can lead to the predominant synthesis of a specific member (or members) of the complex normally produced by that organism.

III.   BIOCHEMICAL ROUTES TO ACTINOMYCIN

The central issue of actinomycin biosynthesis is the assembly of the acylpentapeptide lactone chain, which is formed in a nonribosomal process. Nonribosomal peptide synthesis has been structurally and mechanistically investigated in the case of peptide antibiotics and other biologically active peptides from bacilli and filamentous fungi, and it has been previously described in a series of reviews (8–12). Here, we briefly remind the reader that in this process the constituent amino acids are activated as thioesters via their amino acid adenylates and polymerized on the surface of large multifunctional enzymes consisting of peptide chains hundreds of kilodaltons in size. These peptide synthetases represent protein templates consisting of large repeating units (domains of ca. 100 kDa in size) that show considerable homology to each other in their amino acid sequences (13). It has been shown that each of these domains is responsible for the activation and the incorporation into the peptide of its cognate amino acid. In addition, the modular structure of

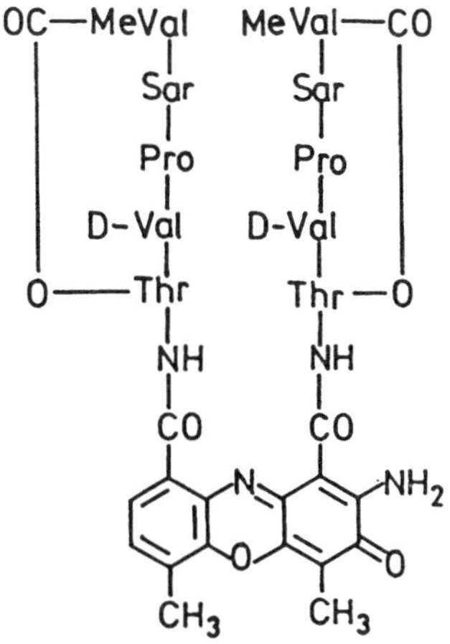

Figure 1 Structure of actinomycin D; Sar and Meval are N-methylglycine and N-methyl-L-valine, respectively.

the peptide synthetases provides additional functions in these enzymes such as methylations, epimerizations, and cyclizations via peptide or ester bonds (12,14).

As can be seen from the structure of the peptide portion of actinomycin D (Figure 1), the actinomycin synthetases responsible for the assembly of the actinomycin molecule would be one of the most complex systems in nonribosomal peptide synthesis, because they would contain a large number of reaction centers responsible for carboxylic acid and amino acid activation, peptide bond formation, N-methylation of amino acids, epimerization of amino acids, and ester bond formation. A prerequisite to the formation of the actinomycin molecule, with its bicyclic ring structure, is synthesis of 4-methyl-3-hydroxyanthranilic acid (4-MHA). 4-MHA is a free intermediate in the cell and serves as the precursor of the chromophoric part of all actinomycins, the phenoxazinone dicarboxylic acid actinocin (15). Formally, actinocin arises by the oxidative condensation of two molecules of 4-MHA. Actually, however, this occurs most probably at the stage of the 4-MHA peptide lactone (16). In any case, 4-MHA is the key substance for actinomycin synthesis, since it is itself a unique secondary metabolite confined to the genus *Streptomyces*. All other building blocks of actinomycin are amino acids from the free cellular pool that also serves primary metabolism (17).

A. Biosynthesis of 4-Methyl-3-Hydroxyanthranilic Acid

4-MHA originates from catabolism of tryptophan. The reaction chain leading from tryptophan to 4-MHA is shown in Figure 2. Biosynthesis of 4-MHA is closely related with

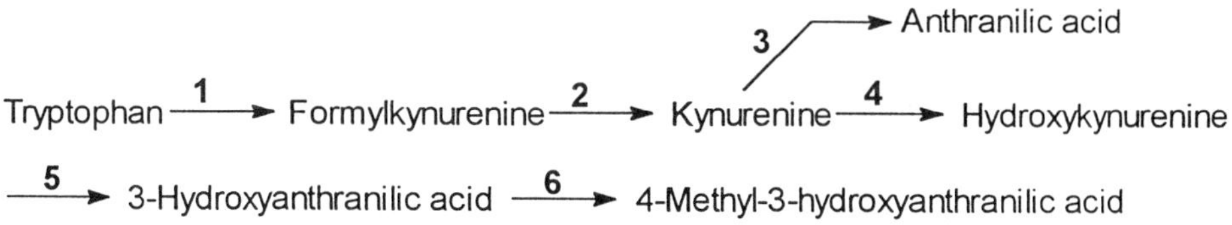

Figure 2 Pathway of catabolism of tryptophan leading to 4-MHA.

primary (housekeeping) metabolism, because it shares with the latter some of the reactions necessary for degradation of tryptophan. Tryptophan, when fed to streptomycetes, is degraded to anthranilic acid (18). In addition, there is a pathway via hydroxykynurenine that appears to be destined for the synthesis of 4-MHA. The evidence for this is that actinomycin-producing *Streptomyces parvulus* contains isoforms of several of the enzymes involved in that pathway. Two forms of kynurenine formamidase have been partially purified, one of which appears to be involved in actinomycin biosynthesis (19, and see further below). Kynureninase and hydroxykynureninase, two distinct enzymes, differ from each other in their affinities for kynurenine and hydroxykynurenine as substrates (20). The data indicate that hydroxykynureninase, an enzyme with high preference for hydroxykynurenine as substrate when compared with kynurenine, is involved in the synthesis of 3-hydroxyanthranilic acid (3-HA). 3-HA is well known as an intermediate in the catabolism of tryptophan, and in eukaryotes it serves as precursor of nicotinic acid (21). In the actinomycin-producing streptomycetes, 3-HA is the ultimate precursor of 4-MHA. Jones (22) has described a 3-HA-methylating enzyme that introduces the methyl-group from *S*-adenosyl-L-methionine into the 4-position of the benzene ring of 3-HA. The enzyme has been purified to homogeneity from *S. antibioticus* and is the only enzyme yet known that can introduce a C–C bond in an aromatic nucleus (23,24). The enzyme does not methylate 3-hydroxykynurenine, which leaves no doubt about the intermediacy of 3-HA in the formation of 4-MHA. From its structure, 3-HA would be quite adequate to form a phenoxazinone, but in the process of 4-MHA peptide formation, it is probably too weak as a substrate for the 4-MHA-activating enzyme when compared with 4-MHA (25).

B. Phenoxazinone Synthase

Phenoxazinone synthase (PHS) was first identified in extracts of *S. antibioticus* by Katz and Weissbach (15). The enzyme was shown to catalyze the oxidative condensation of two molecules of 2-aminophenol and its derivatives to yield the relevant phenoxazinone (Figure 3). Thus, the enzyme can catalyze the condensation of 3-HA or 4-MHA to yield cinnabarinic acid or actinocin, respectively, and will also function with 3-HA or 4-MHA peptides to yield actinocinyl peptides (26). At one time, it was thought that the actinocinyl peptides were intermediates in the acm biosynthetic pathway, but the work of Keller and coworkers, described in this chapter, argues strongly for the condensation of 4-MHA pentapeptides as the ultimate or penultimate step in the process.

Phenoxazinone synthase was purified to homogeneity by Choy and Jones (27). These workers confirmed the oxygen requirement for PHS activity (Figure 3) and also demonstrated that the enzyme exists in two forms in *S. antibioticus*. A large form, L,

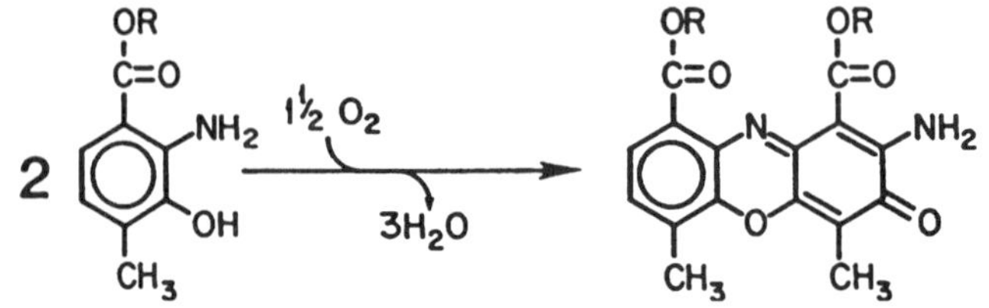

Figure 3   The reaction catalyzed by phenoxazinone synthase.

appears to be a homohexamer, whereas a small form, S, is a homodimer. The regulation of the large and small forms of PHS will discussed further below.

Begley and coworkers have examined the mechanism of PHS action. They proposed that the formation of the phenoxazinone ring occurs via a series of three consecutive two-electron aminophenol oxidations (28). The reaction sequence involves the conversion of the 2-aminophenol to a quinone imine intermediate, which reacts with a second molecule of 2-aminophenol. The resulting intermediate undergoes two additional two-electron oxidations to yield the phenoxazinone ring. Begley and coworkers (28) also demonstrated a copper requirement for PHS and subsequently showed that the enzyme is a member of the blue copper family of oxidases (29). This latter finding has been confirmed by sequencing of the cloned gene for PHS and comparison of the amino acid sequence of the protein with other members of the blue copper family (30).

In *S. antibioticus*, PHS is believed to catalyze the ultimate or penultimate step in the acm pathway. It is not yet known whether the enzyme plays a corresponding role in other acm producers, as it has not yet been detected in any of those organisms. This point will be discussed in greater detail below.

C. Actinomycin Synthetases

I. Actinomycin Synthetase I

Dissection of the various catalytic activities that are characteristic for peptide synthetases, such as activation as adenylates and thioesters, permitted the identification of the various enzymes and enzyme activities involved in the assembly of the actinomycin peptide backbone. As the first enzyme of that multienzyme system, a 4-MHA-activating enzyme from actinomycin C–producing *S. chrysomallus* was isolated, which has later been designated actinomycin synthetase I (ACMS I) (31). It is a 45 kDa protein that catalyzes the synthesis of adenylyl-4-MHA from 4-MHA and ATP (Figure 4). It does not form an enzyme–acyladenylate complex, does not charge itself with 4-MHA in thioester linkage, and differs from other activating enzymes such as coumarate: coenzyme A ligase (32,33) or luciferase (34). The enzyme has broad substrate specificity with respect to various structurally related benzene carboxylic acids. Other aromatic carboxylic acids such as pyridine, quinoline, or quinoxaline carboxylic acids are not activated by the enzyme (25,35,36).

The *S. chrysomallus* enzyme displays different activities in the presence of a number of different benzene carboxylic acids tested as substrates (Table 2). The value of K_{eq}, the equilibrium constant of the adenylate formation reaction, was increased when substituents such as an amino-, hydroxyl-, or methyl-groups in the 4-position were present, compared with benzoic acid alone. The same substituents in the 3-position resulted in a less pronounced response of the enzyme, whereas substituents in the 2-position were

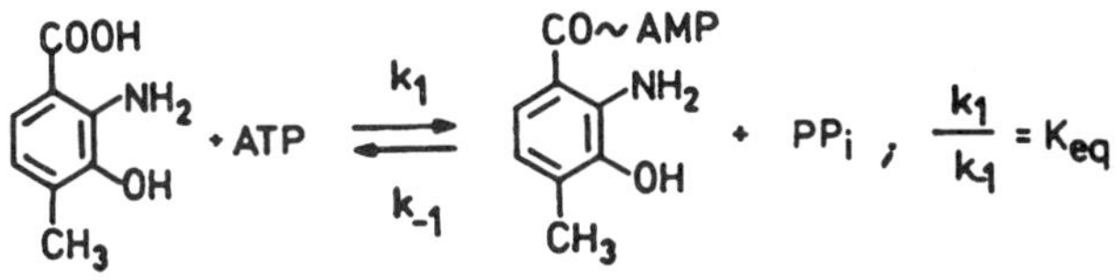

Figure 4 Formation of 4-methyl-3-hydroxyanthranilic acid adenylate catalyzed by ACMS I. K_{eq} is the reaction equilibrium constant.

Table 2   Equilibrium Constants (K_{eq}) of Various Aromatic Carboxylic acids in the Activation Reaction Catalyzed by ACMS I

Substrate	$K_{eq} \times 10^3$
4-Methyl-3-hydroxyanthranilic acid	—[a]
4-Methyl-3-hydroxybenzoic acid	3.2
3-Hydroxyanthranilic acid	0.58
Benzoic acid	0.01
2-Aminobenzoic acid	0.015
3-Aminobenzoic acid	0.001
4-Aminobenzoic acid	1.04
2-Hydroxybenzoic acid	0
3-Hydroxybenzoic acid	0.17
4-Hydroxybenzoic acid	0.41
2,3-Dihydroxybenzoic acid	0.004
3-Toluic acid	0.21
4-Toluic acid	0.54

[a] The equilibrium constant of adenyl-4-MHA formation was not determined due to the instability of 4-MHA in prolonged incubations.

much less effective (Table 2). On the other hand, combinations of substituents in the 4- and 3-positions (as in 4-methyl-3-hydroxybenzoic acid, 4-MHB) or 3- and 2-positions (as in 3-HA) led to a drastic increase of enzyme activity (25).

Kinetic constants of ACMS I, such as K_m and k_{cat}, revealed that 4-MHA, the natural substrate, has the lowest K_m (0.4 µM) among the substrates tested (Table 3). K_m values for 3-HA and 4-MHB were more than one order of magnitude higher than that of 4-MHA, indicating a stimulatory kinetic effect of the combination of 2-amino-, 3-hydroxy-, and 4-methyl-groups when compared with 2-amino, 3-hydroxy (3-HA), or 3-hydroxy-, 4-methyl (4-MHB) substituents. Also, the substrate specificity of the enzyme as expressed by k_{cat}/K_m is highest for 4-MHA, which is important in view of the extremely low concentration of 4-MHA in the cells of actinomycin-producing streptomycetes (31,37). This might also explain why 4-MHA, and not 3-HA, is incorporated in the peptide chain. It has been speculated that this is a mechanism for detoxifying the cell from 3-HA, because both 3-HA and 4-MHA are toxic and methylation of 3-HA would convert the aminophenol into a better substrate for being incorporated into the antibiotic (25).

Jones (24) found that ACMS I from *S. antibioticus* differed with respect to its substrate specificity significantly from ACMS I of *S. chrysomallus*. Here, the enzyme showed

Table 3   Kinetic Constants of ACMS I with Various Substrates

Substrate	K_m (fM)	k_{cat} (min⁻¹)	k_{cat}/K_m (min⁻¹fM⁻¹)
4-Methyl-3-hydroxyanthranilic acid	0.4	0.19	0.47
4-Methyl-3-hydroxybenzoic acid	5	0.44	0.066
3-Hydroxyanthranilic acid	18	0.32	0.018

strongest preference for anthranilic acid and to a lesser but still significant extent for benzoic acid, both of which were poorly utilized by the *S. chrysomallus* enzyme. In the presence of 3-HA and 4-MHA, both enzymes displayed comparable activities. The specific activities of the pure enzymes, although measured at different conditions, were of the same order of magnitude (about 6 and 13 nkat per mg pure protein, for the *S. chrysomallus* and *S. antibioticus* enzymes, respectively). The finding that the *S. antibioticus* enzyme is most active, with respect to V_{max}, with anthranilic acid might explain why in *S. antibioticus* externally added tryptophan is a strong inhibitor of actinomycin synthesis (26). Presumably, the anthranilate formed from tryptophan acts as a competitive inhibitor of the 4-MHA incorporation into the actinomycin peptide. It has also been shown that ACMS I of *S. antibioticus* can activate phenoxazinone dicarboxylic acids such as cinnabarinic acid or actinocin (24). Whether this has relevance for the mechanism of actinomycin peptide formation is not clear. In summary, the different substrate specificities of the two enzymes possibly may be correlated with different regulatory mechanisms of actinomycin synthesis in *S. chrysomallus* and *S. antibioticus*.

Strong evidence for the involvement of ACMS I in actinomycin biosynthesis came from the finding that feeding structural analogs of 4-MHA such as 4-methyl-3-hydroxy-benzoic acid, 3-hydroxybenzoic acid, *p*-toluic acid, or *p*-aminobenzoic acid to cells of actinomycin-producing *S. chrysomallus* and *S. antibioticus* resulted in the formation of new compounds instead of actinomycin (38). These carboxylic acids had previously been shown to be efficiently activated by purified ACMS I (see Table 2 and Refs. 25 and 31). The new compounds were monocyclic acylpentapeptide lactones (actinomycin half molecules) containing the corresponding 4-MHA analog at their amino-terminal ends (Figure 5). This indicated that 4-MHA had been replaced in each case through competition by the administered precursor. These findings also suggested that formation of the phenoxazinone takes place after incorporation of 4-MHA into the peptide chain, presumably

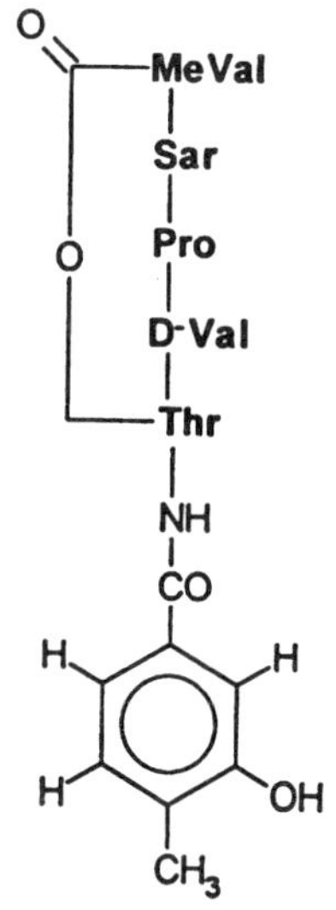

Figure 5   Structure of an actinomycin half molecule. 4-Methyl-3-hydroxybenzoyl pentapeptide lactone, a structural analog of 4-MHA pentapeptide lactone, accumulates in cultures of actinomycin-producing streptomycetes when fed 4-MHB.

through oxidative condensation of two 4-MHA pentapeptide lactones. Further support for this assumption comes from the finding that a 4-MHA pentapeptide lactone can be isolated from cultures of an actinomycin-producing *Streptomyces cucumerosporus* (39), where it accumulated as a minor product.

2. Actinomycin Synthetases II and III

Multifunctional protein thiol templates, actinomycin synthetases II and III (ACMS II and III), are peptide synthetases responsible for the assembly of 4-MHA and the constituent amino acids of the pentapeptide rings of actinomycins (40). They were first detected in protein extracts of *S. chrysomallus* and *S. parvulus* by their ability to bind covalently all of the amino acids present in the peptide chains of actinomycin as thioesters with concomitant consumption of ATP. After separation of the two enzymes, it was demonstrated that ACMS II is responsible for the activation of L-threonine and L-valine or L-isoleucine as thioesters via the corresponding adenylates, that is, amino acids in positions 1 and 2 of the pentapeptide lactone ring, whereas ACMS III activates proline, glycine, and valine, the corresponding amino acids in positions 3, 4, and 5 of the pentapeptide lactone ring. In the presence of *S*-adenosyl-L-methionine, thioester-bound glycine and valine become *N*-methylated, yielding covalently bound sarcosine and *N*-methyl-L-valine, respectively (Figure 6). This indicates that ACMS III harbors catalytic activities that are responsible for the *N*-methylation of covalently bound amino acid residues. The same mechanism of *N*-methylation had been described earlier in the case of fungal peptide synthetases

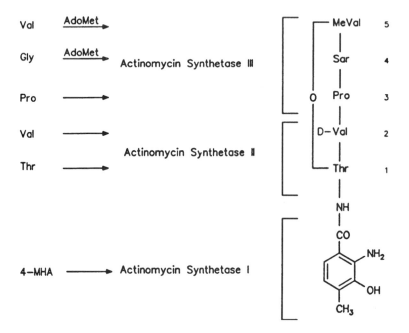

Figure 6 Assembly of 4-MHA and the five constituent amino acids in the synthesis of 4-MHA pentapeptide lactone D. The corresponding actinomycin D arises by oxidative condensation of two of these 4-MHA pentapeptide lactone moieties, catalyzed by phenoxazinone synthase. Sar = sarcosine (*N*-methylglycine); MeVal = *N*-methyl-L-valine.

involved in the biosyntheses of fungal N-methyl amino acid–containing enniatins or cyclosporin A (41,42). As in the case of the fungal enzymes, the N-methyltransferase domains are integral parts of the *Streptomyces* synthetase.

The occurrence of N-methylated peptide bonds is characteristic of peptide lactones and cyclodepsipeptides from streptomycetes and fungi. No such structures are observed in peptide antibiotics from the bacilli. Monoclonal antibodies directed against the N-methyltransferase domain of enniatin synthetase strongly cross-reacted with ACMS III but not ACMS II, confirming the presence of N-methyltransferase domain(s) in ACMS III (Billich A, Zocher R, and Keller U, unpublished results). Further characterization revealed that ACMS II is a polypeptide chain of 280 kDa, whereas ACMS III has a size of 480 kDa (43; Stindl A and Keller U, unpublished results). Both enzymes contain 4'-phosphopantetheine as a characteristic cofactor of peptide synthetases, which, in contrast to the situation in fatty acid synthase or type II polyketide synthetase (PKS) systems (44), is not restricted to the acyl carrier protein (ACP) but is present as the principal carrier in each domain responsible for the incoming amino acids as well as for the corresponding peptidyl intermediate (45). It is now known that each amino acid–activating domain of a peptide synthetase contains one 4'-phosphopantetheine arm to which the corresponding amino acid will be attached in thioester linkage after its activation as amino acyl adenylate (11).

Although ACMS I, II, and III contain all necessary sites for activation of 4-MHA and the five amino acids, total cell-free synthesis of 4-MHA pentapeptide lactone with these three enzymes has not yet been accomplished. Data from the one of our laboratories (UK) indicate that at least ACMS I and ACMS II are functionally intact, which allows the formation and accumulation of reaction intermediates on the surface of ACMS II when substrates are present. However, these intermediates were not found to be further transferred to ACMS III. Nevertheless, analysis of the peptide intermediates formed covalently bound to ACMS II in the additional presence of ACMS I enabled the establishment of the mechanisms of initiation, elongation, and epimerization in 4-MHA pentapeptide lactone formation up to position 2 in the peptide ring sequence.

D. Initiation of Actinomycin Synthesis

The site of initiation of acylpeptide synthesis is located on ACMS II. ACMS II contains three distinct sites for covalent binding of 4-MHA, L-threonine, and L-valine as thioesters (43,46). Evidence was obtained that at least the sulfhydryl-group responsible for covalent binding of 4-MHA belongs to a covalently attached 4'-phosphopantetheine cofactor. To bind threonine and valine as thioesters, ACMS II has to activate both amino acids as adenylates with consumption of ATP (40). By contrast, 4-MHA-adenylate is formed by ACMS I and subsequently thioesterified to ACMS II. Initiation occurs by N-acylation of enzyme-bound threonine with 4-MHA. This has been shown by incubation of ACMS II with threonine, ACMS I, and *p*-toluic acid, a structural analog of 4-MHA used as model substrate, where covalently bound *p*-toluyl-L-threonine was formed in an ATP-dependent manner. The same result was obtained when chemically synthesized *p*-toluyl-adenylate was present in the reaction mixture instead of both ACMS I and *p*-toluic acid, confirming that free adenylyl-4-MHA is involved in the process of 4-MHA peptide formation and that covalent binding of 4-MHA to ACMS II is independent of ACMS I. Under optimal conditions, all the threonine became acylated with *p*-toluic acid, which indicates

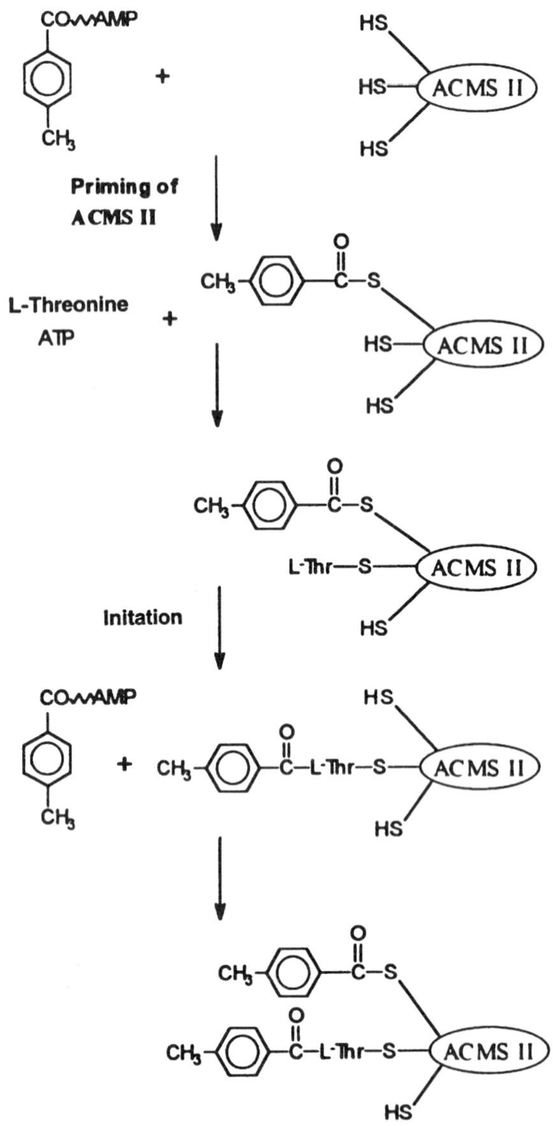

Figure 7   Scheme of initiation of 4-MHA peptide formation on ACMS II using the model substrate *p*-toluic acid. (After Stindl and Keller, unpublished results, 1993.)

that the site to which 4-MHA-threonine is bound is identical to the site that is responsible for the previous covalent binding of threonine (Figure 7). Concomitantly, the 4-MHA site became filled with *p*-toluic acid in these experiments for a next round of initiation, as was revealed by the finding that besides *p*-toluyl-L-threonine, a nearly equimolar amount of *p*-toluic acid was found to be attached to the enzyme (Stindl and Keller, unpublished results; see scheme in Figure 7).

That ACMS II binds 4-MHA (or its structural analog *p*-toluic acid) as thioester led Stindl and Keller (43) to probe ACMS II with soluble thioesters of *p*-toluic acid in the presence of threonine in order to see if these would be incorporated into *p*-toluyl-threonine, as had been the case when chemically synthesized p-toluyl-adenylate was used. During investigation of fatty acid synthase from yeast (47) or of erythromycin synthesis in *Saccharopolyspora* sp. (48), short fatty acyl-N-acetylcysteamine thioesters were used as model substrates and efficiently incorporated in the long-chain fatty acids or the erythronolide, respectively. Acyl-N-acetylcysteamine thioesters have partial structural similarity with the corresponding acyl coenzyme A thioesters.

Several p-toluyl thioesters structurally related to p-toluyl coenzyme A were shown to be accepted by ACMS II in acylation reactions. These were p-toluyl coenzyme A thioester, toluyl pantetheine thioester, and p-toluyl-cysteaminyl-β-alanine (Figure 8). ACMS II did not accept p-toluyl-N-acetylcysteamine thioester or p-toluylcysteamine thioester as substrates. Apparently, these were too short for recognition by the enzyme, whereas the longer p-toluyl thioesters appeared to mimic the carrier arm of the enzyme to which p-toluic acid was bound in synthesis conditions. This arm is likely to be 4'-phosphopantetheine. Sequence data from other peptide synthetases indicate that such 4'-phosphopantetheine arms also operate in the case of threonine and valine. Thus, one has to expect a total of three such carrier arms on ACMS II. It remains to be seen whether future analysis of the sequence of ACMS II will confirm this expectation.

E.   Elongation

The first elongation step in actinomycin peptide synthesis is transfer of 4-MHA-threonine to the amino-group of the covalently bound valine in the valine domain of ACMS

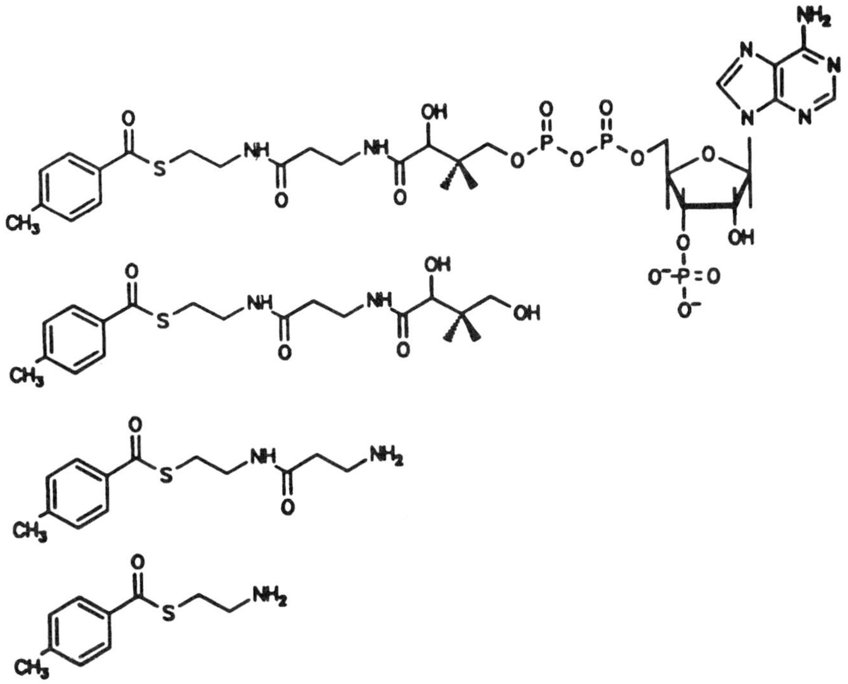

Figure 8   Some structures of p-toluic acid thioesters structurally related to p-toluic acid:coenzyme A thioester (top). With the exception of p-toluyl-cysteamine thioester, all of these compounds were active as model substrates in initiation of acylpeptide synthesis.

II, as revealed by the formation of *p*-toluyl-L-threonyl–L-valine and *p*-toluyl-L-threonyl–D-valine in experiments involving *p*-toluic acid, L-threonine, and L-valine (46). Characteristically, the threonine site was filled exclusively with *p*-toluyl-L-threonine, as revealed by the absence of threonine covalently bound to the enzyme. Similarly, the absence of L-valine in these conditions provides strong evidence that the valine site of ACMS II is also the site to which *p*-toluyl-L-threonyl–L-valine was attached during synthesis of the growing peptide chain. The same authors showed that in the absence of ACMS I, ACMS II also can catalyze condensation of threonine with valine without *p*-toluic acid. This results in the formation of the diastereomer pair L-threonyl–L-valine and L-threonine–D-valine in equimolar ratio. Under these conditions, both threonine and valine were found to be present on the enzyme's surface, indicating that this reaction did not go to completion when aromatic carboxylic acid was missing. Under these same conditions, isoleucine, which can replace valine in vivo and in vitro, reacts poorly with threonine. Only when *p*-toluic acid was present was isoleucine efficiently incorporated in the acyl-L-threonyl–L-isoleucine and acyl-L-threonyl–D-allo-isoleucine dipeptides. These data clearly indicate a pronounced stimulation of overall reactivity of substrates when the *N*-terminus of the growing peptide is acylated with *p*-toluic acid.

F.   Epimerization

The mechanism of amino acid epimerization in actinomycin synthesis differs from that of racemizations by single amino acid–activating enzymes of nonribosomal peptide synthesis such as gramicidin S synthetase I, where D- or L-phenylalanine are equally well accepted in the process of overall peptide synthesis (8,49,50). Investigation of the mechanism of valine epimerization during the synthesis of the diastereomer pair L-threonyl–L-valine and L-threonyl–D-valine (and, of course, of the corresponding *p*-toluyl-dipeptides) revealed that this occurs at the stage of peptide-bound L-valine. ACMS II accepts L-valine, but not D-valine, in the activation step, and all the valine attached to the enzyme after activation has the L-configuration. This rules out the possibility that valine is epimerized prior to incorporation into L-threonyl–L-valine. In contrast, evidence for the epimerization after formation of the peptide bond between threonine and valine came from radiotracer experiments with 2,3-^{3}H-valine. Comparison of the two radioactive dipeptides formed on ACMS II revealed loss of 50% of the tritium label in the L-threonyl–D-valine when compared with the amount of radioactivity present in the L-threonyl–L-valine diastereomer. Earlier in vivo data by Mason et al. (51) had shown that the radioactive D-valine in actinomycin D obtained after 2,3-^{3}H-valine feeding had lost label exclusively at carbon C2, whereas label at carbon C3 was retained. These findings strongly suggest that L-threonyl–D-valine is derived from L-threonyl–L-valine by proton abstraction catalyzed by a dipeptidyl epimerase function on ACMS II. Additional confirmation for this hypothesis came from the finding that during epimerization radioactive water was formed, which makes removal of the hydrogen via hydride shift unlikely. By contrast, this observation supports the intermediacy of a carbanion structure at C2 of valine, which would explain the loss of a proton during inversion. In addition, release of tritium from C2 of valine in those experiments depended on the presence of both ATP and threonine; this leaves no doubt that for epimerization the formation of the peptide bond between threonine and valine was necessary. Epimerization proceeds independently of the addition of cofactors such as NAD, FAD, or pyridoxalphosphate. Spectral analysis of ACMS II revealed no absorption in the far ultraviolet and visible range, indicating the absence of all of those cofactors from the enzyme. Thus, this mechanism of peptide epimerization is novel and may operate in the syntheses of large numbers of nonribosomally as well as ribosomally synthesized peptides that have D–amino acids at internal or carboxy-terminal positions of their chains (46). Whether in the case of actinomycin synthetase II the two dipeptides are located on the same or two different sulhydryl-groups remains to be seen. All currently available data on the initiation and first elongation steps of 4-MHA pentapeptide synthesis are summarized in Figure 9.

G.   Further Elongations and Termination

As yet, no transfer of acyl-L-threonyl–D-valine from ACMS II to ACMS III has been accomplished in a cell-free system. It is conceivable that this must be the next step after epimerization in the reaction chain of 4-MHA pentapeptide lactone formation, by enabling the formation on ACMS III of the peptide bond between D-valine and proline in the pentapeptide lactone ring (see Figure 5). It follows, therefore, that no data are available concerning the termination of acylpeptide lactone synthesis. Formation of dioxopiperazines between sarcosine and N-methylvaline and between proline and sarcosine are the only events that have been observed as yet beyond the stage of MHA-threonyl–D-valine formation (40; Stindl A and Keller U, unpublished results). Work to establish a cell-free system for actinomycin synthesis as well as the cloning and sequencing of the ACMS genes is therefore necessary to clarify the late steps of this most interesting type of peptide synthesis, catalyzed by the actinomycin synthetases I, II, and III.

IV.   GENETICS AND REGULATION OF ACTINOMYCIN BIOSYNTHESIS

A.   Mutations in the Actinomycin Pathway

The availability of well-characterized mutants was essential to the isolation and analysis of the genes involved in antibiotic production and morphological differentiation in *Streptomyces coelicolor* (e.g., 52,53). Unfortunately, only a few mutants blocked in the acm pathway have been isolated to date. Polsinelli et al. (54) isolated auxotrophs of *S. antibioticus* by ultraviolet (UV) irradiation of spores. They found that auxotrophs requiring amino acids not found in the acm pentapeptide chain synthesized acm on minimal medium supplemented with the relevant amino acid(s), in amounts similar to the levels of synthesis observed with the parental strain. In contrast, auxotrophs requiring amino acids that are present in acm synthesized significantly reduced amounts of the antibiotic on minimal medium containing the amino acid(s). No difference in growth rate was observed when auxotrophs requiring amino acids that were absent from the acm pentapeptide chain were compared with auxotrophs requiring an amino acid that is present in acm. The authors interpreted these results to mean that *S. antibioticus* utilizes amino acids in the exogenous and endogenous pools in a differential fashion. Their studies supported the conclusion that *S. antibioticus* uses exogenous amino acids efficiently to support protein synthesis (i.e., growth) but does not use the exogenous pool efficiently for the synthesis of actinomycin.

Troost and Katz (55) isolated mutants of *S. parvulus* by treatment of spores with UV light alone or in combination with 8-methoxypsoralen. An important class of mutants produced by this treatment accumulated 4-methyl-3-hydroxyanthranilic acid (4-MHA). These studies provided convincing evidence for the function of 4-MHA as an

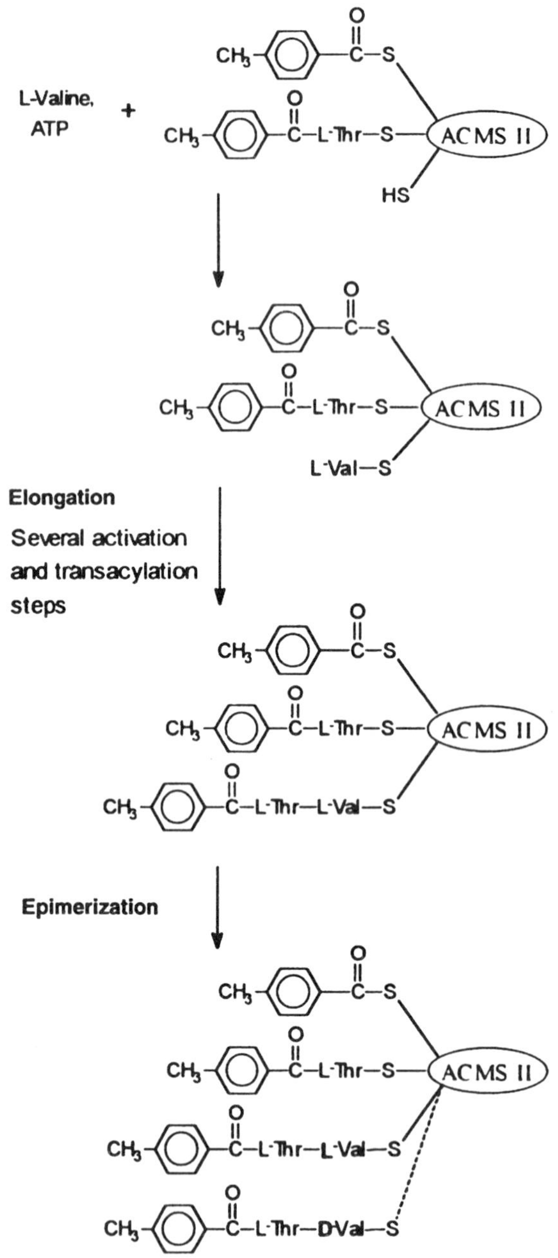

Figure 9   Scheme of elongation and epimerization of 4-MHA peptide synthesis.

intermediate in acm biosynthesis and led to the proposal of a pathway for the production of the antibiotic. As discussed above, actinomycin synthetase I functions to activate 4-MHA as the first step in the formation of the acm pentapeptide chain.

Using procedures similar to those described in the preceding paragraphs, Haese and Keller (18) isolated three classes of acm mutants from *S. chrysomallus*. The mutant classes were distinguished by their ability to generate actinomycin-producing progeny in crosses involving protoplast fusion. Some of the mutants of class I were shown to be blocked at some step in the acm pathway prior to the production of 4-MHA. Thus, these mutants synthesized small amounts of acm when they were fed 4-MHA. The lesion in class I did not appear to affect the production or activities of tryptophan pyrrolase (tryptophan oxygenase), kynurenine formamidase, or kynureninase, and the authors speculated that at least some of the class I mutants were defective in either kynurenine hydroxylase or the enzyme that methylates 3-hydroxyanthranilic acid. Mutants of all three classes contained reduced amounts of ACMS I as compared with the parental strain, but the reduction was greatest for classes II and III (<20% of the wild-type specific activity). Class I mutants contained ACMS I levels that were 40–70% of those observed for the wild-type strain. Class I mutants manifested near-wild-type specific activities for ACMS II and III. Class III mutants had reduced ACMS II and III specific activities, but the levels observed for those of class III were significantly higher than the class II levels. Because ACMS II and III activities appeared to decrease coordinately in class II mutants, Haese and Keller (18) argued that the mutations in that class affected the regulation of the expression of acm synthetases II and III. The role of the locus represented by class III was not determined in that study, but the authors speculated that the mutations in that class influenced the expression of ACMS I and that class III may be a subset of class I.

In more recent studies, Keller and coworkers have isolated additional class I mutants of S. chrysomallus. Two of these lack ACMS III but still have wild-type levels of ACMS I and II. Other mutants lack ACMS II and III. These findings suggest that the acm synthetase genes are located at the locus represented by class I mutants (Keller U, unpublished results).

Mapping studies performed with the S. chrysomallus mutants indicated that the loci were chromosomally linked but not clustered. If the class I–III mutations do occur in genes of the acm biosynthetic pathway, this result would stand in stark contrast to those obtained for essentially all other antibiotic pathways that have been analyzed in Streptomyces; antibiotic production genes appear to be organized in clusters in other systems that have been characterized to date (e.g., 56).

Ochi and Katz (57) presented evidence for the involvement of a plasmid in acm biosynthesis. These workers observed that acriflavine or novobiocin treatment of S. antibioticus or S. parvulus resulted in the loss of the ability to produce actinomycin. That ability could be restored by crossing acm⁻ and acm⁺ strains, but not by crossing an acm⁻ strain with another nonproducer. The facts that the mutagens used in these experiments were known curing agents and that the acm⁺ progeny could not be obtained from crosses of the acm⁻ strains led Ochi and Katz to propose the involvement of an extrachromosomal genetic element in the regulation of the synthesis of acm. Additional support for this hypothesis was obtained in studies suggesting that one or more of the loci required for acm production were not linked to any of four auxotrophic markers present in acm⁺ and acm⁻ strains used in recombination experiments (58). Moreover, Ochi (59) demonstrated that a doubly auxotrophic acm⁻ strain of S. parvulus could be transformed at low frequency to actinomycin production using DNA from an acm⁺ strain with complementary nutritional requirements. In a companion study (60), Ochi demonstrated that acm⁻ mutants produced by acriflavine or novobiocin treatment of S. antibioticus contained wild-type levels of phenoxazinone synthase and kynurenine formamidase but were unable to accumulate 4-MHA or to convert 4-MHA to actinomycin. Thus, if a plasmid is involved in acm production, the relevant loci would appear to be required for the production of 4-MHA and for its ultimate conversion to acm. The acm⁻ mutants produced by the curing agents were also shown to be less resistant to acm than the parental strain, but this phenotype did not appear to be plasmid-dependent (60). No further evidence in support of plasmid involvement in acm biosynthesis has been reported, but it is interesting to note that *S. antibioticus* has been shown to contain a giant linear plasmid (Kinashi H, unpublished results) and such a plasmid has been definitively shown to bear the genes responsible for the production of methylenomycin by *S. coelicolor* (61).

B.   Catabolite Regulation of Actinomycin Production

Catabolite repression, the repression of enzyme synthesis by specific metabolites when cells are grown in media containing rapidly metabolizable substrates along with other carbon or energy sources, is mediated by several different mechanisms in bacteria and unicellular eukaryotes (62). The best characterized of these mechanisms involves the phosphoenolpyruvate-dependent carbohydrate phosphotransferase system (PTS), which functions in the enteric bacteria. The PTS regulates the uptake of substrates, the generation of cytoplasmic inducers for catabolite-regulated pathways, and the modulation of the synthesis of cAMP, which is required for catabolite repression in the enterics. Available evidence indicates that *Streptomyces* do not contain cAMP, although contrary to earlier reports, recent studies do confirm the presence of a PTS in members of the genus (63). The role of the PTS in catabolite repression in *Streptomyces* has not been determined.

Like many other antibiotics, for example, bacitracin (64,65), enniatin (66), and novobiocin (67), actinomycin synthesis is subject to catabolite repression. When actinomycin-producing streptomycetes are grown on media containing glucose and a relatively noninterfering carbon source (e.g., galactose), acm production is delayed until essentially all the glucose in the medium is utilized. Phenoxazinone synthase and ACMS I appear to be subject to catabolite control in *S. antibioticus* (24,68). Catabolite control of PHS production will be discussed in greater detail below.

C.   Regulation of the Enzymes of the Actinomycin Pathway

As has been discussed, actinomycin biosynthesis is connected to the pathway of tryptophan catabolism. The regulation of three of the enzymes involved in the conversion of tryptophan into precursors of acm has been studied by Katz and coworkers. Tryptophan oxygenase catalyzes the conversion of tryptophan to *N*-formylkynurenine. Foster and Katz (69) showed that the activity of the enzyme in *S. parvulus* increased significantly just prior to the onset of acm production. These studies were conducted using media containing L-glutamate, and that amino acid was almost completely consumed before actinomycin synthesis was initiated in *S. parvulus*. The addition of glutamate to cultures that had consumed the amino acid originally present in the medium (and that had initiated acm production) inhibited both antibiotic biosynthesis and the increase in tryptophan oxygenase activity normally observed. These workers developed a chemically defined medium lacking L-glutamate and showed that this medium (and spent medium obtained after the consumption of L-glutamate by the mycelium) would support acm production by mycelium at a stage of growth that should have been too early for acm production. The results argue against the synthesis of an inducer during the period in which L-glutamate is consumed, and for the regulation of tryptophan oxygenase via catabolite repression involving metabolites of glutamic acid.

Katz (70) and Brown et al. (19,71) demonstrated the presence of two forms of kynurenine formamidase in *S. parvulus*. Kynurenine formamidase catalyzes the conversion of N-formylkynurenine to kynurenine. The higher-molecular-weight form of the enzyme (form I, M_r = 42,000) was synthesized constitutively in S. *parvulus* and was present at only low levels in the mycelium. The other form of the enzyme (form II, M_r = 25,000) appeared in the mycelium just prior to the initiation of acm biosynthesis and was essentially undetectable in young cultures that did not produce the antibiotic. Brown et al. (71) examined the levels of the two forms of kynurenine formamidase in an acm⁻ mutant obtained initially in the studies of Troost and Katz (55) described earlier. They observed that the mutant, designated AM8, contained only low levels of kynurenine formamidase activity, and that only enzyme form I was present in these mutants. Thus, like tryptophan oxygenase, the synthesis of kynurenine formamidase II appears to be required for acm production, and that enzyme appears to play a specific role in the catabolism of tryptophan to produce intermediates in the acm pathway.

Extracts of S. *parvulus* contain enzyme activities that convert kynurenine and hydroxykynurenine to anthranilate and 3-hydroxyanthranilate, respectively (20). 3-Hydroxyanthranilate is the immediate precursor of 4-MHA in the acm pathway. Both the kynureninase and the hydroxykynureninase activities were inducible by growth of the organism in the presence of tryptophan. In the absence of tryptophan, only one of the two activities, the hydroxykynureninase, increased immediately prior to the onset of acm production. Elevated levels of hydroxykynureninase were maintained for the duration of acm production by S. *parvulus*. The acm⁻ mutant, AM8, which contained only form I of kynurenine formamidase, contained lower than wild-type levels (up to 30 times less) of hydroxykynureninase as well. Taken together, the results of the studies of Katz and coworkers argue strongly for the requirement of specific enzymes of tryptophan catabolism for acm production, and for the regulation of those enzymes, some of them possibly coordinately, by factors that trigger acm biosynthesis.

D.   Regulation of Phenoxazinone Synthase

In S. *antibioticus*, phenoxazinone synthase (PHS) catalyzes the ultimate or penultimate step in the acm biosynthetic pathway, the oxidative condensation of two molecules of 3-hydroxyanthraniloyl pentapeptide to yield actinomycin or actinomycinic acid (It is not yet known when the lactone rings of the acm pentapeptide chains are formed.) PHS was first identified by Katz and Weissbach (15) and was purified to homogeneity by Choy and Jones (27). PHS exists in two forms in S. *antibioticus*, a large form, L, a homohexamer and a small form, S, a homodimer (27). L and S do not appear to be interconvertible, but their production by S. *antibioticus* is developmentally regulated. Young cultures, not producing acm, contain S predominantly, whereas older, antibiotic-producing cultures contain primarily L (27). The biochemical basis for the existence of the two PHS forms has yet to be determined. The PHS subunit was originally estimated to have an M_r of 88,000, but studies of the cloned *phs* gene indicate an actual M_r of 70,000 for the protein (30).

To date, the gene for PHS, *phs*A, is the only gene in the acm pathway to be cloned. *phs*A is present on a ca. 2.3 kb SphI fragment and encodes a protein of 642 amino acids (30,72). The transcription start site for the gene has been established, and −10 and −35 promoter elements have been identified. A ca. 300 bp fragment of *phs*A, containing the −10 and −35 regions and the transcription start, promotes the expression of a promoterless *xyl*E gene in the streptomycete promoter probe vector pIJ2843. The promoter region of *phs*A contains several sequence elements that may be involved in regulating the expression of the gene. These include six pairs of direct repeats, two pairs of inverted repeats, and two sequences (TNTNAN) that have been implicated in catabolite control of gene expression in other streptomycetes (73).

In growing *S. antibioticus* cultures, *phs*A is not expressed constitutively. Rather, *de novo* synthesis of the enzyme is initiated after about 9 hr of growth on acm production medium (74). The specific activity of the enzyme increases after its synthesis begins and reaches a plateau at about the time acm begins to accumulate in the growth medium. Using the cloned gene as a probe, it was possible to demonstrate that the increase in PHS specific activity in growing *S. antibioticus* cultures is due in part to a transcriptional regulatory mechanism. Thus, the concentration of *phs*A mRNA in growing cultures increases concomitantly with the increase in enzyme specific activity (75).

PHS production has also been shown to be subject to catabolite repression. Repression of PHS synthesis was first observed in the experiments of Marshall et al. (74), and the phenomenon was studied in detail by Gallo and Katz (68). These workers showed that the synthesis of PHS was repressed by glucose in *S. antibioticus* cultures growing in a chemically defined medium with galactose as the alternative carbon source. PHS synthesis in such cultures did not begin until the glucose in the medium was consumed, and no galactose was utilized until the glucose supply was depleted. Other carbon sources were more or less effective than glucose at repressing PHS synthesis; those compounds that supported the most rapid rates of growth were the most effective repressors. Jones (75) provided evidence that glucose repression of PHS production in *S. antibioticus* was mediated via a transcriptional mechanism. Thus, the concentration of *phs*A mRNA was lower in cultures grown on glucose as compared with cultures of the same age grown on galactose. An increase in the concentration of *phs*A mRNA was observed in glucose-grown cultures when the glucose in the medium was depleted. Marshall et al. (74) and Gallo and Katz (68) argued that the increase in PHS specific activity observed in *S. antibioticus* cultures grown on galactose (see above) is due to the release of the *phs* gene from catabolite repression, reflecting the fact that galactose is not a completely nonrepressing carbon source.

Hsieh and Jones (30) have examined the cloned *phs*A promoter to determine whether its function is subject to catabolite control. As indicated above, a ca. 300 bp fragment of *phs*A, containing the putative promoter elements, promotes expression of the *xyl*E gene in the promoter probe vector pIJ2843 in *S. antibioticus*. This construct was used to examine the effects of glucose on expression of the *phs*A promoter. In these studies, the expression of *xyl*E from the *phs*A promoter was examined in *S. antibioticus* transformants grown on galactose, glucose, or galactose plus glucose. These experiments revealed that the cloned promoter was most active when transformants were grown on galactose, and that its activity was significantly decreased in glucose-grown cultures. The level of *xyl*E expression observed when transformants were grown on galactose plus glucose was essentially the same as that obtained for growth on glucose alone. It is noteworthy that the levels of endogenous PHS activity in the *S. antibioticus* transformants in question paralleled exactly the levels of *xyl*E expression. These results are consistent with the conclusion that the cloned 300 bp promoter fragment from *phs*A possesses at least some of the sequence elements required to mediate the glucose response in *S. antibioticus*. The specific sequences required for catabolite repression of *phs*A have not been identified.

The studies reported by Jones (75) indicated that *phs*A expression was regulated in part at the level of transcription. However, a posttranscriptional mechanism was also implicated in *phs*A regulation. It was observed that PHS was significantly more resistant to degradation by intracellular proteases than most other proteins synthesized by *S. antibioticus*. Thus, at a time when many, if not most, mycelial proteins were being degraded,

PHS was not broken down. The specific activity of PHS in growing S. antibioticus increases in part, therefore, because the total amount of mycelial protein decreases while the amount of PHS remains constant or increases. This observation may explain how acm-producing cultures of S. antibioticus can maintain the required levels of PHS activity at a time when the rates of macromolecular synthesis in the mycelium have decreased significantly as compared with those of younger cultures (76). It will be of interest to determine whether other acm enzymes also demonstrate a greater resistance to proteolytic degradation than most mycelial proteins.

In initial cloning experiments, phsA was identified by virtue of its expression in a heterologous host, Streptomyces lividans (72). In those same experiments, two other fragments of the S. antibioticus genome were cloned that transformed S. lividans with concomitant production of PHS activity. These fragments, 1.8 and 4.3 kb in size, were shown not to encode the PHS subunit; rather, they served to activate a silent phs gene in S. lividans (77). That silent gene, phsB, was subsequently cloned, and shown, in vitro at least, to encode a protein with the properties of the PHS subunit (78). The two activator fragments also evoked PHS production when they were used to transform a variety of other streptomycetes (77). More recently, the function of one of the two fragments, the 4.3 kb activator, has been examined in greater detail. Fawaz and Jones (79) isolated a ca. 700 bp fragment from the 4.3 kb activator that retained the ability to activate the silent phs gene in S. lividans. Sequencing of that fragment revealed several potential open reading frames (ORFs) but the G+C distribution in those ORFs was uncharacteristic of streptomycete genes. No transcription products from the active sequence could be detected, and no proteins corresponding to the sizes of the predicted products of the ORFs were detected in a streptomycete coupled transcription–translation system with the active fragment as a template. Polymerase chain reaction (PCR) cloning was used to further localize the active region of the 700 bp fragment, and a product of 249 bp was obtained that retained the ability to activate the silent phs gene in S. lividans. Interestingly, a 243 bp fragment, almost identical in sequence to the 249 bp fragment from S. antibioticus, was obtained by the PCR using S. lividans total DNA as a template (79). Preliminary evidence has been obtained for the function of the 249 and 243 bp fragments in protein binding (Fawaz F, and Jones GH, unpublished results). The role of the 249 bp activator fragment (and of the 1.8 kb activator, which has not been further characterized) in acm biosynthesis is unknown at this point.

Two final points regarding the function and regulation of PHS deserve mention. First, the analysis of the sequence of the phsA promoter revealed a striking similarity in the −10 and −35 regions to the P2 promoter of the agarase gene of S. coelicolor. That promoter is recognized by an RNA polymerase holo-enzyme containing an alternative sigma factor, σ^E (80,81). In vitro transcription experiments demonstrated that the similarity of the two promoters was more than skin deep and that phsA is also recognized by RNA polymerase containing σ^E (Jones GH, Paget M, Chamberlin L, and Buttner M, unpublished results). In more recent studies, the sigE gene was identified in S. antibioticus, and a null mutation in that gene was constructed. Surprisingly, the null mutation did not abolish the ability of the mutant to produce PHS (Jones GH, Paget M, Chamberlin L, and Buttner M, unpublished results). Thus, the transcription experiments described above may reflect a relaxed specificity of the holo-enzyme containing σ^E in vitro rather than the requirement of σ^E for transcription of the phsA promoter in vivo. It is nevertheless significant that even though the S. antibioticus strain containing the null mutation in sigE continued to produce PHS, it did not produce acm. ACMS I levels were reduced by 90% in the mutant (Jones GH, Paget M, Chamberlin L, and Buttner M, unpublished results).

Thus, one or more promoters required for acm production appears to depend on *sig*E for transcription in *S. antibioticus*.

Second, it is curious and perplexing that whereas PHS can be easily detected in *S. antibioticus* and almost certainly plays a key role in acm production in that organism, repeated attempts to detect the enzyme in two other acm producers, *S. chrysomallus* and *S. parvulus*, have failed. It may be that PHS is present in those organisms but has more stringent substrate requirements than the corresponding enzyme in *S. antibioticus* and, thus, cannot be detected with the usual assays. Alternatively, the acm chromophore might be synthesized nonenzymatically in acm producers other than *S. antibioticus*. It is noteworthy that preliminary results of gene disruption experiments suggest that an intact *phs*A gene is required for acm production in *S. antibioticus* (Jones GH, unpublished results).

E.   A Possible Role for Guanosine Tetraphosphate (ppGpp) in the Regulation of Actinomycin Biosynthesis

There is abundant evidence for the function of guanosine tetraphosphate (ppGpp) as a mediator of the stringent response to amino acid, carbon, or energy starvation in *Escherichia coli* (82). The *rel*A and *spo*T loci encode proteins that catalyze the synthesis of ppGpp, in concert with other enzymes, and SpoT is also involved in the degradation of ppGpp (82–85). The stringent response to amino acid starvation has been demonstrated in streptomycetes (86), and in several members of the genus, the intracellular concentration of ppGpp increases dramatically just prior to the onset of antibiotic biosynthesis (87,88).

Ochi (89) demonstrated the occurrence of the stringent response in an actinomycin-producing strain of *S. antibioticus* and isolated several thiopeptin-resistant mutants that displayed a relaxed phenotype when subjected to amino acid starvation. In *S. antibioticus* and several other strains, the relaxed mutants were shown to contain an altered ribosomal protein L11 and thus were assigned to the *rel*C class of mutations by analogy with the *E. coli* system (90). One of the *S. antibioticus* mutants, designated *rel*C49, was examined in detail by Ochi, and it was demonstrated that, in addition to its relaxed phenotype, *rel*C49 was completely unable to synthesize actinomycin (89). The mutant contained reduced levels of phenoxazinone synthase, but the levels of kynurenine formamidase were unaffected by the *rel* mutation. The *rel*C49 mutant also contained significantly reduced levels of ppGpp, and unlike in the parental strain, no increase in ppGpp concentration was observed during nutritional shiftdown of the mutant cultures (89). The results suggested the possibility that ppGpp plays a role in the initiation of actinomycin biosynthesis in *S. antibioticus*.

In a subsequent study, Kelly et al. (91) demonstrated that, like several other streptomycetes, a burst of ppGpp production (or accumulation) preceded the initiation of acm biosynthesis. It was also shown that the decreased level of PHS observed in the *rel*C49 mutant was due to an effect of the mutation at the level of the mRNA for the enzyme. Thus, there was a direct correlation between PHS specific activity and the concentration of *phs* mRNA; *phs* mRNA levels in the mutant were 14–25% of those observed in the parental strain and did not increase during the course of growth of the mutant on acm production medium. Kelly et al. (91) also reported that one of the other enzymes in the acm pathway, ACMS I, was completely absent from the *rel*C49 mutant.

Though the foregoing results are consistent with a role for ppGpp in initiating acm biosynthesis, their interpretation is complicated by the fact that the *rel*C49 mutant is not completely devoid of ppGpp. As an approach to the isolation of true "spotless" mutants,

Jones (92) has undertaken the characterization of enzymes involved in ppGpp synthesis in S. antibioticus. A pppGpp synthetase has been purified from S. antibioticus, and crude mycelial extracts of that organism have been shown to convert pppGpp to ppGpp (92). The pppGpp synthetase, designated guanosine pentaphosphate synthetase I (GPSI), has several properties that are reminiscent of the RelA protein from E. coli. Thus, GPSI will catalyze the formation of pppGpp from ATP and GTP in the presence of methanol. However, GPSI differs from the RelA protein in several important respects. First, whereas RelA utilizes both GTP and GDP as substrates, GDP was shown to be a poor substrate for GPSI. Second, the activity of the RelA protein is stimulated by ribosomes and uncharged tRNA in a codon-dependent fashion. No stimulation of GPSI activity by ribosomes could be demonstrated, but it was observed that synthetic mRNA (polyuridylic acid) and tRNA (charged or uncharged) did stimulate the enzyme. The level of stimulation observed with mRNA plus tRNA was greater than the maximal level obtained with either RNA alone (93). Finally, it was found that the activity of GPSI could be stimulated by mild proteolysis of the enzyme with trypsin (93). Levels of stimulation comparable to those achieved with methanol or RNAs were obtained by trypsin activation. No effect of trypsin on the activity of the RelA protein could be demonstrated.

The gene for GPSI has been cloned and shown to encode a protein with an M_r of 79,000 (94). Surprisingly, the deduced amino acid sequence of GPSI bore no similarity to the sequences of the RelA or SpoT proteins from E. coli, or to proteins of similar function from other bacteria. Rather, the GPSI protein sequence bears a striking similarity to that of polynucleotide phosphorylase (PNPase) from E. coli (94). Indeed, polymerization and phosphorolysis assays performed using purified GPSI demonstrated that the enzyme does function as a polynucleotide phosphorylase, at least in vitro (94). dCDP, which inhibits the activity of E. coli PNPase, also inhibited the PNPase activity of GPSI; however, the pppGpp synthetase activity of GPSI was not inhibited by dCDP. This result suggests the intriguing possibility that GPSI is a bifunctional enzyme with both PNPase and pppGpp synthetase activities, and this possibility raises the question whether there may be a heretofore unappreciated connection between ppGpp metabolism and mRNA degradation in bacteria.

Since GPSI is neither a RelA or SpoT homolog, it is relevant to ask whether the latter protein species exist in S. antibioticus. To answer this question, a DNA probe, corresponding to a conserved region of known RelA/SpoT protein sequences, was synthesized via the PCR. That probe, obtained using primers designed by Mervyn Bibb of the John Innes Institute, was first used to identify hybridizing fragments in restriction digests of total S. antibioticus DNA and was utilized subsequently in colony hybridization experiments to clone a ca. 7 kb fragment containing the sequences of interest. Preliminary DNA sequencing results indicate that the gene of interest is almost identical to a RelA/SpoT homolog identified in S. coelicolor (95,96). The role of the product of the cloned relA/spoT homolog in S. antibioticus has not been determined. Disruption of the gene in question in S. coelicolor failed to produce a consistent effect on actinorhodin production in one study (95) but abolished actinorhodin production (but not production of undecylprodigiosin or calcium-dependent antibiotic) in a second study (96).

V. CONCLUSIONS AND PROSPECTS

At the biochemical level, the development of a cell-free system capable of synthesizing actinomycin from the relevant precursors remains to be achieved. In the absence of such a system, several relevant questions, some of which have been listed above, remain unanswered. The cloning and overexpression of the acm genes should allow the isolation of sufficient quantities of the relevant enzymes to permit the construction of appropriate in vitro systems for acm production. Cloned acm genes will also be necessary for the genetic manipulation of the acm pathway and the preparation of modified actinomycins.

It will also be apparent to the reader that many important questions related to the regulation of actinomycin biosynthesis remain unanswered. The cloning of the genes for the acm enzymes other than PHS will facilitate the subsequent analysis of the relevant regulatory mechanisms, especially if, as is likely, it turns out that the pathway genes are clustered and the cluster also contains one or more regulatory genes. The mechanism of self-resistance to acm has also not been determined, and there may be coordinate regulation of the expression of the resistance determinant(s) and one or more of the biosynthetic genes. It will be of particular interest to determine whether enzymes in the biosynthetic pathway other than PHS are subject to catabolite repression, and to elucidate the specific mechanisms by which catabolite repression of the acm pathway is effected, since there is evidence, as indicated above, that cAMP is not involved. Thus, the mechanism of glucose repression of PHS and acm production may be novel among the bacteria. At the level of transcription, there is the interesting possibility that alternative sigma factors may play a role in regulating acm production, and since ppGpp is thought to act at the level of transcription, at least in some systems (see Ref. 81), it is possible that RNA polymerase or some accessory transcription factor might be the target for ppGpp action in *S. antibioticus*. The creation of "spotless" mutants by inactivation of the gene for GPSI and for the putative RelA/SpoT homolog should shed considerable light on the role of ppGpp in the initiation of acm biosynthesis. In addition, the cloning of the RelA/SpoT homolog described above will make it possible to determine, via Southern blotting, whether *S. antibioticus* contains yet another RelA/SpoT-related sequence.

There is, thus, much interesting and important work yet to be done on the acm pathway and on antibiotic synthesis and morphological differentiation in other streptomycetes. One can but hope that funding agencies around the globe will see the value of continuing this work and will provide the funds to support it.

ACKNOWLEDGMENT

This chapter is dedicated to the memory of Edward Katz, whose pioneering work on the physiology, biochemistry, and genetics of actinomycin biosynthesis laid the foundation for many of the studies described herein.

REFERENCES

1. Katz E. Actinomycin. Gottlieb D, Shaw PD. eds. Antibiotics II. New York: Springer-Verlag, 1976:276–341.
2. Meienhofer J, Atherton E. Structure-activity relationships in the actinomycins. Adv Appl Microbiol 1973; 16:203–300.
3. Hollstein U. Actinomycin: Chemistry and mechanism of action. Chem Rev 1974; 74:625–652.
4. Okumura Y. Peptidolactones. Vining LC. ed. Biochemistry and Genetic Regulation of Commercially Important Antibiotics. Reading, Massachusetts: Addison-Wesley, 1983:147–178.

5. Brockman H, Bohnsack G, Franck B, Gröne H, Muxfeldt H, Süling C. Zur Konstitution der Actinomycine. Angew Chem 1956; 8:70–71.

6. Johnson AW, Mauger AB. The isolation and structure of actinomycins II and III. Biochem J 1959; 73:535–538.

7. Katz E, Goss WA. Controlled biosynthesis of actinomycin with sarcosine. Biochem J 1959; 73:459–465.

8. Kurahashi K. Biosynthesis of small peptides. Annu Rev Biochem 1974; 43:445–459.

9. Kleinkauf H, von Döhren H. Biosynthesis of peptide antibiotics. Annu Rev Microbiol 1990; 41:59–289.

10. Kleinkauf H, von Döhren H. Nonribosomal biosynthesis of peptide antibiotics. Eur J Biochem 1990; 192:1–5.

11. Marahiel M. Multidomain enzymes involved in peptide synthesis. FEBS Lett 1992; 307:40–43.

12. Stachelhaus T, Marahiel MA. Modular structure of genes encoding multifunctional peptide synthetases required for non-ribosomal peptide synthesis. FEMS Microbiol Lett 1995; 125:3–14.

13. Turgay M, Krause M, Marahiel MA. Four homologous domains in the primary structure of GrsB are related to domains in a superfamily of adenylate-forming enzymes. Mol Microbiol 1992; 6:529–546.

14. Haese A, Schubert M, Herrmann M, Zocher, R. Molecular characterization of the enniatin synthetase gene encoding a multifunctional enzyme catalyzing N-methyldepsipetide formation in *Fusarium scirpi*. Mol Microbiol 1993; 7:905–914.

15. Katz E, Weissbach H. Biosynthesis of the actinomycin chromophore: Enzymatic conversion of 4-methyl 3-hydroxyanthranilic acid to actinocin. J Biol Chem 1962; 237:882–886.

16. Keller U. Peptidolactones. Vining LC, ed. Genetics and Biochemistry of Antibiotic Production. Toronto, New York: Heinemann-Butterworths, 1994:71–94.

17. Katz E, Weissbach H. Effect of chloromycetin and penicillin on the incorporation of amino acids into actinomycin and protein by *Streptomyces antibioticus*. Biochem Biophys Res Commun 1962; 8:186–190.

18. Haese A, Keller U. Genetics of actinomycin C production in *Streptomyces chrysomallus*. J Bacteriol 1988; 170:1360–1368.

19. Brown DA, Hitchcock MJ, Katz E. Evidence for a constitutive and inducible form of kynurenine formamidase in an actinomycin-producing strain of *Streptomyces parvulus*. Arch Biochem Biophys 1980; 202:18–22.

20. Troost T, Hitchcock, MJM, Katz E. Distinct kynureninase and hydroxykynureninase enzymes in an actinomycin-producing strain of *Streptomyces parvulus*. Biochim Biophys Acta 1980; 612:97–106.

21. Gaertner FH, Cole, KW, Welch, GR. Evidence for distinct kynureninase and hydroxykynureninase activities in *Neurospora crassa*. J Bacteriol 1971; 108:902–909.

22. Jones GH. Actinomycin synthesis in *Streptomyces antibioticus*: Enzymatic conversion of 3-hydroxyanthranilic acid to 4-methyl-3-hydroxyanthranilic acid. J Bacteriol 1987; 169:5575–5578.

23. Fawaz F, Jones GH. Actinomycin synthesis in *Streptomyces antibioticus*: Purification and properties of 3-hydroxyanthranilate-4-methyltransferase. J Biol Chem 1988; 263:4602–4606.

24. Jones GH. Combined purification of actinomycin synthetase I and 3-hydroxyanthranilic acid 4-methyltransferase from *Streptomyces antibioticus*. J Biol Chem 1993; 268:6831–6834.

25. Keller U, Schlumbohm W. Purification and characterization of actinomycin synthetase I, a 4-methyl-3-hydroxyanthranilic acid: AMP ligase from *Streptomyces chrysomallus*. J Biol Chem 1992; 267:11745–11752.

26. Salzman L, Weissbach H, Katz E. Enzymatic synthesis of actinocinyl peptides. Arch Biochem Biophys 1969; 130:536–546.

27. Choy HA, Jones GH. Phenoxazinone synthase from *Streptomyces antibioticus*: Purification of the large and small enzyme forms. Arch Biochem Biophys 1981; 211:55–65.

28. Barry CE III, Parmesh G, Nayar PG, Begley T. Phenoxazinone synthase: Mechanism for the formation of the phenoxazinone chromophore of actinomycin. Biochem 1989; 28:6323–6333.
29. Freeman JC, Nayar PG, Begley TP, Villafranca JJ. Stoichiometry and spectroscopic identity of copper centers in phenoxazinone synthase: A new addition to the blue copper oxidase family. Biochem 1993; 32:4826–4830.
30. Hsieh C-J, Jones GH. Nucleotide sequence, transcriptional analysis and glucose regulation of the phenoxazinone synthase gene (*phsA*) from *Streptomyces antibioticus*. J Bacteriol 1995; 177:5740–5747.
31. Keller U, Kleinkauf H, Zocher R. 4-Methyl-3-hydroxyanthranilic acid (4-MHA) activating enzyme from actinomycin producing *Streptomyces chrysomallus*. Biochem 1984; 23:1479–1484.
32. Knobloch K-H, Hahlbrock K. Isoenzymes of p-coumarate:CoA ligase from cell suspension cultures of *Glycine max*. Eur J Biochem 1975; 52:311–320.
33. Lozoya E, Hoffmann H, Douglas C, Schulz W, Scheel D, Hahlbrock K. Primary structure and catalytic properties of isoenzymes encoded by the two 4-coumarate:CoA ligase genes in parsley. Eur J Biochem 1988; 176:661–667.
34. de Wet JR, Wood KV, DeLuca M, Helinski DR, Subramani S. Firefly luciferase gene: Structure and expression in mammalian cells. Mol Cell Biol 1987; 7:725–737.
35. Glund K, Schlumbohm W, Bapat M, Keller U. Biosynthesis of quinoxaline antibiotics: Purification and characterization of the quinoxaline-2-carboxylic acid activating enzyme from *Streptomyces triostinicus*. Biochem 1990: 29:3522–3527.
36. Schlumbohm W, Keller U. Chromophore activating enzyme involved in the biosynthesis of the mikamycin B antibiotic etamycin from *Streptomyces griseoviridus*. J Biol Chem 1990; 265:2156–2161.
37. Weissbach H, Redfield B, Beaven V, Katz E. 4-Methyl-3-hydroxyanthranilic acid, an intermediate in actinomycin biosynthesis. Biochem Biophys Res Commun 1965; 19:524–530.
38. Keller U. Acyl pentapeptide lactone synthesis in actinomycin-producing streptomycetes by feeding with structural analogs of 4-methyl-3-hydroxyanthranilic acid (4-MHA). J Biol Chem 1984; 59:8226–8231.
39. Hanada M, Sugawara K, Nishiyama Y, Kamei H, Hatori M, Konishi M. Protactin, a new metabolite and a possible precursor of the actinomycins. J Antibiot 1992; 45:20–28.
40. Keller U. Actinomycin synthetases: Multifunctional enzymes responsible for the synthesis of the peptide chains of actinomycin. J Biol Chem 1987; 262:5852–5856.
41. Zocher R, Keller U, Kleinkauf H. Enniatin synthetase, a novel type of multifunctional enzyme catalyzing depsipeptide synthesis in *Fusarium oxysporum*. Biochem 1982; 21:43–48.
42. Zocher R, Nihira T, Paul E, Madry N, Peeters H, Kleinkauf H, Keller U. Biosynthesis of cyclosporin A: Partial purification and properties of a multifunctional enzyme from *Tolypocladium inflatum*. Biochem 1986; 25:550–553.
43. Stindl A, Keller U. The initiation of peptide formation in the biosynthesis of actinomycin. J Biol Chem 1993; 268:10612–10620.
44. Hopwood DA, Sherman, DH. Molecular genetics of polyketides and its comparison to fatty acid biosynthesis. Annu Rev Genet 1990; 24:37–66.
45. Schlumbohm W, Stein T, Ullrich C, Vater J, Krause M, Marahiel MA, Kruft V, Wittmann-Liebold B. An active serine is involved in covalent substrate amino acid binding at each reaction center of gramicidin S synthetase. J Biol Chem 1991; 266:23135–23141.
46. Stindl A, Keller U. Epimerization of the D-valine portion in the peptide chain of actinomycin. Biochem 1994; 33:9358.
47. Lynen F. Yeast fatty acid synthase. Meth Enzymol 1980; 14:17–33.
48. Cane DE, Yang C. Macrolide biosynthesis. 4. Intact incorporation of a chain-elongation intermediate into erythromycin. J Am Chem Soc 1987; 109:1255.

49. Vater J, Kleinkauf, H. Gramicidin S-synthetase: A further characterization of phenylalanine racemase, the light enzyme of gramicidin S-synthetase. Biochim Biophys Acta 1976; 429:1062–1072.

50. Gocht M, Marahiel MA. Analysis of core sequences in the D-Phe activating domain of the multifunctional peptide synthetase TycA by site-directed mutagenesis. J Bacteriol 1994; 176:2654–2662.

51. Mason KT, Shaw GJ, Katz E. Biosynthetic studies with L-[2, 3-^{3}H$_2$]valine as precursor of the D-valine moiety in actinomycin. Arch Biochem Biophys 1977; 180:509–513.

52. Malpartida F, Hopwood DA. Physical and genetic characterization of the gene cluster for the antibiotic actinorhodin in Streptomyces coelicolor A3(2). Mol Gen Genet 1986; 205:66–73.

53. Chater KF. Genetics of differentiation in Streptomyces. Annu Rev Microbiol 1993; 47:685–713.

54. Polsinelli M, Albertini A, Cassani G, Ciferri O. Relation of biochemical mutations to actinomycin biosynthesis in Streptomyces antibioticus. J Gen Microbiol 1965; 39:239–246.

55. Troost T, Katz E. Phenoxazinone biosynthesis: Accumulation of a precursor, 4-methyl-3-hydroxyanthranilic acid, by mutants of Streptomyces parvulus. J Gen Microbiol 1979; 111:121–132.

56. Martin JF, Liras P. Organization and expression of genes involved in the biosynthesis of antibiotics and other secondary metabolites. Annu Rev Microbiol 1989; 43:173–206.

57. Ochi K, Katz E. The possible involvement of a plasmid(s) in actinomycin synthesis by Streptomyces parvulus and Streptomyces antibioticus. J Antibiot 1978; 31:1143–1148.

58. Ochi K, Katz E. Genetic analysis of the actinomycin producing determinants (plasmid) in Streptomyces parvulus using the protoplast fusion technique. Can J Microbiol 1980; 26:1460–1464.

59. Ochi K. Protoplast fusion permits high frequency transfer of a Streptomyces determinant which mediates actinomycin synthesis. J Bacteriol 1982; 150:592–597.

60. Ochi K. Control of the actinomycin biosynthetic pathway and actinomycin resistance of Streptomyces spp. J Bacteriol 1982; 150:598–603.

61. Kinashi H, Shimaji M, Sakai A. Giant linear plasmids in Streptomyces which code for antibiotic biosynthesis genes, Nature 1987; 328:454–456.

62. Saier MH Jr. A multiplicity of potential carbon catabolite repression mechanisms in prokaryotic and eukaryotic microorganisms. New Biologist 1991; 3:1137–1147.

63. Titgemeyer F, Walkenhorst J, Reizer J, Stuiver MH, Cui X, Saier MH Jr. Identification and characterization of phosphoenolpyruvate:fructose phosphotransferase systems in three Streptomyces species. Microbiol UK 1995; 141:51–58.

64. Haavik HI. Studies on the formation of bacitracin by Bacillus licheniformis: Effect of glucose. Gen Microbiol 1974; 81:383–390.

65. Haavik HI. Studies on the formation of bacitracin by Bacillus licheniformis: Role of catabolite repression and organic acids. J Gen Microbiol 1974; 84:321–326.

66. Audhya RK, Russell DW. Enniatin production by Fusarium sambucinum: Primary and secondary metabolism. J Gen Microbiol 1975; 86:327–332.

67. Kominek LA. Biosynthesis of novobiocin by Streptomyces niveus. Antimicrob Agents Chemother 1972; 1:123–134.

68. Gallo M, Katz E. Regulation of secondary metabolite biosynthesis: Catabolite repression of phenoxazinone and actinomycin formation by glucose. J Bacteriol 1971; 109:659–667.

69. Foster JW, Katz E. Control of actinomycin D biosynthesis in Streptomyces parvullus: Regulation of tryptophan oxygenase activity. J Bacteriol 1981; 48:670–677.

70. Katz E. Kynurenine formamidase isoenzymes in Streptomyces parvulus. Hayaishi O, Ishimura Y, Kido R, eds. Amsterdam: Elsevier/North Holland Biomedical Press, 1980:159–177.

71. Brown D, Hitchcock MJM, Katz, E. Purification and characterization of kynurenine formamidase activities from Streptomyces parvulus. Can J Microbiol 1986; 32:465–472.

72. Jones GH, Hopwood DA. Molecular cloning and expression of the phenoxazinone synthase gene from *Streptomyces antibioticus*. J Biol Chem 1984; 259:14151–14157.

73. Mattern, SG, Brawner, ME, Westpheling J. Identification of a complex operator for galP1, the glucose-sensitive, galactose-dependent promoter of the *Streptomyces* galactose operon. J Bacteriol 1993; 175:1213–1220.

74. Marshall R, Redfield B, Katz E, Weissbach, H. Changes in phenoxazinone synthase activity during the growth cycle of *Streptomyces antibioticus*. Arch Biochem Biophys 1968; 123:317–323.

75. Jones GH. Regulation of phenoxazinone synthase expression in *Streptomyces antibioticus*. J Bacteriol 1985; 163:1215–1221.

76. Jones GH. RNA synthesis in *Streptomyces antibioticus*: In vitro effects of actinomycin and of transcriptional inhibitors from 48 hr cells. Biochem 1976; 15:3331–3341.

77. Jones GH, Hopwood DA. Activation of phenoxazinone synthase expression in *Streptomyces lividans* by cloned DNA sequences from *Streptomyces antibioticus*. J Biol Chem 1984; 259:14158–14164.

78. Madu AC, Jones GH. Molecular cloning and in vitro expression of a silent phenoxazinone synthase gene from *Streptomyces lividans*. Gene 1989; 84:287–294.

79. Fawaz F, Jones GH. Activation of phenoxazinone synthase expression in *Streptomyces lividans*: Characterization of the activator fragment from *Streptomyces antibioticus*. Microbiol UK 1994; 140:1051–1058.

80. Buttner MJ, Smith, AM, Bibb, MJ. At least three different RNA polymerase holoenzymes direct transcription of the agarase gene (*dagA*) of *Streptomyces coelicolor* A3(2). Cell 1988; 52:599–607.

81. Lonetto M, Brown KL, Rudd K, Buttner MJ. Analysis of the *Streptomyces* coelicolor *sigE* gene reveals a new sub-family of eubacterial RNA polymerase σ factors involved in the regulation of extracytoplasmic functions. Proc Natl Acad Sci USA 1994; 91:7573–7577.

82. Cashel, M, Rudd KE. The stringent response. Neidhardt FC, Ingraham JL, Low KB, Magasanik B, Schechter M, Umbarger HE, eds. *Escherichia coli* and *Salmonella typhimurium*: Cellular and Molecular Biology, Vol. 2. Washington, D.C.: American Society for Microbiology, 1987:1410–1438.

83. Pedersen FS, Kjelgaard. Analysis of the *relA* gene product of *Escherichia coli*. Eur J Biochem 1977; 76:91–97.

84. Xiao HM, Kalman K, Ikehara K, Zemel S, Glaser G, Cashel, M. Residual guanosine 3′, 5′-bispyrophosphate synthetic activity of *relA* mutants can be eliminated by *spoT* null mutations. J Biol Chem 1991; 266:5980–5990.

85. Hernandez VJ, Bremer H. *Escherichia coli* ppGpp synthetase II activity requires *spoT*. J Biol Chem 1991; 266:5991–5999.

86. Takano E, Bibb MJ. The stringent response, ppGpp and antibiotic production in *Streptomyces coelicolor* A3(2). Actinomycetol 1994; 8:1–16.

87. Simuth J, Hudec J, Chau HT, Danyi O, Zelinka J. The synthesis of highly phosphorylated nucleotides, RNA and protein by *Streptomyces aurofaciens*. J Antibiot 1979; 32:53–58.

88. Strauch E, Takano E, Bayliss HA, Bibb MJ. The stringent response in *Streptomyces coelicolor* A3(2). Mol Microbiol 1991; 5:289–298.

89. Ochi K. A *rel* mutation abolishes the enzyme induction needed for actinomycin synthesis by *Streptomyces antibioticus*. Agric Biol Chem 1987; 51:829–835.

90. Ochi K. *Streptomyces relC* mutants with an altered ribosomal protein ST-L11 and genetic analysis of a *Streptomyces griseus relC* mutant. J Bacteriol 1990; 172:4008–4016.

91. Kelly KS, Ochi K, Jones GH. Pleiotropic effects of a *relC* mutation in *Streptomyces antibioticus*. J Bacteriol 1991; 173:2297–2300.

92. Jones GH. Purification and properties of ATP:GTP 3′-pyrophosphotransferase (guanosine pentaphosphate synthetase) from *Streptomyces antibioticus*. J Bacteriol 1994; 176:1475–1481.

93. Jones GH. Activation of ATP:GTP 3′-pyrophosphotransferase (guanosine pentaphosphate synthetase) from *Streptomyces antibioticus*. J Bacteriol 1994; 176:1482–1487.

94. Jones, GH. Guanosine pentaphosphate synthetase I from *Streptomyces antibioticus* is also a polynucleotide phosphorylase. J Bacteriol 1996 (in press).

95. Chakraburtty R, White J, Takano E, Bibb M. Cloning, characterization and disruption of a (p)ppGpp synthetase gene (*relA*) of *Streptomyces coelicolor*. Mol Microbiol 1996; 19:357–368.

96. Martinez-Costa OH, Arias P, Romero NM, Parro V, Mellado RP, Malpartida F. A *relA/spoT* homologous gene from streptomyces coelicolor A3(2) controls antibiotic biosynthetic genes. J Biol Chem 1996; 271:10627–10634.

12

Vancomycin and Other Glycopeptides

Thalia I. Nicas and Robin D. G. Cooper
Lilly Research Laboratories, Eli Lilly and Company, Indianapolis, Indiana

I. INTRODUCTION

When vancomycin [1] (Figure 1) was isolated at Eli Lilly and Co. in the early 1950s (1), it was the first example of the presently large family of naturally occurring glycopeptide antibiotics. Vancomycin has been in clinical use now for more than 35 years, and recently there has been renewed interest in this class of antibiotics (see, for example, Ref. 2). Over the past 20 years, vancomycin use has increased steadily, and it is now the first line of therapy against serious infections due to staphylococci and enterococci. As the importance of vancomycin as an agent to treat resistant Gram-positive bacteria has increased, resistance to vancomycin has also made its first appearance, affording potentially serious clinical consequences. Though a number of glycopeptides was discovered, only one other, teicoplanin [2] (Figure 2), is currently used in human medicine (3). Avoparcin [3] (Figure 3),one of several glycopeptides shown to promote growth activity in farm animals (4,5), has been used in Europe as a feed additive in poultry and cattle.

Vancomycin was introduced in 1958 as a therapy for the treatment of infection due to Gram-positive bacteria. Emergence of resistance to penicillin as well as erythromycin and tetracycline made it a welcome alternative for the treatment of *Staphylococcus aureus*. In the 1960s, new drugs, first methicillin and later the cephalosporins, displaced vancomycin in this role, and for a time it was used sparingly, primarily in penicillin-allergic patients. In the last 15 years, however, vancomycin has made a dramatic resurgence. The primary cause for the increased use of vancomycin is the emergence of methicillin-resistant staphylococci. These pathogens are often resistant to many classes of antibiotics, and currently vancomycin is the only reliable therapy available in most of the world (6). Other factors that encouraged its use were the recognition of *Staphylococcus epidermidis* and the enterococci as important pathogens in the hospital setting. Indeed, the increasing prevalence and importance of hospital-acquired infections due to Gram-positive bacteria have been major trends in hospitals over the last decade (7). This, coupled with ever-increasing antibiotic resistance, has made vancomycin a critically important drug. Vancomycin is also used as an oral treatment for pseudomembranous colitis caused by *Clostridium difficile*, a pathogen that emerges during antibiotic therapy, especially with the β-lactam antibiotics.

A remarkable property of vancomycin has been the long delay in the emergence of resistance in susceptible species. The unusual mechanism of activity of vancomycin is often cited as the reason that mutational resistance is essentially unknown. The first well-documented reports of vancomycin resistance appeared only in 1988 (8,9). Resistance appeared in the enterococci, and it was mediated by plasmids carrying nine new genes, probably the most complex mechanism of resistance seen to date (10,11).

As use of vancomycin has grown, interest in the glycopeptide class has increased. Systematic efforts to find new naturally occurring glycopeptides have been successful, although none of these has yet to be developed clinically, primarily because they have not been found to show any substantive improvements over vancomycin or teicoplanin. A new development over the past few years has been interest in semisynthetic glycopeptides (12,13). At least two of these are currently approaching clinical trials, and they have demonstrated that activity of the class can be expanded to include vancomycin-resistant enterococci and even some Gram-negative bacteria.

II. STRUCTURE AND CLASSIFICATION

The glycopeptide antibiotics form a group of natural products readily defined by their chemical structure and biological properties. The term "dalbaheptide" has been proposed for the group (14). Lipopeptide antibiotics, such as daptomycin, and lipoglycopeptides, such as ramoplanin, are structurally and mechanistically distinct (15). The essential distinguishing feature of the dalbaheptide or glycopeptide class is a linear heptapeptide backbone in which the side chains of at least five of the amino acids are linked together such that the peptide backbone is held in a rigid conformation (16–18) (Figure 4). Amino acids 2, 4, and 6 are the same in all glycopeptide antibiotics, and these residues are linked to each other through ether bonds to afford the characteristic triphenylether system. Amino acids 5 and 7 are also invariant, and they are linked through a carbon–carbon bond to give a diphenyl moiety. Sugar moieties are not present on all dalbaheptides, and indeed some highly active members of the group have none; these are often referred to as "glycopeptide aglycones" (19–21), an oxymoron that makes the proposed "dalbaheptide" name all the more attractive.

Amino acids 1 and 3 may be either aliphatic or aromatic. These amino acids can be used to divide the glycopeptides into structural types (13,16–18).

The vancomycin type (group I) is defined generally by the presence of aliphatic amino acids, leucine (R_4, R_5 = H or methyl, Figure 4) and asparagine in positions 1 and 3, although there can be a certain flexibility at amino acid 3: aspartic acid and glutamine residues have been observed. Vancomycin, eremomycin, the chloro-orienticin, or A82846, group, and the recently discovered balhimycin (22) are members of this class. They may also differ in the level of halogenation: X and Y can be either chlorine or hydrogen.

The actinoidin type, which includes avoparcin, has aromatic residues at positions 1 and 3 (group II). Synmonicin (23) is the sole representative of a third distinct type, with an aliphatic amino acid (methionine) at position 3 and an aromatic amino acid at position 1; it is sometimes grouped with the actinoidin type as a member of group II. In the ristocetin type (group III), aromatic amino acids are present in both positions 1 and 3 but have an ether linkage joining these two amino acids (Figure 5). Other examples of this class are actaplanin and A41030.

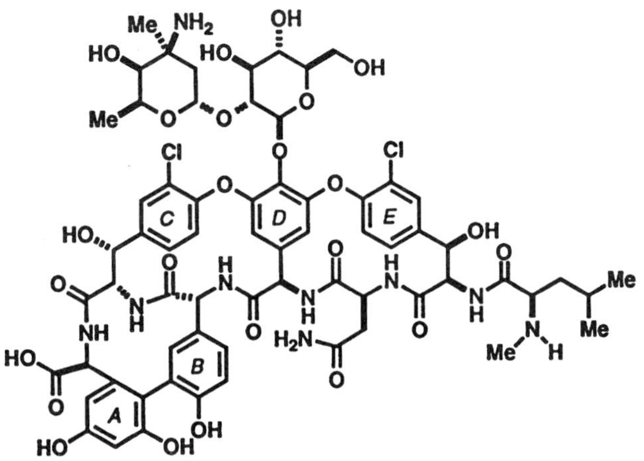

Figure 1   Vancomycin.

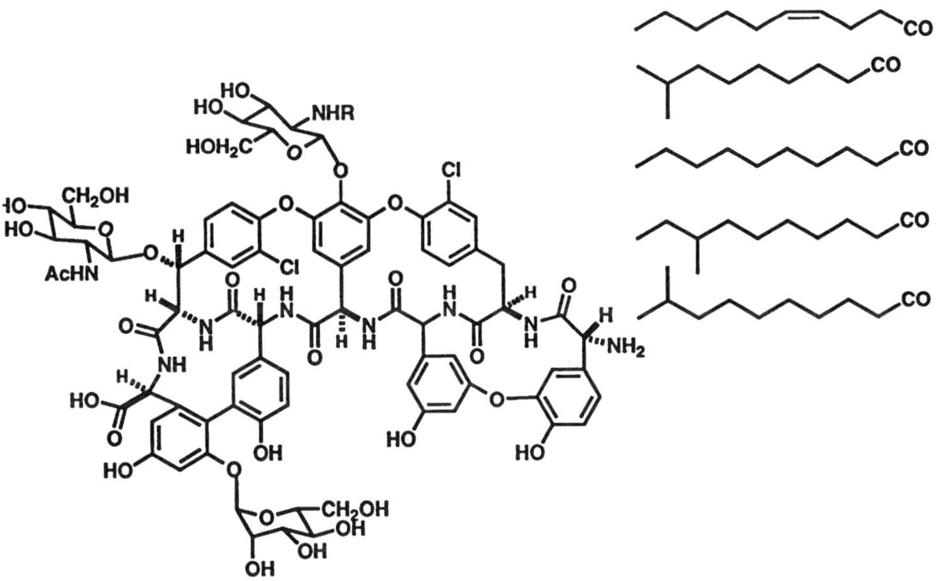

Figure 2   Teicoplanin.

The teicoplanin group could be considered a subgroup of the ristocetin type. The peptide structure is the same as the ristocetin type, but whereas in ristocetin the sugars are not substituted, in the teicoplanin type (group IV) the amino-group of the sugar linked to amino acid 4 is acylated with fatty acids, and the sugar linked to amino acid 6 is acylated. Other members of this subgroup include ardacin, kibdelin, A84575, and parvodicin.

The sugars of glycopeptides show considerable variation in structure, quantity, and site of substitution (19). Sugars can be important determinants of biological activity, and they clearly influence antibacterial activity, toxicity, and pharmacodynamic properties

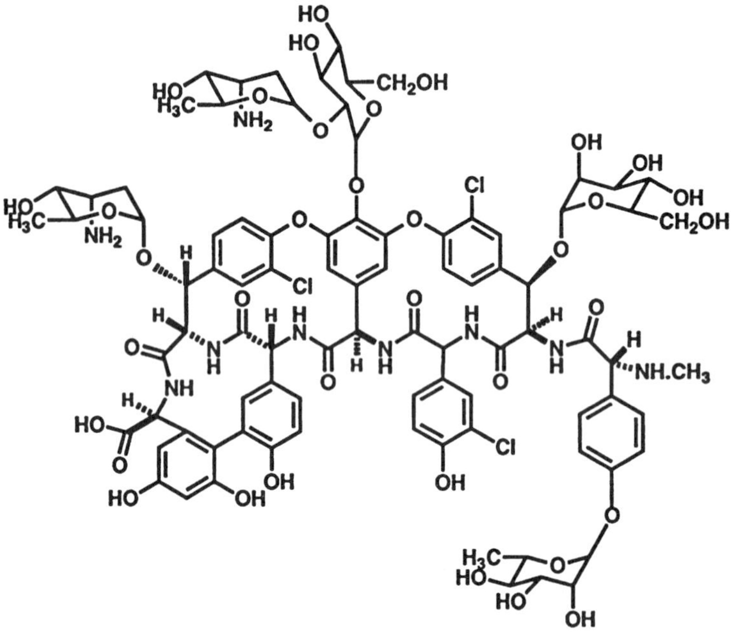

Figure 3　Avoparcin.

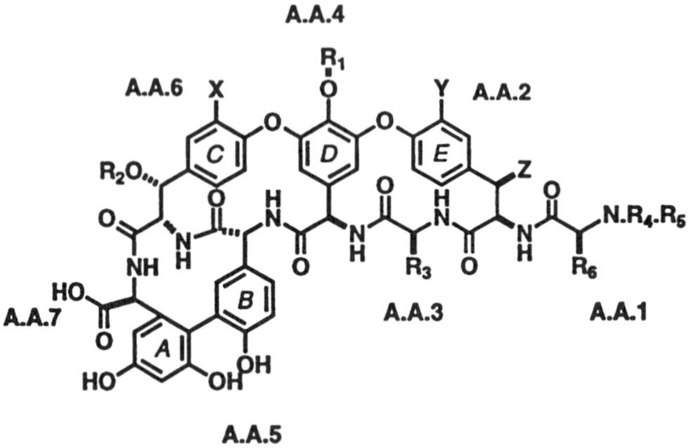

Figure 4　Generalized glycopeptide structure. Numbering scheme for the seven amino acids of the hexapeptide core is shown. (Based on Refs. 16–18.)

(12,24). Much of the challenge in structural elucidation of glycopeptide antibiotics is due the presence of rare 2,3,6 trideoxy-3-amino-hexopyranose building units, some unique to these antibiotics.

III.　BIOSYNTHESIS OF GLYCOPEPTIDE ANTIBIOTICS

The biosynthesis of vancomycin and other glycopeptide antibiotics has not been extensively studied. Examination of the structure and analogy to other peptide antibiotics has

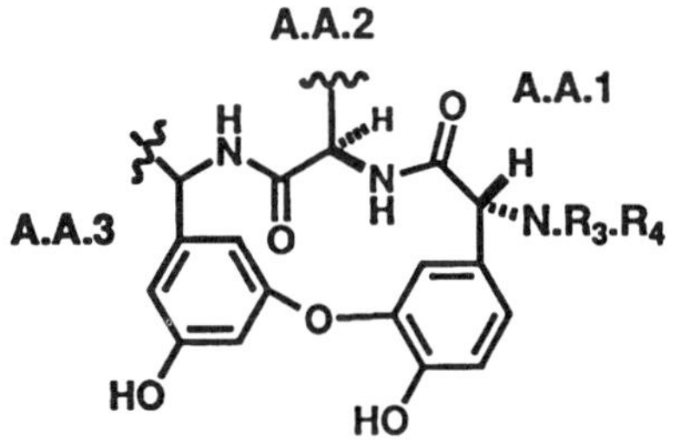

Figure 5   Amino acids 1–3 of ristocetin-type glycopeptides, showing ether linkage between amino acids 1 and 3. (Adapted from Ref. 16.)

led reviewers to suggest the following steps (17,25): (a) synthesis of the atypical amino acids; (b) assembly of the amino acids through a multienzyme thiotemplate mechanism; (c) formation of the ether and carbon–carbon bonds linking the amino acid side chains; (d) glycosylation. Although the final core structure is extensively modified, the order of the modification with respect to synthesis of the peptide backbone is unknown. However, it can be inferred from the observation that during fermentation the relative ratios of dechloro to monochloro to dichloro remain constant that the halogenation happens at the initial amino acid level before incorporation into the heptapeptide chain.

There is only limited experimental evidence at present for the overall proposed biosynthesis scheme. Studies with radiolabeled amino acids have established that for vancomycin synthesis, D-tyrosine is the precursor of D-p-hydroxyphenylglycine and β-hydroxy-m-chlorotyrosine, with the overall pathway being m-tyrosine →β-hydroxytyrosine → 3-hydroxy-3-(p-hydroxyphenyl)pyruvate → p-hydroxymandelate → p-hydroxyphenylglyoxylate → p-hydroxyphenylglycine (Figure 6), and that acetate is the precursor of the two m,m'-dihdroxyphenylglycine moieties (26). Similar results have been found in precursor studies of aridicin (27,28).

One sugar transferase, the glucosyltransferase, for vancomycin synthesis has been characterized (25,29). The enzyme recognized cores of the vancomycin type, even when fully or partially deglycosylated, but failed to recognize the actaplanin core or a modification of the vancomycin core with rearrangements within the peptide backbone. In studies of aridicin (27), it has been shown that mannose is the first sugar added, followed by N-acylglucosamine. For teicoplanin-producing cultures, there is some evidence that the mannosylation step may occur by way of a nonspecific enzyme that is not part of the biosynthetic pathway (27,30). This sugar addition occurs whether or not the other sugars are present, and Actinoplanes teichomyceticus cultures may also mannosylate the aridicin aglycone.

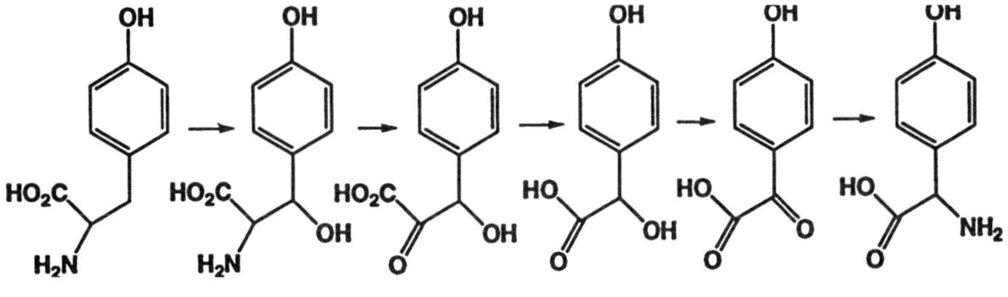

Figure 6   Proposed pathway for synthesis of phenyl glycine from tyrosine. (Based on data from Refs. 25–27.)

The pathways for biosynthesis of the unusual sugars found in glycopeptide antibiotics have not been studied. However, it would be expected that there will be considerable overlap with the aminosugar biosynthesis occurring in the macrolide and aminoglycoside antibiotics.

The sulfonated glycopeptide A47934 (21) has been studied by the generation and analysis of blocked mutants (31). Although other strains produce analogs of A47934 identical except for the sulfonation (20), the data indicate that for A47934 sulfonation is not a terminal step.

Teicoplanin is an antibiotic complex where individual components differ in the fatty acid attached to the glucosamine amino-group (Figure 2) (32). Fatty acids incorporated reflect those of the cell medium. Linoleic acid supplied in growth medium is also incorporated (32).

The overall lack of knowledge of glycopeptide antibiotic biosynthesis is somewhat surprising given the importance of the class. Zmijewski and Fayerman (25) have suggested that some of the reasons for this limited progress have been lack of blocked mutants, the wide range of producing genera with the subsequent difficulties in intergeneric gene expression and the need for specific genetic methodologies for each, and lack of known linked resistance genes. Whereas for other antibiotic classes resistance genes have proven a useful handle for finding biosynthetic genes (33,34), this has not been the case with glycopeptides. Whereas plasmid-encoded resistance genes have recently been found in enterococci, the same genes could not be identified in the vancomycin- or teicoplanin-producing strains (35,36). The teicoplanin resistance genes from A. *teichomyceticus* identified by Moroni et al. and Sosio et al. (37,38) appear to encode an unrelated mechanism of resistance, and they may prove to be a useful starting point.

IV. MODE OF ACTION

A. Molecular Basis of Glycopeptide Activity

Vancomycin and other glycopeptide antibiotics exert their antibacterial effect by inhibition of the synthesis of peptidoglycan, the principal component of the bacterial cell wall. The mechanism of action has been extensively studied, and excellent reviews of both the biochemical and molecular bases of action are available (39,40). Still, new insights continue to develop, especially now that resistance has emerged (41).

The action of this group of antibiotics is unusual in that the primary interaction is not with a protein or protein complex, but with the precursor substrate for peptidoglycan synthesis. Peptidoglycan consists of a sugar backbone of alternating N-acetylglucosamine and N-acetylmuramic acid, cross-linked through peptide bridges. Nucleotide-linked precursors consisting of UDP-N-acetylmuramyl-L-alanyl–Disoglutamyl–L-lysine[or *meso*-diaminopimelic acid]–D-alanyl–D-alanine and UDP-N-acetylglucosamine are assembled in the cytoplasm. These precursors are joined and transferred to a lipid carrier in a process that also results in the translocation of the lipid-linked disaccharide pentapeptide to the outside of the cytoplasmic membrane (Figure 7). The observation that vancomycin and ristocetin could interact with peptidoglycan precursors led to the proposal the glycopeptides act by forming a complex that blocks cell wall biosynthesis (42,43). Subsequent work supports this mechanism (39,40). This interaction results in the inhibition of incorporation of the precursors into peptidoglycan, blocking the transglycosylation that adds the disaccharide–pentapeptide precursor to the sugar backbone (Figure 7). Transpeptidation, the cross-linking of the subterminal alanine to the lysine or diaminopimelate, may

Peptidoglycan

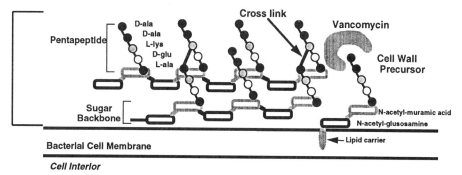

Figure 7 Peptidoglycan and vancomycin action. Vancomycin interacts with the terminal D-alanyl–D-alanine residues of the peptidoglycan precursor, shown as the membrane-associated lipid–disaccharide pentapeptide. Binding of vancomycin prevents both transglycosylation to the sugar backbone and transpeptidation. (Based on data reviewed in Ref. 39.)

also be inhibited (39). In susceptible cells treated with vancomycin, accumulation of the UDP-*N*-acetylmuramyl-pentapeptide is observed (39). Gram-negative cells are resistant to glycopeptides because the antibiotic is unable to cross the outer membrane to reach the site of peptidoglycan assembly. Recent semisynthetic glycopeptides have some limited ability to disrupt and cross the outer membrane (44).

Binding studies with acetyl-D-alanyl–D-alanine and other model peptides, especially the nuclear magnetic resonance (NMR) studies of Williams and coworkers (40), have clarified the nature of the interaction. The vancomycin peptide backbone assumes a cup-shaped form, held rigid by the cross-linking between amino acid side chains. The cavity forms a pocket into which the D-alanyl–D-alanine fits snugly to form a complex stabilized by five sets of hydrogen bonds (Figure 8). Difference in affinity of binding of model peptides can be measured and, in some cases, related to antibacterial activity (45).

This molecular mechanism is part of what makes the glycopeptide class attractive as antibacterial agents. The interaction with the precursor is highly specific, and as no eukaryotic analog of D-alanyl–D-alanine is present in mammalian cells, no basis for mechanism-based toxicity is present. The mechanism also seems to be one for which mutational resistance should be relatively difficult to achieve, as the D-alanyl–D-alanine-containing pentapeptide is the result of several synthetic steps in precursor formation, and it is involved in several steps of wall synthesis.

This rather unusual mechanism of action has some interesting research implications. The receptor–ligand type interaction provides an interesting small-molecule model for protein–ligand interactions (46). The affinity of glycopeptides for D-alanyl–D-alanine can be exploited both in searching for new glycopeptides and for purifying and isolating compounds (see section below).

B. Recently Elucidated Elements of Glycopeptide Activity: Dimerization and Membrane-Interacting Side Chains

It is likely that elements besides affinity for the peptidyl-D-ala–D-ala sequence play a role in glycopeptide antibiotic activity. Williams and colleagues have suggested a role for

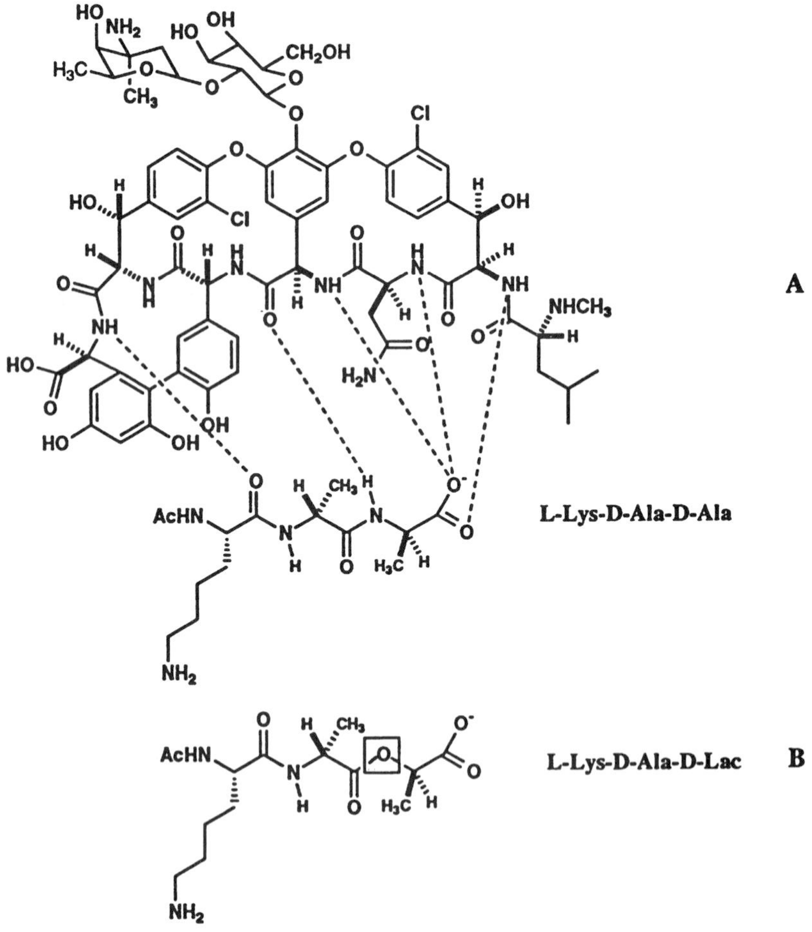

Figure 8   Interaction of vancomycin and cell wall precursor. (A) Interaction of vancomycin and lysyl-D-alanyl–D-alanine. Dashed lines represent hydrogen bonds. (B) The lysyl-D-alanyl–D-lactate ligand found in glycopeptide-resistant enterococci. The change from an amide to an ester linkage is indicated by the square. Note that this change eliminates a key hydrogen-bonding site. (Based on data reviewed in Refs. 40 and 45.)

dimerization. NMR studies have been used to characterize glycopeptide dimers (47–49). Asymmetrical "back-to-back" homodimers are formed through hydrophobic interactions between aromatic rings 4 and 6, and through a series of hydrogen bonds between opposing backbones (Figure 9). Recent studies have shown that for some glycopeptides, affinity for the bacterial cell wall precursor may be enhanced by as much as 10-fold by dimerization (50). A role for dimerization in the activity of glycopeptides has been proposed, and offered as a partial explanation for the activity of certain vancomycin-like glycopeptides, such as eremomycin and A82846B, that possess excellent antimicrobial activity despite relatively weak binding to synthetic ligands (41,50,51).

The lipid side chain of glycopeptides such as teicoplanin [2] (Figure 2) and some semisynthetic glycopeptides (2) may also serve to enhance activity by enhancing affinity

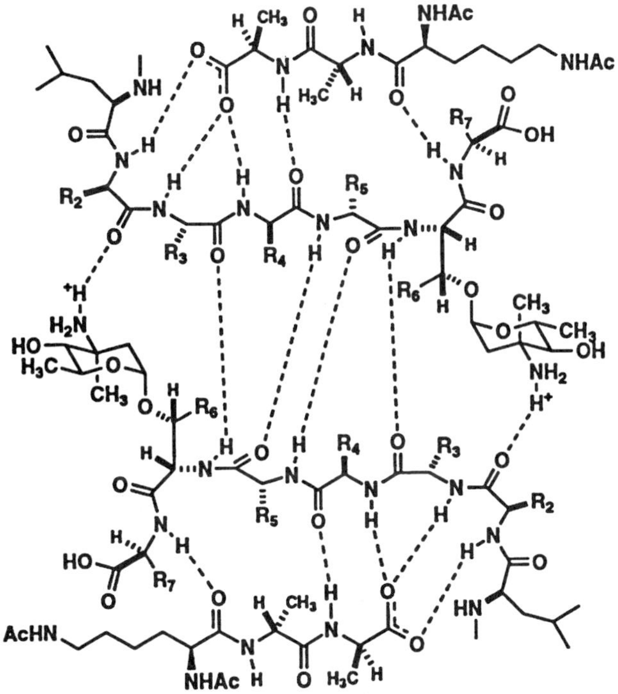

Figure 9 Hydrogen bonding network of glycopeptide dimer with bound lysyl-D-alanyl–D-alanine. Side-chain residues of amino acids are represented by R_2 to R_7. The dashed lines represent hydrogen bonds. (Adapted from Refs. 47–51.)

for the cell envelope (41,50). Both dimerization and lipophilic interactions may be regarded as a means of enhancing binding affinity and subsequent antimicrobial activity by preferential localization of antibiotic near its target at the site of cell wall biosynthesis.

V.   RESISTANCE

A.   Glycopeptide Resistance Due to Emergence of Resistance Genes

1.   The Emergence of Transferable High-Level Glycopeptide Resistance

The emergence of resistance to vancomycin was first documented in *Enterococcus faecium* and *Enterococcus faecalis* in 1988, more than 30 years after the introduction of vancomycin. Resistance was plasmid-mediated and transferable to other enterococci. Two distinct phenotypes were noted in early studies: one termed "VanA" afforded high-level resistance to both vancomycin and teicoplanin; the second, "VanB," afforded resistance to vancomycin only (36,52,53). Subsequent studies have indicated both forms have a similar mechanism of resistance but are genetically distinct (54–57). VanA resistant enterococci are cross-resistant to all naturally occurring glycopeptide antibiotics so far examined (58; Nicas TI, unpublished results) (Table 1). This newly emergent resistance has spurred several areas of research: the molecular basis of resistance has been intensively studied; new targets for antimicrobial agents have emerged from studies of both the

Table 1   Activity of Some Naturally Occurring Glycopeptides Against a Typical VanA
Enterococcus and Its Plasmid-Cured Glycopeptide-Sensitive Derivative

Glycopeptide	MIC for resistant Enterococcus faecium isolate 180 (μg/ml)	MIC for sensitive Enterococcus faecium isolate 180-1 (μg/ml)
Vancomycin	1000	1
Teicoplanin	250	0.06
Avoparcin	>100	2
Ristocetin	1000	2
LY264826 (A82846B)	125	0.25
Eremomycin	500	1
Orienticin A	>1000	1
Actaplanin	500	1
Actinoidin	>100	8

Data from Ref. 58 and unpublished results of Nicas TI.

mechanism of resistance and the regulation of resistance genes; and our knowledge of the
basics of peptidoglycan wall biochemistry has been challenged and expanded. Most critical, however, is the concern over spread of resistance to methicillin-resistant staphylococci, creating an essentially untreatable pathogen. This specter has fueled new interest
in novel agents for Gram-positive bacteria.

Acquired resistance to glycopeptides occurs by one of the most complex and
unusual mechanisms seen to date. The molecular basis of VanA glycopeptide resistance
has been intensively studied and is well understood, largely through work in the laboratories of Courvalin and Walsh (10,36,59). Essentially, the bacteria have reengineered
their cell wall, making a new precursor, in which the terminal D-alanine is replaced with
D-lactate. This alteration, resulting in an ester rather than amide linkage of the terminal
moiety, affords the loss of one of the key hydrogen bonds in complex formation with vancomycin (59,60) (Figure 8B). This results in binding that is at least 1000-fold weaker,
affording resistance.

2.   Molecular Mechanism of Resistance

The genes encoding resistance in VanA enterococci have been found on Tn*1546*, a
transposon related to Tn3 (61). The transposon includes nine genes, five of which are
required for resistance. These include *van*A, *van*H, and *van*X, encoding functions essential to formation of resistant precursor, and *van*R and *van*S, encoding a two-component
regulatory system. The most evident new protein in glycopeptide-resistant enterococci is
a 39 kDa protein, the *van*A gene product. The function of the protein was first inferred
from its homology to the *ddl* gene product, the ligase that forms D-alanyl–D-alanine. Biochemical studies showed that the enzymatic activity of the VanA protein is ligation of D-
alanine and D-2-hydroxy acids (62). Studies of the precursor isolated from resistant cells
established that its natural substrate is D-lactate (63–65). D-lactate is synthesized by oxidation of pyruvate by the *van*H gene product (60). A dipeptidase that degrades D-
alanyl–D-alanine is encoded by the *van*X gene, and this is also essential for resistance
(66). The *van*Y gene product, a carboxypeptidase that removes the terminal D-alanine

from the native precursor, is also present but not required for resistance (67). The *vanZ* gene product is of unknown function, but alone it is sufficient to confer low-level resistance to teicoplanin (68). All of the genes essential for resistance have been suggested as possible targets for new therapeutic agents (36,59). The VanA protein, the D-alanine:D-lactate ligase, is probably the most attractive of these.

3.   Regulation of Expression of Resistance

In VanA and VanB resistance, expression of resistance generally requires induction (8,52,53,58). VanA isolates are inducible by vancomycin and other glycopeptides and, in some cases, by other cell wall active agents (69,70). Sequencing of the regulatory genes *vanS* and *vanR* of the VanA resistance genes has shown similarity to two-component signal-transducing regulatory systems that sense and respond to environmental stimuli (71,72). These induction systems have been suggested as possible targets for agents to overcome glycopeptide resistance (71,72). In VanB isolates, teicoplanin does not act as an inducer, but cells induced to express resistance are resistant to teicoplanin as well (52). However, clinical isolates with VanB genotypes and constitutive expression of resistance to both teicoplanin and vancomycin are known (e.g., 73,74). Resistant strains can give rise to vancomycin-dependent isolates; these strains are believed to have lost the native ligase function and require the inducible ligase gene product for viability (75–77).

4.   Origin of Resistance Genes

The origin of the resistance genes of VanA and VanB enterococci remains unknown. Hybridization studies and, more recently, sequence analysis of ligase genes has shown that not only are the *vanA* and *vanB* genes of distinct origin, but they are also not closely related to the ligase genes of the intrinsically resistant lactic acid bacteria (54). No genes closely related to the glycopeptide resistance genes have been found in the glycopeptide-producing species (34,54), nor is G + C content high enough to suggest an origin in the actinomycetes or mycobacteria (57,61). Whereas the average G + C content of Tn*1546* is similar to that of the enterococci, the base composition of the nine genes within the transposon varies, perhaps suggesting origins in different species (57,61). The sudden appearance of such a complex scheme for resistance, complete with auxiliary functions and an elaborate regulatory system, suggests that the resistance genes are borrowed from another source where the genes serve some other function in modulating wall composition (10). However, the source remains elusive.

The use of the glycopeptide avoparcin at low levels as a growth promotant in livestock feed in Europe has afforded speculation that resistant enterococci originated in poultry. Although recent studies have demonstrated VanA resistant isolates in farm animals (78,79), especially poultry receiving avoparcin (80), there is little evidence from either the geography or history of glycopeptide resistance outbreaks that supports this view. The emergence of vancomycin resistance followed two trends: (a) rapidly increasing use of vancomycin and teicoplanin in medical practice for the treatment of methicillin-resistant staphylococci; and (b) the use of vancomycin orally in patients as an unabsorbed topical agent to treat C. *difficile* enterocolitis. This latter use exposes gut organisms such as the enterococci to vancomycin, and it could promote the exchange of resistance genes and selection of resistant organisms.

B.   New Insights into Cell Wall Synthesis

Before the advent of glycopeptide-resistant enterococci, the existence of cell wall precursors with pentapeptide structures ending in moieties other than D-alanine was not appreciated. However, it is now apparent that such alternative structures are responsible for intrinsic resistance to glycopeptides in several bacterial species. *Enterococcus gallinarum*, *Enterococcus casseliflavus*, and *Enterococcus flavescens* show low-level intrinsic resistance to vancomycin (54,81). These organisms have cell wall precursors containing D-alanyl–D-serine (82,83). Some lactic acid bacteria such as leuconostocs, pediococci, and some species of lactobacilli are intrinsically resistant to high concentrations of glycopeptides. Recently, it has been shown that these bacteria also have D-alanyl–D-lactate or other unusual wall components (82,84).

C.   Resistance in Staphylococci

A different form of glycopeptide resistance has also been documented in several species of staphylococci. Resistance is relatively uncommon in *S. aureus*, but it has been shown in the coagulase-negative staphylococci (85–88). In staphylococci, resistance emerges more readily after exposure to teicoplanin than to vancomycin (89,90). Most coagulase-negative staphylococci, especially *Staphylococcus haemolyticus*, are less sensitive to teicoplanin than vancomycin, and isolates resistant to teicoplanin can arise during treatment (91–93). Strains resistant to teicoplanin often retain susceptibility to vancomycin (94,95). The mechanism of resistance in clinical isolates of staphylococci has not been elucidated as yet, but it is clearly not related to the VanA and VanB resistance observed in enterococci (54,96,97). Altered cell wall precursors are not present (97). Resistance levels are typically relatively low (minimum inhibitory concentrations (MICs) 16–64 µg/ml). Resistance does not appear to be transferable, but such glycopeptide-resistant staphylococci are emerging as a clinical problem.

D.   Implications of Glycopeptide Resistance on Treatment of Gram-Positive Infections

The transferable nature of VanA and VanB resistance raises the possibility of its transfer to other more serious pathogens such as *S. aureus* or *Streptococcus pneumoniae*. The VanA genes are on a transposon, and they have been found on many different enterococcal plasmids (54). The VanB genes generally are found in the chromosome, but they may be transferable among enterococci as part of a mobile genetic element (98). At least one lab has successfully transferred VanA-type resistance into *S. aureus* in laboratory experiments (99); the implications of this form of resistance in staphylococci are truly ominous. Staphylococci are the most common causes of hospital-acquired infection, and for the increasingly prevalent methicillin-resistant staphylococci, vancomycin is the only consistently effective therapeutic option. This spread may be inevitable, and the possibility underlines the urgent need for new agents.

VI.   DISCOVERY OF GLYCOPEPTIDE ANTIBIOTICS

Vancomycin has proved to be a very useful agent. The unique mechanism of action and limited potential for resistance development made the pursuit of new agents of the class very attractive to the pharmaceutical industry. Few classes of antibiotics have been sought out as systematically and successfully as the glycopeptide antibiotics.

A. Producing Organisms

All of the naturally occurring glycopeptide antibiotics discovered to date are fermentation products of actinomycetes. More than 30 glycopeptide-producing strains have been reported (19). As is often seen with metabolites, a single strain typically produces a complex of several closely related substances, so that the total number of structural variants in the class is well over 100. These products are made by a diverse selection of actinomycetes, including both rare and common genera. About half of the producing organisms identified belong the relatively uncommon genera *Actinoplanes* and *Amycolatopsis*.

B. Targeted Discovery of Glycopeptides

Whereas vancomycin and other early glycopeptides were discovered in general screening programs, more highly targeted programs are responsible for the proliferation of new discoveries through the mid 1980s. Teicoplanin emerged from screens designed to select for cell wall synthesis inhibitors. The comprehensive approach to discovery, isolation, and structure determination of glycopeptide antibiotics reported by investigators at Smith-Kline-French Laboratories (100) included attention to selection of cultures and growth conditions to optimize elaboration of secondary products. The relatively high representation of nonstreptomycete "rare-actino" among the glycopeptide producers identified may reflect a trend to use unusual microorganisms in screening to improve the chances of isolating novel compounds (20,100).

The most important innovation leading to enhanced discovery of glycopeptides, however, is the introduction of mechanism-based screening (101). Vancomycin acts by binding the D-Ala–D-Ala terminus of cell wall precursor. Peptides that include D-Ala–D-Ala can be used both as affinity ligands or specific inhibitors to help detect vancomycin-like antibiotics.

As vancomycin acts by binding the D-Ala–D-Ala terminus of cell wall precursor, its activity can be reversed by adding peptide terminating in D-Ala–D-Ala (43). This ability of Lys–D-Ala–D-Ala to antagonize the antibacterial activity of glycopeptides was found to be a sensitive and highly specific way to detect the glycopeptide antibiotic class (101). As described by the Smith-Kline-French group, fermentation broths were tested in disk diffusion assay with and without added Lys–D-Ala–D-Ala; reduction of zone size in the presence of Lys–D-Ala–D-Ala was indicative of the presence of a vancomycin-like antibiotic. The D-Ala–D-Ala binding affinity for the class was also applied to affinity chromatography in the purification and identification of screen leads. D-Ala–D-Ala coupled to activated agarose support could be used for efficient one-step separation from fermentation broths (100). The Smith-Kline-French group reported the discovery of glycopeptides at the rate of 1 per 320 cultures screened. This efficient and successful approach yielded a number of novel entities including kibdelin, ardacin, and parvodicin.

Affinity methods have also been used successfully by the Merrell Dow Lepetit Research Group (102). Fermentation broths were applied to columns with D-Ala–D-Ala-based affinity resins. After elution and neutralization, samples were tested for activity. The advantage of this approach is that the affinity step also concentrates antibiotic, allowing great sensitivity. The approach yielded several novel structures, A42867 and A40926. Both Lilly and Lepetit Research Laboratories have also used a solid phase competitive binding assay (103,104), in which a peptide ending in D-Ala–D-Ala is coupled to a carrier protein attached hydrophobically to the surface of a polystyrene well. Fermentation broths containing glycopeptides competitively inhibit the binding of labeled vancomycin or teicoplanin. This assay is specific, but no more sensitive than conventional antimicrobial assays (19).

Lilly scientists have taken a different approach by using antibody to glycopeptide as a means of detecting structurally related antibiotics (19). This approach has also been highly successful, yielding glycopeptides in 0.5% of 5100 cultures screened, with about 1 in 5 of these affording a novel structure. Examples of both ristocetin and vancomycin structural types were found. A82846 (the complex including LY264826), A84850, A84575, and A80407 are new entities found using this approach.

C.   Outlook for Discovery of New Glycopeptides

Despite the sensitivity and specificity of ligand-based approaches, some of the most active glycopeptides show relatively weak ligand binding (50,105) and were discovered by other methods. Recent work by Williams and coworkers (41,50) has highlighted the involvement of elements other than affinity to peptide precursor in determining the relative activity of glycopeptides. Affinity methods, of course, would also be unable to detect structural variants of glycopeptides that might have activity against vancomycin-resistant enterococci where resistance is mediated by an altered peptidoglycan precursor (10,35). Such variants have not been found in nature, but they have been generated in semisynthetic studies (2), as discussed below. Several labs, notably that of Evans as well as those of Rao and others, have approached the total synthesis of vancomycin (for reviews, see Refs. 106 and 107). Though total synthesis represents an exciting academic challenge, there is no likelihood it will supplant fermentation. Semisynthetic approaches, however, are proving to be very interesting means of generating glycopeptides with novel activity.

VII.   STRUCTURE–ACTIVITY RELATIONSHIPS AND MODULATION OF ACTIVITY BY CHEMICAL MODIFICATION

A.   Recent Advances in the Structure–Activity Relationships of the Glycopeptide Antibiotics

The variety of naturally occurring glycopeptide antibiotics has facilitated gaining an understanding of the structure–activity relationships (SARs) within the class. A recent review (12) has extensively discussed the SARs of the vancomycin group of antibiotics. The complexity of the glycopeptide molecule has limited its amenability to chemical modification, and until recently, most efforts at modification of the structure failed to improve activity (12). However, recent efforts to modulate the activity of this group of antibiotics by chemical modification are now yielding impressive results. Perhaps the most interesting developments are extension of the spectrum of glycopeptide antibiotics to include vancomycin-resistant enterococci as seen in certain *N*-alkyl derivatives explored by Lilly scientists (12), and the Gram-negative activity and enhanced potency afforded by certain carboxamide derivatives explored by the scientist of the Lepetit Research Center (13).

B. N-Alkyl Derivatives

Substitution of eremomycin has been explored by Pavlov et al. (108,109). Though these efforts did not result in more active compounds, they illustrate the problem of selective reaction. Eremomycin [4a] (A82846A; Figure 10) has three basic nitrogen atoms; nevertheless, a selective acylation reaction of the amino-group of AA-1 was accomplished using standard procedures to yield either the N-Boc [4b] or the N-Cbz [4c] derivatives. Carbamoylation also gave the N-carbamate at AA-1 [4d]; however, on further reaction, the disubstituted derivative [4e] in which the second group was located on the disaccharide of AA-4 could be obtained. Nitrosation also gave the AA-1 derivative [4f], in the case of both eremomycin and vancomycin. Reductive alkylation of the N-NO compound yielded the AA-4, AA-6 dialkylated product [4g]. As is shown in Table 2, the N-NO compound [4f] did retain most of its antibacterial activity against methicillin-resistant S. aureus, whereas the carbamoyl compounds [4b–e] were devoid of activity.

Further work studied the alkylation of eremomycin with alkyl and arylalkyl halides (109). The most reactive halides (methyl iodide and allyl iodide) reacted initially at the N-Me group of AA-1, resulting in both the tertiary [4h,4i] and quaternary derivatives [4j,4k], followed then by alkylation of the carboxyl-group [4m]. With the bulkier benzyl chloride, no quaternary compound was observed, alkylation now affording the tertiary derivative, followed by esterification and then by reaction at the amino-group of the disaccharide of AA-4 [4n]. As shown in Table 3, alkylations on AA-1 with a small alkyl-group had little effect on activity; both the tertiary and quaternary derivatives [4h,4j]

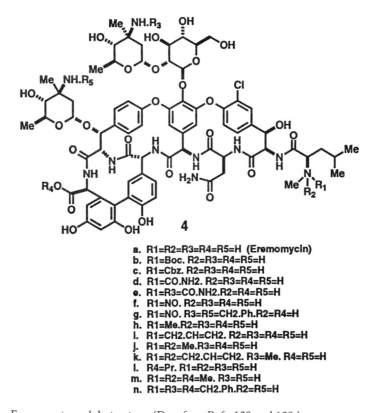

a. R1=R2=R3=R4=R5=H (Eremomycin)
b. R1=Boc. R2=R3=R4=R5=H
c. R1=Cbz. R2=R3=R4=R5=H
d. R1=CO.NH2. R2=R3=R4=R5=H
e. R1=R3=CO.NH2.R2=R4=R5=H
f. R1=NO. R2=R3=R4=R5=H
g. R1=NO. R3=R5=CH2.Ph.R2=R4=H
h. R1=Me.R2=R3=R4=R5=H
i. R1=CH2.CH=CH2. R2=R3=R4=R5=H
j. R1=R2=Me.R3=R4=R5=H
k. R1=R2=CH2.CH=CH2. R3=Me. R4=R5=H
l. R4=Pr. R1=R2=R3=R5=H
m. R1=R2=R4=Me. R3=R5=H
n. R1=R3=R4=CH2.Ph.R2=R5=H

Figure 10   Eremomycin and derivatives. (Data from Refs. 108 and 109.)

Table 2   Activity of Eremomycin Derivatives

| Compound[a] | MRSA[b] (25 isolates) | |
	MIC$_{50}$ (µg/ml)[c]	MIC$_{90}$ (µg/ml)[c]
4f	2	4
4g	4	8
4d	16	32
4e	>32	>32
4c	>32	>32
4b	>32	>32
Eremomycin 4a	0.5	1

[a] See Figure 10.

[b] MRSA = methicillin-resistant *S. aureus*.

[c] MIC$_{50}$ and MIC$_{90}$ (concentration required to inhibit 50% and 90% of isolates) against methicillin-resistant *S. aureus*.

Table 3   Activity of Eremomycin Derivatives from Figure 10 Against Representative Gram-Positive Bacteria

| Organism | MIC (µg/ml) | | | | | | |
	4a	4i	4j	4k	4l	4m	Vancomycin
Staphylococcus aureus Oxford	0.5	0.5	0.5	4	2	0.25	2
Staphylococcus epidermidis	0.125	0.125	0.5	1	0.5	0.25	2
Staphylococcus sanguis	0.5	0.25	1	2	0.5	0.25	2
Staphylococcus saphrophyticus	1	1	4	4	4	0.5	2
Enterococcus faecalis	1	0.5	1	1	0.5	0.5	8

Data from Ref. 109.

possessed somewhat superior activity to vancomycin and comparable activity to eremomycin. However, the overall size of the functionality on this nitrogen did appear to play a role: the quaternary compound having one methyl-group and two allyl-groups [4k] was less active than the compound having three methyl-groups [4j], and it was also less active than the parent eremomycin [4a]. Esterification of the carboxyl-group of eremomycin, that is, [4l], caused little change in the activity. These compounds were inactive against both vancomycin-resistant enterococci and Gram-negative organisms.

It had been noted that N-alkylation of vancomycin produced derivatives that were more active and had longer serum elimination half-lives than vancomycin (e.g., [5a] in Figure 11) (110). The regiochemistry of the alkylation was also critical: the alkylation on the disaccharide of amino acid 4 displayed higher potency than that on the N-Me leucine of amino acid 1 (110). When this chemistry was applied to A82846B, where there are now three potential sites of reaction, it was again observed that the derivatization of amino acid 4 was critical and that monoalkylation was preferred for enhancement of

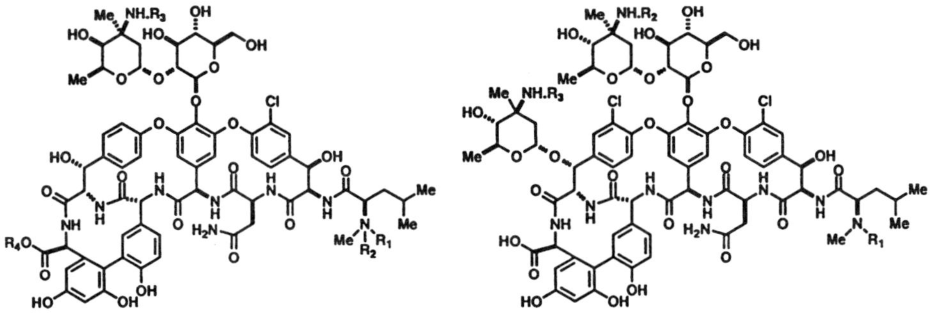

a. R1=R2=H (Vancomycin)
b. R1=H, R2=C10H21

a. R1=R2=R3=H. (A82846B)
b. R1=R3=H, R2=C8H17.
c. R1=R3=H, R2=p-Cl.Phenyl.CH2.
d. R1=R3=H. R2=Diphenyl.CH2

Figure 11   N-alkyl derivatives of vancomycin [5] and A82846B [6]. (Data from Refs. 12 and 110–113.)

activity (12). Such compounds showed both interesting activity and alterations in pharmacokinetics (110).

After the isolation of vancomycin-resistant enterococci, Lilly scientists screened many naturally occurring and semisynthetic glycopeptides against a panel of clinical isolates. The N-alkyl derivatives were the only compounds that showed interesting activity (12,111). Certain A82846B derivatives were the most active and demonstrated a dramatic improvement over vancomycin. The best of these compounds included the N-octyl [6b] and the N-p-chlorobenzyl [6c] (Figure 11) side chains on amino acid 4 of A82846B (Table 4). It was later discovered that further modification of the alkyl-group leads to the synthesis o f compounds with high potency against the vancomycin-resistant strains of enterococciof both VanA and VanB phenotypes. These new compounds retain excellent activity against methicillin-resistant S. aureus (MRSA), methicillin-resistant S. epidermidis (MRSE), and the pneumococci (12,112–114) (Table 4). Recently, related

Table 4   MICs of N-Alkyl Derivatives Against Representative Isolates

	MIC (µg/ml)					
Organism	Vancomycin 5a	A82846B 6a	5b	6b	6c	6d
Staphylococcus aureus	0.5	0.25	0.13	0.5	0.13	0.004
Streptococcus pneumoniae	0.5	0.25	0.13	0.13	0.25	0.13
Enterococcus faecium, vancomycin sensitive	1	0.5	0.5	1	1	0.13
E. faecium, VanA	512	32	4	2	2	0.5

Data from Refs. 12 and 110–112.

compounds with consistent potency against vancomycin-resistant enterococci have been reported (112–114). Highly active side chains include biphenyl (LY307599) and chloro-biphenyl (LY333328). MICs for VanA enterococci are typically 0.5 to 1 µg/ml. The reported compounds had the unusual property of bactericidal activity against some enterococci, good activity against MRSA and coagulase-negative staphylococci (MICs 0.06–0.5 µg/ml), and remarkable potency against streptococci (MICs 0.002–0.008 µg/ml).

C. Amide Modifications of Carboxyl-Group

The Lepetit group has carried out extensive studies on modifications of teicoplanin with some of their most interesting compounds emerging from amide modifications of the terminal carboxyl-group (13,115–119). This group has also noted that removal of sugars, especially the removal of the mannosyl moiety or of all the sugars from teicoplanin, enhanced in vitro activity but did not improve in vivo efficacy (116,120).

The aglycones have provided an interesting starting point for further modification. The condensation of amines with teicoplanin [7a] (Figure 12), the pseudoaglycones [7b,7c], and its aglycone [7d] furnished a series of new amide derivatives that exhibited improved activity over the parent molecule. From a variation in both the lipophilicity and isoelectric point of the side chain, it was observed that the best improvement in activity was obtained when basic amino-groups were included in the side chain (119,121). One of these derivatives, mideplanin [7e] (MDL 62,873; Figure 13), has been investigated more extensively (123). A summary of its in vitro activity compared with those of

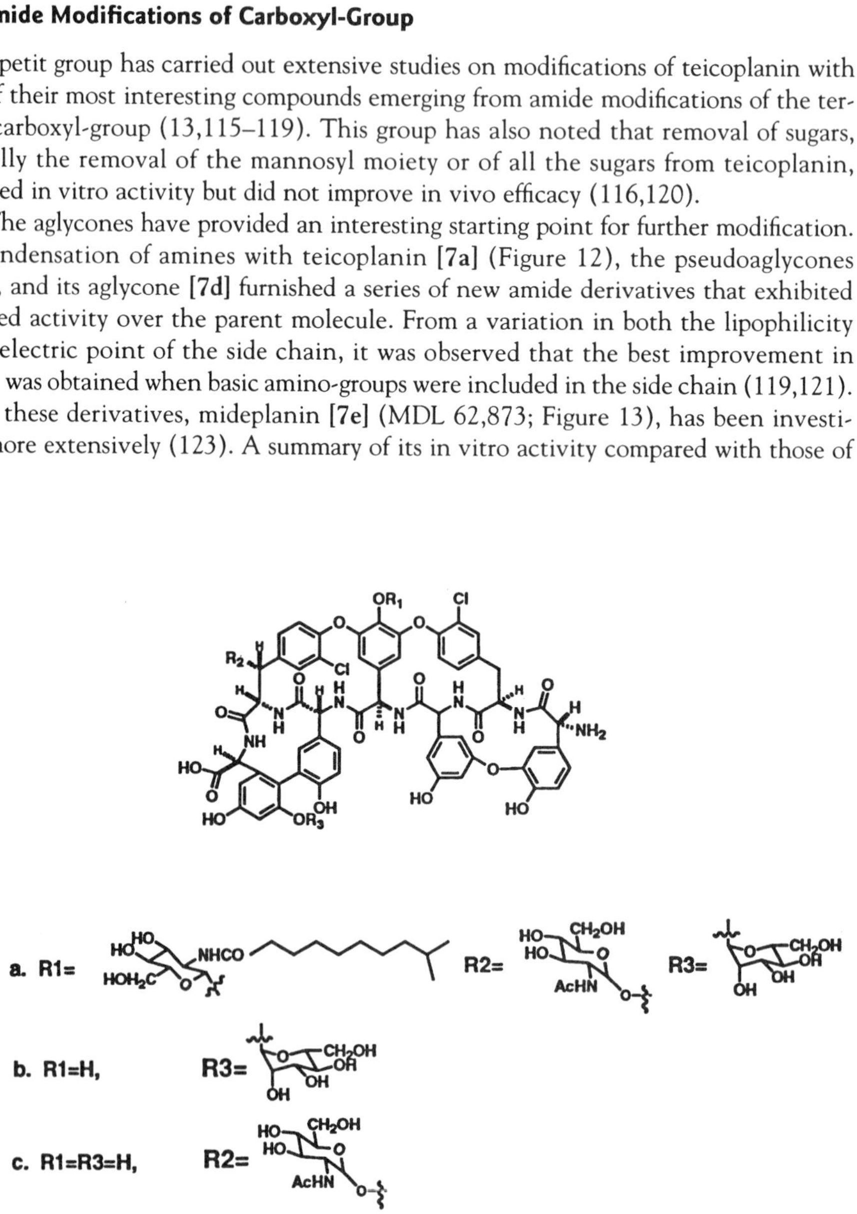

Figure 12 Teicoplanin-related aglycones and pseudoaglycones. (Adapted from Ref. 13.)

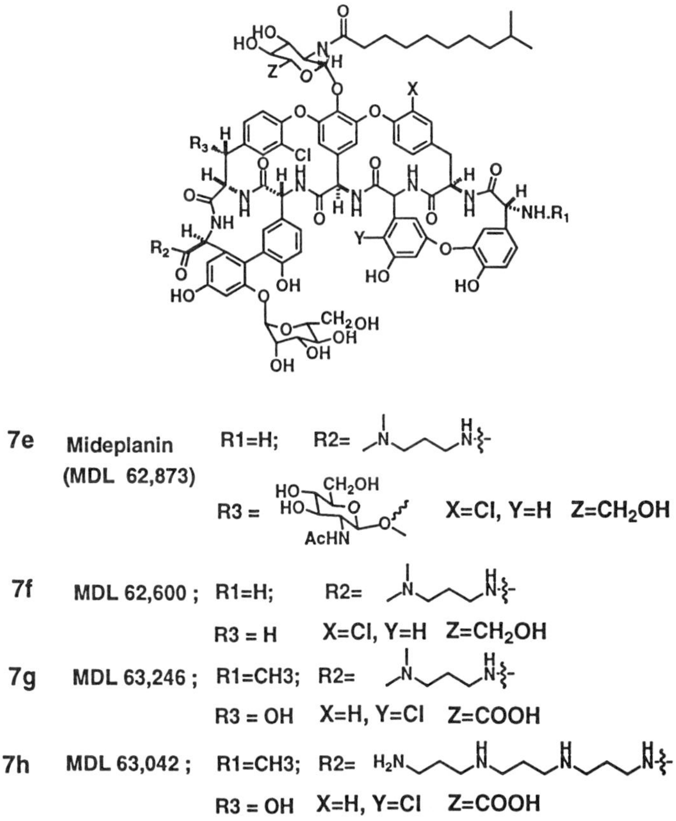

Figure 13   Amide derivatives of teicoplanin A40926. (Adapted from Ref. 122.)

teicoplanin and vancomycin is shown in Table 5. Activity in a mouse septicemia model correlated with in vitro susceptibility of staphylococci and streptococci. Mideplanin has considerable improvements over teicoplanin, especially against the coagulase-negative staphylococci, against which teicoplanin is somewhat weak and inconsistent. However, this new compound has no improvement against the vancomycin and teicoplanin VanA resistant enterococci.

Reductive removal of the sugar unit on amino acid 6 from mideplanin resulted in a compound MDL 62,600 [7f], which now began to show some activity against VanA enterococci, albeit of insufficient magnitude to be considered clinically useful (MICs against five isolates in the range 16–32 µg/ml) (118). Using an alternative natural glycopeptide, A40926, as starting material, a series of amide derivatives were synthesized on a nucleus with the sugar on amino acid 6 removed but with the hydroxyl substitution retained. Two examples of these compounds are MDL 63,246 [7g] and MDL 63,042 [7h]; the in vitro activity of these compounds is shown in Table 6.

Although the overall activity of these compounds is very similar to that of mideplanin, they show some interesting activity against the VanA enterococci, with MDL 63,042 having a MIC_{90} against 20 strains of 16 µg/ml. Recent studies with MDL 63,246 have confirmed its broad Gram-positive activity and efficacy in animal models of septicemia and endocarditis (124,125).

Table 5   Activity of Mideplanin[a]

Organism (no.)	MIC$_{90}$ (MIC range)					
	Mideplanin **7e**		Teicoplanin **7a**		Vancomycin	
Staphylococcus aureus (20)	0.5	(0.25–0.5)	0.5	(0.25–0.5)	2	(0.5–4)
Staphylococcus epidermidis (25)	0.25	(0.06–0.5)	8	(0.25–32)	2	(1–2)
Staphylococcus haemolyticus (34)	2	(0.125–4)	32	(0.25–64)	2	(0.5–4)
Enterococcus faecalis (31)	0.5	(0.06–0.5)	0.5	(0.125–0.5)	2	(0.5–4)
Streptococcus pneumoniae (9)	0.25	(0.06–0.25)	0.06	(<0.03–0.06)	0.5	(0.25–0.5)

[a] *In vitro* activity against multiple strains of Gram-positive bacteria expressed as the MIC$_{90}$ (concentration required to inhibit 90% of isolates) and range of MIC, in µg/ml.
Data from Refs. 13 and 123.

Table 6   Activity of Mideplanin, MDL63,246, and MDL 63,042

Organism (no.)	MIC$_{90}$ (MIC range)[a]		
	Mideplanin **7e**	MDL 63,246 **7g**	MDL 63,042 **7h**
Staphylococcus aureus (20)	0.5 (0.25–0.5)	0.25 (0.125–0.5)	0.125 (<0.03–0.125)
Staphylococcus epidermidis (25)	0.25 (0.06–0.5)	0.25 (<0.03–0.5)	0.25 (<0.03–0.25)
Staphylococcus haemolyticus (34)	2 (0.125–4)	1 (0.125–2)	0.5 (0.06–1)
Enterococcus faecalis (31)	0.5 (0.06–0.5)	1 (0.125–1)	0.25 (0.03–0.25)
E. faecium (13)	0.5 (0.06–0.5)	0.5 (0.06–1)	0.25 (0.06–0.5)
E. faecium (VanB) (25)	0.5 (0.125–0.5)	0.5 (0.125–0.5)	0.5 (0.125–0.5)
E. faecium (VanA) (20)		32 (4–64)	16 (0.5–32)
Streptococcus pneumoniae (9)	0.25 (0.06–0.25)	<0.03	<0.03

[a] *In vitro* activity against multiple strains of Gram-positive bacteria expressed as the MIC$_{90}$ (concentration required to inhibit 90% of isolates) and range of MIC, in mg/ml.
Data from Refs. 13 and 124–126.

Similar derivatives were also reported on the aglycone of teicoplanin (13,126). The two most interesting ones again had amide side chains having amino-functionality as shown in Figure 14. The activities of these are shown in Table 7 compared with that of mideplanin. A striking property of these derivatives is their unusual activity against Gram-negative organisms, in sharp distinction to mideplanin and all the other glycopeptides (Table 7). This appears to be related to the ability of the cationic side chain to promote permeability of the Gram-negative outer membrane (44). MDL 62,708 [**7i**] (Figure 14) demonstrated a rapid bactericidal activity against *Escherichia coli*. This activity could also be demonstrated in an in vivo septicemia model in mice against an *E. coli* challenge (126).

An alternative approach to enhancing activity of vancomycin-like glycopeptides is under study by Griffin and colleagues (127). The overall objective is eventually to build a molecule that will have catalytic as well as binding activity. Vancomycin derivatives

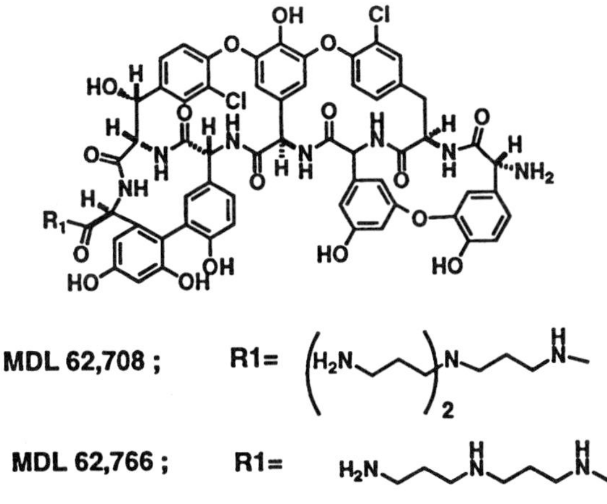

Figure 14 Amide modifications of dalbaheptide aglycones. (Adapted from Ref. 13.)

Table 7 Activity of Amide Modifications of the Carboxyl of Dalbaheptide Aglycones Compared with That of Teicoplanin

Organism (no.)	MIC range (µg/ml)		
	MDL 62,766 **7j**	MDL 62,708 **7i**	Teicoplanin
Staphylococcus aureus (1)	0.06	0.125	0.5
Escherichia coli (7)	0.5–4	1–8	>64
Enterobacter cloacae (2)	4–8	64	>64
Serratia marcescens (2)	8	8	>64
Pseudomonas (5)	2–64	8–64	>64

Data from Refs. 13, 122, and 126.

bearing propyl-, histmanyl-, and 3-aminopropyl-groups attached to the C-terminus have been reported. To date, the group has successfully taken a first step in this direction by making derivatives capable of catalytic carbamate hydrolysis. The group has also reported amide derivatives of vancomycin (128), which included some of peptidyl type, for example, the L-Ala–L-Ala amide, but no biological activity was given.

D.   Nucleus Variations

Although the glycopeptides are a large and reasonably diverse group of naturally occurring antibiotics, all the differences in the heptapeptide binding pocket have been limited to amino acids 1 and 3. Furthermore, these changes have been somewhat limited. Recently, a chemical methodology has been developed that could allow a far more systematic investigation of the effect on binding and activity that can be realized by changes in this part of the molecule (129–131).

Reduction of teicoplanin aglycone [**7d**] with sodium borohydride in aqueous alcohol solution resulted in a specific reductive cleavage of the amide bond between amino

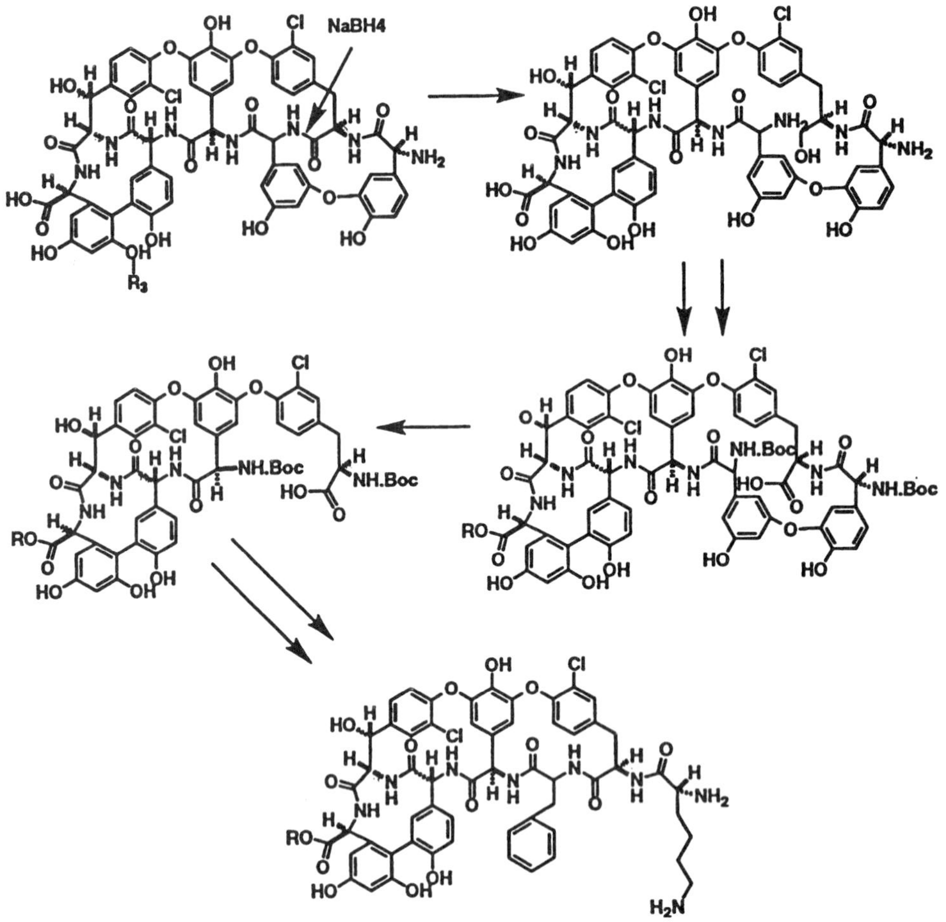

Figure 15 Derivation of amino acid core modifications of glycopeptides. (Adapted from Ref. 122.)

acids 2 and 3. After protection of the two amino-groups as their Boc carbamates, reoxidation of the resultant alcohol-group gave the carboxylic acid [8] (Figure 15). This compound could now be subjected to a double Edman degradation, where the removal of both amino acids 1 and 3 resulted. This new pentapeptide [9] represented a synthon from which heptapeptides varying at the amino acids 1 and 3 could be generated. Other glycopeptides such as vancomycin, vancomycin aglycone, ristocetin, and teicoplanin all underwent this chemical process. Interestingly the des-methylleucine vancomycin (hexapeptide) was resistant to this procedure.

Reconstruction of a heptapeptide nucleus was accomplished by initially synthesizing selectively N-protected pentapeptide, via the differentially N,N'–protected derivative) [9]. Coupling with N-Boc protected L-phenylalanine; removal of the Boc group and ring closure resulted in the cyclic hexapeptide. A final acylation with suitably protected D-lysine and removal of the protecting groups yielded a new glycopeptide aglycone [13] in which amino acids 1,3 were now D-phenylalanine and L-lysine, respectively. This new derivative had activity comparable to that of the original teicoplanin aglycone, with some interesting additional activity against a teicoplanin-resistant strain of E. faecalis. Overall, this methodology will allow the synthesis of highly novel compounds, and it is a very promising approach to modulation of activity of glycopeptide antibiotics.

E. Future Prospects

The highly specific and elegant interaction between the glycopeptide antibiotics and their molecular target, the D-alanyl–D-alanine moiety of peptidoglycan precursor, once afforded speculation that this was an entity optimized by evolution (132). As our knowledge expands and chemical modifications of both older and newly discovered natural products are explored, it now seems that the potential of the class for highly potent and broad-spectrum activity is greater than might have been previously imagined. New compounds are not likely to be exempt from the toxicities found in the glycopeptide class, and this, as well as their pharmacodynamic complexity, could remain a restriction to their future development. Some of the most interesting semisynthetic molecules now being reported are intrinsically complex to make, and cost may limit the attractiveness of development. Nonetheless, the class provides an instructive example of the effectiveness of the marriage of natural product research and medicinal chemistry applied to new medical needs.

ACKNOWLEDGMENTS

We thank Richard C. Thompson for his help with figures and thoughtful comments. We thank Adriano Malabarba, Marion Merrell Dow Research Institute, Lepetit Center, for copies of manuscripts prior to publication.

REFERENCES

1. McCormick MK, Stark WM, Pittenger GE, Pittenger RC, McGuire GM, eds. Antibiot Annu 1955; 606.
2. Nagarajan R, ed. Glycopeptide Antibiotics. New York: Marcel Dekker, 1994:423.
3. Speller D, Greenwood D. Teicoplanin, clinical use and laboratory correlation. J Antibiot Ther 1988; 21 Suppl A:441.
4. MacGregor R. Growth promoters and their importance in ruminant livestock production. Haresign W, Cole DJA, eds. Recent Advances in Ruminant Nutrition, Vol. 2. London: Butterworths, 1988:308–322.
5. Moughan PJ, Stevens EVJ, Reisma ID, Rendel J. The effect of avoparcin on the ileal and faecal digestibility of nitrogen and amino acids in the milk-fed calf. Animal Prod 1989; 49:63–71.
6. Gaynes RP, Culver DH, Horan TC, Henderson TS, Tolson JS, Martone WJ, National Nosocomial Infection Surveillance System. Trends in methicillin-resistant Staphylococcus aureus in United States hospitals. Infect Dis Clin Prac 1994; 6:452–455.
7. Banerjee SN, Emori TG, Culver DH, Gaynes RP, Jarvis WR, Horan T, Edwards JR, Tolson J, Henderson T, Martone WJ, National Nosocomial Infection Surveillance System. Secular trends in nosocomial primary bloodstream infections in the United States, 1980–1989. National Nosocomial Infection Surveillance System. Am J Med 1991; 91:86S–89S.
8. Leclercq R, Derlot E, Duval J, Courvalin P. Plasmid-mediated resistance to vancomycin and teicoplanin in Enterococcus faecium. N Eng J Med 1988; 319:157–161.
9. Uttley AHC, Collins CH, Naidoo J, George RC. Vancomycin-resistant enterococci. Lancet 1988; 1:57–58.

10. Arthur M, Courvalin C. Genetics and mechanisms of glycopeptide resistance in entero-cocci. Antimicrob Agents Chemother 1993; 37:1563–1571.

11. Walsh CT, Fisher SL, Park IS, Wu Z. Bacterial resistance to vancomycin: Five genes and one missing hydrogen bond tell the story. Chem Biol 1996; 3:21–28.

12. Nagarajan R. Structure-activity relationships of vancomycin-type glycopeptide antibiotics. J Antibiot 1993; 46:1181–1195.

13. Ciabatti R, Malabarba A. Glycopeptide antibiotics and their structural modifications. La Chimica e L'industria 1994; 76:300–304.

14. Parenti F, Cavelleri B. Proposal to name the vancomycin-ristocetin like glycopeptides as dal-baheptides. J Antibiotics 1989; 42:1882–1883.

15. Reynolds P, Somner EA. Comparison of the target sites and mechanisms of action of gly-copeptide and lipoglycopeptide antibiotics. Drugs Exp Clin Res 1990; 16:385–389.

16. Yao RC, Crandall LW. Glycopeptides: Classification, occurrence, and discovery. Nagarajan R, ed. Glycopeptide Antibiotics. New York: Marcel Dekker, 1994:1–28.

17. Lancini GC, Cavelleri B. Glycopeptide antibiotics of the vancomycin group. Kleinkauf H, van Döhren H, eds. Biochemistry of Peptide Antibiotics. Berlin: Walter de Gruyter, 1990: 160–178.

18. Cavelleri B, Parenti F. Glycopeptides (dalbaheptides). Encyclopedia of Chemical Technol-ogy, Vol. 2. New York: John Wiley and Sons, 1992:995–1018.

19. Sztaricskai F, Pelyvás-Ferenczik I. Chemistry of carbohydrate components. Nagarajan R, ed. Glycopeptide Antibiotics. New York: Marcel Dekker, 1993:105–193.

20. Boeck LD, Mertz FP, Clem GM. A41030, a novel complex of novel glycopeptide antibiotics produced by a strain of *Streptomyces virginiae*: Taxonomy and fermentation studies. J Antibiot 1985; 38:1–8.

21. Boeck LD, Mertz FP. A47934, a novel glycopeptide-aglycone antibiotic produced by a strain of *Streptomyces toyacaensis*: Taxonomy and fermentation studies. J Antibiot 1986; 39:1533–1540.

22. Nadkarni SR, Patel MV, Chatterjee S, Vijayakumar EKS, Desikan KR, Blumach J, Ganguli BN. Balhimicin, a new glycopeptide antibiotic produced by *Amycolatopsis* sp. Y-82,21022. J Antibiot 1994; 47:335–341.

23. Verma AK, Goel AK, Rao A, Venkateswarlu A, Sitrin RD. Glycopeptide antibiotics. US Patent 4,742,045; 1988.

24. Coller BS, Granlick HR. Studies on the mechanism of ristocetin-induced platelet agglutina-tion. Effects of structural modification of ristocetin and vancomycin. J Clin Invest 1977; 60:302–312.

25. Zmijewski MA Jr, Fayerman JT. Glycopeptide antibiotics. Vining LC, Stuttard C, eds. Genet-ics and Biochemistry of Antibiotic Production. Boston: Butterworth-Heineman, 1994:71–83.

26. Hammond DJ, Williamson MP, D H W, Boeck LD, Marconi GG. On the biosynthesis of vancomycin. J Chem Soc (Chem Comm) 1982; 344–346.

27. Chung SK, Oh YK, Taylor P. Biosynthetic studies of aridicin antibiotics. I. Labeling patterns and overall pathways. J Antibiot 1986; 39:652–659.

28. Chung SK, Taylor P, Oh YK. Biosynthetic studies of aridicin antibiotics. II. Microbial trans-formations and glycosylations by protoplasts. J Antibiot 1986; 39:642–651.

29. Zmijewksi MA Jr, Briggs B. Biosynthesis of vancomycin: Identification of TDP-glucose agly-cosyl-vancomycin glucosyltransferase from *Amycolatopsis orientalis*. FEMS Microbiol Lett 1989; 59:129–133.

30. Borghi A, Ferrari P, Gallo GG. Microbial de-mannosylation and mannosylation of teicoplanin derivatives. J Antibiot 1991; 44:1444–1451.

31. Zmijewski MA Jr, Briggs B, Logan R, Boeck LD. Biosynthetic studies on antibiotic A47934. Antimicrob Agents Chemother 1987; 31:1497–1501.

32. Borghi A, Duncan E, Zerelli LF, Lancini GC. Factors affecting the normal and branched-chain acyl moieties of teicoplanin components produced by *Actinoplanes teichomyceticus*. J Gen Microbiol 1991; 137:587–592.

33. Cundliffe E. How antibiotic-producing organisms avoid suicide. Annu Rev Microbiol 1989; 42:207–233.

34. Piepersberg W. Pathway engineering in secondary metabolite–producing Actinomycetes. Crit Rev Biotechnol 1994; 14:251–285.

35. Dutka-Malen S, Molinas C, Arthur M, Courvalin P. Molecular basis for vancomycin resistance in Enterococcus faecium BM4147. Mol Gen Genet 1990; 224:364–372.

36. Courvalin P. Resistance of enterococci to glycopeptides. Antimicrob Agents Chemother 1990; 34:2291–2296.

37. Moroni MC, Granozzi C, Lorenzetti R, Parenti F, Sosio M, Denaro M. Cloning of a DNA region of Actinoplanes teichomyceticus conferring teicoplanin resistance. FEBS Lett 1989; 253:108–1121.

38. Sosio M, Lorenzetti R, Robbiatti F, Denaro M. Nucleotide sequence to a teicoplanin resistance gene from Actinoplanes teichomyceticus. Biochim Biophys Acta 1991; 1089: 401–403.

39. Reynolds PE. Structure, biochemistry, and mechanism of action of glycopeptide antibiotics. Eur J Clin Microbiol Infect Dis 1989; 8:789–803.

40. Barna JCJ, Williams DH. The structure and mode of action of glycopeptide antibiotics of the vancomycin group. Annu Rev Microbiol 1984; 38:339–357.

41. Beauregard DA, Williams DH, Gwynn MN, Knowles DJC. Dimerization and membrane anchors in the extracellular targeting of vancomycin group antibiotics. Antimicrob Agents Chemother 1995; 39:781–785.

42. Chatterjee AN, Perkins HR. Compounds formed between nucleotides related to the biosynthesis of bacterial cell wall and vancomycin. Biochem Biophys Res Commun 1966; 24:489–494.

43. Nieto M, Perkins HR, Reynolds PE. Reversal by a specific peptide (diacetyl-α-γ-L-diamobu-tyryl-D-alanyl-D-alanine) of vancomycin inhibition in intact bacteria and cell-free preparations. Biochem J 1972; 126:139–149.

44. Hancock REW, Farmer S. Mechanism of uptake of deglucoteicoplanin amide derivatives across outer membranes of Escherichia coli and Pseudomonas aeruginosa. Antimicrob Agents Chemother 1993; 37:453–456.

45. Williams DH, Waltho JP. Molecular basis of the activity of antibiotics of the vancomycin group. Biochem Pharm 1988; 17:133–141.

46. Williamson MP, Williams DH, Hammond SJ. Interactions of vancomycin and ristocetin with peptides as a model for protein binding. Tetrahedron 1984; 40:569–573.

47. Groves P, Searle MS, Mackay JP, Williams DH. The structure of an asymmetric dimer relevant to the mode of action of glycopeptide antibiotics. Structure 1994; 2:747–754.

48. Prowse WG, Kline AD, Skelton MA. An NMR study of the asymmetric homodimer of the antibiotic glycopeptide A82846B complexed with its pentapeptide ligand. Biochem 1995; 34:9632–9644.

49. Waltho JP, Williams DH. Aspects of molecular recognition: Solvent exclusion and dimerization of the antibiotic ristocetin when bound to a model bacterial cell-wall precursor. J Am Chem Soc 1989; 111:2475–2480.

50. Mackay JP, Gerhard U, Beauregard DA, Maplestone RA, Williams DH. Dissection of the contribution toward dimerization of glycopeptide antibiotics. J Am Chem Soc 1994; 116:4573–4580.

51. Mackay JP, Gerhard U, Beauregard DA, Westwell MS, Searle MS, Williams DH. Glycopeptide antibiotic activity and the possible role of dimerization: A model for biological signaling. J Am Chem Soc 1994; 116:4581–4590.

52. Williamson R, Al-Obeid S, Shlaes JH, Goldstein FW, Shlaes DM. Inducible resistance to vancomycin in Enterococcus faecium D366. J Infect Dis 1989; 159:1095–1104.

53. Shlaes DM, Bouvet A, Devine C, Shlaes JH, Al-Obeid S, Williamson R. Inducible, transferable resistance to vancomycin in Enterococcus faecalis A256. Antimicrob Agents Chemother 1989; 33:198–203.

54.   Dutka-Malen S, Leclercq R, Coutant V, Duval J, Courvalin P. Phenotypic and genotypic heterogeneity of glycopeptide resistance determinants in gram-positive bacteria. Antimicrob Agents Chemother 1990; 34:1875–1879.

55.   Evers S, Reynolds P, Courvalin P. Sequence of the *vanB* and *ddl* genes encoding D-alanine:D-lactate and D-alanine:D-alanine ligases in vancomycin-resistant *Enterococcus faecalis* V583. Gene 1994; 140:97–102.

56.   Quintiliani R Jr, Evers S, Courvalin P. The *vanB* gene confers various levels of self-transferable resistance to vancomycin in enterococci. J Infect Dis 1993; 167:1220–1223.

57.   Evers S, Sahm DF, Courvalin P. The *vanB* gene of vancomycin-resistant *Enterococcus faecalis* is structurally related to genes encoding D-Ala:D-Ala ligases and glycopeptide-resistance proteins VanA and VanC. Gene 1993; 124:143–144.

58.   Nicas TI, Wu CYE, Hobbs JNJr, Allen NE. Characterization of vancomycin resistance in *Enterococcus faecium* and *Enterococcus faecalis*. Antimicrob Agents Chemother 1989; 33:1121–1124.

59.   Walsh CT. Vancomycin resistance: Decoding the molecular logic. Science 1993; 261:308–309.

60.   Bugg TH, Wright GD, Dutka-Malen S, Arthur M, Courvalin P, Walsh CT. Molecular basis for vancomycin resistance in *Enterococcus faecium* BM4147: Biosynthesis of a depsipeptide peptidoglycan precursor by vancomycin resistance proteins VanA and VanH. Biochem 1991; 30:10408–10415.

61.   Arthur M, Molinas C, Depardieu F, Courvalin P. Characterization of Tn*1546*, a Tn3-related transposon conferring glycopeptide resistance by synthesis of depsipeptide peptidoglycan precursors in *Enterococcus faecium* BM4147. J Bacteriol 1993; 175:117–121.

62.   Bugg TH, Dutka-Malen S, Arthur M, Courvalin P, Walsh CT. Identification of vancomycin resistance protein VanA as a D-alanine:D-alanine ligase of altered substrate specificity. Biochem 1991; 30:2017–2021.

63.   Allen N, Hobbs JN Jr, Richardson JM, Riggin RM. Biosynthesis of modified peptidoglycan precursors by vancomycin-resistant *Enterococcus faecium*. FEMS Microbiol Lett 1992; 98:109–116.

64.   Handwerger S, Pucci MJ, Volk KJ, Liu J, Lee MS. The cytoplasmic peptidoglycan precursor of vancomycin-resistant *Enterococcus faecalis* terminates in lactate. J Bacteriol 1992; 174:5982–5984.

65.   Messer J, Reynolds P. Modified peptidoglycan precursors produced by glycopeptide-resistant enterococci. FEMS Microbiol Lett 1992; 1992:195–200.

66.   Reynolds PE, Depardieu F, Dutka-Malen S, Arthur M, Courvalin P. Glycopeptide resistance mediated by enterococcal transposon Tn*1546* requires production of VanX for hydrolysis of D-alanyl-D-alanine. Mol Microbiol 1995; 13:1065–1070.

67.   Wu Z, Wright GD, Walsh CT. Overexpression, purification and characterization of vanX, a D-, D-dipeptidase which is essential for vancomycin resistance in *Enterococcus faecium* BM4147. Biochem 1995; 34:2455–2463.

68.   Arthur M, Depardieu F, Molinas C, Reynolds P, Courvalin P. The *vanZ* gene of Tn*1546* from *Enterococcus faecium* BM4147 confers resistance to teicoplanin. Gene 1995; 15:87–92.

69.   Handwerger S, Kolokathis A. Induction of vancomycin resistance in *Enterococcus faecium* by inhibition of transglycosylation. FEMS Microbiol Lett 1990; 90:167–170.

70.   Allen NE, Hobbs J Jr. Induction of vancomycin resistance in *Enterococcus faecium* nonglycopeptide antibiotics. FEMS Microbiol Lett 1995; 132:107–114.

71.   Arthur M, Molinas C, Courvalin P. The VanS-VanR two-component regulatory system controls synthesis of depsipeptide peptidoglycan precursors in *Enterococcus faecium* MB4147. J Bacteriol 1992; 174:2582–2591.

72.   Wright GD, Holman TR, Walsh CT. Purification and characterization of VanR and the cytosolic domain of VanS: A two-component regulatory system required for vancomycin resistance in *Enterococcus faecium* BM4147. Biochem 1993; 32:5957–5963.

73. Hayden MK, Trenholme GM, Schultz JE, Sahm DF. In vivo development of teicoplanin resistance in a VanB *Enterococcus faecium* isolate. J Infect Dis 1993; 167:1224–1227.

74. Handwerger S, Skoble J, Discotto L, Pucci M. Heterogeneity of the vanA gene cluster in clinical isolates of enterococci from the northeastern United States. Antimicrob Agents Chemother 1995; 39:362–368.

75. Fraimow HS, Jungkind DL, Landers DW, Deslo DR, Dean JL. Urinary tract infections with an *Enterococcus faecalis* isolate that requires vancomycin for growth. Ann Intern Med 1994; 121:22–26.

76. Rosato A, Pierre J, Billot-Klien D, Buu-Hoi A, Gutmann L. Inducible and constitutive expression of resistance to glycopeptides and vancomycin dependence in glycopeptide-resistant *Enterococcus avium*. Antimicrob Agents Chemother 1995; 39:830–833.

77. Woodford N, Johnson AP, Morrison D, Hastings FGM, Elliott TSJ, Worthington A, Stephenson JRJ, Chin AT, Tolley TL. Vancomycin-dependent enterococci in the United Kingdom. J Antimicrob Chemother 1994; 36:1066.

78. Klare I, Heier H, Claus H, Teissbrodt R, Witte W. *vanA*-mediated high-level glycopeptide resistance in *Enterococcus faecium* from animal husbandry. FEMS Microbiol Lett 1995; 127:165–172.

79. Bates J, Jordans JZ, Griffiths DT. Farm animals as a putative reservoir for vancomycin-resistant enterococcal infections in man. J Antimicrob Chemother 1994; 34:507–516.

80. Witte W, Klare I. Animal production as a potential reservoir of glycopeptide resistant *E. faecium*. Can J Infect Dis 1995; 6 Suppl C:275C.

81. Vincent D, Minkler P, Bincziewski B, Etter L, Shlaes DM. Vancomycin resistance in *Enterococcus gallinarum*. Antimicrob Agents Chemother 1992; 36:1392–1399.

82. Billot-Klein D, Gutmann L, Sablé S, Guittet E, van Heijenoort J. Modification of peptidoglycan precursors is a common feature of the low-level vancomycin-resistant VANB-type Enterococcus D366 and of the naturally glycopeptide-resistant species *Lactobacillus casei*, *Pediococcus pentosaceus*, *Leuconostoc mesenteroides*, and *Enterococcus gallinarum*. J Bacteriol 1994; 175:2398–2405.

83. Reynolds PE, Snaith HA, Maguire AJ, Dutka-Malen S, Courvalin P. Analysis of peptidoglycan precursors in vancomycin resistant *Enterococcus gallinarum* BM4174. Biochem J 1994; 301:5–8.

84. Handwerger S, Pucci MJ, Volk KJ, Liu J, Lee S. Vancomycin-resistant *Leuconostoc mesenteroides* and *Lactobacillus casei* synthesize cytoplasmic peptidoglycan precursors that terminate in lactate. J Bacteriol 1994; 174:5982–5984.

85. Haverkorn M. Glycopeptide sensitivity of staphylococci. J Infect 1993; 27:335–345.

86. Schwalbe RS, Stapleton JT, Gilligan PH. Emergence of vancomycin resistance in coagulase-negative staphylococci. N Eng J Med 1987; 316:927–931.

87. Biavasco F, Giovanetti E, Montanari M, Varaldo PE. Development of in-vitro resistance to glycopeptide antibiotics: Assessment in staphylococci of different species. Antimicrob Agents Chemother 1991; 27:71–79.

88. Goldstein F, Coutrot A, Seiffer A, Acar JF. Percentages distributions of teicoplanin- and vancomycin-resistant strains among coagulase-negative staphylococci. Antimicrob Agents Chemother 1990; 34:899–900.

89. Watanakunakorn C. In-vitro selection of resistance to *Staphylococcus aureus* to teicoplanin and vancomycin. J Antimicrob Chemother 1990; 25:69–75.

90. Watanakunakorn C. In-vitro induction of resistance in coagulase-negative staphylococci to vancomycin and teicoplanin. Antimicrob Agents Chemother 1988; 22:321–324.

91. Froggatt JW, Johnston JL, Galetto DW, Archer GL. Antimicrobial resistance in nosocomial isolates of *Staphylococcus haemolyticus*. Antimicrob Agents Chemother 1989; 33:460–466.

92. Aubert G, Passot S, Lucht F, Dorche G. Selection of vancomycin- and teicoplanin-resistant *Staphylococcus haemolyticus* during teicoplanin treatment of *S. epidermidis* infection. J Antimicrob Chemother 1990; 25:491–493.

93. Sanyal DAP, Johnson GRC, Cookson BD, Williams AJ. Peritonitis due to vancomycin-resistant *Staphylococcus epidermidis*. Lancet 1991; 337:54.

94. Kaatz GW, Seo SM, Dorman NJ, Lerner SA. Emergence of teicoplanin resistance during therapy of *Staphylococcus aureus* endocarditis. J Infect Dis 1990; 162:103–108.

95. Shlaes DM, Shlaes JH. Teicoplanin selects *Staphylococcus aureus* that is resistant to vancomycin. Clin Infect Dis 1995; 20:1071–1073.

96. Daum RS, Gupta S, Sabbagh R, Milewski WM. Characterization of *Staphylococcus aureus* isolates with decreased susceptibility to vancomycin and teicoplanin: Isolation and purification of a constitutively produced protein associated with decreased susceptibility. J Infect Dis 1992; 166:1066–1072.

97. O'Hare MD, Reynolds PE. Novel membrane proteins present in teicoplanin-resistant, vancomycin sensitive, coagulase negative *Staphylococcus* sp. J Antimicrob Chemother 1992; 30:752–768.

98. Quintiliani RJ, Courvalin P. Conjugal transfer of the vancomycin resistance determinant vanB between enterococci involves the movement of large genetic elements from chromosome to chromosome. FEMS Microbiol Lett 1994; 119:359–364.

99. Noble WC, Virani Z, Cree RG. Co-transfer of vancomycin and other resistance genes from *Enterococcus faecalis* NCTC 12201 to *Staphylococcus aureus*. FEMS Microbiol Lett 1992; 72:195–198.

100. Jeffs PW, Nisbet LJ. Glycopeptide antibiotics: A comprehensive approach to discovery, isolation, and structure determination. Actor P, Daneo Moore L, Higgins ML,.Salton MRJ, Shockman GD, eds.Antibiot Inhib Bact Cell Surf Assemb Funct. Washington DC: American Society for Microbiology. 1988; 509–530.

101. Rake JB, Gerber R, Mehta RJ, Newman DJ, Oh YK, Phelen C, Shearer NC, Sitrin RD, Nisbet LJ. Glycopeptide antibiotics: A mechanism-based screen employing a bacterial cell wall receptor mimetic. J Antibiot 1986; 39:58–67.

102. Cassini G. Glycopeptides: Antibiotic discovery and mechanism of action. Bushell ME, Grafe U, eds. Bioactive Metabolites from Microorganisms, Vol. 27. Amsterdam: Elsevier, 1980: 221–235.

103. Corti A, Rurali C, Borghi A, Cassini G. Solid-phase enzyme-receptor assay (SPERA): A competitive-binding assay for glycopeptide antibiotics of the vancomycin class. Clin Chem 1985; 31:1606–1610.

104. Mahoney DF, Baisden DK, Yao RC. A peptide-binding chromogenic assay for glycopeptide antibiotics of the vancomycin class. J Ind Microbiol 1989; 4:43–47.

105. Good VM, Gwynn MN, Knowles DJC. MM 45289, a potent glycopeptide antibiotic which interacts weakly with diacetyl-L-Lysyl-D-alanyl-D-alanine. J Antibiot 1990; 43:550–555.

106. Rao AVR, Gurjar MK, Reddy KL, Rao AS. Studies directed toward the synthesis of vancomycin and related cyclic peptides. Chem Rev 1995; 95:2135–2167.

107. Evans DA, DeVries KM. Approaches to the synthesis of the vancomycin aglycones. Nagarajan R, ed. Glycopeptide Antibiotics. New York: Marcel Dekker, 1994:63–101.

108. Pavlov AY, Berdnikova TF, Olsfyeva EN, Lazko EI, Malkova V, Probrazhenskaya MN, Probrazjenskaya GD. Synthesis and biological activity of derivatives of glycopeptide antibiotics eremonycin and vancomycin nitrosated, acylated or carbamylated at the *N*-terminal. J Antibiot 1993; 46:1731–1739.

109. Pavlov AY, Olsfyeva EN, Berdnikova TF, Malkova V, Probrazhenskaya MN. Modification of glycopeptide antibiotic eremomycin by the action of alkyl halides and study on antibacterial activity of the compounds obtained. J Antibiot 1994; 47:225–232.

110. Nagarajan R, Schabel AA, Occolowitz JL, Counter FT, Ott JL, Felty-Duckworth AM. Synthesis and anti-bacterial activity of N-alkyl vancomycins. J Antibiot 1989; 42:63–72.

111. Nicas TI, Cole CT, Preston DA, Schabel AA, Nagarajan R. Activity of glycopeptides against vancomycin-resistant gram-positive bacteria. Antimicrob Agents Chemother 1989; 33: 1477–1481.

112. Nicas TI, Mullen DL, Flokowitsch JE, Preston DA, Snyder NS, Zweifel MJ, Wilkie SC, Rodriguez MJ, Thompson RC, Cooper RDG. Semisynthetic glycopeptide antibiotics derived from LY264826 active against vancomycin-resistant enterococci. Antimicrob Agents Chemother 1996; 40:2194–2199.

113. Nicas TI, Flokowitsch JE, Preston DA, Mullen DL, Grissom-Arnold J, Snyder NJ, Zweifel MJ, Wilkie SC, Rodriguez MJ, Thompson RC, Cooper RDG. Semisynthetic glycopeptides active against vancomycin-resistant enterococci: Activity against staphylococci and streptococci in vitro and in vivo. Abstracts of the Thirty-fifth Interscience Conference on Antimicrobial Agents and Chemotherapy. Washington, D.C.: American Society for Microbiology, 1995: Abstract F249.

114. Cooper RDG, Snyder NJ, Zweifel MJ, Staszak MA, Wilkie SC, Nicas TI, Mullen DL, Butler TF, Rodriguez MJ, Huff BE, Thompson RC. Reductive alkylation of glycopeptide antibiotics: Synthesis and antibacterial activity. J Antibiot 1996; 49:575–581.

115. Malabarba A, Ferrari P, Cietto G, Pallanza R, Berti M. Synthesis and biological activity of N63-carboxypeptides of teicoplanin and teicoplanin aglycone. J Antibiot 1989; 42:1800–1816.

116. Malabarba A, Trani A, Tarzia G, Ferrari P, Pallanza R, Berti M. Synthesis and biological evaluation of de(acetylglucosaminyl)didehydrodeoxy derivatives of teicoplanin antibiotics. J Med Chem 1989; 32:783–788.

117. Malabarba A, Ciabatti R, Kettenring J, Scotti R, Candiani G, Pallanza P, Berti M, Goldstein B. Reductive hydrolysis of the 59,60-amide bond of teicoplanin antibiotics: A key step from natural to synthetic glycopeptides. J Med Chem 1994; 37:2988–2990.

118. Malabarba A, Ciabatti R, Kettenring J, Ferrari P, Scotti R, Goldstein BP, Denaro M. Amides of de-acetylglucosaminyl-deoxy teicoplanin active against highly glycopeptide-resistant enterococci. Synthesis and antibacterial activity. J Antibiot 1994; 47:1493–1506.

119. Malabarba A, Trani A, Strazzolini P, Cietto B, Ferrari P, Tarzia G, Pallanza R, Berti M. Synthesis and biological properties of N63-carboxamides of teicoplanin antibiotics. Structure-activity relationships. J Med Chem 1989; 32:2450–2460.

120. Malabarba A, Strazzolini P, Depaoli A, Landi M, Berti M, Cavalleri B. Teicoplanin, antibiotics from Actinoplanes teichomyceticus nov. sp. 7. Chemical degradation: Physico-chemical and biological properties of acid hydrolysis products. J Antibiot 1984; 37:988–999.

121. Altomare C, Carotti A, Cellamare S, Carrieri A, Ciabatti R, Malabarba A, Newman DJ, Oh YK, Phelen C, Shearer MC, Sitrin RD, Nisbet LJ. Lipophilicity of teicoplanin antibiotics as assessed by reversed phase high-performance liquid chromatography: Quantitative structure-property and structure-activity relationships. J Pharm Pharmacol 1994; 46:994–999.

122. Malabarba A. Modulation of the antibacterial activity of glycopeptide antibiotics by chemical derivatization. On the Frontier of Anti-Bacterial Discovery. New York: Strategic Research Institute L.P., 1995.

123. Berti M, Candiani G, Borgonovi M, Landini P, Ripamonti F, Scotti R, Cavenaghi L, Denaro M, Goldstein BP. Antimicrobial activity of MDL 62,873, a semisynthetic derivative of teicoplanin, in vitro and in experimental infections. Antimicrob Agents Chemother 1995; 36:446–452.

124. Goldstein BP, Candiani G, Arain TM, Romanò G, Ciciliato I, Berti M, Abbondi M, Scotti R, Mainini M, Ripamonti F, Resconi A, Denaro M. Antimicrobial activity of MDL 63,246, a new semisynthetic glycopeptide antibiotic. Antimicrob Agents Chemother 1995; 39:1580–1588.

125. Kenny MT, Brackman MA, Dulworth JK. In vitro activity of the semisynthetic glycopeptide amide MDL 63,236. Antimicrob Agents Chemother 1995; 39:1589–1590.

126. Malabarba A, Ciabatti R, Kettenring J, Scotti R, Candiani G, Pallanza R, Berti M, Goldstein B. Synthesis and antibacterial activity of a series of basic amides of teicoplanin and deglucoteicoplanin with polyamines. J Med Chem 1992; 35:4054–4060.

127. Shi Z, Griffin JA. Catalysis of carbamate hydrolysis by vancomycin and semisynthetic derivatives. J Am Chem Soc 1993; 115:6482–6486.

128. Sundram UM, Griffin JH. General and efficient method for the solution- and solid-phase synthesis of vancomycin carboxamide derivatives. J Org Chem 1995; 60:1102–1103.

129. Malabarba A. International Patent WO9426780; 1994.

130. Malabarba A, Ciabatti R, Maggini M, Ferrari P, Colomobo L, Denaro M. Structural modifications of the active site in teicoplanin and related glycopeptides 2: Deglucoteicoplanin-derived tetrapeptide. J Org Chem 1996; 61:2151–2157.

131. Malabarba A, Ciabatti R, Kettinring J, Ferrari P, Vékey K, Bellasio E, Denaro M. Structural modifications of the active site in teicoplanin and related glycopeptides 1: Reductive hydrolysia of the 1,2 and 2,3 peptide bonds. J Org Chem 1996; 61:2137–2150.

132. Williams DH, Maplestone RA. Why are secondary metabolites biosynthesized? Sophistication in the inhibition of cell wall biosynthesis by vancomycin group antibiotics. Secondary Metabolites: Their Function and Evolution, Ciba Foundation Symposium 171. Chichester: John Wiley and Sons, 1992:45–63.

13
Thiopeptide Antibiotics

Todd M. Smith, Ya-Fen Jiang, and Heinz G. Floss
University of Washington, Seattle, Washington

I. INTRODUCTION

The thiopeptide antibiotics comprise a class of naturally occurring, structurally diverse sulfur-rich peptides. They are produced by a wide variety of microorganisms and are distinct from another group of sulfur-rich peptide antibiotics known as lanthionine antibiotics (1). Thiostrepton and nosiheptide (Figure 1) are the archetypal compounds of the thiopeptide family; examples of the structural diversity within this family, however, can be observed in the micrococcins (2), thiocillins (3), glycothiohexide α (4), GE2270 A (5), cyclothiazomycin (6), and berninamycin (7). Micrococcins and thiocillins are produced by *Micrococcus* spp. and *Bacillus* spp. GE2270 A is formed by a fungus, *Planobispora rosea*. Thiostrepton is produced by *Streptomyces laurentii* (8), *Streptomyces azureus* (9), and *Streptomyces hawaiiensis* (10), and nosiheptide by *Streptomyces actuosus* and *Streptomyces antibioticus* (11).

A common architectural feature of thiopeptide antibiotics that distinguishes them from other thiazole- or dihydrothiazole-containing compounds, such as bleomycin (12), bacitracin (13), or microcin B17 (14), is the presence of a macrocyclic ring system that is joined to a side-chain "handle" by a tetrahydropyridine or hydroxypyridine moiety. Within the macrocycle, a variable number of thiazole, thiazoline, or oxazole rings are present as well as other modified amino acids such as dehydroalanine and dehydrobutyrine. In many thiopeptides (thiostrepton, siomycins (15), and thiopeptins (16)), an extra loop structure is formed by joining the amino-terminus of the peptide to a threonine residue through a modified quinaldic acid. Nosiheptide and glycothiohexide α differ in that the extra loop is created by joining a cysteine residue to a hydroxyglutamic acid residue through a modified indolic acid. In the case of glycothiohexide α the modified indole has an additional cross-link to a 3-hydroxyl-group on a glutamic acid residue. This antibiotic also differs from other known thiopeptides in that it is glycosylated (4). The micrococcins, thiocillins, and berninamycins lack an extra loop structure; the latter also contains some oxazoles instead of thiazoles. GE2770 A and the related amythiamicins (17) are more divergent. They contain additional modifications and amino acids, like β-hydroxyphenylalanine or proline residues, that are not found in other thiopeptides a dihydro-oxazole in the side chain, N-methyl amides, and alkylated thiazole rings. The amino acids and other residues in cyclothiazomycin are arranged in two large ring sys-

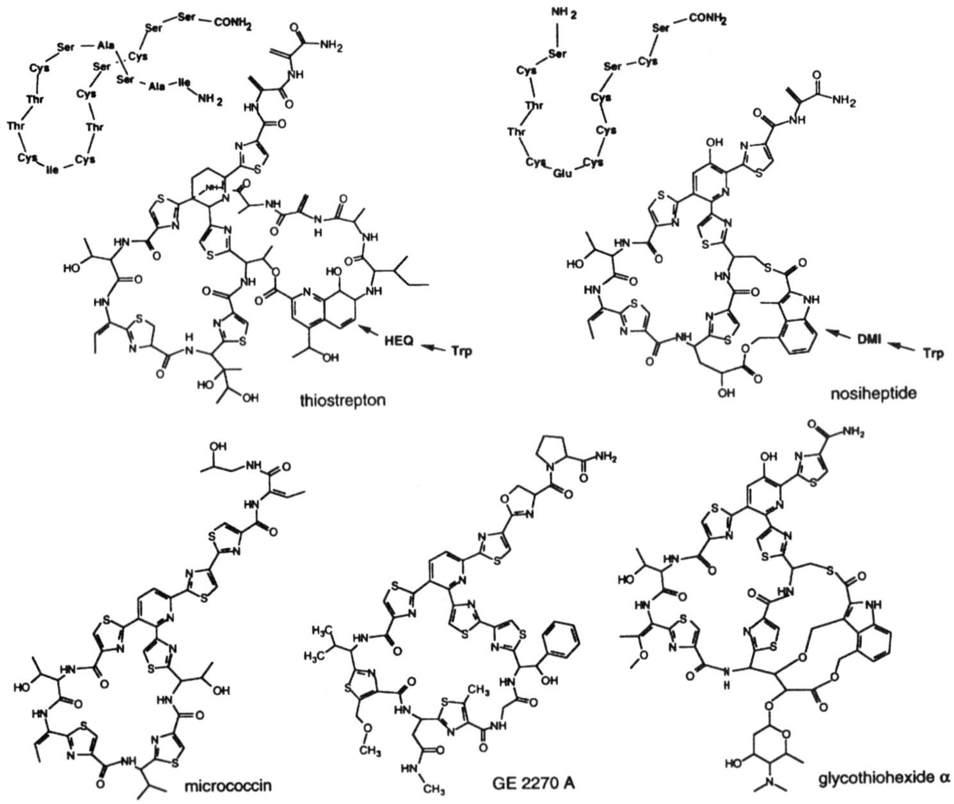

Figure 1 Structures of thiopeptide antibiotics. The amino acids incorporated into thiostrepton and nosiheptide are represented as peptide chains, and the quinaldic (thiostrepton) and indolic acid (nosiheptide) moieties are shown to arise from tryptophan.

tems, which presumably results in a very different three-dimensional structure and biological activity compared with those of the other thiopeptide antibiotics. In fact, this compound was discovered in a pharmacological screen for renin inhibitors (6).

A.   Mechanism of Action

Thiopeptide antibiotics, with the exception of cyclothiazomycin, inhibit protein synthesis in bacteria. They are primarily used in agriculture and veterinary medicine (11); their low solubility prevents utilization in human medicine. Thiostrepton is also employed extensively as a research tool in actinomycete molecular biology. The thiostrepton resistance gene from *S. azureus (tsr)* was one of the first streptomycete genes cloned (18) and is found in many streptomycete cloning vectors (19). Most thiopeptide antibiotics inhibit protein synthesis by binding to the 50S ribosomal subunit, forming a complex with the 23S rRNA and ribosomal protein L11 (20,21) in the region of the ribosome known as the GTPase-associated center. This is the region where elongation factors EF-G and EF-Tu bind. At this site, the effects of specific thiopeptide antibiotics on ribosome function can be remarkably different. For example, thiostrepton has been shown to inhibit EF-G- and EF-Tu-catalyzed GTP hydrolysis, whereas micrococcin stimulates GTP hydrolysis (20). Chemical and nuclease probes were used to show that thiostrepton protects the N1 position of A 1067, whereas micrococcin renders it more reactive (22). The specific mechanism of action for nosiheptide is currently unknown, but it is known that nosiheptide is cross-resistant with, but less potent than, thiostrepton (21). GE2270 A and the amythiamicins, interestingly, inhibit protein synthesis by binding directly to EF-Tu (23,24).

Associated with the thiopeptide antibiotic mode of action is their involvement in the stringent response, a process observed in bacteria during amino acid starvation that results in the synthesis of a pyrophosphate (PP$_i$) adduct of guanosine diphosphate (GDP) or guanosine triphosphate (GTP), guanosine 5',3'-triphosphate diphosphate (pppGpp) or guanosine 5',3'-diphosphate diphosphate (p)ppGpp (25). In some streptomycetes, there is a correlation between high (p)ppGpp levels and the onset of differentiation and antibiotic production (26), but there is no direct evidence that high concentrations of (p)ppGpp are required to initiate antibiotic production (27). Synthesis of (p)ppGpp requires an uncharged tRNA and protein L11. Mutants of *Streptomyces coelicolor* that cannot synthesize (p)ppGpp (*rel*, or relaxed mutants) have been found to either be lacking protein L11 or have altered forms of it (28,29). Consistent with these observations, it has been found that sublethal concentrations of thiopeptin inhibit (p)ppGpp synthesis (30). When thiopeptin binding is blocked by the action of *tsr*, (p)ppGpp can be synthesized, even in the presence of high levels of thiopeptin.

Until recently, it was believed that the only activity of thiopeptide antibiotics was their involvement with processes at the GTPase center of the 50S ribosomal subunit. This view has changed with the discovery that thiostrepton, at low concentrations (<10^{-9} M), can induce the expression of at least eight proteins in *Streptomyces lividans* (31,32). One of these proteins, TipA$_L$, a product of the *tipA* gene, is a thiostrepton-specific recognition protein that acts as an autogenous transcriptional activator of its own gene (32). Other thiopeptides have been discovered by virtue of their ability to bind the *tipA* gene product and activate expression of a kanamycin resistance gene under control of the *tipA* promoter (33–35). The *tipA* gene produces two proteins, TipA$_L$ and TipA$_S$. TipA$_S$ is produced from the same open reading frame as TipA$_L$ by translation from an alternate in-frame initiation codon. Both proteins bind to thiostrepton, and their functions are unknown. The N-terminal region of TipA$_L$ shows some homology to MerR, a transcriptional activator of the *merT* and *merR* genes, which are involved in mercury resistance (32). MerR is a member of a family of two-component regulatory proteins found in bacteria. In these proteins, the N-terminal portion binds DNA and activates transcription; the C-terminal portion binds the regulatory molecule (36). Since both TipA$_L$ and TipA$_S$ bind thiostrepton, it has been hypothesized that TipA$_L$ activates transcription of the *tipA* gene and TipA$_S$ negatively regulates this activation. The ratio of TipA$_S$ to TipA$_L$ in the presence of thiostrepton is 20:1. An interesting aspect of this binding is that thiostrepton becomes covalently attached to TipA$_S$ by forming a bond between a cysteine residue on TipA$_S$ and one of the dehydroalanine residues in thiostrepton (37). This observation raises new questions about the binding of thiostrepton to ribosomes, as well as its role in inducing gene expression in *S. lividans*. None of the other thiostrepton-induced proteins have been characterized.

B.   Mechanism of Resistance

Resistance to thiopeptide antibiotics can be generated by a variety of mechanisms. In the producing streptomycetes, there are genes coding for enzymes that methylate the 2'-OH of adenosine 1067 in the 23S rRNA (38,39). This methylation confers resistance to thiopeptides by preventing antibiotic binding. Three of these genes have been cloned: the thiostrepton resistance genes from *S. azureus* (*tsr*) (18) and *S. laurentii* (*tsnR*) (40), and the nosiheptide resistance gene from *S. actuosus* (*nshR*) (41). Comparison of the nucleotide and deduced amino acid sequences of these genes (40,42,43) showed that they are highly similar.

The rRNA methyltransferases encoded by the thiopeptide-resistance genes appear to form a distinct family of methyltransferase enzymes that has many members and is widespread in nature. Recent searches of the thiopeptide methyltransferase sequences against the nonredundant protein database at the National Center for Biotechnology Information (NCBI), using BEAUTY (44) and blastp (45), identified 13 similar protein sequences from eight bacteria, most of which were deposited in the database as a result of bacterial genome sequencing projects. A multiple alignment of these amino acid sequences revealed two regions of high similarity (Figure 2). In addition to the bacterial sequences, one human sequence, TRP-185 (47), was also identified as containing the two

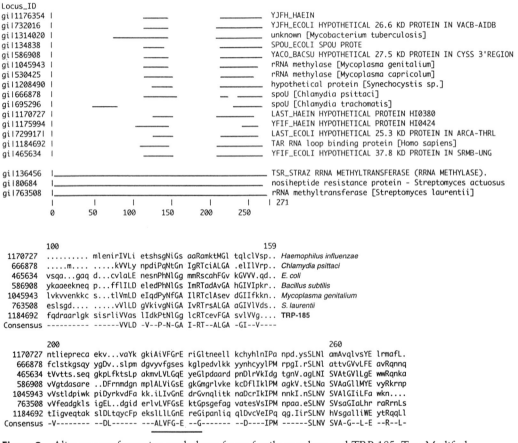

Figure 2 Alignments of putative methyltransferase family members and TRP-185. Top: Modified output from BEAUTY (44) showing a graphical representation of the pairwise alignments for each amino acid sequence with the *S. laurentii* protein sequence (bottom line). The locus ID (sequence ID number used by the Entrez browser at NCBI) is displayed to the left, and the definition line from the GenBank file is displayed to the right. Bottom: Multiple alignment of the highly similar regions for selected amino acid sequences. The putative *S*-adenosyl-L-methionine binding site (46) is underlined.

highly similar regions found in the bacterial amino acid sequences. This protein is particularly interesting because it binds to the stem loop that forms the TAR region in human immunodeficiency virus (HIV) RNA. Like the *tsr* gene product (48), TRP-185 is highly specific for a particular sequence of the loop in the stem loop structure. From this observation, it can be concluded that the two similar regions in this family of proteins are involved in RNA loop binding and sequence recognition. There is also speculation that a portion of the second region contains the S-adenosyl-L-methionine binding site (46). If this is true, it is possible that HIV RNA is methylated in the TAR region.

Other organisms have evolved different strategies for resistance to thiopeptide antibiotics. The *Bacillus* and *Micrococcus* species, which produce micrococcin, contain ribosomes that are sensitive to the thiopeptides in vitro. In vivo, these bacteria are resistant to micrococcin-type antibiotics and sensitive to thiostrepton (49). In this case, resistance is thought to be conferred by a binding or transport protein that is specific for micrococcin (49). Mutants of *Bacillus* spp. have been identified that are resistant to several thiopeptides. Some of these mutants produce altered forms of ribosomal protein L11 (50), and in one species, *Bacillus megaterium*, L11 was absent (51). Currently, the only known mechanism of resistance operating in the producing streptomycetes is through the actions of the rRNA methyltransferase.

II. BIOSYNTHESIS OF THIOPEPTIDE ANTIBIOTICS

A. Fermentation

An important aspect of biosynthetic experiments involves producing the compound of interest, which requires careful management of bacterial strains as well as optimization of growth conditions. In feeding experiments, growth conditions must be compatible with the isolation and subsequent analysis of the desired compound. Optimum production of nosiheptide and thiostrepton requires frequent reisolation, every 8–12 months, of high-producing *S. actuosus* (nosiheptide) and *S. laurentii* (thiostrepton) strains. This is done by sonicating a spore suspension at sufficient energy to produce a 90% kill rate and plating the resulting suspension to isolate pure cultures. Typically, 10 colonies are picked and grown in duplicate small-scale (100 ml cultures) fermentations, and relative yields of antibiotic are determined by high-performance liquid chromatography (HPLC) (52,53). The highest-producing strains are then stored as spore suspensions in 15% glycerol, or as culture suspensions in 20% glycerol (52). Feeding studies with *S. actuosus* required the development of a defined media (52). During this process, it was discovered that glucose provides the best carbon source for growth and production. Other carbon sources, sucrose, maltose, lactose, and glycerol, supported growth but resulted in low yields of nosiheptide. Additionally, high concentrations of ammonia, phosphate, tryptophan, and cysteine inhibited nosiheptide production. High yields of thiostrepton (ca. 10 g/liter) can be produced by *S. laurentii* if the pH of the culture is monitored during production and additional nutrients are added when the glucose is depleted, as observed by a sudden increase in pH (54).

B. Building Blocks

Previous studies have determined which amino acids are incorporated into thiostrepton (55) and nosiheptide (56) by feeding isotopically labeled amino acids to the producing organisms and observing their incorporation by nuclear magnetic resonance (NMR). From these experiments, it was determined that the thiazole (dihydrothiazole) residues are formed from cysteine and the next amino acid, presumably by attack of the cysteine sulfhydryl on the carbonyl of the next amino acid followed by dehydration. Oxidation of the dihydrothiazole yields the thiazole ring. The dehydroalanine and dehydrobutyrine residues are formed by dehydration of serine and threonine, respectively. A condensation between two dehydroalanine residues and the carboxyl-group of an adjacent cysteine has been proposed to give the tetrahydropyridine (thiostrepton) and pyridine (nosiheptide) groups, generating at the same time the central macrocycle (Figure 3). Using these data, the amino acids giving rise to these two antibiotics can be represented as linear peptides as shown in Figure 1. Similar results have been obtained for berninamycin (7).

Of biochemical interest are the origins of the quinaldic acid moiety in thiostrepton and the indolic acid moiety in nosiheptide. Feeding experiments have established that both structures are biosynthesized from tryptophan (55,56) (Figure 1). In the case of the quinaldic acid moiety, tryptophan is converted to a free intermediate 4-(1-hydroxyethyl)-2-quinolinecarboxylate (HEQ). The first step of this transformation has been identified as methylation of the 2-position in tryptophan (57). 2-Methyltryptophan then undergoes a ring expansion in which the C2–N bond in the indole ring is cleaved and the nitrogen is reconnected to the α-carbon of the side chain (Figure 4). Attachment of HEQ to the backbone of thiostrepton then requires two additional steps: activation of the carboxyl-group and ester formation with the side-chain hydroxyl of a threonine; and joining of the carbocylic ring of HEQ to the amino-terminal isoleucine, presumably through epoxidation of the 7,8 double bond in HEQ followed by ring opening of the epoxide with the amino-group of isoleucine.

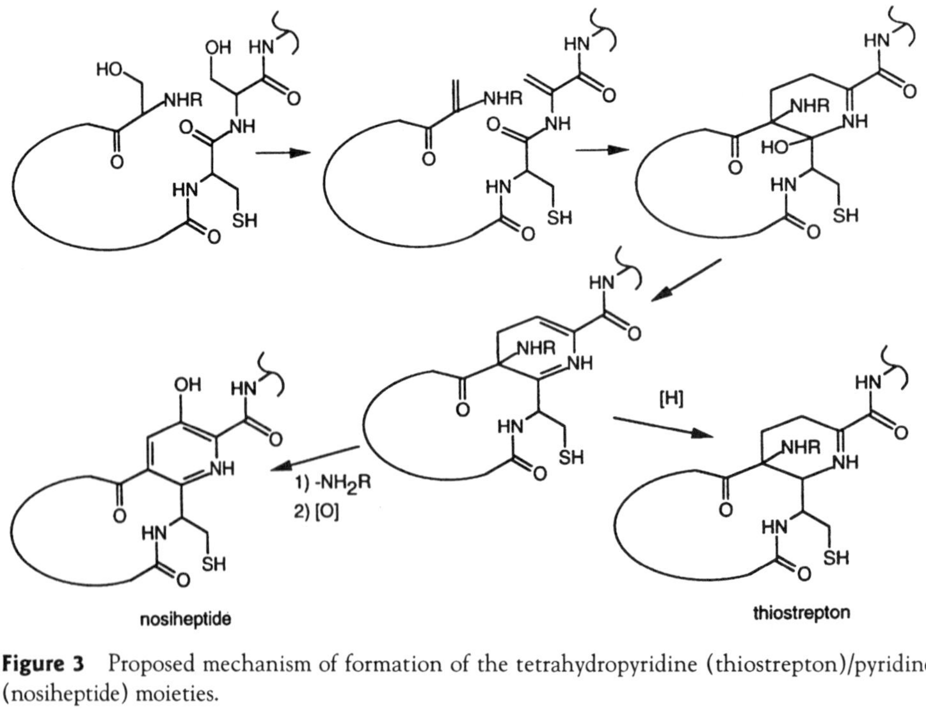

Figure 3 Proposed mechanism of formation of the tetrahydropyridine (thiostrepton)/pyridine (nosiheptide) moieties.

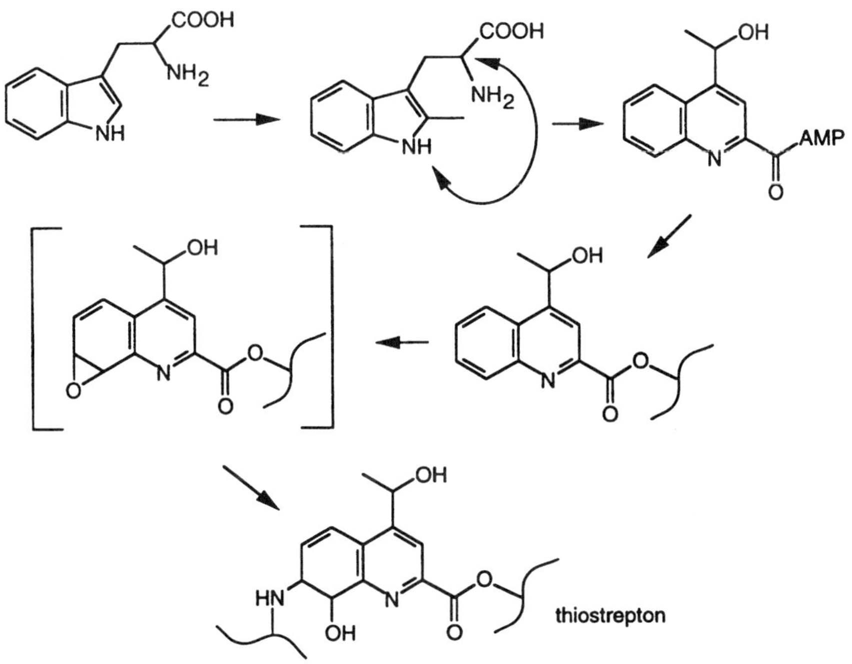

Figure 4 Proposed pathway for the biosynthesis of HEQ, and attachment to the backbone of thiostrepton.

The conversion of tryptophan into the free intermediate, 3,4-dimethyl-2-indole-carboxylate (DMI), the precursor of the modified indolic acid in nosiheptide, is equally interesting. Feeding doubly ^{13}C-labeled tryptophan established that the indole 2-car-boxyl-group arises by an intramolecular migration from the carboxyl-group of tryptophan (Figure 5) (58). Loss of the α-carbon and the amino-group yields the free intermediate, 3-methylindole-2-carboxylate (3-MI), which is methylated in the 4-position to yield DMI. DMI is attached to the backbone of nosiheptide by two ester linkages. The first is a thioester formed between the carboxyl-group of DMI and the side-chain sulfhydryl of a cysteine residue. The second ester is formed between the γ-carboxyl-group of the hydroxyglutamic acid residue and the 4-methyl-group of DMI. This second attachment requires activation of the 4-methyl-group either through oxidation to a hydroxymethyl-group, or to a resonance-stabilized carbocation (59) (Figure 5). It is unknown whether the oxygen atoms in the ester are both derived from glutamic acid or if one comes from molecular oxygen. Interestingly, even though HEQ and DMI are quite different in structure, their biosynthesis and attachment to thiostrepton and nosiheptide share many common features. The biosynthesis of both compounds involves methylation and intramolecular rearrangement reactions. Both molecules are attached to the antibiotics through an ester linkage with their carboxyl-groups on one side, and the other side of each molecule is attached by way of an oxidized intermediate.

Clearly, numerous biosynthetic reactions are required to synthesize thiopeptide antibiotics. The amino acid compositions of thiostrepton and nosiheptide were determined by feeding experiments, but these studies could not provide information about the

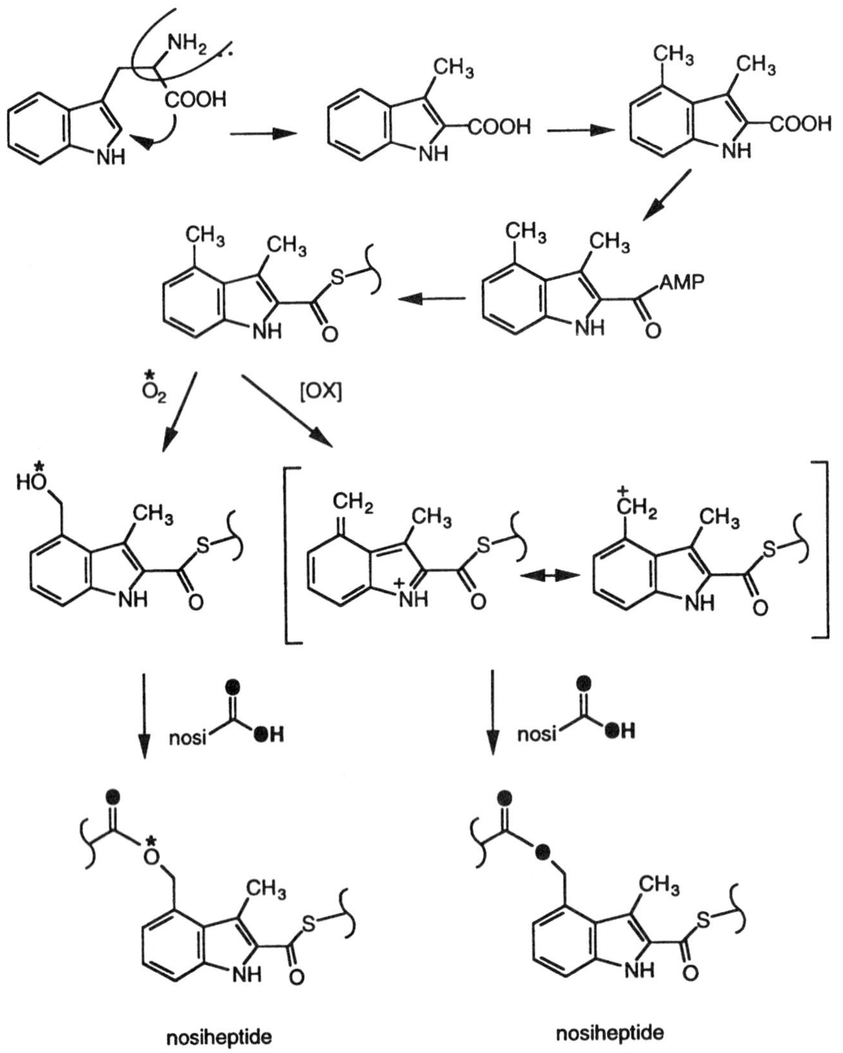

Figure 5   Proposed pathway for the biosynthesis of DMI, and alternative mechanisms for oxidation of the benzylic carbon during attachment to the backbone of nosiheptide. Asterisks show the incorporation of an ^{18}O label fed as $^{18}O_2$. The oxygens derived from glutamate ($RC^{18}O_2^-$) are filled in.

details of thiopeptide biosynthesis. For example, it is unknown whether the peptide backbone is encoded by an mRNA that is translated to give a precursor peptide, which is later modified, or if a peptide is formed and modified nonribosomally by a complex of enzymes. Answers to these questions can only be obtained by studying the biochemistry and genetics of thiopeptide formation in producing organisms.

C.   Thiopeptide Antibiotic Biosynthesis: Ribosomal or Nonribosomal?

A first question that needs to be resolved is whether thiostrepton, and by analogy nosiheptide, is synthesized by a ribosomal or a nonribosomal process. Preliminary experiments conducted to determine the mode of biosynthesis suggest that these compounds are produced via a nonribosomal pathway. When cultures of S. *actuosus* were treated with chloramphenicol at concentrations that inhibit ribosomal protein synthesis (60,61), *de novo* production of nosiheptide was detected (62). Similar results were obtained for thiostrepton production in S. *azureus* (62). With S. *laurentii*, however, the data have been inconclusive. Hybridization experiments also support the possibility of nonribosomal biosynthesis. Oligodeoxynucleotides derived from the amino acid sequences represented in either thiostrepton or nosiheptide failed to hybridize to any homologous sequences under a variety of conditions when used to probe Southern blots of genomic DNA from the respective producing organisms (62).

Additional arguments can be made in favor of a nonribosomal biosynthesis by comparing the structures of thiopeptide antibiotics. For example, thiostrepton-like antibiotics all have one dihydrothiazole ring that is in the same position as one of the thiazole rings in nosiheptide-like antibiotics. This modification can be best explained by the lack of a functional oxidative activity in a peptide synthetase domain (see below). A ribosomal pathway would require that producers of the thiostrepton-like antibiotics lack an enzyme that would oxidize one of the dihydrothiazoles to a thiazole ring, while requiring that these producers have enzymes that oxidize the other dihydrothiazoles. Hence, each modifying enzyme would have to recognize a specific dihydrothiazole. Although the available evidence for nonribosomal synthesis of thiostrepton and related antibiotics is only suggestive, such a process has considerable appeal. Conclusive evidence awaits the cloning of the genes that encode the biosynthetic machinery.

D. Model for Thiopeptide Biosynthesis

If it is assumed that thiostrepton and nosiheptide are formed by a nonribosomal process, then the most probable mode of biosynthesis is the thiotemplate pathway. This pathway is extensively used by numerous microorganisms, both prokaryotic and eukaryotic, to produce an extremely diverse group of compounds (12). In thiotemplate biosynthesis, peptides are assembled by large (100–1400 kDa) multifunctional enzymes called peptide synthetases, which activate amino acids and convert them to enzyme-bound thioesters in a reaction requiring adenosine triphosphate (ATP) and releasing inorganic pyrophosphate (PP$_i$) (12). The amino acid thioester is formed with a 4'-phosphopantetheine arm (63), which is also involved in transferring the growing peptide chain to catalytic sites in a process similar to fatty acid and polyketide biosynthesis (64). Thiotemplate peptide synthetases are also known to catalyze a wide range of additional reactions, which appear to be "programmed" by insertion of functional motifs within peptide synthetase domains (65), thus providing a mechanism for structural modifications to occur on the peptide backbone in precise locations.

By comparison with other bacterial thiotemplate enzymes (65), one can conjecture that thiostrepton may be synthesized by four peptide synthetases. Similarly, nosiheptide would be synthesized by three peptide synthetases. It is also possible that backbone structures of these antibiotics are formed by a single multifunctional polypeptide in a fashion similar to cyclosporin biosynthesis (66). These enzymes would catalyze the reactions required for formation of the peptide backbone (amino acid activation, attachment to a pantetheine arm, and transpeptidation), as well as additional reactions such as thiazole (dihydrothiazole) (Figures 6 and 7), dehydroalanine, and dehydrobutyrine formations. The peptide synthetases could also form a large biosynthetic complex that would maintain a conformation of the peptide backbone favorable for formation of the macrocycle and tetrahydropyridine moiety as well. These multifunctional enzymes would also be

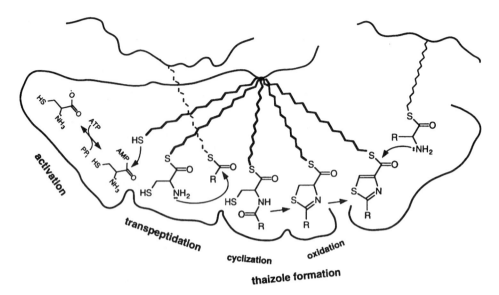

Figure 6   Proposed domain for cysteine activation, transpeptidation, and conversion to a thiazole. Cysteine is first activated to its acyl adenylate and attached to a pantetheine arm through a thioester linkage. In the transpeptidation reaction, the amino-group of cysteine attacks the carbonyl of the next amino acid, transferring the growing peptide chain to the cysteinyl-pantetheine arm. This step is followed by cyclization and oxidation reactions to give the thiazole ring. Finally, the thiazole-containing peptide is transferred to the next pantetheine arm through a transpeptidation reaction with the n_{i-1} amino acid.

responsible for forming the carboxy-terminal amide using the amino-group from serine (55) (Figure 8).

Other reactions, such as oxidations of isoleucine to dihydroxyisoleucine or gluta-mate to hydroxyglutamate, could also be carried out by the peptide synthetases or may be catalyzed by separate modifying enzymes. The quinaldic acid and indolic acid moieties are most likely biosynthesized in separate pathways, since isotopically labeled HEQ and DMI, fed to cultures of S. *laurentii* or S. *actuosus*, are efficiently incorporated into the respective antibiotics (56,55). Incorporation of each compound requires at least two enzymatic reactions, one of which is expected to be activations of the carboxylate-group in a manner similar to other enzymatic activations occurring in the biosynthesis of pep-tide secondary metabolites (see below). In all, there are likely to be more than 70 reac-tions required to assemble thiostrepton, with the majority (more than 60) probably cat-alyzed by peptide synthetases (Table 1).

To design an effective strategy for cloning the thiostrepton biosynthetic genes, it is useful to have an estimate of the amount of DNA required to encode the biosynthetic enzymes (Table 1). The peptide synthetases would be expected to make up the largest portion of the thiostrepton biosynthetic gene cluster. From the DNA sequences of pep-tide synthetase–encoding genes (65), it is estimated that each domain is encoded in 3–4 kilobases (kb) of DNA—one domain per amino acid assembled in the compound. The 18 amino acids assembled in thiostrepton would thus require 54–72 kb of DNA. When other possible enzymatic activities are included, approximately 18 for cyclizations, dehydra-tions, and termination, 78–96 kb of DNA may be required to produce the peptide syn-

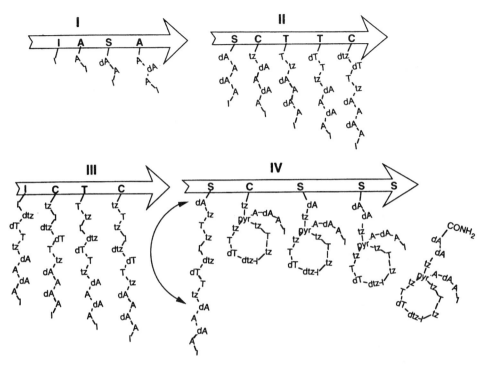

Figure 7 Hypothetical thiostrepton peptide synthetase complex. Shown in the arrows representing the peptide synthetases are the amino acids activated. In the growing polypeptide, the amino acids are shown as their proposed modified counterparts. Synthetase I catalyzes the assembly of the first four amino acids. Synthetase II assembles and modifies the next five amino acids, and synthetase IV releases the modified peptide precursor. Abbreviations: dA, dehydroalanine; dT, dehydrothreonine; tz, thiazole; dtz, dihydrothiazole; pyr, tetrahydropyridine.

thetase complex. Additional enzymes, oxidases, HEQ biosynthesis, attachment, and resistance genes would add approximately 18 kb more to the estimate, to give a total of 97–115 kb of DNA in the putative thiostrepton biosynthetic cluster. Though this may appear to be a large amount of DNA devoted to the production of a secondary metabolite, it is not uncommon for biosynthetic clusters to be of this size. For example, the genes that encode the polyketide synthetases and other enzymes required for the biosynthesis of the antibiotic avermectin are located in a cluster that extends over 90 kb in the *Streptomyces avermitilis* chromosome (67).

III. PROGRESS TOWARD CLONING THE BIOSYNTHETIC MACHINERY

A. Analysis of the DNA Flanking the *S. laurentii tsn*R Gene

As a first step in identifying the genes coding for thiostrepton biosynthesis, the thiostrepton-resistance gene from *S. laurentii* was cloned. This gene then served as a probe to isolate large DNA fragments from cosmid libraries of *S. laurentii* DNA (40). Smaller DNA fragments subcloned from the resulting cosmid clones were used to carry out a disruption analysis of the DNA flanking *tsn*R in order to test for the possibility that it contained

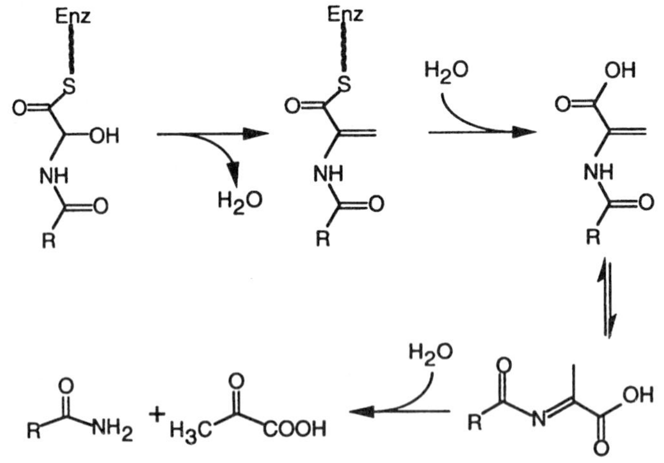

Figure 8   Proposed termination reaction and release of the thiopeptide from the peptide synthetase complex.

Table 1   Estimated Size of the Thiostrepton Biosynthetic
Gene Cluster

Enzyme(s) (no.)	Protein size (kDa)	DNA (kb)
Peptide synthetases (3–4)	1700–2000	54–72
Dehydratases (7)	277	8.4
Thiazoline/thiazole (5)	356	10.8
Pyridine ring		
Cyclase	25–50	1.2
Dehydratase	25–50	1.2
Reductase	25–50	1.2
Racemase	25–50	1.2
Quinaldic acid formation		
Methylase	50	1.4
Transaminase	50	1.4
Mutase	50	1.4
Quinaldic acid attachment		
Adenylyltransferase	47	1.3
Acyltransferase	50	1.4
Oxidase	50	1.4
Dihydroxyisoleucine		
Dehydrogenase	50	1.4
Oxidase	50	1.4
Epoxide hydrolase	50	1.4
Resistance and regulatory genes		6.0
Total		**97–115**

thiostrepton biosynthesis genes. Only 2 of the strains (14 total) resulting from the insert-directed mutagenesis failed to produce thiostrepton. The 2 nonproducers contained insertions in regions found to have homology with the *spc* and *S10* operons of *Escherichia coli* (discussed below). It is quite possible that the phenotypes observed in these mutants were due to pleiotropic effects, rather than to disruptions in biosynthetic genes. If thiostrepton is synthesized by large peptide synthetases, then it could be expected that the genes encoding these enzymes would have open reading frames (ORFs) of 12–18 kb, and they should be easily disrupted by insert-directed integration.

A partial DNA sequence analysis of the region flanking *tsn*R was also carried out. It was hoped that sequence data obtained within this region could be used to identify the nature of the genes flanking *tsn*R, similar to a strategy used by MacNeil and coworkers (67) to determine the putative organization of the genes encoding the polyketide synthetases that generate the aglycone of avermectin. If peptide synthetase genes are linked to *tsn*R, it is reasonable to expect that some of the highly conserved domains found in these genes (65) would be present within the library of partial sequence data from *S. laurentii*. When the sequence analysis was done, with both nucleotide and deduced amino acid sequences, similarities were identified instead to proteins found in ribosomal protein operons as well as to the RNA polymerase β′ subunit (*rpo*C) from *E. coli* and other bacteria. Since these are essential genes, both amino acid and nucleotide sequences are highly conserved among different species.

The organization of the putative ribosomal protein genes identified in *S. laurentii* parallels the organization of similar genes in other bacteria. Of particular interest was the similarity to the actinomycete *Mycobacterium leprae* (Figure 9). Alignments of *M. leprae* and *S. laurentii* DNA sequences indicate that putative *S. laurentii* genes encoding EF-G and EF-Tu are located next to *tsn*R. When *S. laurentii* (proximal to *tsn*R), *M. leprae*, *E. coli*, and *Micrococcus luteus* DNA sequences are compared (Figure 9), striking overlaps are observed. All of these bacteria show a similar arrangement of EF-G and EF-Tu. The *rpo*BC genes in *M. leprae* closely align with the putative *rpo*C gene in *S. laurentii*. A comparison of the DNA from *S. laurentii* (distal to *tsn*R), and similar regions in *M. luteus*, *E. coli*, and *Mycoplasma capricolum* also shows a high degree of conservation for the genes in the *spc* and *S10* operons (Figure 9). In *E. coli*, the ribosomal protein operons (*spc*, *str*, and *S10*) (70) are arranged in the same apparent order observed in *S. laurentii*. In *M. luteus*, the *spc* and *str* operons are also believed to be closely linked (73).

It is unclear why the *S. laurentii tsn*R gene would be clustered with ribosomal protein operons. Its location is intriguing considering the mode of action of thiostrepton, the binding of which to 23S rRNA blocks the functions of EF-G and EF-Tu (22). One possibility is that *tsn*R evolved in a cluster with the genes for EF-G and EF-Tu. However, when the nucleotide sequences for DNA fragments containing the *S. laurentii*, *S. actuosus*, and *S. azureus* resistance-encoding genes are compared, this hypothesis is not supported. The only DNA sequence similarity observed between these species is confined to the 800–900 nucleotide (nt) regions encoding the resistance genes. Furthermore, when the DNA sequences flanking the resistance genes from *S. actuosus* (2326 nt) (43) and *S. azureus* (1521 nt) (42) were used to search the nucleic acid databases, they failed to detect any genes from ribosomal protein operons. In *S. actuosus*, the 2326 nt fragment contains one ORF (*orf*699) immediately preceding *nsh*R (43), which was found, by Southern blot, to be nearly ubiquitous in *Streptomyces* spp. Two other ORFs, *orf*B and *orf*C, have been identified downstream from *nsh*R, and they appear to be unique to nosiheptide producers (75). The amino acid sequence deduced from *orf*C is similar to peptide sequences deduced from *ent*D (76), *sfp* (77), and *gsp* (78) (Strohl W, personal communi-

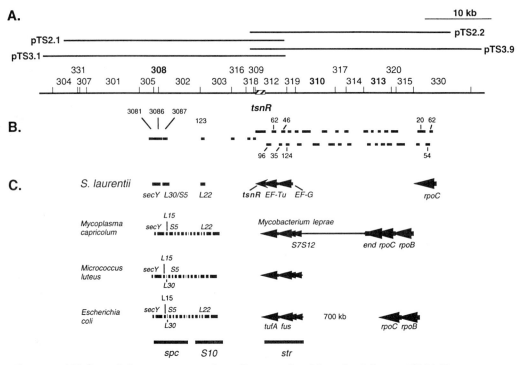

Figure 9   (A) Cosmid clones containing the *tsnR* gene isolated from the *S. laurentii* DNA libraries, and DNA sequence coverage. (B) The *tsnR* gene is shown as a hatched box, and the *Bam*HI fragments are numbered. Cosmids cloned in SuperCos (pTS2.1 and pTS2.2), and pOJ446 (68) (pTS3.1 and pTS3.9) are shown above the map. For simplicity, only the *Bam*HI sites are shown. The numbers above each *Bam*HI fragment denote subclones. (B) Mapped contigs representing a total of 14.8 kb of partial sequence data. (C) Comparison of DNA flanking the *S. laurentii tsnR* gene with homologous DNA from other species, *Mycobacterium leprae* (69), *E. coli* (70,71), *Micrococcus luteus* (72,73), and *Mycoplasma capricolum* (74). Shown at the bottom is a map of the *spc*, *S10*, and *str*, ribosomal-protein operons in *E. coli* (70).

cation), suggesting that these genes may play some yet undefined role in peptide antibiotic biosynthesis. However, there is no direct evidence that either *orf*B or *orf*C is involved in nosiheptide biosynthesis. In fact, nosiheptide production is observed in strains of *S. actuosus* when a 3.0 kb region of DNA containing *orf*B and *orf*C is deleted (79). Finally, a partial sequence analysis (approximately 200 nt every 2–3 kb), extending 30–40 kb in either direction, of the DNA flanking *nsh*R failed to identify any significant similarities to any previously identified genes (79). One would expect that if the thiopeptide biosynthetic gene clusters evolved from a common ancestor, which included an rRNA methyltransferase as the mechanism of resistance, there would be some similarity in the DNA surrounding the resistance genes between different producers; yet none is observed. Additionally, these particular rRNA methyltransferases appear to be unique to thiopeptide-producing streptomycetes (75). It is quite probable that the location of the *S. laurentii tsnR* gene within a cluster of ribosomal operons is unique to this species. There is a possibility that multiple alleles of the *tsnR* gene exist in *S. laurentii*, similar to the situation observed in *S. azureus* (62). However, only one copy of this gene could be detected with three different *tsnR*-like gene probes under a variety of conditions. It remains a mystery why the *S. laurentii tsnR* gene should be clustered with ribosomal protein operons when preliminary data suggest that the *S. actuosus*, and possibly *S. azureus*, resistance genes are not. These data suggest that either biosynthetic genes in an antibiotic-producing microorganism are not always clustered with genes for self-resistance, or other unknown mechanisms of resistance to thiostrepton are operating within *S. laurentii* analogous to the tylosin producer, *Streptomyces fradiae* (80). In that organism, four genes that confer resistance to tylosin have been identified, two of which are clustered with the biosynthetic genes and the other two of which are not.

B. 3,4-Dimethylindole-2-Carboxylate- and 4-(1-Hydroxyethyl)-2-Quinolinecarboxylate-Activating Enzymes

As a complement to the genetic studies and to develop an alternative cloning strategy, it was important to begin a biochemical analysis of thiopeptide production. By studying reactions catalyzed in cell-free extracts, information can be obtained about the types of enzymes that synthesize thiostrepton and related antibiotics. If these enzymes are purified, protein sequences can be determined, from which DNA probes can be prepared and used to clone biosynthetic genes. For several reasons, the most logical place to begin was to look for enzymes that activate the carboxyl-groups of 4-(1-hydroxyethyl)-2-quinolinecarboxylate (HEQ) in *S. laurentii*, and of 3,4-dimethyl-2-indolecarboxylate (DMI) in *S. actuosus*. HEQ and DMI are free intermediates in the biosynthesis of thiostrepton and nosiheptide. There are numerous examples of enzymes that activate carboxylic acids to their acyl adenylates; several of these have been characterized in the biosynthesis of peptide-based secondary metabolites [3-methyl-4-hydroxyanthranilic acid (81,82); quinoxaline-2-carboxylic acid (83); 3-hydroxypicolinic acid (84); D-lysergic acid (85)], and they appear to be cytosolic, stable, and easily assayed. The conversion of carboxylic acids to their acyl adenylates requires ATP, and it produces inorganic pyrophosphate (PP_i) in a reversible reaction that can be monitored by measuring the incorporation of ^{32}P into ATP when the substrate, ATP, Mg^{2+}, and $[^{32}P]PP_i$ are incubated with the activating enzyme (81).

Activating enzymes from *S. laurentii* and *S. actuosus* were enriched 5- to 10-fold and catalyzed ATP/$^{32}PP_i$ exchange reactions that depended on either DMI (*S. actuosus*) or HEQ (*S. laurentii*), Mg^{2+}, and ATP (Figure 10) (86). HEQ-dependent exchange activity was not observed in extracts of *S. actuosus*, nor was DMI-dependent exchange activity observed in *S. laurentii* extracts. The enzyme from *S. actuosus* was specific for DMI and its analog 3-methylindole-2-carboxylate (3-MI), both of which can be incorporated into nosiheptide (58). The *S. laurentii* enzyme is highly selective for the stereoisomer of HEQ

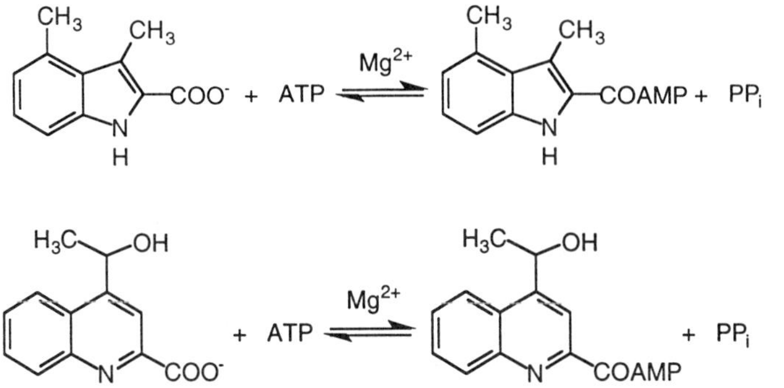

Figure 10   ATP-dependent activation reactions for HEQ and DMI.

found in thiostrepton, but it also showed activity with the des-methyl analog, 4-hydroxy-methyl-2-quinolinecarboxylate (HMQ). Additionally, the methyl ester of HEQ was found to be a competitive inhibitor of the ATP/PP$_i$ exchange reaction catalyzed by the *S. laurentii* enzyme. Finally, the native molecular weight of the HEQ-activating enzyme was estimated by gel permeation chromatography and photoaffinity labeling to be 47 ± 4 kDa (Smith TM, unpublished results, 1993). These values are in good agreement with the molecular weights determined for other carboxylate-activating enzymes involved in the biosynthesis of peptide-based secondary metabolites.

These data demonstrate that *S. actuosus* and *S. laurentii* contain enzymes that activate DMI (*S. actuosus*) and HEQ (*S. laurentii*) to their corresponding acyl adenylates, a reaction believed to be necessary for their attachment to the peptide backbones of nosiheptide and thiostrepton, respectively. The ultimate proof that formation of an acyl adenylate is a requirement for attachment will require additional experimentation—for example, inactivation of the genes encoding these enzymes and subsequent demonstration that DMI or HEQ are not incorporated into the antibiotics.

C.   Identification of Peptide Synthetase Domain Sequences in Thiopeptide Producer DNA

In addition to a classical biochemical approach (described above), a strategy based on conserved sequence motifs found in peptide synthetase proteins has also been employed (87). In this approach, oligodeoxynucleotide probes were derived from highly conserved amino acid sequences in peptide synthetase domains and used as primers to amplify DNA fragments from *S. laurentii* and *S. actuosus* DNA by polymerase chain reaction (PCR). The resulting PCR products were cloned and sequenced, and the deduced amino acid sequences were found to be highly similar to the expected regions of peptide synthetases. These clones then served as probes to isolate cosmids from both *S. laurentii* and *S. actuosus* DNA libraries. One cosmid isolated from the *S. laurentii* library contains a 23 kb *Bam*HI fragment that appears, by partial DNA sequence analysis, to contain three distinct peptide synthetase domains. Similar results have been obtained with cosmid clones isolated from *S. actuosus* DNA libraries. When these clones were hybridized with DNA probes containing domain sequences, 11 putative domains were identified and mapped within a 55 kb region, with an average spacing of approximately 3 kb between hybridizing regions. Partial DNA sequence analysis of these regions shows the presence of the expected conserved motifs. These preliminary data suggest that there are genes encoding peptide synthetases in *S. laurentii* and *S. actuosus*. Gene disruption experiments will be necessary to provide direct evidence that the cloned genes are involved in thiopeptide biosynthesis.

IV.   SUMMARY

It is proposed that thiostrepton and nosiheptide are synthesized by the thiotemplate pathway, making them some of the largest and most complicated antibiotics thought to be produced by large multifunctional enzymes. These enzymes possibly join the amino acids as well as catalyze additional reactions, such as dehydrations and thiazole and tetrahydropyridine ring formations. If this model is correct, the genes encoding the thiostrepton biosynthetic enzymes should be located in a cluster approximately 100 kb in size and would contain at least 18 domains similar to those found in other peptide synthetases (65).

The initial strategy for cloning thiostrepton and nosiheptide biosynthetic genes, using the common approach of first cloning the gene for self-resistance and then using that gene to isolate larger DNA fragments that might contain biosynthetic genes (88), was unsuccessful. DNA flanking the S. *laurentii tsn*R gene was unexpectedly discovered to contain sequences that are similar to genes found in ribosomal protein operons. A similar arrangement, however, is not observed in the DNA flanking the S. *actuosus nsh*R gene or, probably, the S. *azureus tsr* genes. The observation that the S. *laurentii tsn*R gene is uniquely clustered within a region of DNA that appears to be highly conserved among divergent bacteria raises interesting questions about the origins of thiopeptide resistance genes and their role in biosynthesis. One possibility is that the resistance genes were contained in transposons or insertion sequences that were located on plasmids containing the biosynthesis genes. Alternatively, it is possible that there are multiple resistance mechanisms to thiopeptide antibiotics within the producing organisms, and genes that encode such other mechanisms could indeed be clustered with the biosynthetic genes.

These results have made it necessary to explore alternative paths in order to clone thiopeptide biosynthetic genes. Hence, as a first step in the biochemical analysis of thiostrepton and nosiheptide biosynthesis, activities of enzymes that specifically catalyze HEQ- (thiostrepton) and DMI- (nosiheptide) dependent ATP/PP$_i$ exchange reactions were identified. PCR amplification of fragments from the DNA of producing organisms has resulted in the identification of sequences that are highly similar to known peptide synthetases. Future experiments directed toward expression of particular genes, such as the HEQ or DMI adenylate synthetases, or inactivation of thiopeptide biosynthesis will be designed to provide more direct evidence that thiopeptide biosynthesis genes have been cloned.

ACKNOWLEDGMENTS

We would like to thank William Strohl for his help and collaboration. We also thank Paul Shipley and Stepanka Storkova for their assistance. This work was supported by NIH research grant AI20264 (to HGF) and a National Research Service Award GM 07750 (to TMS).

REFERENCES

1. Jack RW, Tagg JR, Ray B. Bacteriocins of gram-positive bacteria. Microbiol Rev 1995; 59:171–200.
2. Walker J. Total structure of the polythiazole-containing antibiotic micrococcin P. A ^{13}C nuclear magnetic resonance study. J Chem Soc (Chem Comm) 1977; 706–870.
3. Shoji J, Hinoo H, Wakisaka Y, Koizumi K, Mayama M, Matsuura S, Matsumoto K. Isolation of three new antibiotics, thiocillins I, II, and III, related to micrococcin P. J Antibiot 1976; 29:366–374.
4. Northcote PT, Siegel M, Borders DB, Lee MD. Glycothiohexide alpha, a novel antibiotic produced by "*Sebekia*" *sp.*, LL-14E605. III. Structural elucidation. J Antibiot 1994; 47:901–908.
5. Kettenring J, Colombo L, Ferrari P, Tavecchia P, Nebuloni M, V'ekey K, Gallo GG, Selva E. Antibiotic GE2270 A: A novel inhibitor of bacterial protein synthesis. II. Structure elucidation. J Antibiot 1991; 44:702–715.
6. Aoki M, Ohtsuka T, Yamada M, Ohba Y, Yoshizaki H, Yasuno H, Sano T, Watanabe J, Yokose K, Seto H. Cyclothiazomycin, a novel polythiazole-containing peptide with renin inhibitory

activity. Taxonomy, fermentation, isolation and physico-chemical characterization. J Antibiot 1991; 44:582–588.

7. Lau RCM, Rinehart KL. Biosynthesis of berninamycin: Incorporation of ^{13}C-labeled amino acids. J Am Chem Soc 1995; 117:7606–7610.

8. Trejo WH, Dean LD, Pluscec J, Meyers E, Brown WE. *Streptomyces laurentii*, a new species producing thiostrepton. J Antibiot 1977; 30:639–643.

9. Vandeputte J, Dutcher JD. Thiostrepton, a new antibiotic. II. Isolation and chemical characterization. Antibiot Annu 1955–1956; 560–561.

10. Cron MJ, Whitehead DF, Hooper IR, Heineman B, Lein J. Braymycin, a new antibiotic. Antibiot Chemother 1953; 6:63–67.

11. Benazet F, Cartier M, Florent J, Godard C, Jung G, Lunel J, Mancy D, Pascal C, Renaut J, Tarridec P, Theilleux J, Tissier R, Dubost M, Ninet L. Nosiheptide, a sulfur-containing peptide antibiotic isolated from *Streptomyces actuosus* 40037. Experientia 1980; 36:414–416.

12. Kleinkauf H, von Döhren H, eds. Biochemistry of Peptide Antibiotics. Berlin: Walter de Gruyter, 1991.

13. Ishihara H, Shimura K. Further evidence for the presence of a thiazoline ring in the isoleucylcysteine dipeptide intermediate in bacitracin biosynthesis. FEBS Lett 1988; 226:319–323.

14. Yorgey P, Lee J, Kordel J, Vivas E, Warner P, Jebaratnam D, Kolter R. Posttranslational modifications in microcin B17 define an additional class of DNA gyrase inhibitor. Proc Natl Acad Sci USA 1994; 91:4519–4523.

15. Tori K, Tokura K, Okabe K, Ebata M, Otsuka H, Lukacs G. Carbon-13 NMR studies of peptide antibiotics, thiostrepton and siomycin A: The structure relationship. Tetrahed Lett 1976; 3:185–188.

16. Hensens OD, Albers-Schönberg G. Total structure of the highly modified peptide antibiotic components of thiopeptin. J Antibiot 1983; 36:814–831.

17. Shimanaka K, Takahashi Y, Iinuma H, Naganawa H, Takeuchi T. Novel antibiotics, amythiamicins. III. Structure elucidations of amythiamicins A, B and C. J Antibiot 1994; 47:1153–1159.

18. Thompson CJ, Ward JM, Hopwood DA. DNA cloning in *Streptomyces*; resistance genes from antibiotic-producing species. Nature 1980; 286:525–527.

19. Hopwood DA, Bibb MJ, Chater KF, Kieser T. Plasmid and phage vectors for gene cloning and analysis in *Streptomyces*. Meth Enzymol 1987; 153:116–166.

20. Cundliffe E, Thompson J. Concerning the mode of action of micrococcin upon bacterial protein synthesis. Eur J Biochem 1981; 118:47–52.

21. Cundliffe E, Thompson J. The mode of action of nosiheptide (multhiomycin) and the mechanism of resistance in the producing organism. J Gen Microbiol 1981; 126:185–192.

22. Egebjerg J, Douthwaite S, Garrett RA. Antibiotic interactions at the GTPase-associated centre within *Escherichia coli* 23S rRNA. EMBO J 1989; 8:607–611.

23. Anborgh PH, Parmeggiani A. New antibiotic that acts specifically on the GTP-bound form of elongation factor Tu. EMBO J 1991; 10:779–784.

24. Shimanaka K, Iinuma H, Hamada M, Ikeno S, Tsuchiya KS, Arita M, Hori M. Novel antibiotics, amythiamicins. IV. A mutation in the elongation factor Tu gene in a resistant mutant of *B. subtilis*. J Antibiot 1995; 48:182–184.

25. Cashel M, Rudd KE. The stringent response. Neidhardt FC, ed. *Escherichia coli* and *Salmonella typhimurium*: Cellular and Molecular biology. Washington, D.C.: American Society for Microbiology, 1987:1410–1438.

26. Ochi K. Metabolic initiation of differentiation and secondary metabolism by *Streptomyces griseus*: Significance of the stringent response (ppGpp) and GTP content in relation to A factor. J Bacteriol 1987; 169:3608–3616.

27. Chakraburtty R, White J, Takano E, Bibb M. Cloning, characterization and disruption of a (p)ppGpp synthetase gene (*relA*) of *Streptomyces coelicolor* A3(2). Mol Microbiol 1996; 19:357–368.

28. Ochi K. A relaxed (rel) mutant of *Streptomyces coelicolor* A3(2) with a missing ribosomal protein lacks the ability to accumulate ppGpp, A-factor and prodigiosin. J Gen Microbiol 1990; 136:2405–2412.

29. Ochi K. *Streptomyces relC* mutants with an altered ribosomal protein ST-L11 and genetic analysis of a *Streptomyces griseus relC* mutant. J Bacteriol 1990; 172:4008–4016.

30. Ochi K. The *tsr* gene-coding plasmid pIJ702 prevents thiopeptin from inhibiting ppGpp synthesis in *Streptomyces lividans*. FEMS Microbiol Lett 1989; 52:219–223.

31. Murakami T, Holt TG, Thompson CJ. Thiostrepton-induced gene expression in *Streptomyces lividans*. J Bacteriol 1989; 171:1459–1466.

32. Holmes DJ, Caso JL, Thompson CJ. Autogenous transcriptional activation of a thiostrepton-induced gene in *Streptomyces lividans*. EMBO J 1993; 12:3183–3191.

33. Yun BS, Hidaka T, Furihata K, Seto H. Microbial metabolites with *tip*A promoter inducing activity. II. Geninthiocin, a novel thiopeptide produced by *Streptomyces* sp. DD84. J Antibiot 1994; 47:969–975.

34. Yun BS, Hidaka T, Furihata K, Seto H. Promothiocins A and B novel thiopeptides with a *tip*A promoter inducing activity produced by *Streptomyces* sp. SF2741. J Antibiot 1994; 47:510–514.

35. Yun BS, Hidaka T, Furihata K, Seto H. Microbial metabolites with *tip*A promoter inducing activity. III. Thioxamycin and its novel derivative, thioactin, two thiopeptides produced by *Streptomyces* sp. DP94. J Antibiot 1994; 47:1541–1545.

36. Summers AO. Untwist and shout: A heavy metal-responsive transcriptional regulator. J Bacteriol 1992; 174:3097–3101.

37. Chiu ML, Folcher M, Griffin P, Holt T, Klatt T, Thompson CJ. Characterization of the covalent binding of thiostrepton to a thiostrepton-induced protein from *Streptomyces lividans*. Biochem 1996; 35:2332–2341.

38. Cundliffe E. Thiostrepton and related antibiotics. Hahn EF, ed. Mechanism of Action of Antibacterial Agents. New York: Springer-Verlag, 1979:329–342.

39. Thompson J, Cundliffe E. Resistance to thiostrepton, siomycin, and sporangiomycin in actinomycetes that produce them. J Bacteriol 1980; 142:455–461.

40. Smith TM, Jiang Y-F, Shipley P, Floss HG. The thiostrepton-resistance-encoding gene in *Streptomyces laurentii* is located within a cluster of ribosomal protein operons. Gene 1995; 164:137–142.

41. Dosch DC, Strohl WR, Floss HG. Molecular cloning of the nosiheptide resistance gene from *Streptomyces actuosus* ATCC 25421. Biochem Biophys Res Commun 1988; 156:517–523.

42. Bibb MJ, Ward JM, Cohen SN. Nucleotide sequences encoding and promoting expression of three antibiotic resistance genes indigenous to *Streptomyces*. Mol Gen Genet 1985; 199:26–36.

43. Li Y, Dosch DC, Strohl WR, Floss HG. Nucleotide sequence and transcriptional analysis of the nosiheptide-resistance gene from *Streptomyces actuosus*. Gene 1990; 91:9–17.

44. Worley KC, Wiese BA, Smith RF. BEAUTY: An enhanced BLAST-based search tool that integrates multiple biological information resources into sequence similarity search results. Genome Res 1995; 5:173–184.

45. Altschul SF, Gish W, Miller W, Myers E, Lipman DJ. Basic local alignment search tool. J Mol Biol 1990; 215:403–410.

46. Koonin EV, Rudd KE. SpoU protein of *Escherichia coli* belongs to a new family of putative rRNA methylases. Nucl Acids Res 1993; 21:5519.

47. Wu-Baer F, Lane WS, Gaynor RB. The cellular factor TRP-185 regulates RNA polymerase II binding to HIV-1 TAR RNA. EMBO J 1995; 14:5995–6009.

48. Bechthold A, Floss HG. Overexpression of the thiostrepton-resistance gene from *Streptomyces azureus* in *Escherichia coli* and characterization of recognition sites of the 23S rRNA A1067 2'-methyltransferase in the guanosine triphosphate center of 23S ribosomal RNA. Eur J Biochem 1994; 224:431–437.

49. Dixon PD, Beven JE, Cundliffe E. Properties of the ribosomes of antibiotic producers: Effects of thiostrepton and micrococcin on the organisms which produce them. Antimicrob Agents Chemother 1975; 7:850–855.

50. Wienen R, Ehrlich R, Stöffler-Meilicke M, Stöffler G, Smith I, Weiss D, Vince R, Pestka S. Ribosomal protein alterations in thiostrepton- and micrococcin-resistant mutants of *Bacillus subtilis*. J Biol Chem 1979; 254:8031–8041.

51. Cundliffe E, Dixon P, Stark M, Stöffler G, Ehrlich R, Stöffler-Meilicke M, Cannon M. Ribosomes in thiostrepton-resistant mutants of *Bacillus megaterium* lacking a single 50S subunit protein. J Mol Biol 1979; 132:235–252.

52. Houk DR. Studies on the biosynthesis of the modified-peptide antibiotic, nosiheptide. Ph.D. dissertation, The Ohio State University, 1986.

53. Smith TM. Genetic and biochemical studies of thiostrepton biosynthesis in *Streptomyces laurentii*. Ph.D. dissertation, University of Washington, 1993.

54. Suzuki T, Yamane T, Shimizu S. Mass production of thiostrepton by fed-batch culture of *Streptomyces laurentii* with pH-stat modal feeding of multi-substrate. Appl Microbiol Biotechnol 1987; 25:526–531.

55. Mocek U, Zeng Z, O'Hagan D, Zhou P, Fan L-DG, Beale JM, Floss HG. Biosynthesis of the modified peptide antibiotic thiostrepton in *Streptomyces azureus* and *Streptomyces laurentii*. J Am Chem Soc 1993; 115:7992–8001.

56. Mocek U, Knaggs AR, Tsuchiya R, Nguyen T, Beale JM, Floss HG. Biosynthesis of the modified peptide antibiotic nosiheptide in *Streptomyces actuosus*. J Am Chem Soc 1993; 115:7557–7568.

57. Frenzel T, Zhou P, Floss HG. Formation of 2-methyltryptophan in the biosynthesis of thiostrepton: Isolation of S-adenosylmethionine:tryptophan 2-methyltransferase. Arch Biochem Biophys 1990; 278:35–40.

58. Houck DR, Chen L-C, Keller PJ, Beale JM, Floss HG. Biosynthesis of the modified peptide antibiotic nosiheptide in *Streptomyces actuosus*. J Am Chem Soc 1988; 110:5800–5806.

59. Yost GS. Mechanisms of 3-methylindole pneumotoxicity. Chem Res Toxicol 1989; 2:273–279.

60. Hurst A. Biosynthesis of the antibiotic nisin by whole *Streptococcus lactis* organisms. J Gen Microbiol 1966; 44:209–220.

61. Ingram I. A ribosomal mechanism for the synthesis of peptides related to nisin. Biochim Biophys Acta 1970; 224:263–265.

62. Woodman RH. Molecular and biochemical studies on thiopeptide antibiotics. Ph.D. dissertation, The Ohio State University, 1991.

63. Marahiel MA. Multidomain enzymes involved in peptide synthesis. FEBS Lett 1992; 307:40–43.

64. Hopwood DA, Sherman DH. Molecular genetics of polyketides and its comparison to fatty acid biosynthesis. Annu Rev Genet 1990; 24:37–66.

65. Stachelhaus T, Marahiel MA. Modular structure of genes encoding multifunctional peptide synthetases required for non-ribosomal peptide synthesis. FEMS Microbiol Lett 1995; 125:3–14.

66. Weber G, Schorgendorfer K, Schneider SE, Leitner E. The peptide synthetase catalyzing cyclosporine production in *Tolypocladium niveum* is encoded by a giant 45.8-kilobase open reading frame. Curr Genet 1994; 26:120–125.

67. MacNeil DJ, Occi JL, Gewain KM, MacNeil T, Gibbons PH, Ruby CL, Danis SJ. Complex organization of the *Streptomyces avermitilis* genes encoding the avermectin polyketide-synthase. Gene 1992; 115:119–125.

68. Bierman M, Logan R, O'Brien K, Seno ET, Rao RN, Schoner BE. Plasmid cloning vectors for the conjugal transfer of DNA from *Escherichia coli* to *Streptomyces spp*. Gene 1992; 116:43–49.

69. Honor'e N, Bergh S, Chanteau S, Doucet PF, Eiglmeier K, Garnier T, Georges C, Launois P, Limpaiboon T, Newton S, Niang K, del Portillo P, Ramesh GR, Reddi P, Ridel PR, Sittisom-

but N, Wu-Hunter S, Cole ST. Nucleotide sequence of the first cosmid from the *Mycobacterium leprae* genome project: Structure and function of the *Rif-Str* regions. Mol Microbiol 1993; 7:207–214.

70. Lindahl L, Zengel JM. Ribosomal genes in *Escherichia coli*. Annu Rev Genet 1986; 20:297–326.

71. Medigue C, Viari A, Henaut A, Danchin A. *Escherichia coli* molecular map (1500 kbp): Update II. Mol Microbiol 1991; 5:2629–2640.

72. Ohama T, Yamao F, Muto A, Osawa S. Organization and codon usage of the streptomycin operon in *Micrococcus luteus*, a bacterium with a high genomic G+C content. J Bacteriol 1987; 169:4770–4777.

73. Ohama T, Muto A, Osawa S. Spectinomycin operon of *Micrococcus luteus*: Evolutionary implications of organization and novel codon usage. J Mol Evol 1989; 29:381–395.

74. Ohkubo S, Muto A, Kawauchi Y, Yamao F, Osawa S. The ribosomal protein gene cluster of *Mycoplasma capricolum*. Mol Gen Genet 1987; 210:314–322.

75. Li Y, Dosch DC, Woodman RH, Floss HG, Strohl WR. Transcriptional organization and regulation of the nosiheptide resistance gene from *S. actuosus*. J Indust Microbiol 1991; 8:1–12.

76. Armstrong SK, Pettis GS, Forrester LJ, McIntosh MA. The *Escherichia coli* enterobactin biosynthesis gene, *entD*: Nucleotide sequence and membrane localization of its protein product. Mol Microbiol 1989; 3:757–766.

77. Grossman TH, Tuckman M, Ellestad S, Osburne MS. Isolation and characterization of *Bacillus subtilis* genes involved in siderophore biosynthesis: Relationship between *B. subtilis sfpo* and *Escherichia coli entD* genes. J Bacteriol 1993; 175:6203–6211.

78. Borchert S, Stachelhaus T, Marahiel MA. Induction of surfactin production in *Bacillus subtilis* by *gsp*, a gene located upstream of the gramicidin S operon in *Bacillus brevis*. J Bacteriol 1994; 176:2458–2462.

79. Jiang Y-F, Storkova S, Smith TM, Floss HG. Manuscript in preparation.

80. Zalacain M, Cundliffe E. Cloning of *tlrD*, a fourth resistance gene, from the tylosin producer, *Streptomyces fradiae*. Gene 1991; 97:137–142.

81. Keller U, Kleinkauf H, Zocher R. 4-Methyl-3-hydroxyanthranilic acid activating enzyme from actinomycin-producing *Streptomyces chrysomallus*. Biochem 1984; 23:1479–1484.

82. Jones GH. Combined purification of actinomycin synthetase I and 3-hydroxyanthranilic acid 4-methyltransferase from *Streptomyces antibioticus*. J Biol Chem 1993; 268:6831–6834.

83. Glund K, Schlumbohm W, Bapat M, Keller U. Biosynthesis of quinoxaline antibiotics: Purification and characterization of the quinoxaline-2-carboxylic acid activating enzyme from *Streptomyces triostinicus*. Biochem 1990; 29:3522–3527.

84. Schlumbohm W, Keller U. Chromophore activating enzyme involved in the biosynthesis of the mikamycin B antibiotic etamycin from *Streptomyces griseoviridus*. J Biol Chem 1990; 265:2156–2161.

85. Keller U, Han M, Stöffler-Meilicke M. D-Lysergic acid activation and cell-free synthesis of D-lysergyl peptides in enzyme fraction from the ergot fungus *Claviceps purpurea*. Biochem 1988; 27:6164–6170.

86. Smith TM, Priestley ND, Knaggs AR, Nguyen T, Floss HG. 3,4-Dimethylindole-2-carboxylate and 4-(1-hydroxyethyl)quinoline-2-carboxylate activating enzymes from the nosiheptide and thiostrepton producers, *Streptomyces actuosus* and *Streptomyces laurentii*. J Chem Soc (Chem Comm) 1993; 21:1612–1614.

87. Turgay K, Marahiel MA. A general approach for identifying and cloning peptide synthetase genes. Pept Res 1994; 7:238–241.

88. Chater K. The improving prospects for yield increase by genetic engineering in antibiotic-producing *Streptomyces*. Bio/Technol 1990; 8:111–121.

14

Lipopeptide Antibiotics Produced by *Streptomyces roseosporus* and *Streptomyces fradiae*

Richard H. Baltz

Lilly Research Laboratories, Eli Lilly and Company, Indianapolis, Indiana

I. INTRODUCTION

Streptomyces roseosporus NRRL11379 produces A21978C, a complex of acidic lipopeptide antibiotics (1). The cyclic depsipeptide portion (Figure 1a) contains 13 amino acids cyclized to form a 10-amino-acid ring. The A21978C factors contain different 10-, 11-, 12-, or 13-carbon fatty acids attached to the amino-group of the terminal L-Trp (1). The fatty acid side chains are readily removed by incubation with *Actinoplanes utahensis* (2), and the cyclic peptide can be reacylated at the amino-terminus of Trp to produce semisynthetic acyl, aroyl, and extended peptide derivatives (3). The n-decanoyl analog of A21978C, LY146032 or daptomycin, is a potent antibiotic active against Gram-positive bacteria, including methicillin-resistant *Staphylococcus aureus*, methicillin-resistant *Staphylococcus epidermidis*, vancomycin-resistant enterococci, and penicillin-resistant *Streptococcus pneumoniae* (see Section IV). *Streptomyces fradiae* A54145 also produces a complex of cyclic lipopeptides containing 13 amino acids with a 10-amino-acid ring (4,5). The A54145 complex is similar to daptomycin in that different factors contain various long-chain fatty acids attached to the N-terminal Trp (Figure 1b). A54145 differs from daptomycin in that the cyclic peptide is variable in positions 12 and 13, and all four possible peptides are observed in normal fermentations (4,5).

In addition to the N-terminal Trp, A54145 contains some amino acids identical or similar to those in daptomycin in other positions, including the position 4 Thr, which participates in the ester linkage that closes the ring. A54145 factors have in vitro antibacterial properties similar to those of daptomycin (see Section IV). The fatty acyl side chains of A54145 can be removed by incubation with *A. utahensis* (6), and the N-terminal Trp can be reacylated (6), just as with the daptomycin nucleus (2,3).

The similarities in the structures of these two lipopeptides suggest that the biosynthetic pathways may have evolved from a common ancestral pathway. Thus, the study of the structural organization and physical map locations of the biosynthetic genes may provide insights into the evolution of these complex lipopeptide pathways. Further, the diversity in amino acid sequence in these related molecules suggests that further modification of the peptide portion of these cyclic peptides may generate as yet unknown, but related antibiotics—some of which may prove to be superior to either of the parent molecules. In this chapter, I summarize what is known about the genetics, biosynthesis, mode of action, and antibacterial activity of these antibiotics. I also speculate on how the activities of these molecules may be further altered by modifying the genes encoding the multienzyme peptide synthetases involved in determining the amino acid sequences of the peptide portion of the molecules.

II.   BIOSYNTHESIS OF LIPOPEPTIDES

A.   Daptomycin Biosynthesis

S. roseosporus produces A21978C, a complex of lipopeptide antibiotics highly active against Gram-positive bacteria (1). The A21978C complex was separated into three major factors, C_1, C_2, and C_3, and three minor factors, C_4, C_5, and C_0 (Table 1). All six factors contain an identical 13-amino-acid core cyclic peptide, containing 11 common L– or D–amino acids and 2 unusual amino acids, 3-methyl glutamic acid (3mGlu), and the L-tryptophan metabolite L-kynurenine (L-Kyn). Enzymatic studies employing glutamine synthetase and L-glutamic acid decarboxylase established that the stereochemistry of the glutamate analog as L-*threo*-3-methyl glutamic acid (1). The linear sequence of the peptide core was established as L-Trp–L-Asn–L-Arg–L-Thr–Gly–L-Orn–L-Asp–D-Ala–L-Asp–Gly–D-Ser–L-3mGlu–L-Kyn. The cyclic depsipeptide is formed by an ester linkage between L-Kyn and the L-Thr hydroxyl-group (Figure 1). The factors C_1, C_2, and C_3 were shown to contain *anteiso*-undecanoyl (C11), *iso*-dodecanoyl (C12), and *anteiso*-tridecanoyl (C13) side chains, respectively. The minor components C_0, C_4, and C_5 contain C10, C12, and C12 fatty acids (1). The ratios of factors C_1, C_2, and C_3, which are normally about 1:1.5:1, can be modulated by adding different branched-chain amino acids to the fermentation medium. Factor C_2 can be increased by adding valine to the fermentation, whereas factors C_1 and C_3 can be increased by adding isoleucine (7). The authors concluded that the branched-chain amino acids served as precursors to provide the branched-chain fatty acid primers for the biosynthesis of the fatty acid side chains of the A21978C factors.

Daptomycin, which contains the C10 fatty acid decanoic acid, is normally produced by *S. roseosporus* in trace amounts. Huber et al. (8) have shown that decanoic acid mixed 1:1 (v:v) in methyl oleate can be fed continuously to fermenters at rates that avoid the accumulation of decanoic acid, which is normally toxic to *S. roseosporus*. Under these conditions, *S. roseosporus* A21978.65 produced over 900 μg/ml of daptomycin directly, and less than 400 μg/ml of factors containing other fatty acid side chains. The process was modified for large-scale production, and daptomycin yields of >1000 μg/ml representing 77% of total A21978C factors have been reported (9). High yields of daptomycin can also be produced by feeding caproic acid (10). This process is much simpler and less costly than the process that combines enzymatic removal of the fatty acid side chains and chemical reacylation with decanoic acid (see Section III).

B.   A54145 Biosynthesis

The cyclic lipopeptide antibiotic complex A54145 is produced by *S. fradiae* A54145 (NRRL 18158). The complex has eight factors composed of four different cyclic peptides

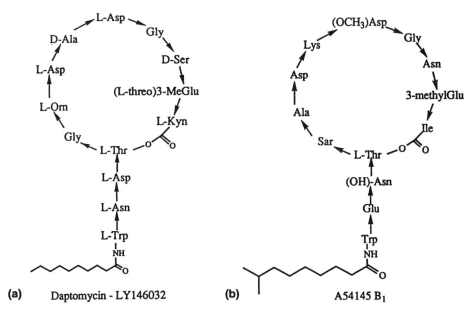

(a)   Daptomycin - LY146032   **(b)**   A54145 B₁

Figure I   Structures of daptomycin and A54145B₁. Daptomycin (a) contains an *N*-decanoyl side chain. The A21978C factors produced in standard fermentations contain the fatty acyl side chains shown in Table 1. A54145B₁ (b) is the most abundant factor produced in standard fermentations. The other A54145 factors are shown in Table 2.

Table I   Lipopeptide A21978C Factors Produced by *S. roseosporus*

Factor	Fatty acid
C_0	Unidentified (10 carbon)
C_1	anteiso-Undecanoyl
C_2	iso-Dodecanoyl
C_3	anteiso-Tridecanoyl
C_4	Unidentified (12 carbon)
C_5	Unidentified (12 carbon)

Data from Ref. 1.

and three different lipid side chains (4,5). The major peptide nucleus has the sequence Trp–Glu–hAsn–Thr–Sar–Ala–Asp–Lys–OmAsp–Gly–Asp–3mGlu–Ile (where hAsn = hydroxy Asn, OmAsp = hydroxymethyl Asp, and 3mGlu = 3-methyl Glu). The peptide is cyclized by an ester linkage between the carboxy-group of Ile and the Thr hydroxy-group. The four different peptide structures are identical in the first 11 amino acids, but have 3mGlu or Glu at position 12 and Ile or Val at position 13. The different peptide structures coupled with three different possible lipid side chains account for the eight factors identified in fermentation broths (Table 2). (Presumably, the four missing factors were present in such low amounts that they were not observed by the high-performance liquid chromatography [HPLC] system used.)

Table 2 Lipopeptide A54145 Factors Produced by
S. fradiae NRRL18158

| Factor | Amino acid at position: | | Fatty acid |
	12	13	
A	Glu	Ile	8-Methylnonanoyl
A_1	Glu	Ile	*n*-Decanoyl
B	3mGlu	Ile	*n*-Decanoyl
B_1	3mGlu	Ile	8-Methylnonanoyl
C	3mGlu	Val	8-Methyldecanoyl
D	Glu	Ile	8-Methyldecanoyl
E	3mGlu	Ile	8-Methyldecanoyl
F	Glu	Val	8-Methyldecanoyl

Data from Ref. 4.

   S. fradiae NRRL 18158 produces >1 mg/m of A54145 factors in a glucose-fed complex medium (4). Factors A and B_1, which differed from each other at position 12, were the most abundant factors produced. Factor A, containing Glu at position 12, was synthesized more rapidly than B_1 early in the fermentation, then stopped accumulating at about 135 hr. Factor B_1, containing 3mGlu, continued to be synthesized up to 180 hr, and it was the most abundant factor at the end of the fermentation. Since A54145 is synthesized by a thiotemplate mechanism by a large multisubunit peptide synthetase (see below), the accumulation of factors A and B_1 suggests several possibilities. One is that early accumulation of factor A and late accumulation of factor B_1 are due to a precursor–product relationship between factor A and factor B_1, and that the methylation of Glu occurs after the peptide is synthesized. A second possibility is that Glu is converted to 3mGlu in the cytoplasm, and that the peptide synthetase can accept either amino acid for incorporation. The change in rates of biosynthesis of factors A and B_1 would reflect the relative availability of Glu and 3mGlu during the course of the fermentation—the latter predominating late in the fermentation. A third possible explanation is that methylation of Glu occurs after binding to the peptide synthetase. In this case, the relative amounts of factors A and B_1 could be influenced by the level of methyl donor, presumably S-adenosyl methionine, during the fermentation. Late accumulation of factor B_1 would reflect a higher level of methyl donor late in the fermentation. The cloning and sequence analysis of genes involved in A54145 biosynthesis, coupled with gene disruption analysis, should shed light on this question.
   The substitution of Val for Ile at position 13 is a simpler problem. In this case, factors containing Val are normally produced in very low quantities, and they are not detectable until 90 hr in the fermentation (4). However, the ratios of the different A54145 factors containing Ile or Val can be altered by feeding the amino acid precursors (11). The feeding of Val had two effects. It caused an increase in factors containing Val at position 13 from 10 to 54%, and it caused the accumulation of nearly 100% of factors containing 8-methylnonanoyl side chains. The feeding of Ile caused a reduction in factors containing Val at position 13 from 10 to 0%, and it caused an increase in factors containing the 8-methyldecanoyl side chain. These results indicate that the peptide synthetase module that catalyzes the binding and addition of amino acid for position 13 has

relatively loose substrate specificity, and can bind, activate, and couple Val or Ile to the growing chain. Furthermore, the enzyme that carries out the formation of the ester bond with Thr at position 4 can tolerate Val or Ile as substrates in the ring closure reaction. The distribution of fatty acid side chains can also be modulated by feeding different fatty acids. Continuous feeding of ethyl caprate increased the factors containing the *n*-decanoyl side chain from 13 to 82% at the expense of factors containing 8-methyl-nonanoyl or 8-methyldecanoyl side chains. The addition of methyl oleate, decyl aldehyde, or decyl alcohol gave a similar response. The feeding of other shorter-chain fatty acids led to the production of novel derivatives containing shorter side chains. For example, feeding of hexanoic acid resulted in 96% of factors containing C6, and feeding nonanoic acid gave 100% of factors containing C9. Therefore, the enzymatic step involved in the coupling of the fatty acid to the amino-group of Trp is indiscriminant in its specificity for fatty acids with chain lengths of C6 to C11.

C. Peptide Synthetase Structure and Function

Like many other linear and cyclic peptide secondary metabolites, daptomycin and A54145 are produced by a nonribosomal thiotemplate mechanism. The peptide synthetases involved in these processes are generally very large, being composed of one or more multienzyme subunits (12–19), and contain about 125 kDa per amino acid incorporated. By analogy, the peptide synthetases for daptomycin and A54145 should be about 1.6 mDa in size. Wessels et al. (20) have been studying the peptide synthetases involved in daptomycin and A54145 biosynthesis. They identified high-molecular-weight proteins from transition phase or early stationary phase cultures of S. *roseosporus* and S. *fradiae* that reacted to antibodies prepared against the *Streptomyces chrysomallus* actinomycin synthetase 2 or to antibodies prepared against the SGTTG sequence conserved in adenylate-forming enzymes. Their data suggest that the daptomycin and A54145 synthetases have similar structures. Each multienzyme appears to have three subunits, two of about 700 kDa and one about 250 kDa. The 250 kDa subunit of the daptomycin synthetase was purified and shown to activate L-Kyn. This suggests that the 250 kDa subunits contain the two domains responsible for the addition of the final two amino acids. A number of other amino acids were activated by the larger subunits, and the data indicated that only L–amino acids were activated, so that epimerizations must occur on the peptide synthetase as observed with other peptide synthetases. Also, N-methylation of Gly must occur on the enzyme, since Gly but not sarcosine (Sar) was activated by the A54145 synthetase. Further work is needed to define what domains are associated with the individual high-molecular-weight subunits. Gene disruption studies may be particularly useful, since they would eliminate the need to purify the individual subunits to homogeneity.

III. ENZYMATIC AND CHEMICAL MODIFICATION OF LIPOPEPTIDES

To study the structure–activity relationships of the fatty acyl side chains, it was desirable to have a method to remove the natural fatty acids from the A21978C complex of antibiotics. The fatty acid side chains could not be removed chemically without significant destruction to the peptide core. However, the side chains were readily removed by incubation of the complex with a culture of A. *utahensis* (2,3). Enzymatic deacylation resulted in complete loss in antibacterial activity (2). Deacylation also occurred with A21978C complex containing *tert*-butoxycarbonyl (*t*-BOC)-protected amino function of the side chain of Orn. Deacylation occurred most efficiently with *A. utahensis* cultures grown for 65 to 85 hr, and conversion efficiencies of ~85% were achieved in 2 hr incubation at pH 7.0–8.0. Conversion rates of >600 µg/ml per hr were achieved. Deacylase activity was also observed with three other *Actinoplanes* strains and a strain of *Streptosporangium roseum*.

The ability to block the amino function of Orn, then deacylate the *t*-BOC-protected nucleus, has facilitated the development of many A21978C analogs containing modifications at the *N*-terminal Trp. Semisynthetic derivatives containing novel fatty acyl, aroyl, and extended peptide side chains were readily deblocked by trifluoroacetic acid treatment (3). Subsequent biological studies identified the *n*-decanoyl derivative, daptomycin, as a candidate for clinical development (see Section IV).

Similar studies have shown that the ε*N*-BOC-L-Lys-protected A54145 complex can be deacylated by *A. utahensis*, the *N*-terminus of Trp reacylated with different fatty acids, and the protected Lys deblocked to give novel semisynthetic antibiotics for in vitro and in vivo testing (6). Several of these derivatives are discussed in Section IV.

IV.   ANTIBACTERIAL ACTIVITY OF DAPTOMYCIN, A54145, AND RELATED LIPOPEPTIDES

A.   In Vitro Studies

Table 3 summarizes the in vitro antibacterial activity of daptomycin against Gram-positive bacteria. Daptomycin is very active against most Gram-positive pathogens, including strict anaerobes, enterococci, staphylococci, and streptococci. Daptomycin is active against antibiotic-resistant pathogens, including methicillin-resistant *S. aureus* and *S. epidermidis*, penicillin-resistant *S. pneumoniae*, and vancomycin-resistant *Enterococcus faecalis* and *Enterococcus faecium* (Table 4). This reflects its novel mechanism of action, which differs from that of β-lactam and glycopeptide antibiotics (see Section V). Daptomycin is bactericidal in Gram-positive pathogens, including enterococci (26,36–38), and the rate of killing is dose-dependent (39–43). Antibacterial activity of daptomycin is calcium-dependent, and the presence of serum or albumin decreases the bactericidal activity of daptomycin (36,44–46). Daptomycin is >90% bound to albumin in serum or in media containing physiological concentrations of albumin (46–48). This work will be discussed in Section IV.C in relation to daptomycin clinical trials. Daptomycin shows synergy with streptomycin (38), gentamicin (49), and tobramycin (49) in its bactericidal activity against enterococci. It also shows synergy with imipenen, amikacin, netilmicin, and fosfomycin in its bactericidal effects on methicillin-sensitive and -resistant strains of *S. aureus* and *S. epidermidis* (50). Interestingly, daptomycin seems to protect experimental animals against tobramycin and gentamicin renal toxicity (51–54).

The in vitro antibacterial activities of the A54145 factors are similar to those of the A21978C factors, and minimal inhibitory concentrations (MICs) ranged from 0.5 to 32 µg/ml against various strains of *S. aureus*, *S. epidermidis*, *Streptococcus pyogenes*, and enterococci (55). Table 5 shows in vitro activities of a series of A54145A derivatives containing different fatty acid side chains compared with those of a comparable series of A21978C derivatives, including daptomycin. The A21978C series were generally 2- to 16-fold more active when comparisons are made between compounds containing identical fatty acid side chains. However, A54145A containing C14 chain length was at least

Table 3 *In Vitro* Antibacterial Activity of Daptomycin Against Gram-Positive Bacteria

Microorganism (no. of strains)	MIC$_{50}$ (µg/ml)	References
Actinomyces spp. (12)	0.25	21
Bifidobacterium spp. (10)	0.5	21
Clostridium difficile (170)	0.12	21–23
Clostridium perfringens (40)	0.25, 4.0	21, 24
Corynebacterium jeikeium (18)	0.12	24
Enterococcus faecalis (199)	0.5–2.0	23–27
Enterococcus faecium (10)	4.0	25
Eubacterium aerofaciens (10)	1.0	21
Eubacterium lentum (10)	4.0	21
Lactobacillus acidophilus (13)	2.0	21
Lactobacillus casei (18)	1.0	21
Lactobacillus plantarum (18)	1.0	21
Lactococcus spp. (32)	0.5	28
Leuconostoc spp. (13)	0.5	28
Listeria monocytogenes (57)	1.0–8.0	24, 25, 29–31
Pediococcus (6)	0.5–1.0	28
Peptostreptococcus anaerobius (16)	0.12	21
Peptostreptococcus asaccharolyticus (32)	0.12	21
Peptostreptococcus magnus (11)	0.12	21
Peptostreptococcus micros (12)	0.12	21
Peptostreptococcus prevotii (9)	0.12	21
Peptostreptococcus productus (9)	0.12	21
Propionibacterium acnes (43)	0.5, 4.0	21, 24
Staphylococcus aureus (436)	0.25–0.5	23–25, 29, 30, 32
Staphylococcus epidermidis (335)	0.25–0.5	23–25, 29, 30, 32
Staphylococcus haemolyticus (50)	0.25	30–32
Staphylococcus hominis (20)	0.25	32
Staphylococcus saprophyticus (20)	0.25	32
Streptococcus agalactiae (37)	0.13–0.5	24–26, 32
Streptococcus avium (10)	1.0	25
Streptococcus bovis (10)	0.25	24
Streptococcus lactis (2)	0.25	21
Streptococcus pneumoniae (91)	0.06–0.5	24–26, 29, 30
Streptococcus pyogenes (60)	0.06–0.25	24, 26, 32
Streptococcus sangius (7)	0.5	31

as active as daptomycin. The A54145A derivatives have not been studied extensively for their activity against an extended set of Gram-positive bacteria because of their disappointing in vivo activities, discussed below.

B. In Vivo Studies

Many derivatives of A21978C have been examined for their in vivo activities against *S. aureus* and *S. pyogenes* using mouse protection tests (3). Generally, derivatives containing relatively short-chain fatty acid side chains (C6–C9) were less active than daptomycin (C10) and derivatives containing C11–C14. However, compounds containing C11–C14 were progressively more toxic to mice as the side chain length increased (see Table 6 for

Table 4 *In Vitro* Antibacterial Activity of Daptomycin Against Antibiotic-Resistant Pathogens

Microorganism (no. of strains)	Antibiotic resistance[a]	MIC or MIC$_{50}$[b]	References
Enterococcus faecalis (2)	Van[S] Erm[S]	2	33
Enterococcus faecalis (1) BM4166	Van[R] Erm[R]	2	33
Enterococcus faecalis (1)	Van[S] Erm[S]	0.5	34
Enterococcus faecalis (1)	Van[R] Erm[R]	0.5	34
Enterococcus faecium (1)	Van[S] Erm[S]	2	33
Enterococcus faecium (1)	Van[S] Erm[R]	2	33
Enterococcus faecium (1)	Van[R] Erm[S]	2	33
Enterococcus faecium (1)	Van[R] Erm[R]	2	33
Staphylococcus aureus (240)	Mcn[S]	0.12–0.5	24–27, 29, 32, 35
Staphylococcus aureus (261)	Mcn[R]	0.25–0.5	24–27, 29, 32, 35
Staphylococcus epidermidis (189)	Mcn[S]	0.12–0.25	23, 24, 26, 27, 29, 32, 35
Staphylococcus epidermidis (176)	Mcn[R]	0.25	23, 24, 26, 27, 29, 32, 35
Staphylococcus haemolyticus (60)	Ocn[S]	0.25, 0.5	31, 32
Staphylococcus haemolyticus (85)	Ocn[R]	0.25, 0.5	31, 32
Streptococcus pneumoniae (10)	Pen[R]	0.5	25

[a] Van, vancomycin; Erm, erythromycin; Mcn, Methycillin; Ocn, oxacillin; Pen, penicillin;[S], sensitive;[R], resistant.
[b] MIC is given for single isolates; MIC$_{50}$ is given for multiple isolates.

Table 5 *In Vitro* Activities of Related Lipopeptide Antibiotics Against Gram-Positive Pathogens

Cyclic peptide nucleus	Lipid side chain	MIC (µg/ml)		
		S. aureus	*S. epidermidis*	*E. faecalis*
A21978C	Nonanoyl	8	8	128
A21978C	Decanoyl	0.5	0.5	16
A21978C	Undecanoyl	0.25	0.5	2
A21978C	Dodecanoyl	0.5	0.5	4
A21978C	Tetradecanoyl	0.5	2	0.5
A54145A	Nonanoyl	32	16	128
A54145A	Decanoyl	8	4	64
A54145A	Undecanoyl	2	2	16
A54154A	Dodecanoyl	1	1	4
A54145A	Tetradecanoyl	0.25	0.5	2

Data from Refs. 3 and 55.

typical results). Calculation of the relative therapeutic index (mouse lethal dose/efficacious dose [LD$_{50}$/ED$_{50}$]) suggests that the C10 derivative (daptomycin) is superior to the others. By comparison, the A54145 derivatives were generally much less active in the mouse ED$_{50}$ tests, but they showed similar levels of toxicity in the mouse LD$_{50}$ tests. Thus, the relative therapeutic indexes of the A54145 derivatives are roughly 100-fold lower than that of daptomycin. For example, the dodecanoyl derivative of A54145A, which was only 2-fold less active than daptomycin in vitro against *S. aureus* and *S. epi-*

Table 6 Comparison of *In Vivo* Activities of Selected Lipopeptide Antibiotics Against *S. pyogenes*

Compound	Mouse ED_{50}	Mouse LD_{50}	Relative therapeutic index (LD_{50}/ED_{50})
A21978C$_1$	0.064	>600	>9,375
A21978C$_2$	0.03	175	5,833
A21978C$_3$	0.032	75	2,344
A21978C heptanoyl	1.49	>600	>402
A21978C octanoyl	0.65	>600	>923
A21978C nonanoyl	0.14	>600	>4,286
A21978C decanoyl	0.03	600	20,000
A21978C undecanoyl	>0.06	450	<7,500
A21978C dodecanoyl	0.05	144	2,880
A54145A nonanoyl	10.06	>500	>47
A54145A decanoyl	5.0	>500	>100
A54145A undecanoyl	1.6	>500	>313
A54145A dodecanoyl	1.2	321	268
A54145F decanoyl	10.08	>500	>46
A54145B decanoyl	0.94	28	30

Data from Refs. 3 and 55. See Table 1 for A21978C$_1$, C$_2$, and C$_3$ structures.

dermidis and 4-fold more active against *E. faecalis*, (Table 5) had a relative therapeutic index against *S. pyogenes* 75-fold lower than that of daptomycin (Table 6). The data suggest that the mouse toxicity is determined primarily by the fatty acid side chain length, and the in vivo antibacterial activity is determined by a combination of the amino acid sequence of the depsipeptide and the fatty acid side chain length.

Daptomycin-treated *Clostridium difficile* colitis was examined in a hamster model (56). Daptomycin was equal in in vitro activity to vancomycin, but it was 100 times as active as vancomyin in vivo in this model. The authors suggested that the difference in in vivo efficacy may be due to the bactericidal activity of daptomycin. Daptomycin has also been shown to treat *S. aureus* endocarditis in a rabbit model, and these studies will be discussed in Section IV.D in the context of the human clinical studies.

C. Clinical Studies

Daptomycin was shown to be well tolerated in normal human volunteers when given intraveniously in a 30 or 60 min infusion at 1 or 2 mg/kg every 24 hr (41,57). Woodworth et al. (58) also studied the safety, pharmacokinetics, and disposition of daptomycin in healthy volunteers. They showed that in single intravenous doses infused over 30 min, daptomycin was well tolerated at 0.5 to 6.0 mg/kg per day. An average of 96.4% of daptomycin was bound to protein in the serum. About 78% of radiolabeled daptomycin was recovered in the urine, but about one-third of the radioisotope was present in uncharacterized metabolites lacking antibacterial activity. The relatively long serum half life ($T_{1/2}$) of ~8 hr and the high serum levels of daptomycin achieved at doses of 4 or 6 mg/kg indicated that adequate antibacterial levels can be achieved at 95% serum binding. Direct tests of serum samples for antibacterial activity against *S. aureus* and *E. faecalis* confirmed this. The authors cautioned that the high protein binding and large molecular size of daptomycin may limit the distribution of daptomycin out of the plasma, and so daptomycin treatment of deep-seated infections, such as bone infections and endocarditis, may have limited effectiveness.

At a dose of 2 mg/kg every 24 hr, daptomycin was shown to be effective in treating a variety of Gram-positive infections (59). In another study, daptomycin given at a dose of 3 mg/kg every 12 hr was shown to be effective in treating Gram-positive bacteremias and endocarditis caused by Gram-positive pathogens (including *E. faecalis*) other than *S. aureus* (60). Only two of seven patients with *S. aureus* endocarditis had successful outcomes. Five patients were discontinued from the study because of adverse effects. In another study, daptomycin at 2 mg/kg once a day failed to treat two very seriously ill patients with Gram-positive infections (61). It was suggested in the latter two studies that higher doses of daptomycin would be required to treat *S. aureus* endocarditis and severely ill patients. However, the occasional adverse effects noted at a dose of 3 mg/kg every 12 hr seemed to preclude raising the dose further, and clinical trials were stopped.

Rybak et al. (46), during the clinical evaluation of a higher-dose regimen of daptomycin, observed that within a group of intravenous drug abusers, daptomycin peak serum concentrations were lower and volumes of distribution were higher than those reported in healthy volunteers. They also noted that serum albumin levels tended to be low in this group. They noted that patient-specific variability that may lead to lower than expected peak daptomycin concentrations, as exemplified by intravenous drug abusers, coupled with high serum binding, may impair the efficacy of the drug, and this may have contributed to some failures in clinical trials. They also showed that the bactericidal activity of daptomycin is greater in exponentially growing *S. aureus* cultures than in stationary phase cultures, and that this may be an additional factor in the poor efficacy of daptomycin in treating *S. aureus* endocarditis.

Lee et al. (62) studied serum binding in six human volunteers given an intravenous infusion of daptomycin at 3 mg/kg, and demonstrated that the average binding was 90%. They noted that the total serum concentration of daptomycin was about 30 µg/ml 30 min after infusion. However, the unbound daptomycin dropped to 0.37 µg/ml by 12 hr. This was below the MIC for enterococci and close to the MIC for staphylococci. They suggested that the serum binding may have been part of the reason that clinical failures were observed in the once-a-day protocol using 2 mg/kg, and that higher daptomycin concentrations at more frequent dosing intervals would be needed to maintain adequate unbound concentrations of daptomycin.

D.   Postclinical Studies

Hanberger et al. (45) showed that in the presence of physiological concentrations of albumin and Ca^{2+}, the MICs and postantibiotic effects (PAEs) of daptomycin increased about two-fold against *S. aureus* and *E. faecalis*. This effect appears to be due to the binding of daptomycin to albumin, which has been shown to be >90% in other studies. However, the PAEs at clinically achievable concentrations were still >6 hr. The authors suggested that the low dose concentrations achieved in the suspended clinical trials of daptomycin may not have been sufficient to eradicate the susceptible infecting organisms, but the failure may also have been due to insufficient Ca^{2+} concentrations at the infectious foci, thus reducing daptomycin antibacterial activity.

Garrison et al. (44) set up an in vitro model to assess the effects of serum albumin on the killing rate of an *S. aureus* strain isolated from a patient unsuccessfully treated by daptomycin in a clinical trial. High and low dose regimens were tested in the model. They showed that the killing rate was reduced 3-fold in the presence of albumin in the high-dose daptomycin simulation and 10-fold in the low-dose simulation. They concluded that the presence of albumin can dramatically decrease the activity of daptomycin against S. aureus, and that the magnitude of the loss is related to daptomycin concentration. They also concluded that larger daily doses of daptomycin than those used in the early clinical trials of daptomycin (2 mg/kg per day; see Section IV.C) are more likely to be successful in the management of bacteremia and endocarditis in humans.

In an attempt to understand the treatment failures in the phase II clinical trial of daptomycin, Lamp et al. (47) carried out studies to explore the effects of inoculum size, growth phase, and pH on the bactericidal activity of daptomycin in serum. They noted that S. aureus endocarditis represents an infection characterized by a high bacterial inoculum, impaired host defense, and low metabolic activity in a nutritionally deficient environment. They showed that the MICs of daptomycin increased by 3- to 4-fold when inoculum size was increased from 5×10^5 to 1×10^7 colony forming units (CFU). They also confirmed earlier reports (39,40,42,44–46) that daptomycin shows an increase in bactericidal activity as the concentration increases. They demonstrated that daptomycin activity was lower at pH 6.4 than at pH 7.4 or 8.0, and that daptomycin maintained bactericidal activity against stationary phase cells. Daptomycin showed 91% protein binding in these studies. Perhaps significantly, they showed some differences in serum bactericidal activity of daptomycin that were not predicted by MICs, suggesting that unexplained S. aureus strain differences may adversely affect the outcome of daptomycin treatment. They suggested that, if lipopeptides similar to daptomycin are to be developed, serum-binding studies, concentration-dependent killing studies against bacteria in exponential and stationary growth phases, and studies on pH effects may help determine appropriate target concentrations in serum to treat difficult Gram-positive infections.

Ramos et al. (63) compared daptomycin, vancomycin, and a combination of ampicillin plus gentamicin for the treatment of experimental enterococcal endocarditis in rabbits. Daptomycin at 20 mg/kg body weight twice a day intramuscularly was superior to vancomycin or ampicillin–gentamicin in treating an aminoglycoside-resistant penicillin-resistant strain of E. faecalis. The daptomycin therapy reduced the average vegetation bacterial concentrations from 10^9 CFU/g of vegetation in controls to ~10^4 CFU/g of vegetation after 6 days of treatment. An identical dose of vancomycin given intravenously reduced the bacterial counts to ~10^6 CFU/g of vegetation. Daptomycin at the same dose was equivalent to vancomycin or ampicillin–gentamicin in treating experimental endocarditis caused by a strain of Enterococcus raffinosus that is sensitive to aminoglycosides but resistant to penicillin. Curiously, parallel in vitro studies showed that daptomycin bactericidal activity against both of these strains was not reduced in the presence of 50% rabbit serum. The in vivo results clearly established that, at the dose tested, daptomycin is efficacious in treating enterococcal endocarditis in the rabbit model.

Kaatz et al. (64) compared the efficacy of daptomycin to those of teicoplanin and vancomycin in a rabbit model for S. aureus endocarditis. They used a dose of daptomycin (8 mg/kg of body weight intravenously every 8 hr) that produced peak serum levels of 40 to 60 µg/ml daptomycin, which was moderately above the peak concentrations tested in human clinical trials. Daptomycin was 97% bound to rabbit serum proteins and 96% bound to human serum controls. Daptomycin was as good as, or superior to, teicoplanin and vancomycin in reducing bacterial counts and sterilizing vegetations in the left-side endocadium caused by three different strains of S. aureus. Daptomycin was also as efficacious as vancomycin or high-dose teicoplanin in reducing bacterial counts in the spleen and kidneys. However, some of the isolates derived from one of the three strains that sur-vived daptomycin treatment showed diminished susceptibility to daptomycin. Since dap-tomycin-resistant mutants were not observed upon direct plating of *S. aureus* strains on 2, 5, or 10 times the MIC of daptomycin ($<10^{-10}$ with all three strains), the authors sug-gested that resistance to daptomycin may require multiple mutations, which might occur during prolonged exposure to subinhibitory concentrations of daptomycin. The nature of the mutation(s) is unknown, and its relevance to the clinical use of daptomycin or a related lipopeptide is a potential concern. The results, however, demonstrated that the high protein binding and large molecular weight of daptomycin do not limit its distribu-tion to tissues such as spleen, kidney, and heart.

Caron et al. (65) studied the effects of daptomycin alone and in combination with gentamicin in a rabbit endocarditis model using a highly vancomycin-resistant strain of *E. faecium*. They showed that daptomycin and gentamicin are synergistic in vitro and in vivo in the endocarditis model. They demonstrated that daptomycin alone, given at a dose chosen to reproduce the serum levels obtained in the human clinical trials at the 3 mg/kg twice-per-day dose, was only marginally effective in reducing bacterial counts in cardiac vegetations. A higher dose was more effective at reducing bacterial counts in veg-etations, but it did not eliminate bacteria in the vegetations. The higher dose in combi-nation with gentamicin further reduced bacterial counts in vegetations, and this eradi-cated the *E. faecium* in five of nine rabbits. The authors also demonstrated that daptomycin penetrated the cardiac tissue effectively and was distributed homogeneously. The concentrations achieved at the higher dose of daptomycin alone should have been sufficient to treat endocarditis. They suggested that the lack of efficacy at this dose may be due to daptomycin binding to other components of the cardiac vegetation, or to a pos-sible lower Ca^{2+} concentration in cardiac tissue relative to serum. They concluded that the levels of daptomycin needed to treat *E. faecium* endocartitis are probably not safely achievable in humans. They suggested that future lipopeptide clinical candidates should undergo analysis of protein binding and its consequences on in vivo efficacy. They also suggested that tests be conducted with difficult-to-treat bacterial infections using animal models, and that toxicity tests be carried out before embarking on future clinical trials with this class of antibiotics.

Voorn et al. (66) studied the treatment of a cloxacillin-tolerant strain of *S. aureus* and a nontolerant derivative in a rat endocarditis model. In vitro studies showed that the tolerant strain was also tolerant to the glycopeptides vancomycin and teicoplanin, but not to daptomycin. In vivo studies showed that daptomycin was significantly more effec-tive than vancomycin or teicoplanin at reducing bacterial numbers in endocardial vege-tations when the drugs were administered twice a day. The authors pointed out that dap-tomycin is distributed homogeneously throughout the vegetation (65), whereas teicoplanin is not (67). This may help explain the greater efficacy of daptomycin com-pared with those of glycopeptides.

V.   MECHANISM OF ACTION

A.   Effects on Macromolecular Biosynthesis

Eliopoulos et al. (36) have shown that $A21978C_1$ (see Table 1) requires Ca^{2+} at about 50 mM for full antibacterial activity. Activity diminished by about 100-fold as Ca^{2+} concen-tration was reduced to ~4 mM. They also showed that $A21978C_1$ does not bind to peni-cillin-binding proteins and does not inhibit DNA or RNA synthesis in *E. faecalis* when added at 4 μg/ml, which is above the MIC. A21978C$_1$ at 100 μg/ml did not inhibit protein synthesis, but it resulted in about 50% inhibition of peptidoglycan biosynthesis as measured by incorporation of radiolabeled Ala. However, no inhibition of peptidoglycan biosynthesis was observed at A21978C$_1$ concentrations of 5 or 10 μg/ml. They indicated that their data did not rule out peptidoglycan biosynthesis as the target, but that there may be additional sites of antimicrobial action.

Allen et al. (68) showed that LY146032 (daptomycin) inhibited peptidoglycan biosynthesis in S. aureus and Bacillus megaterium. In S. aureus, 50% inhibition of incorporation radiolabeled Ala into cell wall was achieved with 25 μg/ml daptomycin, which is substantially higher than the MIC. They also showed that daptomycin inhibited incorporation of UDP-N-acetylmuramyl-pentapeptide and UDP-N-acetylglucosamine into peptidoglycan by a cell-free particulate fraction of B. megaterium at 100 μg/ml daptomycin. Incorporation was not inhibited at 10 μg/ml. Inhibition of peptidoglycan biosynthesis in S. aureus did not cause the accumulation of UDP-MurNAc-peptide, as would be expected for an antibiotic that interferes with polymerization of peptidoglycan, indicating that daptomycin must interfere with precursor formation. Daptomycin also caused leakage of K$^+$ from B. megaterium and S. aureus when added at relatively high concentrations. The authors noted that daptomycin may have to cross the cytoplasmic membrane to inhibit one or more reactions leading to the biosynthesis of nucleotide-linked sugar peptide precursors, and that the perturbation of membrane function as evidenced by K$^+$ leakage is consistent with this possibility. Studies of Mengin-Lecreulx et al. (69) suggested that daptomycin interferes in peptidoglycan biosynthesis in B. megaterium at some step between glucosamine 6-phosphate and UDP-GlcNAc. However, other studies did not demonstrate that daptomycin inhibited any of the enzymes involved in early steps in peptidoglycan biosynthesis (70).

Alborn et al. (71) have shown that daptomycin at 100 μg/ml causes Ca^{2+}-dependent reduction in membrane potential in S. aureus. They suggest that the ability of daptomycin to collapse membrane potential may explain its inhibitory effects on protein, RNA, DNA, lipid, and peptidoglycan biosynthesis. Allen et al. (70) have shown that daptomycin at 100 μg/ml also causes dissipation of membrane potential in B. megaterium. Daptomycin at 25 μg/ml caused >90% inhibition of uptake of diaminopimelic acid, Glu, and Ala, the amino acid precursors to the pentapeptide in peptidoglycan. They proposed that the target for daptomycin is the energized cytoplasmic membrane, and that the effects of daptomycin on peptidoglycan biosynthesis result from the Ca^{2+}-dependent binding to the cytoplasmic membrane that dissipates the electrical potential, thereby interfering with the uptake of precursors for cell wall biosynthesis. They also suggested that the membrane effects may explain the other effects of daptomycin on macromolecular biosynthesis.

If the primary mechanism of daptomycin bactericidal activity is dissipation of membrane function that indirectly influences peptidoglycan, DNA, RNA, protein, lipid, and teichoic acid biosynthesis, it is not clear why daptomycin is synergistic with aminoglycosides. Uptake and bactericidal activity of aminoglycosides require membrane potential (72,73).

Canepari et al. (74) have shown that at the MIC, daptomycin caused only partial blockage of DNA, RNA, protein, and peptidoglycan biosynthesis in E. faecium. In contrast, it caused >50% inhibition of radiolabeled phosphate into teichoic acid and >90% inhibition of incorporation of radiolabeled glycerol into lipoteichoic acid in 20 min in both S. aureus and in E. faecium. They also showed that daptomycin does not penetrate bacterial cells, but binds reversibly to cell walls and irreversibly to cell membrane in the presence of Ca^{2+}. The irreversible binding to bacterial cell membranes appears to be particularly significant, since daptomycin binds reversibly to mammalian cell membranes. The authors suggested that the primary target for daptomycin is lipoteichoic acid biosynthesis.

In another study, Boaretti et al. (75) have shown that daptomycin at the MIC in the presence of Ca^{2+} causes inhibition of protoplast regeneration in *E. faecium*, whereas vancomycin does not. They showed that daptomycin caused 82% inhibition of lipoteichoic acid biosynthesis in *E. faecium* protoplasts, 40% inhibition of lipid biosynthesis, and only 14, 17, and 23% inhibition of peptidoglycan, DNA, and protein biosynthesis, respectively. They demonstrated Ca^{2+}-dependent tight binding of daptomycin to the cytoplasmic membrane. These data are consistent with the notion that lipoteichoic acid biosynthesis is the primary target of daptomycin at low concentrations.

More recently, Boaretti and Canepari (76) have studied the binding of daptomycin to membrane components in *Enterococcus hirae*. Of the three main membrane components, lipoteichoic acid, lipid, and protein, daptomycin binds to only the protein fraction. The binding was noncovalent, but stable enough to persist through membrane solubilization by nonionic detergent and Bio-Gel chromatography. When the membrane proteins were separated by isoelectric focusing, radiolabeled daptomycin was shown to bind five different proteins ranging in pIs from 5.9 to 6.2. They also studied the patterns of lipids synthesized during treatment of *E. hirae* with daptomycin. Whereas most lipids did not change in relative percentage, the fraction of diglucosyl diacylglycerol increased from 6.4 to 18.7% over 20 min, and three other lipids (phosphatidyl-α-kojibiosyldiacylglycerol, glycerophosphophosphatidyl-α-kojibiosyldiacylglycerol, and glycerophosphokojibiosyl-diacylglycerol) decreased about threefold. Since diglucosyl diacylglycerol is a precursor to the latter three lipids, the authors propose that daptomycin blocks an enzyme involved in the conversion of diglucosyl diacylglycerol to the next intermediate(s) in this part of the lipoteichoic acid biosynthetic pathway. They have not yet shown if this enzyme is one of the membrane-bound daptomycin-binding proteins.

B. Physical Studies

Biophysical studies of Lakey and Lea (77) showed that four A21978C factors increase the conductivity of planar lipid bilayers, and the effect decreases with reduction in lipid side-chain length. The effect was highly dependent on the presence of Ca^{2+}, and it increased roughly proportionately in the range of 2 to 20 mM Ca^{2+}. Their data showed that A21978C factors were not simply functioning as ionophores, but that a more complex membrane interaction was taking place. They raised the possibility that Ca^{2+} is required to neutralize the negative charge on the peptide portion of daptomycin to aid in its penetration into the membrane. They suggested that the membrane interactions are fundamental to the antibacterial action of daptomycin.

Using fluorescence measurements to monitor Kyn, Lakey and Ptak (78) showed that daptomycin interacts with phospholipid bilayers, presumably by inserting the lipid side chain into the nonpolar hydrocarbon layer. In the absence of Ca^{2+}, the peptide portion is still accessible to solvent at the lipid–water interface. When Ca^{2+} is added, the polarity around Kyn falls considerably, suggesting that neutralization of the negative charge on the peptide (daptomycin has four negatively charged amino acids and one positively charged amino acid) facilitates the penetration of the peptide portion of daptomycin into the membrane. Additional studies (79) have shown that Ca^{2+} plays a role in inducing strong antibiotic–phospholipid interactions.

The seemingly conflicting data on the mechanism of action of daptomycin might be reconciled by the following model. At low concentrations, daptomycin primarily inhibits lipoteichoic acid biosynthesis by its Ca^{2+}-dependent insertion into the bacterial membrane and binding to one or more membrane-bound proteins. This action is synergistic with aminoglycosides and some other agents. At higher concentrations, more daptomycin is bound to the membrane, and membrane potential is dissipated. The latter effect may account for the nonspecific inhibition of biosynthesis of DNA, RNA, protein, lipid, and peptidoglycan. It is not clear, however, if the effects on membrane potential have any relevance in the clinical setting, based on the high (~95%) serum binding of daptomycin. Clearly, more work is needed to clarify the mechanism of daptomycin action. Identification of the functions of the daptomycin-binding proteins in E. hirae (76) should be particularly instructive.

IV.   GENETICS OF LIPOPEPTIDE BIOSYNTHESIS

A.   Transposition Mutagenesis in *S. roseosporus*

S. roseosporus is a suitable host for molecular genetic manipulation. McHenney and Baltz (80) have shown that S. roseosporus is relatively nonrestricting for foreign DNA as determined by the bacteriophage host range test (81). DNA can be introduced into S. roseosporus by bacteriophage FP43–mediated transduction (80–83) and by conjugation from *Escherichia coli* (80,81). Transposon Tn5099 (84) was introduced into S. roseosporus on plasmid pCZA213 (85) by conjugation from E. coli S17-1, and transposition mutations were obtained after a temperature shiftup to cure the plasmid [pCZA213 does not replicate above 35°C (85)]. Tn5099 has three attributes that are very useful for genetic mapping and cloning of genes. First, it contains portable restriction endonuclease cleavage sites found infrequently in streptomycetes (i.e., DraI, AseI, and SspI). Thus, the sites of insertion can be readily localized to relatively large chromosomal fragments by pulsed-field gel electrophoresis (PFGE). Also, the relative distances from the ends of the DraI, AseI, and SspI fragments containing Tn5099 can be determined from the PFGE analysis. Since the DraI site is asymmetrically located in Tn5099, additional useful mapping data can be deduced by Southern hybridization analysis. Second, Tn5099 contains an apramycin-resistance gene that can express in streptomycetes and E. coli. Thus, the DNA flanking Tn5099 inserts can be readily cloned along with Tn5099 into E. coli, and the flanking DNA sequence can be determined using primers to the Tn5099 terminal sequences. Third, Tn5099 contains a promoterless xylE gene that encodes catechol dioxygenase. This allows the determination of the direction of transcription in transcribed genes.

Many mutants that influenced daptomycin production or red pigment production were obtained by Tn5099 insertion mutagenesis in S. roseosporus. They included the following: (a) mutants showing reduced or enhanced daptomycin production only; (b) mutants showing reduced or enhanced red pigment formation only; (c) mutants showing enhanced daptomycin and red pigment formation; (d) mutants completely blocked in red pigment formation only; and (e) mutants completely blocked in daptomycin production only (80). The mutants blocked in red pigment production mapped to two different regions on the linear chromosome of S. roseosporus, and one cluster was close to one end of the chromosome (80). Three of the mutants completely blocked in daptomycin biosynthesis mapped to the opposite end of the chromosome, and these are discussed in the following section.

B.   Cloning and Physical Mapping of Lipopeptide Biosynthetic Genes

The DNA flanking three different Tn*5099* insertions in *S. roseosporus* that disrupted dap-tomycin biosynthesis were physically mapped and cloned. The cloned DNA was reintro-duced into *S. roseosporus* and inserted into the chromosome by homologous recombina-tion (86). Two of the cloned DNA segments disrupted daptomycin biosynthesis. These DNAs were partially sequenced, and each contained DNA segments that are highly con-served among peptide synthetase genes. The Tn*5099* inserts in the original mutant strains mapped within about 20 kb of each other. The putative peptide synthetase DNA was used to probe a cosmid library of *S. roseosporus*, and several overlapping cosmids were obtained. Segments of DNA from these cosmids were subcloned into plasmid pRHB146, which is unable to replicate in streptomycetes but can conjugate from *E. coli* S17-1 into streptomycetes. Recombinants obtained by homologous recombination of these plasmids into the chromosome were analyzed for daptomycin production. The pattern of dapto-mycin production and nonproduction suggested that the daptomycin biosynthetic genes span at least 50 kb, starting about 420 kb from one end of the chromosome.

Segments of the cloned *S. roseosporus* peptide synthetase genes were used to probe a cosmid library of *S. fradiae* A54145, and several overlapping cosmids were identified (87). Gene disruption analysis indicates that the A54145 biosynthetic gene cluster maps to a ~50 kb region that starts about 150 kb from the end of the linear chromosome. It will be interesting to determine if the daptomycin and A54145 gene clusters have similar organization and map to the same chromosomal ends relative to other genes. This might be expected if the lipopeptide biosynthetic pathways have diverged from a common ancestral pathway.

VII.   FUTURE DIRECTIONS

Daptomycin is a potent antibiotic that is bacteriocidal for all of the most important Gram-positive pathogens. It has a novel mode of action, which is not yet fully under-stood, but may involve inhibition of lipoteichoic acid biosynthesis. Its mode of action clearly differs from those of other antibiotics used to treat Gram-positive infections. This is a real advantage since daptomycin kills methicillin-resistant *S. aureus*, penicillin-resis-tant *S. pneumonia*, and vancomycin-resistant enterococci. Daptomycin was successful in clinical trials at treating some Gram-positive infections, but it failed to treat staphylo-coccal endocarditis adequately. Elevated doses of daptomycin suggested that it may cause muscle toxicity in some patients, and so the clinical trials were stopped.

Because of the structural complexity of daptomycin, chemical modifications have been limited to the fatty acid side chain. However, comparative studies on the in vivo activities of daptomycin, other A21978C factors, and A54145 factors suggest that the toxicity of this class of molecules is due primarily to the fatty acid side chains, but that the in vivo antibacterial activity is determined primarily by the amino acid structure of the core peptide. Since daptomycin came very close to being successful in clinical trials, it appears that a moderate increase in therapeutic index may be sufficient for a dapto-mycin analog to be a clinically useful antibacterial agent. Thus, the development of a means to modify the peptide structure of daptomycin may allow for the development of a superior daptomycin analog. The recent successes in modifying the surfactin peptide syn-thetase by molecular genetic "module swapping" to produce novel derivatives of surfactin (88) suggest that the peptide portion of daptomycin might be modified by similar meth-ods. The cloning of the genes for daptomycin biosynthesis and for A54145 biosynthesis provide the starting materials to explore this approach to improve the clinically relevant properties of this class of lipopeptide antibiotics.

ACKNOWLEDGMENTS

The author thanks N. Allen and G. Huffman for comments on the manuscript and B. Fogleman for typing the manuscript.

REFERENCES

1. Debono M, Barnhart M, Carrell CB, Hoffman JA, Occolowitz JL, Abbott BJ, Fukuda DS, Hamill RL. A21978C, a complex of new acidic peptide antibiotics: Isolation, chemistry, and mass spectral structure elucidation. J Antibiot 1987; 40:761–777.
2. Boeck L, Fukuda DS, Abbott BJ, Debono M. Deacylation of A21978C, an acidic lipopeptide antibiotic complex, by *Actinoplanes utahensis*. J Antibiot 1988; 41:1085–1092.
3. Debono M, Abbott BJ, Malloy RM, Fukuda DS, Hunt AH, Daupert VM, Counter FT, Ott JL, Carrell CB, Howard LC, Boeck LD, Hamill RL. Enzymatic and chemical modifications of lipopeptide antibiotic A21978C: The synthesis and evaluation of daptomycin (LY146032). J Antibiot 1988; 41:1093–1105.
4. Boeck LD, Papiska HR, Wetzel RW, Mynderse JS, Fukuda DS, Mertz FP, Berry DM. A54145, a new lipopeptide antibiotic complex: Discovery, taxonomy, fermentation and HPLC. J Antibiot 1990; 43:587–593.
5. Fukuda DS, Du Bus RH, Baker PJ, Berry DM, Mynderse JS. A54145, a new lipopeptide complex: isolation and characterization. J Antibiot 1990; 43:594–600.
6. Fukuda DS, DeBono M, Molloy RM, Mynderse JS. A54145, a new lipopeptide antibiotic complex: Microbial and chemical modification. J Antibiot 1990; 43:601–606.
7. Zmijewski M, Briggs B, Occolowitz J. Role of branched chain fatty acid precursors in regulating factor profile in the biosynthesis of A21978C complex. J Antibiot 1986; 39:1483–1485.
8. Huber FM, Pieper RL, Tietz AJ. The formation of daptomycin by supplying decanoic acid to *Streptomyces roseosporus* cultures producing the antibiotic complex A21978C. J Biotechnol 1988; 7:283–292.
9. Huber FM, Pieper RL, Tietz AJ. Dispersal of insoluble fatty acid precursors in stirred reactors as a mechanism to control antibiotic factor distribution. Ho CS, Oldshue JY, eds. Biotechnology Processes. New York: American Institute of Chemical Engineers, 1987:249–253.
10. Huber FM, Pieper RL, Tietz AJ. Process for producing A-21978C derivatives. U.S. Patent 4,885,243; December 5, 1989.
11. Boeck LD, Wetzel RW. A54145, a new lipopeptide antibiotic complex: Factor control through precursor directed biosynthesis. J Antibiot 1990; 43:607–615.
12. Kleinkauf H, von Döhren H. Nonribosomal biosynthesis of peptide antibiotics. Eur J Biochem 1990; 192:1–15.
13. Kleinkauf H, von Döhren H. Bioactive peptides: Recent advances and trends. Kleinkauf H, von Döhren H., eds. Biochemistry of Peptide Antibiotics. New York: de Gruyter, 1990:1–31.
14. Turgay K, Krauss M, Marahiel MA. Four homologous domains in the primary structure of GrsB are related to domains in a superfamily of adenylate-forming enzymes. Mol Microbiol 1992; 6:529–546.
15. Turgay K, Krauss M, Marahiel MA. Four homologous domains in the primary structure of GrsB are related to domains in a superfamily of adenylate-forming enzymes. Mol Microbiol 1992; 6:2743–2744.
16. von Döhren H, Pfeifer E, van Liempt H, Lee Y-O, Pavela-Vraneic M, Schweeke T. The nonribosomal system: What we learn from the genes encoding protein templates. Baltz RH,

Hegeman GD, Skatrud PL, eds. Industrial Microorganisms: Basic and Applied Molecular Genetics. Washington, D.C.: American Society for Microbiology, 1993:159–167.

17. Aharonowitz Y, Bergmeyer J, Cantoral JM, Cohen G, Demain AL, Fink U, Kinghorn J, Kleinkauf H, MacCabe A, Palissa H, Pfeifer E, Schwecke T, Van Liempt H, von Döhren H, Wolfe S, Zhang J. δ(L-α-Aminoadipyl)-L-cysteinyl-D-valine synthetase, the multienzyme integrating the four primary reactions in β-lactam biosynthesis, as a model peptide synthetase. Bio/Technol 1993; 11:807–810.

18. Haese A, Schubert M, Herrman M, Zocker R. Molecular characterization of the enniatin synthetase gene encoding a multifunctional enzyme catalyzing N-methyldepsipeptide formation in *Fusarium scirpi*. Mol Microbiol 1993; 7:905–914.

19. Pavela-Vrancic M, Van Liemt H, Pfeifer E, Freist W, von Döhren H. Nucleotide binding by multienzyme peptide synthetases. Eur J Biochem 1994; 220:535–542.

20. Wessels P, von Döhren H, Kleinkauf H. Biosynthesis of acylpeptidolactones of the daptomycin type: A comparative analysis of peptide synthetases forming A21978C and A54145 Eur J Biochem (in press).

21. Chow AW, Cheng N. In vitro activities of daptomycin (LY146032) and paldimycin (U-70,138F) against anaerobic gram-positive bacteria. Antimicrob Agent Chemother 1988; 32:788–790.

22. Faruki H, Niles AC, Heeren RL, Murray PR. Effect of calcium on in vivo activity of LY146032 against *Clostridium difficile*. Antimicrob Agent Chemother 1987; 31:461–462.

23. Huovinen P, Kotilainen P. In vitro activity of a new cyclic lipopeptide antibiotic, LY146032, against gram positive clinical bacteria. Antimicrob Agent Chemother 1987; 31:455–457.

24. Niu W-W, Neu HC. Activity of mersacidin, a novel peptide, compared with that of vancomycin, teicoplanin, and daptomycin. Antimicrob Agent Chemother 1991; 35:998–1000.

25. Eliopoulos GM, Willey S, Reiszner E, Spitzer PG, Caputo G, Moellering RC. In vitro and in vivo activity of LY146032, a new cyclic lipopeptide antibiotic. Antimicrob Agent Chemother 1986; 30:532–535.

26. Verbist L. In vitro activity of LY146032, a new lipopeptide antibiotic, against gram-positive cocci. Antimicrob Agent Chemother 1987; 31:340–342.

27. Shonekan D, Mildvan D, Handwerger S. Comparative in vitro activities of teicoplanin, daptomycin, ramoplanin, vancomycin and PD127,391 against blood isolates of gram-positive cocci. Antimicrob Agent Chemother 1992; 36:1570–1572.

28. De La Maza L, Ruoff KL, Ferraro MJ. In vitro activities of daptomycin and other antimicrobial agents against vancomycin-resistant gram-positive bacteria. Antimicrob Agent Chemother 1989; 33:1383–1384.

29. Kline MW, Mason EO, Kaplan SL, Lamborth LB, Johnson GS. Comparative in-vitro activity of LY146032 and eight other antibiotics against Gram-positive bacteria isolated from children. J Antimicrob Chemother 1987; 20:203–207.

30. Jorgensen JH, Redding JS, Maker LA. Antibacterial activity of the new glycopeptide antibiotic SKF104662. Antimicrob Agent Chemother 1989; 33:560–561.

31. Low DE, McGeer A, Poon R. Activities of daptomycin and teicoplanin against *Staphylococcus haemolytecus* and *Staphylococcus epidermidis*, including evaluation of susceptibility testing recommendations. Antimicrob Agent Chemother 1989; 33:585–588.

32. Fass RJ, Helsel VL. In vitro activity of LY146032 against staphylococci, streptococci, and enterococci. Antimicrob Agent Chemother 1986; 30:781–784.

33. Leclercq R, Derlot E, Weber M, Duval J, Courvalin P. Transferable vancomycin and teicoplanin resistance in *Enterococcus faecium*. Antimicrob Agent Chemother 1989; 33:10–15.

34. Nicas TI, Wu CYE, Hobbs JN, Preston DA, Allen NE. Characterization of vancomycin resistance in *Enterococcus faecium* and *Enterococcus faecalis*. Antimicrob Agent Chemother 1989; 33:1121–1124.

35. Knapp CC, Washington JA. Antistaphylococcal activity of a cyclic peptide, LY146032, and vancomycin. Antimicrob Agent Chemother 1986; 30:938–939.

36. Eliopoulos GM, Thauvin C, Gerson B, Moellering RC. In vitro activity and mechanism of action of A21978C$_1$, a novel cyclic peptide antibiotic. Antimicrob Agent Chemother 1985; 27:357–362.

37. Jones RN, Barry AL. Antimicrobial activity and spectrum of LY146032, a lipopeptide antibiotic, including susceptibility testing recommendations. Antimicrob Agent Chemother 1987; 31:625–629.

38. Wanger AR, Murray BE. Activity of LY146032 against enterococci with and without high level aminoglycoside resistance, including two penicillinase-producing strains. Antimicrob Agent Chemother 1987; 31:1779–1781.

39. Stratton CW, Liu C, Ratner HB, Weeks LS. Bactericidal activity of daptomycin (LY146032) compared with those of ciprofloxin, vancomycin, and ampicillin against enterococci as determined by kill-kinetic studies. Antimicrob Agent Chemother 1987; 31:1014–1016.

40. Flandrois JP, Fardel G, Carrot G. Early stages of in vitro killing curve of LY146032 and vancomycin for Staphylococcus aureus. Antimicrob Agent Chemother 1988; 32:454–457.

41. Van der Auwera P. Ex vivo study of serum bactericidal titers and killing rates of daptomycin (LY146032) combined or not combined with amikacin compared with those of vancomycin. Antimicrob Agent Chemother 1989; 33:1783–1790.

42. Stratton CW, Weeks LS. Effect of human serum on the bactericidal activity of daptomycin and vancomycin against staphylococcal and enterococcal isolates as determined by time-kill kinetic studies. Diagn Microbiol Infect Dis 1990; 13:245–252.

43. Vance-Bryan K, Larson TA, Rotschafer JC, Toscano JP. Investigation of the early killing of Staphylococcus aureus by daptomycin by using an in vitro pharmacodynamic model. Antimicrob Agent Chemother 1992; 36:2334–2337.

44. Garrison MW, Vance-Bryan K, Larson TA, Toscano JP, Rotchafer JC. Assessment of effects of protein binding on daptomycin and vancomycin killing of Staphylococcus aureus by using an in vitro pharmacodynamic model. Antimicrob Agent Chemother 1990; 34:1925–1931.

45. Hanberger H, Nilsson LE, Maller R, Isaksson B. Pharmacodynamics of daptomycin and vancomycin on Enterococcus faecalis and Staphylococcus aureus demonstrated by studies of initial killing and post antibiotic effect and influence of Ca^{2+} and albumin on these drugs. Antimicrob Agent Chemother 1991; 35:1710–1716.

46. Rybak MJ, Bailey EM, Lamp KC, Kaatz GW. Pharmacokinetics and bactericidal rates of daptomycin and vancomycin in intravenous drug abusers being treated for gram-positive endocarditis and bacteremia. Antimicrob Agent Chemother 1992; 36:1109–1114.

47. Lamp KC, Rybak MJ, Bailey EM, Kaatz GW. In vitro pharmacodynamic effects of concentration, pH, and growth phase on serum bactericidal activities of daptomycin and vancomycin. Antimicrob Agent Chemother 1992; 36:2709–2714.

48. Bush LM, Boscia JA, Kaye D. Daptomycin (LY146032) treatment of experimental enterococcal endocarditis. Antimicrob Agent Chemother 1988; 32:877–881.

49. Watanakunakorn C. In vitro activity of LY146032, a novel cyclic lipopeptide, alone and in combination with gentamicin or tobramycin against enterococci. J Antimicrob Chemother 1987; 19:445–448.

50. Debbia E, Pesce A, Schito GC. In vitro activity of LY146032 alone and in combination with other antibiotics against gram-positive bacteria. Antimicrob Agent Chemother 1988; 32:279–281.

51. Wood CA, Finkbeiner HC, Kohlhepp SJ, Kohnen PW, Gilbert DN. Influence of daptomycin on staphylococcal abscesses and experimental tobramycin nephrotoxicity. Antimicrob Agent Chemother 1989; 33:1280–1285.

52. Beauchamp D, Pellerin M, Gourde P, Pettigrew M, Bergeron MG. Effects of daptomycin and vancomycin on tobramycin nephrotoxicity in rats. Antimicrob Agent Chemother 1990; 34:139–147.

53. Beauchamp D, Gourde P, Simard M, Bergeron MG. Subcellular distribution of daptomycin given alone or with tobramycin in renal proximal tubular cells. Antimicrob Agent Chemother 1994; 38:189–194.

54. Thibault N, Grenier L, Simard M, Bergeron MG, Beauchamp D. Attenuation by dapto-mycin of gentamicin-induced experimental toxicity. Antimicrob Agent Chemother 1994; 38:1027–1035.

55. Counter FT, Allen NE, Fukuda DS, Hobbs JN, Ott J, Ensminger PW, Mynderse JS, Preston DA, Wu CYE. A54145, a new lipopeptide antibiotic complex: Microbiological evaluation. J Antibiot 1990; 43:616–622.

56. Doug M-Y, Chang T-W, Gorbach SL. Treatment of *Clostridium difficile* colitis in hamsters with a lipopeptide antibiotic, LY146032. Antimicrob Agent Chemother 1987; 31:1135–1136.

57. Rothschafer JC, Garrison MW, Rodvold KA. Therapeutic update on glycopeptide and lipopeptide antibiotics. Pharmacother 1988; 8:211–219.

58. Woodworth JR, Nyhart EH, Brier GL, Wolny JD, Black HR. Single-dose pharmacokinetics and antibacterial activity of daptomycin, a new lipopeptide antibiotic, in healthy volunteers. Antimicrob Agent Chemother 1992; 36:318–325.

59. Sexton D, Brown R, McCloskey R, Dowell AR, Daptomycin Study Group. The use of dap-tomycin, a lipopeptide antibiotic, in the treatment of gram positive infections in man. Abstracts of the Interscience Conference on Antimicrobial Agents and Chemotherapy, 1988: A932.

60. Lee BL, Chambers HF, Novak RM, Rodvold KA, Kaatz G, Rybak M, McCloskey R, Zeckel M, Therasse D. Daptomycin versus conventional therapy in the treatment of endocarditis (E) and bacteremia (B). Abstracts of the Interscience Conference on Antimicrobial Agents and Chemotherapy, 1991: A885.

61. Garrison MW, Rotschafer JC, Crossley KB. Suboptimal effect of daptomycin in the treat-ment of bacteremias. South Med J 1989; 82:1414–1415.

62. Lee BL, Sachdeva M, Chambers HF. Effect of protein binding of daptomycin on MIC and antibacterial activity. Antimicrob Agent Chemother 1991; 35:2505–2508.

63. Ramos MC, Grayson ML, Eliopoulos GM, Bayer AS. Comparison of daptomycin, van-comycin, and ampicillin-gentamicin for treatment of experimental endocarditis caused by penicillin-resistant enterococci. Antimicrob Agent Chemother 1992; 36:1864–1869.

64. Kaatz GW, Seo SM, Reddy VN, Bailey EM, Rybak MJ. Daptomycin compared with teicoplanin and vancomycin for therapy of experimental *Staphylococcus aureus* endocarditis. Antimicrob Agent Chemother 1990; 34:2081–2085.

65. Caron F, Kityis, M-D, Gutmann L, Cremieux A-C, Mayiere B, Vallois, J-M, Ozzam SM, Lemeland J-F, Carbon C. Daptomycin and teicoplanin in combination with gentamicin treatment of experimental endocarditis due to a highly glycopeptide-resistant isolate of *Ente-rococcus faecium*. Antimicrob Agent Chemother 1992; 36:2611–2616.

66. Voorn GP, Kuyvenhoven J, Goessens WHF, Schmal-Baues WC, Broeders PHM, Thompson J, Michel MF. Role of tolerance in treatment and prophylaxis of experimental *Staphylococcus aureus* endocarditis with vancomycin, teicoplanin, and daptomycin. Antimicrob Agent Chemother 1994; 38:487–493.

67. Cremieux AC, Maziere B, Valois JM, Ottaviani M, Azanest A, Raffoul H, Bouvet A, Poci-dalo JJ, Carbon C. Evaluation of antibiotic diffusion into cardiac vegetations by qualitative and autoradiography. J Infect Dis 1989; 159:938–944.

68. Allen NE, Hobbs JN, Alborn WE. Inhibition of peptidoglycan biosynthesis in Gram-posi-tive bacteria by LY146032. Antimicrob Agent Chemother 1987; 31:1093–1099.

69. Mengin-Lecreulx D, Allen NE, Hobbs JN, van Heijenoort J. Inhibition of peptidoglycan biosynthesis in *Bacillus megaterium* by daptomycin. FEMS Microbiol Lett 1990; 69:245–248.

70. Allen NE, Alborn WE, Hobbs JN. Inhibition of membrane potential-dependent amino acid transport by daptomycin. Antimicrob Agent Chemother 1991; 35:2639–2642.

71. Alborn, WE, Allen NE, Preston DA. Daptomycin disrupts membrane potential in growing *Staphylococcus aureus*. Antimicrob Agent Chemother 1991; 35:2282–2287.

72. Mates SM, Eisenberg ES, Mandel LJ, Patel L, Kaback HR, Miller MH. Membrane potential and gentamicin uptake in *Staphylococcus aureus*. Proc Nat Acad Sci USA 1982; 79:6693–6697.

73. Eisenberg ES, Mandel LJ, Kaback HR, Miller MH. Quantitative association between electrical potential across the cytoplasmic membrane and early gentamicin uptake and killing in *Staphylococcus aureus*. J Bacteriol 1984; 157:863–867.

74. Canepari P, Boaretti M, del Mar Lleo M, Satta G. Lipoteichoic acid as a new target for activity of antibiotics: Mode of action of daptomycin (LY146032). Antimicrob Agent Chemother 1990; 34:1220–1226.

75. Boaretti M, Canepari P, del Mar Lleop M, Satta G. The activity of daptomycin on *Enterococcus faecium* protoplasts: Indirect evidence supporting a novel mode of action on lipoteichoic acid synthesis. J Antimicrob Chemother 1993; 31:227–235.

76. Boaretti M, Canepari P. Identification of daptomycin-binding proteins in the membrane of *Enterococcus hirae*. Antimicrob Agent Chemother 1995; 39:2068–2072.

77. Lakey JH, Lea EJA. The role of acyl chain character and other determinants on the bilayer activity of A21978C on acidic lipopeptide antibiotic. Biochem Biophys Acta 1986; 859:219–226.

78. Lakey JH, Ptak M. Fluorescence indicates a calcium-dependent interaction between lipopeptide antibiotic LY146032 and phospholipid membranes. Biochem 1988; 27:4639–4645.

79. Lakey JH, Maget-Dana R, Ptak M. The lipopeptide antibiotic A21978C has a specific interaction with DMPC only in the presence of calcium ions. Biochem Biophys Acta 1989; 985:60–66.

80. McHenney MA, Baltz RH. Gene transfer and transposition mutagenesis in *Streptomyces roseosporus*: Mapping of insertions that influence daptomycin or pigment production. Microbiol 1996; 142:2363–2373

81. Baltz RH. Molecular genetic approaches to yield improvement in actinomycetes. Strohl WR, ed. Biotechnology of Industrial Antibiotics, 2nd ed. New York: Marcel Dekker.

82. McHenney MA, Baltz RH. Transduction of plasmid DNA in *Streptomyces* spp. and related genera by bacteriophage FP43. J Bacteriol 1988; 170:2276–2282.

83. McHenney MA, Baltz RH. Transposition Tn*5096* from a temperature-sensitive transducible plasmid in *Streptomyces* spp. J Bacteriol 1991; 1973:5578–5581.

84. Hahn DR, Solenberg PJ, Baltz RH. Tn*5099*, a *xylE* promoter probe transposon for *Streptomyces* spp. J Bacteriol 1991; 173:5573–5577.

85. Solenberg PJ, Baltz RH. Hypertransposing derivatives of the streptomycete insertion sequence IS*493*. Gene 1994; 147:47–54.

86. McHenney MA, Hosted, TJ, DeHoff BS, Rosteck PR Jr, Baltz RH. Molecular cloning and physical mapping of the lipopeptide antibiotic biosynthetic gene cluster from *Streptomyces roseosporus* (manuscript in preparation).

87. Hosted TJ, DeHoff BS, Rosteck PR Jr, Baltz RH. Cloning and sequence sampling of the *Streptomyces fradiae* lipopeptide antibiotic biosynthetic gene cluster (manuscript in preparation).

88. Stachelhaus T, Schneider A, Marahiel MA. Rational design of peptide antibiotics by targeted replacement of bacterial and fungal domains. Science 1995; 269:69–72.

15

Nisin and Related Antimicrobial Peptides

J. Norman Hansen
University of Maryland at College Park, College Park, Maryland

I. NISIN HAS A LONG HISTORY OF INDUSTRIAL USE

Nisin is an antimicrobial peptide that is currently being used worldwide as a food preservative, and it has many other potential industrial applications. Although nisin has become intensely studied during the last few years, it is actually one of the longest-known antimicrobial substances, having been observed in the 1920s (1) and studied since the 1940s (2). An early attempt to find a practical use for nisin involved the treatment of mastitis in dairy herds (3). The results were disappointing because of adverse reactions caused by the nisin preparations, but this appears to have been a consequence of impurities, because nisin is now widely used for the prevention of bovine mastitis, and its use in treatment of bovine mastitis is under development (4–6). It has also been found to be very effective in preventing oral plaque and gingivitis and, therefore, has much potential for dental applications such as in mouthwashes and dentifrices (7). Nisin's effectiveness against many different types of bacteria argues that its potential uses have only begun to be explored.

To date, the most important application of nisin has been as a food preservative, which bodes well for its continued importance. In 1988, nisin was given GRAS (generally recognized as safe) status for certain food applications (8), but it was initially limited to processed cheese spreads, where an enhancement of shelf life had been demonstrated (9). This approval of nisin for food use is a logical consequence of the fact that nisin is produced by *Lactococcus lactis*, which is a food-grade lactic acid bacterium that has a long history of use in the dairy industry as a component of starter cultures. Whereas the initial use of *L. lactis* was unrelated to its nisin production, it is now believed that the presence of nisin can enhance the shelf life of fermented dairy products (10). Indeed, the simple logic that led to the approval of nisin as a food additive leads to the general expectation that the entire panoply of antimicrobial substances produced by food-grade organisms is a rich source for nontoxic, safe, and effective new antimicrobial substances (11). Even the most ardent opponents of the use of food additives characteristically regard a fermented food such as yogurt as natural and unadulterated, even though the fermentation process has introduced thousands of organic compounds that are alien to milk. This attitude is appropriate, since fermented foods have been part of the human food supply since ancient times, and their wholesomeness is assured by long experience. It is therefore appropriate to think of nisin as blazing a trail that can be followed by other substances that are currently being discovered in large numbers (12), many of which are completely unrelated to nisin itself.

Nisin is now approved for use as a food preservative in about 50 countries (10). The variety of the types of foods and beverages in which nisin has been successfully used continues to grow impressively. Most abundant are applications in dairy products (13,14), where nisin can inhibit the outgrowth of spores as well as being bacteriocidal against vegetative cells (15–17), increasing the shelf life of cheeses (18) and ice cream (19).

Nisin has proved useful in a variety of meat products, and this area of use is likely to grow. Nisin has long been considered as a possible alternative to nitrite, which is potentially carcinogenic (20). Accordingly, several studies have examined the possibility of using nisin alone or in combination with nitrite (21–27).

Another area of growing use of nisin is in beer and wine (28,29). It is also proving useful in foods that are particularly subject to bacterial contamination, such as low-acid canned foods that have been pasteurized instead of sterilized, and bakery products that have been baked at moderate temperatures (30).

The discovery that the bacteriocidal effect of nisin can be extended to Gram-negative bacteria by combining nisin with chelating agents such as EDTA (31) has dramatically increased the potential applications of nisin, allowing its use as a decontaminating agent of carcasses and equipment during processing of beef and poultry (32,33).

II. NISIN AND ITS RELATIONSHIP TO OTHER LANTIBIOTICS

A. Nisin Is a Ribosomally Synthesized Peptide that Contains Unusual Residues

Nisin has two features that contribute to its versatility for industrial applications. It is a gene-encoded, ribosomally synthesized antimicrobial peptide, and it contains many unusual residues that are introduced by posttranslational modification. That nisin is gene encoded allows the utilization of powerful genetic engineering methodologies for its study and manipulation. Its unusual residues are important because they confer unique chemical, physical, and biological properties that are unattainable by peptides composed solely of the 20 common amino acids. Unlike ordinary antibiotics, such as penicillin, which is a nonpeptide organic molecule that is synthesized by a complex metabolic pathway, the nisin structure is encoded in a gene. This means that this structure can be conveniently manipulated by mutagenesis of the nisin gene, rather than the laborious synthetic organic chemistry that is required to manipulate the structure of penicillin. Detracting somewhat from the unique character of nisin, this attribute is shared by an enormous variety of other gene-encoded antimicrobial peptides that have been discovered in recent years among eukaryotic organisms, including humans and other mammals. Major categories are magainins (34,35), defensins (36,37), and cecropins (38,39) (see Chapter 6 in this book). It would appear that whatever arguments can be made about exploiting the gene-encoded nature of nisin to construct variants with improved properties can be made equally strongly for all these other peptides. Moreover, since they are found in mammalian tissues, one can argue that they are also nontoxic and safe.

What these other peptides cannot duplicate is the unusual residues that are present in nisin and the other lantibiotics. It is the presence of these unusual residues that will ultimately prove to be the fundamental and unique contribution of these molecules.

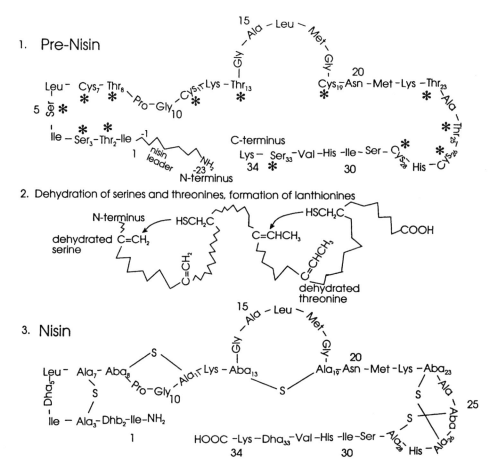

Figure 1   Conversion of prenisin to nisin. (1) The 57-residue sequence of prenisin consists of a leader segment (residues –23 to –1) that is cleaved from the nisin structural region (residues 1–34) during maturation. The serines, threonines, and cysteines that undergo modifications are marked with asterisks. Serines and threonines that undergo dehydrations are at positions 2, 3, 5, 8, 13, 23, 25, and 33. Cysteines are at positions 7, 11, 19, 26, and 28. (2) Serines and threonines are dehydrated to give dehydroalanine (Dha) and dehydrobutyrine (Dhb), respectively. Some of the dehydro residues undergo a Michael-type addition to give lanthionine (Ala–S–Ala) and β-methyllanthionine (Ala–S–Aba), respectively. (3) Structure of mature nisin, showing the locations of the unusual residues.

The general scheme for posttranslational modification of prenisin to form nisin was outlined many years ago by Ingram (40), as represented in Figure 1. The scheme involves dehydration of the alcoholic residues (Ser, Thr) to their corresponding dehydro forms (dehydroalanine [Dha] and dehydrobutyrine [Dhb]). Nisin contains eight serines and threonines that undergo dehydration; however, there is one serine that is not modified. The observation that lactocin S contains three D-serines that arise as a consequence of stereospecific rehydration of dehydroalanine (41), though, suggests the possibility that the "unmodified" serine in nisin is actually a rehydrated dehydroalanine. Subsequent to their dehydration, five of the dehydro residues undergo an intramolecular Michael-type reaction in which a cysteine residue adds to the double bond of the dehydro residue to form a thioether cross-linkage. When this reaction occurs with Dha, lanthionine is formed; when it occurs with Dhb, β-methyllanthionine is formed.

B.　Different Types of Known Lantibiotic Structures

It is the presence of the lanthionine reside that defines the peptide as a lantibiotic (42,43), and several general reviews of lantibiotics are available (11,43–49). Early studies on nisin were performed by Hurst (same person as Hirsch) and coworkers (e.g., 50–53), and the structure was determined by Gross and coworkers (54). The next lantibiotic to be discovered was subtilin (55,56), the structure of which was also determined by Gross and coworkers (57). Another 40 years passed before the discovery of a third lantibiotic, epidermin (42). Since then, the number of known lantibiotics has increased dramatically, and there are now nearly 20 lantibiotics that have been identified, and several others the identifications of which as lantibiotics are still tentative. The rate of discovery is escalating, and lantibiotics are now being reported with a frequency of one every few months. They have been discovered in at least seven different genera of Gram-positive bacteria, and the ease and rate with which they are being found suggests that they are indeed very common. Table 1 shows a list of currently known lantibiotics.

　　Lantibiotics can be categorized according to their structural features (46). The type A lantibiotics are the nisinlike lantibiotics, and these include nisin (76), subtilin (57), Pep5 (60), epidermin (42), and gallidermin (77). Mersacidin (65,78–80) and actagardine (66,81,82) can also be considered as lantibiotics, although they depart somewhat from

Table 1　Currently Known Lantibiotics

Lantibiotic	M_r[a]	Producer organism	Ref.
Nisin	3353	*Lactococcus lactis*	50
Subtilin	3317	*Bacillus subtilis*	58
Epidermin	2164	*Staphylococcus epidermidis*	59
Pep5	3488	*Staphylococcus epidermidis*	60
Epilancin K7	3032	*Staphylococcus epidermidis*	61
Duramycin A	2012	*Streptomyces cinnamoneus*	62
Duramycin B	1951	*Streptomyses cinnamoneus*	62
Duramycin C	2008	*Streptomyces cinnamoneus*	62
Cinnamycin	2041	*Streptomyces cinnamoneus*	63
Ancovenin	1959	*Streptomyces* sp.	64
Mersacidin	1825	*Bacillus subtilis*	65
Actagardine	1890	*Actinoplanes* sp.	66
Lacticin 481	2901	*Lactococcus lactis*	67
Streptococcin AFF 22	2795	*Streptococcus pyrogenes*	68
Salivaricin A	2315	*Streptococcus salilvarius*	69
Lactocin S	3769	*Lactobacillus sake*	70
Carnocin IU 49	4635	*Carnobacterium piscicola*	71
Mutacin II	3245	*Streptococcus mutans*	72–74
Cytolysin	nr	*Enterococcus faecalis*	75

[a] Abbreviation: nr, not reported.

the general description of the group. As a group, lantibiotics are linear cationic (basic) peptides with sizes up to 34 residues that possess sequence homology and similarities in the locations of their lanthionine bridges. The type B lantibiotics, all thus far produced by Streptomycetes, are the duramycin-like lantibiotics, which include duramycin A, duramycin B, duramycin C (62,83–86), cinnamycin (62,63), and ancovenin (64). The duramycin-like peptides are smaller (as few as 19 residues), and less cationic or neutral; and the C-terminal residue is involved in bridge formation, which results in a generally globular shape. In duramycin A, the C-terminal lysine forms a lysinoalanine bridge by reaction with a Dha at position 6. In duramycin B and C, this bridge is not formed, and there is an unreacted Dha residue at position 6. Mersacidin and actagardine do not fit easily into either category (46), and they are now considered as separate, type C lantibiotics. They are small and neutral, but their lanthionine bridges resemble those of nisin. As more lantibiotics are discovered, it seems likely that it may become increasingly difficult to classify them into a small number of categories. For example, several of the lantibiotics have not been assigned to a particular type, and these may represent members of new types. Structures of representative examples of type A, type B, and type C lantibiotics are shown in Figure 2.

Whereas nisin already has several important industrial applications as described above, the potential uses of the other lantibiotics are still being explored. Epidermin and gallidermin are effective in treating a variety of skin infections (42,77). Actagardine inhibits peptidoglycan biosynthesis (66,81,82). Ancovenin can inhibit the angiotensin-converting enzyme and, thus, has potential for use in treatment of high blood pressure (64). Cinnamycin, previously named lanthiopeptin and Ro 09-0198 (87,88), shows antiviral activity against herpes simplex virus, HSV1 (89). Mersacidin has shown activity as an immunosuppressor (62–66,78–90).

The range of biological effects exerted by lantibiotics is amazing. Whereas it is reasonable for an organism like *Lactococcus lactis* to produce antibiotic, that is targeted against other bacteria that occupy its ecological niche (91), it is hard to imagine why *Streptomyces* would be under selective pressure to produce ancovenin, that inhibits mammalian angiotensin-converting enzyme, or why *Actinoplanes* spp. would be under selective pressure to produce actagardine, that inhibits HSV1, which is a human-specific virus. Whatever the answer, it is clear that lantibiotics are capable of exerting an enormous range of biological effects, and that we need to learn more about the relationships between their structures and their properties and functions. Because the lantibiotics are gene encoded, it is possible to perform structure–function studies using mutagenesis; this will enable us to construct new lantibiotics, beginning with the natural forms and altering them to build new constructs with new and altered functions. It may be possible to direct these new molecules toward infectious agents that have become resistant to known antimicrobials or toward infectious agents, such as viruses, against which no treatments are currently available.

C. Nisin: A New Antibiotic Paradigm

I. The Penicillin Paradigm

Although we may not realize it, our concept of the term "antibiotic" is shaped almost entirely by penicillin. This is because of the enormous role that penicillin has played in the history of modern medicine. Prior to the discovery of penicillin, the concept of an antimicrobial drug was shaped in the nineteenth century by Paul Ehrlich's "magic bullet" idea, in which organic chemists would construct molecules that would, like magic, seek

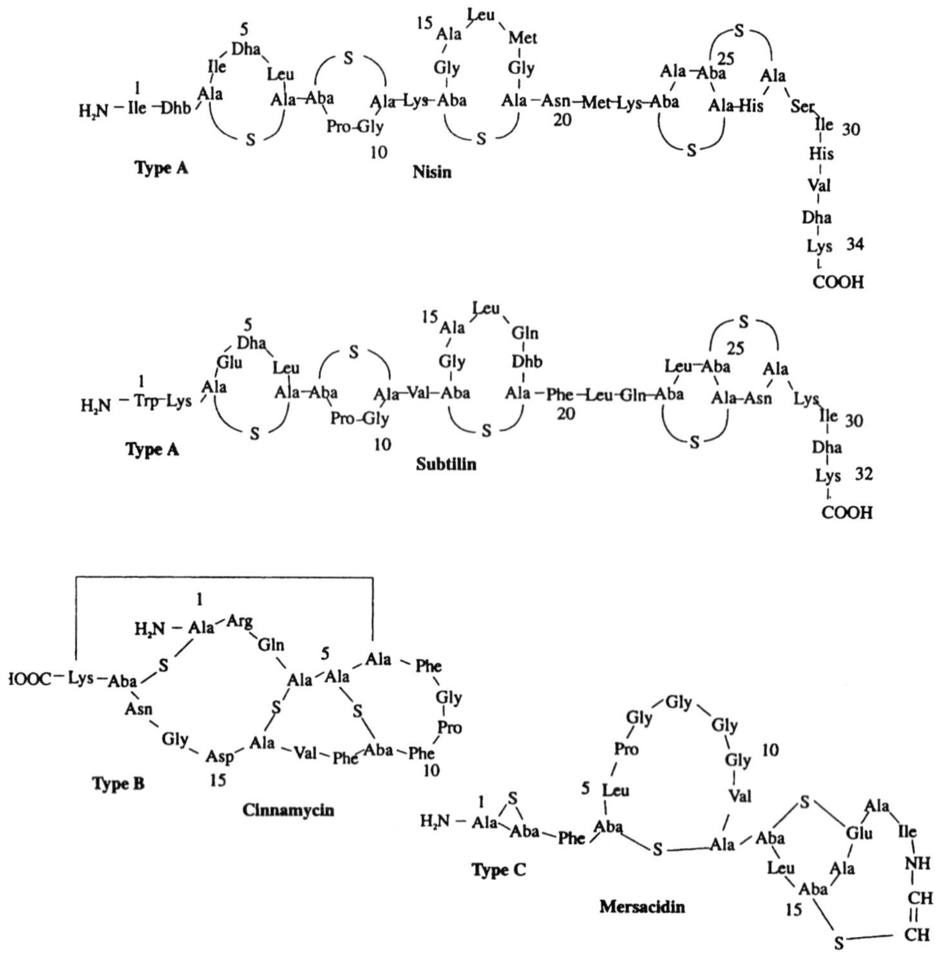

Nisin structure (Type A):

5
Dha
Ile   Leu   S
Ala   15 Ala Leu Met   S
H₂N – Ile –Dhb   Ala–Aba   Ala–Lys–Aba   Gly   Gly   25
Pro–Gly   Ala–Asn–Met–Lys–Aba   Ala–Aba Ala
S   Ala –Asn–Met–Lys–Aba   Ala–His Ser
10   20   Ile 30
Type A   Nisin   S   His
Val
Dha
Lys 34
COOH

Subtilin structure (Type A):

5
Dha
Glu   Leu   S
Ala   15 Ala Leu Gln
H₂N – Trp–Lys   Ala–Aba   Ala–Val–Aba   Gly   Dhb   25
Pro–Gly   Ala –Phe–Leu–Gln–Aba   Leu–Aba Ala
S   Ala–Asn Lys
10   20   Ile 30
Type A   Subtilin   S   Dha
Lys 32
COOH

Cinnamycin structure (Type B):

1
H₂N – Ala–Arg
Gln   5
IOOC–Lys–Aba   S   Ala–Ala   Ala ~ Phe
Asn   S   S   Gly
Gly   Pro
Asp   Ala –Val–Phe–Aba–Phe   10
Type B   15
Cinnamycin

Mersacidin structure (Type C):

Gly
Gly   Gly
Pro   Gly 10
1   S   5 Leu   Val
H₂N – Ala   Aba–Phe   Aba   S——Ala   Aba   S   Ala
Type C   Leu   Ala   Glu Ile
Aba   NH
Mersacidin   15   CH
S —— CH

Figure 2 Primary structures of representative examples of type A (nisin-like) lantibiotics, type B (*duramycin-like*) lantibiotics, and type C (mersacidin-like) lantibiotics.

out and destroy their targets in a highly specific way. With the possible exception of the sulfa drugs, this idea was doomed because no one had the slightest idea of what molecules to construct, or what targets at which to aim them. The serendipitous discovery of penicillin, as a natural product of a living organism with powerful antimicrobial effects, established a wholly new line of thinking. This paradigm acknowledged that biological warfare has been going on among microorganisms for countless millions of years; and that microorganisms have accordingly evolved very sophisticated weapons for attacking each other, as well as for defending themselves from each other. Scientists then spent several decades just going out and looking at Nature's ideas about how to conduct this biological warfare. This has nurtured the pharmacological concept of "rational drug design," or "knowledge-based drug design," which purports to provide a means for a neverending supply of new drugs based on making incremental improvements in known drugs through chemical synthesis of analogs from which the undesirable properties or inadequacies have been alleviated through clever design.

Despite the undeniable success of penicillin, its use has resulted in a Faustian bargain the undesirable elements of which are just now becoming evident. Whereas evolution has produced very sophisticated biological weapons that organisms use to battle each other, these weapons have been in the environment for, perhaps, hundreds of millions of years, and there has been ample time for counter-defenses against these weapons to evolve. Thus, it is never long before these defenses manifest themselves by conferring resistance on the infectious organisms that we are trying to kill; this assures us that each of the antibiotics in our arsenal will begin to fail shortly after it is in widespread use.

What we now have to do is get back to Paul Ehrlich's original idea of making "magic bullets" using our human ingenuity. Nature has now taught us a great deal about how to approach designing antimicrobial agents, what kinds of sensitive targets there are, and how it is possible to destroy these targets in a highly specific way.

There are other problems with the penicillin paradigm. Penicillin, as well as virtually all other antibiotics in current use, is a small organic molecule that has evolved to react in a very specific way with an appropriate biological product. The producer organism has an interest in not being destroyed by its own antibiotic, and so it will construct the molecule (subject to forces of evolution) so that it is relatively nontoxic to itself. However, what is relatively nontoxic to the producer organism, often a mold, may not be nontoxic to us. Moreover, it is appropriate to classify most of these antibiotics as "xenobiotics," meaning that they are alien to our metabolic processes, and it is thus unpredictable how they will be metabolized by our bodies into excretion and other waste products. This alien nature is also responsible for many of the familiar allergic responses that doctors always have to worry about when prescribing antibiotics.

Yet another problem with these antibiotics is the demonstrated dangers caused by their residues in food. Farmers discovered many years ago that liberal use of antibiotics in their livestock feed increased profits because their animals were less subject to bacterial infections, and for reasons that are poorly understood, antibiotic-treated animals gained weight more rapidly and efficiently. This antibiotic use among livestock resulted in antibiotic residues being present in the meat products that consumers purchased from the stores. Everyone agrees that the ubiquitous use of antibiotics in this way has greatly increased the incidence of antimicrobial resistance and, thus, hastened the day when today's antibiotics will be useless. The Food and Drug Administration (FDA) has thus banned antibiotic residues in food, with a concomitant perception among consumers that antibiotic residues in food are dangerous. They are right, partly because of the xenobiotic nature of these residues, and partly because of their contribution to the rise of resistance.

2.   The Nisin Paradigm

Much of the negative attitude about antibiotics arises because the aforementioned problems are inherent in the nature of penicillin and other common antibiotics—namely, they are xenobiotic compounds that have evolved in a context that virtually assures that for every antibiotic, Nature has co-evolved a defense, or resistance, to it. If each and every one of Nature's antibiotic substances conformed to this same general pattern, then we would indeed be in a difficult situation. Fortunately, this is not the case, and nisin is an excellent example of an antibiotic with something very different to offer. First of all, it is a peptide and, therefore, a polymer of amino acids. Peptides are not alien things, and our metabolism has evolved around utilizing polypeptides as food. An antimicrobial peptide such as nisin will be digested in a normal residue-free fashion, unlike penicillin, which persists in the gut and floods out into the tissues, where its fate is problematic.

Nisin has been subjected to rigorous toxicity tests, and it emerged with the excellent results that qualified it for GRAS status, as described in Section I. Although one can conceive of peptides that could be toxic when consumed, it is undeniable that as a class, peptides have as low a likelihood of causing toxic effects as anything in existence. A good illustrative case of this is the sweetener aspartame, which is a dipeptide, instead of being a xenobiotic such as saccharine or cyclamate. The argument that peptides are inherently safe was a major factor in its approval by the FDA, and in its overwhelming acceptance by consumers. A similar attitude appears to persist with respect to nisin, and one can expect that it will be relatively easy to extend this attitude to encompass other antimicrobial peptides.

Another aspect that is central to the nisin paradigm is that it is a gene-encoded peptide, in contrast to penicillin, which is biosynthesized by a complex metabolic pathway. The fact that the pharmaceutical industry has synthesized more than 10,000 structural analogs of penicillin (92–94) obscures the fact that doing organic chemistry on a natural product such as penicillin is extraordinarily difficult and expensive. The difficulty of analog synthesis makes the rounds of hypothesis, synthesis, and testing required for rational design (95,96) very difficult and time consuming. The requirement for organic synthesis in constructing analogs of penicillin and other antibiotics effectively prevents the utilization of the most powerful methodologies of modern biotechnology, namely, recombinant DNA, and in turn, genetic and protein engineering. It does not require deep reflection to realize that, to merge the search for new antimicrobials with modern biotechnology, we must develop antimicrobials that can be structurally manipulated using genetic engineering methods. Although it is theoretically possible to change the structure of an antibiotic by altering the enzymes for its biosynthetic pathway (97), how to genetically engineer structural changes is much more obvious when the antibiotic is, itself, a gene-encoded polypeptide. The fact that gene-encoded antimicrobial polypeptides such as nisin exist in Nature makes progress down this pathway straightforward. Indeed, the abundance of such peptides is vastly greater than would have been imagined just a few years ago. It now appears that we have been so accustomed to thinking of antibiotics as conforming to the penicillin paradigm that the vast number of antibiotics that are better represented by the nisin paradigm were simply not noticed. Now that they have been noticed, as indicated by the several chapters in this book that are devoted to them, it is very likely that they will be subjected to intense scrutiny during the next few years. As a result of these efforts, what we think of as an "antibiotic" will proceed to change; and as increasing numbers of antimicrobial peptides are put into practical use in medical, industrial, and consumer products, the attitudes of people about the risks involved in using these substances will cause fears about antibiotics to recede. As the nisin paradigm begins to supplant the penicillin paradigm, we will see that the opportunities to employ antibiotics in a useful and satisfactory way will expand, instead of contract, as they are doing under the penicillin paradigm.

III. MOLECULAR GENETICS OF NISIN AND OTHER LANTIBIOTICS

A. Organization of Lantibiotic Genes

Our understanding of the molecular genetics of the lantibiotics has progressed rapidly during the last few years, and most of the genes involved in the biosynthesis of nisin, subtilin, epidermin, Pep5, cytolysin, lacticin 481, and lactocin S have been identified. The organization of these genes is generally consistent with the principle that all the genes involved in the biosynthetic pathway of an antibiotic (98) are clustered together in the chromosome or other genetic element and expressed in a coordinated fashion. In the case of the lantibiotics, what is conceived as the "biosynthetic pathway" is very different from that of common antibiotics such as penicillin. Penicillin is biosynthesized in a series of enzyme-catalyzed steps that construct the antibiotic in an incremental fashion from precursor metabolites. In this pathway, genes encode the enzymes that catalyze the biosynthetic steps. In contrast, nisin and the other lantibiotics are derived from posttranslational modifications of a ribosomally synthesized polypeptide; this involves dehydrations of alcoholic residues, thioether formation, translocation to the exterior of the cell, proteolytic cleavage of the leader segment, and release of the mature lantibiotic into the medium as described in Section II. What one accordingly expects to see among the cluster of genes that catalyze the steps of the lantibiotic pathway are the structural gene that encodes the prelantibiotic polypeptide, the genes for proteins that catalyze the posttranslational modification steps just mentioned, and one or more genes for the factor(s) that confer immunity of the producer cell against the antibiotic that it produces.

These expectations are substantially realized for all of the lantibiotics that have so far been characterized at the gene level. The organization that has been found is shown in Figure 3.

When the genes shown in Figure 3 were originally discovered, they were assigned names that were unrelated to function. As more lantibiotic genes were discovered, homologies and functional studies allowed the various classes of lantibiotic genes to be assigned to specific families. The genes have accordingly been renamed so that each representative of a particular gene would have the same name, and a standard nomenclature

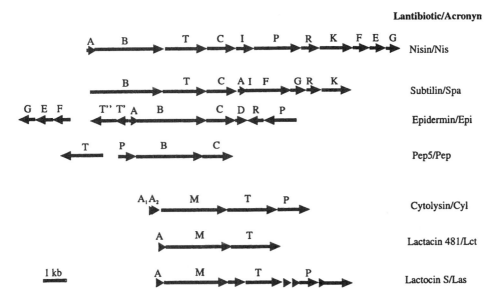

Figure 3 Organization of lantibiotic gene clusters. The direction of the arrows indicates the direction of transcription of the *lan* genes that are identified by letters. The structural gene for each lantibiotic is *lanA*, and the roles of the other genes are described in the text. The standardized (99) nomenclature of the genes is used.

of lantibiotic genes has been established (99). These name changes, such as the change of *spa*S to *spa*A, and *spa*D/*spa*E to *spa*B, have been reviewed and tabulated (100). Accordingly, the *lan* genes are all these genes involved in lantibiotic synthesis, and those of a particular lantibiotic have their specific names, such as the *nis* genes involved in nisin biosynthesis and the *spa* genes involved in subtilin biosynthesis. Other standard names include *lan*A as the lantibiotic structural gene; *lan*T for the transporter gene, which is involved in translocation of the lantibiotic precursor across the cell envelope; *lan*B, which has been implicated in the dehydrations of serines and threonines; *lan*C, which has been implicated in the formation of the thioether cross-linkages; *lan*P, which is responsible for proteolytic cleavage of the prelantibiotic leader segment; and *lan*I, which is responsible for conferring immunity (see Table 2). Several of the lantibiotic gene clusters contain regulatory genes for two-component regulatory systems, called *lan*R (the response regulator) and *lan*K (the sensor kinase). There are several genes that fall outside of this basic nomenclature scheme, such as the M gene, which is a homolog of the C gene, except the M gene is considerably larger than the C gene. Also, there are sometimes several genes involved in immunity or self-protection, such as the F and G genes in the subtilin gene cluster, and the EFG genes in the nisin and epidermin gene clusters. The epidermin cluster has two copies of a T-type gene, each of which possesses a deletion and may therefore not be fully functional. The epidermin cluster contains a unique D-gene, which is responsible for the novel modification at the C-terminus of epidermin (101). There are also circumstances in which it is suspected that there are host functions that supplement the

Table 2   Characteristics of Predicted Gene Products in Lantibiotic Gene Clusters

Gene	Function
*lan*A	Prelantibiotic structural gene
*lan*B	Modification, probably dehydration
*lan*C	Modification, probably thioether formation
*lan*T	Transport during biosynthesis
*lan*I	Immunity
*lan*P	Cleavage of leader segment
*lan*R	Response regulator
*lan*K	Response kinase
*lan*E	Transport/immunity
*lan*F	Transport/immunity
*lan*G	Transport/immunity
*cyl*M	Large homolog of *lan*C
*epi*D	Modification, unique to epidermin
*cyl*A	Cytolysin structural gene (2 required)

The different types of genes found in lantibiotic operons as depicted in Figure 3 are listed, along with the functions gene products that have been attributed to them. Genes denoted with *lan* names are found as homologs in more than one type of lantibiotic operon. Genes such as *epi*D are unique and are found in only one operon. A good review of the lantibiotic gene clusters and their encoded proteins is available (100).

functions of genes found in the lantibiotic cluster. Such an example is the subtilin gene cluster, which lacks a P-type gene, and it has been speculated that the leader segment is cleaved by a protease encoded in the host chromosome outside the *lan* gene cluster.

B.   Homologies and Functional Characteristics of the Lan Proteins

The various families of *lan* genes have characteristic conserved features. The *lanA* genes encode LanA prepeptides that range from 51 to 68 residues, and propeptides (leader removed) from 22 to 37 residues. The most unusual *lanA* genes are the *cylA1* and *cylA2* genes, which are tandem structural genes the products of which are both required for activity (75). Thioether rings and dehydro residues are ubiquitous among the lantibiotics; otherwise, there is little sequence homology among them. Certain lantibiotics such as epidermin/gallidermin and nisin/nisinZ differ by single residues, and these are merely natural structural variants of the same lantibiotic. Otherwise, nisin and subtilin are the most homologous, sharing about 60% identical residues, followed by salivaricin and streptococcin (55% identity), Pep5 and epilancin (35% identity), and lactocin and cytolysin (24% identity). The *lanI* genes, such as *nisI*, *spaI*, and *pepI*, are membrane-bound lipoproteins (102–104). These and other aspects of sequence homologies among the mature lantibiotics and the leader peptides have been reviewed (48,105).

The *lanB* genes encode LanB proteins of about 1000 residues, the homologies of which include about 28% identical residues. They are predominantly hydrophilic with a high level of predicted secondary structure (106). An intact *lanB* gene is essential for lantibiotic production (107–109). LanB is a candidate as the enzyme responsible for dehydration of the serines and threonines to dehydro residues, although biochemical experiments showing this have not yet been performed. LanB has a weak homology to IlvA (106), which is an *Escherichia coli* threonine dehydratase, but this homology does not correspond to conserved regions of the LanB proteins, making the significance of this homology tenuous.

The LanC proteins are about 400 residues long, and they possess 24–32% identity. They contain alternating hydrophilic and hydrophobic regions (110). The hydrophilic segments contain predicted amphipathic helices, which suggests a globular structure with alternating α-helices and β-sheets (100). The LanM proteins are much longer, containing more than 900 residues, but contain a C-terminal domain with 25% sequence identity to the LanC proteins, arguing that they perform LanC functions. Experiments in which part of the *pepC* gene was deleted showed an accumulation of pro-Pep5 that contained dehydro residues and free cysteine sulfhydryl-groups, providing strong evidence that an intact PepC protein is required for thioether bond formation (111).

LanP proteins are responsible for removal of the leader peptide from the prelantibiotic. There are two types of leader peptides, one possessing a subtilisin-like cleavage site, and another containing a Gly–X cleavage site, where X has been found to be Gly, Ala, or Ser. Some of the LanP proteins (PepP, ElkP, LasP) do not possess a signal sequence, so would be confined to the cytoplasm and may function intracellularly, and cleave the leader prior to transport. Others, such as NisP, appear to be extracellular peptidases that cleave the leader after it has traversed the membrane (112). There is some evidence that the LanT protein may participate in cleavage of the leader in some of the lantibiotics, particularly those that are cleaved at the Gly–X sequence. The CylT and LctT proteins contain a domain that corresponds to a protease that can cleave after this Gly–X sequence

(113). A LanP gene has not as yet been found in the subtilin gene cluster, and cleavage of the leader segment may be performed by a host protease. However, deletion of the central portion of the SpaT protein results in precursors being transported without cleavage, suggesting that the SpaT protein may possess proteolytic activity (114).

Whereas all of the prelantibiotics contain leader segments that must be removed during maturation, none of these leader segments possesses a typical *sec*-type signal sequence, and they therefore depend on a non-*sec*-dependent transport system. The LanT proteins possess characteristics of ABC-transporters, which contain an "ATP Binding Cassette," reflecting their requirement for ATP hydrolysis during secretion (115). These are homologous to the *E. coli* HlyB protein, which is used for hemolysin secretion (116), and the multidrug-resistance (*mdr*) proteins that are ubiquitous in eukaryotic cells (116). The relationship between the LanT proteins and other Lan proteins that possess characteristics of ABC-transport proteins is not completely clear. These are the LanE, LanF, and LanG proteins that are found in the *nis*, *epi*, and *spa* operons. Whereas the LanT proteins appear to function as exporters of the lantibiotic peptide as part of the biosynthetic pathway of the lantibiotic, the LanEFG proteins appear to participate in immunity. In this immunity role, they reside in the membrane to presumably intercept incoming molecules of the mature lantibiotic and pump them back out into the medium where they will not harm the producer cell, which can otherwise be killed by its own lantibiotic. In this way, they can supplement the LanI immunity protein, which is the protein that is primarily responsible for immunity (102,104,117).

The expression of the nisin and subtilin gene clusters is regulated by tandem R and K genes, which are homologous to two-component regulators (106,118), where LanR is the response regulator and LanK is the sensor kinase.

IV. ROLE OF THE LEADER SEGMENT IN THE LANTIBIOTIC POSTTRANSLATIONAL MODIFICATION REACTIONS

A. Recognition Signals in the Prelantibiotic Peptide

The feature of nisin and the other lantibiotics that distinguishes them from other antimicrobial peptides is the unusual amino acid residues that they contain. Although our understanding of their role in the functional properties of the lantibiotics is rudimentary, the fact that they persist throughout evolution of the diverse forms of lantibiotics argues that they are important. The series of reactions that occur during posttranslational modifications of the prelantibiotics appear to be unique; they have not been observed in any other system. For the posttranslational modifications to occur, the cell has to possess the proper machinery for performing the modifications, and there has to be a polypeptide substrate that is recognized by the machinery. It is clearly important that this recognition be very specific, in order to prevent introduction of the modifications into ordinary cytoplasmic proteins, which would be lethal to the cell. For example, prenisin contains 57 residues, of which the N-terminal 23 residues are removed during maturation, leaving a 34-residue mature region. The cellular machinery that carries out the modifications must be able to recognize and become engaged with the 57-residue prenisin, whereupon it can initiate the sequence of modification events.

Where in the prenisin are these recognition signals? Are they localized solely in the leader region or solely in the mature region, or distributed between them? It has been suggested that the homologies that exist in the leader region, in which there is a consistent pattern in the hydropathic profiles of nisin, subtilin, and epidermin, indicate that the recognition signals have evolved to perform a common function (44,45,119). The hydropathic profile is not typical of a *sec*-type translocation signal, so that these lantibiotics must be secreted by a non-*sec* secretion pathway. It seems likely that the posttranslational modification reactions are associated with this non-*sec* pathway (119).

The processes of recognition and maturation can be segregated into two distinct categories. One is related to those signals in the prepeptide that determine whether it is recognized and engaged by the modification machinery. The other is related to those signals that are responsible for actually performing the modifications, and for orchestrating them so that the molecule actually acquires its correct, biologically active mature structure. What this implies is that a molecule can possess signals that result in the formation of modified residues, but it might lack the necessary information to acquire the correct, biologically active mature structure. For example, formation of each thioether cross-linkage involves the reaction of a particular cysteine residue with its appropriate dehydro residue partner. Nisin contains eight serines and threonines that undergo dehydration, and there are five cysteines that react to form five specific thioether bridges, to leave three unmodified dehydro residues. Therefore, the process by which the correct cysteine–dehydro partners are selected must be highly directed. This directed selection is probably determined by the same folding and conformation effects that are encountered during disulfide bridge formation in common proteins like ribonuclease. Just as ribonuclease cannot form the correct disulfide bridges if the normal conformation is disrupted (120), disruption of folding information in the prenisin molecule may result in formation of incorrect thioether bridges.

There is evidence that the recognition signals required for the dehydration reactions are distinct from the ones that direct the formation of the correct thioether cross-linkages. Hawkins (121) constructed a chimera consisting of the subtilin leader segment fused to the nisin structural segment and then expressed this construct in a subtilin-producing cell. It was determined that the full complement of posttranslational modifications had occurred, and that all the serines and threonines had undergone modification to dehydro residues (with the exception of a single serine, as is present in natural nisin), all the cysteines had been converted to thioethers, and the leader region had been correctly excised. Despite this, the resulting molecule had no antimicrobial activity against outgrowing bacterial spores, and this inactive product electrophoresed on sodium dodecyl sulfate (SDS) gels with the size of a dimer (121) instead of a monomer, as is observed with nisin produced by *L. lactis* (122).

The lack of activity by this same subtilin–nisin chimera has also been reported by Rintala and coworkers (123). Interestingly, these workers also constructed a mosaic molecule in which the 24-residue leader segment consisted of the first 7 residues corresponding to subtilin, and the next 17 residues from nisin, with this in turn fused to the nisin structural region. This construction resulted in the production of active nisin in *Bacillus subtilis* ATCC 6633 (123). One interpretation of these results is that the leader region is sufficient to cause the posttranslational modifications to occur, but in order for the modifications to form correctly in every detail, it is necessary to have the correct interactions between the leader region and the structural region. Thus, although the subtilin leader can induce the modifications to occur, it cannot provide the correct conformational and folding information to direct each cysteine residue to find its correct dehydro residue partner within the nisin structural region. However, providing a subtilin–nisin mosaic leader does provide the correct information.

Recent work by Chakicherla and Hansen (124) has corroborated this interpretation. We constructed a mosaic consisting of the entire subtilin leader, and the N-terminal portion of the nisin structural region, fused to the C-terminal portion of the subtilin structural region. This mosaic underwent the full complement of posttranslational modifications, and it was fully active, with an activity that was equal to or slightly greater than nisin itself. However, when the reverse mosaic molecule was constructed, which consisted of the N-terminal segment of structural region corresponding to subtilin and the C-terminal segment corresponding to nisin, the processing products were highly heterogeneous, suggesting that the processing reactions had "run amok" (124). This result demonstrates that the C-terminal portion of the structural region is particularly important in orchestrating partner selection during thioether bond formation, and that there must be an important interaction between the N-terminal end of the leader segment and the C-terminal end of the structural region. If it is subtilin-like at the N-terminal end of the leader, it must be subtilin-like at the C-terminal end of the structural region in order for the processing to proceed correctly. What is in between the ends seems to be less important: alterations of the sequence around the Dha_5 residue do not disrupt processing or biological activity of the processing products. This is especially demonstrated by the fact that the subtilin machinery can correctly process a serine residue at position 2 to dehydroalanine. Prenisin has a serine at position 2 of the structural region that undergoes dehydration, but subtilin has a lysine at this position. Even though the subtilin machinery is not accustomed to a serine at position 2, it nevertheless proceeds to flawlessly process it to a dehydro-group (124). Sorting out the interactive and conformational relationships that exist between the N- and C-terminal portions of the leader segment and the N- and C-terminal portions of the structural region is going to be very important in providing us with information about how to go about constructing chimeras and mosaics that will be correctly processed into active mature lantibiotic polypeptides. Table 3 summarizes how these chimeric and mosaic molecules are expressed and processed to active forms in *B. subtilis*.

B.   Engineering of the Lantibiotics

Whereas nearly 20 lantibiotics are known, only a few have been subjected to mutagenesis with a view to structure–function studies and making lantibiotics with novel properties and uses. The lantibiotics that have been engineered include nisin (A and Z) (127–133), subtilin (124,134), gallidermin (135), epidermin (135), and Pep5 (136,137), and the general progress has been reviewed (124,138).

A major hurdle in making lantibiotic mutants has been the need to inactivate or remove the natural gene, and then to express the mutant gene in such a way that the mutant gene product has access to the normal lantibiotic-processing machinery. The genes for some lantibiotics, such as Pep5 and epidermin, are plasmid encoded, whereas others such as nisin and subtilin are chromosomally encoded. For the plasmid systems, replacing the natural gene with a mutant gene has required little more than appropriate restriction digestions and ligations to produce a plasmid with an appropriate complement of a mutant lantibiotic gene and the genes for the processing proteins. In this way, a variety of mutants of Pep5 (136) and epidermin (109) have been constructed. In the subtilin system, a mutagenic host–vector pair was engineered in which the chromosomal copy of the subtilin gene in the host was deleted and replaced by an erythryomycin gene. The vector contained a *cat* gene and a cassette version of the subtilin gene, in which a variety

Table 3 Expression of Nisin/Subtilin Chimeras and Mosaics in *Bacillus subtilis*

Cleavage site	Peptide is processed?	Peptide is secreted into extracellular medium?	Secreted peptide is active?	Ref.
ITSISLCTPGCKTGALMGCNMKTATCHCSIHVSK (Nis$^{1-34}$ Mature structure region) **MSTKDFNLDLVSVSKKDSGASPR** (N$_L$$^{1-23}$ Leader region) Nisin (N$_L$$^{1-23}$–Nis$^{1-34}$)	No	No	Not applicable	123,125
WKSESLCTPGCVTGALQTCFLQTLTCNCKISK (Sub$^{1-32}$ Mature structural region) **MSKFDDFDLDVVKVSKQDSKITPQ** (S$_L$$^{1-24}$ Leader region) Subtilin (S$_L$$^{1-24}$–Sub$^{1-32}$)	Yes	Yes	Yes	126
ITSISLCTPGCKTGALMGCNMKTATCHCSIHVSK (Nis$^{1-34}$ Mature structural region) **MSKFDDFDLDVVKVSKQDSKITPQ** (S$_L$$^{1-24}$ Leader region) (S$_L$$^{1-24}$–Nis$^{1-34}$)	Yes	Yes	No	123,125
ITSISLCTPGCKTGALMGCNMKTATCHCSIHVSK (Nis$^{1-34}$ Mature structural region) **MSKFDDF LDLVSVSKKDSGASPR** (S$_L$$^{1-7}$–Nis$^{8-23}$ Leader region) (S$_L$$^{1-7}$–Nis$^{8-23}$–Nis$^{1-34}$)	Yes	Yes	Yes	123
ITSISLCTPGC VTGALQTCFLQTLTCNCKISK (Nis$^{1-11}$–Sub$^{12-32}$ Mature structural region) **MSKFDDFDLDVVKVSKQDSKITPQ** (S$_L$$^{1-24}$ Leader region) (S$_L$$^{1-24}$–Nis$^{1-11}$–Sub$^{12-32}$)	Yes	Yes	Yes	124
WKSESLCTPGC KTGALMGCNMKTATCHCSIHVSK (Sub$^{1-11}$–Nis$^{12-34}$ Mature structural region) **MSKFDDFDLDVVKVSKQDSKITPQ** (S$_L$$^{1-24}$ Leader region) (S$_L$$^{1-24}$–Sub$^{1-11}$–Nis$^{12-34}$)	Heterogeneous	Yes	Partially	124

of restriction sites had been engineered. This permits the excision of portions of the gene, which can be replaced by appropriate synthetic oligo sequences to give a mutant gene. A double recombination then introduces the mutant into the chromosome while deleting the *erm* gene from the chromosome, whereupon the double recombinants with the mutant subtilin gene are chloramphenicol resistant and erythromycin sensitive (134). A similar cassette strategy has been recently developed for making nisin mutants (128); it is superior to a previously used plasmid system (130).

The idiosyncracies of lantibiotic biosynthesis have slowed progress in understanding the roles of the various residues and regions of the mature lantibiotics. In making mutants, one must not just be concerned with the role of the mutagenized residue in the mature lantibiotic, but also its role in the processing reactions. If a particular residue or structural motif plays a critical role in processing, then its modification may result in altering or aborting the processing reactions, so that the corresponding mature lantibiotic may never appear; thus, its role in the biological activity in the mature lantibiotic cannot be assessed. One observation has been that destruction of the lanthionine rings, by means of changing the serine and cysteine components to alanines, usually results in little or no production of the respective lantibiotic. Accordingly, almost all C-terminal alterations of preepidermin that affected the thioether bridge formation at ring C or D resulted in complete loss of epidermin production (138). This sensitivity of the C-terminal end is reminiscent of the situation with subtilin, in which a C-terminal end that is nisin-like instead of subtilin-like appears to disrupt the subtilin-processing reactions (124).

In contrast, changes in the dehydro residues appears to be tolerated well. A Dhb can be placed into subtilin at position 2, which is ordinarily a lysine (124). Similarly, a glycine at position 18 of nisin can be changed to threonine, which is then dehydrated, although not completely; and the Dha_5 can be changed to Dhb (129,130). Many mutations in the ordinary amino acids have been made among nisin, subtilin, epidermin, and Pep5, with well over 40 having been documented. In almost every case, the activity was reduced somewhat (138). The only instances in which significant increases in activity or in the biological spectrum of activity have been observed were when either one dehydro residue has been changed to another dehydro residue, or the environment around a dehydro residue has been changed. The most dramatic effect has been in subtilin, in which the biological activity of the molecule increases 4- to 6-fold upon making substitutions in residues that immediately flank the Dha_5 residue (124,134).

Mutations have also resulted in increased stability of the lantibiotic molecule, toward both chemical inactivation and inactivation by proteases. Changing the Glu_4 of subtilin to Ile enhances the chemical stability of the Dha_5 residue nearly 60-fold, suggesting that the Glu_4 carboxyl-group may actually participate in the spontaneous modification of the Dha_5, perhaps by general-base catalysis of addition of a water molecule across the double bond (134). With respect to proteases, it seems very likely that a major role of the lanthionine rings is to defeat endolytic proteases, which generally possess a peptide-binding cleft on the surface of the molecule. The lanthionine ring creates a topological barrier to binding in the cleft and, therefore, imparts resistance to cleavage. This accounts for nisin, which contains three lysine residues, being resistant to trypsin, which cleaves at lysine residues (139).

The resistance to proteolytic cleavage that is conferred by the lanthionine rings may ultimately prove very important to the utility of lantibiotics and lantibiotic analogs for pharmacological purposes. Important barriers to the use of peptides for treatment of internal infections as well as external ones are the potential for allergic reactions to the peptide and inactivation of the peptide by proteolytic cleavage. Nisin turns out to have very poor immunogenic properties; this is vexing to the experimentalist who wishes to raise antinisin antibodies as an experimental tool, but it is a blessing to nisin's potential use in circumstances where it could provoke an allergic reaction. This, together with the ability of the lanthionine rings to suppress proteolysis, seems to place nisin, and presumably its structural derivatives, in a special category that is different from ordinary peptides.

C.   The Unusual Chemical Properties of the Dha$_5$ Residue of Subtilin and Nisin

The fact that the dehydro and lanthio residues appear in so many lantibiotic molecules argues that they perform important roles in the biological function of the lantibiotic. Whereas the lanthionines have a clear utility in resisting proteases, the role of the dehydro residues is less apparent. In nisin, the dehydro residues can be changed to alanines without destroying their ability to inhibit vegetative cells, but the ability of both subtilin (140) and nisin (141) to inhibit outgrowing spores is destroyed if Dha$_5$ is changed to alanine. As discussed below, this strongly argues that the mechanism by which these lantibiotics inhibit spore outgrowth is different from the mechanism by which they inhibit growing cells.

To understand the mechanism by which the peptide environment around Dha$_5$ might affect its specificity toward nucleophiles, it is useful to consider the unique chemical environment of dehydro residues. Whereas the dehydro residues can be considered simply as novel amino acid side chains, a close examination of their relationship with the polypeptide backbone reveals that they are much more profound than this. One of the essential structural features of polypeptides is that the peptide backbone consists of a series of flat plates that are articulated at the α-carbons, and the polypeptide chain can swivel freely around the pivot points provided by the α-carbons. The ϕ and ψ angles that are adopted at each α-carbon along the chain are what establish the type of structure into which the polypeptide will fold. However, the ϕ–ψ angles that the flat plates can adopt are restricted by various things, such as clash between the amide-groups and the carbonyl, and the nature of the R-groups at the α-carbons. These restrictions are reflected in the familiar Ramachandran plot (142). A dehydro residue can change the fundamental nature of the peptide unit of the peptide backbone. This is because the peptide units in a normal polypeptide have swivel points at the α-carbons, which allow free rotation within the conformational constraints provided by the R-groups. However, the dehydro residue results in a double bond being placed at the α-carbon. This destroys the asymmetry of the α-carbon, and it also causes the planarity of the peptide bond to be extended into the R-group. This is illustrated in the top part of Figure 4.

One can see that the presence of the dehydroalanine has a profound effect on the polypeptide backbone: The α-carbon swivel point at the dehydro residue has disappeared, because of the new delocalization of electrons that becomes possible because of the dehydro-group. For example, the dehydro residue is conjugated with the adjacent carbonyl on one side, and with the lone pair of the amide nitrogen on the other side. This creates a double-bond character that extends throughout the entire region between R$_{-1}$ and R$_{+1}$, which tends to force all the atoms within this region to become coplanar with the peptide bond. This extended region of planarity is introduced wherever a dehydro residue occurs, as shown in Figure 4. This extended rigid plate swivels at the α-carbons attached to R$_{-1}$ and R$_{+1}$. One can also see that the conjugation of the dehydro electrons with the adjacent carbonyl and delocalization into the plane of the peptide are also responsible for

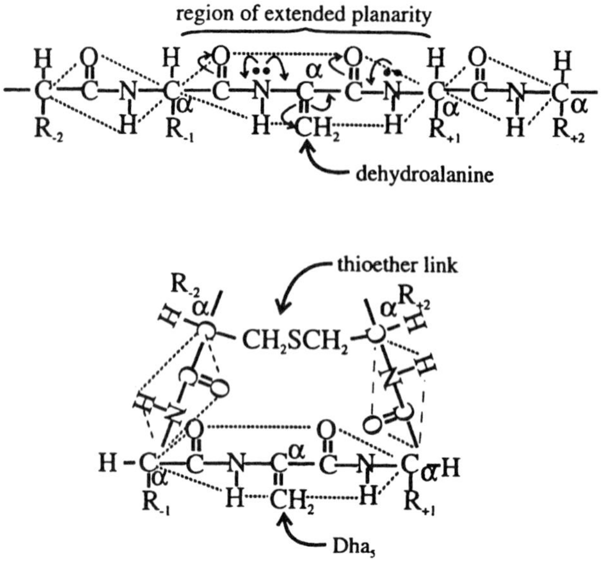

Figure 4 Effect of the Dha residue on the planarity of the peptide backbone. Top: The double bond of the Dha$_5$ residue causes a region of extended planarity that spans across two residues, and the ability of the polypeptide backbone to swivel at the α-carbon of the Dha is lost. Bottom: The thioether link between Dha$_3$ and Cys$_7$ is shown. The region of extended planarity around Dha$_5$ creates an unusual steric configuration in which the ability of nucleophilic agents to approach and add to the double bond of the Dha$_5$ residue is strongly influenced by the size and shape of R$_{-1}$ and R$_{+1}$.

the dehydro-group being a Michael acceptor. Moreover, since the R$_{-1}$- and R$_{+1}$-groups are attached to corners of this planar region, it seems very likely that the nature of R$_{-1}$ and R$_{+1}$ should affect the planar unit and, therefore, the chemical reactivity of the dehydro-group. When seen in this light, the chemical reactivity of the dehydro-group could be quite sensitive to everything about R$_{-1}$ and R$_{+1}$, including their tendency to release and withdraw electrons, any charge that R$_{-1}$ and R$_{+1}$ might have, and steric effects caused by their sizes and shapes.

Now let us consider the effect of the lanthionine ring on this unusual planarity around the Dha$_5$ residue. The bottom part of Figure 4 shows how the thioether cross-link is related to this planar region around the Dha$_5$ residue. The peptide backbone swivels at the α-carbons of the R$_{+1}$ and R$_{-1}$ residues, and the flanking peptide units are twisted upward like butterfly wings that are tethered by their tips. These "wings" span across the region of extended planarity like an awning, and this probably restricts access to the Dha$_5$ by nucleophilic groups, and the electronic and steric properties of R$_{-1}$ and R$_{+1}$ would therefore become very important in determining the reactivity and specificity of the Dha$_5$-group. One can imagine designing a variety of lantibiotic mutants in which these R-groups, as well as other R-groups throughout the peptide, would modulate the reactivity and specificity of the Dha$_5$ residue so that it could be directed toward a variety of different nucleophilic targets. In principle, these could be any nucleophilic targets that are accessible to the lantibiotic, such as those found on viral, enzyme, and bacterial surfaces. Binding to the viral surface could occlude receptor sites, rendering the viral particle noninfectious as well as providing a target for the immune system, which would clear away the inactivated particles. Suitable enzyme targets would be any enzymes that utilize polypeptides as substrates, especially those that have active nucleophiles in their active sites that could react with the dehydro residue. These types of enzymes include proteases and protein kinases, which often play key regulatory roles in metabolic and signal transduction pathways. It is accordingly possible to imagine an array of lantibiotic analogs that could be used to treat a broad range of bacterial and viral infections, and a large variety of regulatory diseases, which could include AIDS and cancer. Infections and regulatory diseases constitute the vast majority of human ailments, and lantibiotics could conceivably be used to treat a great many of these.

Such lantibiotic analogs can be conceptualized as a kind of artificial antibody (44,134). These differ from the antibodies of the immune system: they are much smaller, and they can become covalently attached to their targets (antibodies cannot). Their small size should give them access to targets that exclude antibodies, such as receptors that are hidden in viral crevices; and once the target is reached, it is covalently modified, thus making its inactivation more certain. Because of the conceptual link to antibodies, it is proposed that these lantibiotic analogs be called "lantibodies."

V. MECHANISM OF NISIN/SUBTILIN ANTIMICROBIAL ACTION

Compared with other bacteriocins, nisin and the other lantibiotics have a broad spectrum of action, and they are effective against a wide variety of Gram-positive bacteria, but generally not against Gram-negative bacteria unless the lipopolysaccharide layer (LPS) has been compromised by treatment with chelating agents (143) or by genetic defects (31). The primary site of action is the cytoplasmic membrane of Gram-positive cells, or the inner membrane of Gram-negative cells. Much evidence has been obtained that shows that the type A (nisin-like) lantibiotics form voltage-dependent short-lived pores in the cytoplasmic membrane. However, there also is evidence that nisin and subtilin can become covalently attached to the cell envelope by reacting with a nucleophilic group, such as a sulfhydryl-group. The evidence also supports the idea that these are two separate mechanisms, the pore mechanism and the covalent mechanism, which can act against cells of different types or at different stages of development. We now present the evidence for these two mechanisms.

A. Pore Mechanism

The ability of nisin and other lantibiotics to depolarize membranes and collapse electrochemical and voltage potential gradients has been known for many years (144–150). Whereas an understanding of the mechanism by which lantibiotics achieve this is obviously important, it is becoming perhaps more so because of the mechanistic features that lantibiotics share with the eukaryotic defense molecules such as magainins, defensins, and cecropins. Over the last decade or so, studies of these different classes of molecules have shown that all these molecules function in a generally analogous fashion, with differences in the details of how they exert their effects. In most cases, the agents being studied have been initially shown to interact with membranes to cause leakage of components, collapse of gradients, and cell death through dissipation of critical cell substances and/or cessation of energy metabolism because of the loss of proton-motive forces. Subsequent studies usually include the effects of the agent on natural and artificial vesicles and artificial membranes such as planar black phospholipid bilayers. The conclusion drawn in most cases is that the insertion of the agent molecules into the membrane requires a voltage potential across the membrane that is present in a normal cell as a result of electron transport. Once inserted, ion-conductive pores or channels are formed, which causes collapse of gradients and cessation of cellular functions.

For example, in a review of the bacterially produced lantibiotics (47), Sahl states

> The primary activity of type A lantibiotics is based upon formation of voltage-dependent, short-lived pores in the cytoplasmic membrane. This model is derived from a series of experiments with intact cells, membrane vesicles and planar lipid bilayers [see Refs. 151 and 152]. These studies showed that the peptides rapidly induce leakage of ions and small metabolites from bacterial cells and a collapse of the electrochemical proton gradient. Loss of precursors and energy leads to the cessation of biosynthetic processes and eventually cell death. Type A lantibiotics require a driving force for pore formation which is the proton motive force.

In a completely unrelated paper in that it involves the study of eukaryotic defensins (153), it is stated that

> Defensins are cationic, cysteine-rich peptides (M_r = 3500–4000) found in the cytoplasmic granules of neutrophils and macrophages. These peptides possess broad antimicrobial activity in vitro against bacteria, fungi, tumor cells, and enveloped viruses, and they are believed to contribute to the "oxygen-independent" antimicrobial defenses of neutrophils and macrophages. Pathophysiologic studies in vitro have pointed to the plasma membrane as a possible target for the cytotoxic action of defensins. We report here that defensins form voltage-dependent, weakly anion-selective channels in planar lipid bilayer membranes, and we suggest that this channel-forming ability contributes to their antimicrobial properties observed.

One finds similar statements in other papers on studies of defensins (154), *E. coli*–produced colicin (155), moth-produced cecropin (156), frog-produced magainin (157–159), and lactococcal-produced lactococcin A (160). It would be reasonable to conclude that the same fundamental mechanism is occurring in all cases. However, this simple conclusion would ignore the high specificity of all these agents toward particular target cell types. The significance of this specificity is explored further in Section V.C.

B. Covalent Modification Mechanism

Studies of nisin were initiated in the author's laboratory while doing research on the mechanism of action of inhibition of bacterial spore outgrowth by nitrite. Experiments on nitrite analogs (161–162) and on nitrite itself (164–166) established that modification of sulfhydryl-groups in the membranes of outgrowing bacterial spores would result in inhibition of the outgrowth process at the stage between phase-darkening of germination and the onset of swelling in outgrowth. It was observed that virtually any sulfhydryl-modifying agent could achieve this inhibition. Experiments with labeled iodoacetate established that the sulfhydryl-groups were in the membrane (166), and that nitrite (164) and its analogs (165–167) could inhibit uptake of labeled iodoacetate by the membrane sulfhydryl-groups. It was the speculation by Gross that the natural biological function of the dehydro residues in nisin is to act as sulfhydryl-group modifying agents in a Michael-type reaction (168) that prompted us to test whether nisin could react with the membrane sulfhydryl-groups of outgrowing bacterial spores and, in this way, cause inhibition of spore outgrowth. Whereas it was already known that nisin was effective as an inhibitor of spore outgrowth (16,22,169,170), the mechanism by which it achieved this effect was unknown. We observed that nisin indeed interfered with radioactive iodoacetate uptake into bacterial spores, and it inhibited the spores at exactly the same stage (166), between germination and outgrowth, as did all the other sulfhydryl-modifying agents that we had tried. This provided circumstantial evidence that nisin inhibits spore outgrowth via the same mechanism as nitrite, and that this mechanism involves the modification of membrane sulfhydryl-groups in spores that have undergone germination. We have attempted the obvious next step, which is to treat germinated spores with nisin and recover a membrane component to which the nisin molecule is covalently attached. Experimental attempts to do this did not succeed in recovering such a nisin-modified membrane component. What was recovered was a nisin-modified component of the spore coat (Liu W and Hansen JN, unpublished results).

1.   Dha$_5$ of Nisin Is Critical for Inhibition of Spore Outgrowth

If a covalent-modification mechanism of nisin action is involved in inhibition of spore outgrowth, then mutagenesis to change dehydro residues to non-dehydro residues should destroy the antimicrobial effect. Liu and Hansen performed some experiments with subtilin that shed light on this question (134). Subtilin is an intrinsically unstable molecule in aqueous solution, and we observed that the kinetics of subtilin activity loss was correlated with the disappearance of the Dha$_5$ nuclear magnetic resonance (NMR) resonance peak (134). We then changed Dha$_5$ to Ala, and we found that the Dha5A-subtilin was completely inactive toward inhibition of spore outgrowth, which suggests that an intact Dha$_5$ is necessary for the molecule to possess biological activity.

2.   Nisin with Dha$_5$ Changed to Ala Is Active Against Vegetative Cells

Additional studies of the Dha5A-subtilin variant produced the observation that spores germinated in the presence of the variant proceeded through outgrowth without any signs of inhibition, but when they reached the vegetative stage of growth, they lysed (140). Moreover, it was observed that subtilin with a normal Dha$_5$ would also lyse the cells when added during vegetative growth, and that the specific activity of subtilin with a normal Dha$_5$ was the same as Dha5A-subtilin. We concluded that the mechanism by which subtilin halted spore outgrowth (without lysis) was different from the mechanism by which subtilin killed vegetative cells (with lysis). That subtilin could exert its biological effects by more than one mechanism was not completely unexpected (171). Now that it has been explicitly observed, workers who are performing structure–function studies of lantibiotics will constantly need to be concerned about the effects of their assay system on the interpretations of their results. For example, if Liu and Hansen had been using the conventional assay that employs growing cells, they would have missed the observation that Dha$_5$ is a critical residue for the activity of subtilin against outgrowing spores.

C.   The Nisin/Subtilin Mechanism Compared with the Defensin Mechanism

The history of experience with antibiotics that conform to the penicillin paradigm is that they come in many structural forms and have many strategies for destruction of their targets. Some of these, such as penicillin itself, target the cell wall. Others interfere with membranes, and a large number are known to enter the cell and interfere with a variety of functions, very frequently the protein biosynthetic machinery, as is the case with antibiotics such as chloramphenicol, erythromycin, and streptomycin. Early studies with proteinaceous antibiotics such as the bacteriocins did not force us to revise this viewpoint, since they also are directed toward a wide variety of targets (172).

Now the nisin-like lantibiotics and the enormous variety of eukaryotic defense proteins have appeared on the scene. Despite the apparent multiple mechanisms of subtilin and the surprising array of biological effects exerted by the various types of lantibiotics as described in Section II, these defense proteins are generally cationic (i.e., basic) polypeptides that contain amphipathic helices, and they kill cells by entering the cytoplasmic membrane, causing the collapse of chemical and voltage gradients, the dissipation of the cell's resources, and the eventual death of the cell. That a polypeptide could do this is not remarkable. What is remarkable is the exquisite specificity with which this effect can be achieved by the various individual defense peptides toward different target cell types. For example, magainins can destroy bacteria, fungi, protozoa (35,173), and even eukaryotic tumor cells (174), but they do not harm the somatic cells (34) or erythrocytes (175) of the frog. Similarly, cecropins have powerful antimicrobial effects, but they do not harm erythrocytes (176). This kind of specificity is not something that one automatically expects, as evidenced by the tendency of researchers to use artificial membranes and other generic model systems to study the ability of these substances to cause permeability increases. They would not do this if their reflexive expectation were that a given defense peptide is highly specific for the membrane from a particular type of cell. Instead, the picture that is emerging is that each cell type has a membrane that differs from those of other, even very closely related, cell types such as may be found within a single eukaryotic organism, and that these differences are sufficient to permit highly selective targeting by the defense peptides. A clue to the source of this selectivity is that cecropins are not very effective in permeabilizing bilayers that have a positive surface charge or contain cholesterol, which is consistent with the known insensitivity of eukaryotic cells to cecropins (156).

Although we are accustomed to the idea that protein–protein interactions are highly specific, we are not so accustomed to the idea that polypeptides are highly specific with respect to the type of membrane that they can enter to assemble into a pore or channel. The accumulating evidence that defense peptides have such specificity allows us to consider how to exploit this capability in a useful way. Nature has already demonstrated that defense peptides are extremely versatile, in that they are employed by virtually all types of organisms, and that today's defense peptides are of ancient evolutionary origin (177). Indeed, these defense peptides were probably the main form of immunity that organisms possessed prior to the evolution of the adaptive immune system (178). It seems very likely that acquiring an understanding of the specificity of the defense peptides for their targets would give rise to our ability to design and construct polypeptides that are targeted in ways that we find useful. Inasmuch as there appears to be great commonality in the underlying mechanisms of interactions by nisin-like lantibiotics and the panoply of defense peptides, the ease and flexibility with which the bacterially produced lantibiotics can be constructed and synthesized seems to position them as a model system for studying the basic principles of specificity of membrane targeting and the mechanism of induction of membrane permeability and cell destruction.

VI.   INDUSTRIAL PRODUCTION OF NISIN

A.   Nisin Manufacture

At present, Aplin and Barrett in England is the only industrial producer of nisin. Nisin is produced by the fermentation of a proprietary strain of *Lactococcus lactis*, on a skim-milk-based medium. The origin of the strain has not been reported, but it was in use prior to the development of recombinant DNA methods, so that it must have been derived using classical genetic methods. The manufacturing process involves dewatering of the culture by a drying process that involves spraying onto a rotating heated drum. The resulting tan-colored powder is marketed as Nisaplin, and it contains about 2% nisin by weight with a specific nisin activity of 1 million IU/g. If one assumes that the original culture medium consisted of 2% dissolved skim milk powder, which was converted to nisin in 2% yield, the culture medium would contain about 400 mg of nisin per liter. The production of this industrial strain is probably at least 50 times better than typical wild-type laboratory strains, such as L. lactis ATCC 11454. It is reasonable to expect that our knowledge of the nisin operon would permit the engineering a dramatic increase in the expression of nisin, probably by manipulating the promoters to increase expression of the nisA structural gene, as well as by modification of critical transport proteins. Nisin is ordinarily produced in late growth phases (50,119), but it may be possible to alter the regulation of the expression of the nisin genes so that nisin would be produced continuously, which could lead to higher production levels. Subtilin is similarly produced during late growth phases in Bacillus subtilis, with production being greatest in relatively late stationary phase (126). Since this is a stage at which the metabolism of the cell is greatly reduced, it seems likely that one could obtain much higher production levels if the regulation of expression could be altered so that production during log-phase growth would occur. It seems likely that as we learn to increase production of one lantibiotic, we will gain insight about how to increase production of the others.

Assays of nisin are done using Streptococcus cremoris, which is very sensitive to nisin (52). Nisin activity was originally measured in "Reading Units," because the work was performed at the University of Reading. Mattick and Hirsch (51) compared unknown nisin solutions with a purified standard that was stored frozen in 0.05 N HCl. Activity was determined in the manner of a minimum inhibitory concentration, and "the titre of the substance is taken as the dilution of the last tube in which growth is not visible" (51). The term "Reading Units" has been changed to "International Units," or IU/ml, but the numerical values are not changed. A more recent description of the nisin assay is given by Hurst (179), in which a nisin that was purified by ultracentrifugation was used as a standard. The standard most readily available today is Nisaplin, which consistently has an activity of about 1 million IU/g. Because Nisaplin is 2% nisin, pure nisin should have an activity of about 50 million IU/g. Highly purified nisin is obtained from Nisaplin by a proprietary purification process developed by AMBI, Inc., Tarrytown, NY, to give nisin preparations that consist of a white fluffy powder that is about 98% pure nisin. About 12–15% of the preparation appears to be a structural variant of nisin that contains an undehydrated serine instead of a dehydroalanine at position 33. It is this purified form that is used for pharmacological formulations, under the name of Ambicin N.

B.   Production of Nisin and Other Lantibiotics in Genetically Engineered Heterologous Strains, such as *Bacillus subtilis* 168

In Section IV, the role of the leader segment of the prelantibiotic polypeptide in orchestrating the posttranslational modifications was discussed. Although studies of the mechanism of posttranslational modification reactions and how the leader segment participates in and orchestrates this process are still in their early stages, certain principles are already clear. First, there seems to be some specificity between the host modification enzymes and the lantibiotic precursor that they can process. Accordingly, it is not possible to simply express the prenisin gene in subtilin-producing *Bacillus subtilis* 168, and have the subtilin-processing enzymes flawlessly perform modifications to produce active nisin. However, it is possible to produce nisin if one constructs a mosaic prenisin in which the leader segment combines appropriate portions from both prenisin and presubtilin. If this is done, it is possible to produce nisin from *B. subtilis* ATCC 6633 (see Section IV). Moreover, Liu and Hansen (180) have successfully transferred the ability to produce subtilin from *B. subtilis* ATCC 6633 to *B. subtilis* 168. This is an important achievement, because *B. subtilis* is an important industrial organism that has been groomed to produce a wide variety of biological products, and all of these industrial strains have been derived from strain 168. The genetic information and methodologies that are available for strain 168 are superb, and the fact that strain 168 has been adapted to produce a lantibiotic suggests that it is only a matter of time and effort to engineer 168 to produce copious amounts of subtilin. If strain 168 can produce subtilin, why not the other lantibiotics? This would be an advantage, because the *L. lactis* that is used for commercial production of nisin was obtained using classical genetic selection techniques long before the advent of genetic engineering, and the genetic basis for its efficient production of nisin is not known. It is reasonable to suppose that current knowledge about the structure and sequence of the nisin operon could be exploited to enable the construction of a high-production strain of *L. lactis* using genetic engineering methods. However, a disadvantage of *L. lactis* is that it is a fastidious organism that can only be grown in a complex medium such as milk. The fact that production of active extracellular nisin requires the orchestrated expression of several genes, including the production of proteins involved in the posttranslational modifications and translocation, suggests that it may be important to coordinate their expression both temporally and quantitatively. It is therefore probable that simply expressing the nisin gene in a high-copy plasmid with a strong promoter in a nisin-producing strain of *L. lactis* will not suffice to construct an efficient nisin producer. Unless increased production of the precursor of nisin is coordinated with an increase in the enzymes involved in modification and secretion, these enzymes may be overwhelmed and unable to perform their functions, leaving some of the nisin either incompletely or inaccurately processed. These concerns have some foundation in that the expression of plasmids that contained mutations in the nisin structural genes was found to result in production of heterologous forms of nisin that differed in the extent of conversion of threonine to dehydrobutyrine (130), and further, studies of the expression of peptides consisting of fusions between the subtilin leader and alkaline phosphatase showed that the alkaline phosphatase was not subjected to modification when expressed from a multi-copy plasmid (114).

An alternative is to transfer nisin production into a heterologous bacterial strain that is better suited for industrial production than is *L. lactis*. An attractive candidate is *B. subtilis* 168, for the reasons just stated. Section IV describes some of the results from attempts to convert *B. subtilis* to a nisin producer. So far, all of the attempts to achieve this conversion have involved expressing the prenisin gene in a strain of *B. subtilis* that is capable of making subtilin, and entrusting the task of carrying out the posttranslational modifications in prenisin to the subtilin machinery. Whereas this was achievable by the stratagem of constructing mosaic molecules in order to make the prenisin more recognizable, what has not yet been attempted is to move the entire nisin machinery from *L. lactis* into *B. subtilis*. This would address the question of whether the inability of *B. subtilis* to process prenisin is a consequence of the differences in the components of the modification machinery, or of the differences in the host cell. For example, if the posttranslational machinery is localized in the cell envelope, the structure of the envelope may influence the function of the machinery. If this is the case, then transfer of the nisin machinery to B. subtilis would not help, since the nisin components would have to operate in the environment of the subtilin envelope. On the other hand, the inability to achieve perfect heterologous recognition may be due to structural differences in the modification machinery, with no effect exerted by the cell envelope. If the former is the case, then conversion B. subtilis 168 to a general producer of lantibiotics will be difficult. If the latter is true, then producing essentially any lantibiotic by the same highly efficient industrial organism should be possible. If it is possible, then the prospects of lantibiotics achieving their potential for practical use will be bright, because to manufacture a lantibiotic, it will not be necessary to optimize production in each lantibiotic host, as is being done at present (127,181,182). Generating the availability of bulk quantities of a variety of lantibiotics at moderate cost will be a key step in bringing these interesting and versatile molecules into the common use that they deserve.

ACKNOWLEDGMENTS

The author's research on lantibiotics is being supported by NIH grant AI24454, and AMBI, Inc., Tarrytown, NY.

DEDICATION

The author dedicates this chapter to the memory of Andre "Bundy" Hurst (previously known as A. Hirsch), whose studies of nisin and its role in cells spanned nearly 50 years. It was Hurst's conviction that nisin was a potentially important biological material that caused him to nurture its development during the early 1940s, and he continued studies of nisin during subsequent decades. It was he who provided sufficient quantities of nisin to permit the structural studies performed by Erhard Gross, without which identification of the nisin gene would have been impossible. The author was fortunate to have spent a day in intense conversation about nisin with Bundy Hurst, and then he exchanged many telephone calls and letters with him, in which Hurst was extremely supportive of the new direction that nisin research had taken and provided constructive criticism about some of my manuscripts. Although illness prevented Bundy from attending, he was delighted when the first international meeting about nisin was held in Bonn in 1991, which was 47 years after his first nisin publication. Because of my interest in continuing the nisin research that he was forced to abandon, Bundy called me his "spiritual son," which confers on me a responsibility to be mindful of the history of nisin, as well as of the present and the future that it portends.

REFERENCES

1. Rogers LA, Wittier EO. Limiting factors in the lactic fermentation. J Bacteriol 1928; 16:211–229.
2. Mattick ATR, Hirsch A. A powerful inhibitory substance produced by group N streptococci. Nature 1944; 154:551–552.

3. Taylor JI, Hirsch A, Mattick ATR. The treatment of bovine Streptococcal and Staphylococcal mastitis with nisin. Vet Rec 1949; 61:197–198.

4. Sears PM, Smith BS, Rubino SD, Kulisek E, Gusik S, Blackburn P. Non-antibiotic approach to treatment of mastitis in the lactating dairy cow. J Dairy Sci 1991; 74:203.

5. Broadbent JR, Chou YC, Gillies K, Kondo JK. Nisin inhibits several gram-positive, mastitis-causing pathogens. J Dairy Sci 1989; 72:3342–3345.

6. Sears PM, Smith BS, Stewart WK, Gonzalez RN, Rubino SD, Gusik SA, Kulisek ES, Projan SJ, Blackburn P. Evaluation of a nisin-based germicidal formulation on teat skin of live cows. J Dairy Sci 1992; 75:3185–3190.

7. Howell TH, Fiorellini JP, Blackburn P, Projan SJ, de la Harpe J, Williams RC. The effect of a mouthrinse based on nisin, a bacteriocin, on developing plaque and gingivitis in beagle dogs. J Clin Periodontol 1993; 20:335–339.

8. Food and Drug Administration. Nisin preparation: Affirmation of GRAS status as a direct human food ingredient. Fed Reg 1988; 53:11247–11251.

9. Zottola EA, Yezzi TL, Ajao DB, Roberts RF. Utilization of cheddar cheese containing nisin as an antimicrobial agent in other foods. Intl J Food Microbiol 1994; 24:227–238.

10. Delves-Broughton J, Blackburn P, Evans RJ, Hugenholtz J. Applications of the bacteriocin, nisin. Antonie van Leeuwenhoek 1996; 69:193–202.

11. Hansen JN. Nisin as a model food preservative. Clydesdale FM, ed. CRC Critical Reviews in Food Science and Nutrition. Boca Raton, Florida: CRC Press, 1994:69–93.

12. Vandamme EJ. The search for novel microbial fine chemicals, agrochemicals and biopharmaceuticals. J Biotechnol 1994; 37:89–108.

13. McClintock M, Serres LMJJ, Hirsch A. Mocquot G. Action inhibitrice des streptocoques producteurs de ninine sur le developpement des sporules anaerobies dans le fromage de Gruyere Fondue. J Dairy Res 1952; 19:187–193.

14. Delves-Broughton J. Nisin and its uses as a food preservative. Food Technol 1990; 44:100–117.

15. Scott VN, Taylor SL. Effect of nisin on the outgrowth of *Clostridium botulinum* spores. J Food Sci 1981; 46:117–126.

16. Scott VN, Taylor SL. Temperature, pH, and spore load effects on the ability of nisin to prevent the outgrowth of *Clostridium botulinum* spores. J Food Sci 1981; 46:121–126.

17. Somers EB, Taylor SL. Antibotulinal effectiveness of nisin in pasteurised processed cheese spreads. J Food Prot 1987; 50:842–848.

18. Roberts RF, Zottola EA. Shelf-life of pasteurized process cheese spreads made from cheddar cheese manufactured with a nisin-producing starter culture. J Dairy Sci 1993; 76:1829–1836.

19. Dean JP, Zottola EA. Use of nisin in ice-cream and effect on the survival of *Listeria monocytogenes*. J Food Prot 1996; 59:476.

20. Benedict RC. Biochemical basis for nitrite-inhibition of *Clostridium botulinum* in cured meat. J Food Prot 1980; 43:877–891.

21. Taylor SL, Somers EB. Evaluation of the antibotulinal effectiveness of nisin in bacon. J Food Prot 1985; 48:949–952.

22. Taylor SL, Somers EB, Krueger LA. Antibotulinal effectiveness of nisin-nitrite combinations in culture and chicken frankfurter emulsions. J Food Prot 1985; 48:234–239.

23. Caserio G, Ciampella M, Gennari M, Barluzzi AM. Utilization of nisin in cooked sausages and other cured meat products. Ind Aliment 1979; 18:12–19.

24. Caserio G, Stecchini M, Pastore M, Gennari M. The individual and combined effects of nisin and nitrite on the spore germination of *Clostridium perfringens* in meat mixtures subjected to fermentation. Ind Aliment 1979; 18:894–898.

25. Rayman MK, Aris B, Hurst A. Nisin: A possible alternative or adjunct to nitrite in the preservation of meats. Appl Environ Microbiol 1981; 41:375–380.

26. Rayman K, Malik N, Hurst A. Failure of nisin to inhibit outgrowth of *Clostridium botulinum* in a model cured meat system. Appl Environ Microbiol 1983; 46:1450–1452.

27. Calderon C, Collins-Thompson DL, Usborne WR. Shelf-life studies of vacuum-packaged bacon treated with nisin. J Food Prot 1985; 48:330–333.

28. Daeschel MA, Jung D-S, Watson BT. Controlling wine malolactic fermentation with nisin and nisin-resistant strains of *Leuconostoc oenos*. Appl Environ Microbiol 1991; 57:601–603.

29. Breuer B, Radler F. Inducible resistance against nisin in *Lactobacillus casei*. Arch Microbiol 1996; 165:114–118.

30. Jensen I, Baird L, Delves-Broughton J. The use of nisin as a preservative in crumpets. J Food Prot 1994; 57:874–877.

31. Stevens KA, Klapes NA, Sheldon BW, Klaenhammer TR. Antimicrobial action of nisin against *Salmonella typhimurium* lipopolysaccharide mutants. Appl Environ Microbiol 1992; 58:1786–1788.

32. Mahadeo M, Tatini SR. The potential use of nisin to control *Listeria monocytogenes* in poultry. Lett Appl Microbiol 1994; 18:323–326.

33. Cutter CN, Siragusa GR. Decontamination of beef carcass tissue with nisin using a pilot-scale model carcass washer. Food Microbiol 1994; 11:481–489.

34. Zasloff M. Magainins, a class of antimicrobial peptides from *Xenopus* skin: Isolation, characterization of two active forms, and partial cDNA sequence of a precursor. Proc Natl Acad Sci USA 1987; 84:5449–5453.

35. Zasloff M, Martin B, Chen HC. Antimicrobial activity of synthetic magainin peptides and several analogues. Proc Natl Acad Sci USA 1988; 85:910–913.

36. Rice WG, Ganz T, Kinkade JM Jr, Selsted ME, Lehrer RI, Parmley RT. Defensin-rich dense granules of human neutrophils. Blood 1987; 70:757–765.

37. Valore EV, Ganz T. Posttranslational processing of defensins in immature human myeloid cells. Blood 1992; 79:1538–1544.

38. Siden I, Boman HG. *Escherichia coli* mutants with an altered sensitivity to cecropin D. J Bacteriol 1983; 154:170–176.

39. Gudmundsson GH, Lidholm DA, Asling B, Gan R, Boman HG. The cecropin locus. Cloning and expression of a gene cluster encoding three antibacterial peptides in *Hyalophora cecropia*. J Biol Chem 1991; 266:11510–11517.

40. Ingram L. A ribosomal mechanism for synthesis of peptides related to nisin. Biochim Biophys Acta 1970; 224:263–265.

41. Skaugen M, Nissenmeyer J, Jung G, Stevanovic S, Sletten, K, Abildgaard, CIM, Nes, IF. *In vivo* conversion of L-serine to D-alanine in a ribosomally synthesized polypeptide. J Biol Chem 1994; 269:27183–27185.

42. Allgaier H, Jung G, Werner RG, Schneider U, Zahner H. Epidermin: Sequencing of a heterodetic tetracyclic 21-peptide amide antibiotic. Eur J Biochem 1986; 160:9–22.

43. Nes IF, Tagg JR. Novel lantibiotics and their pre-peptides. Antonie van Leeuwenhoek 1996; 69:89–97.

44. Hansen JN. Antibiotics synthesized by post-translational modification. Annu Rev Microbiol 1993; 47:535–564.

45. Hansen JN. The molecular biology of nisin and its structural analogs. Hoover D, Steenson L, eds. Bacteriocins of Lactic Acid Bacteria. New York: Academic Press, 1993:93–120.

46. Jung G. Lantibiotics: A survey. Jung G, Sahl H-G, eds. Nisin and Novel Lantibiotics. Leiden, The Netherlands: ESCOM, 1991:1–34.

47. Sahl H-G. Gene-encoded antibiotics made in bacteria. Marsh J, Goode JA, eds. Antimicrobial Peptides, Ciba Foundation Symposium 186. Chichester, England: John Wiley and Sons, 1994:27–53.

48. Sahl H-G, Jack RW, Bierbaum G. Biosynthesis and biological activities of lantibiotics with unique post-translational modifications. Eur J Biochem 1995; 230:827–853.

49. De Vos WM, Kuipers OP, van der Meer JR, Siezen RJ. Maturation pathway of nisin and other lantibiotics: Post-translationally modified antimicrobial peptides exported by grampositive bacteria. Mol Microbiol 1995; 17:427–437.

50. Hurst A. Nisin. Adv Appl Microbiol 1981; 27:85–123.

51. Mattick ATR, Hirsch A. Further observations on an inhibitory substance (nisin) from lactic streptococci. Lancet 1947; 2:5–12.

52. Hirsch A. The assay of the antibiotic nisin. Intl J Food Microbiol 1950; 4:70–83.

53. Hirsch A. Growth and nisin production of a strain of *Streptococcus lactis*. J Gen Microbiol 1951; 5:208–221.

54. Gross E, Morell JL. The structure of nisin. J Am Chem Soc 1971; 93:4634–4635.

55. Stubbs JJ, Feeney RE, Lewis JC, Feustel IC, Lightbody HD, Garibaldi JA. Subtilin production in submerged cultures. Arch Biochem 1947; 14:427–435.

56. Feeney RE, Garibaldi JA, Humphreys EM. Nutritional studies on subtilin formation by *Bacillus subtilis*. Arch Biochem Biophys 1948; 17:435–445.

57. Gross E, Kiltz HH, Nebelin E. Subtilin 6: The structure of subtilin. Hoppeseyler's Z Physiol Chem 1973; 354:810–812.

58. Gross E. Subtilin and nisin: The chemistry and biology of peptides with alpha, beta-unsaturated amino acids. Walter R, Meienhofer J, eds. Peptides: Chemistry, Structure, and Biology. Ann Arbor, Michigan: Ann Arbor Science, 1975:31–42.

59. Schnell N, Entian KD, Schneider U, Gotz F, Zahner H, Kellner R, Jung G. Prepeptide sequence of epidermin, a ribosomally synthesized antibiotic with four sulphide-rings. Nature 1988; 333:276–278.

60. Kellner R, Jung G, Josten M, Kaletta C, Entian K-D, Sahl H-G. Pep5: Structure elucidation of a large lantibiotic. Angew Chem Int Ed Engl 1989; 28:616–619.

61. van de Kamp M, van den Hooven HW, Konings RN, Bierbaum G, Sahl H-G, Kuipers OP, Siezen RJ, De Vos WM, Hilbers CW, van de Ven FJ. Elucidation of the primary structure of the lantibiotic epilancin K7 from *Staphylococcus epidermidis* K7. Cloning and characterisation of the epilancin-K7-encoding gene and NMR analysis of mature epilancin K7. Eur J Biochem 1995; 230:587–600.

62. Marki F, Hanni E, Fredenhagen A, van Oostrum J. Mode of action of the lanthionine-containing peptide antibiotics duramycin, duramycin B and C, and cinnamycin as indirect inhibitors of phospholipase A2. Biochem Pharmacol 1991; 42:2027–2035.

63. Kaletta C, Entian KD, Jung G. Prepeptide sequence of cinnamycin (Ro 09-0198): The first structural gene of a duramycin-type lantibiotic. Eur J Biochem 1991; 199:411–415.

64. Wakamiya T, Ueki Y, Shiba T, Kido Y, Motoki Y. The structure of ancovenin, a new peptide inhibitor of angiotensin I converting enzyme. Tetrahedron Lett 1985; 26:665–668.

65. Niu WW, Neu HC. Activity of mersacidin, a novel peptide, compared with that of vancomycin, teicoplanin, and daptomycin. Antimicrob Agents Chemother 1991; 35:998–1000.

66. Malabarba A, Pallanza R, Berti M, Cavalleri B. Synthesis and biological activity of some amide derivatives of the lantibiotic actagardine. J Antibiot (Tokyo) 1990; 43:1089–1097.

67. Piard JC, Kuipers OP, Rollema HS, Desmazeaud MJ, De Vos WM. Structure, organization, and expression of the *lct* gene for lacticin 481, a novel lantibiotic produced by *Lactococcus lactis*. J Biol Chem 1993; 268:16361–16368.

68. Tagg JR, Wannamaker LW. Streptococcin A-FF22: Nisin-like antibiotic substance produced by a group A *Streptococcus*. Anitmicrob Agents Chemother 1978; 14:31–39.

69. Ross KF, Ronson CW, Tagg JR. Isolation and characterization of the lantibiotic salivaricin A and its structural gene salA from *Streptococcus salivarius* 20P3. Appl Environ Microbiol 1993; 59:2014–2021.

70. Mortvedt CI, Nissen-Meyer J, Nes IF. Purification and amino acid sequence of lactocin S, a bactericin produced by *Lactobacillus sake* L45. Appl Environ Microbiol 1991; 57:1829–1834.

71. Stoffels G, Sahl H-G, Gudmundsdottir A. Carnocin UI49, a potential biopreservative produced by *Carnobacterium piscicola*: Large scale purification and activity against various gram-positive bacteria including *Listeria* sp. Intl J Food Microbiol 1993; 20:199–210.

72. Novak J, Caufield PW, Miller EJ. Isolation and biochemical characterization of a novel lantibiotic mutacin from *Streptococcus mutans*. J Bacteriol 1994; 176:4316–4320.

73. Novak J, Kirk M, Caufield PW, Barnes S, Morrison K, Baker J. Detection of modified amino-acids in lantibiotic peptide mutacin-II by chemical derivatization and electrospray-ionization mass spectroscopic analysis. Anal Biochem 1996; 236:358–360.

74. Chikindas ML, Novak J, Driessen AJ, Konings WN, Schilling KM, Caufield PW. Mutacin II, a bactericidal lantibiotic from *Streptococcus mutans*. Anitmicrob Agents Chemother 1995; 39:2656–2660.

75. Gilmore MS, Segarra RA, Booth MC, Bogie CP, Hall LR, Clewell DB. Genetic structure of the *Enterococcus faecalis* plasmid pAD1–encoded cytolytic toxin system and its relationship to lantibiotic determinants. J Bacteriol 1994; 176:7335–7344.

76. Gross E, Morrell JL. The structure of nisin. J Am Chem Soc 1971; 93:4634–4635.

77. Kellner R, Jung G, Horner T, Zahner H, Schnell N, Entian KD, Gotz F. Gallidermin: A new lanthionine-containing polypeptide antibiotic. Eur J Biochem 1988; 177:53–59.

78. Kogler H, Bauch M, Fehlhaber H-W, Griesinger C, Schubert W, Teetz V. NMR-spectroscopic investigations on mersacidin. Jung G, Sahl H-G, eds. Nisin and Novel Lantibiotics. Leiden, The Netherlands: ESCOM, 1991:159–170.

79. Brotz H, Bierbaum G, Markus A, Molitor E, Sahl H-G. Mode of action of the lantibiotic mersacidin: Inhibition of peptidoglycan biosynthesis via a novel mechanism? Antimicrob Agents Chemother 1995; 39:714–719.

80. Bierbaum G, Brotz H, Koller KP, Sahl H-G. Cloning, sequencing and production of the lantibiotic mersacidin. FEMS Microbiol Lett 1995; 127:121–126.

81. Kettenring JK, Malabarba A, Vekey K, Cavalleri B. Sequence determination of actagardine, a novel lantibiotic, by homonuclear 2D NMR spectroscopy. J Antibiot (Tokyo) 1990; 43:1082–1088.

82. Malabarba A, Landi M, Pallanza R, Cavalleri B. Physico-chemical and biological properties of actagardine and some acid hydrolysis products. J Antibiot (Tokyo) 1985; 38:1506–1511.

83. Navarro J, Chabot J, Sherrill K, Aneja R, Zahler SA, Racker E. Interaction of duramycin with artificial and natural membranes. Biochem 1985; 24:4645–4650.

84. Sheth TR, Henderson RM, Hladky SB, Cuthbert AW. Ion channel formation by duramycin. Biochim Biophys Acta 1992; 1107:179–185.

85. Fredenhagen A, Fendrich G, Marki F, Marki W, Gruner J, Raschdorf F, Peter HH. Duramycins B and C, two new lanthionine containing antibiotics as inhibitors of phospholipase A2. Structural revision of duramycin and cinnamycin. J Antibiot (Tokyo) 1990; 43:1403–1412.

86. Fredenhagen A, Marki F, Fendrich G, Marki W, Gruner J, Van Oostrum J, Raschdorf F, Peter HH. Duramycin B and C, two new lanthionine-containing antibiotics as inhibitors of phospholipase A2, and structural revision of duramycin and cinnamycin. Jung G, Sahl H-G, eds. Nisin and Novel Lantibiotics. Leiden, The Netherlands: ESCOM, 1991:131–140.

87. Kessler H, Seip S, Wein T, Steuernagel S, Will M. Structure of cinnamycin (Ro 09-0198) in solution. Jung G, Sahl H-G, eds. Nisin and Novel Lantibiotics. Leiden, The Netherlands: ESCOM, 1991:76–90.

88. Shiba T, Wakamiya T, Fukase K, Ueki Y, Teshima T, Nishikawa M. Structure of the lanthionine peptides nisin, ancovenin, and lanthiopeptin. Jung G, Sahl H-G, eds. Nisin and Novel Lantibiotics. Leiden, The Netherlands: ESCOM, 1991:113–122.

89. Naruse N, Tenmyo O, Tomita K, Konishi M, Miyaki T, Kawaguchi H, Fukase K, Wakamiya T, Shiba T. Lanthiopeptin, a new peptide antibiotic. Production, isolation and properties of lanthiopeptin. J Antibiot (Tokyo) 1989; 42:837–845.

90. Chatterjee S, Chatterjee DK, Jani RH, Blumbach J, Ganguli BN, Klesel N, Limbert M, Seibert G. Mersacidin, a new antibiotic from *Bacillus*. *In vitro* and *in vivo* antibacterial activity. J Antibiot (Tokyo) 1992; 45:839–845.

91. Hurst A, Collins-Thompson D. Food as a bacterial habitat. Adv Microb Ecol 1979; 3:79–133.

92. Hedge PJ, Spratt BG. Resistance to beta-lactam antibiotics by re-modelling the active site of an *E. coli* penicillin-binding protein. Nature 1985; 318:478–480.

93. Spratt BG. Resistance to antibiotics mediated by target alterations. Science 1994; 264:388–393.

94. Kelly JA, Moews PC, Knox JR, Frere JM, Ghuysen JM. Penicillin target enzyme and the antibiotic binding site. Science 1982; 218:479–481.

95. Bruice TC, Mei HY, He GX, Lopez V. Rational design of substituted tripyrrole peptides that complex DNA by both selective minor-grove binding and electrostatic interaction with the polyphosphate backbone. Proc Natl Acad Sci USA 1992; 89:1700–1704.

96. Kuntz ID. Structure-based strategies for drug design and discovery. Science 1992; 257:1078–1082.

97. Hopwood DA, Malpartida F, Kieser HM, Ikeda H, Duncan J, Fujii I. Prediction of "hybrid" antibiotics by genetic engineering. Nature 1985; 314:642–644.

98. Marlpartida F, Hopwood DA. Molecular cloning of the whole biosynthetic pathway of a *Streptomyces* antibiotic and its expression in a heterologous host. Nature 1984; 309:462–464.

99. De Vos WM, Jung G, Sahl H-G. Definitions and nomenclature of lantibiotics. Jung G, Sahl H-G, eds. Nisin and Novel Lantibiotics. Leiden, The Netherlands: ESCOM, 1991:457–463.

100. Siezen RJ, Kuipers OP, De Vos WM. Comparison of lantibiotic gene clusters and encoded proteins. Antonie van Leeuwenhoek 1996; 69:171–184.

101. Kupke T, Stevanovic S, Sahl H-G, Gotz F. Purification and characterization of EpiD, a flavoprotein involved in the biosynthesis of the lantibiotic epidermin. J Bacteriol 1992; 174:5354–5361.

102. Kuipers OP, Beerthuyzen MM, Siezen RJ, De Vos WM. Characterization of the nisin gene cluster *nis*ABTCIPR of *Lactococcus lactis*. Requirement of expression of the *nis*A and *nis*I genes for development of immunity. Eur J Biochem 1993; 216:281–291.

103. Reis M, Eschbach-Bludau M, Iglesias-Wind MI, Kupke T, Sahl H-G. Producer immunity towards the lantibiotic Pep5: Identification of the immunity gene *pep*I and localization and functional analysis of its gene product. Appl Environ Microbiol 1994; 60:2876–2883.

104. Klein C, Entian KD. Genes involved in self-protection against the lantibiotic subtilin produced by *Bacillus subtilis* ATCC 6633. Appl Environ Microbiol 1994; 60:2793–2801.

105. Devos WM, Kuipers OP, Vandermeer JR, Siezen RJ. Maturation pathway of nisin and other lantibiotics: Posttranslationally modified antimicrobial peptides exported by gram-positive bacteria. Mol Microbiol 1995; 17:427–437.

106. Gutowski-Eckel Z, Klein C, Siegers K, Bohm K, Hammelmann M, Entian KD. Growth phase-dependent regulation and membrane localization of SpaB, a protein involved in biosynthesis of the lantibiotic subtilin. Appl Environ Microbiol 1994; 60:1–11.

107. Klein C, Kaletta C, Schnell N, Entian KD. Analysis of genes involved in biosynthesis of the lantibiotic subtilin. Appl Environ Microbiol 1992; 58:132–142. [Published erratum appears in Appl Environ Microbiol 1992; 58:1795.]

108. Chung YJ, Hansen JN. Determination of the sequence of *spa*E and identification of a promoter in the subtilin (*spa*) operon in *Bacillus subtilis*. J Bacteriol 1992; 174:6699–6702.

109. Augustin J, Rosenstein R, Wieland B, Schneider U, Schnell N, Engelke G, Entian KD, Gotz F. Genetic analysis of epidermin biosynthetic genes and epidermin-negative mutants of *Staphylococcus epidermidis*. Eur J Biochem 1992; 204:1149–1154.

110. Engelke G, Gutowski-Eckel Z, Mann MH, Entian K-D. Biosynthesis of the lantibiotic nisin: Genomic organization and membrane localization of the NisB protein. Appl Environ Microbiol 1992; 58:3730–3743.

111. Meyer C, Bierbaum G, Heidrich C, Reis M, Suling J, Iglesias-Wind MI, Kempter C, Molitor E, Sahl H-G. Nucleotide sequence of the lantibiotic Pep5 biosynthetic gene cluster and functional analysis of PepP and PepC. Eur J Biochem 1995; 232:478–489.

112. van der Meer JR, Polman J, Beerthuyzen MM, Siezen RJ, Kuipers OP, De Vos WM. Characterization of the *Lactococcus lactis* nisin A operon genes *nis*P, encoding a subtilisin-like serine protease involved in precursor processing, and *nis*R, encoding a regulatory protein involved in nisin biosynthesis. J Bacteriol 1993; 175:2578–2588.

113. Havarstein LS, Diep DB, Nes IF. A family of bacteriocin ABC transporters carry out proteolytic processing of their substrates concomitant with export. Mol Microbiol 1995; 16:229–240.

114. Izaguirre G, Hansen JN. Submitted.

115. Fath MJ, Kolter R. ABC transporters: Bacterial exporters. Microbiol Rev 1993; 57:995–1017.

116. Chung YJ, Steen MT, Hansen JN. The subtilin gene of *Bacillus subtilis* ATCC 6633 is encoded in an operon that contains a homolog of the hemolysin B transport protein. J Bacteriol 1992; 174:1417–1422.

117. Reis M, Sahl H-G. Genetic analysis of the producer self-protection mechanism ("immunity") against Pep5. Jung G, Sahl H-G, eds. Nisin and Novel Lantibiotics. Leiden, The Netherlands: ESCOM, 1991:320–330.

118. Engelke G, Gutowski-Eckel Z, Kiesau P, Siegers K, Hammelmann M, Entian KD. Regulation of nisin biosynthesis and immunity in *Lactococcus lactis* 6F3. Appl Environ Microbiol 1994; 60:814–825.

119. Buchman GW, Banerjee S, Hansen JN. Structure, expression, and evolution of a gene encoding the precursor of nisin, a small protein antibiotic. J Biol Chem 1988; 263:16260–16266.

120. Creighton TE. Intermediates in the refolding of reduced ribonuclease A. J Mol Biol 1979; 129:411–431.

121. Hawkins G. Investigation of the site and mode of action of the small protein antibiotic subtilin and development and characterization of an expression system for the small protein antibiotic nisin in *Bacillus subtilis*. Dissert Abs Internatl 1991; 52:655B.

122. Liu W, Hansen JN. Some chemical and physical properties of nisin, a small-protein antibiotic produced by *Lactococcus lactis*. Appl Environ Microbiol 1990; 56:2551–2558.

123. Rintala H, Graeffe T, Paulin L, Kalkkinen N, Saris PEJ. Biosynthesis of nisin in the subtilin producer ATCC 6633. Biotech Lett 1993; 15:991–996.

124. Chakicherla A, Hansen JN. Role of the leader and structural regions of prelantibiotic peptides as assessed by expressing nisin-subtilin chimeras in *Bacillus subtilis* 168, and characterization of their physical, chemical, and antimicrobial properties. J Biol Chem 1995; 270:23533–23539.

125. Au: pls give 125 (see Table 3)

126. Banerjee S, Hansen JN. Structure and expression of a gene encoding the precursor of subtilin, a small protein antibiotic. J Biol Chem 1988; 263:9508–9514.

127. Dodd HM, Horn N, Hao Z, Gasson MJ. A lactococcal expression system for engineered nisins. Appl Environ Microbiol 1992; 58:3683–3693.

128. Dodd HM, Horn N, Gasson MJ. A cassette vector for protein engineering the lantibiotic nisin. Gene 1995; 162:163–164.

129. Kuipers OP, Yap WMGJ, Rollema HS, Beerthuyzen MM, Siezen RJ, De Vos WM. Expression of wild-type and mutant nisin genes in *Lactococcus lactis*. Jung G, Sahl H-G, eds. Nisin and Novel Lantibiotics. Leiden, The Netherlands: ESCOM, 1991:250–259.

130. Kuipers OP, Rollema HS, Yap WM, Boot HJ, Siezen RJ, De Vos WM. Engineering dehydrated amino acid residues in the antimicrobial peptide nisin. J Biol Chem 1992; 267:24340–24346.

131. Kuipers OP, Rollema HS, De Vos WM, Siezen RJ. Biosynthesis and secretion of a precursor of nisin Z by *Lactococcus lactis*, directed by the leader peptide of the homologous lantibiotic subtilin from *Bacillus subtilis*. FEBS Lett 1993; 330:23–27.

132. Rollema HS, Kuipers OP, Both P, De Vos WM, Siezen RJ. Improvement of solubility and stability of the antimicrobial peptide nisin by protein engineering. Appl Environ Microbiol 1995; 61:2873–2878.

133. Kuipers OP, Rollema HS, Beerthuyzen MM, Siezen RJ, De Vos WM. Protein engineering and biosynthesis of nisin and regulation of transcription of the structural *nisA* gene. Intl Dairy J 1995; 5:785–795.

134. Liu W, Hansen JN. Enhancement of the chemical and antimicrobial properties of subtilin by site-directed mutagenesis. J Biol Chem 1992; 267:25078–25085.

135. Ottenwalder B, Kupke T, Gnau V, Metzger J, Jung G, Gotz F. Isolation and characterization of genetically engineered gallidermin and epidermin analogues. Second International Workshop on Lantibiotics, November 20–24, 1994. Arnhem, The Netherlands.

136. Bierbaum G, Reis M, Szekat C, Sahl H-G. Construction of an expression system for engineering of the lantibiotic Pep5. Appl Environ Microbiol 1994; 60:4332–4338.

137. Bierbaum G, Szekat C, Josten M, Heidrich C, Kempter C, Jung G, Sahl H-G. Engineering of a novel thioether bridge and the role of modified residues in the lantibiotic Pep5. Appl Environ Microbiol 1996; 62:385–392.

138. Kuipers OP, Bierbaum G, Ottenwalder B, Dodd HM, Horn N, Metzger J, Kupke T, Gnau V, Bongers R, van den Bogaard P, Kosters H, Rollema HS, De Vos WM, Siezen RJ, Jung G, Gotz F, Sahl H-G, Gasson MJ. Protein engineering of lantibiotics. Antonie van Leeuwenhoek 1996; 69:161–170.

139. Jarvis B, Mahoney RR. Inactivation of nisin by alpha-chymotrypsin. J Dairy Sci 1969; 52:1448–1450.

140. Liu W, Hansen JN. The antimicrobial effect of a structural variant of subtilin against outgrowing *Bacillus cereus* T spores and vegetative cells occurs by different mechanisms. Appl Environ Microbiol 1993; 59:648–651.

141. Chan WC, Dodd HM, Horn N, Maclean K, Lian LY, Bycroft BW, Gasson MJ, Roberts GC. Structure-activity relationships in the peptide antibiotic nisin—role of dehydroalanine. Appl Environ Microbiol 1996; 62:2966–2969.

142. Dickerson RE, Geis I. The Structure and Action of Proteins. New York: Harper and Row, 1969.

143. Stevens KA, Sheldon BW, Klapes NA, Klaenhammer TR. Nisin treatment for inactivation of *Salmonella* species and other gram-negative bacteria. Appl Environ Microbiol 1991; 57:3613–3615.

144. Ruhr E, Sahl H-G. Mode of action of the peptide antibiotic nisin and influence on the membrane potential of whole cells and on cytoplasmic and artificial membrane vesicles. Anitmicrob Agents Chemother 1985; 27:841–845.

145. Sahl H-G, Grossgarten M, Widger WR, Cramer WA, Brandis H. Structural similarities of the staphylococcin-like peptide Pep-5 to the peptide antibiotic nisin. Anitmicrob Agents Chemother 1985; 27:836–840.

146. Bierbaum G, Sahl H-G. Induction of autolysis of staphylococci by the basic peptide antibiotics Pep 5 and nisin and their influence on the activity of autolytic enzymes. Arch Microbiol 1985; 141:249–254.

147. Bierbaum G, Sahl H-G. Autolytic system of *Staphylococcus simulans* 22: Influence of cationic peptides on activity of N-acetylmuramoyl-L-alanine amidase. J Bacteriol 1987; 169:5452–5458.

148. Sahl H-G, Kordel M, Benz R. Voltage-dependent depolarization of bacterial membranes and artificial lipid bilayers by the peptide antibiotic nisin. Arch Microbiol 1987; 149:120–124.

149. Schuller F, Benz R, Sahl H-G. The peptide antibiotic subtilin acts by formation of voltage-dependent multi-state pores in bacterial and artificial membranes. Eur J Biochem 1989; 182:181–186.

150. Jack R, Benz R, Tagg J, Sahl H-G. The mode of action of SA-FF22, a lantibiotic isolated from *Streptococcus pyogenes* strain FF22. Eur J Biochem 1994; 219:699–705.

151. Sahl H-G. Pore formation in bacterial membranes by cationic lantibiotics. Jung G, Sahl H-G, eds. Nisin and Novel Lantibiotics. Leiden, The Netherlands: ESCOM, 1991:347–358.

152. Benz R, Jung G, Sahl H-G. Mechanism of channel-formation by lantibiotics in black lipid membranes. Jung G, Sahl H-G, eds. Nisin and Novel Lantibiotics. Leiden, The Netherlands: ESCOM, 1991:359–372.

153. Kagan BL, Selsted ME, Ganz T, Lehrer RI. Antimicrobial defensin peptides form voltage-dependent ion-permeable channels in planar lipid bilayer membranes. Proc Natl Acad Sci USA 1990; 87:210–214.

154. Hill CP, Yee J, Selsted ME, Eisenberg D. Crystal structure of defensin HNP-3, an amphiphilic dimer: Mechanisms of membrane permeabilization. Science 1991; 251:1481–1485.

155. Wilmsen HU, Pugsley AP, Pattus F. Colicin N forms voltage and pH dependent channels in planar lipid bilayer membranes. Eur Biophys J 1990; 18:149–158.

156. Christensen B, Fink J, Merrifield RB, Mauzerall D. Channel-forming properties of cecropins and related model compounds incorporated into planar lipid membranes. Proc Natl Acad Sci USA 1988; 85:5072–5076.

157. Duclohier H, Molle G, Spach G. Antimicrobial peptide magainin I from *Xenopus* skin forms anion-permeable channels in planar lipid bilayers. Biophys J 1989; 56:1017–1021.

158. Cruciani RA, Barker JL, Durell SR, Raghunathan G, Guy HR, Zasloff M, Stanley EF. Magainin 2, a natural antibiotic from frog skin, forms ion channels in lipid bilayer membranes. Eur J Pharmacol 1992; 226:287–296.

159. Westerhoff HV, Juretic D, Hendler RW, Zasloff M. Magainins and the disruption of membrane-linked free-energy transduction. Proc Natl Acad Sci USA 1989; 86:6597–6601.

160. van Belkum MJ, Kok J, Venema G, Holo H, Nes IF, Konings WN, Abee T. The bacteriocin lactococcin A specifically increases permeability of lactococcal cytoplasmic membranes in a voltage-independent, protein-mediated manner. J Bacteriol 1991; 173:7934–7941.

161. Hansen JN, Levin RA. Effect of some inhibitors derived from nitrite on macromolecular synthesis in *Bacillus cereus*. Appl Microbiol 1975; 30:862–869.

162. Custer MC, Hansen JN. Lactoferrin and transferrin fragments react with nitrite to form an inhibitor of *Bacillus cereus* spore outgrowth. Appl Environ Microbiol 1983; 45:942–949.

163. Hynes WL, Friend VL, Ferretti JJ. Duplication of the lantibiotic structural gene in M-type-49 group-A *Streptococcus* strains producing streptococcin-A-M49. Appl Environ Microbiol 1994; 60:4207–4209.

164. Buchman GW, Hansen JN. Modification of membrane sulfhydryl groups in bacteriostatic action of nitrite. Appl Environ Microbiol 1987; 53:79–82.

165. Morris SL, Hansen JN. Inhibition of *Bacillus cereus* spore outgrowth by covalent modification of a sulfhydryl group by nitrosothiol and iodoacetate. J Bacteriol 1981; 148:465–471.

166. Morris SL, Walsh RC, Hansen JN. Identification and characterization of some bacterial membrane sulfhydryl groups which are targets of bacteriostatic and antibiotic action. J Biol Chem 1984; 259:13590–13594.

167. Morris SL, Levin RA, Wright-Wilson C, Hansen JN. Effect of S-nitrosothiol structure on inhibition of germination and outgrowth of *Bacillus cereus* spores. Chambliss G, Vary JC, eds. Spores VII. Washington, D.C.: American Society for Microbiology, 1978:85–89.

168. Gross E, Morrell JL. The presence of dehydroalanine in the antibiotic nisin and its relationship to activity. J Am Chem Soc 1967; 89:2791–2792.

169. Gaggero C, Moreno F, Lavina M. Genetic analysis of microcin H47 antibiotic system. J Bacteriol 1993; 175:5420–5427.

170. Ramseier HR. The action of nisin on *Clostridium botulinum*. Arch Mikrobiol 1960; 37:57–94.

171. Hansen JN, Chung YJ, Liu W, Steen MJ. Biosynthesis and mechanism of action of nisin and subtilin. Jung G, Sahl H-G, eds. Nisin and Novel Lantibiotics. Leiden, The Netherlands: ESCOM, 1991:287–302.

172. Tagg JR, Dajani AS, Wannamaker LW. Bacteriocins of Gram-positive bacteria. Bacteriol Rev 1976; 40:722–756.

173. Soravia E, Martini G, Zasloff M. Antimicrobial properties of peptides from *Xenopus* granular gland secretions. FEBS Lett 1988; 228:337–340.

174. Cruciani RA, Barker JL, Zasloff M, Chen HC, Colamonici O. Antibiotic magainins exert cytolytic activity against transformed cell lines through channel formation. Proc Natl Acad Sci USA 1991; 88:3792–3796.

175. Cuervo JH, Rodriguez B, Houghten RA. The magainins: Sequence factors relevant to increased antimicrobial activity and decreased hemolytic activity. Pept Res 1988; 1:81–86.

176. Steiner H, Andreu D, Merrifield RB. Binding and action of cecropin and cecropin analogues: Antibacterial peptides from insects. Biochim Biophys Acta 1988; 939:260–266.

177. Qu Z, Steiner H, Engstrom A, Bennich H, Boman HG. Insect immunity: Isolation and structure of cecropins B and D from pupae of the Chinese oak silk moth, *Antheraea pernyi*. Eur J Biochem 1982; 127:219–224.

178. Flajnik M. Primitive vertebrate immunity: What is the evolutionary derivation of molecules that define the adaptive immune system? Marsh J, Goode JA, eds. Antimicrobial Peptides, Ciba Foundation Symposium 186. Chichester, England: John Wiley and Sons, 1994:224–236.

179. Hurst A. Biosynthesis of the antibiotic nisin by whole *Streptococcus lactis* organisms. J Gen Microbiol 1966; 44:209–220.

180. Liu W, Hansen JN. Conversion of *Bacillus subtilis* 168 to a subtilin producer by competence transformation. J Bacteriol 1991; 173:7387–7390.

181. Matsusaki E, Endo N, Sonomoto K, Ishizaki A. Purification and identification of a peptide antibiotic produced by *Lactococcus lactis* IO-1. J Faculty Agricult Kyushu Univ 1995; 40:73–85.

182. Mortvedt-Abildgaard CI, Nissen-Meyer J, Jelle B, Grenov B, Skaugen M, Nes IF. Production and pH-dependent bactericidal activity of lactocin S, a lantibiotic from *Lactobacillus sake* L45. Appl Environ Microbiol 1995; 61:175–179.

16

Cationic Peptides

Robert E. W. Hancock
University of British Columbia, Vancouver, British Columbia, Canada

Timothy John Falla
University of Leeds, Leeds, England

I. INTRODUCTION

It has been often observed that no new classes of antibiotics have been developed since the introduction of the first quinoline, nalidixic acid, in 1962. However, over the past decade scientists have discovered that one of nature's most persistent approaches against bacteria involves cationic peptides. For example, cationic peptides are the major mechanism of defense against microbes in insects and plants, a predominant local defense at host surfaces including the skins of amphibians and mucosa of mammals, and the major proteinaceous species of the dedicated antimicrobial defense cells of mammals—namely, neutrophils. These peptides have a variety of structures and functions that include antibacterial (Gram-positive and -negative), antifungal, antiviral, antiendotoxin, and anticancer activities. Thus, they present perhaps the most profound example of convergent evolution, in which a variety of different peptides have evolved to a common set of functions.

Cationic peptides were traditionally isolated from natural sources or synthesized by solid phase or solution phase chemistry. Moreover, they have recently been synthesized by recombinant DNA methods in bacteria (1), insect cells (2), and plants (3,4). The fact that cationic peptides are produced naturally by certain bacteria (e.g., see Chapter 17), as well as the newly discovered ability to synthesize virtually any peptide by recombinant means in bacteria (1), clearly merits the use of the term "antibiotic" for these compounds. Thus, cationic peptides represent not only the first new class of antibiotic in the past 30 years, but the world's first genetically engineering antibacterials.

II. OCCURRENCE OF CATIONIC PEPTIDES IN NATURE

Recently, we reviewed the natural cationic peptides in depth and identified 145 sequences that have been isolated from nature (5). Some of these are listed according to structural class in Tables 1 and 2. Cationic peptides are ubiquitous in nature; they have been identified in bacteria, fungi, plants, insects, crustaceans, amphibians, mammals, and humans.

Table 1   Examples of Cationic Peptides

Mammalian defensins (NP-1)	VVCACRRALCLPRERRAGFCRIRGRIHPLCCRR
β-Defensins (BNBD5)	EVVRNPQSCRWNMGVCIPISCPGNMRQIGTCFGPRVPCCR
Insect defensins (Sapecin)	ATCDLLSGTGINHSACAAHCLCRGNRGGYCNGKAVCVCRN
Tachyplesins (Tachyplesin)	RRWCFRVCYRGFCYRKCR
Thionins (Rabbitwood)	KSCCRNTWARNCYNVCRIPGTISREICAKKCDCKIISETTCPS-DYPK
Loops (Bactenicin)	RLCRIVVIRVCR
α-Helical (Cecropin A)	KWKFKKIEKMGRNIRDGIVKAGPAIEVIGSAKAI
Histidine-rich (Histadin 2)	MKFFVALILALMLSMTGADSHAKRHHGYKRKFHEKHHSHRGY-RSNYLYDN
Tryptophan-rich (Indolicidin)	ILPWKWPWWPWRR
Proline-rich (Bac 5)	PFRPPIRRPPIRPPFYPPFRPPIRPPIFPPIRPPFRPPLRFP

Generally speaking, these compounds provide relatively nonspecific defenses against microbes (Table 3). Even those compounds elicited by bacteria are known to function as bacteriocins that kill other bacteria, presumably as a mechanism of competition for an ecological niche.

A. Mammals

A variety of peptides are involved in the mammalian oxygen-independent antimicrobial defense mechanism. Defensins are a family of small (29–35 amino acids) arginine- and cysteine-rich peptides that have been isolated from a variety of mammals, including rats, rabbits, and humans (6,7). Six human defensins have been identified, four of which, human neutrophil peptides (HNP-1,2,3,4), were purified from polymorphonuclear leukocytes and two of which, human defensins (HD-5 and 6), have been detected in the intestinal Paneth cells by *in situ* hybridization. Mouse defensins, cryptidins, are also found in the Paneth cells of the small intestine. All six human defensins share sequence homology that includes six cysteine residues forming three disulfide bridges. This results in a β-pleated sheet secondary structure. Defensins, although capable of killing a wide range of bacteria, fungi, and viruses, are more active against Gram-positive than Gram-negative bacteria. In addition to their permeabilization of biological membranes, these peptides also exhibit chemotactic and endocrine regulatory activities (8).

Human defensins are synthesized as 94- to 100-amino-acid preprodefensins that contain a conserved 19-amino-acid *N*-terminal signal sequence that targets the peptide to the endoplasmic reticulum. This is followed by an anionic propiece, proposed to balance the cationic charge of the defensin (9).

A subset of defensins, the β-defensins, have been isolated from bovine neutrophils (10). A unique consensus sequence distinguishes these defensins from those described above, although both contain the characteristic three disulfide bridges. Tracheal antimicrobial peptide (TAP) isolated from the bovine respiratory tract also contains the triple disulfide motif but is specifically expressed in the respiratory tract (11). This peptide is active against Gram-negative and -positive bacteria and yeast.

A distinct family of peptides, termed the cathelicidins, has been isolated from mammalian neutrophils; these include the bovine peptides bactenecin 5 (Bac5) (12) and indolicidin (13), the porcine PR-39 (14), and the rabbit peptide CAP18 (15). These

```
BAC5         METQRASLSLGRCSLWLLLLGLVLPSASAQALSYREAVLRAVDQFNERSSEANLYRLLELDPTPNDDLDPGTRKPVSFRVKETDCPRT
INDOLICIDIN  MQTQRASLSLGRWSLWLLLLGLVYPSASAQALSYREAVLRAVDQLNELSSEANLYRLLELDPPPKDNEDLGTRKPVSFRVKETVCPRT
CAP18        METHKHGPSLAWWSLLLLLLGLLMPPAIAQDLTYREAVLRAVDAFNQOSSEANLYRLLSMDPQOLEDAKPYTPOPVSFTVKETECPRT


BAC5         SQQPLEQCDFKENGLVKQCVGTVTLDPSNDQFDINCNELQSVRFRPPIRRPPIRPPFYPPFRPPIRPPIFPPIRPPFRPPLGPFPGRR
INDOLICIDIN  IQQPAEQCDFKEKGEVKQCVGTVTLDPSNDQFDINCNELQSVILPWKWPWWPWRR
CAP18        TWKLPEQCDFKEDGLVKECVGTVTRYQAWDSFDIRCNRAQESPEPTGLRKRLRKFRNKIKEKLKKIGQKIQGFVPKLAPRTDY
```

Figure I   Alignment of Bac5, indolicidin, and CAP18 proregion sequences. Sequence variation from Bac5 is denoted by underlining in the indolicidin and CAP18 prosequences. Cleaved antimicrobial domains are indicated by bold lettering. (Reproduced by permission of Zanetti et al. (16).)

peptides contain a highly conserved propiece that is also homologous to the cysteine-rich protease inhibitor cathelin (16,17). The antimicrobial N-terminal region of these proforms is cleaved by elastase. An alignment of the deduced proforms of Bac5, indolicidin, and CAP18 is presented in Figure 1.

B.   Amphibians

Frog skin and frog gastric mucosa are rich in peptides, and many of them have antimicrobial activity (18,19). One of the first antimicrobial peptides to be isolated from this source was bombinin from the species of frog *Bombina variegata* (20). This and subsequently isolated, related bombinins display a high level of antibacterial activity against staphylococci (21).

A family of amphipathic α-helical peptides, the magainins, has been identified in the African clawed frog (*Xenopus laevis*) (22). Magainin has a broad range of antimicrobial activity against Gram-positive and Gram-negative bacteria (23–25), fungi (24), and protozoa (23,24).

These peptides have been well characterized, and the analysis of many synthetic analogs has developed an understanding of the components required for biological activity (22,26). The cloning of the cDNA for magainin and other related amphibian peptides (PGLa, PGO, and xenopsin) has revealed that all are produced as precursor molecules, the signal peptides of which share considerable homology (23,27–30).

Cationic peptides have also been isolated from other species of frogs. For example, cationic peptides termed brevinins have been isolated from *Rana brevipoda* and *Rana esculenta*—brevinin-1 and brevinin-1E, respectively (31,32). These 24-amino-acid peptides both possess single C-terminal disulfide bonds and two prolines. Also, dermaseptin has been isolated from the South American frog *Phyllomedusa sauvagii*. This peptide has no homology with other amphibian peptides, but due to its amphipathic nature, it permeabilizes membranes in a similar fashion (19).

C.   Insects

Upon infection, insects can produce a wide range of antimicrobial peptides, which are synthesized in the fat body and/or haemocytes and secreted into the haemolymph. Such peptides include cecropins (33), and defensin-like peptides such as sapecin and phormicin (34,35). Cecropins are highly amphipathic peptides containing 31–39 residues that form voltage-dependent channels in lipid membranes (36). They were initially isolated from the silk moth *Hyalophora cecropia* (37) and have subsequently been isolated from the flesh fly (sarcotoxin I) and *Drosophila* (38,39). Cecropins are distinct from other insect cationic peptides in that they contain no cysteine residues and fail to lyse eukaryotic cells (33),

Table 2 Structural Classes of Cationic Peptides

Class of peptide	Structural motifs	Sources	Examples
Mammalian defensins	3 β-strands 3 disulfides	Rat, rabbit, guinea pig, human neutrophils, rabbit alveolar macrophages, human, mouse Paneth cells	MCP, NP, HNP, GNCP, rat NP, cryptidins
β-defensins	3 disulfides β-stranded	Bovine neutrophils, trachea	TAP, BNBD
Insect defensins	3 disulfides 2 β-strands 1 α-helix	Dragonfly, blowfly, flesh fly	Phormicin, sapecin, sarcotoxin, royalisin
Tachyplesins	2 disulfides 2 β-strands	Pig leukocytes, crabs, amaranth plants, maize, turnip	Protegrins, polyphemusins, tachyplesins, Ac-AMP, 1AFP2, MBIP-1
Thionins	3 disulfides structure unknown	Maize, radish, rabbitwood, barley lead, rape, crambe	Mj-AMP1, trionin, crambin
α-Helical	amphipathic α-helix	Fruit fly, bees, frogs, toads, cattle	Bombolitin, bombinin, cecropins, magainins, melittin, dermaseptin
Loops	1 disulfide structures unknown	Bovine neutrophils, pit viper	Bactenicin, toxin 1
Histidine-rich	structures unknown	Primates, humans	Histadins
Tryptophan-rich	poly-L-proline II	Bovine neutrophils	Indolicidin
Proline-rich	poly-L-proline II	Fruit fly, honey bee, bovine neutrophils	Drosocin, abaecin, apidaecin, Bac5, Bac7

although they retain activity against Gram-negative and -positive bacteria in micromolar concentrations (37). Interestingly, cecropin-like peptides have now been isolated from the pig intestine (40). This latter peptide, cecropin P1, however, differs from the insect forms by not containing an amidated C-terminus and also in its tertiary structure (41).

Defensins have also been isolated from a variety of insect species (34,35). They share an array of six cysteine residues resulting in a tertiary structure containing three disulfide bridges but forming a structure that is distinct from mammalian defensins (42). These peptides instead share amino acid sequence homology and tertiary structure homology with royalisin from bees and charybdotoxin and defensin from scorpions (43–45).

Sapaecin, an insect defensin isolated from the flesh fly *Sacrophaga peregrina*, consists of 40 amino acids including the conserved six cysteine residues (46) and is most active against Gram-positive bacteria (35).

A number of well-characterized novel antimicrobial peptides have been isolated from the honeybee (*Apis mellifera*). These include abaecin (47), the apidaecins (48), and hymenoptaecin (49). The apidaecins are a family of small (18 residues) proline-rich peptides, isolated from the haemolymph of the honeybee, which have activity against Gram-negative and plant-associated bacteria (48). Apidaecin precursors consist of cassettes of tandemly repeated sequences of the mature peptide preceded by dipeptides that are cleaved to produce the mature peptide (50). These precursors retain antibacterial activity, although the increasing dipeptide content reduces activity. Abaecin is a 34-amino-acid proline-rich peptide that has sequence homology with the apidaecins but has a different antibacterial spectrum and a delayed antibacterial effect (47). Hymenoptaecin, larger than the other bee-derived peptides at 93 residues, does not contain a high proline content nor the characteristic cysteine residues of defensins (49). This peptide has been shown to be active against the inner and outer membranes of Gram-negative bacteria (49).

D. Crustaceans

Tachyplesins (I, II, and III) are a class of antimicrobial peptides produced in the haemocytes of the horseshoe crabs *Tachypleus tridentatus*, *Tachypleus gigas*, and *Carcinoscorpius rotundicauda* (51–53). Two tachyplesin analogs, polyphemusin I and II, have also been isolated from the horseshoe crab *Limulus polyphemus* (52). Tachyplesins (17 amino acids) and polyphemusins (18 amino acids) contain four cysteine residues and subsequently form a rigid structure containing two disulfide linkages, which results in a stable structure resistant to low pH and high temperature (51). These peptides have activity against Gram-negative and -positive bacteria and fungi (51).

E. Microbes

Bacterial antibiotic proteins have been studied for many years since their initial discovery in the 1920s. Common among Gram-negative bacteria are the colicins; rarer are the peptide bacteriocins such as microcin B17. Among Gram-positive bacteria, peptide bacteriocins are the most commonly isolated. Of these, the cationic type A antibiotics such as nisin (54) and Pep 5 (55) isolated from *Lactococcus lactis* and *Staphylococcus epidermidis*, respectively, are the most characterized. These peptides contain such unusual amino acids as lanthionine, 3-methyllanthionine, and dehydrobutyrine (55,56). The mode of action of these peptides is by the formation of transient voltage-dependent pores in the cytoplasmic membrane (57,58). Such activity causes ion leakage from the cell and a breakdown in the electropotential across the cell membrane, resulting in death. Fungi, such as *Rhizomucor pusillus*, have also been shown to produce antibacterial peptides. *R. pusillus* produces sillucin, a defensin-like peptide active against Gram-positive bacteria (59).

F. Plants

Thionins are specific cationic peptides produced by plants in response to infection. For example, barley produces a leaf-specific thionin, BTH6 (60). In addition, other cysteine-rich basic peptides belonging to the superfamily of peptides that includes thionins and mammalian and insect defensins have been isolated from the seeds of plants. These contain generally between 30 and 50 amino acids and between four and eight cysteine residues. Examples of such peptides include Ac-AMP (61) and Mj-AMP (62). Plant-derived peptides are most active against Gram-positive bacteria and fungi. IC_{50} (concentration inhibiting 50% of fungi) values for Ac-AMP against a broad spectrum of fungi are 2 to 10 μg/ml, and for Mj-AMP2, 0.5 to 20 μg/ml against 13 plant pathogenic fungi (61,62).

III. ANTIMICROBIAL ACTIVITIES

A. Antibacterial Activities

It is a little difficult to assess the relative activities of cationic peptides compared with those of other antibacterial agents, for two basic reasons. The first is that many investigators working on cationic peptides utilize nonstandard assays. The appropriate method of measuring antibacterial activities is to determine a minimal inhibitory concentration (MIC) by either the broth dilution method, in which 10^3-10^4 bacteria are inoculated into a row of tubes containing serial twofold dilutions of antibiotics (63), or the agar dilution procedure, which involves incorporation of dilutions of the antibiotic into plates and subsequent spotting of 10^3-10^4 organisms onto the surfaces of the plates (64). In contrast, cationic peptides are often tested by measuring zones of clearance on plates spread with bacteria after inoculation of peptides into wells cut into the agar or onto paper discs (65), or by measuring the concentration of peptide killing 50% of bacteria in killing assays. The former method suffers from diffusion limitations of peptides, whereas the latter suffers from an uncertain relationship to MIC. Furthermore, the activities of cationic peptides tend to be reduced in media of high ionic strength or with high divalent cation concentrations.

With the foregoing general comments, cationic peptides have just moderate antibacterial activities compared with those of conventional antibiotics (Table 4). Nevertheless, cationic peptides do have certain highly desirable activities. First, they tend to have broad-spectrum activity that can encompass both Gram-negative and Gram-positive bacteria, although different cationic peptides often preferentially affect one or the other. Second, their activities do not appear to be compromised by resistance mechanisms that commonly appear in the clinic. Thus, common resistance mechanisms, such as methicillin resistance in *Staphylococcus aureus,* intrinsic antibiotic resistance in

Table 3   Roles of Cationic Peptides in Nature

Peptide	Host	Function	Mechanism
Pep5	*Straphylococcus epidermidis*	Antibacterial	Membrane disruption
Rs-AFP	Radish seeds	Antifungal	Cause hyperbranching and swelling of hyphae
Cecropins	Silk moth	Antibacterial	Membrane disruption
Tachyplesins	Horseshoe crab	Antibacterial, antifungal	Membrane disruption
Magainins	African clawed frog	Antibacterial, antifungal, antiprotozoal	Membrane disruption
Defensins	Human	Antibacterial, antifungal, antiviral	Membrane disruption

Pseudomonas aeruginosa, β-lactam resistance due to chromosomal β-lactamase derepression in *Enterobacter cloacae* or plasmid-encoded TEM β-lactamase in *Escherichia coli,* and tetracycline efflux in *E. coli,* have no effect on the MIC of cationic peptides (66). Furthermore, they themselves do not tend to select resistant mutants, although some bacteria, such as *Burkholderia cepacia* tend to be naturally resistant.

Despite their modest MICs, cationic peptides can kill bacteria potently at or around the MIC, in contrast to most conventional antibiotics. Thus, a cecropin–melittin hybrid peptide can cause 3–4 orders of magnitude of killing of *P. aeruginosa* in 20 min at the MIC, whereas other potent antipseudomonal antibiotics generally cause less than one order of magnitude of killing at the analogous concentration (Figure 2).

The detailed mechanism of action of cationic peptides is described in Section IV.C. The most prominent effect on cells is the formation of channels in or disruptions of the cytoplasmic membrane. Thus, these molecules appear to kill by a physical method that takes advantage of the specific composition of bacterial membranes. In contrast, most

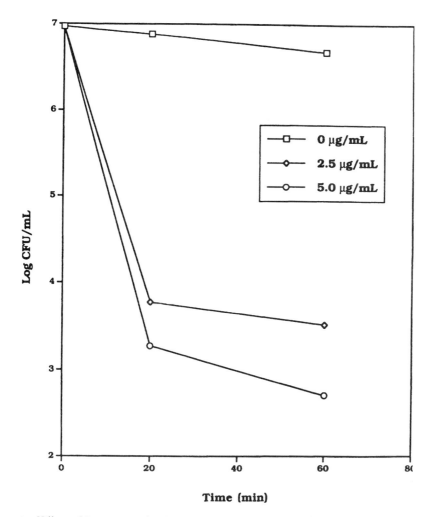

Figure 2   Killing of *P. aeruginosa* by the cationic peptide CEME. (From Ref. 67.)

conventional antibiotics are enzyme inhibitors that act on specific enzyme targets in bacteria (e.g., β-lactams acting on transpeptidases). This may explain many of the more desirable features of the cationic peptides, as described above, for example, (a) lack of resistance development, since it is difficult to fundamentally alter membrane composition, and (b) rapid killing, since the action is physical rather than catalytic.

Another feature of the mechanism of action that can be exploited is the ability of cationic peptides to break down the outer membrane barrier of Gram-negative bacteria. This barrier has been shown to limit the uptake of, and thus cellular susceptibility to, most conventional antibiotics, since its permeabilization by, for example, EDTA or specific mutations leads to reduced MICs for such antibiotics. In the same way, cationic peptides tend to be synergistic with certain conventional antibiotics, suggesting that they may be useful in the clinic in combination with such antibiotics. In keeping with these suggestions, Darveau et al. (68) demonstrated that magainin was synergistic with cefpirome in mouse protection experiments. The clinical implications of cationic peptides as antibiotic and antiendotoxic agents is discussed further in Sections II.B and IV.C.3.

B. Antiendotoxin Activities

Endotoxin is synonymous with lipopolysaccharide (LPS), a complex glycolipid that is an integral part of the outer membranes of Gram-negative bacteria (Figure 3). More specifically, endotoxin is the lipid A portion of LPS, which is the most membrane-proximal portion of the LPS making up the outer monolayer of the outer membrane. Endotoxin is a potent inducer of the cytokines interleukin 1 (IL1), tumor necrosis factor (TNF), and interleukin 8 (IL8). The presence of endotoxin in the body leads to a wide variety of physiological effects mediated in part by this vigorous cytokine response. These responses range from beneficial effects, such as fever response and tumor necrosis, to toxic effects,

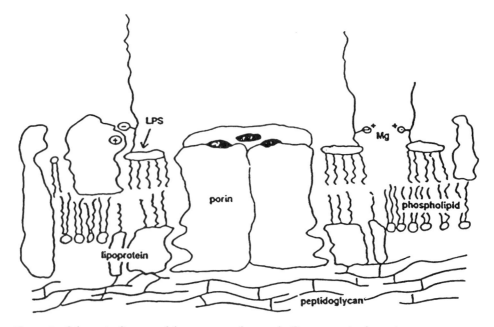

Figure 3   Schematic diagram of the outer membrane of a Gram-negative bacteria.

including toxic or septic shock. It has been observed in the clinic that patients with Gram-negative bacterial blood infections can die even under circumstances where antibiotic treatment clears the infection. It is generally accepted that high endotoxin levels play an important role in determining lethality. One of the complicating factors is the tendency of antibiotics to promote LPS release both through lysis of bacteria and nonlytic mechanisms (69). Thus, it is of great interest to develop either antibiotics that do not enhance the release of LPS or treatments that neutralize released LPS.

LPS molecules contain several phosphate moieties in addition to the unique acidic octasaccharide, 2-keto-3-deoxyoctanate. Thus, they are strongly negatively charged, a charge that is neutralized in part by divalent cations such as Mg^{2+} and Ca^{2+}. As described below, such anionic residues are the site of initial interaction of cationic peptides with bacterial outer membranes. Indeed, it has been clearly demonstrated that cationic peptides bind to bacterial LPS with an affinity that is at least three orders of magnitude higher than the divalent cations (1,71,72). Such binding prevents LPS from interacting with macrophages to elicit a TNF response both in vitro and in vivo (72,73). Consequently, cationic peptides are protective in a mouse endotoxic shock model (74). Thus, unlike other antibiotics, which promote endotoxin release and consequent endotoxic shock, cationic peptides neutralize endotoxin and prevent endotoxic shock.

C. Antifungal Activity

Mammalian defensins kill *Candida albicans* within minutes in vitro (75). The action of such peptides involves four distinct steps: primary binding, postbinding events, permeabilization, and secondary binding to internal macromolecules (76). Other cationic peptides having antifungal activity include the tachyplesins and polyphemusins, which have MIC values against *C. albicans* of 3.1 and 6.3 µg/ml, respectively (52). Not surprisingly, those peptides isolated from plants have a broad range of antifungal activity against plant pathogenic fungi. For example, Rs-AFP, the antifungal peptide isolated from radish seed, has MIC values as low as 0.3 µg/ml against certain plant pathogenic fungi (77). The plant peptides Mj-AMP and Ac-AMP cause a delay in growth of the fungal hyphae without changing mycelial morphology, whereas Rs-AFP causes a hyperbranching and swelling of the hyphae (61,62,77). However, these peptides show little or no activity against plant, insect, or human cells. Thionins cause a permeabilization of the plasmalemma around the hyphal tips (78).

D. Antiviral Activity

Several of the defensins have been found to neutralize herpes simplex virus (HSV) in tissue culture media (79). For example, rat NP-1 (50 µg/ml) caused direct viral neutralization, reducing HSV type 1 plaque forming units/ml by 90% in 60 min, and >99.9% of input viral titer was inactivated within 1 hr by 75 µg/ml guinea pig defensin at 37°C (80).

E. Other Properties

In addition to the killing of the microorganisms described above, certain cationic peptides have been associated with the killing of parasites. Killing of *Giardia lamblia* has been demonstrated with indolicidin, cryptidins 2 and 3, and NP-2 (81). These peptides reduced the viability of the protozoal trophozoites by three orders of magnitude in 2 hr. The binding and lysis of the cells appears to involve charge interactions, as NaCl, Ca^{2+}, and Mg^{2+}

all inhibited killing. In addition, magainin analogs disrupted the morphological integrity and motility of several parasites, including *Entamoeba histolytca* and *Trypanosoma cruzi* (82). The latter was killed by 100 μg/ml of the magainin analog magainin B.

Other properties may exist for cationic peptides within the host. For example, sapaecin, the insect defensin, has been found to stimulate cell proliferation of *Sarcophaga* embryo cells. This perhaps indicates a dual role of antimicrobial agent and developmental hormone for this peptide in the flesh fly (83). Indeed, Magainin Pharmaceuticals, Inc., Plymouth Meeting, PA has claimed to have available cationic peptides that promote reepithelialization of damaged corneas.

Much work has been carried out on the potential for cationic peptides as anticancer agents. This has been most extensively studied with the magainins. An ovarian cancer murine model (84) showed the elimination of 99% of tumor cells after two injections of a magainin analog. In this study there was only mild damage caused to surrounding tissue, which indicates a higher susceptibility of malignant cells to these compounds.

F.   Immunogenicity, Toxicity, and Stability

There has been no detailed examination of immunogenicity of cationic peptides. However, the general consensus in the field is that they are weakly immunogenic or nonimmunogenic. This could be due to clonal deletion during development, because of the importance of peptides in nonspecific host defenses at mucosal surfaces, and their secretion by neutrophils at sites of inflammation, resulting in their recognition as "self" antigens.

Although many cationic peptides are antimicrobial to some extent, their propensity to be toxic to mammalian cells varies greatly. For example, Schluesener et al. (85) found that although indolicidin and, to a lesser extent, bactenecin are strongly cytotoxic to T lymphocytes, the defensins HNP-1, HNP-2, and HNP-3 did not affect the proliferation or viability of the T lymphocytes. On the other hand, the cationic peptides melittin and charyldotoxin are the potent toxins of bee and scorpion venom, respectively.

The issue of stability in vivo has not been addressed in detail. Clearly proteases, which are found in all body fluids, provide the potential for cleavage. One approach to overcoming such problems has involved synthesis of peptides with all D–amino acids; such peptides are not protease susceptible and often have equal activity to that of the L-form peptides (see Section IV.B).

IV.   BIOCHEMICAL BASIS FOR ANTIBACTERIAL ACTIVITIES

A.   Common Themes, Different Structures

All known cationic peptides share two properties: a high proportion of basic amino acids that are protonated and, thus, positively charged at neutral pH; and a high proportion of hydrophobic amino acids. These tend to distribute themselves through the three-dimensional structure of the peptide so as to create an amphipathic molecule having a hydrophilic, positively charged face and a hydrophobic face. However, the secondary and tertiary folding patterns of such peptides are quite diverse. For this reason, we consider the cationic peptides to be one of the finest arguments for convergent evolution, in which a variety of peptides have converged toward a common function, namely, defense against microbes.

The basic amino acids include arginine (pI = 10.8) and lysine (pI = 9.5), which are protonated and thus positively charged at pHs below their pI values. In addition, histidine has a pI of 7.6, rendering it only partially positively charged at neutral pH. However, at acidified sites in the body, including the upper gastrointestinal tract, the interior of phagocytic cell phagolysosomes, or some infection sites, histidine would be strongly positively charged. Nevertheless, with a few exceptions, histidines are relatively uncommon in cationic peptides. In contrast, cationic peptides usually contain four to nine positive residues that can comprise exclusively arginine (in defensins and thionins) or lysine (in cecropins or magainins) residues, or a mixture of the two. The acidic amino acids glutamate and aspartate are sometimes found in cationic peptides, but not more than two residues per peptide. The remaining (uncharged) residues often exclude several amino acids for a given peptide. Overall nonpolar (hydrophobic) residues usually exceed polar (hydrophilic) residues by a ratio of 2:1. Despite this high proportion of hydrophobic residues, the cationic peptides tend to be soluble in water, buffer, or acidified aqueous solutions due to their ability to fold and aggregate to mask their hydrophobic faces.

Despite their thematic similarities (i.e., their amphipathic nature), cationic peptides offer a range of secondary and tertiary folding patterns. The two most pronounced structural classes are the β-stranded and α-helical classes. The β-stranded class includes the defensins. The mammalian defensins have been crystallized (HNP-3) and studied by two-dimensional nuclear magnetic resonance (NMR) techniques (HNP-1, NP-2, NP-5) with rather similar results. They comprise two antiparallel β-strands with a short stretch of triple-stranded β-sheet (Figure 4). The β-strands are connected by short β-turn regions, and the entire structure is stabilized by three disulfide bridges. Despite some sequence variations, within a given class of defensins the positions of cysteines, the disulfide bonding patterns, and the positions of charged residues are strongly conserved. At least three classes of defensins exist, the mammalian defensins, β-defensins, and insect defensins (Table 2). Although not structurally well characterized, the plant thionins may make up another class of defensins. Only one other class has been examined structurally, namely, the insect defensins. These compounds have a different disulfide bonding array than do the mammalian defensins. The structure of the insect defensin, sapecin, has been defined by NMR and shown to contain two extended (β-stranded) regions, a short stretch of α-helix, and a flexible loop (87). However, the structurally characterized defensins all retain the characteristic hydrophobic surface and hydrophilic, positively charged surface. NMR evidence suggests that, in solution, defensins dimerize to mask the hydrophobic surface (88). It has also been demonstrated that tachyplesin adopts an amphipathic β-structure, in this case with two antiparallel β-strands stabilized by two disulfide bridges.

The second major structural class studied is the α-helical class. Interestingly, such structures tend to be rather disorganized in aqueous solution, but they become α-helical structured upon entering a membrane environment or exposure to nonpolar solvents (89,90). The predominant structures observed upon interaction with membranes are helix–bend–helix with a 9–16 amino acid amphipathic α-helix, a 2–4 residue bend, and a 11–14 amino acid amphipathic but more hydrophobic α-helix, as demonstrated by two-dimensional NMR of cecropins A and B, melittin, the magainins, and a synthetic cecropin–melittin hybrid (89,91–93). A small variation is provided by mammalian cecropin P1, which comprises an uninterrupted amphiphilic helix for 24 amino acids, bounded by 2–4 residues at the N- and C-termini.

Several cationic peptides are rich in proline, and specific peptides within this group have been demonstrated to adopt a poly-L-proline II helical structure (94–96). In the

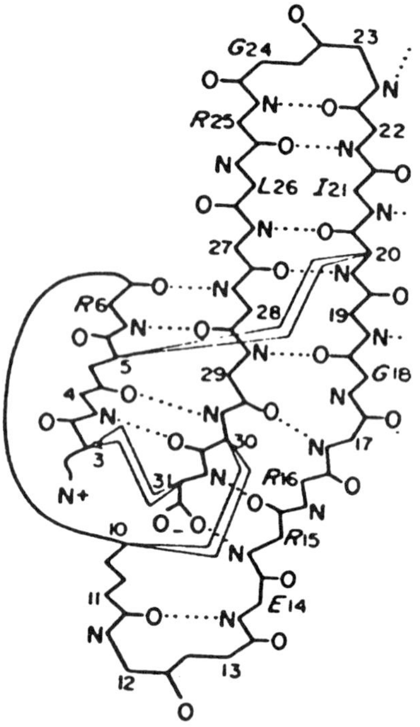

Figure 4 Model of the mammalian defensin structure. The triple-stranded antiparallel β-sheet structure of an HNP-3 monomer. The disulfide bonds are represented as "lightning bolts." Charged residues are indicated as R = arginine and E = glutamate. (Reproduced by copyright permission of Hill et al. (86). © American Association for the Advancement of Science.)

case of the proline/arginine-rich peptides, bactenecin 5 and PR-39, this structure is unaffected by the presence of lipid vesicles (95,96). However, in the case of the proline/tryptophan-rich peptide indolicidin, the assumption of this specific helical structure is greatly increased in the presence of negatively charged liposomes (94). Other peptides form loops due to single disulfide bonds, or they have extremely high histidine or tryptophan contents (Table 3). We anticipate that these will have a variety of structures.

B. Structure–Activity Relationships

The influence of substitutions or deletions of specific amino acids on the activity of the cationic peptides has been investigated in detail in several studies. The following principles seem to apply: (a) There is considerable specificity in how the changes in amino acid sequence influence activity (97,98). For example, introduction of a turn-promoting proline at positions 4 or 8 in the first α-helical segment of cecropins had a substantial effect on activity against *Micrococcus luteus*, lesser effects on activities against *Bacillus megaterium* and *P. aeruginosa*, and no effect on activity against *E. coli*. Furthermore, even conservative substitutions (changing selected amino acids to ones with similar physical properties) can substantially influence function. (b) For the α-helical peptides, changes that increase the tendency to form an α-helix in aqueous solution (i.e., prior to interacting with membranes) tend to increase activity (97–100). (c) There is no clear relationship between the numbers of positive charges and activity, and the position of specific positive charges is important (98). (d) Enantiomers (i.e., all D–amino acids vs. all L–amino acids) of the structured peptides have equal activity (101), showing that chirality is not important. (e) Decreased ability of cationic peptides to bind to bacteria or to lyse liposomes correlates to some extent with decreased MIC (99). However, this correlation is not absolute. For example, one can design peptides that bind extremely well to Gram-negative bacteria but have little or no antibiotic activity (66; Hancock REW and Gough M, unpublished data). Furthermore, it must be noted that some cationic peptides that are potent mediators of liposomal lysis are potent toxins but relatively weak antibacterial agents. (f) For the disulfide-bonded peptides, reduction of the cysteine disulfides destroys activity. (g) Finally, there is no absolute correlation between peptide size and antibacterial potency. For example, reduction in size of cecropin–melittin hybrids from 26 to 14 amino acids did not influence activity so long as these compounds maintained an α-helical structure (102).

It must be stressed, however, that we do not at present have a set of design rules that will create the perfect peptide antibiotic. For example, although amphipathicity and α-helicity favor activity, a perfectly amphipathic α-helix (Lys–Ala–Ala–Lys–Ala–Ala–Ala–Lys) was a potent hemolysin.

C.   Interactions with Membranes

The primary mechanism of action of cationic peptides is probably through the generation of channels in membranes. These can range from ordered channels through to so-called multistate channels. It must be stressed that we do not know in detail the basis for membrane target selectivity. For example, although they both fall into the amphipathic α-helical class, moth cecropins are strongly antibacterial and demonstrate minimal eukaryotic selectivity (i.e., toxicity), whereas melittin from bee venom is a weak antibacterial compound but a potent toxin. The primary basis for selectivity has been reported to be the target lipid composition (see below).

A secondary mechanism of action is a detergent-like effect (103). However, it is unclear whether this merely represents the cooperative accumulation of multistate channels or gross multimerization of cationic peptides in the membrane, and whether this mechanism is relevant to bacterial cell killing, since it has only been demonstrated in nondefinitive experiments in eukaryotic cell lines and model liposomes (103). In contrast, the lysis of bacteria—often at concentrations exceeding the MIC—probably arises from the triggering of autolytic enzymes (104). With these caveats, it is worth considering how cationic peptides interact with membranes.

1.   Model Systems

The process of interaction of the peptides with lipid layers can be modeled as shown in Figure 5. The peptides initially present in solution as aggregates are present in the form of dimers (e.g., defensins) (88) and/or conformers (e.g., cecropins are relatively unstructured in solution). Interaction with the negatively charged head groups of lipids occurs in a cooperative, rapid process involving progressive binding and alignment of positive charges of the peptide with lipid head groups (105–107). The extent of binding corresponds to the zeta potential of the lipids involved, leading one to conclude that it is electrostatic in nature (106,107). Lipid composition is important: binding to liposomes composed of negatively charged lipids is extremely fast, but binding to zwitterionic lipids is slower and can demonstrate negative cooperativity (107).

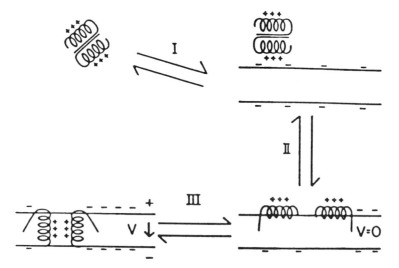

Figure 5 Tentative model for the interaction of cecropins with a lipid bilayer membrane. Aggregates adsorb to the bilayer–water interface by electrostatic forces (I). Only a dimer is sketched for the sake of simplicity, but larger aggregates are likely to occur. The next step (II) would be insertion of the hydrophobic segment into the membrane core. Upon application of voltage (positive on the side of the peptide addition), a major conformational rearrangement takes place (III), which results in channel formation. This rearrangement could be insertion of the positively charged amphipathic helix into the membrane or opening of preformed, closed channels. (Reproduced by copyright permission from Christensen et al. (36). © The National Academy of Sciences of the United States of America.)

It is uncertain whether at this point the permeability of the target lipid membrane changes. However, it seems credible that the phenomenon of leakiness (usually assessed by carbofluorescein leakage from liposomes) may occur in part at this stage. Furthermore, it is probable that the cationic peptide undergoes a change in conformation and aggregation state as a result of this interaction.

The next event is the insertion of the cationic peptide into the membrane. This occurs at a critical concentration of peptide that depends on the nature of the peptide and the target membrane, as well as on the fluidity of the membrane and the existence and size of the transmembrane electrical potential. Although insertion can occur into membranes with little or no transmembrane potential, it seems likely that the membrane potential of living cells (oriented interior negative) is always an important factor in peptide insertion. In addition, it has been demonstrated in planar lipid bilayer model membrane experiments (in which the "membrane potential" is provided as an applied voltage) that this potential must be oriented positive on the cis side (where the cationic peptides are added) and negative on the trans side of the membrane (toward which the cationic peptides move as they enter the membrane). This results in an observable increase in conductance as the peptides enter the membrane and form channels (36,94,108–111). Reversal of the voltage actually causes peptides to leave the membrane (36). It is relevant to the issue of toxicity that bacterial cytoplasmic membranes bear large transmembrane electrical potential gradients, $\Delta\psi$ (up to –140 mV), whereas eukaryotic membranes have gradients of only about –20 mV or less.

The process of insertion causes changes in phase and/or motion of the lipids of the target membrane (112). However, the lipid composition can dramatically influence the possibility of insertion, and positively charged phospholipids and cholesterol decreased the formation of membrane channels by cecropin by 5- to 60-fold (36). Indeed, this may explain, in addition to the difference in $\Delta\psi$, the selectivity of cationic antibacterial peptides for bacteria over eukaryotes, since the former lack cholesterol, which is abundant in eukaryotic membranes, whereas anionic phosphatidyl glycerol and cardiodipin, major components of bacterial membranes, represent excellent target lipids.

The process of insertion can also cause a conformational change in the cationic peptides (e.g., from unstructured to α-helical), for example, with melittin (113) and magainins (90,114). In many cases, the peptides are thought to end up spanning the membrane bilayer (41,102,113) in multimeric complexes. Other peptides are too short to span the bilayer and presumably must form aggregates to permit transmembrane channel formation (102,114,115).

Generally speaking, cationic peptides form multistate channels, and planar lipid bilayer experiments demonstrate a substantial range of channel sizes, with single-channel conductances (which reflect size) varying from 10 to 2000 pS (94,108–110,116) and lifetimes ranging from milliseconds to seconds (110). This behavior is similar to that observed for alamethicin (117), for which it has been proposed that application of a voltage induces alamethicin monomers to span the membrane, and that these monomers associate and disassociate with various rate constants, leading to aggregates of different sizes and lifetimes. Each aggregate contains a variable number of monomers arrayed like staves of a barrel around a central axis, and oriented with the hydrophilic portion of the monomer facing inward toward the channel interior and the hydrophobic face adjacent to the membrane interior. Thus, the size of the aggregates would decree the size of the channel. These channels are water filled and tend to be weakly selective for chloride over sodium ions.

In specific instances, for example, the cecropins, the channels formed are more defined (118). In this case, the actual channel forming unit has been modeled at atomic-level resolution. Two arrangements of six dimers have been proposed to account for the two discrete conductance increments (0.4 and 1.9 nS) reported by Christensen et al. (36).

2. Bacterial Cytoplasmic Membranes

As discussed above, cationic peptides can form channels in model bilayers. Thus, it seems likely that their primary antibacterial action is to disrupt the integrity of bacterial cytoplasmic membranes. This would have the effect of permitting leakage of ions and small metabolites, and destroying the ability of bacteria to maintain a transmembrane proton gradient (proton-motive force) with consequent loss of ability to generate adenosine triphosphate and transport substrates (see Ref. 119 for review of cytoplasmic membranes).

Bacteria maintain, across their cytoplasmic membranes, a proton-motive force of approximately −170 mV (120), comprising an electrical potential gradient $\Delta\psi$ (oriented interior negative) and a proton chemical gradient ΔpH (oriented interior alkaline). Treatment of cells with any of several different cationic peptides (e.g., magainins, nisin, or Pep5) leads to destruction of $\Delta\psi$ at concentrations approaching the MIC, as assessed using the cationic lipid-soluble probe triphenyl phosphonium (121,122). Evidence suggests that this decrease of proton-motive force occurs as a sigmoidal function of peptide concentration, indicating that peptides act in a cooperative fashion on cytoplasmic membranes (121). Other data favoring the hypothesis that destruction of cytoplasmic membrane integrity is the primary basis of the activity of cationic peptides against bacteria include the demonstration that mastoporan and melittin cause K^+ leakage in Gram-positive bacteria (123).

3. Bacterial Outer Membranes

Only Gram-negative bacteria have outer membranes, and it is clear that the interaction of an antibiotic with outer membranes cannot directly lead to cell death. However, outer membranes are discussed separately here for two reasons. First, the cationic peptides include molecules that are rare among antibiotics in having better activities against Gram-negative than Gram-positive bacteria (normally, the influence of the outer membrane on penetration of antibiotics decreases activity). Second, the interaction of cationic peptides with the outer membranes of Gram-negative bacteria explains two of the pharmaceutically interesting properties of these molecules, namely, their "enhancer" and antiendotoxin properties.

Cationic peptides, like other polycationic antibiotics, traverse the outer membrane using a process termed self-promoted uptake (124); in contrast, small hydrophilic antibiotics such as β-lactams diffuse through the water-filled channels of porin proteins (125). Self-promoted uptake (Figure 6) involves the initial interaction of cationic peptides with the negatively charged, divalent-cation-binding sites of the surface glycolipid lipopolysaccharide (LPS). Since the cationic peptides have an affinity for LPS that is three orders of magnitude higher than the native divalent cations, Mg^{2+} or Ca^{2+} (70), they competitively displace these cations. This causes a distortion of outer membrane structure that has been visualized in the electron microscope as induction of outer membrane blebs (70), and a consequent permeabilization of the membrane to probe molecules, including lysozyme and the hydrophobic probe 1-*N*-phenyl-napthylamine (71,126). By analogy with other polycations, this distortion of the membrane is proposed to lead to enhanced ability of the cationic peptide to promote its own uptake (hence the term self-promoted uptake). The basic features of this uptake system have been demonstrated for interaction of both the α-helical (66) and β-structured cationic peptides (70).

The ability of cationic peptides to act in synergy with certain classical antibiotics (68) can be explained by their ability to disrupt outer membrane integrity, promoting the uptake of antibiotics across this barrier. Interestingly, the most potent cationic peptides do not have this "enhancer" activity for most antibiotics, presumably since they kill cells

Table 4 MICs of Selected Cationic Peptides Compared with Conventional Antibiotics

	MIC[a](µg/ml)				
Organism	CP-29[b]	CP-11c[c]	Gentamicin	Ceftazidime	Polymyxin
Pseudomonas aeruginosa	4	8	0.3	0.5	0.3
Escherichia coli	2	2	0.3	0.3	0.1
Staphylococcus aureus	16	8	2	2	>64
Candida albicans	32	8	>64	>64	>64

[a] MIC values were determined by the broth dilution method (63).

[b] CP-29 is a cecropin/mellitin hybrid cationic peptide (Hancock, Gough, and Farmer, unpublished data).

[c] CP-11c is an extended helix cationic peptide (Falla, T., Hancock, R. E. W., unpublished data).

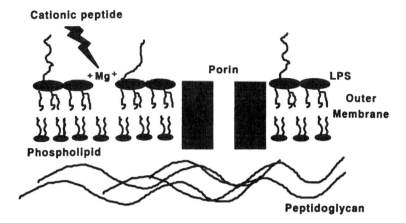

Figure 6 Schematic diagram of the self-promoted uptake model. Cationic antibiotics disrupt the Mg^{2+} cross-bridges, displace the Mg^{2+} ions, and cause perturbation of the lipid bilayer. Further disruption of the outer membrane results in uptake of normally excluded compounds.

at concentrations equal to their permeabilizing concentrations (66). This is analogous to the situation for the polycationic antibiotic polymyxin B, which is not an enhancer, whereas its deacylated derivative PMBN (which interacts weakly with cytoplasmic membranes but strongly with outer membranes) is a potent enhancer of antibiotic activity (127).

The antiendotoxin activity of cationic peptides is also related to the above uptake mechanism. Endotoxin is in fact LPS, or more precisely the lipid A portion of LPS. As mentioned above, cationic peptides bind to polyanionic LPS (70,128,129). The binding is of high affinity and cooperative (70). This binding can neutralize the ability of LPS to induce TNF in macrophage cell lines or in a murine model, and it reduces endotoxin mortality in galactosamine-sensitized mice (130,131).

V. PRODUCTION METHODS

A. Natural Sources

As described in Section II, cationic peptides are very widely distributed in nature. Recovery from these sources involves a wide range of methods. One effective procedure is extraction with 30% acetic acid, which tends to solubilize cationic peptides and precipitate many globular proteins. This is usually followed by a variety of chromatographic procedures often including reverse phase HPLC or FPLC as the final step in purification. However, purification from natural sources is rarely a practical alternative for commercial purposes, since yields tend to be relatively low. For example, a single rabbit will permit the recovery of only 200 mg of rabbit defensins. The one exception is the production of cationic lantibiotic peptides such as nisin from bacteria and commercial production of nisin by fermentation of *Lactococcus lactis* (see Chapter 15).

B. Protein Chemical

A very convenient laboratory-scale procedure for making peptides is the use of automated peptide synthesizers using t-boc or f-moc chemistry (132). However, the expense of reagents and the limited capacities of these automated synthesizers has limited the scale and, thus, the industrial relevance of this method. An alternative is provided by solution phase chemistry, which is, unfortunately, less conductive to automation.

C.   Recombinant Procedures

One potential advantage of the peptide nature of cationic peptides is their potential ability to be synthesized recombinantly, since they can be directly encoded by DNA. There are certainly some limitations to this, since nonnatural amino acids (e.g., in the antibiotics) and many modifications (e.g., carboxyl-terminal amidation) are difficult to introduce recombinantly. As with the protein chemical procedures, however, one is not limited to "natural" cationic peptides.

The first attempt to synthesize cationic peptides recombinantly appears in the patent literature (133). A sequence encoding cecropin was fused to a portion of the *ara*C gene of *E. coli.* Although few details were provided, it is clear that this method was not optimized: although cecropin could be manufactured recombinantly, it had poor potency (i.e., 5 μg of recombinant cecropin gave a clearing zone diameter against *E. coli* of 5 mm, whereas 1 μg of authentic cecropin gave a clearing diameter of 7 mm). Furthermore, the patent claimed that virtually any fusion partner would work to support the production of cecropins, whereas it is now evident that this is not the case. Subsequently, it was demonstrated that cecropin could be synthesized as a fusion with a protein A–like, IgG-binding domain, using baculovirus vector in an insect cell line (2). After affinity purification of the fusion protein and cleavage of cecropin from its carrier using cyanogen bromide, the cecropin could be recovered in its amidated form. The yields were 600 μg/ml of haemolymph, of which 70% was amidated, indicating that this method may be cost prohibitive given the expense associated with animal cell culture.

Piers et al. (1) have developed a procedure for the synthesis of cationic peptides in bacteria. The main feature is inclusion of an anionic stabilizing fragment in the fusion protein to counteract the cationic peptide portion. This anionic fragment could be the carrier protein itself if the fusion protein was expressed in *S. aureus,* but for expression in *E. coli* an extra anionic sequence equivalent to the pre pro sequence from the gene for human defensin (which sequence stabilizes defensin during its synthesis in human cells; 134) is needed. Additional elements were the inclusion of a methionine residue immediately adjacent to the cationic peptide sequence, to permit removal of the cationic peptide by CNBr cleavage, and a carrier sequence that, when desired, could be tailored to enhance affinity purification of the resultant fusion. The general nature of the fusion protein is demonstrated in Figure 7. We believe this system offers significant advantages in the production of cationic peptides. An interesting side note is that the successful production of antibacterial cationic peptides by molecular genetic means makes these cationic peptides the first recombinant antibiotics.

VI.   AN EXCITING FUTURE

Cationic peptides do not have as potent activities against the most susceptible bacteria as do other antibiotics. Furthermore, the spectrum of cationic peptides includes some of the most potent toxins (e.g., bee venom and scorpion toxin), so that toxicity will always be a closely observed issue. In addition, being peptides, they are potentially susceptible to host

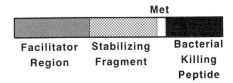

Figure 7   Schematic diagram of a protein A–cationic peptide fusion protein. Met represents the position of the methionine residue used to cleave the peptide with cyanogen bromide.

peptidases and proteases, and innovative approaches will have to be applied to overcome this problem (e.g., the use of D–amino acids). However, activity, toxicity, and pharmacology are issues with every compound used in medicine.

With these reservations, we believe that cationic peptides offer an exciting future. They represent a "natural" solution to infection, since they mimic the anti-infective defense systems of several eukaryotes. Their activities cover a far broader spectrum than do those of other antibiotics. Indeed, they offer the potential for organ-specific therapy directed against the major bacterial and fungal infections of a given body site. In addition, the most active cationic peptides have activities against some of the more refractory antibiotic-resistant pathogens (e.g., *Pseudomonas aeruginosa* and methicillin-resistant *Staphylococcus aureus*) that are equivalent to those observed for the antibiotics tailored for use against those pathogens. Indeed, that they do not seem to induce antibiotic resistance and are effective against most bacteria resistant to conventional antibiotics are important features of cationic peptides. In addition, their potential to act in synergy with conventional antibiotics and to neutralize endotoxin released by these antibiotics makes them an attractive candidate for use in combination therapy.

ACKNOWLEDGMENT

The authors' own research on polycationic peptides was supported by the Canadian Bacterial Diseases Network.

REFERENCES

1.   Piers KL, Brown MH, Hancock REW. Recombinant DNA procedures for producing small antimicrobial cationic peptides in bacteria. Gene 1993; 134:7–13.
2.   Hellers M, Gunne H, Steiner H. Expression of post-translational processing of prececropin A using a baculovirus vector. Eur J Biochem 1991; 199:435–439.
3.   Jaynes JM, Nagpala P, Destefano-Bettran L, Huang JCH, Kim JH, Denny T, Cetiner S. Expression of a Cecropin B lytic peptide analog in transgenic tobacco confers enhanced resistance to bacterial wilt caused by *Pseudomonas solanacearum*. Plant Sci 1993; 43–53.
4.   Mitra A, Zhang Z. Expression of a human lactoferrin cDNA in tobacco cells produces antibacterial protein(s). Plant Physiol 1994; 106:971–981.
5.   Hancock REW, Falla T, Brown MM. Cationic bactericidal peptides. Poole RK, ed. Advances in Microbial Physiology, 2nd ed. London: Academic Press, 1995:137–175.
6.   Couto MA, Harwig SSL, Cullor JS, Hughes JPÊ, Lehrer RI. eNAP, a novel cysteine-rich bactericidal peptide from equine leukocytes. Infect Immun 1992; 60:5042–5047.

7. Eisenhauer PB, Lehrer RI. Mouse neutrophils lack defensins. Infect Immun 1992; 60:3446–3447.

8. Lehrer RI, Ganz T, Selsted ME. Defensins: Natural peptide antibiotics from neutrophils. ASM News 1990; 56:315–318.

9. Michaelson D, Rayner J, Cuoto M, Ganz T. Cationic defensins arise from charge-neutralized propeptides: A mechanism for avoiding leukocyte autocytotoxicity. J Leukocyte Biol 1992; 51:634–639.

10. Selsted ME, Tang YQ, Morris WL, McGuire PA, Novotny MJ, Smith W, Henschen AH, Cullor JS. Purification, primary structures and antibacterial activities of beta-defensins, a new family of antimicrobial peptides from bovine neutrophils. J Biol Chem 1993; 268:6641–6648.

11. Diamond G, Zasloff M, Eck H, Brasseur M, Maloy WL, Bevins CL. Tracheal antimicrobial peptide, a cysteine-rich peptide from mammalian tracheal mucosa: Peptide isolation and cloning of a cDNA. Proc Natl Acad Sci USA 1991; 88:3952–3956.

12. Gennaro R, Skerlaray B, Romeo D. Purification, composition and activity of two bactenecins, antibacterial peptides of bovine neutrophils. Infect Immun 1989; 57:3142–3146.

13. Selsted ME, Novotny MJ, Morris WL, Tang YQ, Smith W, Cullor JS. Indolicidin, a novel bactericidal tridecapeptide amide from neutrophils. J Biol Chem 1992; 267:4292–4295.

14. Agerberth B, Lee JY, Bergman T. Carlquist M, Boman HG, Mutt V, Jornvall H. Amino acid sequence of PR-39: Isolation from pig intestine of a new member of the family of proline-arginine-rich antibacterial peptides. Eur J Biochem 1991; 202:849–854.

15. Larrick JW, Morgan JG, Palings I, Hirata M, Yen MH. Complementary DNA sequence of rabbit CAP18—a unique lipopolysaccharide binding protein. Biochem Biophys Res Commun 1991; 179:170–175.

16. Zanetti M, Del Sal G, Storici P, Schneider C, Romeo D. The cDNA of the neutrophil antibiotic Bac5 predicts a pro-sequence homologous to a cysteine proteinase inhibitor that is common to other neutrophil antibiotics. J Biol Chem 1993; 268:522–526.

17. Levy O, Weis J, Zarember K, Ooi CE, Elsbach P. Antibacterial 15-kDa protein isoforms (p15s) are members of a novel family of leukocyte proteins. J Biol Chem 1993; 268:6058–6063.

18. Bevins CL, Zasloff M. Peptides from frog skin. Annu Rev Biochem 1990; 59:395–414.

19. Lazarus LH, Attila M. The toad, ugly and venomous, wears yet a precious jewel in his skin. Prog Neurobiol 41:473–507.

20. Csordas A, Michl H. Isolation and structure of a hemolytic polypeptide from the defensive secretion of European Bombina species. Monatsh Chem 1970; 101:182–189.

21. Simmaco M, Barra D, Chiarini F, Noviello L, Melchiorri P, Kreil G, Richter K. A family of bombinin-related peptides from the skin of *Bombina variegata*. Eur J Biochem 1991; 199:217–222.

22. Chen HC, Brown JH, Morell JL, Huang CM. Synthetic magainin analogues with improved antimicrobial activity. FEBS Lett 1988; 236:462–466.

23. Zasloff M. Magainins, a class of antimicrobial peptides from *Xenopus* skin: Isolation, characterization of two active forms, and partial cDNA sequence of a precursor. Proc Natl Acad Sci USA 1987; 84:5449–5453.

24. Zasloff M, Martin B, Chen HC. Antimicrobial activity of synthetic magainin peptides and several analogues. PNAS 1988; 85:910–913.

25. Levison M, Pitsaki PG, May PL, Johnson CC. The bactericidal activity of magainins against *Pseudomonas aeruginosa* and *Enterococcus faecium*. J Antimicrob Chemother 1993; 32:577–585.

26. Cuervo JH, Rodriquez B, Houghten RA. The Magainins: Sequence factors relevent to increased antimicrobial activity and decreased hemolytic activity. Pept Res 1988; 1:81–86.

27. Hoffmann W, Richter K, Kreil G. A novel peptide designated PYLa and its precursor as predicted from cloned mRNA of *Xenopus laevis*. EMBO J 1983; 2:711–714.

28. Moore KS, Bevins CL, Brasseur MM, Tomassini N, Turner K, Eck H, Zasloff M. Antimicrobial peptides in the stomach of *Xenopus laevis*. J Biol Chem 1991; 266:19851–19857.

29. Sures L, Crippa M. Xenopsin: the neurotensin-like octapeptide from *Xenopus* skin at the carboxyl terminus of its precursor. Proc Natl Acad Sci USA 1984; 81:380–384.

30. Terry AS, Poulter L, Williams DH, Nutkins JC, Giovannini MG, Moore CH, Gibson BW. The cDNA sequence for prepro-PGS (prepro-magainins) and aspects of the processing of this polypeptide. J Biol Chem 1988; 263:5745–5751.

31. Morikawa N, Hagiwara K and Nakajima T. Brevinin-1 and -2, unique antimicrobial peptides from the skin of the frog *Rana brevipoda porsa*. Biochem Biophys Res Commun 1992; 189:184–190.

32. Simmaco M, Mignogna G, Barra D, Bossa F. Novel antimicrobial peptides from skin secretion of the European frog *Rana esculenta*. FEBS Lett 1993; 324:159–161.

33. Steiner H, Hultmark D, Engström A, Bennich H, Boman HG. Sequence and specificity of two antibacterial proteins involved in insect immunity. Nature 1981; 292:246–248.

34. Lambert J, Keppi E, Dimarcq JL, Wicker C, Reichhart JM, Dunbar B, Lepage P, Van DA, Hoffman J, Fothergill J, Hoffman D. Insect immunity: Isolation from immune blood of the dipteran *Phormia terranovae* of two insect antibacterial peptides with sequence homology to rabbit lung macrophage bactericidal peptides. Proc Natl Acad Sci USA 1989; 86:262–266.

35. Matsuyama K, Natori S. Molecular cloning of cDNA for sapacin and unique expression of the sapecin gene during the development of *Sacrophaga peregrina*. J Biol Chem 1988: 263:17117–17121.

36. Christensen B, Fink J, Merrifield RB, Mauzerall D. Channel forming properties of cecropins and related model compounds incorporated into planar lipid membranes. Proc Natl Acad Sci USA 1988; 85:5072–5076.

37. Hultmark D, Engström A, Bennich H, Kapur R, Boman HG. Insect immunity: Isolation and structure of cecropin D and four minor antibacterial components from *Cecropia pupae*. Eur J Biochem 1982; 127:207–217.

38. Okada M, Natori S. Ionophore activity of sarcotoxin I, a bactericidal protein of *Sarcophaga peregrina*. Biochem J 1985; 229:453–458.

39. Samakovlis C, Kimbrell DA, Kylsten P, Engström A, Hultmark D. The immune response in *Drosophila*: Pattern of cecropin expression and biological activity. EMBO J 1990; 9:2969–2976.

40. Lee J-Y, Boman A, Sun CX, Anderson M, Jornvall H, Mutt V, Boman HG. Antibacterial peptides from pig intestine: Isolation of a mammalian cecropin. Proc Natl Acad Sci USA 1989; 86:9159–9162.

41. Sipos D, Andersson M, Ehrenberg A. The structure of the mammalian antibacterial peptide cecropin P1 in solution, determined by proton-NMR. Eur J Biochem 1992; 209:163–169.

42. Hoffmann JA, Hetru C. Insect defensins: Inducible antibacterial peptides. Immun Today 1992; 13:411–415.

43. Bontems F, Roumestand C, Gilguin B, Menez A, Toma F. Refined structure of charybdotoxin: Common motifs in scorpion toxins and insect defensins. Science 1991; 254:1521.

44. Cociancich S, Goyffon M, Bontems F, Bulet P, Bouet F, Menez A, Hoffmann J. Purification and characterization of scorpion defensin, a 4KDa antibacterial peptide presenting structural similarities with insect defensins and scorpion toxins. Biochem Biophys Res Commun 1993; 194:17–22.

45. Fujiwara S, Imai J, Fujiwara M, Yaeshima T, Kawashima T, Kobayashi K. A potent antibacterial protein in royal jelly. Purification and determination of the primary structure of rayalısın. J Biol Chem 1990; 265:11333–11337.

46. Kuzuhara T, Nakajima Y, Matsuyama K, Natori S. Determination of the disulphide array in sapecin, an antibacterial peptide of *Sarcophaga peregrina* (flesh fly). J Biochem 1990; 107:514–518.

47. Casteels P. Possible applications of insect antibacterial peptides. Isolation and characterization of abaecin, a major antibacterial response peptide in the honeybee (*Apis mellifera*). Res Immun 1990; 141:940–942.

48. Casteels P, Ampe C, Jacobs F, Vaeck M, Tempst P. Apidaecins: Antibacterial peptides from honeybees. EMBO J 1989; 8:2387–2391.

49. Casteels P, Ampe C, Jacobs F, Tempst P. Functional and chemical characterization of Hymenoptaecin, an antibacterial polypeptide that is infection-inducible in the honeybee (*Apis mellifera*). J Biol Chem 1993; 268:7044–7054.

50. Casteels-Josson K, Capaci T, Casteels P, Tempst P. Apidaecin multipeptide precursor structure: A putative mechanism for amplification of the insect antibacterial response. EMBO J 1993; 12:1569–1578.

51. Nakamura T, Furunaka H, Miyata T, Tokunaga F, Muta T, Iwanaga S, Niwa M, Takao T, Shimonishi Y. Tachyplesin, a class of antimicrobial peptide from the hemocytes of the horseshoe crab (*Tachypleus tridentatus*): Isolation and chemical structure. J Biol Chem 1988; 263:16709–16713.

52. Miyata T, Tokunaga F, Yoneya T, Yoshikawa K, Iwanaga S, Niwa M, Takao T, Shimonishi Y. Antimicrobial peptides isolated from horseshoe crab hemocytes, tachyplesin II, and polyphemusins I and II: Chemical structures and biological activity. J Biochem 1989; 106:663–668.

53. Muta T, Fujimoto T, Nakajima H, Iwanaga S. Tachyplesins isolated from hemocytes of Southeast Asian horseshoe crabs (*Carcinoscorpius rotundicauda* and *Tachypleus gigas*): Identification of a new tachyplesin III, and a processing intermediate of its precursor. J Biochem 1990; 108:261–266.

54. Hurst A. Nisin. Adv Appl Microbiol 1981; 27:85–123.

55. Kaletta C, Entian KD, Kellner R, Jung G, Reis M, Sahl HG. Pep5, a new lantibiotic: Structural gene isolation and prepeptide sequence. Arch Microbiol 1989; 152:16–19.

56. Weil HP, Beck-Sickinger AG, Metzger J, Stevanovic S, Jung G, Josten M, Sahl HG. Biosynthesis of the lantibiotic Pep5: Isolation and characterization of a prepeptide containing dehydroamino acids. European J Biochem 1990; 194:217–223.

57. Sahl HG. Pore formation in bacterial membranes by cationic lantibiotics. Jung G, Sahl HG, eds. Nisin and Novel Lantibiotics. Leiden: ESCOM, 1991:347–348.

58. Benz R, Jung G, Sahl HG. Mechanism of channel-formation by lantibiotics in black lipid membranes. Jung G, Sahl HG, eds. Nisin and Novel Lantibiotics. Leiden: ESCOM, 1991:359–372.

59. Bradley WA, Somkuti GA. The primary structure of sillucin and antimicrobial peptide from *Mucor pusillus*. FEBS Lett 1979; 97:81–83.

60. Bohlmann H, Clausen S, Behnke S, Giese H, Hiller C, Reimann-Philipp U, Schrader G, Barkholt V, Apel K. Leaf-specific thionins of barley—a novel class of cell wall proteins toxic to plant pathogenic fungi and possibly involved in the defence mechanism of plants. EMBO J 1988; 7:1559–1565.

61. Broekaert WF, Marlen W, Terras FR, De Bolle MF, Proost P, Van Damme J, Dillen L, Claeys M, Rees SB, Vanderleyden J, et al. Antimicrobial peptides from *Amaranthus caudatus* seeds with sequence homology to the cysteine/glycine-rich domain of chitin-binding proteins. Biochem 1992; 31:4308–4314.

62. Cammue BP, De Bolle MF, Terras FR, Proost P, Van Damme J, Rees SB, Vanderleyden J, Broekaert WF. Isolation and characterization of a novel class of plant antimicrobial peptides from *Mirabilis jalapa L.* seeds. J Biol Chem 1992; 267:2228–2233.

63. Amsterdam D. Susceptibility testing of antimicrobials in liquid media. Lorian V, ed. Antibiotics in Laboratory Medicine, 3rd ed. Baltimore: Williams and Wilkins, 1991:72–128.

64. Barry AL. Procedures and theoretical considerations for testing antimicrobial agents in agar media. Lorian V, ed. Antibiotics in Laboratory Medicine, 3rd ed. Baltimore: Williams and Wilkins, 1991:1–14.

65. Acar JF, Goldstein FW. Disk susceptibility test. Lorian V, ed. Antibiotics in Laboratory Medicine, 3rd ed. Baltimore: Williams and Wilkins, 1991:17–48.

66. Piers KL, Brown MH, Hancock REW. Improvement of outer membrane-permeabilization and lipopolysaccharide-binding activities of an antimicrobial cationic peptide by C-terminal modification. Antimicrob Agents Chemother 1994; 38:2311–2316.

67. Piers K. The bacterial production of antimicrobial cationic peptides and their effects on the outer membrane of Gram-negative bacteria. PhD thesis, University of British Columbia, 1993.

68. Darveau RP, Cunningham MD, Seachord CL, Cassiano-Clough L, Cosand WL, Blake J, Watkins CS. Beta-lactam antibiotics potentiate magainin 2 antimicrobial activity in vitro and in vivo. Antimicrob Agents Chemother 1991; 35:1153–1159.

69. Goto H, Nakamura S. Liberation of endotoxin from Escherichia coli by addition of antibiotics. Japan J Med 1980; 50:35–43.

70. Sawyer JG, Martin NL, Hancock REW. Interaction of macrophage cationic proteins with the outer membrane of Pseudomonas aeruginosa. Infect Immun 1988; 56:693–698.

71. Piers KL, Hancock REW. The interaction of a recombinant cecropin/melittin hybrid peptide with the outer membrane of Pseudomonas aeruginosa. Mol Microbiol 1994; 12:951–958.

72. Lin Y, Kohn FR, Kung AH, Ammons WS. Protective effect of a recombinant fragment of bactericidal/permeability increasing protein against carbohydrate dyshomeostasis and tumor necrosis factor-alpha elevation in rat endotoxaemia. Biochem Pharm 1994; 47:1553–1559.

73. Rogy MA, Moldawer LL, Oldenburg HS, Thompson WA, Montegut WJ, Stackpole SA, Kumar A, Pulladino MA, Marra MN, Lowry SE. Anti-endotoxin therapy in primate bacteremia with HA-1A and BPI. Ann Surg 1994; 220:77–85.

74. Gough MA, Hancock REW, Kelly NM. Anti-endotoxin activity of cationic peptide antibiotics. Infect Immun 1996; 64:4922–4927.

75. Selsted ME, Szklarek D, Ganz T, Lehrer RI. Activity of rabbit leukocyte peptides against Candida albicans. Infect Immun 1985; 49:202–206.

76. Lehrer RI, Szklarek D, Ganz T, Selsted ME. Correlation of binding of rabbit granulocyte peptides to Candida albicans with candidacidal activity. Infect Immun 1985; 49:207–211.

77. Terras FR, Schoofs HM, De Bolle MF, Van Leuven F, Rees SB, Vanderleyden J, Cammue BP, Broekaert WF. Analysis of two novel classes of antifungal proteins from radish (Raphanus sativus L.) seeds. J Biol Chem 1992; 267:15301–15309.

78. Terras FRG, Torrekens S, Van Leuven F, Osborn RW, Vanderleyden J, Cammune BPA, Broekaert WF. Synergistic enhancement of the antifungal activity of wheat and barley thionins by radish and oilseed rape 2S albumins and by barley trypsin inhibitors. Plant Physiol 1993; 103:1311–1319.

79. Daher KA, Selsted ME, Lehrer RI. Direct inactivation of viruses by human granulocyte defensins. J Virol 1986; 60:1068–1074.

80. Eisenhauer PB, Harwig SS, Szlarek D, Ganz T, Selsted M, Lehrer RI. Purification and antimicrobial properties of three defensins from rat neutrophils. Infect Immun 1989; 57:2021–2027.

81. Aley SB, Zimmerman M, Hetsko M, Selsted ME, Gillin FD. Killing of Giardia lamblia by cryptidins and cationic neutrophil peptides. Infect Immun 1994; 62:5397–5403.

82. Huang CM, Chen HC, Zierdt CH. Magainin analogs effective against pathogenic protozoa. Antimicrob Agents Chemother 1990; 34:1824–1826.

83. Komano H, Homma K, Natori S. Involvement of sapecin in embryonic cell proliferation of Sarcophage peregrina (flesh fly). FEBS Lett 1991; 289:167–170.

84. Baker MA, Malog WL, Zasloff M, Jacob L. Anticancer efficacy of magainin 2 and analogue peptides. Cancer Res 1993; 58:3052–3057.

85. Schluesener HJ, Radermacher S, Melms A, Jung S. Leukocytic antimicrobial peptides kill autoimmune T cells. J Neuroimmun 1993; 47:199–201.

86. Hill CP, Yee J, Selsted ME, Eisenburg D. Crystal structure of defensin HNP-3, an amphiphilic dimer: Mechanisms of membrane permeabilization. Science 1991; 251:1481–1485.

87. Hanzawa H, Shimada I, Kuzuhara T, Komano H, Kohda D, Inagaki F, Natori S, Arata Y. 1H nuclear magnetic resonance study of the solution conformation of an antibacterial protein, sapecin. FEBS Lett 1990; 269:413–420.

88. Zhang X, Selsted ME, Pardi A. NMR studies of defensin antimicrobial petides. Resonance assignment and secondary structure determination of rabbit NP-2 and human HNP-1. Biochem 1992; 31:11348–11356.

89. Marion D, Zasloff M, Bax A. A two dimensional NMR study of the antimicrobial petide magainin 2. FEBS Lett 1988; 227:21–26.

90. Bechinger B, Zasloff M, Opella SJ. Structure and interactions of magainin antibiotic peptides in lipid bilayers: A solid-state nuclear magnetic resonance investigation. Biophys J 1992; 62:12–14.

91. Holak TA, Engström A, Kraulis PJ, Lindberg G, Bennich H, Jones TA, Gronenborn AM, Clore GM. The solution conformation of the antibacterial peptide cecropin A: A nuclear magnetic resonance and dynamical simulated annealing study. Biochem 1988; 27:7620–7629.

92. Bazzo R, Tappin MJ, Pastore A, Harvey S, Carver JA, Campbell ID. The structure of melittin A: 1H-NMR study in methanol. Eur J Biochem 1988; 173:139–146.

93. Sipos D, Chandrasekhar K, Arvidsson K, Engström A, Ehrenberg A. Two dimensional proton-NMR studies on a hybrid peptide between cecropin A and melittin. Resonance assignments and secondary structure. Eur J Biochem 1991; 199:285–291.

94. Falla TJ, Karunaratne DN, Hancock REW. Mode of action of the antimicrobial peptide indolicidin. J Biol Chem 1996; 271:19,298–19,303.

95. Cabiaux V, Agerberth B, Johansson J, Homblé F, Goormaghtigh E, Ruysschaert J-M. Secondary structure and membrane interaction of PR-39, a Pro+Arg-rich antibacterial peptide. Eur J Biochem 1994; 224:1019–1027.

96. Raj PA, Edgerton M. Functional domain and poly-L-proline conformation for candidacidal activity of bactenecin 5. FEBS Lett 1995; 368:526–530.

97. Andreu D, Merrifield RB, Steiner H, Boman HG. N-terminal analogues of cecropin A: Synthesis, antibacterial activity, and conformational properties. Biochem 1985; 24:1683–1688.

98. Blondelle SE, Houghten RA. Hemolytic and antimicrobial activities of the twenty-four individual omission analogues of melittin. Biochem 1991; 30:4671–4678.

99. Steiner H, Andreu D, Merrifield RB. Binding and action of cecropin and cecropin analogues: Antibacterial peptides from insects. Biochim Biophys Acta 1988; 939:260–266.

100. Frohlich DR, Wells MA. Peptide amphipathy: A new strategy in design of potential insecticides. Intl J Pept Res 1991; 37:2–6.

101. Wade D, Boman A, Wahlin B, Drain CM, Andreu D, Boman HG, Merrifield RB. All-D amino acid–containing channel-forming antibiotic peptides. Proc Natl Acad Sci USA 1990; 87:4761–4765.

102. Andreu D, Ubach J, Boman A, Wahlur B, Wade D, Merrifield RB, Boman HG. Shortened cecropin A-melittin hybrids. Significant size reduction retains potent antibiotic activity. FEBS Lett 1992; 296:190–194.

103. Bashford CL, Alder GM, Menestrina G, Micklem KJ, Murphy JJ, Pasternak CA. Membrane damage by hemolytic viruses, toxin, complement, and other cytotoxic agents. A common mechanism blocked by divalent cations. J Biol Chem 1986; 261:9300–9308.

104. Chitnis SJ, Prasad KSN, Bhargava PM. Isolation and characterization of autolysis-defective mutants of *Escherichia coli* that are resistant to the lytic activity of seminalplasmin. J Gen Microbiol 1990; 136:463–469.

105. Batenburg AM, Hibbeln JCL, de Kruijff B. Lipid specific penetration of melittin into phospholipid model membranes. Biochim Biophys Acta 1987; 903:155–165.

106. Matsuzaki K, Harada M, Funakoshi S, Fujii N, Miyajima K. Physicochemical determinants for the interactions of magainins 1 and 2 with acidic lipid bilayers. Biochim Biophys Acta 1991; 1063:162–170.

107. Sekharam KM, Bradrick TD, Georghiou S. Kinetics of melittin binding to phospholipid small unilamellar vesicles. Biochim Biophys Acta 1991; 1063:171–174.

108. Kagan BL, Selsted ME, Ganz T, Lehrer RI. Antimicrobial defensin peptides form voltage-dependent ion-permeable channels in planar lipid bilayer membranes. Proc Natl Acad Sci USA 1990; 87:210–214.

109. Hanke W, Methfessel C, Wilmsen HU, Katz E, Jung G, Boheim G. Melittin and a chemically modified trichotoxin form alamethicin-type multistate pores. Biochim Biophys Acta 1983; 727:108–114.

110. Kordel M, Benz R, Sahl HG. Mode of action of the staphylococcin like peptide Pep5: Voltage dependent depolarization of bacterial and artificial membranes. J Bacteriol 1988; 170:84–88.

111. Cociancich S, Ghazi A, Hetru C, Hoffman JA, Letellier LJ. Insect defensin, an inducible antibacterial peptide, forms voltage dependent channels in *Micrococcus luteus*. J Biol Chem 1993; 268:19,239–19,245.

112. Vogel H, Jahnig F. The structure of melittin in membranes. Biophys J 1986; 50:573–582.

113. Smith R, Separovic F, Bennett FC, Cornell BA. Melittin-induced changes in lipid multilayers: A solid-state NMR study. Biophys J 1992; 63:469–474.

114. Williams RW, Starman R, Taylor KMP, Gable K, Beeler T, Zasloff M, Covell D. Raman spectroscopy of synthetic antimicrobial frog peptides magainin 2a and PGLa. Biochem 1990; 29:4490–4496.

115. Agawa Y, Lee S, Ono S, Aoyagi H, Ohno M, Tamguchi T, Anzai K, Kirino Y. Interaction with phospholipid bilayers, ion channel formation, and antimicrobial activity of basic amphiphilic alpha-helical model peptides of various chain lengths. J Biol Chem 1991; 266:20218–20222.

116. Duclohier H, Molle G, Spach G. Antimicrobial peptide magainin I from *Xenopus* skin forms anion-permeable channels in planar lipid bilayers. Biophys J 1989; 56:1017–1021.

117. Boheim G. Statistical analysis of alamethicin channels in black lipid membranes. J Membr Biol 1974; 19:277–303.

118. Durell SR, Raghunathan G, Guy HR. Modelling the ion channel structure of cecropin. Biophys J 1992; 63:1623–1631.

119. Cronan JE, Gennis RB, Maloy SR. In: Ingraham JL, Brookslow K, Magnasanik B, Schaechter M, Umbarger HE, eds. *Escherichia coli* and *Salmonella typhimurium*: Cellular and Molecular Biology. Washington, D.C. 5:31–55: ASM Press, 1987.

120. Bakker EP, Mangerich WE. Inconversion of components of the bacterial proton motive force by electrogenic potassium transport. J Bacteriol 1981; 147:820–826.

121. Juretic D, Chen HC, Brown JH, Morell JL, Hendler RW, Westerhoff HV. Magainin 2 amide and analogues: Antimicrobial activity, membrane depolarization and susceptibility to proteolysis. FEBS Lett 1989; 249:219.

122. Westerhoff HV, Juretic D, Hendler RW, Zasloff M. Magainins and the disruption of membrane-linked free-energy transduction. Proc Natl Acad Sci USA 1989; 86:6597–6601.

123. Katsu T, Kuroko M, Morikawa T, Sanchika K, Yamanaka H, Shinoda S, Fujita Y. Interaction of wasp venom mastoparan with biomembranes. Biochim Biophys Acta 1990; 1027:185–190.

124. Nicas TI, Hancock REW. Outer membrane protein HI of *Pseudomonas aeruginosa*: Involvement in adaptive and mutational resistance to ethylenediaminetetraacetate, polymixin B, and gentamicin. J Bacteriol 1980; 143:872.

125. Hancock REW. Bacterial outer membranes: Evolving concepts. ASM News 1991; 57:175–82.

126. Hancock REW, Wong PG. Compounds which increase the permeability of the *Pseudomonas aeruginosa* outer membrane. Antimicrob Agents Chemother 1984; 26:48–52.

127. Vaara M. Agents that increase the permeability of the outer membrane. Microbiol Rev 1992; 56:395–411.

128. Rana FR, Macias EA, Sultany CM, Modzradowski MC, Blazyk J. Interactions between magainin 2 and *Salmonella typhimurium* outer membranes: Effect of lipopolysaccharide structure. Biochem 1991; 30:5858–5866.

129. David SA, Mathan VI, Balaram P. Interaction of melittin with endotoxic lipid A. Biochim Biophys Acta 1992; 1123:269–274.

130. Fisher CJ Jr, Marra MN, Palardy JE, Marchbanks CR, Scott RW, Opal SM. Human neutrophil bactericidal/permeability-increasing protein reduces mortality rate from endotoxin challenge: A placebo controlled study. Crit Care Med 1994; 22:553–558.

131. Marra M, Thornton MB, Snable JL, Wilde CG, Scott RW. Endotoxin-binding and -neutralizing properties of recombinant bactericidal/permeability-increasing protein and monoclonal antibodies HA-1A and E5. Crit Care Med 1994; 22:559–565.

132. Fields GB, Tian Z, Barany G. In: Grant GA, ed. Synthetic Peptides: A User's Guide. 1992:77–150.

133. Lai J, Lee J-H, Lin Y-L, Ray D, Wilcox G. Method of producing cecropins by microbiological techniques. U.S. Patent 5,206,154; April 27, 1994.

134. Daher KA, Lehrer RI, Ganz T, Kronenberg M. Isolation and characterization of human defensin cDNA clones. Proc Natl Acad Sci USA 1988; 85:7327–7331.

135. Bodansky M, Bodansky A. The practice of peptide synthesis. 284p, Springer Verlag, Berlin, 1994.

17

Rapamycin, FK506, and Ascomycin-Related Compounds

Kevin A. Reynolds
University of Maryland at Baltimore, Baltimore, Maryland

Arnold L. Demain
Massachusetts Institute of Technology, Cambridge, Massachusetts

I. PHARMACEUTICAL ROLE

For years, the only natural product used as an immunosuppressant was the peptide anti-fungal agent cyclosporin A, produced by the fungus *Beauveria nivea*, previously known as *Tolypocladium inflatum* and *Trichoderma polysporum* (1). In recent years, more potent molecules produced by streptomycetes have been discovered, such as rapamycin, FK506, and ascomycin (2–4). Cyclosporin A can cause various side effects such as kidney, nerve, and liver damage, hypertension, diabetes and, abnormal hair growth. FK506 (= tacrolimus) was approved in the United States in 1994 for liver transplants and, although more potent than cyclosporin A, has similar toxicities. Rapamycin (5) is in phase II clinical trials at present and may show different activities and, hopefully, lower toxicity than cyclosporin A and FK506 due to its distinct mode of action.

Immunosuppressants act by intracellularly binding to enzymes, known as immunophilins (Figure 1) (6). As one would expect from the structural similarity of FK506 and rapamycin, they bind to the same enzyme, FK506-binding protein 12 (FKBP12) (7), whereas cyclosporin A binds to a different enzyme, cyclophilin (8). Both immunophilins are rotamases, that is, cis–trans peptidylprolyl isomerases and "protein foldases." When bound in the immunosuppressant–immunophilin complex, the enzyme is inactive and the complex inhibits the action of other enzymes involved in signal-transduction pathways that normally lead to activation of T cells (9,10). Surprisingly, the FK506–FKBP12 complex inhibits the same enzyme as the cyclosporin A–cyclophilin complex, namely, the protein phosphatase, calcineurin. On the other hand, the rapamycin–FKBP12 complex inhibits FRAP (FKBP12–rapamycin associated protein), which is phosphatidylinositol kinase. The latter is also known as RAFT (rapamycin and FKBP12 target), mTOR (mammalian target of rapamycin), or P210.

Inhibition of calcineurin results in T cells that no longer respond to antigen presentation; thus, they no longer can transcribe the interleukin-2 gene and cannot undergo interleukin-2-dependent proliferation. In contrast, inhibition of FRAP acts at a later step

497

of T cell activation. It leads to T cells that cannot respond to interleukin-2 and, thus, do not proliferate (Figure 1). Since calcineurin is required for viability in yeast strains that are sensitive to cyclosporin A and hypersensitive to FK506, the inhibition of calcineurin by the cyclosporin A–cyclophilin complex or by the FK506–FKBP12 complex is responsible for both immunosuppression in humans and antibiotic activity against fungi (11).

II. ISOLATION

Rapamycin (Figure 2) was first reported as an antifungal agent produced by *Streptomyces hygroscopicus* (ATCC 29253, NRRL 5491) in 1975 (12). Since then, it has been shown to have antitumor and immunosuppressant activity (13–17). The structure of rapamycin was confirmed by both x-ray crystallographic (18), chemical degradation, and high-field nuclear magnetic resonance (NMR) spectroscopy studies (19). The major portion of the molecule is a large 31-membered macrolide ring containing three conjugated double bonds. The macrolide structure also contains a heterocyclic moiety that can be isolated as L-pipecolate by either acid- or base-catalyzed hydrolysis. Also contained at C14 and C15 is an unusual α-ketoamide functionality. In this chapter, we have adopted the original carbon numbering system used for rapamycin (20), not the more conventional macrolide numbering system (21,22). Recently, it has been reported that rapamycin is also produced by *Actinoplanes* sp. N902-109 (23).

Ascomycin (Figure 3) was first isolated in 1962 as an antifungal antibiotic of unknown structure from *S. hygroscopicus* subsp. *ascomyceticus* (ATCC 14891, MA6475) (24,25). More than 25 years later, screening programs for novel immunosuppressants resulted in the isolation of ascomycin as immunomycin and FK520 from *S. hygroscopicus* subsp. *ascomyceticus* and subsp. *yakushiaensis* (FERM BP-928, MA6531), respectively (26–28). It has since been confirmed that ascomycin, FK520, and immunomycin are structurally identical (29–31).

Ascomycin is a novel 23-membered macrolide lactone with many structural similarities to rapamycin. In fact, with the exception of the differing oxidation state at C27–C28 and a methoxy substituent at C13, the ascomycin structure, extending from the substituted furan ring through the α-ketoamide functionality and heterocyclic system to the substituted cyclohexane ring, is identical to rapamycin. Both *S. hygroscopicus* subsp. *yakushiaensis* and subsp. *ascomyceticus* produce a minor ascomycin analog (FK523, L-683,795) that has a methyl rather than an ethyl side chain at C21 (Figure 2) (26–28).

Prior to the structural identification of ascomycin, the immunosuppressant agent FK506 (Figure 3) was isolated from *Streptomyces tsukabaensis* (32,33). The structure of this compound is identical to that of ascomycin with the exception that the ethyl side chain at C21 is replaced by an allyl side chain.

III. BIOSYNTHESIS

A. Origin of the Carbon Atoms of the Macrolide Ring

The large 23-membered ring of the ascomycin family and the 31-membered ring of rapamycin are similar to many macrolide antibiotics. The biosynthetic precursors of the carbon backbone of macrolide antibiotics, which include compounds such as erythromycin and tylosin, have been shown to be acetate, propionate, and occasionally

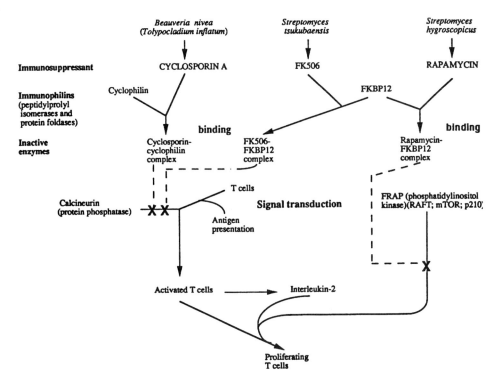

Figure 1 Mode of action of cyclosporin A, FK506, and rapamycin. ✗: inhibition.

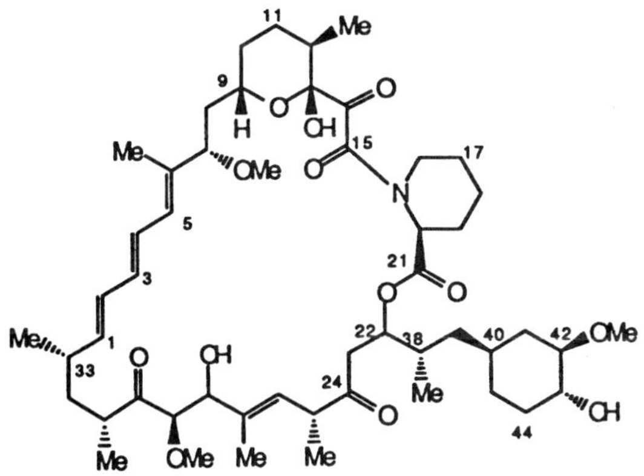

Figure 2 The structure of rapamycin.

butyrate (34). Considerable biochemical and genetic evidence has been obtained to show that macrolide antibiotics and other polyketides are biosynthesized by the condensation of these precursors, activated as malonyl CoA, methylmalonyl CoA, and ethylmalonyl CoA, in a sequential manner with a specific primer unit.

The origin of the macrolide ring of rapamycin has been investigated using ^{13}C-labeled acetate and propionate (20). Monitoring of the isotopic enrichment in the [13]C

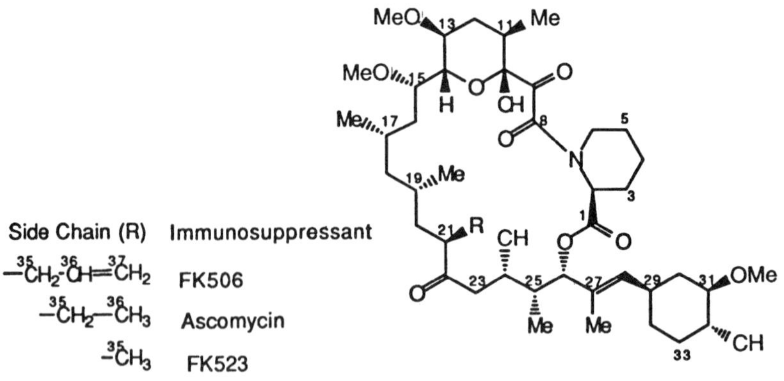

Figure 3   The structure of FK506, ascomycin (immunomycin, FK520), and FK523.

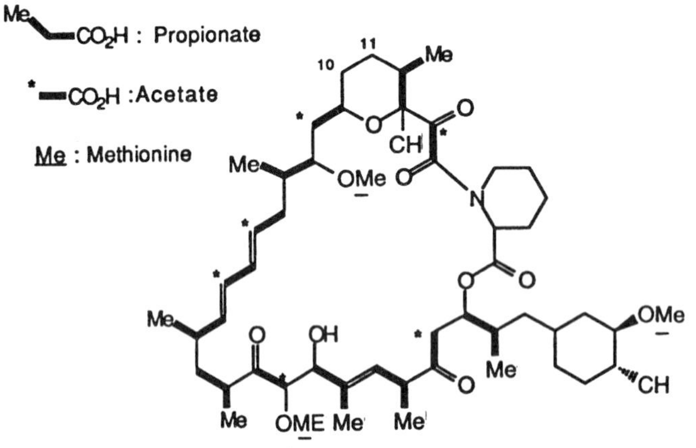

Figure 4   Origin of the carbon backbone of rapamycin.

NMR of rapamycin following incorporation of $[1\text{-}^{13}C_1]$-, $[2\text{-}^{13}C_1]$-, and $[1,2\text{-}^{13}C_2]$ acetate by producing cultures of *S. hygroscopicus* revealed both the location and orientation of six acetate-derived positons (Figure 4). Similar incorporation experiments with $[1\text{-}^{13}C]$propionate and $[2\text{-}^{13}C]$propionate revealed the location and orientation of the seven propionate-derived positions. An efficient incorporation of $^{13}CH_3$ from L-$[^{13}C\text{-}methyl]$methionine into all three methoxy-groups of rapamycin was also observed. The C10 and C11 of the furan ring were predicted to be of acetate origin, although initial analysis suggested that these were not labeled by acetate in these incorporation experiments. However, subsequent revised reassignments of the NMR assignments for rapamycin (21) indicate that these carbons are also enriched in ^{13}C in the feeding studies with ^{13}C-labeled acetate.

A similar set of incorporation studies were conducted to examine the carbon backbone of the ascomycin family of immunosuppressants (30). For all three of these compounds (ascomycin, FK523, and FK506), the three methoxy carbons at C13, C15, and C31 were shown to be derived from methionine. All three immunosuppressants were enriched at C10, C16, C18, C24, and C26 by $[1\text{-}^{13}C]$propionate and at C8 and C22 by $[1\text{-}^{13}C]$acetate (Figure 5). Interestingly, in the acetate incorporation study, no ^{13}C enrich-

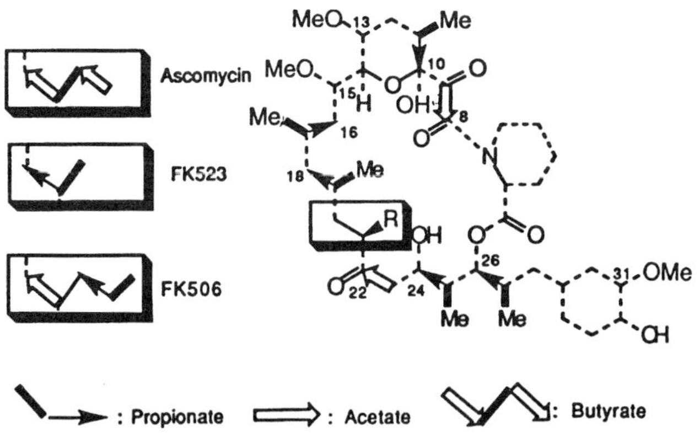

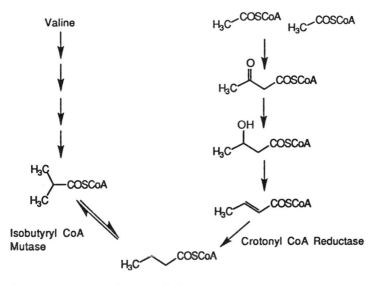

Figure 5   Origin of the carbon backbone of ascomycin, FK506, and FK523.

ment of C12 of the furan ring or C14 was observed. The the C12–C15 of the ascomycin family is, however, almost certainly derived from acetate. In FK523, the three carbons C20, C21, and C35 were shown to be propionate. The four carbons of ascomycin at C20, C21, C35, and C36 were labeled by [1-^{13}C]acetate, although the enrichment at these positions was lower than at other acetate-derived positions, indicating a more direct butyrate precursor. This hypothesis was confirmed by incorporation experiments with [1-^{13}C]butyrate and [4-^{13}C]butyrate, which led to an efficient ^{13}C enrichment at C20 and C36, respectively. Finally, C21 was also shown to be enriched by an incorporation experiment with [2-^{13}C]D/L-valine (30).

These results are consistent with (a) the role of butyrate, presumably activated as ethylmalonyl CoA, as the precursor to C20, C21, C35, and C36 of ascomycin, and (b) two alternative pathways for butyrate formation functioning in *Streptomyces* (Figure 6)

Figure 6   Proposed pathways for butyryl CoA formation in *Streptomyces hygroscopicus* var. *ascomyceticus* (35, 42).

(35). The role of valine as a precursor to butyrate units in streptomycete metabolism has been observed in the biosynthesis of many secondary metabolites, such as tylosin and monensin (36,37). In these pathways, the valine is thought to be degraded to isobutyryl CoA, which is then isomerized to *n*-butyryl CoA. The stereochemistry of this latter isomerization has been investigated in vivo in *Streptomyces cinnamonensis*, the producer of the antibiotic monensin A (38).

The formation of butyrate from two acetyl CoA molecules has not been fully addressed, although it seems to be an operational pathway in many *Streptomyces*. It is possible that two acetyl CoA molecules are condensed together to form an acetoacetyl CoA molecule, which is converted to hydroxybutyryl CoA and subsequently to crotonyl CoA by three enzymes usually associated with the β-oxidation of fatty acids (39,40). An nicotinamide adenine dinucleotide phosphate, reduced form (NAD(P)H)-dependent reductase could then catalyze the conversion of crotonyl CoA to butyryl CoA (39,40). A crotonyl CoA reductase catalyzing this reduction has been purified from *Streptomyces collinus* and characterized (41,42). The gene encoding this enzyme has been cloned and sequenced (42). It is reasonable to suggest that *S. hygroscopicus* subsp. *ascomyceticus* may also have a crotonyl CoA reductase responsible for formation of the butyrate-derived unit of ascomycin from two acetyl CoA molecules. Cell-free extracts of *S. hygroscopicus* subsp. *ascomyceticus* have been shown to exhibit crotonyl CoA reductase activity (Reynolds KA, unpublished results). Furthermore, a 348 bp fragment of *S. hygroscopicus* subsp. *ascomyceticus* DNA has been amplified using oligonucleotide primers based on the *S. collinus* crotonyl CoA reductase sequence. The polymerase chain reaction (PCR) product was cloned and sequenced in *Escherichia coli*, and the predicted amino acid sequence was shown to be 88% identical to a predicted 116-amino-acid residue fragment of the *S. collinus* crotonyl CoA reductase (Reynolds KA, unpublished results) (Figure 7).

It is difficult to predict which of the butyrate pathways (Figure 6) plays a more significant role in ascomycin biosynthesis. The labeling of the butyrate unit (approximately 2.5-fold enrichment) relative to the labeling of the positions directly obtained from acetate (approximately 5-fold enrichment) in the acetate incorporation study, however, suggest that both pathways play a significant role in butyrate production.

The five carbons (C20, C21, C35, C36, and C37) of FK506 have been shown to be labeled by an acetate and a propionate (Figure 5) (30). Presumably, these two building blocks are condensed as CoA thioesters to form a pentanoate/pentenoate starter unit in a process analogous to butyryl CoA formation. The resulting pentanoyl CoA could be incorporated into FK506 either after oxidation to 4-pentenoyl CoA or directly, with formation of the double bond occurring at a later step in the biosynthetic process. A simple

A) TqFALAGGANPICVVSSPqKAEICRsMGAEAIIDRnAEgYkFWKDehTQDPkEWKRFGK

B) ThFALAGGANPICVVSSPrKAEICRRMGAEAIIDRtAEDYrFWKDdgTQDPrEWKRFGK

A) rIRELTGGEDiDIVFEHPGRETFGASVYVTRKGGTItTCASTSGmHEYDNRYLWM

B) kIRELTGGEDvDIVFEHPGRETFGASVYVTRKGGTIvTCASTSGtHEYDNRYLWM

Figure 7 Comparison of predicted partial peptide sequences of the *Streptomyces collinus* crotonyl CoA reductase (A) with a putative crotonyl CoA reductase from *S. hygroscopicus* var. *ascomyceticus* (B).

incorporation study using labeled pentanoic and pentenoic acid should distinguish between these possibilities. The utilization of a pentanoic acid building block in secondary metabolism is unprecedented; only utilization of acetate, propionate, and less commonly, butyrate building blocks have been observed. There has been considerable and unresolved controversy concerning a potential hexanoate building block as the starter unit in the biosynthesis of averufin by *Aspergillus parasiticus* (43–45).

B. Formation and Activation of the Pipecolate-Derived Unit

Pipecolic acid, which is derived from L-lysine, has been shown to be the direct precursor to the heterocyclic ring of both rapamycin and the ascomycin-related family. Radioactive rapamycin was produced by incorporation of both L-[U-14C]lysine and DL-[U-3H]pipecolic acid in a rapamycin-producing culture of *S. hygroscopicus* (strain AY B-1206) in a low-lysine fermentation medium (46). Hydrolysis of the isolated rapamycin afforded radioactive pipecolic acid, clearly demonstrating that radioactivity had been incorporated into this portion of the antibiotic. Unlabeled pipecolic acid reduced the incorporation of radioactive lysine more substantially than unlabeled lysine decreased the incorporation of radioactive pipecolate. This result provided evidence that the pipecolic acid was a more direct precursor to the heterocyclic system of rapamycin than was lysine. A similar conclusion was reached for formation of the heterocyclic moiety of ascomycin using an analogous set of competitive incorporation studies with labeled and unlabeled lysine and pipecolic acid (30). The incorporation of DL-[1-13C]lysine into ascomycin led to a single 80-fold enrichment at the resonance corresponding to C1, confirming the radioactive incorporation results.

Based on studies of pipecolate formation in other systems, a minimum of two alternative biosynthetic pathways for the conversion of lysine to pipecolate can be envisioned (Figure 8) (47–49): (a) cyclization of lysine to form 1-piperideine-6-carboxylate occurring with retention of the α-amino nitrogen atom and ε-deamination (Figure 8, pathway a); (b) cyclization of lysine to 1-piperideine-2-carboxylate proceeding with retention of the ε-amino nitrogen atom and α-deamination (Figure 8, pathway b). To distinguish between these possibilities, incorporation studies with ascomycin using DL-lysine α-15N, and DL-lysine-ε-15N were carried out (30). Mass spectrometric analysis of the resulting ascomycin revealed a high level of 15N enrichment (49%), but only from the experiment utilizing DL-lysine-ε-15N. The level of enrichment was sufficiently high to give a measurable coupling to the natural abundance 13C signals for C2 and C6 of ascomycin, clearly indicating the location of the 15N. These results are consistent with a pathway from lysine to pipecolate involving loss of the α-nitrogen atom (Figure 8, pathway b). The pipecolate pathway in *Streptomyces virginiae* and *Pseudomonas aeruginosa* also proceeds with α-deamination (47,48).

The pipecolate is incorporated into all of these immunosuppressants by formation of an amide linkage with the acyl-group of the growing polyketide chain. It has been suggested that this pipecolate is activated in a manner described for nonribosomally synthesized peptide antibiotics (50). In these processes, the amino acid is generally activated as an acyl adenylate using ATP and subsequently transferred to a cysteine residue of the enzyme to form an amino acid thioester (51). Peptide bond formation occurs by transfer of the activated amino acid on a phosphopantetheine arm to a second component of the enzyme.

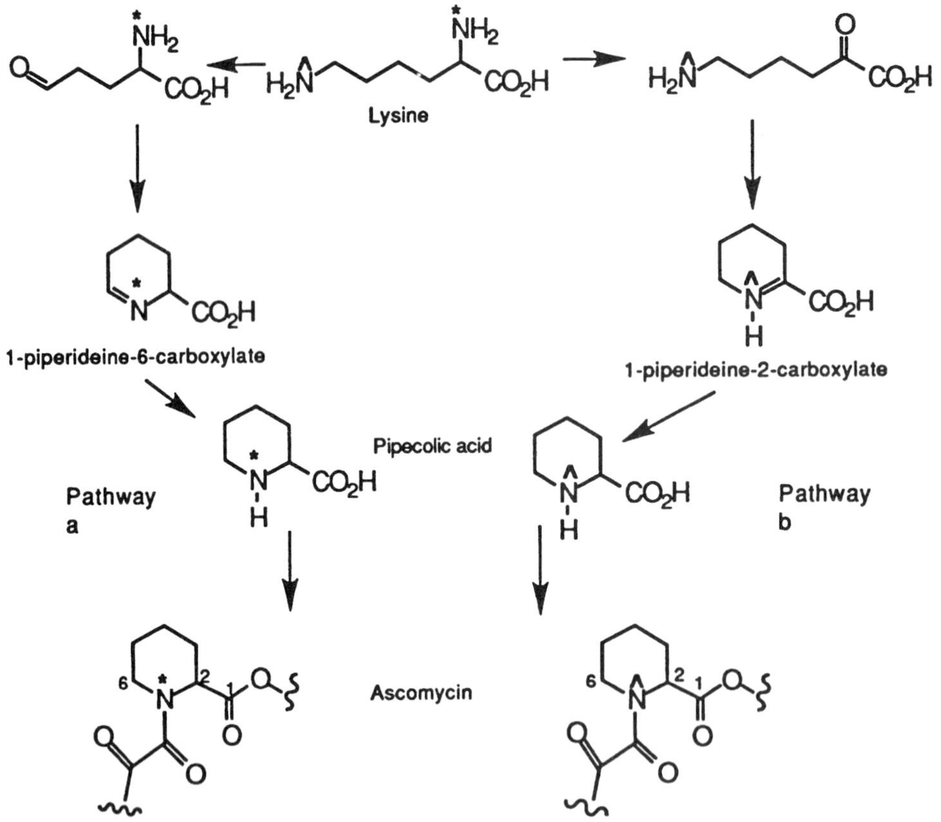

Figure 8 Alternative pathways for conversion of lysine to the pipecolate-derived moiety of ascomycin.

An enzyme likely responsible for activation of L-pipecolic acid as the adenylate deriv-ative during the biosynthesis of ascomycin has been isolated, purified, and characterized from S. *hygroscopicus* subsp. *ascomyceticus* (50). This enzyme was active using the adenosine triphosphate (ATP)–pyrophosphate exchange assay (52) in the presence of pipecolate or pipecolate adenylate. In the presence of ATP and Mg^{2+}, the enzyme was able to bind pipecolate in a form that could be precipitated by trichloroacetic acid. This binding was inhibited by sulfhydryl-group inhibitors. All of these observed properties are consistent with the activation of the carboxylate-group of pipecolate as an adenylate derivative and subsequently as an enzyme-bound thioester derivative. Antibody raised to the purified enzyme was used to follow antigen during the course of fermentation. Maximal levels of antigen were observed when synthesis of ascomycin was maximal. A surprising 10 of 12 ascomycin-nonproducing mutants were shown to lack a detectable pipecolate-activating enzyme in Western blots. It has been suggested that a genetic analysis of ascomycin biosyn-thesis might explain this unusually high number (50). These data are strongly indicative of a role of this enzyme in activating pipecolic acid for ascomycin biosynthesis.

The substrate specificity of the enzyme with a variety of amino acids was tested using the pyrophosphate–ATP exchange assay. Of the amino acids found in proteins,

Table I   The Ability of Proline and Pipecolate Derivatives to Stimulate
ATP–Pyrophosphate Exchange with a Pipecolate-Activating Enzyme Purified
from *Streptomyces hygroscopicus* var. *ascomyceticus*

Pipecolate or proline analog	L-Pipecolate activity (%)
L-Proline	19
L-Hydroxyproline	12
X-Hydroxyproline (X = 1, 2, or 3)	12
trans-3-Methyl-L-proline	19
cis-3-Methylproline	5
cis-3-Methyl-DL-proline	4
cis, *trans*-4-Methylproline	178
cis-4-Methyl-DL-proline	4
trans-4-Aminoproline	6
cis-4-Chloro-L-proline	33
5-Iminoproline hydrogen chloride	16
cis-5-Methyl-DL-proline	25
(+)-Piperazic acid	24
5-Chloropipecolate	32
5-Hydroxypipecolate	7
cis-4-Hydroxy-L-pipecolate	16
trans-4-Hydroxy-D-pipecolate	6
4-Hydroxyallopipecolate	19
Thiazolidone-4-carboxylic acid (thioproline)	4

Source: Ref. 50.

only L-proline was active. A variety of proline and pipecolate acid derivatives were found
to be active with the enzyme (Table 1). It has been noted (50), however, that though
activity in the exchange reaction is presumably necessary for these analogs to be utilized
in ascomycin biosynthesis, it does not guarantee thioester formation or subsequent incorporation into the immunosuppressant macrolide. In other systems, it has been shown
that reaction at the thiol site is often more specific than the exchange reaction (53). Furthermore, many of the compounds active in the exchange reaction are poor inhibitors
(with IC_{50} values in the 0.1–3 mM range) of the binding of pipecolate (K_m of 0.4 µM) to
the enzyme. Accordingly, very high intracellular concentrations of these amino acids
would be needed in a fermentation to produce an ascomycin analog. However, even with
such caveats, it is noted that a prolyl derivative of FK506 has been reported as a minor
component in fermentation broths (54). Furthermore, with whole-cell directed biosynthesis experiments, high levels of proline have resulted in the formation of prolylas-
comyin (prolylimmunomycin) (50), prolylrapamycin, and 27-O-demethylprolylra-
pamycin (23). These results would suggest that there are further opportunities for
obtaining novel immunosuppressants by directed biosynthesis experiments with proline
and pipecolate analogs. Such an approach might be most productive either in a chemically defined medium supplied with minimal lysine or in a mutant deficient in pipecolate
production. Whether such an approach will generate an analog with greater activity is a
separate issue. It is noted that the prolyl analog of ascomycin is considerably less potent
in immunosuppression than ascomycin (54).

C.   Purification and Characterization of Methyltransferases

A methyltransferase (FKMT) catalyzing the conversion of 31-O-desmethyl-FK506 to FK506 has been purified 600-fold with an overall 3% purification from *Streptomyces* sp. MA6858 (ATCC No. 55098) (55). The methyltransferase substrate 31-O-desmethyl-FK506 was obtained by a biotransformation (FK506 and ascomycin have been shown to be desmethylated by *Actinoplanes* sp.) (56). Similarly, a methyltransferase (DIMT) capable of converting desmethylascomycin to ascomycin was purified 140-fold in 2.5% yield from *S. hygroscopicus* subsp. *ascomyceticus* (30).

Both of these enzymes have an absolute requirement for magnesium ions and S-adenosylmethionine (SAM). The enzymes have very similar physical and kinetic properties. FKMT was shown to be able to convert 31-O-desmethylascomycin as effectively as it does 31-O-desmethyl-FK506. By comparison, only 10–20% efficiency has been reported for C31 methylation of the following compounds by either DIMT or FKMT: 15,31-O-bis-desmethylascomycin, 13,31-O-bis-desmethylascomycin, and 13,15,31-O-tris-desmethyl-ascomycin. A variety of 32-substituted-31-O-desmethylated ascomyin analogs were not substrates for either methyltransferase. Neither FKMT or DIMT could catalyze methylation at C13 or C15. The substrate specificity of FKMT with FK506 desmethylated compounds has not been studied, although it has been reasonably suggested that similar results would be obtained (55). These results give a strong indication that other methyltransferases are responsible for the methylation reactions at C13 and C15 of both FK506 and ascomycin. Furthermore, the efficient conversion of 31-O-desmethylascomycin in comparison with those of the bis- and tris-desmethylated compounds would indicate that the methylation at C31 is the last step in both ascomycin and FK506 biosynthesis. This suggestion is substantiated by preliminary indications that in whole-cell incorporation studies with radiolabeled 31-desmethyl- and 15,31-bis-desmethylascomycin, production of labeled ascomycin and 15-O-desmethylascomycin occurred. These experiments also indicate that the enzyme catalyzing C15 methylation has a narrow substrate specificity, as it is unable to react with the C31-methylated substrate.

Utilization of DIMT and microbial desmethylation of both FK506 and ascomycin have allowed investigators to produce a whole series of desmethylated products (56,57). These compounds have all been tested for immunosuppressive activity in an in vitro proliferation assay. This work has clearly demonstrated that the methylation at C15 is critical for full biological activity of ascomycin.

D.   Formation of the (1R, 3R, 4R)-Dihydroxycyclohexanecarboxylic Acid–Derived Unit

The conclusion that methylation at C31 is the last step in FK506 and ascomycin biosynthesis implicates (1R, 3R, 4R)-dihydroxycyclohexanecarboxylic acid (DHCHC) as the putative primer unit for formation of these immunosuppressants as well as rapamycin. The role of shikimic acid as a biosynthetic precursor to this unit has been investigated for both rapamycin and ascomycin (30,58). For the biosynthetic studies with rapamycin, shikimate with a 5- to 10-fold ^{13}C enrichment at all carbons except C1 was obtained from [1-^{13}C]glucose feeding to a fermentation of an amino acid auxotrophic mutant of *Klebsiella pneumoniae* (58). When this compound was added to producing cultures of *S. hygroscopicus*, rapamycin enriched with ^{13}C at C39 and C41–C45 was obtained. No other enrichments were observed, clearly indicating the role of shikimate in formation of the

DHCHC starter unit. Unfortunately, this experiment did not allow the orientation of shikimic acid during incorporation into rapamycin to be clearly determined. However, based on the stereochemical configuration of the rapamycin C42 hydroxy and C43 methoxy substituents, it was suggested that C5 of shikimate gives rise to C42 of rapamycin (Figure 9) (58).

The likely shikimate-derived origin of the substituted cyclohexyl ring of ascomyin has also been demonstrated (30). In this case, incorporation of D-[1-^{13}C]erythrose with *S. hygroscopicus* subsp. *ascomyceticus* produced ascomycin with a single major ^{13}C enrichment at C31. This result is consistent with the pathway (Figure 9) in which erythrose is used to provide shikimate enriched with ^{13}C at C5, which is subsequently utilized to provide the substituted cyclohexane ring of ascomycin. These incorporation studies demonstrate the shikimate origin of the cyclohexane moiety of the immunosuppressants, but they do not determine whether shikimate is incorporated directly or is modified first (58).

Recently, evidence that shikimic acid is converted to DHCHC prior to incorporation into ascomycin has been obtained (59). Two putative intermediates in this conversion to DHCHC, *trans*-4,5-[2-^{2}H]dihydroxycyclohex-1-enecarboxylic acid and *trans*-3,4-dihydroxy-[2,3,4,5,6-^{2}H$_5$]cyclohexa-1,5-dienecarboxylic acid, were successfully incorporated into ascomycin by producing cultures of *S. hygroscopicus*. Furthermore, the fate of the hydrogen atoms attached to the ring of shikimate during this transformation was monitored by incorporation studies with regiospecifically deuterated shikimates. The regio- and stereospecific locations of deuterium labels on the cyclohexyl ring of ascomycin produced in each of these studies were obtained by ^{2}H NMR analysis. The results obtained were consistent with a proposed pathway (Figure 10) that commences with either a syn or anti 1,4-conjugate elimination of the C3 hydroxyl-group and a C6 hydrogen of shikimic acid to produce (3R, 4R)-3,4-dihydroxycyclohexa-1,5-dienecarboxylic acid [1]. A reduction of the Δ^1 double bond of this compound produces (4R, 5R)-4,5-dihydroxycyclohex-2-enecarboxylic acid [2a or 2b], which is subsequently converted to (4R, 5R)-4,5-dihydroxycyclohex-1-enecarboxylic acid [3] by an isomerization of the remaining double bond from the Δ^2 to the Δ^1 position.

Two alternative stereochemical pathways for the conversion of 1 to 3 are consistent with the results from the incorporation studies: a syn reduction of the Δ^1 double

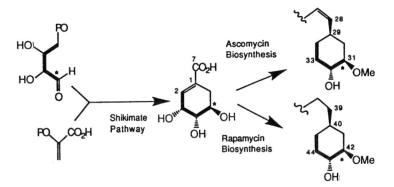

Figure 9 The shikimate origin of the substituted cyclohexyl moiety of rapamycin and ascomycin.

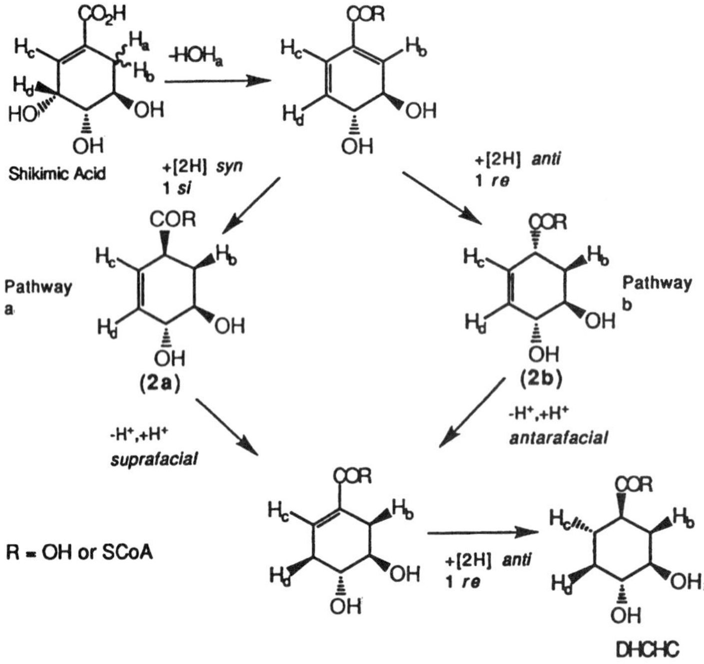

Figure 10   Proposed pathways to DHCHC from shikimic acid in S. *hygroscopicus*.

bond with hydrogen addition to the *si* face of C1 to produce 2a, and a subsequent suprafacial 1,3-allylic rearrangement of 2a to produce 3 (Figure 10, pathway a); an anti reduction of the Δ^1 double bond of 1 with hydrogen addition to the *re* face of C1 (anti addition) to produce 2b, and a subsequent antarafacial 1,3-allylic rearrangement of 2b to produce 3 (Figure 10, pathway b). All previously studied rearrangements of this type (60,61,62), including the interconversion of 2-cyclohexenylcarbonyl CoA and 1-cyclohexenylcarbonyl CoA (41,62–64) have been shown to be suprafacial. In many of these cases, evidence that a single catalytic residue acts as a general acid/base catalyst for the isomerization has been presented. Based on these precedents, a syn reduction of 1 to produce 2a seems to be the more likely pathway (Figure 10, pathway a). In the final step of the proposed pathway, 3 is reduced to DHCHC by an anti addition of hydrogen to the *re* faces of C1 and C2.

A comparison of this pathway to DHCHC with the conversion of shikimic acid to fully reduced cyclohexanecarboxylic acid (CHC) (Figure 11) in S. *collinus* and *Alicyclobacillus acidocaldarius* (62,63,65) has been made (59). The first two steps of each biosynthetic pathway appear on preliminary analysis to be identical: either a syn or anti 1,4-conjugate elimination of shikimate to produce (3R, 4R)-3,4-dihydroxycyclohexa-1,5-dienecarboxylic acid [1] followed by reduction of Δ^1 double bond to produce (4R, 5R)-4,5-dihydroxycyclohex-2-enecarboxylic acid [2]. However, upon closer examination, it has been observed that the double bond reduction of 1 in the CHC pathway proceeds in an anti fashion with addition of hydrogen to the *si* face of C1. By comparison, the proposed Δ^1 double bond reduction of 1 in the DHCHC pathway occurs either in an anti fashion, but with opposite absolute stereochemistry (addition of hydrogen to the *re* face

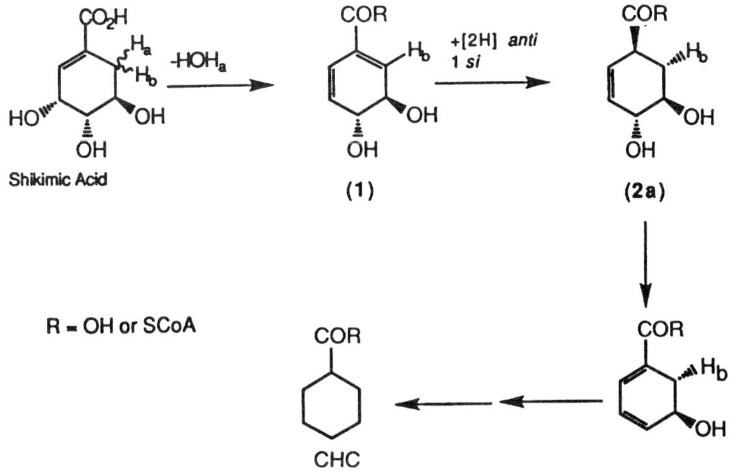

Figure 11   Initial steps in the pathway to CHC from shikimic acid in S. *collinus* and *Alicyclobacillus acidocaldarius*.

of C1) or with syn addition of hydrogen. The biosyntheses of DHCHC and CHC apparently diverge at or before the first intermediate, *trans*-4,5-dihydroxycyclohexa-1,5-dienecarboxylic acid [1]. It could be suggested, based on these stereochemical differences, that the enzymes involved in the reduction of **1** in the CHC and DHCHC pathways are not closely related.

IV.   ANALYSIS OF THE RAPAMYCIN AND FK506 BIOSYNTHETIC GENE CLUSTERS

The macrocyclic erythromycin produced by *Saccharopolyspora erythraea* was the first polyketide shown to be produced by the action of so-called type I polyketide synthases (PKSs), multienzymes in which different sets or modules of enzymatic activities catalyze each successive round of elongation (66,67). Avermectin, produced by *Streptomyces avermitilis*, also appears to be produced by a similar type I PKS (68). Recently, it has been reported that the rapamycin biosynthetic genes in *S. hygroscopicus* were identified by hybridization with the erythromycin PKS genes (22). The formation of the macrocyclic ring of rapamycin appears to be catalyzed by three large multienzyme complexes (Figure 12) (Table 2). Raps1 (encoded by *rapA*) is a 900 kDa a polypeptide containing the appropriate functionality for catalyzing the first four rounds of polyketide extension (successive addition of a propionate, acetate, propionate, and propionate units to the starter unit to extend the carbon skeleton to C28) (Figure 13). Raps2 (encoded by *rapB*) is a 1.07 MDa polypeptide containing the appropriate functionality for catalyzing the next six successive condensations (extending the rapamycin as far as C7). Raps3 (encoded by *rapC*) is a 660 kDa polypeptide containing the appropriate functionality for catalyzing the final four condensations to complete the polyketide portion of the rapamycin ring. Gene disruptions of this putative rapamycin PKS gene cluster using a streptomycete temperate phage vector have resulted in loss of rapamycin production (Leadley PF, personal communication; Hutchinson CR, personal communication). That gene disruptions of an additional

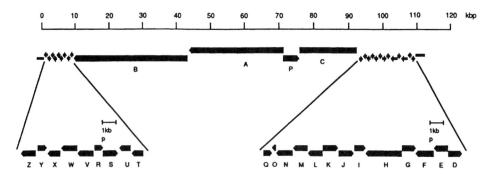

Figure 12   Organization of the rapamycin biosynthetic gene cluster. The direction of transcription and the relative sizes of A, B, C, and P are indicated. Letters at the bottom are defined in Table 2.

PKS gene cluster in *S. hygroscopicus* did not result in loss of rapamycin production both serves as a control experiment and suggests that the strain has a capacity to produce other polyketide products (Hutchinson CR, personal communication).

The giant proteins Raps1, 2, and 3 contribute 70 catalytic functions, making this the largest, most complex multienzyme system identified so far. The integration of four or six modules within a single polypeptide is unprecedented. The PKS polypeptides involved in erythromycin (66,67) or avermectin biosynthesis (68) contain only two or three modules. Finally, *rap*A, B, and C, which are divergently transcribed, differ from both the convergently transcribed *avr* modules (encoding the avermectin PKS), and the *ery* modules (encoding the erythromycin PKS) that appear in a colinear arrangement with the individual catalytic steps involved in erythromycin biosynthesis. Although the data set is small, the type I PKSs exhibit considerable diversity both in the gene arrangements and number of modules contained within each polypeptide. It will be interesting to see if any pattern emerges as more type I PKSs are analyzed.

Interestingly, module 3 of Raps1 and module 6 of Raps2 contain putative ketoreduction sites for C24 and C30, respectively. These reductions, however, are not reflected in the ultimate structure of rapamycin, and it may be that these sites are nonfunctional (22). Alternatively, temporary reduction of these sites may be necessary during the chain elongation process. Oxidation of these sites may be catalyzed by one of the many proteins encoded by the open reading frames (ORFs) surrounding the *raps*A, B, and C.

The Raps modules have a high degree of homology, the most striking instances of which are the extremely conserved ketosynthase domains (69). There is some sequence diversity, however, in the acyltransferase domains. It has been reported that this diversity reflects the specificity of the acyltransferase for an acetate or propionate extender unit (22). It has also been observed that the N-terminus of each multienzyme has a potential amphipathic domain, which may encourage dimerization of the polyketide synthase modules into catalytically active homodimers (69,70).

The loading domain of Raps1 is unusual, containing a coenzyme A ligase and an enoyl CoA reductase functionality (22,69). Recent sequence analysis has indicated a putative acyl carrier protein (ACP) domain between this enoyl reductase and the first ketosynthase domain (Leadley PF, personal communication). By contrast, the erythromycin and avermectin loading domains have an acyltransferase and ACP functionality. In these cases, it seems likely that the appropriate starter units, activated as coenzyme A

Table 2 Deduced Functions of the Open Reading Frames (ORFs) in the Rapamycin Biosynthetic Gene Cluster

Polypeptide	Size (amino acids)	Proposed function[a] (sequence similarities detected)					
Raps 1	8,563	Polyketide synthase					
Loading domain		CoA ligase			ER		ACP
Module 1		KS	AT(P)	DH	ER	KR	ACP
Module 2		KS	AT(A)			KR	ACP
Module 3		KS	AT(P)	DH	ER	KR*	ACP
Module 4		KS	AT(P)	DH		KR	ACP
Raps 2	10,222	Polyketide synthase					
Module 5		KS	AT(A)			KR	ACP
Module 6		KS	AT(P)	DH		KR*	ACP
Module 7		KS	AT(P)	DH	ER	KR	ACP
Module 8		KS	AT(A)	DH		KR	ACP
Module 9		KS	AT(A)	DH		KR	ACP
Module 10		KS	AT(P)	DH		KR	ACP
Raps 3	6,260	Polyketide synthase					
Module 11		KS	AT(A)			KR	ACP
Module 12		KS	AT(A)			KR	ACP
Module 13		KS	AT(P)	DH	ER	KR	ACP
Module 14		KS	AT(A)				ACP
OrfD	383	?					
OrfE	465	?					
OrfF	454	(Membrane transport protein?)					
OrfG	330	(P helix–turn–helix DNA-binding protein?)					
OrfH	872	(Putative regulator of cholesterol oxidase)					
OrfI	260	?					
RapJ	386	Cytochrome P450					
OrfK	341	?					
pL	343	Lysine cyclodeaminase					
apM	317	Methyltransferase					
RapN	404	Cytochrome P450					
RapO	78	Ferredoxin					
RapP	1,541	Pipecolate-incorporating enzyme					
RapQ	211	Methyltransferase					
RapT	264	(Ketoreductase/dehydrogenase)					
OrfU	200	?					
OrfS	399	(Sensory protein kinase)					
OrfR	220	(Response regulator)					
OrfV	437	(Membrane transport protein?)					
OrfW	459	?					
OrfX	235	(ABC-transporter)					
OrfY	204	(Regulators of antibiotic transport complexes?)					
OrfZ	389	?					

[a] Potential polyketide synthase (PKS) activities are indicated as follows: ACP, acyl carrier protein; KS, β-ketoacyl-ACP synthase; AT, acyltransferase incorporating either an acetate (A) or propionate (P) extender unit; KR, β-ketoacyl-ACP reductase; DH, β-hydroxyacyl-thioester dehydratease; ER, enoyl reductase. Activities for Raps 1–3 are colinear with the sequence of each ORF as listed from left to right and top to bottom. Asterisk indicates an activity that may not be functional.
Source: Ref. 22.

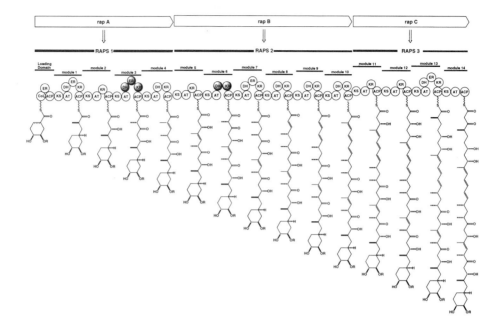

Figure 13 The proposed role of Raps1, Raps2, and Raps3 in biosynthesis of the carbon backbone of rapamycin. Shaded domains are possibly inactive. (Reproduced by kind permission of P. F. Leadley, University of Cambridge.)

thioesters, are transferred to the ACP functionality. In the case of rapamycin, it seems that the starter unit in the form of the free acid is linked to the PKS using a coenzyme A ligase (22,69). Furthermore, the presence of the enoyl reductase activity in the loading domain would suggest that the final reduction step in the conversion of shikimic acid to the substituted cyclohexanecarboxylic acid (DHCHC) (the reduction of (4*R*, 5*R*)-4,5-dihydroxycyclohex-1-enecarboxylic acid [3]) (Figure 10) would occur after this linkage to Raps1. The initial conversion of shikimic acid to [3] (Figure 10) would therefore likely occur at the level of the free acid. The pathway from shikimic acid to cyclohexanecarboxylic acid (CHC) (Figure 11), on the other hand, is thought to occur primarily at the level of a coenzyme A thioester (Reynolds KA, unpublished results). These observations provide further support for the suggestion that the pathways to CHC and DHCHC are very different (59). At this point, the theories concerning chain initiation are unproven.

Compelling evidence has been presented that the enzyme responsible for activating pipecolate in the unusual chain termination and cyclization process in rapamycin biosynthesis is encoded by *rap*P (22,71). It seems likely that the polyketide chain of rapamycin is transferred from Raps3 to the amino-group of an enzyme-bound pipecolyl moiety, which in turn is attacked at the carboxyl functionality by the C22 hydroxyl-group to form the macrolactam ring.

To the right of the PKS genes in Figure 12 are other ORFs to which at least some functions can be assigned (22,71). RapM, RapQ, and RapI likely encode methyltransferases catalyzing at least the three O-methylation steps in rapamycin biosynthesis (22,71). RapJ and RapN gene products resemble P450 enzymes and are likely involved in hydroxylation of C14 and C29 of rapamycin. Use of the cytochrome P450 inhibitor, metyrapone, generated one dehydroxy analog and three deoxo analogs of rapamycin (23). Finally, it has been suggested that *rapL* encodes an enzyme responsible for conversion of lysine to pipecolate. At the fringes of the cluster are genes thought to be involved in regulation or export of rapamycin.

A region of the FK506 gene cluster clustered with the *fkbM* gene, encoding the 31-O-demethyl-FK506 methyltransferase, has also been sequenced and analyzed (72,73). The *fkbM* gene was cloned using oligonucleotide probes designed based on the N-terminal amino acid sequence of the FKMT (55). The *fkbM* gene involved in ascomycin biosynthesis has also been cloned and sequenced in a similar fashion (73; Reynolds KA, unpublished results). Disruption of the *fkbM* gene in the FK506-producing *Streptomyces* sp. MA6548 generated a mutant that produced 31-O-demethyl-FK506 (73). A 32% identity of the deduced amino acid sequence of *fkbM* and *rapI* suggests that *rapI* encodes 39-O-demethyl-rapamycin methyltransferase. Immediately upstream of the FK506 and ascomycin *fkbM* gene lies another open reading frame, *fkbD* (73; Reynolds KA, unpublished results). The deduced amino acid sequence of the *fkbD* gene shows strong homology to streptomycete cytochrome P450 hydroxylases. Disruption of the *fkbD* gene in FK506-producing *Streptomyces* sp. MA6548 resulted in a mutant that produced 9-deoxo-31-O-desmethyl-FK506. This experiment establishes the role of this gene in hydroxylation of C9 of the FK506 macrolactone ring (73). It is unclear at this time which gene product is responsible for oxidation of the C9—OH. The observation that this *fkbD* mutant produces 9-deoxo-31-O-desmethyl-FK506 rather than 9-deoxo-FK506 may indicate that the gene disruption has an effect on expression of the downstream *fkbM*, indicating that these two genes are transcribed. The deduced amino acid sequences of *rapJ* and *fkbD* have 74% identity, suggesting that *rapJ* is involved in the analogous step in rapamycin biosynthesis.

A polyketide synthase gene *fkbA*, immediately preceding this *fkbD*, has also been cloned and sequenced (73). The predicted gene product of *fkbA* is a 630,660 Da protein (6420 amino acids) containing 4 type I PKS modules. A total of 10 PKS modules are predicted to be required for the biosynthesis of the FK506 macrolactone ring. Comparison of *fkbA* with *rapC* reveals the same enzyme activities in the same order. The only difference is that the first module of deduced amino acid sequence of *fkbA* has an additional β-hydroxyacylthioester dehydratase and enoyl reductase, required to reduce C16 of FK506 to methylene (the equivalent carbon in rapamycin is C7 and remains at the oxidation state of an alcohol). The disruption of the *fkbA* resulted in the production of a mutant unable to produce FK506. These results are all consistent with *fkbA* gene product catalyzing the last four condensation steps in FK506 biosynthesis (73).

Upstream of *fkbA* is a peptide synthetase gene (analogous to *rapP*) that is likely responsible for incorporating pipecolate into the polypeptide chain of FK506. The loading domain of FK506 PKS has also been sequenced and shown to contain a coenzyme A ligase, an enoyl reductase, and an ACP domain (analogous to that observed for loading domain of Raps1) (72; Motamedi H, unpublished results).

V. FERMENTATION AND NUTRITION

The rapamycin-producing streptomycete strain AY B-994 isolated from Easter Island (Rapa Nui) soil was first grown on yeast–starch agar (12). The organism was identified as

S. hygroscopicus and deposited as NRRL 5491 and ATCC 29253. The best solid medium for its growth was tomato paste–oatmeal agar. Good carbon sources for growth on agar were D-glucose, D-fructose, D-mannitol, *i*-inositol, starch, and glycerol. Those supporting moderate growth were D-xylose, L-arabinose, L-rhamnose, raffinose, lactose, and D-maltose. The optimum pH and temperature for growth were 6–8 and 25–27°C, respectively. Spores were produced on tomato paste–oatmeal agar after 14 days. Initial studies on rapamycin production were done using a liquid medium containing glucose, oatmeal, enzymatic digest of casein, blackstrap molasses, NaCl, and tap water for inoculum preparation and fermentation. Later studies (13) employed a seed medium containing glucose, soybean meal, $(NH_4)_2SO_4$, $CaCO_3$, and tap water and a large-scale production medium containing glucose, soybean meal, $(NH_4)_2SO_4$, KH_2PO_4, and antifoam.

Rapamycin biosynthetic studies (21) were carried out with a second natural isolate, strain AY B-1206, which produced more rapamycin and less demethoxyrapamycin (Sehgal SN, personal communication). Sporulation was achieved out on a glucose–KNO_3–inorganic salts agar. Fermentation was performed in a liquid medium containing glycerol, leucine, glutamic acid, lysine, yeast extract, and inorganic salts. These media had been developed by Sehgal and Vezina of the Ayerst Research Laboratories (Princeton, NJ). In a later biosynthetic study (56), lysine was replaced by monobasic ammonium phosphate with no negative effects being observed.

Up until 1994, no chemically defined medium had been reported for growth and rapamycin production by strain AY B-1206 or AY B-994. In a study on carbon source nutrition, Kojima et al. (74) began with the yeast extract–containing medium used by Paiva et al. (20) mentioned above. Removal of yeast extract markedly reduced growth and rapamycin production. Addition of glucose, aspartic acid, arginine, and histidine replaced the effect of yeast extract, and thus medium 1 (Table 3) was developed. It was used to determine the effects of various carbon sources as replacements for glucose plus glycerol on growth and rapamycin production. In medium 1, the insoluble $CaCO_3$ of earlier media had been replaced by 100 mM MES (2-[N-morpholino]ethanesulfonic acid) buffer to facilitate observation of growth. The support of growth and rapamycin production by the carbon sources are shown in Table 4. Of 34 carbon sources tested, 19 shown in the table supported growth and rapamycin production. Eight carbon sources failed to support growth. Seven compounds exerted catabolite repression or inhibition; that is, they supported growth but not production of rapamycin. The better carbon sources for rapamycin production are marked with an asterisk in Table 4. After further studies, it was deemed that a mixture of 20 g/liter fructose plus 5 g/liter mannose was the best combination of two carbon sources, and these were chosen for medium 2 (Table 3).

Minerals exert different types of regulatory control of rapamycin biosynthesis. Cheng et al. (75) reported that limitation of phosphate, ammonium, and magnesium was required for optimal production in medium 2. Whereas total growth was maximal at 100 mM K_2HPO_4, production peaked at 5–10 mM. Ammonium chloride supported maximum growth at 25 mM, but a level as low as 5 mM inhibited rapamycin formation. Magnesium sulfate showed its maximum effect on growth at 1 mM but inhibited rapamycin production at levels higher than 0.01 mM. Although it is not uncommon for production of macrolide antibiotics to be under control of nitrogen and phosphate sources, regulation by Mg^{2+} has been only rarely described. In contrast to the negative effects of the above minerals, $FeSO_4$ increasingly stimulated rapamycin production at concentrations up to 0.36 mM with virtually no effect on growth. Medium 3 (Table 3) was devised by virtue of the information obtained from these studies (75).

Table 3 Chemically Defined Media Sequentially Developed for Growth of *Streptomyces hygroscopicus* and Production of Rapamycin[a]

Component	Medium 1	Medium 2	Medium 3	Medium 4
Glycerol	20.0 g	—	—	—
α–D(+)Glucose	10.0 g	—	—	—
DFructose	—	20.0 g	20.0 g	20.0 g
D(+)Mannose	—	5.0 g	5.0 g	5.0 g
Na-L-Aspartate	1.5 g	1.5 g	1.5 g	1.5 g
L-Arginine	0.5 g	0.5 g	0.5 g	0.5 g
L-Histidine•HCl	0.5 g	0.5 g	0.5 g	0.5 g
L-Lysine	—	—	—	10.0 g
Shikimic acid	—	—	—	10.0 g
K_2HPO_4	2.0 g	2.0 g	1.7 g	1.7 g
KH_2PO_4	2.0 g	2.0 g	—	—
NaCl	5.0 g	5.0 g	5.0 g	5.0 g
$ZnSO_4•7H_2O$	60 mg	60 mg	60 mg	60 mg
$MgSO_4•7H_2O$	256 mg	256 mg	2.5 mg	2.5 mg
$MgCl_2•6H_2O$	510 mg	510 mg	—	—
$MnSO_4•H_2O$	12 mg	12 mg	12 mg	12 mg
$FeSO_4•7H_2O$	100 mg	100 mg	100 mg	100 mg
$(NH_4)_6MO_7O_{24}•4H_2O$	18 mg	18 mg	18 mg	18 mg
$Na_2B_4O_7•10H_2O$	10 mg	10 mg	10 mg	10 mg
$CoCl_2•6H_2O$	10 mg	10 mg	10 mg	10 mg
$CuCl_2•2H_2O$	1.3 mg	1.3 mg	1.3 mg	1.3 mg
Na_2SO_4	360 mg	360 mg	360 mg	360 mg
MES buffer	21.3 g	21.3 g	21.3 g	21.3 g
pH (initial)	6.0	6.0	6.0	6.0

[a] All weights are per liter.

The effect of addition of amino acids to medium 3 (which already contains aspartate, arginine, and histidine as nitrogen sources) was studied by Cheng et al. (76). Of 18 amino acids tested at 1 g/liter, only L-lysine showed a marked stimulation of both volumetric and specific rapamycin production. Its effect was maximal at 10 g/liter, the highest concentration examined. Lysine stimulation is probably due to its conversion to pipecolic acid, a precursor of rapamycin (58). Suppression of rapamycin production was observed with L-methionine and L-phenylalanine. Since methionine is a rapamycin precursor (20), it is peculiar that it interferes with rapamycin formation. However, for some unknown reason, methionine often suppresses formation of antibiotics for which it acts as precursor (77–80). One possibility for phenylalanine suppression of rapamycin formation was considered to be feed-back inhibition of shikimic acid formation, since shikimate is a precursor of rapamycin (20). However, in a recent study (81) demonstrating stimulation of rapamycin biosynthesis by exogenous shikimate (57 mM), it was also shown that shikimate does not reverse phenylalanine interference.

Shikimate stimulation had not been observed earlier when tested in complex medium (56). Only upon development of the effective chemically defined medium 3 plus lysine was a shikimate response observed (81). Medium 4 (Table 3) is the most effective chemically defined medium available for rapamycin biosynthesis. However, the very high

Table 4   Ability of Sole Carbon Sources to Support Growth of *Streptomyces hygroscopicus* and Rapamycin production in Chemically Defined Medium 1 Less Glucose and Glycerol[a]

Rapamycin production and good growth	Rapamycin production and moderate growth	Rapamycin production and poor growth	Growth but no rapamycin production	No growth
Soluble starch	*meso*-Erythritol	a-D(+)Melibiose	Sucrose	Dextrin
D(+)Raffinose	D(+)Mannose*	a-L-Rhamnose	a-D-Lactose	Inulin
D(+)Cellobiose*	D(+)Xylose*		D(+)Trehalose	Salicin
Laminarin	D(+)Maltose		Xylitol	L(−)Sorbose
Glycerol	D(+)Galactose*		Propanol	D-Sorbitol
i-Inositol*			Methyloleate	Ethanol
D-Fructose*			Oleate	Sodium acetate
L(+)Arabinose			Sodium acetate	
a-D(+)Glucose				
D-Mannitol*				
Pectin				
D-Ribose				

[a] All sources tested at 30 g/liter. The carbon sources marked with an asterisk gave the best rapamycin production.

cost of shikimate may preclude its routine use. Genetic manipulation should be examined in order to relieve the shikimate-production deficiency of *S. hygroscopicus*.

Very little has been published concerning the nutrition of the FK506- and ascomycin-producing strains. The initial reports on the seed medium for *S. tsukubaensis*, the producer of FK506 (33), indicated use of glycerol, corn starch, glucose, cotton seed meal, corn steep liquor, and calcium carbonate. The production medium contained soluble starch, corn steep liquor, dried yeast, calcium carbonate, and Adekanol (a defoaming agent). *S. hygroscopicus* var. *yakushimaensis* strain No. 7238, producer of ascomycin, showed an optimum temperature of 28°C and utilized D-glucose, sucrose, lactose, maltose, D-trehalose, inositol, inulin, and salicin (27). For inoculum, a seed medium (pH 6.5) containing glycerol, corn starch, glucose, cotton seed meal, dried yeast, corn steep liquor, and calcium carbonate was used. The production medium was made up of glucose, corn steep liquor, dried yeast, gluten meal, wheat germ, calcium carbonate, and Adekanol (28). Byrne et al. (30) grew *S. hygroscopicus* var. *ascomyceticus* strain ATCC 14891 (= MA-6475) (24,25), another ascomycin producer, on slants of ISP (International Streptomyces project) medium, in a seed medium containing glucose, yeast extract, Hy-Case SF, and mineral salts, and a fermentation medium of glucose, glycerol, corn steep liquor, yeast extract, L-tyrosine, lactic acid, and MOPS (3-[N-morpholino]propane-sulfonic acid) buffer.

VI.   CONCLUDING COMMENTS

The discovery of the immunosuppressant effects of rapamycin, FK506, and ascomycin has sparked renewed fervor in secondary metabolic studies, provided a new class of immuno-suppressants, and led to a greater understanding of the immune response. It is impossible to predict what advances and in which directions the field of natural products research will take us in the next century. What is clear, however, is that in an era of combinatorial chemistry and rational drug design, natural products will continue to provide lead compounds for the chemist, biochemist, molecular biologist, and pharmacologist alike.

REFERENCES

1. Dreyfuss M, Härri H, Hofmann H, Kobel H, Pache W, Tscherter H. Cyclosporin A and C; new metabolites from *Trichoderma polysporum*. (Link ex Pers) Rifai. Eur J Appl Microbiol 1976; 3:125–133.
2. Kohsaka M, Kino T, Hatanaka H, Goto T, Okuhara M, Aoki H, Imanaka H. Isolation of immunomodulators from microbial sources. Okami Y, Beppu T, Ogawara H, eds. Biology of Actinomycetes '88. Tokyo: Japan Scientific Societies Press, 1988:195–199.
3. Caulfield CE, Musser, JH Macrocyclic immunomodulators. Annu Rept Med Chem 1989; 25:195–204.
4. Sehgal SN, Chang JY. Rapamycin: A new immunosuppressive macrolide. Transpl Immunol Lett 1990; 7:12–14.
5. Sehgal SN, Molnar-Kimber K, Ocain TD, Weichman BM. Rapamycin: A novel immuno-suppressive macrolide. Med Res Rev 1994; 14:1–22.
6. Liu J. FK506 and cyclosporin: Molecular probes for studying intracellular signal transduction. TiPs 1993; 14:182–188.
7. Siekierka JJ, Hung SHY, Poe M, Lin CS, Sigal NH. A cytosolic binding protein for the immunosuppressant FK506 has peptidyl-prolylisomerase activity but is distinct from cyclophilin. Nature 1989; 341:755–757.
8. Handschumacher RE, Harding MW, Rice J, Drugge RJ, Speicher DW. Cyclophilin: A specific cytosolic binding protein for cyclosporin A. Science 1984; 226:544–547.
9. Liu J, Albers MW, Wandless TJ, Luan S, Alberg DG, Belshaw PJ, Cohen P, MacKintosh C. Klee CB, Schreiber SL. Inhibition of T cell signalling by immunophilin-ligand complex correlates with loss of calcineurin phosphatase activity. Biochem 1992; 31:3896–3901.
10. Schreiber SL, Crabtree GR. The mechanism of action of cyclosporin A and FK506. Immunol Today 1992; 13:136–142.
11. Breuder T, Hemenway CS, Movva NR, Cardenas ME, Heitman J. Calcineurin is essential in cyclosporin A- and FK506-sensitive yeast strains. Proc Natl Acad Sci USA 1994; 91:5372–5376.
12. Vezina C, Kudelski A, Sehgal SN. Rapamycin (AY-22,989), a new antifungal antibiotic 1. Taxonomy of the producing streptomycete and isolation of the active principal. J Antibiot 1975; 28:721–726.
13. Sehgal SN, Baker H, Vezina C. Rapamycin (AY-22,989), a new antifungal antibiotic. 2. Fermentation, isolation and characterization. J Antibiot 1975; 28:727–732.
14. Baker H, Sidorowicz A, Sehgal SN, Vezina C. Rapamycin (AY-22,989), a new antifungal antibiotic. 3. Protection studies in mice. J Antibiot 1978; 31:539–545.
15. Douros J, Suffness M. Novel antitumor substances of natural origin. Cancer Treat Rev 1981; 8:63–87.
16. Eng CP, Sehgal SN, Vezina C. Activity of rapamycin (AY-22,989) against transplanted tumors. J Antibiot 1984; 37:1231–1237.
17. Martel RR, Klicus J, Galet S. Inhibition of the immune response by rapamycin, a new antifungal antibiotic. Can J Physiol Pharmacol 1977; 55:48–51.
18. Swindells NDC, White PS, Findlay JA. The X-ray crystal structure of rapamycin, $C_{51}H_{79}NO_{13}$. Can J Chem 1978; 56:2491–2492.
19. Findlay JA, Radics L. On the chemistry and high field nuclear magnetic resonance spectroscopy of rapamycin. Can J Chem 1980; 58:579–590.
20. Paiva NL, Demain AL, Roberts MF. Incorporation of acetate, propionate, and methionine into rapamycin by *Streptomyces hygroscopicus*. J Nat Prod 1991; 54:167–177.

21. McAlpine JB, Swanson SJ, Jackson M, Whittern DN. Revised NMR assignments for rapamycin. J Antibiot 1991; 44:688–690.

22. Schwecke T, Aparico JF, Molnar I, Konig A, Khaw LE, Haydock SF, Oliynyk M, Caffrrey P, Cortes J, Lester JB, Bohm GA, Staunton J, Leadlay PF. The biosynthetic gene cluster for the polyketide immunosuppressant rapamycin. Proc Natl Acad Sci USA 1995; 92:7839–7843.

23. Nishida H, Sakakibara T, Aoki F, Saito T, Ichikawa K, Inagaki T, Kojima Y, Yamauchi Y, Huang LH, Guadliana MA, Kaneko T, Kojima N, Generation of novel rapamycin structures by microbial manipulations. J Antibiot 1995; 48:657–666.

24. Arai T. Ascomycin and process for its production. U.S. Patent 3,244,592; 1996.

25. Arai T, Koyama Y, Suenaga T, Honda H. Ascomycin, an antifungal antibiotic. J Antibiot(Ser A) 1962; 15:231–232.

26. Dumont FJ, Byrne KM, Sihgal NH, Kaplan L, Monaghan RL, Garrity G. Novel immuno-suppressive agent. European Patent Office publication 0323865; 1989.

27. Hatanaka H, Iwami M, Kino T. FR-900520 and FR-900523, novel immunosuppressants iso-lated from a *Streptomyces*. 1. Taxonomy of the producing strain. J Antibiot 1988; 41:1586–1591.

28. Hatanaka H, Kino T, Miyata S, Inamura N, Kuroda A, Goto T, Tanaka H, Okuhara M. FR-900520 and FR-900523, novel immunosuppressants isolated from a *Streptomyces*. 2. Fermen-tation, isolation and physico-chemical and biological characteristics. J Antibiot 1988; 41:1592–1601.

29. Or YS, Clark RF, Xie Q, McAlpine J, Whittern DN, Henry R, Luly JR. The chemistry of ascomycin: Structure determination and synthesis of pyrazole analogues. Tetrahedron 1993; 49:8771–8786.

30. Byrne KM, Shafiee A, Nielsen J, Arison B, Monaghan RL, Kaplan L. The biosynthesis and enzymology of an immunosuppressant, immunomycin, produced by *Streptomyces hygroscopi-cus* var. *ascomyceticus*. Dev Ind Microbiol 1993; 32:29–45.

31. Morisaki M, Arai T. Identity of immunosuppressant FR900520 with ascomycin. J Antibiot 1992; 45:126–128.

32. Tanaka H, Kuroda A, Marusawa H, Hatanaka H, Kino T, Goto T, Hashimoto M, Taga T. Structure of FK-506: A novel immunosuppressant isolated from *Streptomyces*. J Am Chem Soc 1987; 109:5031–5033.

33. Kino T, Hatanaka H, Hashimoto M, Nishimaya M, Goto T, Okuhara, M, Kohsaka M, Aoki H, Imanaka H. FK-506, a novel immunosuppressant isolated from a Streptomyces. I. Fer-mentation, isolation, and phsico-chemical and biological characteristics. J Antibiot 1987; 40:1249–1255.

34. O'Hagan D. The Polyketide Metabolites. Chichester, England: Ellis Horwood, 1991.

35. Wallace KK, Zhao B, McArthur HAI, Reynolds KA. In vivo analysis of straight-chain and branched-chain fatty acid biosynthesis in streptomycetes. FEMS Lett 1995; 131:227–234.

36. Omura S, Tsuzuki K, Tanaka Y, Sakakibara H, Aizawa M, Lukacs G. Valine as a precursor of n-butyrate unit in the biosynthesis of macrolide aglycone. J Antibiot 1983; 36:614–616.

37. Pospisil S, Sedmera P, Havranek M. Krumphanzl V, Vanek Z. Biosynthesis of monensins A and B. J Antibiot 1983; 36:617–619.

38. Reynolds KA, O'Hagan D, Gani D, Robinson JA. Butyrate metabolism in *Streptomycetes*. Characterization of an intramolecular vicinal interchange rearrangement linking isobutyrate and butyrate in *Streptomyces cinnamonensis*. J Chem Soc Perkin Trans I 1987; 3195–3207.

39. Inui H, Miyatake K, Nakano Y, Kitaoka S. Purification and some properties of short chain-length specific *trans*-2-enoyl CoA reductase in mitochondria of *Euglena gracilis*. J Biochem 1986; 100:995–1000.

40. Maitra SK, Kumar S. Crotonyl coenzyme A reductase activity of bovine mammary fatty acid synthase. J Biochem 1981; 89:1075–1080.

41. Reynolds KA. Comparison of two unusual enoyl CoA reductases in *Streptomyces collinus*. J Nat Prod 1993; 56:175–185.

42. Wallace KK, Bao Z-y, Dai H, DiGate R, Schuler G, Speedie MK, Reynolds KA, Purification of crotonyl CoA reductase from *Streptomyces collinus* and cloning, sequencing and expression of the corresponding gene in *Eschericia coli*. Eur J Biochem 1995; 233:954–962.

43. Townsend CA, Brobst SW, Ramer SE, Vederas JC. Stereochemical features of enoyl thioester reductase in averufin and fatty acid biosynthesis in *Aspergillus parasiticus*. J Am Chem Soc 1988; 110:319–321.

44. Bhatnagar D, Ehrlich KC, Cleveland TE. Oxidation and reduction reactions in biosynthesis of secondary metabolites. Bhatnagar D, Lillehoj EB, Arora DK, eds. Handbook of Applied Mycology, Vol. 5: Mycotoxins in Ecological Systems. New York: Marcel Dekker, 1992: 255–285.

45. Chandler IM, Simpson TJ. Studies of polyketide chain assembly processes: Incorporation of [2-^{13}C]malonate into averufin in *Aspergillus parasiticus*. J Chem Soc Chem Commun 1987; 17–18.

46. Paiva NL, Demain AL, Roberts MF. The immediate precursor of the nitrogen-containing ring of rapamycin is free pipecolic acid. Enz Microb Technol 1993; 15:581–585.

47. Fothergill JC, Guest JR. Catabolism of L-lysine by *Pseudomonas aeruginosa*. J Gen Microbiol 1977; 99:139–155.

48. Reed JW, Purvis, MB, Kingston, DI, Blot A, Gossele F. Biosynthesis of the antibiotics of the virginamycin family. 7. Stereo- and regiochemical studies on the formation of the 3-hydroxypipicolinic acid and pipecolic acid units. J Org Chem 1989; 54:1161–1165.

49. Wickwire BM, Harris CM, Harris TM, Broquist HP. Pipecolic acid biosynthesis in *Rhizoctonia leguminicola*. 1. The lysine, saccharopine, Δ¹-piperidine-6-carboxylate pathway. J Biol Chem 1990; 265:14742–14747.

50. Nielsen JB, Hsu M-j, Byrne KM, Kaplan L. Biosynthesis of the immunosuppressant immunomycin: The enzymology of pipecolate incorporation. Biochem 1991; 30:5789–5796.

51. Kleinkauf H, von Döhren H. Nonribosomal biosynthesis of peptide antibiotics. Eur J Biochem 1990; 192:1–15.

52. Lee S, Lipmann F. Tyrocidine synthetase system. Meth Enzymol 1975; 43:585–602.

53. Katz E, Demain AL. The peptide antibiotics of Bacillus: Chemistry, biogenesis and possible functions. Bacteriol Rev 1977; 41:449–474.

54. Hatanaka H, Kino T, Asano M, Goto T, Tanaka H, Okuhara M. FK 506 related compounds produced by *Streptomyces tsukabaensis* No. 9993. J Antibiot 1989; 42:620–622.

55. Shafiee A, Motamedi H, Chen T. Enzymology of FK-506 biosynthesis. Purification and characterization of 31-O-desmethylFK506 O: Methyltransferase from *Streptomyces sp*. MA6858. Eur J Biochem 1994; 225:755–764.

56. Chen TS, Arison BH, Wicker LS, Inamine ES, Monaghan RL. Microbial transformation of immunosuppressive compounds. I. Desmethylation of FK506 and immunomycin (FR900520) by *Actinoplanes sp*. ATCC53771. J Antibiot 1992; 45:118–123.

57. Shafiee A. Chen TS, Arison BS, Dumont FJ, Colwell L, Kaplan L. Enzymatic synthesis and immunosuppressive activity of novel desmethylated immunomycins (ascomycins). J Antibiot 1993; 46:1397–1405.

58. Paiva NL, Roberts MF, Demain AL. The cyclohexane moiety of rapamycin is derived from shikimic acid in *Streptomyces hygroscopicus*. J Ind Microbiol 1993; 12:423–428.

59. Wallace KK, Reynolds KA, Koch K, McArthur HAI, Brown MS, Wax RG, Moore BS. Biosynthetic studies of ascomyin (FK520): Formation of the (1R,3R,4R)-3,4-dihydroxycyclohexanecarboxylic acid-derived moiety. J Am Chem Soc 1994; 116:11600–11601.

60. Schwab JM, Henderson B. Enzyme catalyzed allylic rearrangements. Chem Rev 1990; 90:1203–1245.

61. O'Sullivan MC, Schwab JM, Zabriskie TM, Helms GL, Vederas JC. Reevaluation of the stereochemical courses of the allylic rearrangement and the double bond reduction catalyzed by the *Brevibacterium ammoniagenes* fatty acid synthase. J Amer Chem Soc 1991; 113:3997–3998.

62. Moore BS, Cho H, Casati R, Kennedy E, Reynolds KA, Mocek U, Beale JM, Floss HG. Biosynthetic studies on ansatrienin A. Formation of the cyclohexanecarboxylic acid moiety. J Am Chem Soc 1993; 115:5254–5266.

63. Moore BS, Poralla K, Floss HG. Biosynthesis of the cyclohexanecarboxylic acid starter unit of ω-cyclohexylfatty acids in *Alicyclobacillus acidocaldarius*. J Am Chem Soc 1993; 115:5267–5274.

64. Reynolds KA, Seaton N, Fox KM, Warner, K, Wang P. Mechanistic studies of a Δ^1,Δ^2-cyclohexenylcarbonyl CoA isomerase catalyzing the penultimate step in the biosynthesis of the cyclohexanecarboxylic acid moiety of ansatrienin A. J Nat Prod 1993; 56:825–829.

65. Reynolds KA, Fox KM, Yuan Z-m, Lam Y. Biosynthesis of ansatrienin: Stereochemical course of the final reduction step leading to the cyclohexanecarboxylic acid moiety. J Am Chem Soc 1991; 1113:4339–4340.

66. Cortes J, Haydock SF, Roberts GA, Bevitt DJ, Leadley PF. An unusually large multifunctional polypeptide in the erythromycin-producing polyketide synthase of *Saccharopolyspora erythraea*. Nature (London) 1990; 348:176–178.

67. Donadio S. Staver MJ, McAlpine JB, Swanson SJ, Katz L. Modular organization of genes required for complex polyketide biosynthesis. Science 1991; 252:675–679.

68. MacNeil DJ, Occi JL, Gewain KM, MacNeil T, Gibbons PH, Ruby CL, Davis SJ. Complex organization of the *Streptomyces avermitilis* genes encoding the avermectin biosynthetic gene cluster. Gene 1992; 115:119–125.

69. Aparico JF, Molnár I, Schwecke T, König A, Haydock SF, Khaw LE, Staunton J, Leadley PF. Organization of the biosynthetic gene cluster for rapamycin in *Streptomyces hygroscopicus*: Analysis of the enzymatic domains in the modular polyketide synthase. Gene 1996;196:9–16.

70. Staunton J, Caffrey P, Aparico JF, Roberts GA, Bethel SS, Leadley PF. Evidence for a double-helical structure for modular polyketide synthases. Nat Struct Biol 1996; 3:188–192.

71. Molnár I, Aparico JF, Haydock SF, Khaw LE, Schwecke T, König A, Staunton J, Leadley PF. Organization of the biosynthetic gene cluster for rapamycin in *Streptomyces hygroscopicus*: Analysis of the genes flanking the polyketide synthase. Gene 1996; 196:9–16.

72. Motamedi H, Cai S, Shafiee A, Elliston KO. Structural organization of a multifunctional polyketide synthase involved in the biosynthesis of the macrolide immunosuppressant FK506 (manuscript in preparation).

73. Motamedi H, Shafiee A, Cai S. Streicher SL, Arison BH, Miller RR. Characterization of methyl transferase and hydroxylase genes involved in the biosynthesis of the immunosuppressant FK506 and FK520. J Bacteriol 1996; 178:5243–5248.

74. Kojima I, Cheng Y, Mohan V, Demain AL. Carbon source nutrition of rapamycin biosynthesis in *Streptomyces hygroscopicus*. J Ind Microbiol 1995; 14:436–439.

75. Cheng YR, Hauck L, Demain AL. Phosphate, ammonium, magnesium and iron nutrition of *Streptomyces hygroscopicus* with respect to rapamycin biosynthesis. J Ind Microbiol 1995; 14:424–427.

76. Cheng YR, Fang A, Demain AL. Effect of amino acids on rapamycin biosynthesis by *Streptomyces hygroscopicus*. Appl Microbiol Biotechnol 1995; 43:1096–1098.

77. Gairola C, Hurley L. The mechanism for the methionine mediated reduction in anthramycin yields in *Streptomyces refuineus* fermentations. Eur J Appl Microbiol 1976; 2:95–101.

78. Uyeda M, Demain AL. Methionine inhibition of thienamycin formation. J Ind Microbiol 1988; 3:57–59.

79. Favret ME, Boeck LD. Effect of cobalt and cyanocobalamin on biosynthesis of A10258, a thiopeptide antibiotic complex. J Antibiot 1992; 45:1809–1811.

80. Lam KS, Veitch JA, Golik J, Krishnan B, Klohr SE, Volk KJ, Forenza S, Doyle TW. Biosynthesis of esperamicin A1, an enediyne antitumor antibiotic, J Am Chem Soc 1993; 115:12340–12345.

81. Fang A, Demain A L. Exogenous shikimic acid stimulates rapamycin biosynthesis in *Streptomyces hygroscopicus*. Folia Microbiol 1995; 40:607–610.

18

Rifamycins

Giancarlo Lancini and Bruno Cavalleri
Lepetit Research Center, Gerenzano, Italy

I. INTRODUCTION

Rifamycins are a family of antibiotics first isolated in Lepetit Research Laboratories as a complex of at least five components, denoted rifomycin A, B, C, D, and E (1). The name was later changed to rifamycins to avoid confusion with the names of other antibiotics. The producing strain was originally named *Streptomyces mediterranei* but, as discussed later, was then classified as *Nocardia* and later as *Amycolatopsis*. Rifamycin B, although less active than the other components, was chosen for development, being more stable, easy to isolate, and soluble at physiological pHs. Moreover, its production resulted in easy purification after the surprising observation (2,3) that it was the only product of the fermentation when barbiturates were added to culture media.

The rifamycin B structure was elucidated by Prelog and coworkers (4) (Figure 1). It was thus revealed that it belonged to a new class of microbial metabolites, characterized by a planar aromatic core spanned by an aliphatic chain, like a handle of a basket. For these compounds, Prelog proposed the name of ansamycin from the Latin "ansa" (handle). Several other ansamycins were later identified (5). Among these, streptovaricins have in common with rifamycins a naphthalene core, an ansa of 17 atoms, and comparable biological activity (6). Other families of ansamycins, such as naphthomycins (7), have a naphthalene ring and a 23-atom aliphatic chain, or a benzene core with an ansa of 15 atoms (e.g., mycotrienin) (8) or 17 atoms (e.g., geldanamycin) (9). All of these are quite different from rifamycins in their biological activities and mechanisms of action.

Development plans for rifamycins were completely changed by another surprising observation: in aqueous solution, rifamycin B spontaneously transforms into more active compounds. Rational chemical reproduction of the spontaneous transformations resulted in the preparation of rifamycins O, S, and SV, through the reactions depicted in Figure 2 (10). These derivatives were microbiologically very active, and among them rifamycin SV was chosen for clinical studies because of its in vivo activity, tolerability, and solubility properties.

An important characteristic of rifamycins is their mechanism of action. These were the first antibiotics found to selectively inhibit RNA synthesis by binding to the bacterial DNA-dependent RNA polymerase (11,12). This aspect, besides being widely exploited for studies of molecular biology, suggested that these antibiotics were particularly suitable for chemical modification.

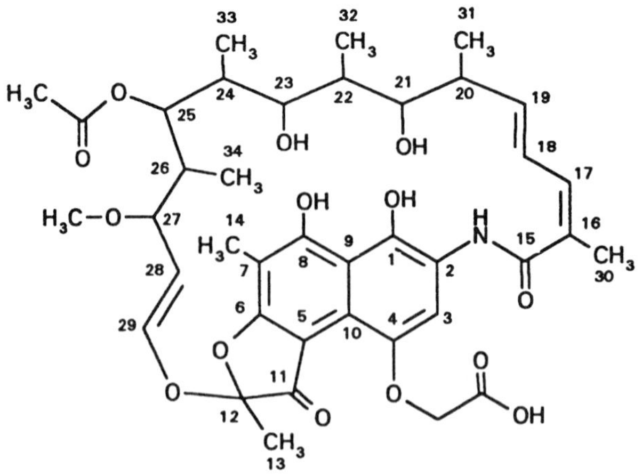

Figure 1   Rifamycin B.

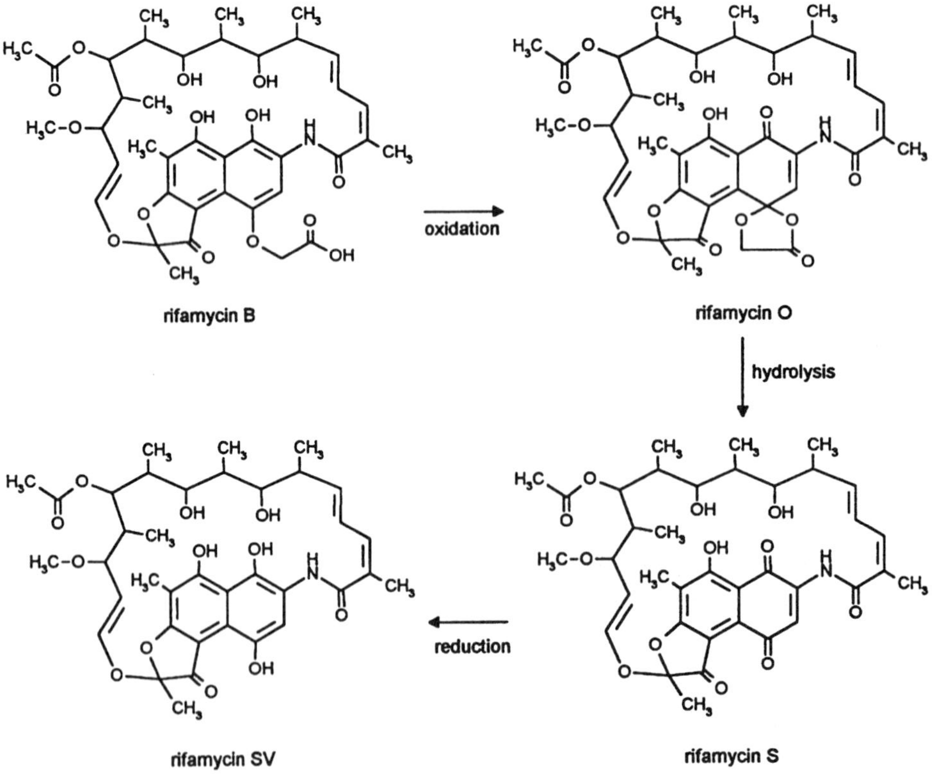

Figure 2   Conversion of rifamycin B into rifamycin O, rifamycin S, and rifamycin SV.

A large program of semisynthesis was then initiated with the aim of obtaining orally active derivatives more efficacious then rifamycin SV in the treatment of tuberculosis. The main result of these efforts was the synthesis of rifampicin, which now is widely used in the treatment of tuberculosis, leprosy, and several other infectious diseases. Other derivatives that have been developed for clinical use include rifamide, rifabutin, rifapentine, and rifaximin. A short account of the properties of the derivatives at present industrially produced is given in Section VI. Structure–activity relationships among the many hundred semisynthetic rifamycins have been reviewed by Sensi and Lancini (12) and Lancini and Zanichelli (13).

II.   MICROORGANISM PRODUCERS OF RIFAMYCINS AND RELATED COMPOUNDS

As far as is known, all strains industrially used today for rifamycin B production derive from the original *Streptomyces mediterranei* described by Margalith and Beretta (14). Further analysis of the fermentation broth of this organism revealed the presence of two other metabolites, rifamycin Y and rifamycin G (Figure 3). A few other soil isolates producing rifamycin B or O (these two compounds are easily interconverted) have been described, as well as strains producing rifamycin S or SV. Other microorganisms have been reported to produce metabolites closely related to rifamycins; these are the tolypomycins, the halomicins, and the 3-methylthio-rifamycin SV. The structures of these products are reported in Figure 4. The microorganisms naturally producing rifamycins or rifamycin-like compounds are listed in Table 1. Novel rifamycins obtained from mutant or recombinant strains are discussed in Sections IV.C and V.B.

III.   BIOLOGY OF *AMYCOLATOPSIS MEDITERRANEI*

A.   Taxonomy

The original strain, isolated from a soil sample collected near St. Raphael (France) was described by Margalith and Beretta (14). It is a typical actinomycete, producing on solid media an aerial mycelium bearing long chains of spores, somewhat twisted. Spores are

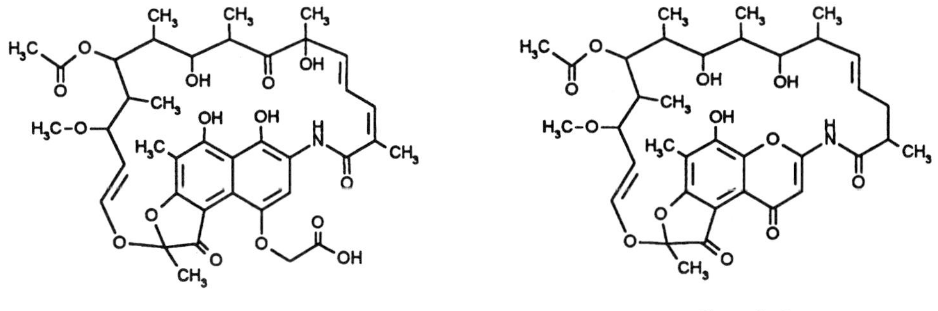

rifamycin Y   rifamycin G

Figure 3   Rifamycin Y and rifamycin G, two inactive metabolites of A. *mediterranei*.

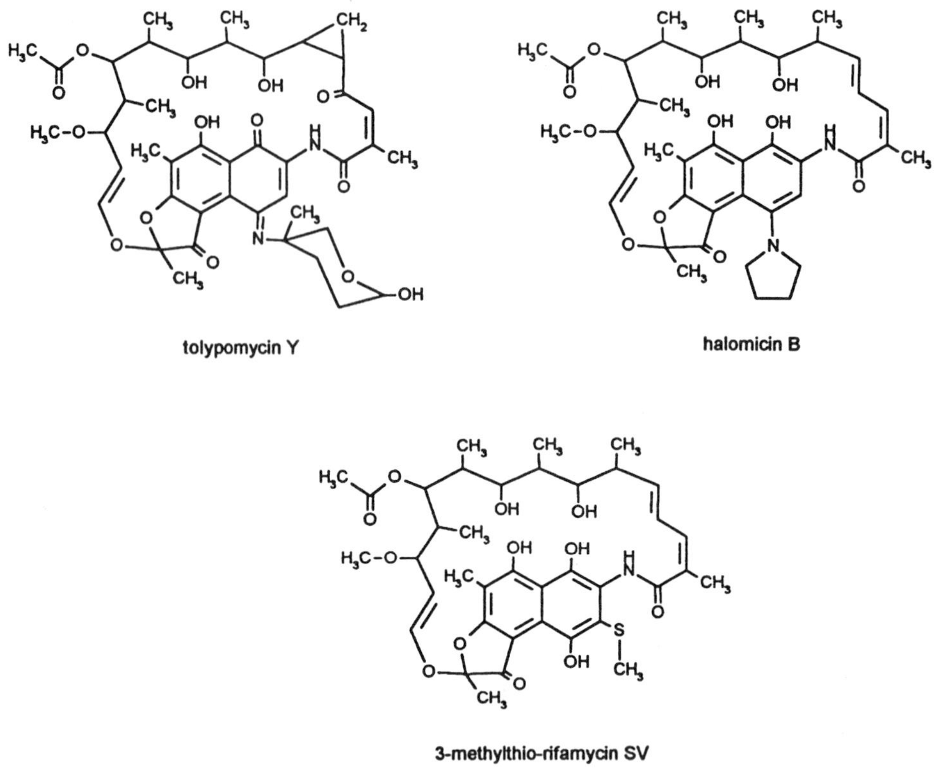

tolypomycin Y

halomicin B

3-methylthio-rifamycin SV

Figure 4   Representative naturally occurring rifamycin-like antibiotics.

Table I   Naturally Occurring Rifamycins and Rifamycin-Like Antibiotics

Producing organism	Product	Ref.
Streptomyces mediterranei[a]	Rifamycins A, B, C, D, and E	1
S. mediterranei[a]	Rifamycin Y	15
Nocardia mediterranea[b]	Rifamycin G	16
Streptomyces 4107 A2	Rifamycins O and B	17
N. mediterranea NT 19	Rifamycin SV	18
Micromonospora lacustris	Rifamycins S, SV, and 3-methylthio-SV	19
Nocardia sp.	Rifamycin B	20
Micromonospora halophytica	Halomicin B	21
	Halomicin A and C	22
Streptomyces tolypophorus	Tolypomycin Y	23
	Rifamycins B and O	24

[a] Renamed as *Nocardia mediterranea* (25) and later as *Amycolatopsis mediterranei* (26).
[b] Renamed as *Amycolatopsis mediterranei*.

nonmotile and ellipsoidal to oblong (0.8–1.0 μm × 3.0–5.0 μm). Colonies are small, compact with a rough surface, and with a yellow to orange color. On the basis of the morphology and the utilization of carbon sources, the authors concluded that it represented a new species of *Streptomyces* and named it *Streptomyces mediterranei*.

The attribution of the organism to the genus *Streptomyces* was later questioned by Thiemann and coworkers (25), who surmised that it could belong to the genus *Nocardia* because of the tendency of the vegetative mycelium to fragment and the scarce presence of aerial mycelium on several media. Analysis of cell wall composition revealed the presence of *meso*-diaminopimelic acid and of arabinose, and the absence of glycine. On this basis, the organism was classified as *Nocardia* and denoted *Nocardia mediterranea*. This name was used for several years in the literature, although some authors preferred the slightly different form *Nocardia mediterranei*.

Further studies on the chemical composition of nocardiae led Lechevalier and coworkers in 1986 to propose two new genera to accommodate nocardioform actinomycetes lacking mycolic acids in their cell wall and not susceptible to typical *Nocardia* phages (26). On this basis the genus *Amycolatopsis* was instituted, to which the rifamycin-producing organism was assigned under the name of *Amycolatopsis mediterranei* (again the form *A. mediterranea* can be sometimes found in the literature). A description of the biochemical properties of the type strain (ATCC 13685 = ISP 5501) is given by the same authors (26).

B. Phage Susceptibility

Clear spots suggesting the presence of actinophages were observed when early A. *mediterranei* strains were grown on agar plates as confluent colonies. Isolation and characterization of the phages was performed by Thiemann and coworkers (27). The first one, denoted phage β, was isolated from lysed cells of the wild-type strain. When a strain resistant to this phage was selected, the presence of infection spots revealed a second phage (phage γ). Three further phages were successively identified (phages 17, 112, and 156), each able to infect a strain resistant to those previously isolated. Since infection can be prevented by addition of calcium-sequestering agents in the culture medium, it was concluded that calcium ions are a necessary cofactor in the infection process.

On the basis of serological characterization, pH stability, and thermal inactivation, phages β, γ, 17, and 112 appear to be mutants deriving from a common ancestor, whereas phage 156 has a different origin. All the phages appear host-specific, since infection was not observed when tested on a number of *Streptomyces* or *Nocardia* strains (28). However, the new taxonomical position of A. *mediterranei* poses the question whether other *Amycolatopsis* species could be sensitive.

The phage-resistant strains did not present any remarkable morphological or biochemical difference from the wild type. However, as described in Section V.C, increased productivity of rifamycin B was associated with phage resistance.

C. Laboratory Media and Culture Conditions

For long-term preservation, early A. *mediterranei* strains were lyophilized and kept in sealed ampoules. At present, the most common method of maintenance is in the form of frozen vegetative mycelium, which avoids the degeneration often observed upon repeated transfers of strains cultured on solid media.

Several media have been proposed for culture on agar surface (29). A suitable minimal medium consists of (g/liter) glucose 10; $(NH_4)_2SO_4$ 2; K_2HPO_4 1; $MgSO_4 \bullet 7H_2O$ 1; $CaCO_3$ 1; NaCl 1; traces of Fe^{2+}, Mn^{2+}, Zn^{2+}; agar 20. As a complete medium, the following can be used (g/liter): yeast extract 4; malt extract 10; glucose 4; agar 20; pH corrected to 7.3 with 1 N KOH. Flask fermentation is usually carried out in two stages. Vegetative cultures are grown in 500 ml flasks containing 100 ml of medium, on rotary shakers at 28°C. As inoculum, a thawed aliquot (2–4 ml/flask) of frozen mycelium is generally used. A suitable medium contains (g/liter) meat extract 5; peptone 5; yeast extract 5; enzymatic hydrolysate of casein 2.5; glucose 20; NaCl 1.5. After incubation for 24–48 hr, the vegetative culture is used to inoculate fermentation cultures, normally also carried out on a rotary shaker in 500 ml flasks but with a reduced volume of the medium (50 or 70 ml), since a high oxygen supply is needed for production. A production medium used in the authors' laboratory consists of (g/liter) glucose 125; propylene glycol 5; $CaCO_3$ 9.5; peanut flour 25; soybean flour 10; $(NH_4)_2SO_4$ 1; $MgSO_4 \bullet 7H_2O$ 1; traces of Fe^{2+}, Cu^{2+}, Zn^{2+}, Mn^{2+}, molybdate. For production of rifamycin B, sodium diethylbarbiturate (1.5–2 g/liter) is required by most strains.

For biochemical or genetic studies, the following minimal medium can be used (g/liter): glucose 90, $(NH_4)_2SO_4$ 15; K_2HPO_4 2; $MgSO_4 \bullet 7H_2O$ 1; $CaCO_3$ 17; trace elements as above.

D.   Genetics

1.   *Mutagenesis*

Generation and selection of mutants played an essential role in the development of strains for industrial production of rifamycins. In addition, auxotrophic mutants and mutants blocked in the rifamycin biosynthetic pathway constituted the basic tools for genetic studies and the elucidation of biosynthetic steps.

Conditions for induction of mutants by exposure to ultraviolet light or by treatment with nitrosoguanidine have been described by Schupp et al. (29). Mycelial suspensions for mutagenic treatment are prepared by shaking samples of a full-grown vegetative culture with quartz pebbles to obtain mycelial fragments about 5 μm long. Ultraviolet irradiation is performed by exposing the suspension of fragmented mycelium to a dose of 600 to 800 ergs/mm², giving a survival of 1.0 to 0.1%. Chemical mutagenesis is performed by treating the mycelium suspended in 0.05 M Tris–maleic acid buffer, pH 9, with 1 mg/ml of nitrosoguanidine for an incubation period of 60 or 120 min.

2.   *Recombination and Linkage Map*

A system of genetic recombination of *A. mediterranei* was described by Schupp, Hütter, and Hopwood in 1975 (29). It was shown that recombination occurs when two marked strains of this microorganism are grown in mixed cultures. Under the conditions used, 1 to 10 recombinants per 10^4 cells of parental genotype were obtained. Because recombinants differing for more than one allele occurred fairly frequently, it was concluded that rather long fragments of the chromosome are transferred, a strong indication that recombination results from a conjugation process. A linkage map was constructed by analyzing the recombination of 14 auxotrophic mutants and 1 streptomycin-resistant strain. The mapping data were combined to give a unique sequence of auxotrophic markers on a circular linkage map. A comparison of this map with the much more complete one of *Streptomyces coelicolor* shows what appears a nonrandom correspondence in the sequence of homologous markers.

Preliminary information on the localization of the genes governing rifamycin production and the use of recombinant strains to produce novel rifamycins are discussed in the following sections.

3. Plasmids

Detection of plasmids possibly present in the standard A. mediterranei ATCC 13685 strain was attempted both by ultracentrifugation of DNA in Cs-ethidium bromide gradient and by selective alkaline denaturation and agarose gel electrophoresis. Both methods gave negative results (30). Evidence that plasmids were not involved in rifamycin production was suggested by the unchanged strain productivity after treatments with curing agents. Moreover, as discussed later, genes controlling some late steps of the antibiotic biosynthesis could be located on the chromosome (31).

It was later found that an extrachromosomal element, denoted pMEA100, was present in an A. mediterranei strain (LBG A3136) closely related to strain ATCC 13685 (32). pMEA100 is a covalently closed circular plasmid of 23.7 kb present in low copy number, which can be isolated only from mycelium grown on agar plates. Whereas it is present in strain LBG A3136 both in the free as well as in the integrated form, in strain ATCC 13685 only an integrated form was detected. Integration in strain LBG A3136 is site-specific, and only one such site was detected in the chromosome (33). The plasmid is self-transmissible, and it is possibly involved in fertility of A. mediterranei.

4. Protoplast Formation and DNA Transformation

Standard procedures for Streptomyces protoplast formation and regeneration were unsuccessfully tried with A. mediterranei. A modified procedure that yields viable protoplasts was developed by Schupp and Divers (34). The primary differences from the standard procedure are in the growth medium, containing a high concentration of mannitol, and in the treatment buffer. The new technique gave satisfactory results when applied to several ansamycin-producing species, although low regeneration yields were observed with some A. mediterranei mutant strains. However, its usefulness appears severely limited, since initial attempts to transform protoplasts with a range of Streptomyces cloning vectors were unsuccessful. More recently, a hybrid plasmid was constructed by cloning a fragment plasmid pA387 (isolated from an Amycolatopsis species) into the Escherichia coli vector pDM10. This hybrid plasmid, termed pRL1, could transform A. mediterranei by electroporation (35).

A different approach to A. mediterranei transformation was investigated by Madon and Hütter (36). They found that intact mycelium of A. mediterranei strain LBG A3136 was transformed with high efficiency in the presence of polyethylene glycol and alkaline cations. Transformation was stimulated by the ionophoric antibiotic valinomycin. A suitable vector, termed pMEA123, was constructed based on the endogenous plasmid pMEA100, into which was placed the erythromycin-resistance gene.

IV. BIOSYNTHESIS OF RIFAMYCINS

A. Origin of the Carbon Skeleton

Preliminary data on the origin of the rifamycins' carbons were obtained by incorporation experiments with ^{14}C- and tritium-labeled precursors. Analysis of the radioactivity of different fragments of the molecule, obtained by chemical degradation, established that pro-

pionate and acetate were incorporated linked head to tail, in agreement with the formation of a polyketide chain (37). However, the data were insufficient to establish the direction of chain growth and which was the chain initiator molecule. The complete precursor alignment was defined by the use of ^{13}C-enriched precursors and nuclear magnetic
resonance (NMR). The study was performed on two intermediates of the biosynthetic
pathway, rifamycin S (38) and rifamycin W (39), rather than on the final product
rifamycin B, since the last does not give a well-defined NMR spectrum. When propionate
^{13}C-labeled in the methyl-group was pulse fed to A. *mediterranei* cultures, semiquantita-
tive analysis of the NMR peak heights of rifamycin S revealed that all seven C-methyls
(two methyls on the aromatic nucleus and five methyls on the ansa) were labeled (38).
With [2-^{13}C]propionate, eight carbons of the ansa chain and of the aromatic moiety of
rifamycin S were enriched. With [carboxy-^{13}C]propionate, again eight carbons were
enriched, all adjacent to a carbon derived from [2-^{13}C]propionate, with the exception of
carbon 29, which was separated from carbon 12 by an oxygen atom. As the only possible
explanation of these results, it was proposed that the polyketide chain is built from eight
propionate units, and that by subsequent modifications, the methyl-group of one of these
is eliminated and the carboxyl and methylene carbon of another unit are split by insertion of an oxygen. Experiments with acetate labeled either in position 1 or 2 revealed the
incorporation of two molecules of this precursor and determined the direction of the
chain growth. All together, the results allowed proposal of the biosynthetic scheme illustrated in Figure 5.

Confirmation that the original polyketide chain comprises eight propionate and
two acetate units was obtained (39) by examining the incorporation of the same precursors into rifamycin W (see Figure 7), an early intermediate in rifamycin B biosynthesis. In
this case, all the intact propionate units were present, the methyl missing in rifamycin S
present as a hydroxymethyl-group (Figure 5).

Further evidence that the chain is built by the usual mechanism of polyketide synthesis was provided by experiments showing that methylmalonate ^{14}C-labeled in the

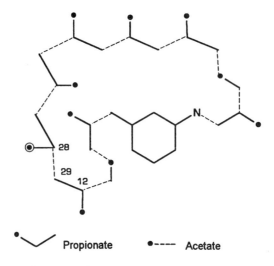

Figure 5 Incorporation of acetate and propionate into rifamycin S and rifamycin W. In rifamycin
S, the circled methyl is missing and the bond between carbon 12 and carbon 29 is interrupted by
the insertion of an oxygen.

methyl-group or [2-^{13}C]malonate gave rifamycin S with the same distribution of labeling as [^{13}C]methyl labeled propionate or acetate, respectively (40).

Seven carbons of the molecule were labeled by neither acetate nor propionate. These appeared to constitute the initiator molecule of the chain. A *meta*-aminobenzoic acid derivative, originating from the aromatic amino acid biosynthetic pathway, was the logical candidate. However, no example of natural *meta*-aminobenzoate was known, and no incorporation was observed when either shikimate or aromatic amino acids were tried as precursors. Nevertheless, the origin of this C$_7$N unit could be established with experiments using as precursors [1-^{13}C]glucose or [1-^{13}C]glycerate (41). The former selectively labeled carbons 1 and 10 of the rifamycin S naphthalene ring, the latter carbons 3 and 8, in full agreement with the origin of the C$_7$N units from cyclization of a product having the carbon skeleton of 3-deoxyheptulosonic acid, the precursor of all aromatic amino acids.

B. Origin of the Chain Initiator Molecule

Experiments with labeled precursors demonstrate that the chain initiator molecule, a C$_7$N unit, is derived from a biosynthetic pathway analogous to that of aromatic amino acids. The product was later identified as 3-amino-5-hydroxybenzoic acid (AHBA) by experiments showing that this compound, in contrast to several other benzoic acid derivatives, restored rifamycin production in a strain blocked in the first step of aromatic amino acids biosynthesis (42). Experiments with auxotrophic mutants blocked in different steps of aromatic amino acids biosynthesis indicated that the rifamycin and aromatic pathways diverged at a step prior to phosphorylation of shikimate (43,44). The problem was recently tackled by Floss and coworkers, who proposed the pathway depicted in Figure 6 for the synthesis of AHBA (45). The basic hypothesis is that 4-deoxy-4-amino-3-deoxy-D-arabinoheptulosonic acid (aminoDAHP) is formed, instead of 3-deoxy-D-arabinoheptulosonic acid (DAHP), by participation of glutamine in the reaction by which

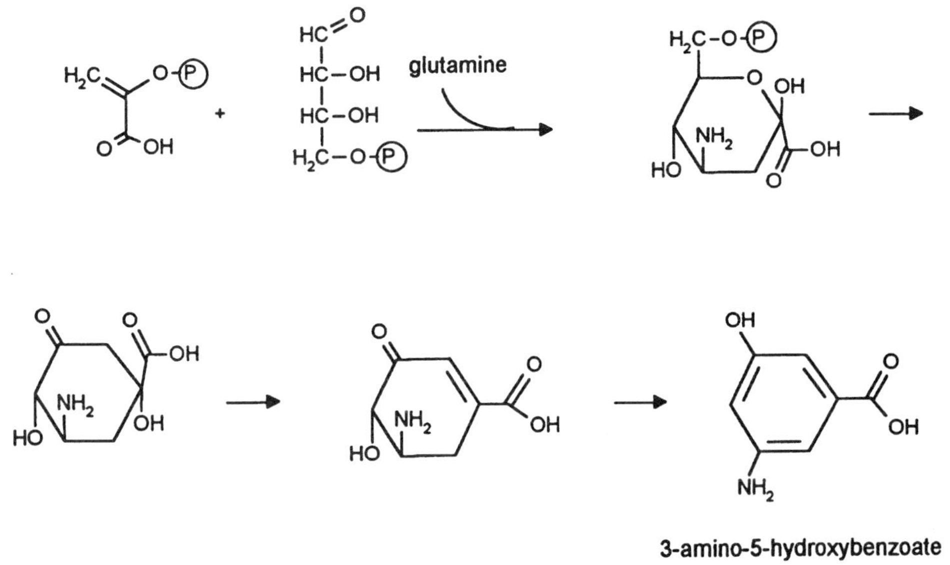

3-amino-5-hydroxybenzoate

Figure 6 Origin of 3-amino-5-hydroxybenzoate, the chain initiator molecule in rifamycin biosynthesis.

phosphoenolpyruvate is condensed with erythrose-4-phosphate to give rise, in primary metabolism, to DAHP. Cyclization of aminoDAHP would then produce the amino analog of dehydroquinic acid, subsequently transformed into AHBA through the intermediate amino-dehydroshikimate. Evidence supporting the validity of this proposal was obtained by synthesizing all these intermediates and showing that they were converted into AHBA by cell-free extracts of *A. mediterranei*. In addition, it was shown that radioactive aminoDAHP could be obtained from radioactive PEP or erythrose-4-phosphate, but not from radioactive DAHP (46).

C.   The Biosynthetic Pathway of Rifamycin B

Combining the results obtained in the Lepetit and Ciba laboratories, it is now possible to depict the pathway leading to the synthesis of rifamycin B, illustrated in Figure 7 (47,48). The earliest identified intermediate in the biosynthesis is protorifamycin I, which was isolated from a blocked mutant and was shown to be a precursor of other intermediates (49). All the subsequent intermediates were also isolated from blocked mutants. The sequence in which each of these is converted into its successor has been mainly established on logical grounds. It appears thus that rifamycin W (39), which derives from protorifamycin I by addition of a hydroxyl-group in position 8, is step-wise oxidized, the hydroxymethyl-group 34 being converted to an aldehyde and then to a carboxyl-group. Evidence for this conversion is the isolation of rifamycin W hemiacetal (50), in which the aldehyde 34 forms an internal hemiacetal with the hydroxyl in position 25, and rifamycin Z (51), in which the carboxyl-group forms a lactone ring with the same hydroxyl. It is not known whether the open or the closed forms or these compounds are the real intermediates. The next intermediate identified is 27-O-demethyl-25-O-deacetylrifamycin S (52,53), the first microbiologically active product of the pathway. Transformation of rifamycin Z into this product involves the elimination of the carbonyl-group 34, the insertion of an oxygen between carbons 12 and 29, and the closure of the furane ring. The order of these reaction is not known; they may occur at the same time. Finally, rifamycin S is made by acetylation at O25 and methylation at O27. It should be noted that rifamycin S and rifamycin SV are easily interconverted, and therefore the isolation of the oxidized (as rifamycin S) or reduced form (as rifamycin SV) of an intermediate depends only on the reducing or oxidizing properties of the isolation medium. The origin of rifamycin B from rifamycin S (or SV) has been demonstrated by several experiments (54,55), and a blocked mutant accumulating rifamycin SV has been obtained from a rifamycin B producer (56).

D.   Further Products of Rifamycin S Transformation

When the original *A. mediterranei* strain is cultured without addition of barbiturate to the medium, rifamycins A, C, D, and E (the so-called rifamycin complex) are produced, together with small amounts of rifamycin B. The chemistry and the biosynthesis of these compounds have never been properly investigated. However, cosynthesis experiments, in which a mutant blocked in an early step of the biosynthesis was grown together with a rifamycin S–producing strain, demonstrated that the members of rifamycin complex are transformation products of rifamycin S (47).

In addition to the rifamycin complex, two other products, rifamycin G and rifamycin Y, are produced. These were not originally noticed, being microbiologically

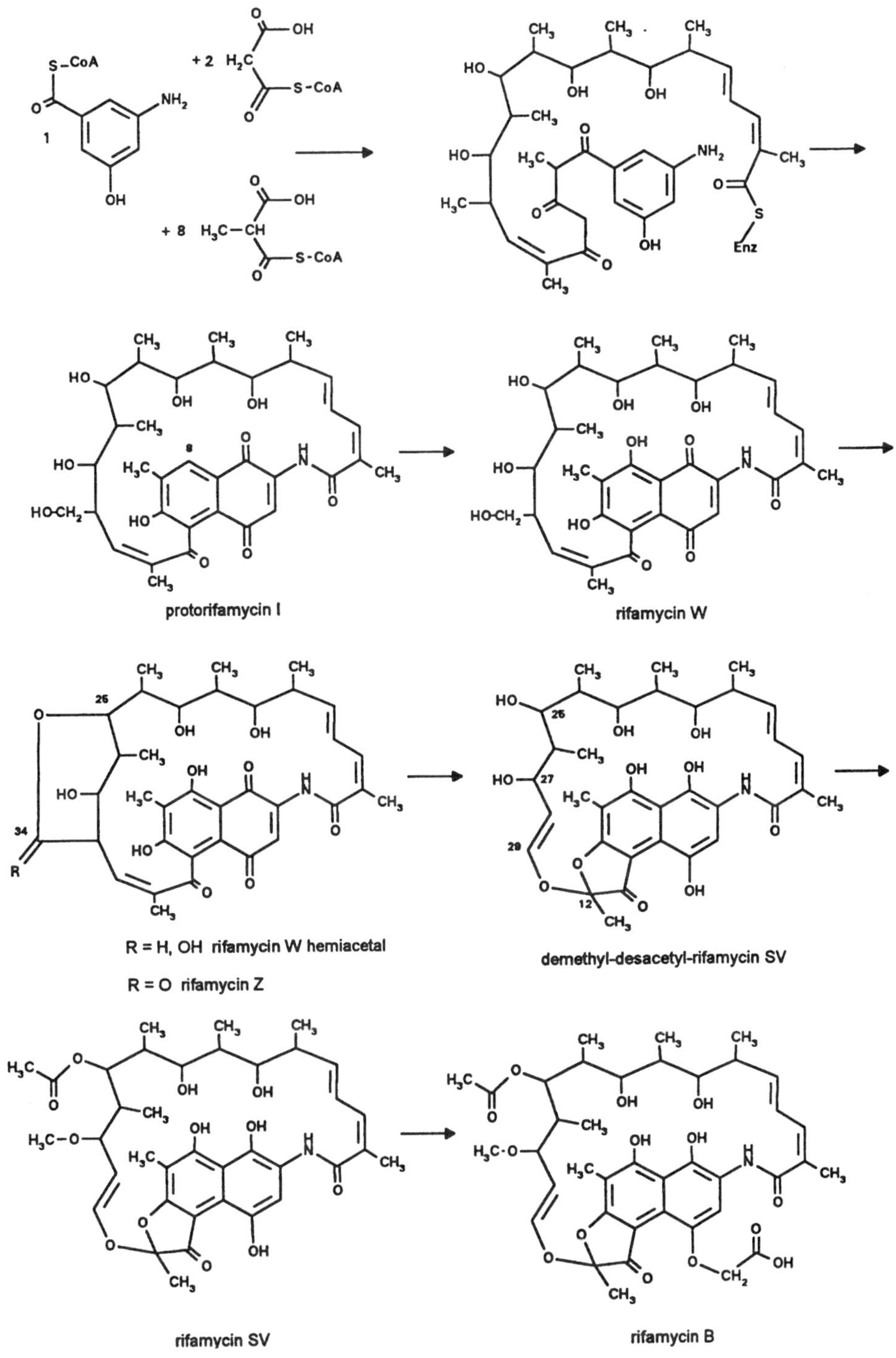

Figure 7 Main steps of rifamycin B biosynthesis.

inactive. Rifamycin G (Figure 3) derives from rifamycin S by substitution of carbon 1 of the latter with an oxygen atom (16). Rifamycin Y (Figure 3) is a product of further oxidation of the rifamycin B ansa chain. It was shown that, in fermentations with early strains, the ratio of rifamycin Y to rifamycin B produced depended on the phosphate concentration in the culture medium (15). High-producing industrial strains at present produce negligible amounts of this derivative.

When cultures of rifamycin S–producing mutants are prolonged beyond the maximum production yields, several transformation products are formed, namely, rifamycin R and the thiazorifamycins P, Q, and Verde (Figure 8). Rifamycin R results from hydroxylation of methyl 30 of rifamycin SV and, thus, is 30-hydroxyrifamycin SV (57). The thiazorifamycins derive from condensation of cysteine with rifamycin S, with formation of an unstable thiazinorifamycin that spontaneously rearranges into the thiazorifamycins (58,59).

E.   The Conversion of Rifamycin S into Rifamycin B and the Role of Barbiturates

A most unusual aspect of A. *mediterranei* fermentation is the drastic change in antibiotic production when diethylbarbituric acid (barbital) is added to the fermentation medium. As observed by Margalith and Pagani (2,3), under these conditions, production of rifamycin A, C, D, and E is reduced to negligible amounts whereas production of rifamycin B is substantially enhanced. The best results were obtained with a concentration of 2 g/liter of barbital, added at the beginning of the fermentation. Several other barbiturates and related compounds were tested. A few of these enhanced production of

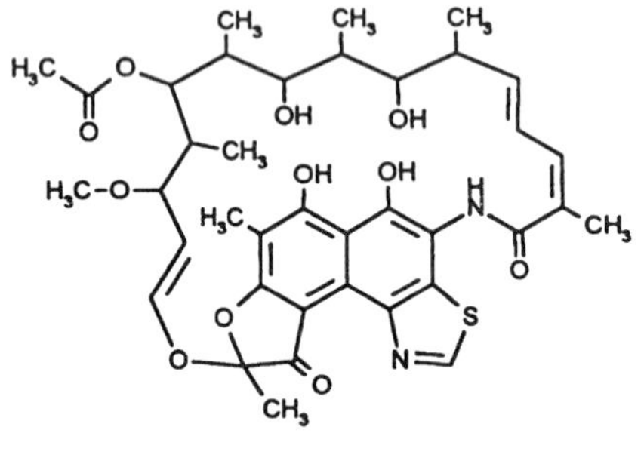

rifamycin P

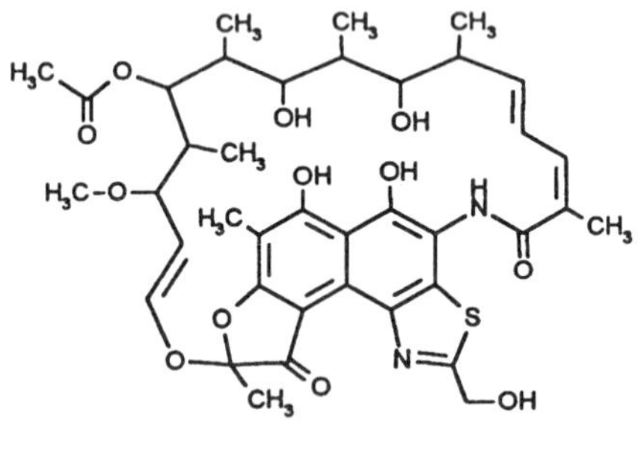

rifamycin Q

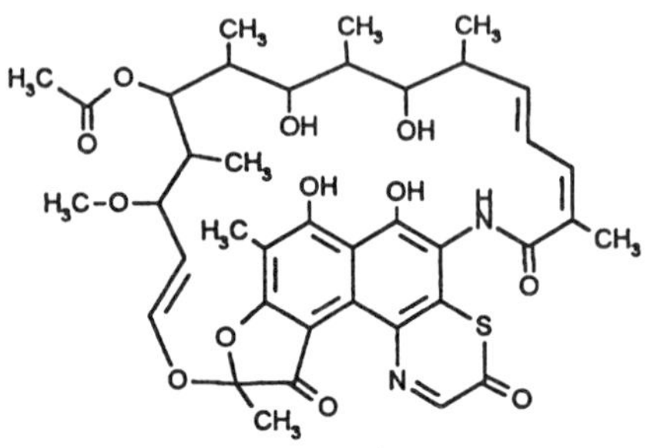

rifamycin verde

Figure 8   Biologically active rifamycins produced by a mutant strain of A. *mediterranei*.

rifamycin B, but none was as effective as barbital. The possibility that barbital could be a specific precursor of rifamycin B was ruled out by adding to the cultures barbital labeled with ^{14}C at different positions of the ring or of the ethyl chains. No radioactivity was detected in rifamycin B. About 10% of the effector was metabolized to metabolically inactive compounds (60). Subsequent studies determined that the biosynthetic step affected by barbital is the conversion of rifamycin SV into rifamycin B (Figure 7). The yields of rifamycin SV in cultures of blocked mutants accumulating this antibiotic are not influenced by barbital, whereas the conversion yield of rifamycin SV into rifamycin B by washed mycelium of A. *mediterranei* is substantially increased by the presence of 2 g/liter of barbital in the growth and incubation media (54,61).

All together, the available data indicate that barbital acts by enhancing the conversion of rifamycin SV to rifamycin B. Since a consistent effect is observed only when barbital is present since the beginning of the culture, it appears that synthesis of one or more enzymes involved, rather than their activity, is affected. It is possible that, on the contrary, barbital inhibits the synthesis or the activity of an enzyme involved in conversion of rifamycin SV into rifamycins A, C, D, and E. However, the observation (16) that the conversion of rifamycin SV into rifamycin G by resuspended mycelium of A. *mediterranei* is not affected by barbital, but no rifamycin G is produced in fermentations with barbital added, gives little credit to this last interpretation.

The conversion of rifamycin SV to rifamycin B can be formally seen as the condensation of a glycolic moiety to the oxygen in position 4 of the former. However, none of the two-carbon compounds tested (^{14}C-labeled glycolic acid, acetic acid, glycine, and so forth) was incorporated into the glycolic moiety of rifamycin B. Of the three-carbon compounds tested, [^{14}C]glycerol was incorporated to a fair extent, whereas no radioactivity from [^{14}C]pyruvate was detected. Experiments with sugars specifically labeled in the different atoms demonstrated that the methylene carbon derives from carbon 1 or 6 and the carboxyl carbon from carbon 2 of glucose, respectively (55). All together, these data suggest that the immediate precursor of the glycolic moiety is a three-carbon molecule, either an intermediate of glycolysis between glyceraldehyde-3-phosphate and phosphoenolpyruvate or a related product. 3-Phosphohydroxypyruvic acid appears as the logical candidate, since the phosphate bond can provide the energy for the condensation with rifamycin SV and the final product can then be easily formed by oxidative decarboxylation.

F.   Regulation of Production

Very little is known of the factors that control rifamycin B biosynthesis. In contrast with what is observed with several antibiotics, production of rifamycin B is not depressed by 2 g/liter of KH_2PO_4 and relatively good yields are obtained in minimal medium containing high concentrations of ammonium ions. Carbon catabolite repression seems also absent, in view of the high concentration of glucose used in high-producing media. However, interpretation of these observations is not simple, since the maximum rate of production is achieved after the levels of these nutrients have been substantially reduced by the initial rapid growth phase. Studies with synthetic media showed that the highest yields were obtained when proline, a typically slowly metabolized amino acid, was partially substituting for ammonium ions.

A regulator factor able to induce the synthesis of rifamycin B in a nonproducing mutant of A. *mediterranei* was isolated from yeast extracts (20). It was named B factor and identified as 3′-(1-butylphosphoryl) adenosine. B factor appears to regulate the production of the rifamycin precursor 3-amino-5-hydroxybenzoic acid, since addition of the latter to the blocked mutant restores production in the absence of the factor. Although originally found in yeasts, B factor was subsequently detected in a producing *Amycolatopsis* strain and, therefore, can be considered as true autoregulator (62,63).

Studies on the production of rifamycin SV by a mutant strain of A. *mediterranei* revealed that, in contrast to rifamycin B, this metabolite inhibits its own synthesis, as well as the growth of the producing organism. The inhibitory effect is not limited to inhibition of the producer RNA polymerase (30).

Possible regulatory mechanisms for rifamycin SV production were investigated by a group of Chinese researchers. These authors observed a stimulation of rifamycin SV yields when nitrates were added to cultures of a *Nocardia* strain producer of this metabolite. It was noticed that production was increased at the expense of lipids (64). However, it appears that this effect is strain-specific, since different results were obtained with a Ciba rifamycin SV–producing strain (30). Further studies indicate an essential role of glutamine synthetase in rifamycin SV biosynthesis, and in fact, high-producing strains were obtained by selecting mutants resistant to glutamylhydrazide, an antagonist of glutamine (64,65).

V. GENETICS OF RIFAMYCIN PRODUCTION

A. Gene Mapping and Cloning

The availability of mutants blocked at various steps of rifamycin biosynthesis allowed the localization of the corresponding genes on the genetic map (31). Analysis of the frequency of recombination between strains carrying both the biosynthetic mutation and other markers revealed that the genes governing the conversion of protorifamycin I into rifamycin W, the conversion of the latter into rifamycin S, and the conversion of rifamycin S into rifamycin B were clustered in a restricted region of the chromosome, between *pro*1 and *str*2. Two *aro*- mutations, believed to constitute the linkage between the primary and the secondary metabolism, mapped in different regions (Figure 9).

The last step in the synthesis of 3-amino-5-hydroxybenzoic acid (AHBA) is the conversion of 5-deoxy-5-amino-dehydroshikimate into AHBA. The gene governing the synthesis of the enzyme catalyzing this reaction (AHBA synthase) has been cloned into and expressed in E. *coli*. The deduced sequence of the enzyme presents homology with a number of pyridoxine-dependent enzymes, and in fact, it was found that it contains a molecule of pyridoxal phosphate in a Schiff-base linkage. It is interesting to note that the gene is flanked by other genes possibly involved in rifamycin biosynthesis, in particular, a gene related to that of erythromycin polyketide synthase (46).

It is not known at present whether these genes map in the same chromosomal region as the previously localized biosynthetic genes.

B. Rifamycin Production by Recombinant Strains

We have seen that by mutagenic treatment one could easily obtain strains accumulating intermediates or novel final products of the biosynthetic pathway. Other novel rifamycins were obtained exploiting the high frequency at which recombinant strains are produced by the conjugation process (transconjugants is a more appropriate term for these strains, since the parental strains are of the same species) (66). From the parental strain, A. *mediterranei* ATCC 13685, a high rifamycin B producer, strain FS 713 was obtained by mutagenic treatment. From this strain a blocked mutant (strain T 191) was then selected,

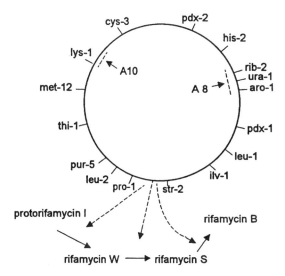

Figure 9 Linkage map of A. *mediterranei*. The genes governing the conversion of protorifamycin I, the earliest identified intermediate, into rifamycin B are located between *str2* and *pro*1. A8 and A10 indicate the location of two genes of the shikimate pathway. The former is involved in the biosynthesis of 3-amino-5-hydroxybenzoate.

which accumulated rifamycin W. A multimarked strain denoted T 104, having an adequate level of rifamycin B productivity, was constructed by crossing a strain carrying a number of selection markers with a high rifamycin B producer. From the parental strains T 191 and T 104 the recombinant strain R 21 was isolated, which produced, besides the common rifamycins B, O, and S, rifamycins W and P, previously isolated from mutant strains, and the new rifamycins 3-hydroxyrifamycin S, 3,31-hydroxyrifamycin S, 16,17-dehydrorifamycin G, rifamycin W lactone, rifamycin W hemiacetal, 30-hydroxyrifamycin W, and 28-dehydromethyl-28,30-dihydroxyrifamycin W (66).

C.   Strain Improvement

Early attempts at strain improvement were aimed at increasing the yields of rifamycin complex. By mutagenic treatment with $MgCl_2$ and random selection, a mutant, ME 83/973, was obtained that produced in flask fermentation a significant increase of fractions C and D of rifamycin complex, or in the presence of barbital, about 500 mg/liter of rifamycin B (2). Among the phage-resistant variants of this strain, a clone producing 660 mg/liter of the antibiotic was selected. Successive isolation of mutants resistant to new phage infections resulted in further yield increases, as shown in Figure 10. No rational explanation was found for this phenomenon. The strains showing higher productivity were practically undistinguishable from the parent strain in their morphological and biochemical properties; however, they often were less stable (28).

Subsequent strain improvement was based on mutagenic treatment and selection. A strain (ATCC 13685) was reported producing, in a suitable medium, 2.2 g/liter (67). A patent issued in 1972 described a strain of *Streptomyces albovinaceous* (ATCC 12951) that gave 4.0–4.5 g/liter of rifamycin B (68), and later, in patent literature (69), yields up to 7 g/liter were reported, resulting from the combination of strain selection and improvement of fermentation conditions. There is no doubt that at present the productivity of

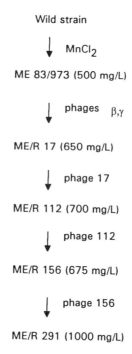

Wild strain

↓ MnCl$_2$

ME 83/973 (500 mg/L)

↓ phages β,γ

ME/R 17 (650 mg/L)

↓ phage 17

ME/R 112 (700 mg/L)

↓ phage 112

ME/R 156 (675 mg/L)

↓ phage 156

ME/R 291 (1000 mg/L)

Figure 10   Step-wise rifamycin yield increase upon selection of phage-resistant strains.

industrial strains is much higher, but the actual values are considered a trade secret and as such are not disclosed.

Yield increase is not the only aim of strain improvement. Isolation of genetically stable strains is one objective of the development work. Strains have also been sought showing lower viscosity, or higher rate of production to reduce the fermentation time and the energy requirement. An interesting result was also the isolation of a mutant strain (ATCC 21789) (selected after treatment with nitrosoguanidine of strain ATCC 13685) producing about 2 g/liter of rifamycin B both in the presence and in the absence of barbiturates in the fermentation medium (67).

Rifamycin B must be converted into rifamycin S for the synthesis of rifampicin. When it was discovered that rifamycin S (or SV) is the last intermediate in rifamycin B biosynthesis, it appeared convenient to isolate a blocked mutant directly producing the former in fermentation. Such a strain (ATCC 21271) was in fact obtained by mutagenic treatment of strain ATCC 13865 and a selection screening based on the different antimicrobial activity of the two products (56). However, improvement of rifamycin SV productivity remained very difficult, and, as far as it is known, industrial production is mainly based on rifamycin B.

VI.   PRODUCTION OF RIFAMYCINS

The state of the art was extensively presented, 10 years after the discovery of rifamycins, by Sensi and Thiemann in their 1967 review (70). These authors carefully examined the significant parameters that govern the fermentation process, such as the composition of some vegetative media, the effect of barbiturates, the composition of complex and synthetic media (effects of inorganic and combined nitrogen sources, vegetative oil addition, and microelements), and the influence of the temperature and aeration patterns. At that time, the maximum yield attained in laboratory experiments was about 1 g/liter, a result obtained mainly by strain improvement. Since then, more than 50 patents have been granted on natural rifamycin production, dealing with new producing strains, methods of fermentation, recovery, and purification. Here we comment on the most relevant advances.

A. Fermentation Media

Industrial producing strains are the result of time-consuming, expensive research. For each new high-producing strain, the medium and the other fermentation parameters must be adjusted to allow the maximal expression of the producing capacity. It is obvious that this kind of information is strictly confidential, and for rifamycin the composition of the media actually used for industrial production is also not known. However, some information can be extrapolated from published laboratory data and patent literature that gives a fairly good idea of the most suitable ingredients and their concentrations.

One medium (designated medium 151b) has been described by Ghisalba et al. (49) that contains (g/liter) glucose 70; glycerol 20; meat meal 30; soybean meal 10; $CaCO_3$ 8; $(NH_4)_2SO_4$ 3; KH_2PO_4 1; trace amounts of Fe^{2+}, Cu^{2+}, Zn^{2+}, Mn^{2+}, Co^{2+}, and $Mo_7O_{24}^{2-}$. This medium differs from those reported by Sensi and Thiemann (70) for the industrial production of rifamycin B mainly in the presence of glycerol as a carbon source.

According to a patent of 1978 (71), addition of 0.2% of n-amyl alcohol to the fermentation medium increased by 2–4 times the yield of rifamycin B (which, however, with the strain used was only 0.7 g/liter). A medium claimed by Sokol and coworkers in a 1982 patent (69) to produce 6 to 7 g/liter of rifamycin B contains (g/liter) peanut meal 25; soybean meal 10; $(NH_4)_2SO_4$ 10; propyleneglycol 5; glucose 110. Glycerol (60 g/liter) was added to the fermentation when the glucose level decreased below 5% of the initial concentration.

The media for rifamycin SV production appear to have similar composition. In the original patent on rifamycin SV production by a mutant strain of *Nocardia mediterranea* (72), yields of about 2 g/liter are reported with a medium containing as carbon sources (g/liter) glucose, 95; glycerol, 40; and propyleneglycol, 5; and peanut meal, soybean meal, and ammonium ions as nitrogen sources.

B. Fermentation Conditions

The optimal fermentation conditions are also related to the strain used and are generally not disclosed in detail by industry. Again, reasonable assumptions may be made based on laboratory and patent data.

I. Temperature

The optimal temperature reported for rifamycin B is 28°C. The effect of variations of the temperature during the fermentation was discussed by Sensi and Thiemann (70). Shifting after 18 hr of fermentation from 28 to 24°C increased the final yields. However, the strain used at that time is certainly different from those used at present, and the authors stated that the effect noted above was strain-specific.

It has been shown that lowering the temperature decreases the rate of glucose consumption. It has often been observed that a lower rate of carbon metabolism results in higher antibiotic production.

2. Aeration and Agitation

A characteristic of A. *mediterranei* fermentations is the very high oxygen requirement in a definite period of the growth–production cycle. The time at which this occurs varies with the strain and the medium composition, but it always coincides with the phase in which glucose is rapidly metabolized. If this demand is not met by an adequate oxygen supply through aeration, very low final yields of rifamycin B are obtained.

The effect of the rate of air supply and the influence of the mechanical and geometric characteristics of the stirring system were investigated by Virgilio et al. (73). An air flow ranging from 0.8 to 1.5 liter/liter/min was found necessary, but it is suggested that this may be reduced in the noncritical phase.

A power input to the stirrer above 3 W/liter was also necessary to satisfy the demand in all phases. Nevertheless, this could be reduced to 1.25 W/liter when turbine impellers of a smaller diameter were used. This can be interpreted taking into account that, at a given power input, the rotational speed is higher when a smaller impeller is used. This results in the formation of smaller bubbles of the flowing air and, thus, a higher rate of oxygen dissolution.

A Polish patent (74) claims that, in rifamycin B production, by decreasing the stirrer circumference speed from 260–310 to 100–20 m/min during vegetative culture and to 160–90 m/min in the production phase, it is possible to prevent mycelium fragmentation and pH drop, to retard sugar consumption, and to decrease the mycelial mass. This leads to a consistent increase of the antibiotic yield.

In several reports and patent disclosures, an air flow of 1 liter/liter/min and a pressure of 0.2 bar is given for fermentation carried out at pilot scale.

C. Reactors

As far as the authors know, industrial fermentations are carried out in conventional bioreactors of 20 to 100 m³ of volume. As usual, these are equipped with turbine stirrers, baffles, air ring spargers, and heating–cooling systems. Computerized apparatuses are used both for in-line monitoring and control of temperature, air flow, dissolved oxygen, and pH and for recording these parameters. In the smaller fermentors, the heating systems is used for *in situ* sterilization. In the larger ones, the medium is conveyed to the fermentors through a flash sterilization system, in which it is heated at 140°C for a few minutes. It seems that little attention has been paid to the bioreactor design. A limited study with an airlift system did not indicate any yield improvement or economic advantage (30). Continuous production of rifamycin B has been investigated using A. *mediterranei* ATCC 21789 immobilized in a dual hollow-fiber bioreactor designed for cultivating aerobic cells. Chung et al. reported (75) production of rifamycin B for at least 50 days continuously with a 22-fold production increase over the batch system when air was used for aeration, and a 30-fold increase with pure oxygen.

D. Fermentation Metabolic Pattern

Rifamycin fermentation appears to be typically monophasic, as reported by many authors. In fact, glucose consumption, mycelial growth, and antibiotic production occur almost at the same time. In the complex media used for industrial production, a consistent lag of about 48 hr is observed before the beginning of the logarithmic growth phase and the appearance of a detectable amount of antibiotic (Figure 11).

A similar delay is observed on a laboratory scale when high-production complex media are used, whereas with less-concentrated chemically defined media the lag phase is shorter. It has been assumed that the growth and production delay is due to the osmotic pressure that arises from the high concentration of glucose and other soluble nutrients. The glucose consumption, initially slow, becomes very fast when mycelium growth starts, and so does nitrogen consumption. At this point, the oxygen demand is highest. The typical pattern of pH variation was reported by Sensi and Thiemann (70). There is an

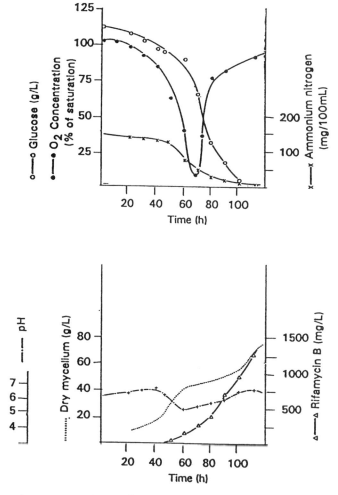

Figure 11 Typical time course of A. *mediterranei* fermentation in an industrial medium.

initial rise from 6.2–6.4 to 6.6–6.7, followed by a sharp decrease to 5.5–5.7 coinciding with the strong metabolic activity phase. Then, the pH rises slowly again until the end of the fermentation.

Continuous pH control of fermentation indicates that the optimal pH range for rifamycin production is 6.2 to 6.4. The presence of $CaCO_3$ in most fermentation media prevents an excessive lowering of the pH value.

The standard duration of early industrial fermentations was about 120 hr. Attempts at extending the production phase by glucose addition were unsuccessful. However, it was later reported that the fermentation can last up to 300 hr by maintaining the pH range between 6.0 and 6.5, and adding batch-wise or continuously carbon and nitrogen sources (30).

With the industrial strains used nowadays, the production of rifamycin Y is negligible, irrespective of the phosphate concentration. The barbiturate may still be needed, in lower amounts, depending on the strain used and the medium composition.

E. Analytical Methods

The main physicochemical properties useful for identification and quantitation of rifamycin B, the final product of industrial fermentation, and of rifamycin SV, which might also be an industrial fermentation product, are listed in Table 2. Some characteristics of rifamycin O and S, the two compounds derived by oxidation of rifamycin B and SV, respectively, are also presented.

Rifamycin B has two acidic functions. As a free acid, it is insoluble in water and moderately soluble in many organic solvents. The disodium salt is freely water-soluble. Rifamycin O and rifamycin S are weak acids, whereas rifamycin SV is strongly acidic.

The analytical methods used for determining the rifamycins concentration in fermentation broth or in the solutions during the extraction process, to monitor the transformation steps and to check the final products, are principally spectrophotometric or chromatographic assays and microbiological assays. Other analytical techniques, such as

Table 2   Physicochemical Properties of Relevant Natural Rifamycins

Compound	Formula	Molecular weight	Melting point, °C	Crystals (solvent)	pK_a	Ultraviolet and visible λ_{max}, nm ($E_{1\,cm}1\%$)	Ref.
Rifamycin B	$C_{39}H_{49}O_{14}N$	755.80	160–164 dec.	Yellow needles (ethyl acetate)	2.5,6.7	223,304,425a (555,275,220)	76
Rifamycin O	$C_{39}H_{47}O_{14}N$	753.79	160 dec.	Pale yellow needles (methanol)	7.9	226,273,370b (365,440,60)	77
Rifamycin S	$C_{37}H_{45}O_{12}N$	695.75	180–182	Orange-yellow (methanol)	7.2	224,317,525c (478,436,68)	10
Rifamycin SV	$C_{37}H_{47}O_{12}N$	697.77	140 dec.	Yellow powder (benzene)d	1.8	223,314,445a (586,322,204)	10

aPhosphate buffer, pH 7.3.
bPhosphate buffer, pH 4.62.
cPhosphate buffer, pH 8.04.
dThe sodium salt is obtained from aqueous solutions (red-orange crystals).

fluorimetric, amperometric, and polarographic methods, have been described (70). Undoubtedly, in several laboratories, rifamycin production during the fermentation and purity in the downstream process are analytically followed by high-performance liquid chromatography (HPLC) methods, but to our knowledge no report on this technique has been published.

For practical purposes, rifamycin B titer in broths and extracts is determined spectrophotometrically. Suitable samples are prepared by extracting the antibiotic from the acidified filtered broth with ethyl acetate and reextracting it into phosphate buffer pH 7.38. Maximal light absorption is read at 425 nm (78).

A more direct method consists of reading the absorption of a sample of the broth diluted with acetate buffer, pH 4.3, against an identical sample diluted with the same buffer containing 0.1% w/v of $NaNO_2$. Nitrous acid oxidizes rifamycin B to rifamycin O, and thus a spectrophotometric determination can be made in which the differential $E_{1\ cm}^{1\%}$ value is 215 at 425 nm (79). For the determination of rifamycin SV, similar methods have been described. The differential absorption between the reduced and oxidized form is $E_{1\ cm}^{1\%} = 156$ at 447 nm (79). These methods can be easily adapted to continuous analyzer systems.

Microbiological methods employ the paper disc–plate assay. For rifamycin B, *Staphylococcus aureus* ATCC 6538 is used as the test microorganism. The agar medium is buffered at pH 5.0, since a low pH enhances the sensitivity of the test, favoring the transformation of the inactive rifamycin B into rifamycins O and S. The dose–response curve is applicable over the range of 0.1–1 µg/ml (80).

For determining rifamycin SV, the preferred test microorganisms are either *Bacillus subtilis* ATCC 6636, which gives a useful dose–response curve from 2 to 12 µg/ml, or *Sarcina lutea*, which is more sensitive and gives a dose–response curve from 0.05 to 0.6 µg/ml.

A simple and very useful technique for identification of rifamycins and for a rapid estimation of their purity is thin-layer chromatography. We report here two convenient systems:

1. Plate: silica gel Merck F254 pretreated with citric acid; solvent methylene chloride–methanol 95:5 (81). R_f values: Rifamycin S = 0.58–0.62; Rifamycin SV = 0.40–0.41; Rifamycin B = 0.24–0.28.
2. Plate: silica gel Merck F254; solvent acetone (unpublished). R_f values: Rifamycin S = 0.72–0.73; Rifamycin O = 0.75–0.76; Rifamycin SV = 0.84–0.86; Rifamycin B = 0.58–0.62.

F. Recovery and Purification

The methods for recovery and purification of rifamycin B employed in the first industrial productions have been described in some detail by Sensi and Thiemann (70). The fermentation broth is filtered at pH 7.5–8.0, and then the antibiotic is extracted with chloroform after acidification to pH 2.0 (although rifamycin B is poorly soluble in this solvent, it is used because it allowed the elimination of most of the barbiturates, which remain largely in the exhaust broth). Rifamycin B is extracted from chloroform into an aqueous solution of phosphate buffer, pH about 7.5, from which it is reextracted into chloroform or into ethyl acetate after acidification to pH 2.0 with sulfuric acid. Upon concentration, the product crystallizes.

To prepare rifamycin S, the solution in the organic solvent is extracted again with phosphate buffer, pH 8.0, and sodium persulfate is added. Thus, rifamycin B is oxidized to rifamycin O, which being insoluble in water precipitates and is collected by filtration. The panel is dissolved in tetrahydrofuran, and rifamycin O is hydrolyzed to rifamycin S with sulfuric acid. Water is then added, and rifamycin S is extracted with chloroform. Upon addition of ethanol and concentration under vacuum, rifamycin S crystallizes and is collected by filtration at a high degree of purity.

Rifamycin S is reduced to rifamycin SV by adding to a methanolic solution an aqueous solution of sodium ascorbate. The solution of rifamycin SV is cleared by filtration, and the sodium salt crystallizes after addition of sodium phosphate solution to pH 7.3.

A laboratory-scale procedure to obtain rifamycin SV from cultures of strains producing rifamycin S consists of adding ascorbic acid to the fermentation broth. The filtrate is acidified to pH 3 and extracted with ethyl acetate. After evaporation of the solvent, the crude product is absorbed on a silica gel column and eluted with acetone. Fractions containing pure rifamycin SV are combined, and the product can be obtained either as a free acid or its sodium salt (56).

The higher concentrations of antibiotic in fermentation broths later obtained allowed simplified procedures of recovery and purification. For example, a filtered broth containing 2.45 g/liter of rifamycin B at alkaline pH was oxidized with a water solution of sodium nitrite. After careful acidification with 10% sulfuric acid, rifamycin O precipitated and was collected by filtration. A 96% yield of the product at 85% purity was obtained (82).

A survey of the literature reveals some interesting features. Technical improvements have been devised for the recovery step. A controlled separation of the chloroform phase by laminar flow of mother solution has been described (83). The use of basic macroreticular ion exchangers, such as cross-linked styrene–divinylbenzene resins, is suggested in a patent for the recovery of both rifamycin B and rifamycin S from aqueous, organic, or mixed solutions (84). A specific desorbant chloroform:methanol:acetic acid:water (84:9.5:5.6:0.9) allows a 85% recovery of rifamycin B from a 0.1% chloroform solution. Direct extraction of rifamycins from fermentation broth by the use of an N-8-14C alkyl lactim is cited in a 1986 patent (85).

Rifamycin SV present in fermentation broths can be oxidized in a >90% yield to the more stable and easily crystallized rifamycin S by aeration of the culture at 60–70°C, after adjusting the pH to 2–3 and the osmotic pressure with an pharmacologically acceptable salt (86).

A critical step in the production of rifamycin S is its transformation from rifamycin B. Essentially, the hydrolysis of rifamycin O presents some disadvantages, such as the strong acidic conditions required (and, as a consequence, expensive acid-resistant equipment), heavy foam formation, and relatively low yields. This stimulated the interest of many research and industrial groups in the development of biochemical transformations using cells and enzymes. A review on this subject by Banerjee et al. (87) also summarizes the knowledge on the biotransformation of rifamycins. Han et al. (88) isolated in 1983 two fungi imperfecti, *Humicola* sp. ATCC 20620 and *Monocillium* sp. ATCC 20621, which could catalyze the conversion of rifamycin B to rifamycin O and to rifamycin S. The reaction proceeds by oxidative cyclization of rifamycin B to rifamycin O, followed by spontaneous hydrolysis of the latter in neutral aqueous medium to give rifamycin S. The enzyme has been characterized as a specific rifamycin-oxidase. Details in view of the industrial application have been subsequently reported, such as (a) the critical parameters for the use in batch of whole cells of *Humicola* (89) or (b) whole cells dried with acetone and immobilized with acrylamide in a fluidized bed reactor (90); (c) the enzyme immobilized on nylon fibers (91) or (d) in a rotary disc reactor (92). In a patent issued in 1982 (93), good yields are reported by using the enzyme within microbial cells, as a cell extract, or in immobilized form. When the oxidation is performed at pH 4–6, rifamycin O is obtained, whereas at pH 7–9, rifamycin S, and in the presence of ascorbic acid, rifamycin SV are obtained, respectively. Due to the mild conditions and the high specificity of the enzyme, rifamycin B (10 mM solution in acetate buffer, pH 5.5) gave rifamycin O in a 96% yield and 98% purity.

The transformation of rifamycin B into rifamycin S also can be performed with the less expensive extracellular enzyme from *Curvularia lunata* var. *aeria* in shake flask or in a batch reactor (94).

VII.   APPLICATIONS

The initial development of rifamycin B was soon abandoned because its transformation product rifamycin SV proved to be more active. This product was introduced by Lepetit into clinical practice in the early 1960s for the treatment of infections by Gram-positive bacteria and of any type of bacterial infections of the biliary tract.

In a few countries, the same indications were covered by a different derivative, namely, the diethylamide of rifamycin B (rifamide) prepared by condensing rifamycin B with diethylamine in the presence of dicyclohexylcarbodiimide. Rifamide has biological properties very similar to those of rifamycin SV.

An intense program of semisynthetic development then was started together with structural evaluation studies, both at Lepetit and at Ciba. Therefore, many hundreds of chemical derivatives were screened for their antibacterial activity, and the synthetic lines were chosen as soon as the main functional characteristics and the intrinsic reactivity and behavior of the molecule were elucidated. From the series of hydrazone derivatives at position 3, a compound emerged with properties decisively better than those of rifamycin SV: rifampicin (Figure 12). A key intermediate in the preparation of rifampicin and a large series of rifamycin derivatives is 3-formyl-rifamycin SV. The starting material is rifamycin S, which by reaction with formaldehyde and a secondary amine, such as diethylamine (a classical Mannich reaction) (95), followed by reduction with sodium ascorbate gives the 3-diethylaminomethyl-rifamycin SV. This is oxidized with MnO_2 in carbon tetrachloride/acetic acid, and reduced again with sodium ascorbate to give 3-formyl-rifamycin SV, which by condensation with 1-amino-4-methylpiperazine gives rifampicin, or 3-(4-methyl-1-piperazinyliminomethyl)-rifamycin SV (96). Rifampicin showed (a) oral absorption; (b) more prolonged therapeutic blood levels; and (c) higher activity in the treatment of mycobacterial and Gram-negative infections. Rifampicin strongly contributed to the eradication of tuberculosis throughout the world, and it is at present widely used for the treatment of tuberculosis and leprosy, generally in combination with other specific drugs. It is also active against some Gram-positive and -negative pathogens, particularly in severe infections caused by staphylococci resistant to β-lactams and infections caused by intracellular bacteria (97,98).

The preparation of new rifamycins, both of natural and chemical origin, has continued since then, and it is still a field of research pursued by many industrial groups. It is

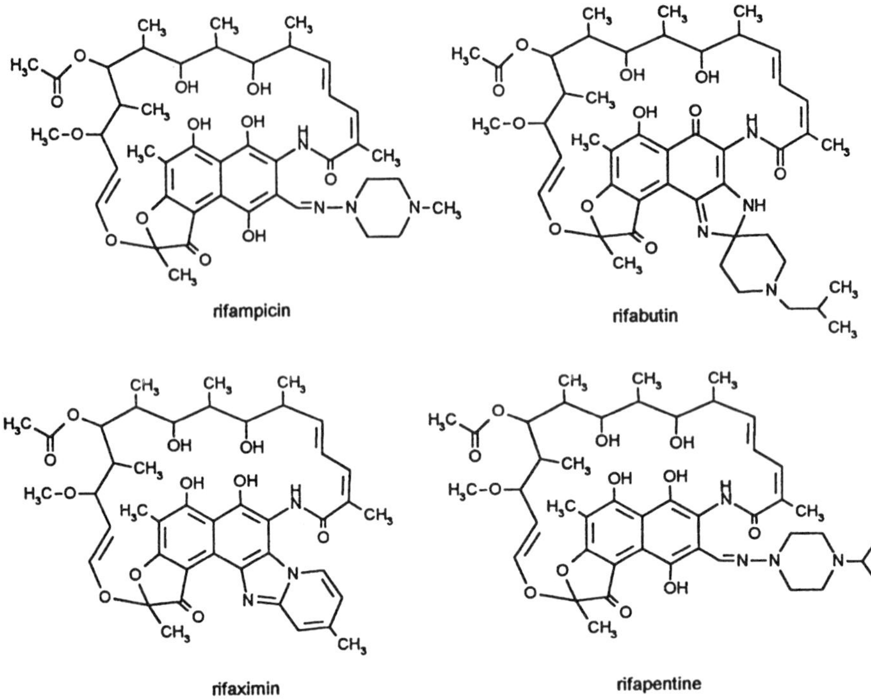

Figure 12 Clinically important rifamycins.

noteworthy, also, the attention that is devoted to the stereoselective construction of rifamycin (99, and references therein) following the first total synthesis of rifamycin S by Kishi's group in 1980 (100). The search for active rifamycins continued with increasing efficiency following the knowledge of the mechanism of action at the molecular level, the chemical structure, and its conformational characteristics. Reviews on semisynthetic rifamycins and their correlation with the biological activity have been published (12,13,101). Structure–activity correlations can be summarized as follows: (a) changes at hydroxyls in position 21 and 23 of the aliphatic ansa chain and 1 and 8 of the naphthalene moiety abolish almost completely the activity (except for the oxidation of hydroxyl-1 to a C=O); (b) inactivation also arises by all the modifications that alter the relative spatial position of the hydroxyls cited above, in agreement with the hypothesis that these form hydrogen bonds with RNA polymerase; (c) minor changes of the ansa chain, such as desacetylation, and partial or complete hydrogenation of the double bonds, do not substantially modify the activity; (d) substitutions at positions 3 and 4 of the naphthalene ring do not modify the intrinsic activity of the molecule but do influence some physicochemical parameters. Therefore, some biological properties such as pharmacokinetics and penetration into bacteria are changed, for example, the penetration into Gram-negative organisms. It has been found that the presence of substituents carrying a carboxyl decreases the antibacterial activity, whereas the presence of basic functions may increase the activity against Gram-negative organisms; (e) oral activity is frequently correlated with the substitutions at position 3, or substitutions that generate a ring between position 3 and 4. However, after rifampicin, only a few rifamycins showed therapeutic characteristics that allow their use in the medical practice; one is rifabutin (Figure 12), characterized by its activity against some strains resistant to rifampicin and a better activity against *Mycobacterium avium*. Rifabutin is the 4-*N*-isobutylspiropiperidyl-rifamycin S (102). The other is rifaximin (4-deoxy-4'-methylpyrido[1'2'-1,2]imidazo[4,5-c]-rifamycin SV) (Figure 12), which is poorly absorbed through the gut and was introduced for the treatment of a variety of gastrointestinal pathogens (103).

Another very interesting compound under clinical evaluation, namely rifapentine (Figure 12), possesses a high degree of activity against atypical mycobacteria and a pharmacokinetic profile that would allow for a long-lasting action. Rifapentine, 3-(4-cyclopentylpiperazyliminomethyl)-rifamycin SV, was the more active among the derivatives in which longer aliphatic moieties replaced the *N*-methyl-group of rifampicin; it also shows particularly favorable pharmacokinetic characteristics (104,105).

Due to their action against DNA-directed RNA polymerase, rifamycins were investigated as potential antiviral and antitumor agents, as potential inhibitors of reverse transcriptases, but it was found that the inhibitory effect on target enzymes is not sufficiently selective. Also recently, rifamycins were discussed for the use against HIV-1 and HIV-2; for the same reasons, no development was possible. Rifamycins appear at present of great interest for the treatment of opportunistic infections caused by mycobacteria in immunocompromised AIDS patients (106). Also, the increasing diffusion of tuberculosis in developed countries due to social events and the still unresolved problem of tuberculosis in undeveloped countries make rifampicin a drug of continuous application.

REFERENCES

1. Sensi P, Margalith P, Timbal MT. Rifomycin, a new antibiotic: Preliminary report. Farmaco Ed Sci 1959; 14:146–147.

2. Margalith P, Pagani H. Rifomycin. XIII. Fermentation and production of rifomycin complex. Appl Microbiol 1961; 9:320–324.

3. Margalith P, Pagani H. Rifomycin. XIV. Production of rifomycin B. Appl Microbiol 1961; 9:325–334.

4. Oppolzer W, Prelog V, Sensi P. Konstitution des Rifamycins B und verwandter Rifamycine. Experientia 1964; 20:336–339.

5. Wehrli W. Ansamycins: Chemistry, biosynthesis and biological activity. Top Curr Chem 1977; 72:21–49.

6. Rinehart KL Jr, Shield LS. Chemistry of the ansamycin antibiotics. Fortschr Chem Org Naturst 1976; 33:231–307.

7. Keller-Schierlein W, Meyer M, Zeeck A, Damberg M, Machinek R, Zähner H, Lazar G. Isolation and structural elucidation of naphthomycins B and C. J Antibiot 1983; 36:484–492.

8. Sugita M, Natori Y, Sasaki T, Furihata K, Shimazu A, Seto H, Otake N. Studies on mycotrienin antibiotics, a novel class of ansamycins. I. Taxonomy, fermentation, isolation and properties of mycotrienins I and II. J Antibiot 1982; 35:1460–1466.

9. DeBoer C, Meulman PA, Wnuk RJ, Peterson DH. Geldanamycin, a new antibiotic. J Antibiot 1970; 23:442–447.

10. Sensi P, Ballotta R, Greco AM, Gallo GG. Rifomycin. XV. Activation of rifomycin B and rifomycin O. Production and properties of rifomycin S and rifomycin SV. Farmaco Ed Sci 1961; 16:165–180.

11. Hartmann GR, Heinrich P, Kollenda MC, Skrobranek B, Tropschung M, Weiss W. Molecular mechanism of action of the antibiotic rifampicin. Angew Chem Int Ed 1985; 24:1009–1074.

12. Sensi P, Lancini GC. Inhibitors of transcribing enzymes: Rifamycins and related agents. Sammes PG, ed. Comprehensive Medicinal Chemistry. Vol. 2. Oxford: Pergamon Press, 1990:793–811.

13. Lancini GC, Zanichelli W. Structure-activity relationships in rifamycins. Perlman D, ed. Structure-Activity Relationships Among the Semisynthetic Antibiotics. New York: Academic Press, 1977:537–600.

14. Margalith P, Beretta G. Rifomycin. XI. Taxonomic study on *Streptomyces mediterranei* nov. sp. Mycopathol Mycol Appl 1961; 13:321–330.

15. Lancini GC, Thiemann JE, Sartori G, Sensi P. Biogenesis of rifamycins. The conversion of rifamycin B into rifamycin Y. Experientia 1967; 23:899–900.

16. Lancini GC, Sartori G. Rifamycin G, a further product of *Nocardia mediterranei* metabolism. J Antibiot 1976; 29:466–468.

17. Sugawara S, Karasawa K, Watanabe M, Hidaka T. Production of rifamycin O by *Streptomyces* 4107 A2. J Antibiot (Ser A) 1964; 17:29–32.

18. Birner J, Hodgson PR, Lane WR, Baxter EH. An Australian isolate of *Nocardia mediterranea* producing rifamycin SV. J Antibiot 1972; 25:356–359.

19. Celmer WD, Sciavolino FC, Routien JB, Cullen WP. U.S. Patent 40,013,789; 1977.

20. Kawaguchi T, Asahi T, Satoh T, Uozumi T, Beppu T. B-factor, an essential regulatory substance inducing the production of rifamycin in a *Nocardia* sp. J Antibiot 1984; 37:1587–1595.

21. Ganguli AK, Szmulewicz S, Sarre OZ, Greeves O, Morton J, McGlotten J. Structure of halomicin B. J Chem Soc Chem Commun 1974; 395–396.

22. Ganguli AK, Liu YT, Sarre OZ, Szmulewicz S. Structures of halomicins A and C. J Antibiot 1977; 30:625–627.

23. Shibata M, Hasegawa T, Higashide E. Tolypomycin, a new antibiotic. I. *Streptomyces tolypophorus* nov. sp., a new antibiotic, tolypomycin-producer. J Antibiot 1971; 24:810–816.

24. Hasegawa T, Higashide E, Shibata M. Tolypomycin, a new antibiotic. II. Production and preliminary identification of tolypomycin Y. J Antibiot 1971; 24:817–822.

25. Thiemann JE, Zucco G, Pelizza G. A proposal for the transfer of *Streptomyces mediterranei* (Margalith and Beretta 1960) to the genus *Nocardia* as *Nocardia mediterranei* comb nov. Arch Mikrobiol 1969; 67:147–155.

26. Lechevalier MP, Prauser H, Labeda DP, Ruan J-S. Two new genera of nocardioform actinomycetes: *Amycolata* gen. nov. and *Amycolatopsis* gen. nov. Int J Syst Bacteriol 1986; 36:29–37.

27. Thiemann JE, Hengeller C, Virgilio A. Rifamycin. XXV. A group of actinophages active on *Streptomyces mediterranei*. Nature 1962; 193:1104–1105.

28. Thiemann JE, Hengeller C, Virgilio A. Buelli O, Licciardello G. Rifamycin. XXXIII. Isolation of actinophages active on *Streptomyces mediterranei* and characteristics of phage-resistant strains. Appl Microbiol 1964; 12:261–268.

29. Schupp T, Hütter R, Hopwood DA. Genetic recombination in *Nocardia mediterranei*. J Bacteriol 1975; 121:128–136.

30. Ghisalba O, Auden JAL, Schupp T, Nüesch J. The rifamycins: Properties, biosynthesis and fermentation. Vandamme E, ed. Biotechnology of Industrial Antibiotics. Basel: Marcel Dekker, 1984:281–327.

31. Schupp T, Nüesch J. Chromosomal mutation in the final step of rifamycin biosynthesis. FEMS Microbiol Lett 1979; 6:23–27.

32. Moretti P, Hintermann G, Hütter R. Isolation and characterization of an extrachromosomal element from *Nocardia mediterranei*. Plasmid 1985; 14:126–133.

33. Madon J, Moretti P, Hütter R. Site-specific integration of pMEA100 in *Nocardia mediterranei*. Mol Gen Genet 1987; 209:257–264.

34. Schupp T, Divers M. Protoplast preparation and regeneration in *Nocardia mediterranei*. FEMS Microbiol Lett 1986; 36:159–162.

35. Lal R, Lal S, Grund E, Eichenlaub R. Construction of a hybrid plasmide capable of replication in *Amycolatopsis mediterranei*. Appl Environ Microbiol 1991; 57:665–671.

36. Madon J, Hütter R. Transformation system for *Amycolatopsis (Nocardia) mediterranei*: Direct transformation of mycelium with plasmid DNA. J Bacteriol 1991; 173:6325–6331.

37. Brufani M, Kluepfel D, Lancini GC, Leitich J, Mesentsev AS, Prelog V, Schmook FP, Sensi P. Über die Biogenese des Rifamycins S. Helv Chim Acta 1973; 56:2315–2323.

38. White RJ, Martinelli E, Gallo GG, Lancini G, Beynon P. Rifamycin biosynthesis studied with ¹³C enriched precursors and carbon magnetic resonance. Nature 1973; 243:273–277.

39. White RJ, Martinelli E, Lancini GC. Ansamycin biogenesis: Studies on a novel rifamycin isolated from a mutant strain of *Nocardia mediterranei*. Proc Natl Acad Sci USA 1974; 71:3260–3264.

40. Karlsson A, Sartori G, White RJ. Rifamycin biosynthesis: Further studies on origin of the ansa chain and chromophore. Eur J Biochem 1974; 47:251–256.

41. White RJ, Martinelli E. Ansamycin biogenesis: Incorporation of [1-¹³C] glucose and [1-¹³C] glycerate into the chromophore of rifamycin S. FEBS Lett 1974; 49:233–236.

42. Ghisalba O, Nüesch J. A genetic approach to the biosynthesis of the rifamycin-chromophore in *Nocardia mediterranei*. IV. Identification of 3-amino-5-hydroxybenzoic acid as a direct precursor of the seven-carbon amino starter-unit. J Antibiot 1981; 34:64–71.

43. Ghisalba O, Nüesch J. A genetic approach to the biosynthesis of the rifamycin-chromophore in *Nocardia mediterranei*. I. Isolation and characterization of a pentose-excreting auxotrophic mutant of *Nocardia mediterranei* with drastically reduced rifamycin production. J Antibiot 1978; 31:202–214.

44. Ghisalba O, Nüesch J. A genetic approach to the biosynthesis of the rifamycin-chromophore in *Nocardia mediterranei*. II. Isolation and characterization of a shikimate excreting auxotrophic mutant of *Nocardia mediterranei* with normal rifamycin-production. J Antibiot 1978; 31:215–225.

45. Kim C-G, Kirschning A, Bergon P, Ahn Y, Wang JJ, Shibaye M, Floss HG. Formation of 3-amino-5-hydroxybenzoic acid, the precursor of mC_7N units in ansamycin antibiotics, by a new variant of the shikimate pathway. J Am Chem Soc 1992; 114:4941–4943.

46. Kirschning A, Bergon P, Wang JJ, Floss HG. Synthesis of 4-amino-3,4-dideoxy-D-*arabino*-heptulosonic acid 7-phosphate, the biosynthetic precursor of C_7N units in ansamycin antibiotics. Carbohydr Res 1994; 256:245–256.

47. Lancini GC, Grandi M. Biosynthesis of ansamycins. Corcoran JW, ed. Antibiotics IV—Biosynthesis. New York: Springer-Verlag, 1981:11–40.

48. Lancini GC. Ansamycins. Rehm HJ, Reed G, eds. Biotechnology, Vol. 4. Weinheim: VCH Verlagsgesellschaft, 1986:431–463.

49. Ghisalba O, Traxler P, Nüesch J. Early intermediates in the biosynthesis of ansamycins. I. Isolation and identification of protorifamycin I. J Antibiot 1978; 31:1124–1131.

50. Traxler P, Schupp T, Fuhrer H, Richter WJ. 3-Hydroxyrifamycin S and further novel ansamycins from a recombinant strain R-21 of *Nocardia mediterranei*. J Antibiot 1981; 34:971–979.

51. Cricchio R, Antonini P, Ferrari P. Ripamonti A, Tuan G, Martinelli E. Rifamycin Z, a novel ansamycin from a mutant of *Nocardia mediterranei*. J Antibiot 1981; 34:1257–1260.

52. Hengeller C, Lancini GC, Sensi P. U.S. Patent 3,473,635; 1973.

53. Lancini GC, Hengeller C, Sensi P. New naturally occurring rifamycins. Progress in Antimicrobial and Anticancer Chemotherapy, Vol. II. Tokyo: University of Tokyo Press, 1970:1166–1173.

54. Lancini GC, Sensi P. Studies on the final steps in rifamycins biosynthesis. Spitzy KH, Haschek H, eds. Proceedings of the Fifth International Congress of Chemotherapy, Vol. I. Wien: Verlag der Wiener Medizinischen Akademie, 1967:41–47.

55. Lancini GC, Gallo GG, Sartori G, Sensi P. Isolation and structure of rifamycin L and its biogenetic relationship with other rifamycins. J Antibiot 1969; 22:369–377.

56. Lancini GC, Hengeller C. Isolation of rifamycin SV from a mutant *Streptomyces mediterranei* strain. J Antibiot 1969; 22:637–638.

57. Martinelli E, Antonini P, Cricchio R, Lancini G, White RJ. Rifamycin R, a novel metabolite from a mutant of *Nocardia mediterranea*. J Antibiot 1978; 31:949–951.

58. Cricchio R, Antonini P, Lancini GC, Tamborini G, White RJ, Martinelli E. Thiazorifamycins. I. Structure and synthesis of rifamycins P, Q and Verde, novel metabolites from mutants of *Nocardia mediterranea*. Tetrahedron 1980; 36:1415–1421.

59. Cricchio R, Antonini P, Sartori G. Thiazorifamycins. III. Biosynthesis of rifamycins P, Q and Verde, novel metabolites from a mutant of *Nocardia mediterranea*. J Antibiot 1980; 33:842–846.

60. Kluepfel D, Lancini GC, Sartori G. Metabolism of barbital by *Streptomyces mediterranei*. Appl Microbiol 1965; 13:600–604.

61. Lancini GC, Hengeller C. U.S. Patent 3,597,324; 1971.

62. Kawaguchi T, Azuma M, Horinouchi S, Beppu T. Effect of B factor and its analogues on rifamycin biosynthesis in *Nocardia* sp. J Antibiot 1988; 41:360–365.

63. Azuma M, Nishi K, Horinouchi S, Beppu T. Ribonucleases catalyze the synthesis of B factor (3′-butylphosphoryl AMP), an inducer of rifamycin production in a *Nocardia* sp. J Antibiot 1990; 43:321–323.

64. Chiao JS, Xia TH, Ni LY, Gu WL, Jin ZK, Mei BJ, Zhang YF. Studies on the metabolic regulation of rifamycin SV biosynthesis. Okami Y, Beppu T, Ogawara H, eds. Biology of Actinomycetes '88. Tokyo: Japan Scientific Societies Press, 1988:412–417.

65. Chiao JS, Xia TH, Mei BG, Jin ZK, Gu WL. Rifamycin SV and related ansamycins. Vining LC, Stuttard C, eds. Genetics and Biochemistry of Antibiotic Production. Boston: Butterworth-Heinemann, 1995:477–498.

66. Schupp T, Traxler P, Auden JAL. New rifamycins produced by a recombinant strain of *Nocardia mediterranei*. J Antibiot 1981; 34:965–970.

67. White RJ, Lancini GC. U.S. Patent 3,871,965; 1975.

68. Archifar. Belgian Patent 805,923; 1972.

69. Tarchominskie Zaklady Farmaceutyczne. Poland Patent 115,340; 1982.

70. Sensi P, Thiemann, JE. Production of rifamycins. Prog Ind Microbiol 1967; 6:21–60.

71. Kanegafuchi Chem KK. Japan Patent 54110-393; 1978.

72. Lancini GC, Hengeller C. U.S. Patent 3,597,324; 1971.

73. Virgilio A, Marcelli E, Agrimino A. Aeration-agitation studies on the rifamycin fermentation. Biotechnol Bioeng 1964; 6:271–283.

74. Tarchominskie Zaklady Farmaceutyczne. Poland Patent 102,110; 1979.

75. Chung BH, Chang HN, Kim IH. Rifamycin B production by *Nocardia mediterranei* immobilized in a dual hollow-fibre bioreactor. Enz Microb Technol 1987; 9:345–349.

76. Sensi P, Greco AM, Ballotta R. Rifomycin. I. Isolation and properties of rifomycin B and rifomycin complex. Antibiot Annu 1960; 1959–1960:262–270.

77. Sensi P, Ballotta R, Greco AM. Rifomycin. V. Rifomycin O, a new antibiotic of the rifomycin family. Farmaco Ed Sci 1960; 15:228–234.

78. Gallo GG, Sensi P, Radaelli P. Rifomicina. VII. Analisi spettrofotometrica della rifomicina B. Farmaco Ed Prat 1960; 15:283–291.

79. Pasqualucci CR, Vigevani A, Radaelli P, Gallo GG. Improved differential spectrophotometric determination of rifamycins. J Pharm Sci 1970; 59:685–687.

80. Füresz S, Scotti R. Rifomycin. IV. Some laboratory and clinical experiences with rifomycin B. Antibiot Annu 1960; 1959–1960:285–292.

81. Ghisalba O, Roos R, Schupp T, Nüesch J. Transformation of rifamycin S into rifamycins B and L. A revision of the current biosynthetic hypothesis. J Antibiot 1982; 35:74–80.

82. Archifar. Belgian Patent 796,018; 1972.

83. Grozn Promavtomatik. SU Pateny 236945; 1987.

84. Dow Chem. U.S. Patent 4,402,877; 1982.

85. GAF Corp. WO Patent 8800-203-A; 1986.

86. Kanegafuchi. Japan Patent J5 4110-391; 1978.

87. Banerjee UC, Saxena B, Christi Y. Biotransformations of rifamycins: Process possibilities. Biotech Adv 1992; 10:577–595.

88. Han MH, Seong B-L, Son H-J, Mheen T-I. Rifamycin B oxidase from *Monocillium* spp., a new type of diphenol oxidase. FEBS Lett 1983; 151:36–40.

89. Seong BL, Son HJ, Mheen TI, Park YH, Han MH. Enzymatic oxidation of rifamycins by a microorganism of the genus *Humicola*. J Ferment Technol 1985; 6:515–522.

90. Lee GM, Choi CY, Park JM, Han MH. Biotransformation of rifamycin B to rifamycin S using immobilised whole cells of *Humicola* spp. in a fluidised bed reactor. J Chem Tech Biotechnol 1984; 35B:3–10.

91. Vohra RM, Vyas VV. Characterization of rifamycin oxidase immobilized on nylon fibers. Biotechnol Tech 1992; 6:61–64.

92. Chung BH, Chang HN, Han MH. Enzymatic conversion of rifamycin B in a rotating packed disk reactor. J Ferment Technol 1986; 64:343–345.

93. Korea Adv. Inst. Sci. Technol. U.S. Patent 4,431,375 A; 1982.

94. Banerjee UC. Transformation of rifamycin B with soluble rifamycin oxidase from *Curvularia lunata*. J Biotechnol 1993; 29:137–143.

95. Maggi N, Gallo GG, Sensi P. Synthesis of 3-formylrifamycin SV. Farmaco Ed Sci 1967; 22:316–325.

96. Maggi N, Pasqualucci CR, Ballotta R, Sensi P. Rifampicin: A new orally active rifamycin. Chemotherapia 1966; 11:285–292.

97. Hobby GL, Lenert TF. The action of rifampicin alone and in combination with other anti-tuberculosis drugs. Am Rev Resp Dis 1970; 102:462–465.

98. Davies AJ, Lewis DA. Rifampicin in non-tuberculous infections. Brit Med J 1984; 289:3–4.

99. Miyashita M, Yoshihara K, Kawamine K, Hoshino M, Irie H. Synthetic studies on polypropionate antibiotics based on the stereospecific methylation of γ, δ-epoxy acrylates by trimethylaluminum. A highly stereoselective construction of the eight contiguous chiral centers of ansa-chains of rifamycins. Tetraedron Lett 1993; 34:6285–6288.

100. Iio H, Nagaoka H, Kishi Y. Total synthesis of rifamycins. 2. Total synthesis of racemic rifamycin S. J Am Chem Soc 1980; 102:7965–7967.

101. Traxler P, Vischer WA, Zak O. New rifamycins. Drugs Fut 1988; 13:845–856.

102. Brogden RN, Fitton A. Rifabutin. A review of its antimicrobial activity, pharmacokinetic properties and therapeutic efficacy. Drugs 1994; 47:983–1009.

103. de Angelis L. L-105. Drugs Fut 1982; 7:260–261.

104. Cricchio R, Arioli V. U.S. Patent 4,002,752; 1977.

105. Mealy NE. DL-473. Drugs Fut 1979; 4:255–256.

106. Havlir DV. *Mycobacterium avium* complex: Advances in therapy. Eur J Clin Microbiol Infect Dis 1994; 13:915–924.

19
Polyene Antibiotics

José A. Gil and Juan F. Martín
University of León, León, Spain

I. INTRODUCTION

A. Present Status of Antifungal Chemotherapy

Over the past several decades, humankind has become free from the attack of many infectious bacteria, thanks to the widespread use of natural and semisynthetic antibiotics. The present clinical scenario is one of a growing number of bacteria that are tolerant or resistant to a wider spectrum of drugs, and therefore, it seems reasonable to look for new antibacterial drugs using new strategies or new screening programs.

In contrast to the advances in antibacterial therapeutics, progress in the treatment of fungal infections has been slow. Amphotericin B, the first commercially significant antifungal drug, has been available for more than 30 years. This polyene macrolide antifungal agent continues to play a major role in the treatment of systemic fungal infections, despite the introduction of newer agents. The absence of new products with antifungal activities in the market can be explained by two facts: (a) the similarity between the biosynthetic pathways of fungal and mammalian or plant cells, which makes it difficult to find nontoxic antifungal agents, and (b) the idea that life-threatening fungal infections were too infrequent to warrant aggressive research. The latter opinion has changed over the past decade, in part due to secondary fungal infections in AIDS patients, and increasing numbers of antifungal compounds have been patented by pharmaceutical companies. However, new approaches and new types of molecules, rather than chemical derivatives, are urgently required, since conditions leading to the emergence of fungal infections (i.e., the increasing number of immunocompromised people) are likely to persist in the future (1).

The discovery of nystatin, the first polyene (tetraene) macrolide antifungal antibiotic, was made in 1950 by Hazen and Brown. Nystatin is effective in vitro against a large number of pathogenic and nonpathogenic fungi and has no effect against some of the common bacteria. Most other polyene macrolides have been described as antifungal agents. However, in the last few years a number of polyene antibiotics with different antibiotic activities were discovered. Facricfungin, a new pentaene macrolide antibiotic produced by *Streptomyces griseus* var. *autotrophicus*, showed bactericidal activity against all species of Gram-positive bacteria examined (2) and (at a concentration of 100 μg per liter) it caused 100% mortality of mosquito larvae (*Aedes aegypti*, Rockefeller strain) and free-living nematodes (*Panagrellus redivivus*).

Until recently, polyene antibiotics were used as antifungal agents, but several functions have been now assigned to polyenes such as immunostimulatory drugs, insecticides, application in AIDS-related fungal infections, and so forth (see Section V).

B. Polyene-Producing Organisms in Nature

The polyene antibiotics are produced by soil actinomycetes, mainly of the genus *Streptomyces*, although the production of polyenes by species of *Streptoverticillum*, *Actinosporangium*, and *Chainia* has been reported. Pisano et al. (3) found a high number of actinomycetes from stuarine sediments that produced antifungal compounds, and the polyene heptaene group was the most common group found.

Recently, a collection of 116 marine sponges, ascidians, and cnidarians was assayed for the presence of antifungal compounds (4). Samples (8.3%) with significant activity against *Candida albicans* were found in this study. The activity of a potent antifungal from the sponge, *Jaspis* sp., was reduced by ergosterol concentrations as low as 10 μg per liter. This ergosterol antagonism is similar to the well-known ergosterol dependence of polyene antifungals, such as amphotericin B, and suggests a common mode of action. It is unclear at this time whether the ability of sponges, ascidians, and cnidarians to produce antifungal metabolites is due to microflora associated with these organisms, as reported in other cases with anticancer agents.

The polyenes are usually formed as mixtures of polyene and nonpolyene products; this situation, common in secondary metabolism, has given rise to great difficulties in separating the different polyene entities and in determining their precise molecular formulas. The identities of many of the polyene antibiotics remain questionable, and caution should be taken in considering all of them as different. For example, tetrafungin, a polyene produced by *Streptomyces albulus* subsp. *tetrafungini*, was compared with nystatin by high-pressure liquid chromatography (HPLC) and it was demonstrated that tetrafungin and nystatin differ qualitatively in, at least, one component, and quantitatively in their relative amounts of common components (5).

Although separation of polyene macrolide antibiotics is difficult, considerable progress has been achieved in their purification by HPLC and in the determination of their complex chemical structure by sensitive analytical methods, such as proton magnetic resonance, x-ray, and mass spectrometry.

II. CHEMICAL STRUCTURE

The polyene macrolides form a subgroup of the macrolide antibiotics containing hydroxylated macrocyclic lactone rings and usually one, or more, sugars. From the biosynthetic point of view, the macrolides are a homogeneous group, being synthesized from acetate, propionate, and other short-chain fatty acids via the polyketide pathway (6,7). The macrolide antibiotics are divided into two subgroups: (a) polyene macrolides (mostly antifungal) and (b) nonpolyene macrolides (antibacterial) antibiotics. Due to the discovery of the antibacterial activity of some polyenes, the strict identification of polyenes as antifungal agents should be avoided. The polyene macrolides have lactone rings of 26–38 carbon atoms, which are much larger than those of the nonpolyene macrolides, except for the axenomycins, which have 34 atoms in the (nonpolyene) macrolide ring (7).

The polyene subgroup has a chromophore formed by a system of three to seven conjugated double bonds in the macrolactone ring. Polyene macrolides are amphipatic molecules containing both a rigid planar lipophilic portion and a flexible hydrophilic polyhydroxylated region. The chromophore accounts for some of the characteristic physical and chemical properties of the polyenes (strong light absorption, photolability, and poor solubility in water) and appears to be responsible for the differences in the mode of action of the polyene and nonpolyene macrolide subgroups. The chromophore gives a typical multipeak ultraviolet visible light absorption spectrum (Figure 1). Polyene macrolides are subdivided into trienes, tetraenes, pentaenes, hexaenes, and heptaenes according to the number of conjugated double bonds in the chromophore (Figure 2). A list of the polyene macrolide antibiotics that are better characterized or are more medically relevant can be found in the reviews of Gil et al. (8) and Martín and McDaniel (9). Some of the new polyenes described after 1983 are given in Table 1.

III. SUGAR AND AMINOSUGAR COMPONENTS

A large number of polyene macrolide antibiotics have an aminosugar (or neutral sugar) moiety that is linked to the macrolide ring by a glycoside bond. In all cases, the aminosugar is attached to a carbon bearing a hydroxyl-group adjacent to the chromophore. Two different aminosugars have been described as components of polyene macrolide antibiotics, namely, mycosamine (3-amino-3,6-dideoxy-D-mannose) and its isomer perosamine (4-amino-4,6-dideoxy-D-mannose) (Figure 3).

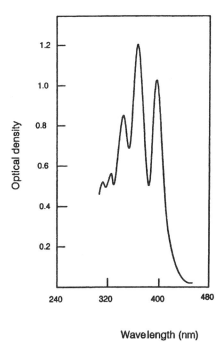

Figure 1   Absorption spectra of candicidin, an aromatic heptaene, produced by *Streptomyces griseus* IMRU3570.

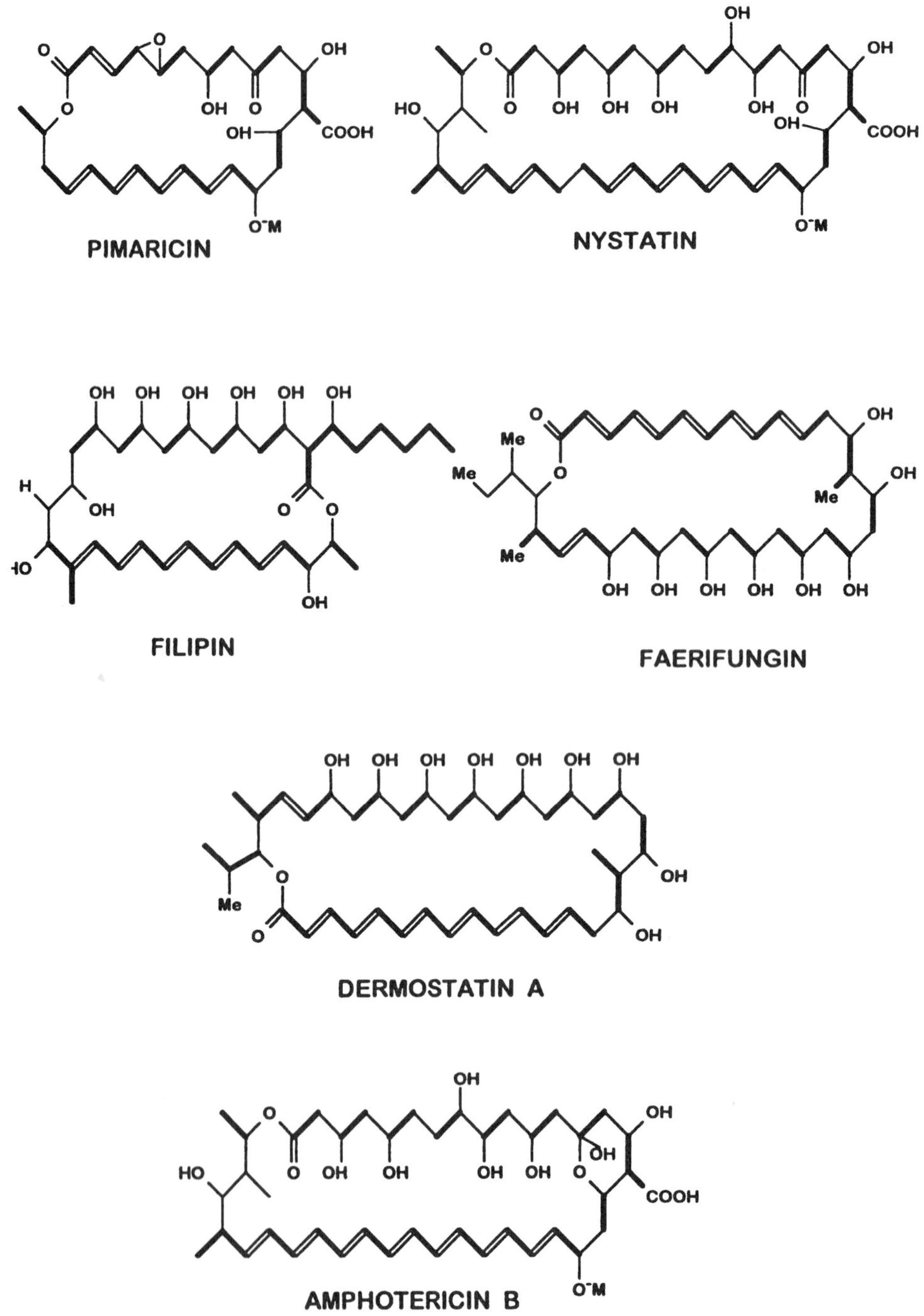

Figure 2 Chemical structure and building units of some polyene macrolide antibiotics. (Data from Refs. 2 and 7.) M, indicates mycosamine and Me a methyl group.

Table 1 Some New Polyenes Described After 1983

Compound	Group	Ref.
Tetrafungin	Tetraene	5
Vacidine	Aromatic heptaene	10
Faeriefungin	Pentaene	2
Trichomycin	Aromatic heptaene	11
YS-822A	Tetraene	12
AB023	Pentaene	13

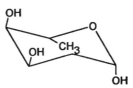

MYCOSAMINE

PEROSAMINE

2,6-DIDEOXY-L-RIBOHEXOPYRANOSE

Figure 3 Chemical structures of the sugar moieties of polyene macrolide antibiotics.

Mycosamine is present in all the aminosugar-containing polyene macrolides described so far, with the exception of the heptaene perimycin (fungimycin), which contains perosamine. Until 1979 it was believed that neutral sugars did not occur in polyene macrolides, but Zielinski et al. (14) isolated the first neutral sugar from nystatin A3, candidinin, and polyfungin B, and identified it as 2,6-dideoxy-L-ribohexopyranose. It is not clear, however, whether this neutral sugar is present in minor components of other polyene antibiotics. This neutral sugar might be a deaminated intermediate in the biosynthesis of the aminated analogs.

The acetylated mycosamine moiety of some heptaenes was identified by chemical ionization and gas chromatography–mass spectrometry (GC–MS) (15).

IV. AROMATIC MOIETIES

Several polyenes belonging to the heptaene subgroup (ascosin, aureofungin, ayfactin, candicidin, heptamycin, levorin, trichomycin, DJ 400 B2, vacidin, etc.) were described as aromatic polyenes, and they have an aromatic *p*-aminoacetophenone moiety (PAAP). Other aromatic heptaenes, including candimycin, DJ 400 B1, and perimycin, have an aromatic *N*-methyl-*p*-aminoacethophenone moiety (*N*-methyl-PAAP) (Figure 4).

An HPLC method for the determination of the aromatic ring of heptaene polyene antibiotics has been developed by Raatikainen et al. (15). The released aromatic moiety of the heptaene polyenes aureofungin, candicidin, candimycin, hamycin, and trichomycin was assayed after alkaline hydrolysis, and the aromatic nature of the individual components of the heptaene complex was demonstrated using radioactivity flow detection for the determination of the incorporation of $[^{14}C]$-*p*-aminobenzoic acid into individual polyene components. The presence of PAAP and *N*-methyl-PAAP in the hydrolysates was determined by HPLC, HPLC–mass spectrometry (HPLC–MS), and GC–MS. Candicidin and hamycin contained only the PAAP residue; aureofungin, previously described as an aromatic heptaene containing PAAP, contained both PAAP and *N*-methyl-PAAP. Trichomycin contained PAAP and some unknown component of molecular weight 179 (15). These results, together with the well-known difficulties in separating the different polyenic entities and in determining their precise chemical structures, suggest that extreme caution should be taken when describing "new" polyenes; the identities of many of the described polyene antibiotics remain questionable.

V. MODE OF ACTION OF POLYENES

In the 1970s great advances were made in understanding the mechanism of action of amphotericin B, candicidin, and nystatin (16,17). The formation of transmembrane pores

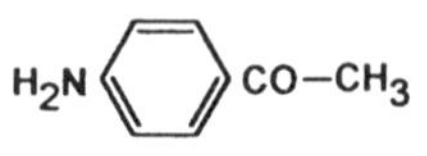

p-aminoacetophenone

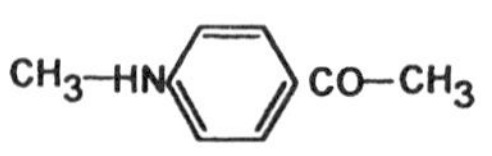

p-N-methylacetophenone

Figure 4   Aromatic moieties present in polyene macrolide antibiotics.

was clearly demonstrated in planar lipid monolayers, in multilamellar phospholipid vesicles, and in pleuroneumonia-like organisms. The fact that fungal membranes contain ergosterol whereas mammalian cell membranes contain cholesterol has generally been considered the basis for the selective toxicity of amphotericin B and nystatin for fungi. For polyene antibiotics with shorter chains, a mechanism of membrane permeability alteration was proposed. However, recent data on the mode of action of polyene unilamellar vesicles have shown that membranes in the gel state (which is not common in cells), even if they do not contain sterols, may be made permeable by polyene antibiotics (18).

Although pore formation is apparently involved in the toxicity of amphotericin B and nystatin, it is not the sole factor that contributes to cell death, since K^+ leakage induced by these antibiotics was shown to be a separate phenomenon from that of their lethal action. The peroxidation of membrane lipids, which has been demonstrated for erythrocytes and C. *albicans* cells in the presence of amphotericin B, may play a determining role in toxicity concurrently with colloid osmotic effects (19).

It has been shown that the action of polyene antibiotics on cells is not always detrimental: at sublethal concentrations, these drugs modify the yeast cell wall (20). Polyene also may stimulate the activity of some membrane enzymes. In particular, some cells of the immune system are stimulated. For example, amphotericin B potently primes macrophages in vitro and in vivo so that they produce large amounts of tumor necrosis factor (TNF) after the secondary stimulation (triggering) by bacterial lipopolysaccharides or a streptococcal preparation used for antitumor immunotherapy (21). Furthermore, polyene antibiotics may act synergistically with other drugs, such as antitumor or antifungal compounds (22,23). This may occur either by an increased incorporation of the drug, under the influence of a polyene antibiotic–induced change of membrane potential, for example, or by a direct interaction of both drugs.

Polyene antibiotics can be also used to enhance several-fold the efficiency of DNA-mediated gene transfer in mammalian cells (24), to inhibit the replication of HIV (25), or to delay the incubation period of a putative prion-caused disease of man (Creutzfeldt–Jakob disease) and animals. At the moment, no therapy is available for the cure of these fatal central nervous system diseases (26).

In contrast to fungicidal antibiotics nystatin and amphotericin B, which show no activity against bacteria, the related faeriefungin showed bactericidal activity against all species of Gram-positive bacteria examined. Minimum inhibitory concentrations (MICs) for these species ranged from 8 to 64 µg/ml, and the MIC for 90% of the isolates tested was 32 µg/ml. Isolates of some fastidious Gram-negative species, including *Neisseria gonorrhoeae*, *Neisseria meningitidis*, and *Haemophilus influenzae*, were slightly sensitive to faeriefungin, with MICs ranging from 16 to 128 µg/ml, but all members of the Enterobacteriaceae and Pseudomonadaceae families, with the exception of *Pseudomonas cepacia*, were completely resistant to faeriefungin at the concentrations tested. Faeriefungin is also active against fungi, nematodes, and mosquito larvae (27).

VI. BIOSYNTHESIS

The three different moieties of polyene macrolides (i.e., the macrolide ring, the aromatic moiety, and the aminosugar moiety) are synthesized by three separate pathways (7). Initial results obtained in the case of candicidin indicated that, at least, the genes involved in the biosynthesis of the aromatic moiety and the macrolide ring are clustered.

A. Biosynthesis of the Aromatic Moiety

The *p*-aminoacetophenone and *N*-methyl-*p*-aminoacetophenone moieties of the polyene (heptaenes) macrolides are synthesized from glucose via the aromatic amino acid pathway. *p*-Aminobenzoic acid (PABA) has been identified as the immediate precursor of the aromatic moiety of candicidin by incorporation of [ring UL^{14}C]PABA and [7-^{14}C]PABA (28,29). There is evidence from biosynthetic studies of several polyketide-derived products with aromatic moieties indicating that aromatic rings are used as primer units in polyketide formation. Light (30) described several examples in which an aromatic cinnamoyl starter unit produced several compounds of the chalcone or stilbene series by addition of malonyl-CoA units or the *p*-coumarate served as an intermediate in the biosynthesis of plant polyketide secondary metabolites, such as flavonoids (31). Another example of an aromatic moiety acting as a starter in the synthesis of aromatic antibiotics is the C$_7$N unit (3-amino-5-hydroxybenzoic acid, an intermediate of the shikimate pathway) involved in the biosynthesis of the macrolactam antibiotic rifamycin (32).

Chorismic acid serves as the branch point intermediate in the biosynthesis of many important aromatic products. These metabolites include anthranilate (required for the end product tryptophan), prephenate (tyrosine and phenylalanine), PABA (folic acid and aromatic polyenes), isochorismate (enterochelin, menaquinone), and *p*-hydroxybenzoate (ubiquinone) (33).

The reactions catalyzed by PABA synthase and anthranilate (*o*-aminobenzoate, OABA) are strikingly similar (Figure 5). In *Escherichia coli*, both enzymes are composed of nonidentical subunits. Component I (M$_r$ ≈ 50,000) of PABA synthase and OABA synthase are the gene products of *pabB* or *trpE*, respectively; component II (M$_r$ ≈ 20,000) of each enzyme is the gene product of *pabA* or *trpG(D)* (34,35). Components I (binding of chorismate) and II (binding of glutamine) of PABA or OABA synthases convert chorismic acid in PABA or OABA, respectively, in presence of glutamine (aminotransferase activity). In each enzyme complex, the component I can function independently, given a high concentration of ammonia and a high pH (aminase activity). This situation was found in *E. coli, Enterobacter aerogenes, Neurospora crassa,* and *Bacillus subtilis* (36–39).

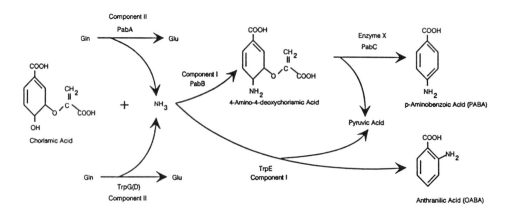

Figure 5   PABA and OABA biosynthesis in *Escherichia coli.*

I. Genetics of PABA Biosynthesis

Genes involved in the biosynthesis of PABA and OABA have been cloned; sequence data revealed similarities between PabB and TrpE, and between PabA and TrpG, suggesting a common ancestor for both enzymes (34,35).

Teng et al. (40) showed that 4-amino-4-deoxychorismic acid is a key intermediate in the biosynthesis of PABA, and later on it was discovered that in *E. coli* and *B. subtilis* three genes are involved in the biosynthesis of PABA instead of the two genes required for OABA biosynthesis (33,41,42). The third gene involved in the biosynthesis of PABA (named *pabC*) encodes an aminodeoxychorismate lyase ($M_r \approx 25,000$) and apparently performs the final aromatization reaction (Figure 5).

Another surprising difference between the genes involved in the biosynthesis of OABA and PABA in *E. coli* is that the genes involved in the biosynthesis of OABA [*trpE* and *trpG*(D)] are located in a single highly regulated operon at 27 min (43), whereas the genes involved in the biosynthesis of PABA are scatered in the chomosome: *pabA* (74 min), *pabB* (40 min), and *pabC* (25 min).

The *Streptomyces griseus* gene (*pabS*) for PABA synthase was cloned in a 4.5-kb BamHI fragment by complementation of a *Streptomyces lividans pab* mutant (JG10) and by resistance to sulfanilamide, and it was one of the first genes involved in antibiotic production cloned from *Streptomyces*. The gene was expressed in several *Streptomyces* species but not in *E. coli* (44). Expression occurred in *E. coli* after in vivo deletion of 1 kb of DNA upstream of the *pab* gene due to recombination between short directed repeats (45). The resulting 3.5 kb fragment could complement mutations in both *pabA* and *pabB* loci of *E. coli*.

The *pab* gene from *S. lividans* was cloned by complementation of *S. lividans* JG10 in a 2.7 kb BamHI:SstI DNA fragment and complemented *pabA* and *pabB E. coli* mutations (46).

The *pab* gene of the candicidin producer *S. griseus* codes for a protein with two domains: a PabA domain at the amino-end, and a PabB domain at the carboxy-end; thus, it has been renamed *pabAB*. The gene contains an open reading frame (ORF) of 2171 nucleotides (nt) coding for a protein of 723 amino acids (45). A similar structure of the *pab* gene was found in *Saccharomyces cerevisiae*, where a 3840 bp DNA fragment from chromosome XIV contains a 2199 bp ORF encoding a 733-amino-acid protein (47). It is very interesting that the *pabAB* gene for candicidin biosynthesis present in *S. griseus* is more similar to the *S. cerevisiae pab* gene than to the primary genes for PABA biosynthesis in *S. lividans*. The *pab* genes of *S. lividans* are organized like those of the primary PABA pathway in *B. subtilis*, with *pabB* upstream of *pabA* (46). Neither *S. griseus* nor *S. lividans* have an ORF corresponding to *pabC* in the region near *pabAB* (*S. griseus*) or *pabB–pabA* (*S. lividans*).

Sequencing of *S. griseus* and *S. lividans pab* genes reveals a different organization of the *pabA* and *pabB* genes, indicating the existence in streptomycetes of two set of genes directing PABA biosynthesis, one for primary and the other for secondary metabolism (48). Similarly, the genes coding for two anthranilate synthases, one for primary and the other one for secondary metabolism (involved in the synthesis of pyocyanin), were cloned from *Pseudomonas aeruginosa* (49).

The *pabAB* from *S. griseus* IMRU 3570 has been used as a probe to find new aromatic polyene–producing *Streptomyces* strains. The *pabAB* gene hybridizes with 6 out of 16 *Streptomyces* strains, and those strains that hybridize turned out to be aromatic polyene

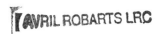

producers (48). The *pab*AB gene was also used as probe to isolate genes involved in the biosynthesis of the candicidin aglycone (see Section VI. B.2.).

2. Biochemical Studies with the PABA Synthase of S. griseus

The PABA synthase from *S. griseus* IMRU 3570, a candicidin producer, was studied in our laboratory (50). This enzyme uses glutamine or ammonia as amino donors for PABA formation and is formed in *S. griseus* only during the antibiotic-producing phase; the enzyme was also synthesized during the production phase of *Streptomyces coelicolor* var. *aminophilus*, producer of the polyene macrolide antibiotic fungimycin (containing *N*-methyl-PAAP). No detectable levels of the enzyme were found in cell-free extracts of nonproducing mutants of *S. griseus* obtained after ultraviolet (UV) mutagenesis, nor in extracts of several other streptomycetes that do not produce aromatic polyene macrolide antibiotics, suggesting that this enzyme is directly involved in candicidin production (50).

The amidotransferase activity of the PABA synthase was partially purified by DEAE-BioGel and Sephacryl S-200 filtrations. The estimated molecular weight of the PABA synthase from *S. griseus* or from *E. coli* carrying the cloned *pab*AB gene was 60,000, which is different from the weight estimated from the sequenced gene (M_r = 77,900). This difference in M_r may be due to an abnormal behavior of the enzyme during gel filtration. PABA synthase purified from *S. lividans* had an M_r of 47,000 (51) and presumably consisted of only the PabB component (475 amino acids, deduced M_r = 51,890) (46). The M_r of the enzyme isolated from *S. lividans* is also comparable to that of the polypeptide encoded by *E. coli pab*B (50,958) (35).

Synthesis of the *S. griseus* PABA synthase was repressed by aromatic amino acids, inorganic phosphate, and PABA, but not by anthranilic acid. In vivo experiments showed that formation of the PABA synthase is also subject to regulation by aromatic amino acids (52).

Asturias et al. (53) used *S. griseus pab*AB as a probe to show that the inhibitory effect of phosphate on candicidin biosynthesis takes place at the transcription level. Inorganic phosphate (7.5 mM) reduced the synthesis of the *pab*AB transcript by 90–95% and, consequently, the formation of PABA synthase and candicidin, but it stimulated two- to threefold total RNA synthesis. Similar results were obtained in *Streptomyces acrimycini* JI2239, another candicidin-producing strain (54).

3. PABA as Starter in Candicidin Biosynthesis

The chemical structure of the aromatic heptaenes shows that the aromatic moiety is covalently linked to the carbon atom of the macrolide ring that supports the lactone bond (see Figure 6). This suggests that cyclization occurs when the polyketide chain formed by polymerization of C_2 and C_3 units, using as starter the aromatic ring, has achieved an adequate length. Supporting the hypothesis that an aromatic moiety is a starter group in polyene macrolide biosynthesis is the fact that cerulenin rapidly inhibits incorporation of PABA into candicidin (6). Rapid inhibition of PABA incorporation into candicidin would not be expected until the pool of macrolide ring is depleted if PABA is attached after the macrolide ring is formed.

Additional evidence supporting the function of PABA as starter unit in the polyketide pathway was provided by the finding of the ORF3 located downstream of *pab*AB with high similarity to *p*-coumarate-CoA ligase, an enzyme involved in activation of aromatic starter units in the biosynthesis of plant polyketides. The ORF3 of the candicidin

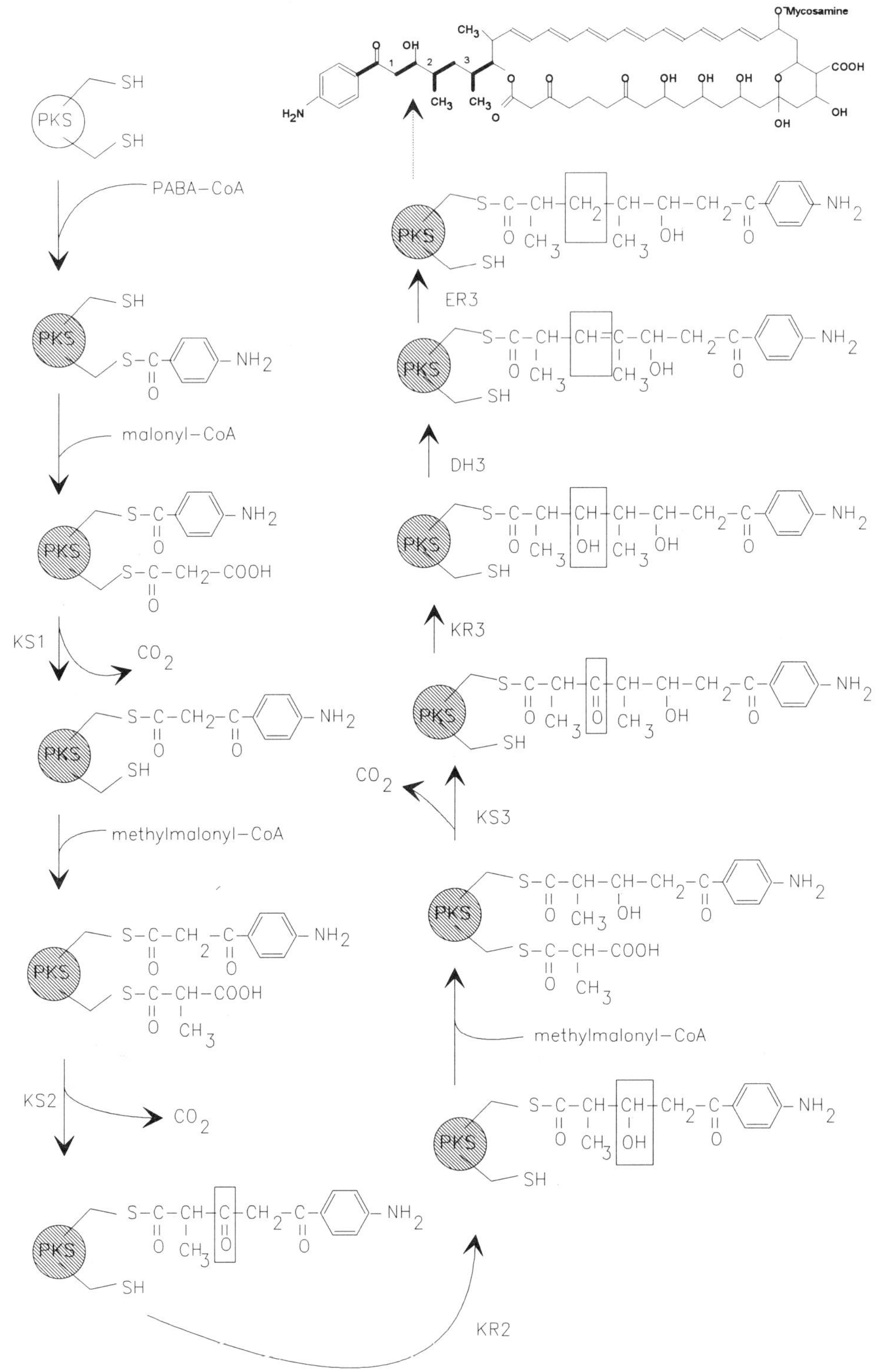

Figure 6 Early steps in the candicidin biosynthetic pathway. KS, ketosynthetase; KR, ketoreductase; DH, dehydratase; ER, enoylreductase.

cluster may code for a PABA-CoA ligase that activates PABA to start the biosynthesis of candicidin. The gene coding for this enzymatic activity was predicted by Martín (7) and was named *pabL* (45; Macias JR, personal communication).

B.   Biosynthesis of the Macrolide Aglycone Ring

The macrolide ring of polyene macrolide antibiotics is formed basically from acetate and propionate. Initial studies by Birch et al. (55) showed that [1-, 2-, and 3-^{14}C]propionate and [1-^{14}C]acetate were incorporated into the nystatin aglycone (nystatinolide), whereas negative results were obtained with [2-^{14}C]mevalonic acid and [methyl-^{14}C]methionine, indicating the absence of C_5 (terpenoid) or C_1 precursor units. Similar precursor incorporations were observed in the biosynthesis of the polyene macrolides lucensomycin (56), amphotericin B (57,58), candicidin (28,29), levorin (59), and fungimycin (60). The lack of incorporation of methyl-groups was also described in amphotericin B (57) and in candicidin (28). All this evidence indicates that the exocyclic methyl-groups in the polyene macrolides (see Figure 2) derive from C3 of propionate rather than from the methyl-group of methionine.

I.   Fatty Acid Polyketide Synthases

The biosynthesis of the macrolide rings of the polyene antibiotics occurs via the polyketide pathway by repeated head-to-tail condensation of acetate and propionate units, as was deduced from experiments through the use of cerulenin, an inhibitor of the condensing reaction of fatty acid (and polyketide) synthesis, which also specifically inhibits the biosynthesis of the polyene macrolide antibiotic candicidin by *S. griseus* (6). Since cerulenin is known to inhibit the condensation of malonyl-CoA subunits in the formation of fatty acids, it was concluded that polyenes are synthesized via the polyketide pathway by condensation steps similar to those occurring in fatty acid biosynthesis. A study in resveratrol and chalcone synthases (plant-specific polyketide synthases [PKSs] involved in the biosynthesis of stilbenes and flavonoids) showed that one of the six conserved cysteines (Cys-169) is the main target of cerulenin; the sequences surrounding the essential cysteine 169, however, revealed no similarity to the active sites of condensing enzymes in other PKSs and in fatty acid biosynthesis, indicating that resveratrol and chalcone synthases represent a group of enzymes that have evolved independently of other condensing enzymes (61).

Most fatty acids (saturated unbranched carbon chain) are synthesized by condensation of an acetyl starter unit with a malonyl unit (extender) to yield a C_4 intermediate, with a concomitant loss of CO_2 during condensation. The distal keto-group of the growing chain is then removed by a cycle of three reactions: ketoreduction, dehydratation, and enoylreduction to give an alkyl function. There are essentially two types of fatty acid synthetases (FAS): (a) FAS type I (typical from vertebrates), in which the different biochemical functions (condensation, ketoreduction, dehydratation, and enoylreduction) are carried out by distinct domains on a large multifunctional polypeptide; and (b) FAS type II (bacteria and high plants), in which the different functions are in different polypeptides (62).

2.   Assembly of Polyketides

Polyketide synthesis may be considered to involve an extension of the limited set of choices made by FAS; therefore, the PKS needs to be more highly programmed than the

FAS. In polyketide synthesis, the β-keto-group formed at each chain-extending step may or may not be retained. The requirement for NADPH (a cofactor in the reduction and hydrogenation steps) should be low in the biosynthesis of the polyenes, since some of them are simply reduced to hydroxyl-groups without undergoing subsequent dehydration and hydrogenation (7). Successive condensation steps result in the formation of the polyketide chain.

Polyketides are formed by a programmed pathway in which one starter unit (typically activated as acetyl-CoA, propionyl-CoA, or p-aminobenzoyl-CoA) and a highly variable number of malonate or methylmalonate (as malonyl-CoA and methylmelonyl-CoA) units are similarly attached together. As mentioned previously, in aromatic polyene biosynthesis the starter units is PABA, activated as p-aminobenzoyl-CoA (Figure 6).

Several gene clusters encoding the enzymes of polyketide synthesis have been cloned (partially or completely). Aromatic polyketides (e.g., tetracyclines, actinorhodine, and anthracyclines) are synthesized by type II PKSs, which are multienzyme complexes similar to FAS type II (63). In contrast, the polyketide chain of macrolide antibiotics such as erythromycin and avermectin are synthesized by PKS type I, consisting of large multifunctional polypeptides similar to FAS type I but composed of repeated units or "modules" with each active site carrying out only one reaction in the assembly and modification of each carbon chain (64,65).

The genes involved in the biosynthesis of candicidin and the antibiotic FR-008 (a heptaene aromatic polyene containing PAAP and a carbohydrate moiety different from mycosamine or perosamine) were cloned separately in two laboratories using a similar strategy. In both cases a pabAB gene from the candicidin producer S. griseus (44,48) was used as a probe to clone the set of genes involved in the biosynthesis of aromatic heptaenes. Hu et al. (66) reported that the DNA of Streptomyces hygroscopicus located downstream of the pabAB gene hybridized strongly with a PKS probe from the erythromycin cluster, and by disruption experiments and hybridizations they showed that the genes encoding the PKS for the FR-008 aglycone cover about 105 kb of the genome, implying enough genetic information for 21 PKS modules. This is precisely the number of condensation steps (4 methylmalonate and 17 malonate units) required to produce the carbon chain of FR-008 or candicidin by condensation of extender units onto a starter unit of p-aminobenzoyl-CoA (Figure 7). Macias (personal communication), by chromosome walking along the S. griseus DNA found by, DNA sequencing, PKS modules located downstream of the pabAB and pabL genes. These two results established that the aglycones of polyene antibiotics of the candicidin family are assembled by modular PKSs. Criado et al. (45) found, upstream of the pabAB gene, a gene coding for a thioesterase possibly involved in the biosynthesis of candicidin. An enzyme with this activity should be needed at the end of the polyketide synthesis to release the macrolide ring from the PKS (62).

3. Reprogramming of Polyketide Synthases: New Antibiotics

The modular organization of the candicidin PKS may be a help in designing new polyene antibiotics with increased activities or reduced toxicities using a variety of techniques. It should be possible to exchange complete ORFs of different PKS clusters, or of whole modules, or to alter specific regions of a PKS gene. This approach was used successfully to probe structure–function relationships in erythromycin biosynthesis (67). Synthesis of erythromycin by Saccharopolyspora erythraea is directed by three large eryA genes, organized in six modules, each governing one condensation cycle (67). Two amino acid sub-

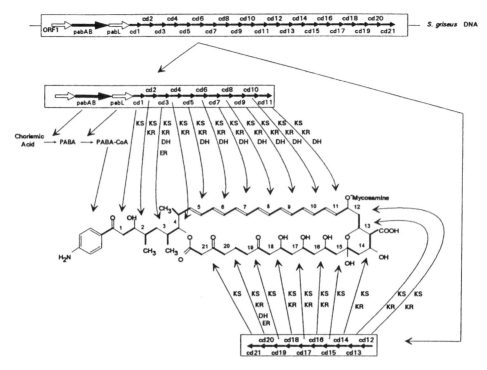

Figure 7   Genetic organization of the candicidin cluster. (Data from Refs. 54 and 65.)

stitutions were introduced in the putative NAD(P)H-binding motif in the proposed enoylreductase domain encoded by *ery*AII (67). The metabolite produced by the resulting strain was identified as delta-6,7-anhydroerythromycin C, formed as a result of the lack of enoylreduction during the fourth cycle of synthesis of the macrolactone. This result demonstrates that a virtually complete novel macrolide can be produced through reprogramming of polyketide synthesis. These kind of experiments will increase our understanding of the programming of a particular PKS system and provide an experimental and theoretical base with which novel biosynthetic pathways may be designed using rational approaches.

4.   Biosynthesis of Polyketide Precursors

The biosynthesis of methylmalonyl-CoA and malonyl-CoA, the building blocks of the macrolide ring, is also being studied. The genes (*mut*A and *mut*B) coding for the methyl-malonyl-CoA mutase from *Streptomyces cinnamonensis* have been cloned. This enzyme catalyzed the conversion of succinyl-CoA into methylmalonyl-CoA, and it represents an important source of building blocks for polyketide antibiotic biosynthesis. The methyl-malonyl-CoA mutase was unable to catalyze the conversion of isobutyryl-CoA into *n*-butyryl-CoA, a possible intermediate in the biosynthesis of methylmalonyl-CoA in streptomycetes (68). The incorporation of a methylmalonyl-CoA unit into the polyketide synthetase leads to a methyl branch in the polyketide backbone, as is observed in many of the structures of polyene antibiotics (see Figure 2). Because several units of methylmalonyl-CoA are needed to build a single molecule of polyene antibiotic (four for the macrolide of candicidin, three for nystatin, or two for lucensomycin), the production of methylmalonyl-CoA may represent a limiting step in the flow of primary metabolites into these antibiotics.

Acetyl coenzyme A carboxylase catalyzes the conversion of acetyl-CoA into malonyl-CoA, the first intermediate of fatty acid and polyketide synthesis. The *E. coli* enzyme is encoded by four subunits located at three different positions on the *E. coli* chromosome. The *accBC* genes lie in a small operon at min 72, whereas *accA* and *accD* are located at min 4.3 and 50, respectively. The *E. coli* accBC operon codes for the biotin carboxyl carrier protein and biotin carboxylase subunits of the acetyl coenzyme A carboxylase enzyme complex (69,70).

The *E. coli* carboxyltransferase component is a complex of two nonidentical subunits, a 35 kDa α-subunit encoded by *accA* and a 33 kDa β-subunit encoded by *accD*. The deduced amino acid sequences of α- and β-subunits show marked sequence similarities to the COOH-terminal and the NH_2-terminal moieties, respectively, of the rat propionyl-CoA carboxylase, a biotin-dependent carboxylase that catalyzes a similar carboxyltransferase reaction (71).

A direct correlation between the levels of transcription of the *E. coli acc* genes and the rate of cellular growth was found (72), suggesting an important role in the primary metabolism of the cell. In *Streptomyces rimosus*, the level of this enzyme is increased in a high oxytetracyline producer mutant, whereas the levels of other enzymes and the adenylate pools in the mycelium did not appear to be correlated with the degree of antibiotic production (73).

The acetyl-CoA carboxylase has been also studied in *Anabaena* (74) and *P. aeruginosa* (75), but in *Anabaena* the *accB* and *accC* are not linked. No information is available about the molecular biology of this enzyme in *Streptomyces*.

C. Biosynthesis of the Macrolide Aminosugars

Many of the naturally occurring secondary metabolites from bacteria and plants are glycosylated, mostly by 6-deoxyhexoses derived from dTDP-glucose (deoxythymidine 5'-diphospho-glucose). 6-Deoxyhexose derivatives are present in a variety of antibiotics from actinomycetes, including macrolides, polyenes, and aminoglycosides, among others.

No in vitro studies have been carried out specifically on the biosynthesis of the aminosugar moieties of polyene macrolide antibiotics; however, the similarity with the biosynthesis of aminosugars of nonpolyene macrolides and bacterial lipopolysaccharides provides some data on the probable biosynthetic pathway.

Genes involved in lipopolysaccharide synthesis in *Salmonella* have been cloned and sequenced (76,77), and genes coding for the biosynthesis of the deoxysugar moiety of streptomycin were also cloned (78). In both cases, pathways for sugar biosynthesis were proposed; all biosynthetic transformations of these sugars occur while they are in the form of nucleoside diphosphate derivatives; the corresponding 4-keto-6-deoxysugar nucleoside diphosphate is as an intermediate, as was described previously (79,80). The 4-keto derivatives are common key intermediates of various metabolic pathways and lead to the formation of new carbohydrates such as epimers, deoxysugars, or branched carbohydrates.

The formation of 4-keto-6-deoxyhexose nucleoside diphosphate from nucleoside diphosphate-glucose is catalyzed by an NAD-dependent nucleoside diphosphate-glucose

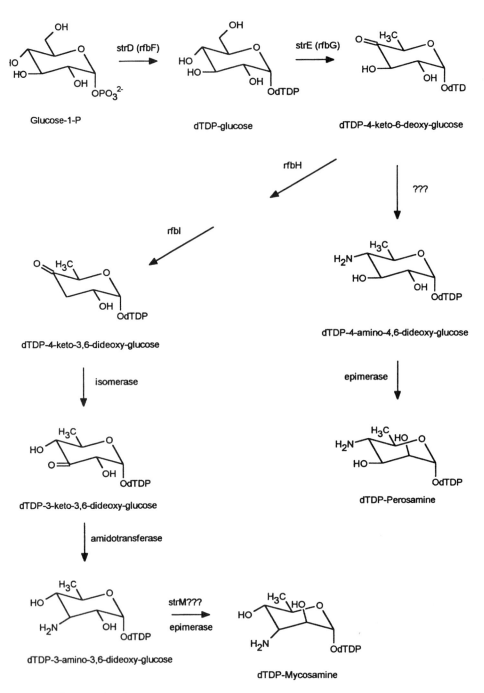

Figure 8   Proposed pathway of biosynthesis of the aminosugar moieties of polyene macrolide antibiotics.

oxidoreductase encoded by strE in S. griseus and rfbG in Salmonella (Figure 8). This enzyme has been purified from S. erythraea, the erythromycin producer (81). The following step seems to be the conversion of dTDP-4-keto-6-deoxy-D-glucose to dTDP-4-keto-3,6-dideoxy-D-glucose, as occurred in Salmonella, and may require the products of genes rfbH and rfbI. The next step in the biosynthesis of mycosamine should be the isomerization of the keto-group to give dTDP-3-keto-3,6-dideoxy-D-glucose. The biosynthesis of dTDP-4-keto-4,6-dideoxy-D-glucose (intermediate in the biosynthesis of perosamine) may take place via similar enzymes, but no isomerization of the keto-group is required.

A further step required for the biosynthesis of both aminosugars is the transfer of an amino-group from L-glutamate to the keto-group by a pyridoxal phosphate–requiring transaminating enzyme (82). The last step is probably the epimerization of glucose to mannose, catalyzed by an enzyme homologous to that encoded by strM (78).

Cloning of the genes involved in the biosynthesis of deoxysugars helps us to clarify their biosynthetic pathway, and it also opens the possibility of using such genes as universal probes for pathways that include the formation of 6-deoxyhexoses. This was proved to be partially true in actinomycetes by Stockmann and Piepersberg (83), who cloned the genes strDE from the streptomycin producer S. griseus. They found that 70% of the 43 strains tested gave positive signals with the probe, and only 63% of them were known to contain 6-deoxyhexoses in their secondary metabolites. The "false" positives probably synthesize some 6-deoxyhexoses of unknown structure, function, and location. On the other hand, no hybridization was found in 8 strains known to produce 6-deoxyhexoses. Streptomyces nodosus (amphotericin B producer; containing mycosamine), Streptomyces noursei (nystatin producer; mycosamine), and Streptomyces coelicolor var. aminophilus (perimicin producer; containing perosamine) are found among the Streptomyces strains giving a positive signal with these probes (81). A positive signal was found in our laboratory between S. griseus DNA (candicidin producer) and the strDE probe (Campelo AB, personal communication), but not with S. hygroscopicus DNA (producer of a heptaene aromatic polyene FR-008, containing PAAP and a carbohydrate moiety different from mycosamine or perosamine) (66).

The attachment of the aminosugar moiety to the macrolide ring seems to take place during the secretion of the polyene. In the biosynthesis of candihexin, it was observed that the intracellular antibiotic consists exclusively of nonglycosylated inactive components, whereas the excreted antibiotic contains a mixture of glycosylated and nonglycosylated components (84). This evidence is consistent with the theory that the macrolide ring acts as a lipid-soluble carrier of the aminosugar during the secretion process (7). Sugar attachment during biosynthesis of the macrolide antibiotic tylosin is also a late step, since mutants blocked in either sugar biosynthesis or in glycosyltransferase reactions are able to form the corresponding aglycone tylonolide (85). Similar results were obtained in the case of erythromycin (86), where the attachment of TDP-mycarose and TDP-desosamine are two of the four late steps of its biosynthesis.

VII. NUTRITIONAL AND ENVIRONMENTAL FACTORS AFFECTING POLYENE MACROLIDE FERMENTATIONS

Nutritional studies of polyene-producing Streptomyces have been carried out with batch cultures, usually in shake flasks, with occasional scale-up to pilot-plant or large-scale fermentors of those polyenes that are produced industrially. In most studies, several nutritional factors or physical parameters are studied, and the combinations giving the highest yields have been selected for further improvement.

A. Carbon Sources

Most polyene antibiotic fermentations have been carried out using glucose as a carbon source. Concentrations of glucose as high as 7.0 to 9.5% have been routinely used (87). Slow feeding of glucose, initially described in penicillin fermentations (88) to bypass the negative effect of high glucose concentrations, resulted in increased synthesis of the polyenes candidin and candihexin (87). Intermittent addition of glucose in amphotericin B fermentations also resulted in a slight increase in the titer of amphotericin. Disaccharides, particularly lactose, were poor substrates for polyene production.

Regulation of secondary metabolites by glucose or other easily assimilated carbon sources (glucose repression) occurs in the biosynthesis of several antibiotics (penicillin, actinomycin, streptomycin, siomycin, bacitracin, etc.) (for a review, see Refs. 89 and 90), but not in the biosynthesis of polyene antibiotics, because glucose is required for their biosynthesis.

Acetate and propionate as their biologically active units, acetyl-CoA and propionyl-CoA, and their carboxylated derivatives, malonyl-CoA and methylmalonyl-CoA, are the building blocks used in the head-to-tail condensation leading to the formation of the macrolide antibiotics. Acetate and propionate do not support antibiotic synthesis by themselves, but supplementation of a glucose basal medium with acetate, propionate, or malonate significantly stimulates candicidin synthesis in batch cultures (91).

Citrate is a positive effector of acetyl-CoA carboxylase (92), the enzyme involved in the biosynthesis of the malonyl-CoA needed for polyketide biosynthesis. However, high levels of citrate were clearly inhibitory for candicidin biosynthesis, apparently due to its metal-chelating properties (91).

Early studies demonstrated that oils and fatty acids stimulated the production of the polyene macrolide antibiotics fungichromin and filipin, but not amphotericin B or candicidin (89). The stimulation of polyene antibiotic biosynthesis by oils might be a simple precursor effect. Catabolism of fatty acids results in a increased pool of acetyl-CoA, which is subsequently used for polyene biosynthesis.

It is not clear at present why oils stimulate the biosynthesis of some polyene macrolides (fungichromin and filipin) and have an inhibitory effect on the biosynthesis of others (89). When ethyl (Z)-16-phenylhexadec-9-enoate, an analog of ethyl oleate, was added to cultures of the fungichromin producer *Streptomyces cellulosae* ATCC 12625, the cultures showed a drastic reduction of fungichromin biosynthesis but produced four new polyene antibiotics (93).

B. Nitrogen Sources

Complex nitrogen sources are the choice for large-scale antibiotic production. A large variety of complex nitrogen sources, including plant (and some animal) proteins, have been used. These include yeast extract, soy peptone, cotton-seed meal, soybean meal, corn meal, casein, corn steep liquor, and distiller's solubles. Soybean meal is a good nitrogen source for producing many polyene macrolides, probably because of its balance of nutrients and slow hydrolysis.

Considerable differences in the ability of different amino acids to support candicidin biosynthesis were founded by Acker and Lechevalier (94). L-Asparagine was the best nitrogen source. L-Histidine, glycine, L-glutamic acid, and L-aspartic acid were next in effectiveness as nitrogen sources. The D-isomers of the amino acids supported negligible growth and no candicidin production.

L-Asparagine is routinely used as unique nitrogen source in a phosphate-limited resting cell system for candicidin production (91). In this system, cells produced candicidin at a constant rate for 36 hr without increase in cell dry weight.

β-Alanine supported a 10-fold higher yield than α-alanine and was the best amino acid source for the production of ayfactin. The explanation for this may be that β-alanine is a component of the pantotheinyl moieties of coenzyme A and the pantotheinyl-protein of fatty acid and polyketide synthases (62) in addition to serving as a nitrogen source. Alternatively, β-alanine may be deaminated by an ω-aminotransferase, giving rise to malonyl semialdehyde, which is a precursor of malonyl-CoA. Inorganic salts are generally poor nitrogen sources for polyene production; however, ammonium salts were acceptable in the case of mycoheptin (95).

There are several reports in the literature that suggest that antibiotic synthesis may be repressed by ammonia and other rapidly utilized nitrogen sources (96). However, there are no detailed studies on the possible nitrogen regulation of the biosynthesis of mycosamine or other aminosugars of polyenes.

C.   Regulation by Aromatic Amino Acids

Candicidin and probably other aromatic polyene macrolides are subject to regulation by aromatic amino acids. The biosynthesis of candicidin was inhibited in vivo by L-tryptophan, L-phenylalanine, and to a lesser degree, L-tyrosine. A mixture of the three aromatic amino acids inhibited candicidin biosynthesis to a greater extent than did each amino acid separately. The inhibitory effect of tryptophan was partially reversed by exogenous PABA, suggesting that this effect is exerted at the PABA synthase level (52). In vitro experiments have clearly shown that PABA synthase activity is insensitive to inhibition by PABA, OABA, or aromatic amino acids. PABA synthase was repressed by aromatic amino acids and PABA, but not by OABA (50). This is a fine example of a regulatory system in which the biosynthesis of a secondary metabolite (candicidin) is regulated by the mechanisms controlling the biosynthesis of primary metabolites, such as aromatic amino acids.

D.   Phosphate Regulation

The biosynthesis of many antibiotics is inhibited in vivo by phosphate (89,91). Antibiotics are synthesized only at concentrations of inorganic phosphate that are suboptimal for growth (from 1 to 50 mM for different antibiotics). Phosphate in the range 0.3–500 mM supports excellent cell growth, whereas 10 mM phosphate often suppresses biosynthesis of antibiotics. The same inhibitory effect is exerted by deoxyribonucleotides, because they are cleaved during uptake by S. griseus cells (97,98).

High phosphate concentration strongly repressed the PABA synthase of S. griseus, the candicidin producer (50). Using an internal fragment of the cloned pabAB gene, specific pabAB mRNA was quantified. When high levels of phosphate (7.5 mM) were added to the culture broth, the formation of specific mRNA for PABA synthase decreased 95%

(53). Repression by phosphate appears to be specific for the transcript of the *pab*AB gene, since total RNA synthesis was stimulated by phosphate.

The molecular mechanism via which many promoters for antibiotic biosynthetic genes are regulated by phosphate is still obscure. Either all promoters contain similar "phosphate" boxes (99), or alternatively, a common regulated DNA-binding protein must occur that in turn is regulated by phosphate. This protein may be a specific σ-factor or a protein interacting with the RNA polymerase (100; Marcos AT, personal communication).

VIII.   SUMMARY AND FUTURE OUTLOOK

Polyene macrolides are synthesized (as are other, better known nonpolyene macrolides) from two- and three-carbon units activated as malonyl-CoA and methylmalonyl-CoA. A few polyene macrolides contain an aromatic moiety that derives from *p*-aminobenzoyl-CoA and is used as starter unit. The different precursor units are condensed by polyketide synthases. Aminosugars, for example, mycosamine or perosamine, are attached glycosidically to the lactone ring.

In the last few years, some of the genes involved in candicidin biosynthesis have been cloned in the authors' laboratory. A gene (*pab*AB) encoding a *p*-aminozoic acid synthase is linked to a gene encoding a putative *p*-aminobenzoyl-CoA ligase, and to the polyketide synthase genes. It is likely that a large amount of genetic information is required for the biosynthesis of these large polyene macrolides (up to 105 kb in candicidin), not even including the genes for synthesis and attachment of the aminosugars. The many modules and enzymatic functions required for the synthesis of these compounds provide interesting tools for reprogramming polyketide synthesis to develop new compounds.

The availability of the cloned genes opens the way for studies on gene expression and regulation by phosphate and other well-known effectors of polyene macrolide biosynthesis.

ACKNOWLEDGMENTS

We thank José Ramón Macías, Ana B. Campelo, and Tobias Kieser for providing data prior to publication. Research in the authors' laboratory was supported by Junta de Castilla y León (Ref. 7/11/92), Iberdrola, CAICYT (BIO93-0831), and Diputación de León (Spain).

REFERENCES

1.   Georgopapadokou NH, Walsh TJ. Human mycosis: Drugs and targets for emerging pathogens. Science 1994; 264:371–372.
2.   Nair MG, Putnam AR, Mishra SK, Mulks MH, Taft WH, Keller JE, Miller JR, Zhu PP, Meinhart JD, Lynn DG. Faerifungin: A new broad-spectrum antibiotic from *Streptomyces griseus* var. *autotrophicus*. J Nat Prod 1989; 52:797–809.

3. Pisano MA, Sommer MJ, Brett BP. Hudson River sediments as a source of actinomycetes exhibiting antifungal activity. Appl Microbiol Biotechnol 1987; 27:214–217.

4. Antonio J, Molinski TF. Screening of marine invertebrates for the presence of ergosterol-sensitive antifungal compounds. J Nat Prod 1993; 56:54–61.

5. Veiga M, Traba MP, Fabregas J. Tetrafungin, a new polyene macrolide antibiotic. II. Taxonomy of the producing organism and comparison with nystatin by means of high performance liquid chromatography. J Antibiot 1983; 36:776–783.

6. Martín JF, McDaniel LE. Specific inhibition of candicidin biosynthesis by the lipogenic inhibitor cerulenin. Biochim Biophys Acta 1975; 411:186–194.

7. Martín JF. Biosynthesis of polyene macrolide antibiotics. Annu Rev Microbiol 1977; 31:13–38.

8. Gil JA, Liras P, Martín JF. The polyenes: Properties, biosynthesis and fermentation. Vandamme EJ, ed. Biotechnology of Industrial Antibiotics. New York: Marcel Dekker, 1983: 513–529.

9. Martín JF, McDaniel LE. Production of polyene macrolide antibiotics. Perlman D, ed. Advances in Applied Microbiology, Vol. 21. New York: Academic Press, 1976:1–52.

10. Sowinski P, Gariboldi P, Czerwinski A, Borowski E. The structure of vacidin A, an aromatic heptaene macrolide antibiotic. I. Complete assignment of the ^{1}H NMR spectrum and geometry of the polyene chromophore. J Antibiot 1989; 42:1631–1638.

11. Komori T. Trichomycin B, a polyene macrolide from *Streptomyces*. J Antibiot 1990; 43:778–782.

12. Hirota H, Itoh A, Ido J, Iwamoto Y, Goshima E, Miki T, Hasuda K, Ohashi Y. YS-822A, a new polyene macrolide antibiotic. II. Planar structure of YS-822A. J Antibiot 1991; 44:181–186.

13. Cidaria D, Borgonovi G, Pirali G. AB023, novel polyene antibiotics. I. Taxonomy of the producing organism, fermentation and antifungal activity. J Antibiot 1993; 46:251–254.

14. Zielinski J, Jereczek E, Sowinski P, Falkowski L, Rudowski A, Borowski E. The structure of a novel sugar component of polyene macrolide antibiotics: 2,6-dideoxy-L-ribohexopyranose. J Antibiot 1979; 32:565–568.

15. Raatikainen O, Auriola S, Tuomisto J. Identification of aromatic moieties and mycosamine in antifungal heptaenes with high-performance liquid chromatography, high-performance liquid chromatography–mass spectrometry and gas chromatography–mass spectrometry. J Chromatogr 1991; 585:247–254.

16. Lampen JO, Arnow PM. Differences in action of large and small polyene antifungal antibiotics. Bull Res Counc Isr 1963; II:286–291.

17. Liras P, Lampen JO. Sequence of candicidine action on yeasts cells. Biochim Biophys Acta 1974; 372:141–153.

18. Bolard J. How do polyene macrolide antibiotics affect the cellular membrane properties? Biochim Biophys Acta 1986; 864:257–304.

19. Cybulska B, Mazerski J, Borowski E, Gary-Bobo CM. Haemolytic activity of aromatic heptaenes. A group of polyene macrolide antifungal antibiotics. Biochem Pharmacol 1984; 1:41–46.

20. Mpona-Minga M, Coulon J, Bonaly R. Effects of subinhibitory dose of amphotericin B on cell wall biosynthesis in *Candida albicans*. Res Microbiol 1989; 140:95–105.

21. Yamaguchi H, Abe S, Tokuda Y. Immunomodulating activity of antifungal drugs. Ann NY Acad Sci 1993; 685:447–457.

22. Valeriote F, Medoff G, Dieckman J. Potentiation of cytotoxicity of anticancer agents by several different polyene antibiotics. J Natl Cancer Inst 1984; 72:435–439.

23. Molowica B, Momsen M, Jenkin HM, Borowski E. Potentiation of antiviral activity of acyclovir by polyene macrolide antibiotics. Antimicrob Agents Chemother 1984; 25:772–774.

24. Hidaka K, An G, Ip P, Kuwana M, Siminovitch L. Amphotericin B enhances efficiency of DNA-mediated gene transfer in mammalian cells. Somat Cell Mol Genet 1985; 11:109–115.

25. Pontani DR, Sun D, Brown JW, Shahied SI, Plescia OJ, Schaffner CP, Lopez-Berestein G, Sarin PS. Inhibition of HIV replication by liposomal encapsulated amphotericin B. Antiviral Res 1989; 11:119–125.

26. Pocchiari M, Schmittinger S, Masullo C. Amphotericin B delays the incubation period of scrapie in intracerebrally inoculated hamsters. J Gen Virol 1987; 68:219–223.

27. Mulks MH, Nair MG, Putnam AR. In vitro antibacterial activity of faeriefungin, a new broad-spectrum polyene macrolide antibiotic. Antimicrob Agents Chemother 1990; 34:1762–1765.

28. Liu CM, McDaniel LE, Schaffner CP. Studies on candicidin biosynthesis. J Antibiot 1972; 25:116–121.

29. Martín JF, Liras P. Rapid incorporation of precursors into candicidin by resting-cells of *Streptomyces griseus*. J Antibiot 1976; 29:1306–1309.

30. Light RJ. Enzymic studies on the polyketide biosynthesis. J Agric Food Chem 1970; 18:260–267.

31. Lozoya E, Hoffmann H, Douglas C, Schulz W, Schell D, Hahlbrock K. Primary structures and catalitic properties of isoenzymes encoded by two 4-coumarate: CoA ligases in parsley. Eur J Biochem 1988; 176:661–667.

32. Ghisalba O, Fuhrer H, Richter WJ, Moss S. A genetic approach to the biosynthesis of the rifamycin chromophore in *Nocardia mediterranei*. III. Isolation and identification of an early aromatic ansamycin precursor containing the seven-carbon amino starter-unit and three initial acetate/propionate-unit of the ansa chain. J Antibiot 1981; 34:58–63.

33. Green JM, Nichols BP. *p*-Aminobenzoate biosynthesis in *Escherichia coli*. Purification of aminodeoxychorismatelyase and cloning of *pabC*. J Biol Chem 1991; 266:12972–12975.

34. Kaplan JB, Nichols BP. Nucleotide sequence of *Escherichia coli pabA* and its evolutionary relationship to *trp(G)D*. J Mol Biol 1983; 168:451–468.

35. Goncharoff P, Nichols BP. Nucleotide sequence of *Escherichia coli pabB* indicates a common evolutionary origin of *p*-aminobenzoate and anthranilate synthetases. J Bacteriol 1984; 159:57–62.

36. Gibson F, Gibson M, Cox GB. The biosynthesis of *p*-aminobenzoic acid from chorismic acid. Biochim Biophys Acta 1964; 82:637–638.

37. Huang M, Gibson F. Biosynthesis of 4-aminobenzoate in *Escherichia coli*. J Bacteriol 1970; 102:767–773.

38. Altendorf KH, Gilch B, Lingens F. Biosynthesis of 4-aminobenzoic acid in *Aerobacter aerogenes*. FEBS Lett 1971; 16:95–98.

39. Kane JF, O'Brien HD. *p*-Aminobenzoate synthase form *Bacillus subtilis*: Amidotransferase composed of nonidentical subunits. J Bacteriol 1975; 123:1131–1138.

40. Teng, CYP, Ganem, B, Doktor SZ, Nichols BP, Bhatnagar RK, Vining LC. Total synthesis of 4-amino-4-deoxychorismic acid: A key intermediate in the biosynthesis of *p*-aminobenzoic acid and L-(p-aminophenyl)alanine. J Am Chem Soc 1985; 107:5008–5009.

41. Nichols BP, Seibold AM, Doktor SZ. *para*-Aminobenzoate synthesis from chorismate occurs in two steps. J Biol Chem 1989; 264:8587–8601.

42. Slock J, Stalhly, DP, Han CY, Six EW, Crawford IP. An apparent *Bacillus subtilis* folic acid biosynthetic operon containing *pab*, an amphibolic *trpG* gene, a third gene required for synthesis of para-aminobenzoic acid, and the dihydropteroate synthase gene. J Bacteriol 1990; 172:7211–7226.

43. Medique C, Viari A, Henaut A, Danchin A. Colibri: A functional data base for the *Escherichia coli* genome. Microbiol Rev 1993; 57:623–654.

44. Gil JA, Hopwood DA. Cloning and expression of a *p*-aminobenzoic acid synthetase gene from the candicidin producer *Streptomyces griseus*. Gene 1983; 25:119–132.

45. Criado LM, Martín JF, Gil JA. The *pab* gene from *Streptomyces griseus*, encoding *p*-aminobenzoic acid synthase, is located between genes possibly involved in candicidin biosynthesis. Gene 1993; 126:135–139.

46. Arhin FF, Vining LC. Organization of the genes encoding *p*-aminobenzoic acid synthases from *Streptomyces lividans*. Gene 1993; 126:129–133.

47. Edman JC, Goldstein AL, Erbe JG. para-Aminobenzoate synthase gene of *Saccharomyces cerevisiae* encodes a bifunctional enzyme. Yeast 1993; 9:669–675.

48. Gil JA, Criado LM, Alegre T, Martín JF. Use of a cloned gene involved in candicidin production to discover new polyene producer *Streptomyces* strains. FEMS Microbiol Lett 1990; 58:15–18.

49. Essar DW, Eberly L, Hadero A, Crawford IP. Identification and characterization of genes for a second anthranilate synthase in *Pseudomonas aeruginosa*: Interchangeability of the two anthranilate synthases and evolutionary implications. J Bacteriol 1990; 172:884–900.

50. Gil JA, Naharro G, Villanueva JR, Martín JF. Characterization and regulation of p-aminobenzoic acid synthase from *Streptomyces griseus*. J Gen Microbiol 1985; 131:1279–1287.

51. Rebollo, A. Expression of the *pab* gene of *Streptomyces griseus* IMRU3570: Genetic and biochemical studies. Ph.D. thesis, University of León, Spain, 1987.

52. Gil JA, Liras P, Naharro G, Villanueva JR, Martín JF. Regulation by aromatic amino acids of the biosynthesis of candicidin by *Streptomyces griseus*. J Gen Microbiol 1980; 118:189–195.

53. Asturias JA, Liras P, Martín JF. Phosphate control of *pabS* gene transcription during candicidin biosynthesis. Gene 1990; 93:79–84.

54. Asturias JA, Martín JF, Liras P. Biosynthesis and phosphate control of candicidin by *Streptomyces acrimycini* JI2236: Effect of amplification of the *pabAB* gene. J Ind Microbiol 1994; 13:183–189.

55. Birch AJ, Holzapfel CW, Rickards RW, Ojerassi C, Suzuki M, Westley J, Dutcher JD, Thomas R. Nistatin. V. Biosynthetic definition of some structural features. Tetrahedron Lett 1964; 1485–1490.

56. Manwaring DG, Rickards RW, Gandiano G, Nicolella V. The biosynthesis of the macrolide antibiotic lucensomycin. J Antibiot 1969; 22:545–550.

57. Perlman RA, Semar JB. Preparation of amphotericin B-¹⁴C. Biotechnol Bioeng 1965; 7:133–137.

58. Linke HAB, Mechlinski W, Schaffner CP. Production of amphotericin B-¹⁴C by *Streptomyces nodosus*. Fermentation and preparation of amphotericin B-¹⁴C-methyl-ester. J Antibiot 1974; 27:155–160.

59. Belousova II, Lishnvskaya EB, Elgari RE. Incorporation of radioactive precursors into levorin and fatty acids by *Actinomyces levoris*. Antibiotiki 1971; 16:184–187.

60. Liu CM, McDaniel LE, Schaffner CP. Fungimycin, biogenesis of its aromatic moiety. J Antibiot 1972; 25:187–188.

61. Lanz T, Tropf S, Marner FJ, Schroder J, Schroder G. The role of cysteines in polyketide synthases. Site-directed mutagenesis of resveratrol and chalcone synthases, two key enzymes in different plant-specific pathways. J Biol Chem 1991; 266:9971–9976.

62. Hopwood DA, Sherman DH. Molecular genetics of polyketide and its comparison to fatty acid biosynthesis. Annu Rev Genet 1990; 24:37–66.

63. Malpartida F, Hallam SE, Kieser HM, Motamedi H, Hutchinson CR, Butler MJ, Sugden DA, Warren M, McKillop C, Bailey CR, Humphreys GO, Hopwood DA. Homology between *Streptomyces* genes coding for synthesis of different polyketides used to clone antibiotic biosynthesis genes. Nature 1987; 325:818–821.

64. Cortes I, Haydock SH, Roberts GA, Bevitt DJ, Lewis PF. An unusually large multifunctional polypeptide in the erythromycin-producing polyketide synthase of *Saccharopolyspora erythraea*. Nature 1990; 348:176–178.

65.   MacNeil DJ, Occi JL, Gewain KM, MacNeil T, Gibbons PH, Ruby CL, Danis SJ. Complex organization of the *Streptomyces avermitilis* genes encoding the avermectin polyketide synthase. Gene 1992; 115:119–125.

66.   Hu H, Bao K, Zhou X, Hopwood DA, Kieser T, Deng Z. Repeated polyketide synthase modules involved in the biosynthesis of a heptaene macrolide by *Streptomyces* sp. FR-008. Mol Microbiol 1994; 14:163–172.

67.   Donadio S, McAlpine JB, Sheldon PJ, Jackson M, Katz L. An erythromycin analog produced by reprogramming of polyketide synthesis. Proc Natl Acad Sci USA 1993; 90:7119–7123.

68.   Birch A, Leiser A, Robinson JA. Cloning, sequencing, and expression of the gene encoding methylmalonyl-coenzyme A mutase from *Streptomyces cinnamonensis*. J Bacteriol 1993; 175:3511–3519.

69.   Karow M, Fayet O, Georgopoulos C. The lethal phenotype caused by null mutations in the *Escherichia coli htrB* gene is suppressed by mutations in the *accBC* operon, encoding two subunits of acetyl coenzyme A carboxylase. J Bacteriol 1992; 174:7407–418.

70.   Li SJ, Cronan JE Jr. The gene encoding the biotin carboxylase subunit of *Escherichia coli* acetyl-CoA carboxylase. J Biol Chem 1992; 267:855–863.

71.   Li SJ, Cronan JE Jr. The genes encoding the two carboxyltransferase subunits of *Escherichia coli* acetyl-CoA carboxylase. J Biol Chem 1991; 267:16841–16847.

72.   Li SJ, Cronan JE Jr. Growth rate regulation of *Escherichia coli* acetyl coenzyme A carboxylase, which catalyzes the first committed step of lipid biosynthesis. J Bacteriol 1993; 175:332–340.

73.   Al Jawadi M, Calam CT. Physiology of a wild strain and high yielding mutants of *Streptomyces rimosus*, producing oxytetracycline. Folia Microbiol Praha 1987; 32:388–401.

74.   Gornicki P, Scappino LA, Haselkorn R. Genes for two subunits of acetyl coenzyme A carboxylase of *Anabaena* sp. strain PCC 7120: Biotin carboxylase and biotin carboxyl carrier protein. J Bacteriol 1993; 175:5268–5272.

75.   Best EA, Knauf VC. Organization and nucleotide sequences of the genes encoding the biotin carboxyl carrier protein and biotin carboxylase protein of *Pseudomonas aeruginosa* acetyl coenzyme A carboxylase. J Bacteriol 1993; 175:6881–6889.

76.   Wyk P, Reeves P. Identification and sequence of the gene for abequose synthase, which confers antigenic specificity on group B salmonellae: Homology with galactose epimerase. J Bacteriol 1989; 171:5687–5693.

77.   Verma N, Reeves P. Identification and sequence of *rfbS* and *rfbE*, which determine antigenic specificity of group A and group D salmonellae. J Bacteriol 1989; 171:5694–5701.

78.   Pissowotzki K, Mansouri K, Piepersberg W. Genetics of streptomycin production in *Streptomyces griseus*: Molecular structure and putative function of genes *strELMB2N*. Mol Gen Genet 1991; 231:113–123.

79.   Lüderitz O, Staub AM, Westphal O. Immunochemistry of O and R antigens of *Salmonella* and related enterobacteriaceae. Bacteriol Rev 1966; 30:192–255.

80.   Ortman R, Matern U, Grisebach H, Stadler P, Sinnwell V, Paulsen H. NADH-dependent formation of thymidine diphosphodihydrostreptose from thymidine diphospho-D-glucose in a cell-free extract from *Streptomyces griseus* and its correlation with streptomycin biosynthesis. J Biochem 1974; 43:265.

81.   Vara J, Hutchinson CR. Purification of thymidine-diphospho-D-glucose 4,6-dehydratase from an erythromycin producing strain of *Saccharopolyspora erythraea* by high resolution liquid chromatography. J Biol Chem 1988; 263:14992–14995.

82.   Matsuhashy M, Strominger JL. Thymidine diphosphate 4-acetamido-4,6-dideoxyhexoses. I. Enzymatic synthesis by strains of *Escherichia coli*. J Biol Chem 1966; 239:2454–2463.

83.   Stockmann M, Piepersberg W. Gene probes for the detection of 6-deoxyhexose metabolism in secondary metabolite-producing streptomycetes. FEMS Microbiol Lett 1992; 90:185–190.

84. Martín JF, McDaniel LE. Candihexin polyene macrolide complex: Physicochemical characterization and antifungal activities of the single components. Antimicrob Agents Chemother 1975; 8:200–208.

85. Baltz RH, Seno ET. Properties of *Streptomyces fradiae* mutants blocked in biosynthesis of the macrolide antibiotic tylosin. Antimicrob Agents Chemother 1981; 20:214–225.

86. Vara J, Lewandowska-Skarbek M, Wang YG, Donadio S, Hutchinson R. Cloning of genes governing the deoxysugar portion of the erythromycin biosynthesis pathway in *Saccaropolyspora erythraea* (*Streptomyces erytheus*). J Bacteriol 1989; 171:5872–5881.

87. Martín JF, McDaniel LE. The submerged culture production of the polyene antifungal antibiotic candidin and candihexin. Dev Ind Microbiol 1974; 15:324–337.

88. Soltero FV, Johnson MJ. Continous addition of glucose for the evaluation of penicillin production by *Penicillium chrysogenum* Q-176. Appl Microbiol 1954; 2:41–44.

89. Martín JF, Demain AL. Control of antibiotic biosynthesis. Microbiol Rev 1980; 44:230–251.

90. Martín JF, Liras P. Organization and expression of genes involved in the biosynthesis of antibiotics and other secondary metabolites. Annu Rev Microbiol 1989; 43:173–206.

91. Martín JF, McDaniel LE. Biosynthesis of candicidin by phosphate limited resting cells of *Streptomyces griseus*. Eur J Appl Microbiol 1976; 3:135–144.

92. Volpe JJ, Vagelos PR. Saturated fatty acids. Biosynthesis and its regulation. Annu Rev Biochem 1973; 42:21–60.

93. Li Z, Rawlings BJ, Harrison PH, Vederas JC. Production of new polyene antibiotics by *Streptomyces cellulosae* after addition of ethyl (Z)-16-phenylhexadec-9-enoate. J Antibiot 1989; 42:577–584.

94. Acker RF, Lechevalier H. Some nutritional requirements of *Streptomyces griseus* 3570 for growth and candicidin production. Appl Microbiol 1954; 2:152–157.

95. Tereshin IM. Polyene Antibiotics: Present and Future. Tokyo: University of Tokyo Press, 1976.

96. Demain AL, Aharanowitz Y, Martín JF. Metabolic control of secondary biosynthetic pathways. Vining LC, ed. Biochemistry and Genetic Regulation of Commercially Important Antibiotics. London: Addison-Wesley Publishing Company, 1983.

97. Martín JF, Demain AL. Effect of exogenous nucleotides on the candicidin fermentation. Can J Microbiol 1977; 23:1334–1339.

98. Martín JF. Control of antibiotic synthesis by phosphate. Ghose TK, Fiechter A, Blakebrough N, eds. Advances in Biochemical Engineering, Vol. 6. Berlin: Springer-Verlag, 1977:105–127.

99. Liras P, Asturias JA, Martín JF. Phosphate control sequences involved in transcriptional regulation of antibiotic biosynthesis. Trends Biotechnol 1990; 8:184–189.

100. Martín JF, Marcos AT, Martin A, Asturias JA, Liras P. Phosphate control of antibiotic Biosynthesis at the transcriptional level. Torriani-Gorini A, Yagil E, Silver S, eds. Phosphate in Microorganisms: Cellular and Molecular Biology. Washington D.C.: ASM Press, 1994:140–147.

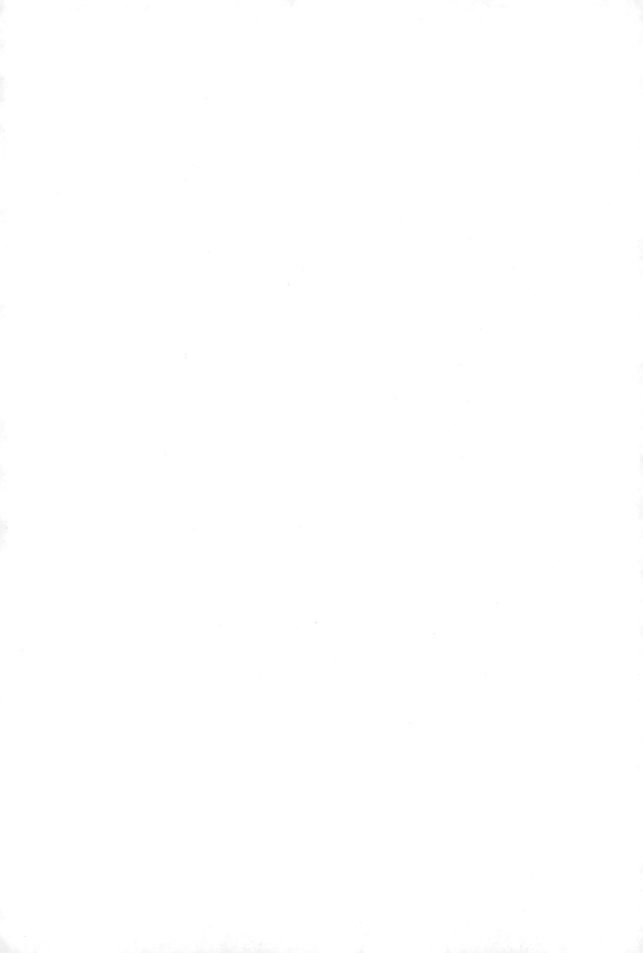

20
Anthracyclines

William R. Strohl, Michael L. Dickens, Vineet B. Rajgarhia,
Anton J. Woo, and Nigel D. Priestley
The Ohio State University, Columbus, Ohio

I. INTRODUCTION

The anthracyclines are among the most intensely studied natural products over the past quarter century, due in part to the mechanisms associated with their antitumor activity and toxicities, and in part to the elusive promise they have afforded researchers. We are now coming up on the twenty-fifth anniversary of the first approval in 1974 of doxorubicin (Figure 1) for use as an anticancer agent. It has been widely stated that the development of antibiotics has been the most important breakthrough in medicine. In a narrower sense, the same could be said for the importance of doxorubicin in cancer chemotherapy. In contrast to most antitumor drugs (including other anthracyclines), doxorubicin displays remarkable activity against a broad range of tumors. To date, doxorubicin has been the most successful and useful anticancer agent developed (1). Nevertheless, it is possible that, as we enter the new millennium, paclitaxel and other recently discovered anticancer agents may displace doxorubicin as the most important antitumor agent on the market. The importance of doxorubicin in cancer chemotherapy, however, particularly to those patients whose lives have been prolonged significantly by its use, will never be in doubt.

In this chapter, we shall describe the historical context of anthracycline discovery, the clinical use of anthracyclines, and molecular aspects of anthracycline activity. We also propose a comprehensive pathway for daunorubicin and doxorubicin biosynthesis, based on published material and our recent experiments with *Streptomyces* sp. strain C5. Support for this pathway is drawn from both classical and molecular genetics and in vivo and in vitro bioconversion of pathway intermediates. It is also clear from the data presented herein and by a variety of laboratories that the daunorubicin, baumycin, and doxorubicin biosynthesis pathways are virtually identical in all producing organisms, with perhaps, at most, minor variations based on growth conditions used.

The structures of the anthracyclines discussed in most detail in this chapter, including daunorubicin (daunomycin), doxorubicin (adriamycin), carminomycin, baumycin A1, pirarubicin, idarubicin, and 4'-epirubicin, are shown in Figure 1. The structures of other important or well-studied anthracyclines, including aclarubicin (aclacinomycin A), nogalamycin, menogaril, steffimycin B, tetracenomycin C, and ε-rhodomycinone are shown in Figure 2.

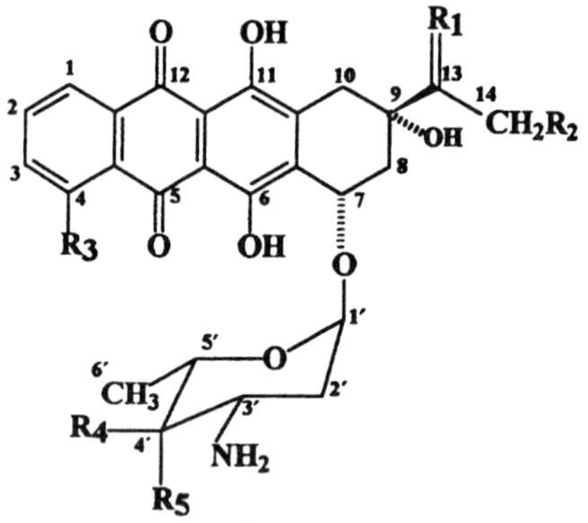

	R_1	R_2	R_3	R_4	R_5
Doxorubicin	=O	—OH	—OCH$_3$	H	—OH
Daunorubicin	=O	—H	—OCH$_3$	H	—OH
Carminomycin	=O	—H	—OH	H	—OH
Idarubicin	=O	—H	—H	H	—OH
Epirubicin	=O	—OH	—OCH$_3$	—OH	—H
Pirarubicin	=O	—OH	—OCH$_3$	H	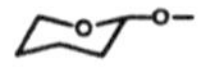
Baumycin A₁	=O	—H	—OCH$_3$	H	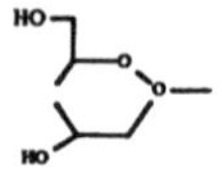
Zorubicin	—NNHCO—⬡ 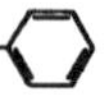	—H	—OCH$_3$	H	—OH

Figure 1 Structures of daunorubicin/doxorubicin family of anthracyclines.

A.   HISTORICAL PERSPECTIVE

In 1950 Hans Brockmann and Klaus Bauer reported the discovery of the first anthracyclines, compounds of the rhodomycin group formed by *Streptomyces purpurascens* (ATCC 25489) (2), a then-new streptomycete isolated from soil obtained from the forest outside of Göttingen. Brockmann and his colleagues worked for several years primarily with two strains. *S. purpurascens* produced not only the glycone, rhodomycin I, but also isorhodomycin and a series of rhodomycinone aglycones, including, for example β-rhodomycinone (10,11-dihydroxycarminomycinone) and ε-rhodomycinone (Figure 2). The rhodomycinones were initially indicated by Brockmann and his colleagues by using Greek letters to indicate their relative chromatographic mobility (3,4). The second anthracycline-producing strain studied by Brockmann and his colleagues, *Streptomyces* sp. DOA 1205, produced primarily pyrromycin and pyrromycinones (4,5). After isolation and characterization of additional similar compounds, Brockmann and Brockmann Jr. (6) named the group of glycosidic derivatives of 7,8,9,10-tetrahydronaphthacene quinones "anthracyclines." The first anthracycline described, β-rhodomycin I (2), displayed strong

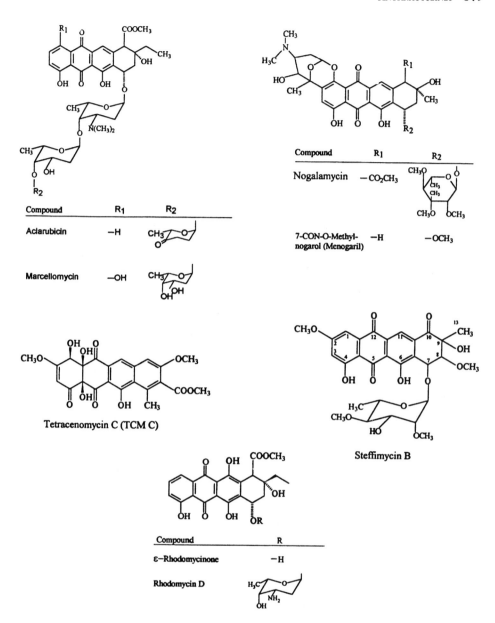

Figure 2 Structures of other important anthracyclines discussed in this chapter.

antibacterial activity against *Staphylococcus aureus* but was of limited clinical use because of its high toxicity.

Researchers for Farmitalia Research Laboratories (now Pharmacia Upjohn) in Milano, Italy, began screening isolates from soil samples for anticancer compounds in the mid 1950s. In 1958 a *Streptomyces* sp., later named *Streptomyces peucetius* (ATCC 29050) (7), was isolated from a random soil sample taken on the grounds of a local tourist attraction, Castel del Monte, in the region of Puglie near the city of Andria in southeastern

Italy (1,4). This organism produced a red-pigmented compound that displayed antibacterial, antifungal, and cytotoxic properties (8–11) and appeared structurally to belong to the newly described class of anthracyclines (6). Named daunomycin, for "Daunia," the ancient name for the region (4), this new compound demonstrated significant anticancer efficacy in initial studies reported in 1963 (10–12). Concurrently, Dubost et al. (13) at Rhône-Poulenc isolated a red antitumor drug from cultures of *Streptomyces coeruleorubidus* that they named rubidomycin, for the French word for "ruby." Rubidomycin (13–15) and daunomycin (7–12) were found to be the same compound, which was renamed the international nonproprietary name, daunorubicin, giving credit to both groups of discoverers (1). Daunorubicin was found to have potent cytotoxic activity in cell cultures, and although it also displayed some organ toxicity, it showed activity against solid and ascites tumors (10,12,15).

As a result of a mutation and screening program at Farmitalia, an *N*-nitroso-*N*-methyl urethane-induced mutant of *S. peucetius* was generated, named *S. peucetius* subsp. *caesius* (ATCC 27952; 16), that produced a 14-hydroxy analog of daunorubicin named adriamycin (named for the Adriatic Sea, located a few kilometers from the site from Castel del Monte), which was initially described in 1969 (16–18). Due to its significant antitumor activity (19), adriamycin (doxorubicin) was approved by the FDA in 1974, only six years after clinical testing had been initiated.

After the discovery of doxorubicin and its inherent antitumor properties, significant efforts were made in laboratories and companies worldwide to discover new anthracycline natural products from different soil isolates. Efforts also have been made to modify existing structures by chemical methods and to synthesize novel anthracyclines *de novo*. Nogalamycin, originally discovered as a product of *Streptomyces nogalater* strain UC-2783 (ATCC 27451) in the early 1960s, was first described in 1968 by researchers at the Upjohn Company (20) (Table 1). Similarly, steffimycin, produced by *Streptomyces steffisbergensis* strain UC-5044 (ATCC 27466), was discovered in the early 1960s (21,22). Carminomycin (4-demethyldaunorubicin) was first described in 1974 as a new anthracycline isolated from *Actinomadura carminata* (23,24). Shortly thereafter, aclacinomycin A (aclarubicin), was described in 1975 as a product of *Streptomyces galilaeus* strain MA-144-M1 (ATCC 31133) (25–29), and baumycins A_1/A_2 were characterized in 1977 as products of *S. coeruleorubidus* strain ME130-A4 (ATCC 31276) (30,31). Table 1 shows most of the major anthracycline-producing actinomycetes (2–107) reported in the literature over the past 30 years and the primary anthracycline products formed by each.

As is the case with most antitumor agents, doxorubicin and daunorubicin display a variety of toxic effects, the worst of which is cumulative cardiotoxicity (108,109). Researchers have used both chemical and biological approaches to find new anthracyclines with a higher efficacy to toxicity index, or possessing a wider range of antineoplastic activities than those of either doxorubicin or daunorubicin. Incredibly, more than 2000 anthracycline analogs have now been isolated or synthesized in laboratories throughout the world in an effort to make a "better doxorubicin," that is, an anthracycline with a higher efficacy to toxicity ratio than doxorubicin (1). Despite all of the efforts, only five new anthracyclines have developed for clinical use worldwide since doxorubicin: idarubicin (4-demethoxydaunorubicin), epirubicin (4′-epidoxorubicin), pirarubicin (tetrahydropyranyldoxorubicin or THP-doxorubicin), zorubicin (rubidazone), and aclarubicin (aclacinomycin A) (1,110,111) (Table 2). Currently, only various formulations of doxorubicin, daunorubicin, and idarubicin are approved for use in the United States (112). Menogaril (7-con-O-methylnogarol), epirubicin, and pirarubicin are currently being tested in the United States under investigational drug status

Table I Anthracycline-Producing Microorganisms

Strains[a]	Major product(s)	Reference(s)
Actinomadura carminata	Carminomycin	23, 24
Actinomadura roseoviolacea 1029-AV1	N-Formyl-13-dihydrocarminomycin; akrobomycin	32, 33
Actinomadura roseoviolacea var. *miuraensis* strain 07	SN-706; rubeomycin derivatives	34
Actinomadura sp. D326	4-Hydroxybaumycins	35
Actinomadura sp. FA-1180	Rubeomycins A and B	36, 37
Actinomadura sp. MG465-yF4	Barminomycins I and II	38
Actinosporangium bohemicum C-36145 (ATCC 31127)	Bohemic acid complex, marcellomycin and ε-pyrromycinone glycosides (4′-O-[2-deoxy-α-L-fucosyl)pyrromycin; musettamycin, marcellomycin	39–43
Ampullariella regularis	Viriplanin A (nogalamycin analog)	44
Streptomyces achromogenes var. *rubradiris*	Protorubradirin, rubradirin	45
Streptomyces atroviolaceus	13-Dihydrocarminomycin	46, 47
Streptomyces avidinii NR0576	Avidinorubicin (nogalamycin analog)	48
Streptomyces bifurcus 23219	Daunorubicin	49
Streptomyces bobili (ATCC 3310)	Cinerubin, rhodomycins X,Y	50
Streptomyces capoamus (ATCC 19006)	Cinerubins	51
Streptomyces chromofuscus	Aranciamycin (2-demethoxysteffimycin)	52
Streptomyces cinereoruber var. *fructofermentans* ETH 6143	Cinerubins	50, 53
Streptomyces coeruleorubidus ME130-A4 (ATCC 31276)	Daunorubicin, baumycins, A,B,C	30, 31
Streptomyces coeruleorubidus strains 8899 and 31723	Daunorubicin, baumycins	13, 14, 54
Streptomyces coeruleorubidus JA10092	13-Dihydrodaunorubicin	55
Streptomyces cosmosus TMF518	Cosmocarcin A, ditrisarubicins A,B	56
Streptomyces diastatochromogenes IMET JA 10081/9	Trypanomycin A$_2$	57
Streptomyces elgreteus UC-5453	Steffimycin B	58
Streptomyces eurythermus H1715MY2	Cinerubin R	59
Streptomyces galilaeus AC-628	1-Hydroxyauramycins, 1-hydroxysulfurmycins	60
Streptomyces galilaeus JA3043	Galirubins, pyrromycin, aklavinone	61, 62
Streptomyces galilaeus MA144-M1 (ATCC 31133)	Aclacinomycin A, aklavinone, pyrromycin, cinerubins	25–29
Streptomyces galilaeus OBB-111 (ATCC 31533)	Auramycins, sulfurmycins	63, 64
Streptomyces galilaeus OBB-731 (ATCC 31615)	Aclacinomycin A, aklavinone	65
Streptomyces galilaeus ATCC 31671	2-Hydroxyaclacinomycin A, 2-hydroxyaklavinone	66, 67
Streptomyces galilaeus S383	Aklaviketone	68
Streptomyces glaucescens GLA.0	Tetracenomycin C	69
Streptomyces glomeratus 3980	Beromycins and nogalamycin	70
Streptomyces griseoruber var. *beromycini* 4620	Beromycins A,B,C; beromycins	71, 72

Table I   Continued

Strains[a]	Major product(s)	Reference(s)
Streptomyces griseoruber	Daunorubicin	73
Streptomyces griseorubiginosus 4915	Cinerubins (pyrromycinone glycosides)	74
Streptomyces griseus IMET JA5142 and JA3933	Leukaemomycins (derivatives of daunorubicin)	75
Streptomyces griseus	Daunorubicin	76
Streptomyces insignis ATCC 31913	Daunorubicin, ε-rhodomycinone	77, 78
Streptomyces melanogenes AC-180	1-Hydroxyauramycins, 1-hydroxysulfurmycins	60
Streptomyces niveoruber ETH 17860, ETH 17403	Cinerubins	50, 53
Streptomyces nogalater ATCC 27451	Nogalamycin	20
Streptomyces olindensis	Retamycin E1,E2	79
Streptomyces olivaceus Tü2353	Elloramycin A	80
Streptomyces peucetius ATCC 29050	Daunorubicin, baumycins	7–12
Streptomyces peucetius subsp. *caesius* (ATCC 27952)	Doxorubicin	16, 17
Streptomyces peucetius subsp. *aureus* (ATCC 31428)	11-Deoxodaunorubicin	81
Streptomyces peucetius subsp. *carminatus* (ATCC 31502)	13-Deoxocarminomycin	82
Streptomyces peucetius subsp. *carneus* (ATCC 21354)	13-Dihydrodaunorubicin; daunosaminil–daunorubicin	83
Streptomyces peucetius subsp. *vinaceus*	4-O-Glucuronides of aklavinone and ε-rhodomycinone	84
Streptomyces purpurascens (ATCC 25489)	Rhodomycin I, isorhodomycin, rhodomycinones	2
Streptomyces ryensis 44 (ATCC 29805)	Ryemycins A_1 and A_2 (pyrromycinone glycosides)	74
Streptomyces steffisbergensis (ATCC 27466)	Steffimycin, steffimycin B	21, 22, 58
Streptomyces tauricus R1A 1417 (ATCC 27470)	Tauromycetins (pyrromycinone glycosides)	85
Streptomyces triangulatus subsp. *angiostaticus*	TAN-1120 (baumycin derivative)	86
Streptomyces violaceochromogenes C73	Cinerubin X	87
Streptomyces violaceus	Rhodomycinone mixture	88
Streptomyces violaceus A262 mutants	β-Rhodomycinone diglycosides; epelycins A–E; obelmycins A–G; yellamycins A–C; alldimycins A–C	89
Streptomyces violochromogenes 1098-AV$_2$	Arugomycin (nogalamycin analog)	90
Streptomyces virginiae MF266-g4 (ATCC 31910)	Decilorubicin (nogalamycin analog)	91, 92
Streptomyces viridochromogenes	Daunorubicin	93
Streptomyces xanthocidicus	Respinomycins A_1, A_2, B, C, D	94
Streptomyces sp. strain ZIMET 43717	Aklanonic acid	95
Streptomyces sp. A21 (ATCC 39235)	Maggiemycin	96, 97
Streptomyces sp. C5 (ATCC 49111)[b]	Daunorubicin, baumycins, ε-rhodomycinone	96, 98
Streptomyces sp. D-788	Daunorubicin, baumycins	99
Streptomyces sp. DOA 1205	Pyrromycin, pyrromycinones	5

Table 1 Continued

Strains[a]	Major product(s)	Reference(s)
Streptomyces sp. HPL Y-11472 (DSM 2658)	Cytorhodin X (9-α-glycoside), ε-rhodomycin	100, 101
Streptomyces sp. I-8	Bisanhydro-ε-pyrromycinone; N_1-pyrromycinone	102
Streptomyces sp. ME505-HEI (ATCC 31273)	Rhodirubins A,B,C,D,E,G	103
Streptomyces sp. 1254	Mutactimycins B,C,D	104
Streptomyces sp. 1683	Rhodomycin B	4
Streptomyces sp. 1725	Dutomycin	105
Streptomyces sp.	Isoquinocycline A	106
Streptosporangium sp.	Figaroic acid complex (carminomycin I)	47
Uncharacterized actinomycete	Rutilantin (pyrromycinone glycoside)	107

[a]ATCC, American Type Culture Collection.

[b]*Streptomyces* sp. strain C5 is a UV-induced mutant of the natural variant, strain V8, of an unspeciated streptomycete HD-1 (96). Other strains derived from HD-1 include strains NZ4, 6-3, R28, 30-8, and the maggiemycin producer A21 (96, 97).

(1,110,113). Additionally, Weiss (1) has listed and briefly described several other doxorubicin analogs that are currently in early phases of testing. Recent efforts in searching for better-suited analogs have been expanded to consider compounds that do not induce the multiple-drug-resistance (MDR) phenotype and for compounds or complexes that can be delivered more specifically to the tumor site (114–116).

Further information on the anthracyclines is available in reviews by Brockmann (3), Vaněk et al. (117), Oki and Yoshimoto (47), White (118), Oki (119), Arcamone (120), White and Stroshane (121), Aubel-Sadron and Londos-Gagliardi (122), Fujiwara and Hoshino (52), Weiss et al. (111), Suarato (110), Grein (123), Strohl et al. (124), Wagner et al. (125), Weiss (1), and Hutchinson (126). Additionally, interest in the chemical, biochemical, and clinical aspects of anthracyclines has spawned at least five books on this topic (4,127–130).

B. Economics and Use of Anthracyclines

In 1988, just as the primary patent held by Farmitalia for doxorubicin was expiring, the world market for doxorubicin was $250 million (131). The U.S. market alone was reported to be $86 million in 1987 (132) and $140 million in 1988 (131). At that point, doxorubicin was the top-selling antitumor drug in the U.S. market (131,132), with a 16.3% market share of all antitumor drugs (132). Because doxorubicin came off patent in 1988, several companies worldwide began to produce this compound generically (Table 3). Pharmacia-Upjohn, the largest producer of doxorubicin, reported 1993 worldwide sales of $156 million (marketed under the trade name, Adriamycin), and their epirubicin (trade name, Pharmorubicin) garnered worldwide sales of about $202 million (133).

Table 2   Anthracyclines Approved or in Advanced Clinical Trials in the United States and Other Countries

Anthracycline	Structure	Status	Indication
Daunorubicin (daunomycin)	Figure 1	Marketed worldwide	Acute leukemias
Doxorubicin (adriamycin)	Figure 1	Marketed worldwide	Several carcinomas, sarcomas, lymphomas
Carminomycin	Figure 1	Marketed in Russia and Eastern Europe	Several carcinomas, sarcomas, lymphomas
Idarubicin	Figure 1	Marketed worldwide	Acute leukemias
Epirubicin (4′-epidoxorubicin)	Figure 1	Marketed worldwide except United States; investigational drug in United States	Several carcinomas, sarcomas, lymphomas
Pirarubicin (THP-doxorubicin)	Figure 1	Marketed in Japan and France; clinical trials in United States	Several carcinomas, sarcomas, lymphomas
Zorubicin (rubidazone)[a]	Figure 1	Marketed in France	Acute leukemias
Aclarubicin (aclacinomycin A)	Figure 2	Marketed in Japan and France	Acute leukemias and non-Hodgkin's lymphomas
Menogaril	Figure 2	Investigational drug in United States	Potentially for several different types of malignancies

[a] Zorubicin is essentially a prodrug form of daunorubicin, since it is metabolized to daunorubicin and daunorubicin derivatives *in vivo*.
Data from Refs. 1 and 110–113.

II. CLINICAL ASPECTS OF ANTHRACYCLINES

A. Efficacy of Anthracyclines

Daunorubicin, doxorubicin, and idarubicin, approved in the United States, aclarubicin (aclacinomycin A), used in Japan and France, epirubicin, used worldwide except in the United States, and carminomycin, used in Russia and throughout eastern Europe (111), are among the most valuable antitumor anthracyclines available. Doxorubicin has been called the most important chemotherapeutic agent available (1,111,116), although its relative importance may subside with time as new drugs with a higher efficacy to toxicity ratio, or which can circumvent the MDR phenotype, become available.

Anthracyclines are known potent antitumor drugs used worldwide for the treatment of a wide variety of neoplasias. Daunorubicin is approved by the U.S. Food and Drug Administration (FDA) for treatment of acute nonlymphocytic leukemia (adults) and acute lymphatic leukemia (adults and pediatric). Daunorubicin also may be effective against chronic myelogenous leukemia, Ewing's sarcoma, neuroblastoma, non-Hodgkin's lymphoma, and Wilms's tumor (113).

Table 3 Anthracyclines Currently Approved for Clinical Use by the U.S. Food and Drug Administration

Trade name	Drug	Company	FDA approval date
Adriamycin PFS	Doxorubicin•HCl	Pharmacia-Upjohn	na[a]
Adriamycin RDF	Doxorubicin•HCl	Pharmacia-Upjohn	na
Rubex	Doxorubicin•HCl	Bristol-Meyers Squibb	04/89
Doxorubicin•HCl	Doxorubicin•HCl	Cetus Ben Venue	03/89
Doxorubicin•HCl	Doxorubicin•HCl	Pharmachemie (NL)	02/95
Doxorubicin•HCl	Doxorubicin•HCl	Gensia	07/95
Doxorubicin•HCl	Doxorubicin•HCl	Fujisawa	10/95
Doxorubicin•HCl	Doxorubicin•HCl	Haimen Pharmaceutical Factory	09/96
Doxil	Doxorubicin•HCl, liposomal	Sequus Pharms	11/95
Cerubidine	Daunorubicin•HCl	Wyeth Ayerst[b]	na
Cerubidine	Daunorubicin•HCl	Rhône-Poulenc Rorer	na
DaunoXome	Daunorubicin citrate, liposomal	NeXstar	04/96
Idamycin	Idarubicin•HCl	Pharmacia-Upjohn	10/90

[a] na = original approval dates were not available in database searched.
[b] Product licensed to Cetus Ben Venue Therapeutics.
Data from Ref. 112.

Doxorubicin is FDA approved in the United States for treatment of acute nonlymphocytic leukemia and acute lymphatic leukemia, Wilms's tumor, neuroblastoma, soft-tissue and bone sarcomas, breast sarcoma, ovarian carcinoma, transitional cell bladder carcinoma, thyroid carcinoma, Hodgkin's disease, non-Hodgkin's lymphoma, gastric carcinoma, and small-cell lung cancer. Doxorubicin also may be useful for treatment of chronic myelogenous leukemia, multiple myeloma, rhabdomyosarcoma, Ewing's sarcoma, Kaposi's sarcoma, and trophoblastic neoplasms, as well as for cancers of the esophagus, endometrium, liver, cervix, islet cell, pancreas, prostate, testes, and head and neck area (113).

Daunorubicin and doxorubicin cannot be given orally, due to their poor adsorption characteristics. Thus, daunorubicin and doxorubicin are given IV in bolus doses often ranging from 20 to 75 mg/m^2, or by continuous infusion over a 48-to-96 hr period. When administered intravenously, doxorubicin is rapidly and widely distributed throughout the body (113).

In recent years, combination chemotherapy, in which doxorubicin or daunorubicin are combined with other antineoplastic drugs, has been used with increasing frequency. One example of a combination therapy regimen would include treatment of breast carcinoma with doxorubicin (60 mg/m^2), cyclophosphamide (600 mg/m^2), and 5-fluorouracil (600 mg/m^2) by intravenous delivery on day 1, and 5-fluorouracil (600 mg/m^2) on day 8, with treatment repeated every 28 days for four courses (113).

Doxorubicin also has been shown to inhibit by ca. 42% the infectivity and replication of human immunodeficiency virus (HIV), the presumed causative agent of acquired immune deficiency syndrome (AIDS) (134), although there are no plans to develop anthracyclines as anti-HIV drugs.

Idarubicin (4-demethoxydaunorubicin), a more lipophilic chemically derived analog, is FDA approved for treatment of acute nonlymphocytic leukemia (113). Idarubicin has the distinct advantage over doxorubicin and daunorubicin that it is bioadsorbed when taken orally. It is the only anthracycline approved for oral delivery (113).

Three new anthracyclines have recently been studied in the United States as investigational drugs. Epirubicin (4'-epidoxorubicin) is a new anthracycline investigational drug with activity against nonlymphocytic leukemia, soft-tissue sarcomas, breast carcinoma, ovarian carcinoma, non-Hodgkin's lymphoma, and small-cell lung cancer (113). Menogaril, produced by the Upjohn Company, is currently approved as an investigational drug that is being studied for its efficacy against a wide variety of malignancies (135). Pirarubicin, a 4'-tetrahydropyranoside semisynthetic derivative of doxorubicin (136), exhibits markedly lower cardiotoxicity than either doxorubicin or epirubicin (137).

Unfortunately, not all forms of cancer are treatable by anthracyclines. For example, colorectal cancers and non-small-cell lung cancer do not respond to currently approved anthracyclines (1). Thus, there is additional impetus to search for new or modified anthracyclines with enhanced pharmacological properties.

B. Molecular Mechanisms of Action

As a group, anthracyclines display the second widest spectrum of activity of any antitumor drugs, second only to the alkylating agents (138). Anthracyclines have been shown to act through their ability to intercalate DNA noncovalently, to inhibit preribosomal DNA and RNA synthesis, to alter cell membranes, and to generate free radicals (quinone action) (109,139). Although free radical formation has not been generally recognized to be related to the antitumor activity of anthracyclines, it is the likely cause of cumulative cardiotoxicity (1,109,115,138), the most serious side effect exhibited by most anthracyclines. It is now clear that the cytotoxic activity of anthracyclines includes a very complex set of interactions between the drug and cellular components (139). It has also become clear that these drug-based interactions are dictated at least in part by the structure of the anthracycline.

The current accepted theory is that the primary activity of anthracyclines on DNA is through topoisomerase II–induced DNA strand breakage (140–143). This specific interaction, however, does not necessarily cover all of the in vitro and in vivo effects observed on DNA by anthracyclines (139), leading researchers to believe that additional, physiologically significant interactions must be taking place (140,144), as discussed below.

Doxorubicin has a very high affinity for DNA (affinity of doxorubicin for targets is DNA > cardiolipin > RNA; 145), which correlates well with the accumulated data that indicate the primary target for activity of anthracyclines is cellular DNA. Additionally, it has been demonstrated that increases of doxorubicin concentration, over three orders of magnitude, directly correlate with increasing DNA binding, DNA damage, and impairment of DNA function (140). As expected, over 80% of doxorubicin has been found to be DNA associated in tumor biopsies, and over 99% of doxorubicin was found to be DNA associated in single cell fluorescence measurements in vitro (140).

The crystal structure of daunorubicin complexed with d(CGTACG), which has been solved to 1.2 Å (146,147) (Figure 3), indicated that the planar aglycone moiety

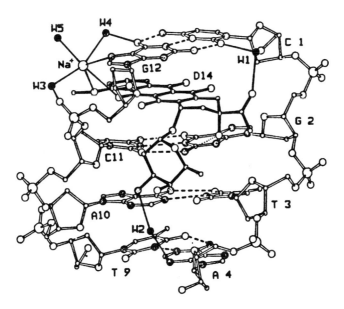

Figure 3   Model of daunorubicin (D14) intercalated into DNA (d-CGTACG) as determined by x-ray crystallographic analysis. As can be observed, the planar portion of the daunorubicin molecule (B- to D-rings) is intercalated between the CG pairs with hydrogen-bond interaction of the 9-hydroxy to base G2 and a water bridge between the 3' N of daunosamine and the N3 of the A4 residue. (From Ref. 146.)

intercalates between the CpG at each end of the molecule with the D-ring protruding into the major groove and that the sugar fits down into the minor groove. Wang et al. (148) have identified three functional components in anthracycline binding to DNA: (a) intercalation into the DNA by rings B–D, causing a distortion in the double helix that may be recognized by DNA-associated enzymes such as topoisomerases I and II, helicase, and polymerases; (b) anchoring of the anthracycline to the DNA by the A-ring. The 9-hydroxy moiety (on the A-ring) of daunorubicin and doxorubicin hydrogen-bonds with a guanine base to anchor the molecule in the double helix, affording specificity (148); and (c) interaction of the aminosugar moiety with the minor groove of a right-handed B-DNA helix (148).

Using DNAse I footprinting at 4°C, Chaires et al. (149,150) showed that doxorubicin intercalated into the stacked base pairs of DNA with a sequence preference for 5'-(A/T)–C–G and 5'-(A/T)–G–C. Very recently, however, Shelton et al. (151) demonstrated, using detailed chemical and enzymatic DNA protection assays, that daunorubicin, ditrirubicin B, and aclarubicin (aclacinomycin A), anthracyclines containing one, two, and three sugars, respectively, all showed a binding preference for 5'-GT-3'. Additionally, they demonstrated that the specificity of this sequence was enhanced if preceded by a run of G residues (151). They also showed that the number of base pairs protected in both chemical and enzymatic protection assays was increased with the increased number of sugar units; the mono-, di-, and trisaccharide anthracyclines protected 3, 4, and 6–8 base pairs, respectively (151). Their protection data were consistent with x-ray crystallographic data on intercalation of the planar aglycone moiety and binding of the hydrophobic, rigid aminosugar moiety in the minor groove of the DNA (151).

The data of Chaires et al. (149,150) and Shelton et al. (151) are consistent from the standpoint that the preferred binding site for anthracyclines is an alternating purine/pyrimidine (e.g., GT), preceded by several G residues (149–151). Significantly, neither the number nor types of sugar side chains appeared to alter the binding site specificity for the anthracyclines tested (151).

When daunorubicin is bound to a hexameric DNA oligonucleotide containing alternating GC bases (e.g., d[CGCGCG]), it has been noted that the 3′-amino-group on the daunosamine sugar moiety is in close proximity to the N2-group of guanine (148). This type of structure is ideal for nucleophilic attack of both amino-groups on a cross-linking agent such as formaldehyde (148). Wang and his coworkers observed in 1991 that formaldehyde could efficiently cross-link daunorubicin, in a sequence-specific fashion (e.g., d[CpG]), to DNA through generation of a methylene bridge between the two N-groups (152) (Figure 4). Covalent alkylation of the DNA molecule in this fashion did not alter the conformation of the DNA–daunorubicin structure (148). Furthermore, Phillips and his colleagues (139,140) showed that after reductive activation by dithiothreitol (or alternatively, xanthine oxidase or NADH dehydrogenase, both of which are present in nuclei; 153), doxorubicin could covalently bind calf thymus DNA and chemically synthesized oligonucleotides in vitro over a period of 24 to 48 hr at physiologically

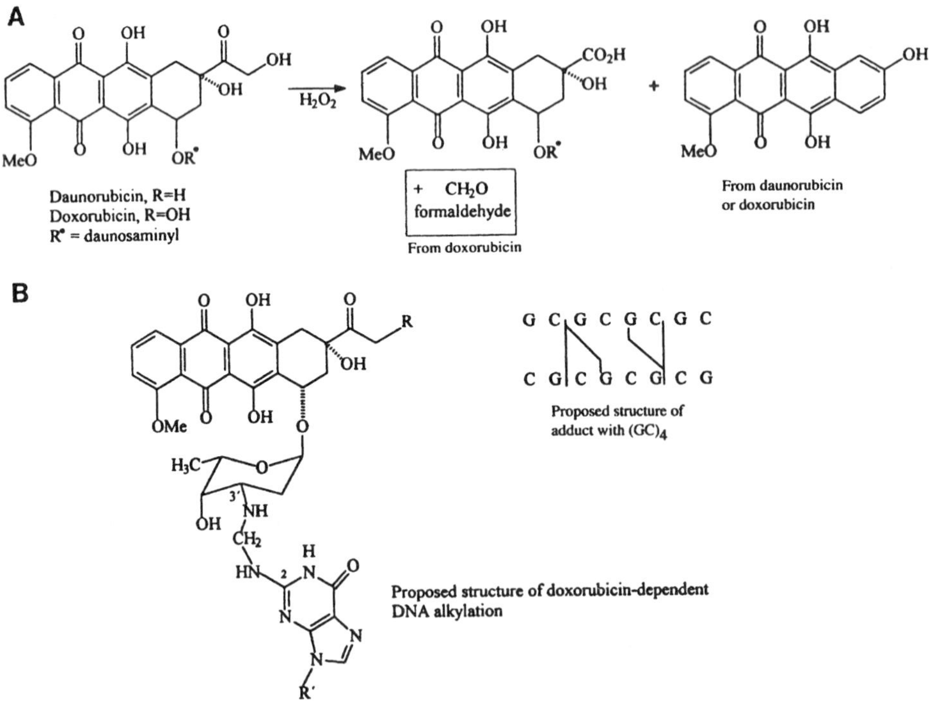

Figure 4   Proposed cross-linkage of daunorubicin to DNA. (A) Formation of formaldehyde from doxorubicin via a H_2O_2-dependent Baeyer–Villager oxidation mechanism. (B) Proposed structure of formaldehyde-dependent daunorubicin/doxorubicin cross-linkage to DNA, and a schematic of how the molecule should covalently link to a p(GC)$_4$ oligonucleotide. (Redrawn and modified from Ref. 144.)

relevant concentrations (e.g., 1 μM). This covalent linkage occurred at p(GpC), possessed an optimal stoichiometry of 1 cross-link per 11 to 20 bp, and was stimulated 5- to 6-fold by the presence of Fe^{3+} (139,140). Consistent with Wang's (148,152) data, they also observed that this cross-linkage involved the N2-group of a guanine residue (140). In contrast, the specifically developed alkylating anthracyclines (2-chloroethyl)-4'-methylsulfonyldaunorubicin (FCE 27726) and (4-demethoxy-3'-deamino-3'-aziridinyl-4'-methylsulfonyldaunorubicin (FCE 28729) cross-linked to the N7-group of guanine in the major groove in vitro and in vivo (154).

It has been hypothesized for several years that reductive activation of doxorubicin, resulting in the quinone methide (155), might be responsible for alkylation of DNA (140). The observation of formaldehyde-dependent DNA alkylation by daunorubicin, coupled with the in vitro data on DNA cross-linking by reductively activated daunorubicin and doxorubicin, generated by Phillips and his colleagues (139,140), has led to a new hypothesis for anthracycline–DNA interaction (144). Very recently, Taatjes et al. (144) tested the ability of daunorubicin and doxorubicin to alkylate DNA after treatment (i.e., activation) with a reducing agent, dithiothreitol, an oxidizing agent, hydrogen peroxide, and the alkylating agent formaldehyde. Incredibly, all three types of anthracycline "activation" resulted in identical DNA–anthracycline adducts (144), leading Taatjes et al. to propose a model for in vivo activation of doxorubicin involving initial reduction of the quinone resulting in the formation, via superoxide, of hydrogen peroxide, which produces formaldehyde via Baeyer–Villiger oxidation of doxorubicin (Figure 4). Nucleophilic addition of the formaldehyde with the 3'-N of daunosamine and 2-N of guanine would result in the expected cross-linkage (144) (Figure 4). Because daunorubicin would not yield formaldehyde from a Baeyer–Villager oxidation reaction, Taatjes et al. (144) proposed that the formaldehyde in that case would come from cellular sources. Indeed, it has been shown that lymphocytic leukemia cells possessed higher intracellular concentrations of formaldehyde than normal cells, and that the breath of patients with tumors has an elevated formaldehyde content (144). If alkylation of DNA by doxorubicin, daunorubicin, and other anthracyclines is found to be a significant reaction in vivo, as proposed recently (139,140,144,148), it will lend credence to the long-hypothesized notion that additional, "unknown" anthracycline–DNA interactions must be taking place (139,140). The fact that there was a good correlation between the ability of alkylating doxorubicin analogs to form interstrand cross-links in DNA and the resultant level of cytotoxicity (156) strongly implicates alkylation and cross-linking of DNA by doxorubicin (153). Such cross-linked anthracycline–DNA adducts would be expected to have a wide range of physiological effects, including inhibition of DNA and RNA polymerases.

One of the significant activities of anthracyclines is the inhibition of topoisomerase II activity (141–143). Topoisomerase II, an enzyme that catalyzes double-strand breakage and religation (157; Figure 5), is a key enzyme in eukaryotic cells involved in chromosomal condensation and structure, segregation of mitotic and meiotic spindles, chromatid separation, and potentially also gene expression. There are two "isoforms" of topoisomerase II, a ca. 170 kDa form known as the α-form, and a ca. 180 kDa form known as the β-form (158), that differ in enzymatic properties and cell-cycle regulation (143). It appears that topoisomerase-α and topoisomerase-β also are encoded by different genes and have different distributions within the cell (143). A model for the topoisomerase II catalytic cycle has recently been proposed by Roca and Wang (159), and supported by data of Sehested and Jensen (160), that includes five steps: (a) reversible binding of an "open" form of topoisomerase II to the DNA to yield an enzyme–DNA complex; (b) interaction of the open form of topoisomerase II with "T" (defined as the DNA segment to be passed through the gate), which maintains the open complex and inhibits strand cleavage; (c) adenosine 5'-triphosphate (ATP)-dependent removal of "T," resulting in double-strand DNA cleavage and formation of a transient "cleavable complex"; (d) religation of the DNA and formation of the "closed" form of topoisomerase II; and (e) release of adenosine 5'-diphospates (ADP) + phosphate (Pi), with concomitant reformation of the "open" form of the enzyme (159,160) (Figure 5). It has been demonstrated that several cytotoxic anticancer agents, including doxorubicin, daunorubicin, etoposide, clerocidin, teniposide, mitoxantrone, and amsacrine, collectively called "topoisomerase poisons," act to trap topoisomerase II in a drug–enzyme–DNA "cleavable complex" stage, between reactions 3 and 4 (see Figure 5). Formation of this cleavable complex inhibits DNA and RNA synthesis, resulting in cessation of cell division (141–143,161,162). Because these drugs trap these cleavable complexes (containing trapped, double-stranded breaks; see Figure 5), they accumulate to high levels in the DNA, resulting in chromosomal abnormalities and inhibition of DNA replication, which trigger cell death via apoptosis (162,163). In the case of several doxorubicin analogs, it has been shown that there is a direct correlation between the number of cleavage sites in the DNA and level of cytotoxicity (164). Thus, topoisomerase II–inhibiting drugs that generate cleavable complexes act by converting topoisomerase II into a "potent physiological toxin" (162).

One consequence of the fact that several antitumor drugs act synonymously to cause stabilization of the cleavable complexes is that these antitumor agents that trap

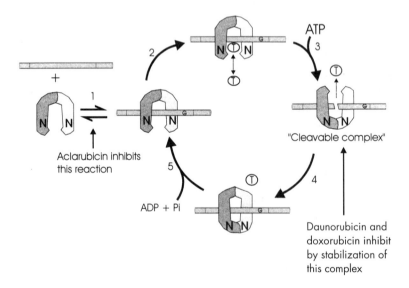

Figure 5   Redrawn and modified model of topoisomerase II catalysis as proposed by Roca and Wang (159). Doxorubicin, daunorubicin, other 10-descarbomethoxy anthracyclines, and other topoisomerase II "poisons" inhibit topoisomerase II activity by stabilization of the "cleavable complex" (i.e., freezing the catalytic cycle between steps 3 and 4), which results in an accumulation of DNA strand breaks, and ultimately, DNA degradation. Aclarubicin and possibly other anthracyclines possessing the 10-carbomethoxy moiety inhibit topoisomerase II by inhibiting reaction 1, namely, the complexation of DNA and the enzyme.

topoisomerase II–DNA in a cleavable complex induce mutations in topoisomerase II, resulting in "altered–topoisomerase II–multidrug resistance" (at-MDR) (143,162,165).

Aclacinomycin A and other anthracyclines possessing a 10-carbomethoxy moiety inhibit topoisomerase II, but not through trapping topoisomerase II in the cleavable complex as found with daunorubicin, doxorubicin, and their analogs (166). Instead, aclarubicin has been shown to inhibit the initial binding of topoisomerase II to the DNA (160,166,167). Jensen et al. (166) demonstrated that aclarubicin and other anthracyclines possessing the 10-carbomethoxy moiety functioned to inhibit topoisomerase II binding to DNA. Other anthracyclines lacking the 10-carbomethoxy moiety, but having 10-hydroxy- or 11-hydroxy-groups (various β-rhodomycin-related glycosides), inhibit topoisomerase II via stabilization of the cleavable complex. Similarly, they showed that at-MDR topoisomerases, resistant to the β-rhodomycins, remained sensitive to anthracyclines possessing the 10-carbomethoxy moiety. It also has been observed that aclarubicin can, via its ability to inhibit topoisomerase II–DNA binding, serve to ameliorate cytotoxic effects exerted by topoisomerase poisons (i.e., drugs that stabilize the cleavable complex) (158,167). This significant difference in anthracycline–topoisomerase II interaction, apparently dictated by the presence or absence of the 10-carbomethoxy moiety, has intrigued researchers and generated suggestions for the use of aclarubicin (or perhaps newly developed 10-carbomethoxy derivatives) as a second line treatment of tumors found to exhibit at-MDR induced by previous treatment with topoisomerase II poisons (167).

Recently, it has been shown that several anthracyclines, including doxorubicin, daunorubicin, and nogalamycin, are exceptional inhibitors of DNA helicases, enzymes responsible for dissociation of double-stranded DNA to single-stranded DNA (168). The most effective anthracyclines in inhibiting helicases were daunorubicin, doxorubicin, and nogalamycin (168). Intercalation of anthracyclines into DNA results in an increase in the stability of the DNA, and also leads to an increase in helix rigidity and in unwinding, deformation, and lengthening of the DNA (168). Bachur et al. (168) have proposed that several of these alterations in the DNA structure may be due to the effects of the anthracyclines on helicases.

C. DuVernay and Crooke's Class I and Class II Anthracyclines

During the 1970s, Duvernay and Crooke divided anthracyclines into two classes based on their effects on DNA and RNA synthesis, as well as overall cytotoxicity (169–174). Class I anthracyclines were typically characterized as being monoglycosylated, 10-descarbomethoxy, 11-hydroxy, 13-keto compounds such as doxorubicin, daunorubicin, and carminomycin (Table 4). According to DuVernay and colleagues (169–174), class I anthracyclines typically interact with DNA in vitro by intercalating between adjacent nucleotide base pairs, usually in G–C-rich regions, and exhibit moderate cytotoxicity. Approximately the same concentrations of these class I antibiotics are required to inhibit DNA, whole cell RNA, and nucleolar RNA synthesis (Table 4).

Class II anthracyclines, on the other hand, were characterized by DuVernay and colleagues to possess a 10(R)-carbomethoxy moiety, to lack the 13-keto-group, and to possess at least two sugar residues (173). These compounds, including aclacinomycin A, marcellomycin, rudolfomycin, and musettamycin, inhibit nucleolar RNA synthesis at concentrations 200- to 1500-fold lower than those required to inhibit DNA synthesis (Table 4). Thus, activity of class II anthracyclines is thought to be due, at least in part, to their abil-

Table 4   Properties of Class I and Class II Anthracyclines Proposed by DuVernay and Crook

Property	Class I	Class II
Structural properties:		
C10 position	10-Descarbomethoxy	10-Carbomethoxy
C13 position	Usually hydroxy or oxo	Never hydroxy or oxo
Sugars	Usually monosaccharide	Usually multiply glycosylated
IC_{50} values (in μM)[a]:		
DNA	0.3–0.8	0.3–2.1
RNA	0.3–0.9	0.03–0.12
No-RNA	6.0–13.1	0.009–0.25
Ratio of IC_{50} values[a]:		
DNA/WC RNA	1.26–1.89	6.53–19.33
DNA/No-RNA	0.93–1.12	170–1256
Mechanism for inhibition of topoisomerase II[b]	Stabilization of cleavable complex	Inhibition of topoisomerase II binding to DNA
Apparent localization within cells	Mostly in the nucleus	Mostly in the cytoplasm
Level of cytotoxicity	Moderate	High
Anthracyclines	Daunorubicin, doxorubicin, carminomycin, rubidazone, 10-descarbomethoxymarcellomycin, 10-descarbomethoxyrudolfomycin	Aclarubicin, cinerubin A, marcellomycin, musettamycin, rudolfomycin, nogalamycin

[a]IC_{50}, concentration of anthracycline required to inhibit synthesis by 50%; No-RNA, nucleolar RNA; WC RNA, whole cell RNA.
[b]In examples thus far tested. This was not proposed by DuVernay and Crooke, but later determined by other investigators (160,166,167).

ity to inhibit nucleolar RNA synthesis (169–174), rather than to act on DNA synthesis. In support of this distinction between class I and class II anthracyclines, Duvernay et al. (170,171,173,174) showed that removal or alteration in stereochemistry of the 10-carbomethoxy moiety of rudolfomycin and marcellomycin significantly decreased their ability to inhibit nucleolar RNA synthesis as well as their cytotoxicity, leading them to suggest that inhibition of nucleolar RNA synthesis was a significant factor in cytotoxicity.

Very recently, another major and very interesting difference has been observed between members of DuVernay and Crooke's class I and class II anthracyclines. As mentioned previously, the class I anthracyclines daunorubicin and doxorubicin are classical topoisomerase II poisons: they arrest the catalytic activity of topoisomerase II in the "cleavable complex" stage (Figure 5). Aclarubicin, a class II anthracycline, on the other hand, inhibits binding of the topoisomerase II to the DNA, rather than acting via stabilization of the "cleavable complex" (160,166,167). Thus, it may prove that DuVernay and Crooke were quite forward-thinking in their classification of anthracyclines into two groups, based primarily on the presence (class II) or absence (class I) of the 10-carbomethoxy moiety. The data may eventually indicate, however, that their observations on the differential inhibition of DNA, RNA, and nucleolar RNA syntheses are effects rather than causes. It is likely that the mechanisms of anthracycline inhibition of DNA-interacting enzymes such as helicases and topoisomerases may be more important differences between class I and class II anthracyclines than are the ratios of inhibition of DNA/RNA synthesis.

D. Quantitative Structure–Activity Relationships (QSARs)

A complex array of properties contribute to the in vivo antitumor activity and toxicity of anthracyclines, including ability to bind DNA, accumulation in tissues (distribution), elimination, and metabolic fate of the drugs. In an effort to find anthracyclines with higher efficacy to toxicity ratios, more than 2000 analogs of daunorubicin, doxorubicin, and other anthracyclines have been synthesized and tested (1). From these tests, some broad generalizations can be made concerning structure–activity relationships.

Daunorubicin/doxorubicin/aklavin (Figure 6) analogs can be classified into six major groups: (a) chemical or bioconverted derivatives of natural glycosides (175); (b) anthracyclines modified in the C9 side chain (175); (c) semisynthetic glycosides of biologically produced aglycones (175); (d) anthracyclines bearing different substitutions in the anthraquinone chromophore (B-, C-, and D-rings) (175); (e) compounds modified in the nonaromatic A-ring (175); and (f) modification in the daunosamine residue or addition of multiple sugar residues.

I. Modifications to the Aglycone Moiety

A series of experiments showed that substitution at the C4 position has a major effect on biological activity, with increased potency correlating with increased hydrophobicity: deoxy (idarubicin) > hydroxy (carminomycin series) > methoxy (daunorubicin, doxorubicin, and analogs) (176,177). A major finding was that chemically synthesized 4-demethoxy analogs of daunorubicin and doxorubicin exhibited 25- to 100-fold and 65- to 200-fold increases in potency, respectively, over the parental molecules, with altered physicochemical properties (175,177,178). One of these, idarubicin, has recently been approved for chemotherapy use in the United States (Table 2).

Also significant with respect to the 4-position is that modification of carminomycin (4-hydroxy) versus daunorubicin (4-methoxy) in the sugar moiety results in far different in vitro and in vivo activities, due to the inherent differences in the parental molecules (179). This could have far-ranging implications in the further development of

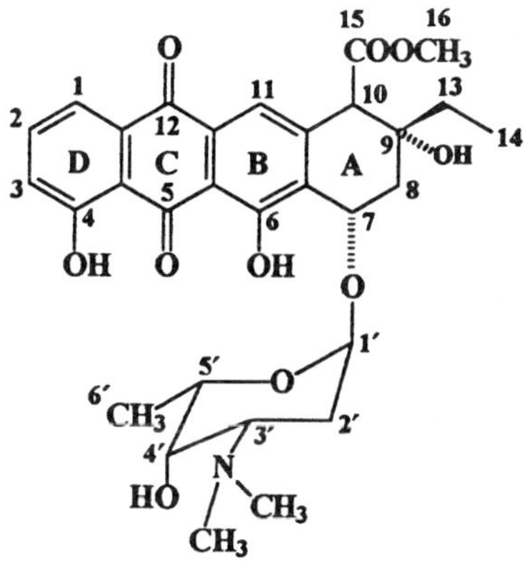

Figure 6 The structure of aklavin, with rings labeled A–D according to conventional practice.

anthracycline analogs: it would seem prudent to test every new analog through a 4-demethoxy (idarubicin-like), 4-hydroxy (carminomycin parent), and 4-methoxy (daunorubicin parent) series.

Modifications in the A-ring yield perhaps the most interesting results. The A-ring of doxorubicin-like anthracyclines contains two asymmetric centers of the aglycone moiety, the most important being at C7. Natural product anthracyclines have the sugar in the C7(S) configuration. C7(R) analogs are not biologically active, thus making chemical synthesis of active glycones more difficult (175).

Modification of C8 to form 8β-methoxydaunorubicin resulted in essentially no change in biological activity (175). This is interesting, since this is the same relative position of steffimycin B occupied by a methoxy moiety.

Inversion of the C9 side chain resulted in only partial reduction in biological activity. The C9 hydroxy-group is considered important because of its potential for 1,3-hydrogen bonding with C7, and also, as previously mentioned (148), for its involvement in binding to a purine residue in the minor groove of DNA (175). O-Methylation of the 9-hydroxy-group resulted in 100-fold less activity in vitro than daunorubicin, and complete cessation of antitumor activity (180). Whereas the 9-hydroxy-group is extremely important due to its role in binding to DNA, the side chain at C9 does not appear to have an impact on in vitro or in vivo activity. Anthracyclines possessing methyl side chains, such as auramycins and feudomycins C and D, or having an isopropyl side chain displayed approximately the same in vitro activities as those having the ethyl side chain (181). Interestingly, however, modification of the side chain of daunorubicin by demethylation of C14 and oxidation of C13, resulting in a carboxy side chain, results in a polar anthracycline that has significant in vitro activity (182). Methylation of the carboxy moiety to the methylester resulted in an analog with in vitro activities approximating those of daunorubicin and doxorubicin (182).

Daunorubicin and doxorubicin have an oxo moiety at C13 (on the side chain at C9) which is reduced to a hydroxy-group in vivo (4), particularly by liver reduced nicotinamide adenine dinucleotide phosphate (NADPH)-dependent carbonyl reductase (183). Similarly, several microorganisms can reduce the C13 oxo moiety of several anthracyclines to hydroxy-groups (184). The effect of the oxidation state at C13 on potency was found to be minor, with both C13 hydroxy (dihydro-derivatives) and C13 deoxy analogs retaining most of the activity of the parental molecules (4). 13-Dihydrodoxorubicin, however, has been reported to be up to 30-fold more cardiotoxic than doxorubicin (185), which suggests that efficacy to cardiotoxicity comparisons on a 13-deoxy derivative of doxorubicin might be worthwhile. Interestingly, the absolute stereochemistry of the enzymatically reduced 13-dihydro analogs is not known (4). Samples of chemically reduced analogs, however, in which there was a mixture of isomers, exhibited the same biological activity as biosynthetic or enzymatically reduced analogs (4), suggesting that the stereochemistry of hydroxy-groups at C13 is not biologically significant. Rubidazone (zorubicin), a semisynthetic analog of daunorubicin in which a benzylhydrazone derivative of the moiety substitutes for the 13-oxo-group, shows greater potency against P388 leukemia and B16 melanoma cell lines than does daunorubicin (182).

As is obvious from the difference in the clinical efficacy of daunorubicin *versus* doxorubicin, hydroxylation at C14 results in greater efficacy and a broader range of antitumor activity (182). Modifications of C14, including 14-azido-, 14-thiocyanato-, 14-bromo-, and 14-acetylthio derivatives of daunorubicin, resulted in markedly lower activities, whereas a 14-acetoxy derivative retained activity comparable to daunorubicin (186);

thus, bromine, sulfur, or nitrogen substitutions at C14 result in low activity, whereas oxygen substitution resulted in strong activity (186). Similarly, modification of C14 to form doxorubicin-14-octanoate resulted in an analog that retained most of the activity of the parental molecule. The doxorubicin-14-octanoate, however, is rapidly degraded by esterases to doxorubicin, whence the similar activity (182).

Other than the requirement for glycosylation with the proper stereochemistry, the most obvious biological effects in A-ring modifications are noted with substitutions at C10. As mentioned previously, the presence at C10 of a 10(R)-carbomethoxy moiety results in anthracyclines of the class II type, that is, those similar to aklavin, aclacinomycin A, musettamycin, rudolfomycin, and marcellomycin, which appear to inhibit nucleolar RNA synthesis preferentially (169–174). Similarly, anthracyclines possessing the 10-carbomethoxy moiety inhibit topoisomerase II binding to DNA, whereas those lacking this side chain trap the topoisomerase II–DNA complex in the "cleavable complex" (160). Comparison of the biological activities of 10(S)-methoxy and 10(R)-methoxy derivatives of daunorubicin revealed that the stereochemistry at this position is critical for biological activity (174). 10(S) derivatives completely lacked biological activity, whereas 10(R) derivatives were nearly as potent as the parental molecule (173–175). Similarly, 10-decarbomethoxylation of aclarubicin resulted in an analog that displayed a 2- to 8-fold decrease in in vitro activities compared with that of aclarubicin (187), and 10-decarbomethoxylation of nogalamycin, marcellomycin, and rudolfomycin resulted in a 5- to 10-fold decrease in potency (170,188).

Hydroxylation modulates activity of anthracyclines in a position-dependent manner. Hydroxylation at C2 of aclarubicin resulted in a decrease of cytotoxicity in vitro, but increased biological activity in vivo (176,181), whereas hydroxylation at C1 or C11 markedly increased cytotoxicity (181). Similarly, 10,11-dihydroxy analogs appear to have high levels of cytotoxicity. The best example is that of oxaunomycin, a 10-hydroxy derivative of 13-deoxycarminomycin, which was shown to have much higher (ca. 100-fold) cytotoxicity than doxorubicin against cultured L1210 leukemia cells (189). Oxaunomycin displayed the unique characteristic of preferentially inhibiting DNA synthesis at a concentration lower than that required to inhibit RNA synthesis (189).

Anthracyclines lacking the 6-hydroxy-group (e.g., α_2-rhodomycinone glycosides), or those that are 6-O-methylated (i.e., 6-O-methyldaunorubicin), exhibit substantially lowered cytotoxicity, indicating the importance of the 6-hydroxy to cytotoxic activity (180,181). Similarly, methylation of the 11-hydroxy-group of daunorubicin also dramatically decreases activity on HeLa cells. In a series of experiments on O-methylated derivatives, Zunino et al. (180) showed that methylation decreased activity in the following order: daunorubicin > 9-O-methyldaunorubicin > 11-O-methyldaunorubicin > 6-O-methyldaunorubicin > 6,9-dimethoxydaunorubicin > 6,11-dimethoxydaunorubicin.

Methylation at other positions also has been shown to decrease the potency of anthracyclines. For example, methylation at C1, C2, or C3 generally decreases activity with respect to parental anthracyclines (182). Similarly, chlorination at any of these positions resulted in decreased in vitro activities (182).

2. Sugar Modifications

The sugar moieties of anthracyclines are extremely important for both in vitro and in vivo activities. Anthracyclinones, that is, aglycones lacking the sugar moieties, are not biologically active. In general, within the aclarubicin series, disaccharides and trisaccharides were found to be more potent than monosaccharides in vitro, although the length of the sugar chain did not appear to have any bearing on in vivo activity (181).

Most natural anthracyclines contain 2'-deoxyhexoses, a structure that lends susceptibility to acid hydrolysis (190). Tsuchiya and Takagi (190) have synthesized 2'-fluoro derivatives in an effort to stabilize the anthracycline in the presence of acids. Their results indicated that 2'-R configuration was required for biological activity, and that substitutions at 3' caused a dramatic decrease in the activity of the 2'-fluoro derivatives (190).

N,N-Dimethyl sugar derivatives (e.g., containing rhodosamine in place of daunosamine) of daunorubicin and doxorubicin are approximately 10-fold more active against L1210 leukemia cells than are the parental compounds (175), indicating that modification of sugar increases potency. Similarly, N-demethyl derivatives of aclarubicin are less cytotoxic than the parental molecule (175,191). Compounds containing the N,N-dimethylated sugar, however, are typically more cardiotoxic than N-demethyl analogs, probably due to increased accumulation of the compound in the heart (192,193). The only exception to this was that the N-demethyl derivative of betaclamycin A was much more cytotoxic than betaclamycin A (191). Conversely, N-L-leucyldaunorubicin exhibited much lower accumulation by heart muscle and, therefore, lowered cardiotoxicity (193).

Modification of the sugar moiety yields important differences in efficacy and cardiotoxicity. For example, as compared with doxorubicin containing daunosamine (3-amino-2,3,6-trideoxy-L-lyxohexose) as the sugar moiety, synthesis of the L-*arabino* form of the sugar (3-amino-2,3,6-trideoxy-L-arabinohexose; L-acosamine), giving 4'-epidoxorubicin, and the 4'-deoxy analog (L-*threo* configuration; named esorubicin) resulted in novel anthracyclines with excellent pharmacological properties (175,194). As mentioned previously, epirubicin is now on the market worldwide (except in the United States) as an alternative to daunorubicin treatment of adult myelogenous leukemia and to doxorubicin treatment of soft-tissue sarcomas, breast carcinoma, ovarian carcinoma, non-Hodgkin's lymphoma, and small-cell lung cancer (113). Esorubicin has been tested clinically, and early studies have indicated that esorubicin displays not only lower cardiotoxicity than doxorubicin, but also reduced antitumor activity (111).

4'-Substituted doxorubicin analogs have shown strong biological activity in many studies. As detailed in Section V.I, another modification of the 4'-hydroxy-group has resulted in a new, clinically useful anthracycline. Pirarubicin, a 4'-tetrahydropyranyl derivative of doxorubicin, currently used clinically in France and Japan (it is still an investigational drug in the United States), appears to have similar efficacy to doxorubicin, with significantly less cardiotoxicity (137).

Since DNA–drug interactions are critical to the activity of anthracyclines, Arcamone and his colleagues at Farmitalia carried out an important set of experiments to determine the binding efficiency of 27 different anthracyclines to DNA, with an eye on structure–activity relationships (4,175). As indicated in Table 5, modifications in the C9 side chain, in the D-ring, and at C4' were tolerated, whereas a variety of other modifications resulted in substantially lower affinity to DNA (175). In vivo data were generally found to agree with the affinity measurements—that is, those compounds in the high relative affinity group possessed similar dose optima and toxicity to daunorubicin and doxorubicin, whereas those compounds in the medium affinity group generally required 5-fold greater dosages to yield similar effects. Those compounds in the low affinity group were found to vary widely in their effects, mostly due to in vivo metabolism and other uncontrollable parameters.

Table 5 Affinity of Substituted Anthracyclines for DNA as Measured by Equilibrium Dialysis

Grouping[a]	Anthracyclines
High affinity anthracyclines (K_{app} value >80% of doxorubicin value)	Doxorubicin, daunorubicin, 4'-epidaunorubicin, 4'-epidoxorubicin, 4'-deoxydaunorubicin, 4'-deoxydoxorubicin, 4-demethoxydaunorubicin, 9-deacetyl-9-hydroxymethyl-daunorubicin, 13-dihydrodoxorubicin
Medium affinity anthracyclines (K_{app} value 50–80% that of doxorubicin)	14-Morpholinodaunorubicin, 9-deoxydaunorubicin, 9,10-anhydrodaunorubicin, 9-deacetyldaunorubicin, 3',4'-diepi-daunorubicin, 4'-O-methyldaunorubicin, 4'-O-methyldoxorubicin, 6'-hydroxydaunorubicin, 3',4'-diepi-6'-hydroxy-daunorubicin, doxorubicin-14-O-glycolate, 9-deoxydoxorubicin
Low affinity anthracyclines (K_{app} value <50% that of doxorubicin)	3'-Epidaunorubicin, 1',4'-diepidaunorubicin (β-anomer), 4'-epi-4'-O-methyldaunorubicin, 9-deacetyl-9-epidaunorubicin, 1'-epidoxorubicin, (β-anomer of doxorubicin), doxorubicin-14-octanoate, 3',4'-diepi-6'-hydroxydoxorubicin, N-acetyl-doxorubicin

[a] K_{app} value is the affinity constant for anthracyclines to calf thymus DNA under standardized conditions (see Ref. 175).

General lipophilicity of drugs is widely accepted as an important parameter of drug activity (175). As defined by retention time in reverse phase high-performance liquid chromatography (HPLC) using acetonitrile:water (35:65; buffered with Tris, pH 7.0) as the mobile phase, the lipophilic index (log K') for several anthracyclines were found to be 3',4'-epidaunorubicin, 0.77; 4-demethoxydaunorubicin, 0.69; daunorubicin, 0.48; 4-demethoxydoxorubicin, 0.33; 4'-deoxydoxorubicin, 0.30; 4'-O-methyldoxorubicin, 0.26; 4'-epidoxorubicin, 0.14; and doxorubicin, 0.016 (175). These data indicated that potent anthracyclines possessed a wide range of lipophilic indices; the only trend observed was that cytotoxic potency appeared to increase with increased lipophilicity, but without an effect on antitumor efficacy (175).

E. Tumor Resistance to Anthracyclines

One of the problems with administration of anthracyclines as antitumor drugs is the *de novo* acquisition of drug resistance, including the induction of the multiple-drug-resistance (MDR) phenotype. MDR is the term given to the resistance developed by tumor cells to structurally and mechanistically diverse antineoplastic drugs (195). The classical form of MDR involves the active extrusion of the drugs from the tumor cells (196), although additional mechanisms for MDR are now known, as described below.

The different mechanisms of MDR observed in tumor cells can be classified into (a) P-glycoprotein-mediated (165,197,198); (b) multidrug resistance protein (MRP)–mediated (199,200); (c) lung resistance protein (LRP)–mediated (201); and (iv) topoisomerase II–mediated (at-MDR) (143,162,165,167,196). By far, the most important resistance mechanism is that mediated by P170, a member of the transmembrane, multidrug resistance exporter protein family (165,197,198).

Classical multidrug resistance involves P-glycoprotein, or P170 (also called Pgp and gp170), a cell membrane–spanning glycoprotein of about 170 kDa molecular weight (glycosylated protein of 1280 amino acids in length), encoded by the *MDR1* gene in humans (165,197,198). P170 belongs to a superfamily of "ABC" (ATP-binding cassette) proteins, all of which are ATP-hydrolyzing proteins involved in transport (200). P170 contains, from N-terminus to C-terminus, 12 predicted membrane-spanning domains: six, followed by an internal ATP-binding site, followed by six additional membrane-spanning domains and a C-terminal ATP-binding site (198). It is thought that the two halves of P170 are derived from a gene duplication event (198). P170 is a drug-inducible protein that functions as an energy-dependent efflux pump that extrudes a wide range of drugs out of the tumor cell. Thus, induction of P170 by one antitumor drug generates cross-resistance to an entire class, including anthracyclines, epipodophyllotoxins, vinca alkaloids, and actinomycin D (196). Levels of expression of P170 correlate directly with drug levels and inversely with therapeutic efficacy in human tumors, as would be expected from its proposed mechanism of action (196,197). Classical MDR is reversible, as has been demonstrated in P388/ADR (murine p388 leukemia cell line resistant to adriamycin) by combination therapy with verapamil, a calcium channel blocker that is implicated in the inhibition of energy-dependent efflux of the drug (195,197).

A second type of ABC-transporter, multidrug resistance protein (MRP), was discovered in 1992 to confer resistance to doxorubicin in small-cell lung cancer cells. MRP also conferred resistance to other antitumor drugs and was found to be a member of the ABC superfamily of efflux proteins (199,200). MRP is encoded by the *MRP* gene in humans and, though, like P170, a member of the ABC superfamily, contains only 15% sequence identity with P170 (199,200). MRP is an N-glycosylated, 1531-amino-acid protein of about 190 kDa in size (199,200). The current hypothesis has the protein spanning the membrane in an 11 or 12 + 6 arrangement, that is, from N-terminus to C-terminus, there are 11 or 12 membrane-spanning domains, followed by the internal ATP-binding domain, followed by an additional 6 membrane-spanning domains (200).

Other membrane proteins have recently been implicated in possible MDR functions, although additional research will be needed to verify their roles, if any. These other proteins include lung resistance protein (LRP), which does not belong to the family of transporters such as P170 and MRP (201), and P95, a protein of the ABC-transporter superfamily implicated in multidrug resistance in lung cancer (202).

Additionally resistance can be mediated through the primary target of anthracyclines, topoisomerase II, a critical protein involved in regulating the three-dimensional structure of double-stranded DNA. As mentioned previously, 10-descarbomethoxy anthracyclines, such as doxorubicin, daunorubicin, and carminomycin, function by binding to the binary DNA–topoisomerase II complex, leading to an irreversible ternary complex (167). Cell lines with altered topoisomerase II or that express only low levels of topoisomerase II activity display cross-resistance to drugs such as anthracyclines, epipodophyllotoxins, and amsacrine, all of which are topoisomerase II poisons (203). As stated previously, class II anthracyclines having the 10-carbomethoxy-group, such as aclarubicin, are not subject to at-MDR (167). In fact, aclarubicin has been used in some experiments to quench the effect of topoisomerase II poisons (167).

F. Side Effects and Cumulative Cardiotoxicity

Anthracyclines in general cause a wide range of side effects, including nausea and vomiting, gastrointestinal disturbances, myelosuppression, hepatotoxicity, and cumulative cardiotoxicity (4). The most destructive side effect of anthracyclines is cumulative cardiotoxicity, which limits lifetime dosages of daunorubicin to 500–600 mg/m^2 and doxorubicin to 550 mg/m^2. Incidence of significant cardiomyopathy caused by doxorubicin treatment is 7, 15, and 30–40% at 550, 600, and 700 mg/m^2, respectively (113). There are three recognizable forms of cardiotoxicity: (a) acute or subacute cardiotoxicity, which usually occurs after a single dose or course of anthracycline therapy; (b) chronic cardiotoxicity, which is defined as cardiotoxicity that occurs within one year of initial treatment; and (c) late-onset cardiotoxicity, or cardiotoxicity that occurs after one year of the original treatment, and often after a prolonged asymptomatic period (204). Unfortunately, late-onset cardiotoxicity can cause early death of patients who have survived childhood cancer via chemotherapy treatments (204). Thus, cardiotoxicity is not only a significant short-term problem, but a long-term problem as well.

The mechanisms for anthracycline-induced cardiotoxicity have been studied intensely for over a quarter of a century, and still the exact mechanisms are not clear. The single most described cause for cardiotoxicity is the generation of free radicals by the quinone redox cycling (109,205,206) of anthracyclines, especially when complexed with iron (205,206). Most anthracyclines undergo biotransformation by quinone action to a semiquinone free radical, which can redox cycle with molecular oxygen to generate a cascade of reactive oxygen species, including superoxide, hydrogen peroxide, and hydroxyl radical (Figure 7). Additionally, free radicals can be formed by intramolecular reduction

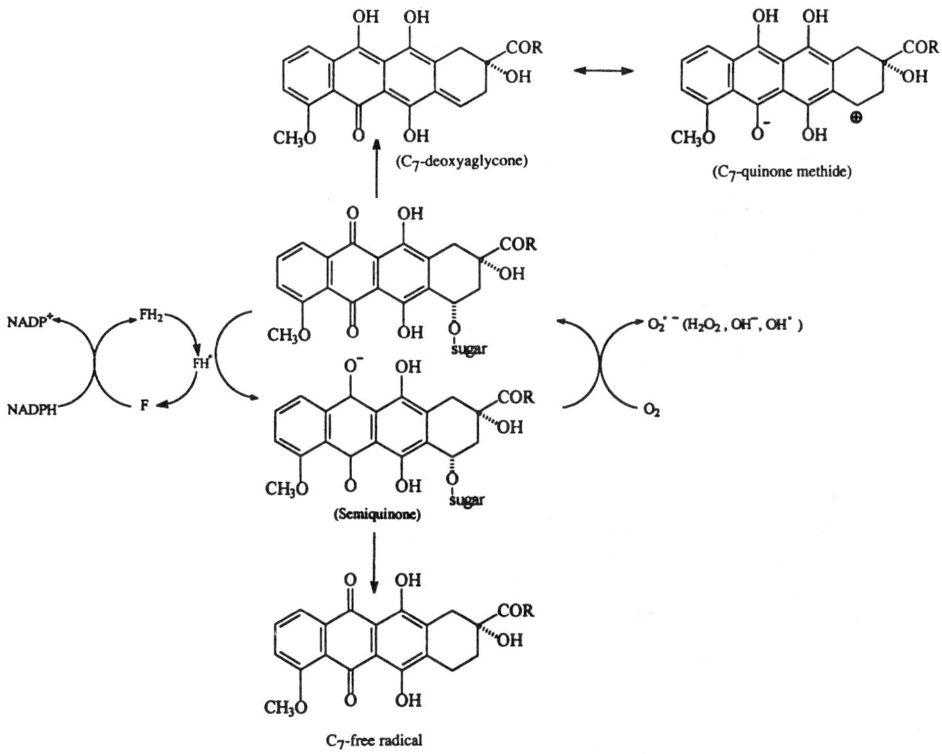

Figure 7 Proposed mechanism for formation of free radicals and potential alkylating agents by anthracyclines in the presence of redox enzymes (flavoproteins [F]), which reduce the anthracycline in a one-electron step to the semiquinone. The C$_7$-quinone methide, a potential alkylating agent, is a tautomer of the deoxyaglycone produced from this reaction. (Redrawn and modified from Ref. 206.)

of chelated iron (109,206). Though these free radicals do not appear to be involved in antitumor activity, they are strongly implicated in anthracycline cardiotoxicity (109). Heart muscle, in particular, has a large number of mitochondria, but low concentrations of protective enzymes, where these potentially cardiotoxic free radicals can be generated. The heart also has low levels of antioxidant enzymes that normally degrade free radicals, allowing for the accumulation of these toxic factors (205). Free radicals generated by anthracyclines cause lipid peroxidation and affect various cellular membranes leading to cell death (205,206).

Detection of cardiotoxicity is via endomyocardial biopsy as well as serial radionuclide angiocardiography (165). Endomyocardial biopsy remains the technique that provides the best linear correlation with cardiac toxicity and power of predicting onset of early cardiac failure. Serial radionuclide angiocardiography also has been used in adults, although the technique is not as accurate in children due to the anatomical considerations that make the image less clear (205).

Certain structure–function factors are known to increase cardiotoxicity by anthracyclines. For example, C13 hydroxy metabolites generated by reduction of anthracyclines such as doxorubicin and daunorubicin, a common physiological reaction (183), are considerably more cardiotoxic than the parental molecules (165,185). *N,N*-dimethyl doxorubicin confers much higher cardiotoxicity than doxorubicin (192,193). Conversely, *N*-L-leucyldaunorubicin exhibited much lower accumulation by heart muscle (193). Interestingly, and significantly, the 4′-tetrahydropyranyl derivative of doxorubicin, pirarubicin, is much less cardiotoxic than either doxorubicin or epirubicin (4′-epidoxorubicin) (137). These studies indicate that the structure of the sugar moiety of class I anthracyclines has a significant impact on their cardiotoxicity.

In recent years, there has been a significant push to develop drugs that would ameliorate cardiotoxic side effects caused by anthracyclines (1,207). In a significant recent development, dexrazoxane (trade name Zinecard), a Pharmacia-Upjohn product, has been approved for use as a cardioprotective agent in combination therapy with doxorubicin. Zinecard, a derivative of ethylenediaminetetraacetic acid (EDTA), apparently undergoes hydrolysis intracellularly, with the resulting activated molecule effective in chelating iron, thus blocking iron-dependent doxorubicin-conferred free radical formation (208,209).

G. New Approaches for Delivery of Anthracyclines

As mentioned previously in this chapter, there are two major problems associated with antitumor anthracycline therapy. First, the drugs typically become concentrated in leukocytes, which leads to undesired localization in kidney, liver, spleen, heart, and bone marrow, resulting in the respective organ-toxicity side effects, the most serious of which is cardiomyopathy. This first problem is due to the inherent lack of tissue specificity associated with all antitumor drugs. Second, the clinical usefulness of anthracyclines as antitumor agents is limited by the development of acquired multidrug resistance (MDR), as detailed in the previous sections. One of the reasons that MDR is induced is the very high levels of drug that need to be used to obtain effective levels at the tumor site. Thus, one of the major strategies to improve the pharmacokinetics of antitumor anthracyclines is to target the drugs more specifically to the tumor sites, both to prevent or minimize damage to other tissues and to limit the dosage to prevent MDR induction (115,116).

There are two basic approaches toward targeting of anthracyclines to tumors. In the first approach, known as a passive method, the anthracyclines are encapsulated within polymers such as liposomes or lipoproteins, the intent of which is to alter the pharmaco-logical properties of the drug so that it can be delivered more directly to the tumor (116,210).

Four types of liposome-mediated delivery of drugs have been used to direct drugs more specifically to their biological targets: (a) natural targeting, the most generalized and least appealing for anthracyclines, in which the particle would be administered into the blood and the drug would predominantly be distributed to phagocytic cells; (b) administration of the liposomes directly into the anatomical region of interest; (c) phys-ical targeting of liposome-mediated drug using pH-sensitive or magnetic liposomes; or (d) ligand-mediated targeting of the liposome–drug complex. In this final approach, antibod-ies, hormones, lectins, or similar such targeting agents are incorporated into the lipo-somes to direct them to the target tissue (210).

Liposome-mediated targeting has been used widely in efforts to direct doxorubicin more specifically to tumors, thereby reducing toxic side effects, including bone marrow suppression, nephrotoxicity, and especially cardiotoxicity, and to lessen the chance for drug resistance mediated by the P170 MDR protein (210). Two new liposomal drugs intro-duced to the market within the past year are liposomal-doxorubicin (Sequus, Inc., Menlo Park, CA "Doxil") and liposomal-daunorubicin (NeXstar, Inc., San Dimas, CA "Dauno-Xome"), both approved for the treatment of AIDS-related Kaposi's sarcoma. Clinical stud-ies have shown that these drugs are highly active against Kaposi's sarcoma (211).

In the second, more "active," approach, the anthracyclines are conjugated to mol-ecules as prodrugs that target tumor cell membrane receptors. In this approach, the anthracyclines may be conjugated to hormones, transferrin, other drugs, or specific anti-bodies (116,212). One of the most widely described examples of this is the conjugation of doxorubicin to the monoclonal antibody (MAb) known as BR96-DOX (212). This anthracycline–MAb conjugate was shown in 1993 to cure 70% of treated rats previously grafted with human lung carcinoma (212).

A more sophisticated strategy for specific delivery of the drug to the tumor surface is antibody-directed enzyme prodrug therapy (ADEPT) first described in 1987 (see refer-ence 213) (Figure 8). In the ADEPT approach, a tumor-specific monoclonal antibody

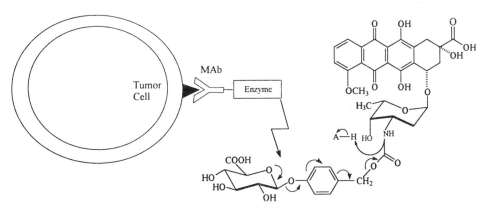

Figure 8 Example of ADEPT (antibody-directed enzyme prodrug therapy) strategy. In the ADEPT approach, the antitumor-antibody-linked cleavage enzyme is allowed to bind to the tumor, fol-lowed by treatment with the inactive prodrug. Only in the region of the tumor, in which the pro-drug is activated by cleavage of the susceptible bond and self-immolation of the side chain, is the active drug released. (Redrawn and modified from Ref. 115.)

conjugated with a specific hydrolase is first injected so that it can localize to the tumor. Then a prodrug of the anthracycline conjugated to a side chain containing a bond hydrolyzable by the MAb-linked hydrolase is injected (115,116,213–220). Only when the prodrug reaches the tumor and is cleaved specifically by the MAb-linked hydrolase does it become active (Figure 8). The potential benefits of this strategy are obvious, but the limitations include possible immunogenicity of the enzyme–MAb conjugate, nonspecific activation of the prodrug by unbound (circulating) enzyme–MAb conjugate, and optimization of the pharmacology of the active drug (116,213). Examples (216–220) of ADEPT strategies used thus far in attempts to target anthracyclines are shown in Table 6. The ADEPT approach, which is still relatively new, has been undergoing considerable scrutiny in recent years, with hopes that it may provide more specific targeting of doxorubicin and other anthracyclines to tumors (116,213).

III. INDUSTRIALLY IMPORTANT ANTHRACYCLINES

The most widely investigated anthracycline-producing organisms include

1. *Streptomyces peucetius* strains ATCC 29050 and 27952, daunorubicin- and doxorubicin-producing strains, respectively, studied in detail by C. Richard Hutchinson and his colleagues at Wisconsin, as well as by the researchers at Pharmacia-Upjohn, by Jung-Joon Lee and his colleagues at the Korea Institute of Science and Technology, and by Ho Coy Choke in Malaysia
2. *Streptomyces* sp. strain C5 (ATCC 49111), a daunorubicin and baumycin producer originally isolated and studied by the research group at the Frederick Cancer Research Center, but now studied almost exclusively by our laboratory
3. *Streptomyces galilaeus* MA-144-M1, an aclacinomycin-producing strain studied in great detail by Oki and his colleagues
4. *Streptomyces* sp. D788 and *Streptomyces coeruleorubidus* ME130-A4 (ATCC 31276), baumycin- and daunorubicin-producing strains isolated and characterized by Yoshimoto and his colleagues
5. *Streptomyces griseus* JA5142, a daunorubicin-producing strain studied by Klaus Eckardt, Christina Wagner, and their colleagues in Jena, Germany
6. *Streptomyces nogalater* (ATCC 27451), a nogalamycin producer isolated by researchers at Upjohn in the 1960s, and now studied by Mäntsälä and his colleagues in Finland

Table 6   Examples of ADEPT Strategies Used to Treat Tumors with Anthracyclines

Drug	Prodrug	Enzyme	Ref.
Doxorubicin	7-(Phenylacetamido)cephalosporin-doxorubicin	Type II β-lactamase	216
Daunorubicin	*N*[4(α-D-Galactopyranosyl)-benzyloxycarbonyl]-daunorubicin	α-Galactosidase	217
Epirubicin	Epirubicin glucuronide	β-Glucuronidase	218
Doxorubicin	Doxorubicin-glucuronide	β-Glucuronidase	217
Doxorubicin	Doxorubicin phosphate	Alkaline phosphatase	219
Doxorubicin	Doxorubicin-phenoxyacetamide	Penicillin amidase	220

A. Carminomycin–Daunorubicin–Doxorubicin–Baumycin Group

Anthracyclines of the carminomycin–daunorubicin–doxorubicin–baumycin group are 7-O-(α-L-daunosaminyl) glycosides of 10-descarbomethoxy-11-hydroxy aglycones (Figure 1). Daunorubicin is produced by a wide range of taxonomically distinct streptomycetes. The following 13 independently isolated strains are known to produce daunorubicin or its close derivatives: *S. peucetius* (7–12), *Streptomyces bifurcus* strain 23219 (49), *S. coeruleorubidus* strains ME130-A4 (30,31), 8899 (13,14,54), 31723 (13,14,54), and JA10092 (55), *Streptomyces griseoruber* (73), *S. griseus* IMET JA5142 (75), a patented *S. griseus* strain (76), *Streptomyces insignis* ATCC 31913 (77,78), *Streptomyces viridochromogenes* (93), *Streptomyces* sp. C5 (ATCC 49111) (96,98), and *Streptomyces* sp. D788 (99). Most of these strains also have been shown to produce baumycins, and we will make the case in this chapter that the genetic capability for baumycin production is probably present in all daunorubicin-producing strains; hence, we believe that baumycins are the true end products in these so-called "daunorubicin-producing" strains, not daunorubicin. Additionally, *Streptomyces triangulatus* subsp. *angiostaticus* (86) was shown to produce the angiostatic natural product TAN-1120, a daunorubicin-based baumycin-like molecule. Whether this strain also accumulates daunorubicin as a product was not stated (86).

Most of these strains, including *Streptomyces* sp. strain C5 (96), *S. peucetius* (124), and *S. insignis* (77), also accumulate large quantities of ε-rhodomycinone, a daunorubicin pathway intermediate. Wagner et al. (125) have put forth the theory that ε-rhodomycinone is not a common intermediate in daunorubicin biosynthesis pathways, but a shunt product. They base their conclusions on the ability of 11-hydroxylase to utilize a variety of different substrates besides aklavinone, which is considered by most researchers to be the "natural" substrate for this enzyme (221–226). The evidence presented in this chapter most strongly supports the notion that ε-rhodomycinone is a direct intermediate of daunorubicin and doxorubicin biosynthesis.

The leukaemomycins produced by *S. griseus* IMET JA5142 were studied in depth by the research group in Jena (68,95,125,227–229). Based on chromatographic evidence, it has been shown that the leukaemomycins are derivatives of daunorubicin-related glycosides as follows: leukaemomycin A, a mixture of daunomycinone-related aglycones; B$_1$, rubomycin B (4'-rhodinosyldaunorubicin); B$_2$, 4'-daunosaminyldaunorubicin; C, daunorubicin; and D, 13-dihydrodaunorubicin (4). Similarly, the antibiotics named rubidomycin by researchers at Rhône-Poulenc (13–15), rubomycin C, and antibiotic B-35251-C are also daunorubicin-related glycosides (117).

Carminomycin, 4-demethyldaunorubicin (23), and various 4-hydroxybaumycin analogs, are produced by *Actinomadura carminata* (23,24), *Actinomadura roseoviolacea* strains 1029-AV1 (32,33) and 07 (34), and the unspeciated *Actinomadura* strains D326 (35) and MG465-yF4 (38). These are essentially baumycin- and daunorubicin-producing strains lacking 4-O-methyltransferase, as described later in this chapter. This concept is supported by the accumulation of carminomycin and its analogs by the daunorubicin-nonproducing mutant strain, *S. peucetius* subsp. *carminatus* (82).

These compounds are all produced by the same pathway and are metabolically linked in substrate–product relationships (see Section V.G). The carminomycin series of anthracyclines contain a 4-hydroxy moiety, whereas daunorubicin and doxorubicin derivatives contain 4-methoxy moieties. Doxorubicin and 13-dihydrodoxorubicin (doxorubicinol or adriamycinol) are 14-hydroxylated analogs of daunorubicin and 13-dihydro-daunorubicin, respectively.

Epirubicin (4′-epidoxorubicin), a semisynthetic analog of doxorubicin in which the natural aminosugar, daunosamine (3-amino-2,3,6-trideoxy-L-lyxohexose), is modified to a 4′-epi analog (3-amino-2,3,6-trideoxy-L-arabinohexose) (110), was first placed into clinical trials in July 1977 (230). 4′-O-Tetrahydropyranyl-doxorubicin (THP-doxorubicin or pirarubicin), a structural analog of baumycin A_1 (Figure 1) (136,231), is produced by Meiji Seika (USA), Inc. Idarubicin (4-demethoxydaunorubicin) (Figure 1) is synthesized chemically (110).

B.   Aclacinomycin Group

The aclacinomycin group of anthracyclines (Figure 2), produced by various strains of *Streptomyces galilaeus* (Table 1), exhibits the greatest variety of sugar components. The primary aglycones within this group are aklavinone (ethyl side chain; 27–29), auramycinone (methyl side chain; 63,64), and sulfurmycinone (acetonyl side chain; 63,64). Isotope labeling experiments on daunomycinone (the aglycone moiety of daunorubicin) and aklavinone (aglycone moiety of aclarubicin) biosynthesis have shown that they are formed from one propionate and nine C_2 units derived from malonyl-SCoA (232–234). To our knowledge, the derivation of the methyl and acetonyl side chains on auramycin and sulfurmycin, respectively, have not been published; nevertheless, it would be expected that the methyl side chain of auramycin is derived from an acetyl starter moiety, whereas the acetonyl side chain of the sulfurmycins is probably derived either from two acetyl units, butyryl-SCoA, or β-hydroxybutyryl-SCoA.

The aclacinomycins were first discovered in the late 1970s with the initial purification and description of 19 different aclacinomycin-like metabolites from cultures of *S. galilaeus* strain MA-144-M1 (ATCC 31133) (27). Subsequently, aclacinomycin A (aclarubicin) was purified from this strain and characterized in detail (28,29). Aclacinomycin A and its closest analogs are triglycosides of aklavinone, a 4-hydroxy-10-carbomethoxy-11-deoxy-13-deoxy-anthracyclinone (Figure 2). The first sugar is rhodosamine (3-dimethylamino-2,3,6-trideoxy-L-lyxohexose), the second is deoxyfucose, and the third is variable, with cinerulose A as the moiety in aclacinomycin A (28,29).

Based on the knowledge obtained from the daunorubicin/doxorubicin biosynthesis pathways of *S. peucetius* and *Streptomyces* sp. strain C5, it is apparent that the primary differences in aclacinomycin production from daunorubicin production are the following: (a) *dnrF/dauF* homolog, encoding aklavinone 11-hydroxylase (223–226), is missing; (b) *dauP/dnrP* homolog, encoding the 10-carbomethoxy esterase function (65,235–239), is lacking; (c) *dauK/dnrK* homolog, encoding anthracycline 4-O-methyltransferase (236–243) activity, is lacking; (d) *doxA* homolog, encoding C13 and C14 oxidation functions (239,244), is missing; and (e) the expected genes encoding thymidine 5′-diphospho (TDP)-daunosamine N-methyltransferase as well as those encoding synthesis and attachment of the additional sugars, missing from the daunorubicin-producing strains, are present.

Mutagenesis of *S. galilaeus* MA-144-M1 resulted in a mutant strain that synthesized 2-hydroxy-aclacinomycin and various other 2-hydroxy derivatives (66,67). This strain was later shown to be mutated in the *aknA* gene (*dpsE* homolog) encoding polyketide reductase (245,246), a fact that assisted greatly in the characterization of polyketide reductase function (245,247).

C.   Pyrromycin and Rhodomycin Groups

Anthracyclines belonging to the pyrromycin group, produced primarily by strains of *S. galilaeus* (25–29,60,62,63,248), *S. purpurascens* (3,5), and *Actinosporangium bohemicum* C-36145 (ATCC 31127) (39–43), are identified as glycosides of 1-hydroxy, 10-carbomethoxy, 11-deoxy aglycones (29,52,56). Cinerubins, anthracyclines produced by several different streptomycete strains (50,52,53,59,74,87), are pyrromycinone triglycosides in which the first two sugars are rhodosamine and deoxyfucose; the third sugar is variable (52).

The rhodomycin group of anthracyclines, produced by *S. purpurascens* (12) and *S. coeruleorubidus* (10), are glycosides of 4,6,7,10,11-hydroxy aglycones, which contain one of more rhodosamine moieties (52). In some rhodomycins, sugars are attached at both the C7 and C10 positions, and some other rhodomycins possess 1-hydroxy-groups (3,4,52).

D.   Nogalamycin Group

Nogalamycin (Figure 2), produced by *Streptomyces nogalater* (20), is synthesized from 10 acetyl moieties as determined by ^{13}C nuclear magnetic resonance (NMR) analysis after labeling with [1,2-^{13}C]acetate (249). Nogalamycin is unique among anthracyclines because it contains a dimethylamino sugar, connected to C1 and C2 of the anthracyclinone, and nogalose, a neutral sugar, connected to position C7 (52) (Figure 2). Discovered at Upjohn in the early 1960s, nogalamycin was found to have antibacterial activity as well as in vitro cytotoxic activity against cultured L1210 leukemia cells (20), but because it was found to have poor activity against solid tumors in vivo, testing was halted (135). Nevertheless, analogs of nogalamycin were developed in the search for a derivative possessing a higher efficacy to toxicity ratio. As a result of chemical modification studies, it was discovered that acid methanolysis of nogalamycin resulted in the replacement of nogalose with a methoxy moiety. One of the products of such treatment, the semisynthetic monosaccharide derivative originally called 7-con-O-methylnogarol (135), was found to have excellent clinical characteristics. This derivative, later renamed menogaril, preferentially inhibits RNA synthesis, and preferentially intercalates adenine–thymine-rich (AT-rich) DNA sequences (135), suggesting that it has a somewhat different mechanism of action from other anthracyclines. Menogaril, currently an investigative antitumor drug in the United States, has modest activity against a variety of cancers (250). Its greatest strength is that menogaril, like idarubicin, is orally active, which may be of benefit for treatment of cancers within certain age groups (250).

E.   Steffimycin Group

The steffimycins (Figure 2), produced by *S. steffisbergensis* strain UC-5044 (21,22,58) and *Streptomyces elgreteus* strain UC-5453 (58), are unique in that they contain C2 and C8 methoxy groups (Figure 2). Like nogalamycin, steffimycin is synthesized from 10 acetate equivalents (249), instead of 9 acetyl moieties and a propionyl-SCoA starter unit (as per daunorubicin (232–234)). Although steffimycin was discovered in the early 1960s, and thus has been available for more than 30 years, it has never been studied intensely due to its initial borderline activity against P388 murine leukemia cell cultures (22).

F. Tetracenomycin and Elloramycin

Tetracenomycin C and elloramycin are produced by *Streptomyces glaucescens* GLA.0 (69) and *Streptomyces olivaceus* strain Tü2353 (80), respectively. Both tetracenomycin and elloramycin are characterized by their tetracyclic structure, within which is the 2,3-dihydro-1,4-anthraquinone chromophore. Whereas the tetracyclic nature of these antibiotics makes them related to both tetracyclines and anthracyclines, the partly unsaturated A-ring makes them more similar to some anthracyclines such as aranciamycin and akrobomycin (251). Only a few members of this group of antibacterial and antitumor antibiotics have been discovered (251). Interestingly, and antithetical to anthracyclines of the daunorubicin or aclarubicin groups, aglycones of this group (e.g., tetracenomycin C) appear to have greater activity against L1210 leukemia cells in vitro than the glycosylated form, elloramycin A (251).

The information gleaned from molecular, biochemical, and chemical studies on tetracenomycin have been critical for understanding not only type II polyketide synthases (PKSs) (126,252–255), but also for helping to characterize several important biochemical reactions (e.g., methyltransferases (256), cyclases (256–258), oxygenases (259)) that occur in daunorubicin biosynthesis as well as biosynthesis of many antibiotics. Though this antibiotic has become one of the primary models for type II PKS reactions due to the pioneering work of C. R. Hutchinson and his colleagues (126,252–255), it is not a commercially viable drug.

Elloramycin (80), like tetracenomycin, is not a candidate for commercialization. However, the polyketide biosynthesis genes for elloramycin have recently been cloned (260). As expected, the elloramycin biosynthesis gene cluster is fairly similar in structure to the tetracenomycin biosynthesis gene cluster (260).

IV. GROWTH, FERMENTATION, AND DOWNSTREAM PROCESSING

A. Defined Medium Studies

Dekleva et al. (261) developed an optimized minimal medium for growth and daunorubicin production by *S. peucetius* strain ATCC 29050, which included 0.5 mM Mg^{2+}, 1 mM phosphate, 10 mM nitrate, 125 mM glucose, and microelements. Ammonia appeared to repress anthracycline biosynthesis by *S. peucetius*, and maltose and fructose were found to be the best carbon sources supporting anthracycline production (261). It was later shown that glucose and fructose typically stimulated acidogenesis (primarily in the form of pyruvate and 2-oxoglutarate) by *S. peucetius*, suggesting that alternative sugar sources such as maltose were also preferable for growth of this organism (262). Such glucose-mediated acidogenesis is relatively common among streptomycetes (262).

It is apparent, however, that glucose does not act to repress anthracycline biosynthesis by either *S. peucetius* (261) or *Streptomyces* sp. strain C5 (Strohl WR and Dekleva ML, unpublished results), as considerable glucose remains in the media during the production phase. Inorganic phosphate, on the other hand, suppressed anthracycline biosynthesis in *S. peucetius* (261).

B. Methods for Growing Anthracycline-Producing Streptomycetes

The anthracycline-producing strains, *Streptomyces* sp. strain C5, *S. insignis*, *S. nogalater*, and *S. steffisbergensis*, grow well and sporulate readily on R2YE (regeneration-yeast extract; 263) solid medium. On the other hand, *S. peucetius* ATCC 29050 grows well on plates of R2YE, YS (yeast extract 0.3%, soluble starch 1.0%, agar 1.5%, pH 7.2) agar, or

ISP4 (Difco, Detroit, Michigan) solid media, but sporulates well only on the latter two. *S. galilaeus* ATCC 31133 also grows well on plates of R2YE, ISP4, or YS but typically sporulates well only on ISP4 or YS agar.

For routine biochemical investigations, we have found that NDYE (nitrate-defined plus yeast extract) medium (227,241,264), modified from NDM (nitrate-defined medium) medium (261) by addition of yeast extract and MOPS (3-[N-Morpholino] propane sulfonic acid) buffer, is the best soluble medium for routine growth and analysis of *Streptomyces* sp. strain C5. This strain grows poorly and produces little or no anthracyclines in YEME (yeast extract-malt extract) (263) or TSB (trypicase soy broth; Difco) media. *S. peucetius* also grows well in NDYE when the glucose is replaced with maltose (262). Alternatively, *S. peucetius* may be grown in either R2YE or APM (anthracycline production medium) medium (265), particularly when the culture is used as a seed for larger-scale fermentations.

S. galilaeus ATCC 31133 grows poorly and does not produce anthracyclines in either NDM or NDYE media. It does, however, produce a small quantity of anthracyclines in YEME, but our limited experience in cultivating this strain has shown that YS medium (described above) appears to yield the highest titer of anthracyclines. Other labs have found SGM (streptomycete growth medium) medium (119) to be suitable for antibiotic production by *S. galilaeus* ATCC 31133, or E1 medium (266) for *S. galilaeus* ATCC 31615, but neither of those has been used in our laboratory.

For small-scale cultivation of *S. insignis*, our laboratory has observed moderate anthracycline production in GYE (glucose-yeast extract) medium consisting of 6.25% cerelose, 1.25% yeast extract, 0.33% NaCl, and 0.625% $CaCO_3$, pH 7.2 (78). Additional media useful for cultivation and fermentation of *S. insignis* also have been described previously (77,78).

S. nogalater grows well and produces nogalamycin in a variety of media, including YEME (although amounts are low and are reduced further when the strain is transformed with high copy number plasmids), E1 (266), and TYG (tryptone, yeast extract, glucose) media (267). Additionally, a variety of rich seed media (10,16) have been described for the fermentation of this organism. *S. steffisbergensis* grows well and produces ample quantities of steffimycins when grown in R2YE medium. It also grows well in YEME, but antibiotic production in this medium is very erratic, ranging from none to moderate. TYG has also been utilized as a production medium in the cultivation of this strain (268). *S. purpurascens* grows well and produces ample quantities of rhodomycin in R2YE medium. It also produces moderate quantities of anthracyclines in NDYE, but very small amounts in YEME. Other media that may be useful for cultivating this and other anthracycline-producing streptomycetes are described by Shirling and Gottlieb (269).

S. coeruleorubidus strains are typically grown in YS seed medium for antibiotic production, and fermentations are carried out in a wide variety of media, including one described by Blumauerová et al. (55) containing 3.5% soluble starch, 3.0% soybean meal, 0.3% NaCl, and 0.3% $CaCO_3$. Growth of *S. coeruleorubidus* in other fermentation media gives a wide range of results, as described by Blumauerová et al. (55) and Yoshimoto et al. (270). The medium used for baumycin isolation from this strain contained 4% sucrose, 2.5% soybean meal, 0.25% NaCl, 0.32% $CaCO_3$, 0.0005% $CuSO_4 \cdot 5H_2O$, 0.0005% $MnCl_2 \cdot 4H_2O$, and 0.0005% $ZnSO_4 \cdot 7H_2O$, pH 7.4 (30).

For most of these organisms, the best anthracycline titers are reached after 5–7 days of growth, although some (such as *S. peucetius* and *S. galilaeus*) require up to 10 days to reach high titers. All of the strains require considerable aeration (i.e., shaking the flasks on the order of 250 rpm), and most of the strains are grown between 28 and 30°C. We routinely incorporate springs in Erlenmeyer flasks for shake-flask culture growth of anthracycline-producing streptomycetes (261). This description of media is not intended to be all-inclusive for each strain listed or for all anthracycline-producing organisms; rather, it is a guide to the types of conditions used to grow anthracycline-producing strains. Additional media for cultivating various anthracycline-producing organisms can be found in reviews by Oki (119) and Hutchinson (126; which lists many media used for cultivating *S. peucetius*).

C.   Production Media and Conditions

Since McGuire and his colleagues at the Frederick Cancer Research Center described in detail the development of fermentation processes and strain improvements that increased titers of daunorubicin from 10–30 mg/liter to over 200 mg/liter (96–98,121,271,272), very little has been published on process, media, and strain development for maximal titer production in commercial fermentations. It is probable that titers of daunorubicin and doxorubicin in commercial processes reach levels of greater than 1 g/liter, but actual data are not public due to the proprietary nature of the processes involved. What has been published mainly describes fermentations for *S. peucetius*, *S. coeruleorubidus*, and *Streptomyces* sp. strain C5, isolated at the Frederick Cancer Research Center. Excellent reviews of these processes can be found in articles by Blumauerová et al. (55), Grein (83,123), McGuire et al. (271), and White and Stroshane (121).

For anthracycline production by *S. peucetius*, the seed medium used is typically APM (265) (although R2YE has also been used). After 24–48 hr of growth, the culture (10–20% inoculum) is transferred to GPS (glucose-Proflo-salts) production medium (262) for 7–10 days at 30°C with aeration at 1 liter air/1 liter culture vol/min and stirring/shaking at 250–300 rpm. It was originally assumed that only *S. peucetius* var. *caesius* ATCC 27952 could produce doxorubicin in fermentations, but recent results have suggested that doxorubicin can be produced as well in cultures of *S. peucetius* ATCC 29050 that contain highly buffered medium (15 g/liter MOPS) and in young seed cultures (126; Hutchinson CR, personal communication). Buffering counteracts acidification effects observed with glucose as the carbon source, which are detrimental to anthracycline and, in particular, doxorubicin production (126,262).

Recent work by Nakamura and Yoshimoto (273) indicates that daunorubicin production is greatly increased by iron salt levels in the fermentations (273). They found that addition of 10 mM ferric salts stimulated daunorubicin production by *Streptomyces* sp. D788 at least fourfold, without increasing the concentration of the accumulated pathway intermediate, D788-1 (10-carboxy-13-deoxycarminomycin) (273).

For small-scale stirred tank fermentations of *Streptomyces* sp. strain C5, our lab typically uses a seed inoculum grown in NDYE for 24–48 hr to inoculate 10 liter fermentors (5% [v/v] inoculum) of SC (streptomycete-Connors) production medium consisting of (in g/liter): glucose, 22.5; yeast extract, 8.0; malt extract, 20; NaCl, 2.0; MOPS, 10; $MgSO_4$, 0.1; $FeSO_4 \cdot 7H_2O$, 0.01; $ZnSO_4 \cdot 7H_2O$, 0.01; and MAZU (Mazer, Inc., Gurnee, IL) DF60P antifoam, 1.2 ml; adjusted to pH 7.3. Fermentors are typically run at 250–300 rpm with aeration at 10 liter/liter/min for 5–7 days at 30°C prior to harvesting for anthracycline purification.

D.   Genetic Manipulation of Anthracycline-Producing Strains

Despite exhaustive attempts to observe cryptic plasmids in the anthracycline-producing strains *S. peucetius* ATCC 29050, ATCC 27952, and ATCC 21354, *S. galilaeus* ATCC

31133, *S. coeruleorubidus* ATCC 23900 and ATCC 31276, and *Streptomyces* sp. C5, none were found (274). A temperate bacteriophage, however, was isolated from *S. galilaeus* ATCC 31133 after plating on *S. peucetius* strain ATCC 29050 (274). The phage, φSPK1, was shown to possess a wide host range but was not further studied due to the availability of wide-host-range streptomycete vectors (274).

S. peucetius ATCC 29050 (275), *Streptomyces* sp. strain C5 (275), and *S. galilaeus* (245) can be transformed with several different common streptomycete plasmids and transfected with φC31-related bacteriophages. Of the three strains, *S. galilaeus* is by far the easiest to protoplast, transform, and regenerate. Nevertheless, there is no evidence for significant restriction barriers between any of these strains and *Streptomyces lividans* TK24, and clones of actinorhodin biosynthesis genes made in the common streptomycete vectors pIJ922, pIJ61, and pIJ350 are stable in all of these strains (245,275). Plasmid pIJ101–derived plasmids (e.g., pIJ702) are introduced by transformation at a high frequency ($>10^6$/μg of DNA) and are stably maintained in all three strains (275). Lower frequencies ($\leq 10^3$/μg of DNA) are obtained, however, when the medium copy number plasmid pIJ61 (SLP1 derivative) is introduced into *S. peucetius* and *Streptomyces* sp. strain C5, or when low copy number SCP2* derivatives (e.g., pIJ922, pIJ941, pKC505) are introduced into *S. galilaeus* (275).

In a recent paper, Ylihonko et al. (276) reported that the transformation frequency for *S. nogalater*, using classical methods (263), was 1 transformant per 10 μg of DNA (276), which is unacceptably low. We have found that pIJ101 derivatives (e.g., pIJ702, pIJ486) could be introduced into both *S. nogalater* ATCC 27451 and *S. steffisbergensis* ATCC 27466 at reasonable frequencies ($>10^3$/μg of DNA), but only when these streptomycetes were grown for protoplasting in YEME medium modified by addition of mannitol in place of the glucose (Dickens ML and Strohl WR, unpublished data). Additionally, we have found that when transformed with the high copy number plasmid pIJ486 (277), neither *S. steffisbergensis* nor *S. nogalater* produce anthracyclines (Dickens ML, DeSanti CL, and Strohl WR, unpublished results). It is probable that the high copy number plasmids inhibit, by an unknown mechanism, transcription of anthracycline biosynthesis genes in these strains.

Other than conditions specified above, the protoplast transformation conditions described by Lampel and Strohl (275) are still followed in our laboratory for most anthracycline-producing strains. No technique has yet been published for electroporation of anthracycline-producing streptomycetes.

E. Methods for Purification of Anthracyclines

Since the principles followed in the original methods for purification of daunorubicin are still applicable, it is worthwhile to review the original purification process described by Cassinelli and Orezzi (9). Daunorubicin was first extracted from *S. peucetius* cake using acetone: 0.1 N H_2SO_4 (4:1 v:v), followed by neutralization and evacuation to remove the acetone (9). By raising the pH of the extract to 8.6, followed by shaking with *n*-butanol, the glycosides were transferred to the organic phase. The organic phase was reextracted into 0.1 N H_2SO_4 to remove lipophilic compounds (including an antifungal polyene also produced by *S. peucetius* that remained in the organic phase). The pH of the acidified aqueous phase was raised again to 8.6, and then it was reextracted with chloroform, followed by concentration of the organic extract (9). The crude daunorubicin•HCl was recovered from the concentrate by addition of methanolic HCl and ethyl ether, and the antibiotic was purified by cellulose column chromatography using a mobile phase of 0.1 M phosphate buffer (pH 5.4) with elution by *n*-butanol in the same buffer. Approximately 5–15 mg of daunorubicin were recovered per liter of fermentation broth extracted, results that are typical for wild-type strains (9).

Daunorubicin was extracted from cultures of *S. insignis* by adjusting the broth to pH 8.5 and adding 10× volume of *n*-butanol (78). After filtering, the filtrate was adjusted to pH 1.5 with ethanolic HCl and concentrated. Crude daunorubicin precipitated by addition of an excess of heptane (10× vol) was then extracted 2–3 times with acidic water (pH 2.5). These acid extracts were washed with chloroform, the pH was adjusted to pH 8.5, and then they were reextracted with chloroform. These extracts were washed 2–3 times with water and then dried (78).

One factor that is sometimes ignored in publications describing daunorubicin purification is that most, if not all, daunorubicin-producing strains produce significant quantities of baumycins. Thus, the total amount of "daunorubicin" is present in the form of "higher glycosides," namely, baumycins, which are readily converted to daunorubicin upon mild hydrolysis with oxalic acid. Therefore, for isolation of daunorubicin from whole broth, the broth is first treated with excess oxalic acid (in our laboratory, 30 mg of oxalic acid per ml of culture broth [final concentration] is typically used) to hydrolyze the acid-labile bond of the baumycin side chain. Since oxalic acid is self-buffering at pH 1.3, it prevents total hydrolysis of the glycones to aglycones (which can be a problem when using mineral acids). Additionally, oxalic acid can be added as a solid, which obviates the need for volume corrections (121).

The methods used in our laboratory for purifying daunorubicin and other daunosamine-based glycosides from shake flasks and small-scale fermentation samples involve raising the pH of the entire broth to 8.5 using 5 M NaOH and extracting 2–3 times with an equal volume of chloroform:methanol (9:1). The increase in pH effectively neutralizes the charged amino-group of the daunosamine sugar, which allows the molecule to enter the organic phase of the mixture. Since this procedure will not hydrolyze baumycins, these compounds must be treated with oxalic acid (typically 30 mg/ml) and heated at 55°C for 45 min. This effectively liberates only monoglycosylated products, which are recovered by raising the pH to 8.5 and extracting 2–3 times with chloroform:methanol (9:1) (oxalic acid treatment also can be performed directly on the whole broth). Alternatively, for extraction of anthracyclines containing a charged carboxyl-group (e.g., 10-carboxy-13-deoxycarminomycin and 10-carboxy-13-deoxydaunorubicin), the pH of the broth must be decreased to 2.5 to effectively neutralize this group. Since decreasing the pH will impart a charge to the amino-group of the sugar, the extraction must be carried out using polar organic solvents, such as *n*-butanol, which are not miscible with water.

Nakamura and Yoshimoto (273) recently described a new method for purification of daunorubicin from fermentation broth. They added phosphoric acid to the fermentation broth (1:3 ratio) to acidify the broth to pH 1.5, and they stirred that mixture for 2 hr. The acidified broth was filtered, the filtrate was applied to a column containing HP-20 resin, and the anthracyclines were eluted with a linear gradient of 15–50% acetone. Daunorubicin eluted in nearly pure form at about 30% acetone (273).

Aglycones can be isolated after total hydrolysis of the glycones based on their strongly hydrophobic characteristics. This treatment involves heating the glycone extract in the presence of 0.4 M HCl at 95°C for 1 hr (240). An alternative protocol described by Arcamone (4) involves mild hydrolysis of monoglycosylated glycones (e.g., doxorubicin, daunorubicin, carminomycin) with 0.1 M HCl at 100°C for 20 min, resulting in recovery of the aglycone moiety as well as the aminosugar, daunosamine (4). After cooling to room temperature, the hydrolyzed extract can be extracted with chloroform:methanol (9:1), followed by column or thin-layer chromatography (TLC).

For larger extractions, such as those carried out at Rhône-Poulenc, the whole broth may be acidified to pH 1.5 with sulfuric acid without heating. After filtering, the spent cake is discarded and the filtrate is extracted by manipulating the pH and extracting with various solvents (121). For descriptions of methods for large-scale daunorubicin purification, Pandey et al. (278) compared three different extraction processes used at the Frederick Cancer Research Center (FCRC), and the review by White and Stroshane (121) compared in detail the processes developed at FCRC with those used at Rhône-Poulenc.

Once extracts have been dried, final purification can be carried out with simple column chromatography using such column matrices as silica gel (279) or Sephadex LH-20 (Pharmacia), TLC with silica gel plates, or by HPLC using various solvent systems and columns. Our lab has found that for general TLC analysis, a solvent system consisting of chloroform:methanol:acetic acid:water (80:20:16:6) adequately separates glycones (244), and one consisting of chloroform:heptane:methanol (10:10:3) separates aglycones (280). For HPLC analysis of glycones, we commonly use a C_{18} reverse phase column with a solvent system of methanol:water (65:35), pH 2.0, with phosphoric acid (244,281). Anthracyclinones are separated and analyzed by C_{18} reverse phase HPLC using a solvent system of methanol:water:glacial acetic acid (65:30:5), pH 2.5 (222).

If, on the other hand, the goal is to isolate baumycins, rubeomycins, and 4-hydroxybaumycins having acid-labile residues at C4', care must be taken to extract only under neutral conditions (121). A detailed purification protocol was provided for the original isolation of the baumycins by Takahashi et al. (31). In their extraction procedures, the mycelia and broth were first separated and then extracted with acetone and chloroform, respectively. The orange pigments extracted by these solvents were precipitated with n-hexane and separated by silica gel TLC and Sephadex LH-20 chromatography to yield pure baumycins (31).

For nogalamycin and steffimycin B, anthracyclines that do not contain an aminosugar moiety, extraction and purification has been carried out using several different methods. Nogalamycin has been purified by extracting fermentation broths adjusted to pH 6–7 directly with ethyl acetate, followed by treatment of the extract with dilute HCl, after which the nogalamycin enters into the aqueous phase. Adjustment of the aqueous phase to pH 7.4 and extraction with ethyl acetate again gives the crude antibiotic. Evaporation and crystallization from methanol or methylene chloride/ether yields the pure anthracycline (20). Nogalamycin also has been purified by adjusting fermentation broths to pH 2 and filtering. The filtered cake was washed with water, and the filtrate was extracted with n-butanol. After evaporation of the solvent, the crude antibiotic was resuspended in water and adjusted to pH 7.0. Extraction with dichloromethane yielded a residue that could be chromatographed on silica gel (267). More recently, Ylihonko et al. (266) developed an extraction process that can be used for both nogalamycin and aclacinomycin A; it involves extraction of mycelia with methanol and reextraction of both broth and methanol extract with chloroform. Chloroform extracts were purified by silica gel chromatography using chloroform:acetic acid (200:1) for aglycones and gradients of chloroform:methanol:acetic acid (200:0:1 to 200:20:1) for glycosides (266). The extraction methods described above also can be used to purify steffimycin B, with final steps including a combination of TLC and silica gel chromatography (22,267).

For aklavinone glycosides such as aclacinomycin A and cinerubin A, the methods of Oki (28,119) have also been used, whereby the mycelia and broth are separated, the mycelia extracted with acetone whereas the broth is extracted with ethyl acetate. Once the solvents have been evaporated, the extracts are combined and reextracted with toluene. Glycosides are separated from aglycones by addition of acetate buffer, pH 3.5, whereby the aglycones remain in the toluene layer (28,119). Alternatively, for small samples, Niemi et al. (65) extracted mycelia directly with mixtures of toluene:methanol:0.1 M sodium phosphate buffer, pH 7.0 (1:1:0.5). Aglycones of this mixture were extracted from the toluene phase with 0.1 M HCl, followed by hydrolysis of the anthracyclines in the aqueous phase for 30 min in boiling water. The resulting aglycones were then be reextracted with toluene (65).

F.   Biological Transformation of Anthracyclines

In animal studies, two major types of anthracycline metabolism have been noted. The first is the NADPH-dependent liver microsomal reductive glycosidase activity, which converts anthracyclines such as doxorubicin and daunorubicin into their respective 7-deoxyaglycones (282–284). This NADPH-dependent reductive deglycosylation is the major anthracycline-deactivating mechanism in mammals. According to Arcamone (4), neither steffimycin nor nogalamycin appear to be good substrates for this microsomal reductive glycosidase. In a comprehensive study, Yoshimoto et al. (283) showed that several redox enzymes of rat liver, including microsomal NADPH-cytochrome P450 reductase, xanthine oxidase, cytochrome c reductase, and DT diaphorase, were capable of reductively deglycosylating a wide variety of anthracyclines. Aclarubicin and daunorubicin were among the most sensitive anthracyclines to reductive deglycosylation by these enzymes, whereas pirarubicin and doxorubicin were relatively resistant (283). Two trends were observed: (a) the greater the size and number of glycoside residues, the less sensitive the anthracyclines; and (b) increased hydroxylation on the aglycone moiety decreased the sensitivity to reductive deglycosylation (283).

Bacterial enzymes from several sources also have been shown to carry out the reductive deglycosylation of several anthracyclines (184,268,284–288). An enzyme capable of catalyzing reduced nicotinamide adenise dinucleotide (NADH)-dependent reductive deglycosylation of steffimycin was partially purified from *Aeromonas hydrophila* (286). The enzyme was acidic, had an M_r of ca. 35,000, and was strongly inhibited by oxygen but not by cyanide or EDTA (i.e., it did not appear to be electron-transport related) (286).

The second major type of reductive metabolism of anthracyclines is the reduction of 13-oxo anthracyclines to their 13-dihydro analogs (182,183,244,287–293). This keto reduction reaction at C13 appears to be carried out by a wide variety of microbial reductases with broad or low substrate specificity (184,244,287–293). In a potential application of this reductive reaction, Marek et al. (291) demonstrated that immobilized mycelia of *Streptomyces aureofaciens* strain B-96 can reduce daunorubicinone to 13-dihydrodaunorubicinone.

We have found recently that *S. lividans* TK24 (the most widely used host for cloning of anthracycline biosynthesis genes and one of the major cloning strains used in *Streptomyces* research), as well as *Streptomyces* sp. strain C5, *Streptomyces coelicolor* A3(2), and *S. peucetius* ATCC 29050 all carry out the 13-oxo reduction of doxorubicin, daunorubicin, carminomycin, and idarubicin (as well as their aglycones) to the respective 13-hydroxy species (244; Dickens ML and Strohl WR, unpublished data). It is presumed at this time that perhaps multiple enzymes can carry out this reduction.

Forrest et al. (183) isolated and sequenced a gene from liver encoding an NADPH-dependent carbonyl (i.e., 13-oxo-anthracycline) reductase. The enzyme belonged to a class of secondary alcohol oxidoreductases and was related to the *Streptomyces* sp. strain C5 ketoreductase encoded by *orf*1 (280; renamed in this chapter to *dauU*). Interestingly, Forrest et al. (183) indicated that the liver enzyme also catalyzed reduction of the anthracycline quinone as well.

Another type of common bioconversion reaction is the *N*-acetylation of daunorubicin or doxorubicin to the *N*-acetyl analogs (287,288,293). Recently, Scotti and Hutchinson (243) described the immobilization of carminomycin 4-*O*-methyltransferase and the use of the immobilized enzyme to bioconvert carminomycin to daunorubicin. Similarly, we recently reported cloning of the *Streptomyces* sp. strain C5 daunorubicin 14-hydroxylase in *S. lividans* TK24 and use of the recombinant strain to bioconvert daunorubicin to doxorubicin (244). This latter reaction will be described in more detail in Section V.G.

In a twist on the normal bioconversion type of experiments, Cassinelli et al. (294) found that addition of sodium barbiturate to the *S. peucetius* fermentation medium resulted in incorporation of that molecule into baumycins naturally produced by the streptomycete. The result was production of a series of barminomycin-like molecules (FCE21424, FCE24366, FCE24367) that were found to possess interesting in vitro activity against P388 ascitic leukemia cells. The barbiturate was attached to the baumycin side chain (294). For additional information on microbial transformation of anthracyclines, see the detailed reviews by Marshall (287) and Gräfe et al. (288) describing the various biotransformation reactions.

V.   DAUNORUBICIN AND DOXORUBICIN BIOSYNTHESIS

A.   Structure of Daunorubicin and Doxorubicin Biosynthesis Gene Clusters

Stutzman-Engwall and Hutchinson cloned five distinct, nonoverlapping regions of DNA from *S. peucetius* ATCC 29050, four of which were also found in *S. peucetius* subsp. *caesius* (295). According to hybridization experiments (295), three of these clusters also were found in *Streptomyces* sp. strain C5, A21, NZ5, and 6-3 (all related strains from the Frederick Cancer Research Center; 96). In addition to daunorubicin, *S. peucetius* produces polyenes with antifungal activities (9,118); the biosynthetic pathway of the polyene antibiotics also might be encoded by one of the five clusters. The daunorubicin/doxorubicin gene cluster of *S. peucetius* was subsequently found to be the group IV gene cluster (296).

The combined map of the daunorubicin/doxorubicin biosynthesis gene clusters of *S. peucetius* ATCC 29050, which has been sequenced virtually in its entirety (223,225,238,242,265,297–303; Hutchinson CR, personal communication), and of *Streptomyces* sp. strain C5, which has been approximately 65% sequenced (236,237,244,280,304; Dickens ML, Ye J, and Woo AJ, unpublished data), is shown in Figure 9. Additionally, the location of the four complete and two partial genes of the daunorubicin gene cluster of *S. griseus* JA3933 that have been sequenced (305) is also indicated in Figure 9. The known and proposed functions for each gene, characterized either from *S. peucetius*, *Streptomyces* sp. strain C5, or for a few, from *S. griseus*, are described in Table 7. In a recent agreement between the Strohl and Hutchinson laboratories, the names for the daunorubicin biosynthesis genes of *S. peucetius* use the prefix *dnr* and their homologs from *Streptomyces* sp. strain C5 utilize the prefix *dau*. Genes shown to

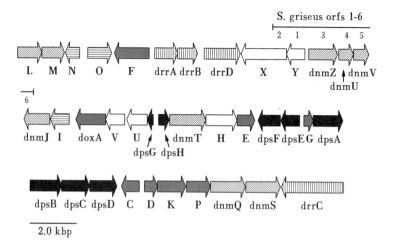

Figure 9   Daunorubicin/doxorubicin gene cluster of *Streptomyces* sp. strain C5 and *S. peucetius* ATCC 29050. By agreement between the Hutchinson and Strohl laboratories, the prefix *dnm* denotes TDP-daunosamine biosynthesis genes, *dps* denotes genes encoding polyketide synthase reactions, and *drr* denotes resistance genes. For all other genes, the prefixes are *dau* for those genes from *Streptomyces* sp. strain C5 and *dnr* for those genes from *S. peucetius*. The location of the TDP-daunosamine biosynthesis genes isolated and sequenced by Krügel et al. (305) from *S. griseus* are noted by a bar. In *S. peucetius* there is an insertion sequence located between *dnmS* and *drr*C. Refer to Table 7 for gene functions and comparison of "old" gene names with new ones.

be involved in TDP-daunosamine biosynthesis in both clusters, including *dnm*S, the gene encoding the glycosyltransferase that condenses TDP-daunosamine with ε-rhodomycinone to form rhodomycin D, are now designated by the prefix *dnm* (for daunosamine), and those genes involved in polyketide biosynthesis use the prefix *dps* (daunorubicin polyketide synthase), as first adopted by Grimm et al. (299) (Table 7). The gene encoding daunorubicin 14-hydroxylase, which confers the ability to synthesize doxorubicin and is now also known to catalyze reactions involved in daunorubicin biosynthesis, is called *dox*A (244).

Over a 20 kbp continuous region, the daunorubicin gene clusters of *Streptomyces* sp. strain C5 and *S. peucetius* are 93% identical at the DNA level. Where data on genes from both strains are available, most of the amino acid sequences of the deduced gene products are >95% identical. Similarly, the DNA, gene organization, and products of the sequenced *S. griseus* daunorubicin biosynthesis genes are also greater than 90% identical with those from *S. peucetius* and *Streptomyces* sp. strain C5. With the knowledge that *S. peucetius* and *Streptomyces* sp. strain C5 are very different organisms (312), isolated from completely different parts of the world, it is probable that most, and conceivably all, of the streptomycetes that accumulate the products daunorubicin, baumycin, and ε-rhodomycinone have highly conserved anthracycline biosynthesis gene clusters. Most notable among the additional strains expected to have such highly conserved "daunorubicin" biosynthesis gene clusters as shown in Figure 7 are the *S. coeruleorubidus* strains isolated by researchers at Rhône-Poulenc (13,14,54), *S. coeruleorubidus* ME130-A4 (ATCC 31276) (30,31), *S. griseus* strains JA3933 and JA5142 (75,305), *S. insignis* ATCC 31913 (77,78), and *Streptomyces* sp. D788 (99).

Other anthracycline biosynthesis genes have also been cloned and sequenced, including the PKS gene clusters of the aclarubicin-producing strain, *S. galilaeus* ATCC 31133 (246,255,313) and the nogalamycin-producing strain, *S. nogalater* (276) (Figure 10), and four complete and two partial genes from the rhodomycin-producing strain, *S. purpurascens* (65,235). Additionally, in recent work, blocked mutants of the early reactions in the aclarubicin-producing *S. galilaeus* ATCC 31615 have been made (314), with the accumulated intermediates (e.g., 2-hydroxyaklanonic acid, aklanonic acid methyl ester, aklavinone) as expected from previous data obtained with blocked mutants of the aclarubicin producer *S. galilaeus* ATCC 31133 (66,67,124,245) and the daunorubicin-producing strains *S. griseus* (68,95,125,227,228,315–317) and *Streptomyces* sp. C5 (124,221,222).

B. Linkage of Primary Metabolism with Anthracycline Production

Dekleva and Strohl (264) showed that for *Streptomyces* sp. strain C5, the carbons from glucose flowed primarily through the Embden–Meyerhof–Parnas glycolysis pathway into ε-rhodomycinone, an important intermediate in daunorubicin and doxorubicin biosynthesis. The oxidative pentosephosphate pathway was present and found by labeling patterns to contribute approximately 30% of the carbon from glucose (264). Interestingly, of several intermediary metabolic enzymes tested, only phosphoenol*pyruvate carboxylase (PEPC) increased significantly during anthracycline biosynthesis (318). The increase in PEPC activity suggests that it may play a role in providing carbon for tricarboxylic acid cycle replenishment and, hence, energy conservation during anthracycline biosynthesis (318).

The source of propionyl-SCoA in daunorubicin- and doxorubicin-producing streptomycetes is not known. In other organisms in which propionyl-SCoA is an important precursor for antibiotic biosynthesis, it is derived via, at least, the catabolism of valine through the action of L-valine dehydrogenase (319).

C. Anthracycline Polyketide Synthases: Biosynthesis of Aklanonic Acid

Aklanonic acid is synthesized via the condensation of nine C_2 units derived from malonyl-SCoA on a propionyl starter moiety (124,126,236,247,299,304,310). Malonyl-SCoA, the primary precursor of anthracyclinone biosynthesis, is synthesized in *Streptomyces* sp. strain C5 by acetyl-SCoA carboxylase (318), as expected from the results of ^{13}C-labeling experiments (232–234).

The PKS gene clusters of *Streptomyces* sp. strain C5 (304), *S. peucetius* ATCC 29050 (299), *S. galilaeus* ATCC 31133 (246,255), and *S. nogalater* ATCC 27451 (276) are compared in Figure 10. The actinorhodin PKS gene cluster of *S. coelicolor* A3(2) (320) is included for comparative purposes. All anthracyclines are synthesized via type II PKSs, that is, PKS gene clusters encoding multiple mono- or bifunctional gene products. One of the aspects that makes the daunorubicin/doxorubicin PKS gene cluster interesting is that these anthracyclines are primed with propionyl starter units instead of the acetyl starter units that are commonly used, making them unique among aromatic PKSs. Thus, the properties and gene structures and functions that confer the propionyl starter moiety might also be expected to be unique. Although this has not yet been fully addressed, there are some interesting similarities and differences between daunorubicin/doxorubicin

Table 7 Description of Genes, with Newly Designated Names, Within the Daunorubicin/Doxorubicin Biosynthesis Gene Clusters of *Streptomyces peucetius* ATCC 29050 and *Streptomyces* sp. Strain C5

Gene[a]	Previous designations[b]			Function and comments	Reference(s)[c]
	Hutchinson	Strohl	Krügel		
dnmL	dnrL	dauL		TDP-Glucose thymidylyltransferase that generates dTDP-glucose	302
dnmM	dnrM	dauM		TDP-Glucose 4,6-dehydratase; non-functional gene in S. peucetius	302, 306
dnrN/dauN	nc	nc		Transcriptional activator	300
dnrO/dauO	nc	nc		Transcriptional repressor; possible regulator of dnrR	300
dnrF/dauF	nc	nc		Aklavinone 11-hydroxylase	223–226
drrA	nc	nc		ATP-binding hydrophilic protein probably involved in anthracycline export	265
drrB	nc	nc		Hydrophobic, membrane spanning protein probably functioning in export	265
drrD	dnrW	dauW		New and only partially characterized resistance gene	H
dnrX/dauX	nc	orfS2	orf2	Unknown	
dnrY/dauY	nc	orfS1	orf1	Unknown	
dnmZ	dnrZ	orfS3	orf3	Involved in unknown reaction in TDP-daunosamine biosynthesis	H
dnmU	dnrU	orfS4	orf4	TDP-4-Keto-6-deoxyglucose 3,5-epimerase	H, S
dnmV	dnrV	orfS5	orf5	TDP-4-Keto-6-deoxyhexulose reductase	H, S
dnmJ	dnrJ	dauJ	orf6	Addition of N-function to TDP-hexulose	307, 308
dnrI/dauI	nc	nc		Transcriptional activator for structural genes	298, 309
doxA	orf	nc		Daunorubicin 14-hydroxylase, 13-deoxyanthracycline hydroxylase, and 13-dihydroanthracycline oxidase	244
dnrV/dauV	orf10	orfA		Unknown	
dnrU/dauU	orf9	orf1		Unknown	
dpsG	nc	dauA–orfG		Acyl carrier protein for polyketide synthase	280, 299, 304
dpsH	dnr–ORF7	orf2, dauZ		Unknown; possible role in polyketide assembly	280, 310, H
dnmT	orf7	orf3		Unknown function in TDP-daunosamine biosynthesis	280, H

dnrH/dauH	orf6	nc	Glycosyltransferase, probably for second "sugar"	280, H
dnrE/dauE	dnrH	nc	Aklaviketone reductase	280
dpsF	nc	dauA–orfF	Polyketide cyclase involved in aklanonic acid formation	299, 304
dpsE	nc	dauB	Polyketide reductase	299, 304
dnrG/dauG	orf8	dauA–orfE	12-Deoxyaklanonic acid oxygenase	299, 304
dpsA	nc	dauA–orfA	Polyketide synthase: Keto-acyl synthase-α subunit (possesses active site —SH)	299, 304, 310
dpsB	nc	dauA–orfB	Polyketide synthase: Keto-acyl synthase-β subunit	299, 304, 310
dpsC	nc	dauA–orfC	Homolog of KASIII but lacking active site; may function to assist in propionyl-SCoA starter unit selection	299, 304, 310
dpsD	nc	dauA–orfD	Acyl-SCoA:ACP acyltransferase of unknown specificity; appears to assist in specifying propionyl-SCoA starter unit selection	299, 304, 310
dnrC/dauC	nc	nc	Aklanonic acid methyltransferase	237, 238
dnrD/dauD	nc	nc	Aklanonic acid methyl ester cyclase	237, 238, 311
dnrK/dauK	nc	nc	Anthracycline 4-O-methyltransferase	237, 239–243
dnrP/dauP	nc	nc	Rhodomycin D 16-methylesterase	237–239
dnmQ	dnrQ	dauQ	Involved in unknown reaction in TDP-daunosamine biosynthesis	301
dnmS	dnrS	dauS	TDP-daunosamine:ε-rhodomycinone glycosyltransferase	301
drrC	nc	nc	Resistance gene of unknown mechanism	303

[a] Daunorubicin/doxorubicin biosynthesis gene names agreed to by the Strohl and Hutchinson laboratories. In the cases where two gene designations are given, the first is for the S. peucetius homolog and the second is for the Streptomyces sp. strain C5 homolog.

[b] nc, name not changed from previous designation.

[c] H, Hutchinson CR, personal communication; S, Strohl WR, unpublished data.

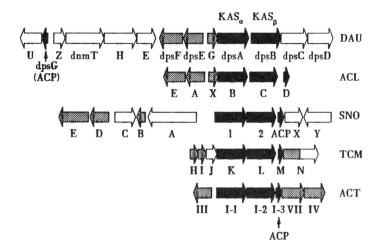

Figure 10   Comparison of the polyketide synthase (PKS) genes from the daunorubicin-producing strain *Streptomyces* sp. strain C5 (DAU; the daunorubicin PKS gene cluster from *S. peucetius* ATCC 29050 is identical), the aclarubicin producer *S. galilaeus* ATCC 31133 (ACL), and the nogalamycin producer *S. nogalater* ATCC 27451 (SNO), the tetracenomycin producer *S. glaucescens* GAO (TCM), and the actinorhodin producer *S. coelicolor* (ACT). Key: KS$_\alpha$ genes (example, *dps*A), large solid arrows; KS$_\beta$ genes (example, *dps*B), shaded arrows; acyl carrier protein (ACP) genes (examples, *dps*G, *act*I-3), short solid arrows; cyclases (example, *dps*F), left slanted arrows; polyketide reductases (example, *dps*E), right slanted arrows; oxygenases/mono-oxidases, dotted arrows. The daunorubicin biosynthesis genes *dps*C and *dps*D are involved in starter unit selection as described in the text. All other unfilled arrows are genes (except possibly *dps*H) hypothesized not to be involved with polyketide assembly. Note that the only gene cluster in which the gene encoding acyl carrier protein (ACP) is not directly downstream of those encoding KS$_\alpha$ and KS$_\beta$ is the daunorubicin biosynthesis cluster.

PKS gene clusters and those encoding aromatic polyketides primed with acetyl starter units.

The structures of the *Streptomyces* sp. strain C5 (304) and *S. peucetius* ATCC 29050 (299) daunorubicin type II PKS gene regions (which share 93.1% sequence identity) differ significantly from those of other known type II PKS gene clusters (Figure 10). Reading left from a divergently transcribed promoter region are *dps*E and *dps*F, encoding polyketide reductase and polyketide cyclase, respectively (Figure 10). Reading right from this sequence are five genes in an operon (299,304): (a) *dau*G (encoding 12-deoxyaklanonic acid oxygenase); (b) *dps*A (ketoacylsynthase; KS$_\alpha$); (c) *dps*B (the ketoacylsynthase homolog that makes up the putative heterodimeric partner; KS$_\beta$). This is described elsewhere as chain length factor (CLF; 321), but there is evidence now that this protein alone does not confer chain length (310,322; Hutchinson CR, personal communication); (d) *dps*C (a homolog of *Escherichia coli* KASIII that lacks the active-site Cys residue). This gene product, thought to have perhaps a structural role, contains a putative coenzyme A–binding site (304); and (e) *dps*D (an acyltransferase speculated, but not proven, to function as propionyl-SCoA:ACP-SH acyltransferase; 236,299,304) (Figure 10). In both *S. peucetius* and *Streptomyces* sp. strain C5, the gene encoding the acyl carrier protein (ACP), *dps*G, is located about 6.8 kbp upstream of the genes encoding the daunorubicin KS$_\alpha$ and KS$_\beta$ (236,299,304) (Figures 9 and 10).

The most significant deviations of the daunorubicin/doxorubicin PKS gene clusters from other type II PKS gene clusters are the presence of two genes directly downstream of the KS_α and KS_β not found in other type II PKS gene clusters, and the obvious absence of a gene encoding ACP directly 3′ of the genes encoding KS_β (236,299,304). We have shown recently that disruption of dpsD or dpsC and dpsD still allowed the biosynthesis of daunorubicin and 13-dihydrodaunorubicin in mutants of Streptomyces sp. strain C5. In addition to these "normal," expected products, we also found that the dpsCD mutant strains (SC5-VR5, SC5-VR6, SC5-VR7) accumulated substantial quantities of feudomycin C and feudomycinone C (Rajgarhia VB, Priestley ND, and Strohl WR, unpublished data), compounds that are initiated with an acetyl starter unit (323). As far as we can tell from detailed chromatographic analysis, neither feudomycin C nor its aglycone are produced by the parental strain, Streptomyces sp. strain C5.

Additionally, we have shown that a minimal PKS gene cluster containing only dpsA (KS_α), dpsB (KS_β), dauG (12-deoxyaklanonic acid oxygenase), dpsF (cyclase), dpsG (ACP), dpsE (polyketide reductase PKR), and dauI (transcriptional activator) conferred on both S. lividans TK24 and S. coelicolor CH999 the ability to produce ample quantities of aklanonic acid (310), the first stable chromophore of the daunorubicin/doxorubicin biosynthesis pathways (Figure 11). Interestingly, we also observed in the mass spectroscopy data substantial levels of products that would have been derived from a methyl-side-chain derivative of aklanonic acid (Rajgarhia VB and Strohl WR, unpublished data), indicating that both acetyl and propionyl moieties were being incorporated as starter units into products by this recombinant strain.

These experiments together indicate two parallel, and overlapping, aspects of daunorubicin PKS function: (a) the products of the two downstream genes (dpsCD) are not required for formation of the polyketide precursor initiated with propionyl-SCoA; and (b) in the absence of dpsCD, the PKS complex is "sloppier," namely, it accepts both acetyl and propionyl starter units. This suggests that the presence of dpsCD ensures that

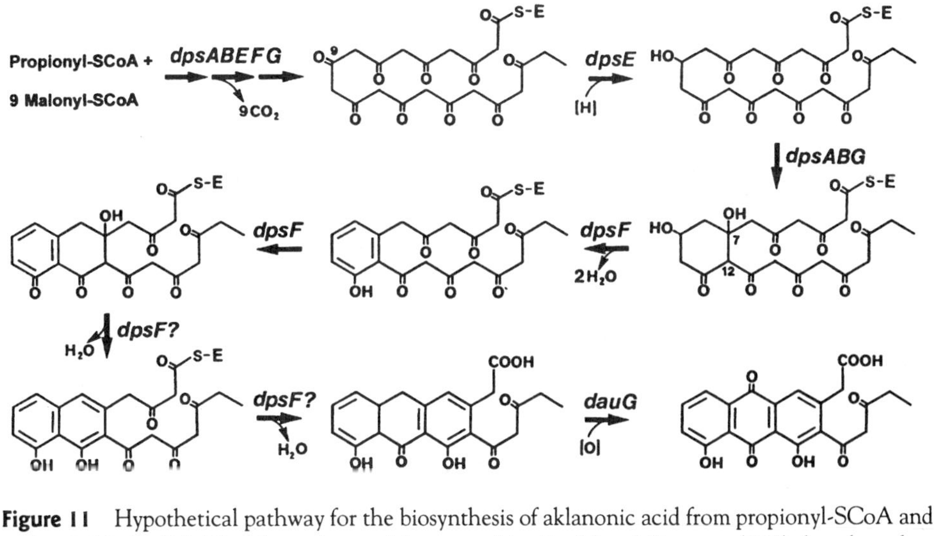

Figure 11   Hypothetical pathway for the biosynthesis of aklanonic acid from propionyl-SCoA and malonyl-SCoA. (Modified from the model proposed by Strohl and Connors (247), based on data obtained by Rajgarhia and Strohl (310), and influenced by results obtained with heterologous PKS functions as shown in other laboratories (126,245,252–255,321,324).)

the propionyl starter moiety is utilized. What evolutionary advantage this selection may have is not known, but at least in these strains, the functions encoded by *dps*C and *dps*D have been maintained.

Our current hypothesis is that the daunorubicin PKS is normally primed with propionyl-SACP as a result of the functions of the *dps*C and *dps*D gene products, which together catalyze the following reaction: propionyl-SCoA + ACP-SH → propionyl-SACP + CoASH. The propionyl moiety would then be transferred to the putative heterodimeric $KS_{\alpha\beta}$ to form a propionyl-S-KS intermediate, freeing up the ACP-SH to accept a malonyl moiety. In the absence of the *dps*CD gene products, we postulate that the daunorubicin/doxorubicin PKSs can accept propionyl-SCoA as the priming substrate that would be transferred directly to the enzyme. Our data suggest that in the absence of *dps*CD, acetyl-SCoA or, perhaps, acetyl-SACP can substitute freely for propionyl-SCoA.

Interestingly, the PKS gene cluster encoding aclacinomycin A, an anthracycline also primed with a propionyl moiety, is more analogous to the PKS gene clusters for actinorhodin biosynthesis and other aromatic polyketides (Figure 10). In this case, the genes encoding KS_α, KS_β, and ACP are linked, just as they are in actinorhodin biosynthesis (Figure 10). It is interesting in this respect that several strains known to accumulate anthracyclines containing ethyl-type side chains (i.e., produced from propionyl starter moieties) also produce, or have been mutated to produce, anthracyclines with methyl side chains (i.e., products formed with acetyl starter units) (60,63,102,323,325). Included in these strains are *S. galilaeus* ATCC 31133 (325), for which much of the PKS gene cluster is known (Figure 10), and a mutant of the baumycin- and daunorubicin-producing *S. coeruleorubidus* ME130-A4 (323). If, as predicted earlier, this strain has a PKS gene arrangement similar to that in *Streptomyces* sp. C5 and *S. peucetius* (including *dps*C and *dps*D homologs), then it is probable that either or both of these genes are nonfunctional in the mutant strain accumulating methyl-side-chain anthracyclines. This would explain how a mutation in this strain could generate the different side chains. It currently is not known whether *S. galilaeus* ATCC 31133 has *dps*CD homologs, but their absence would explain how the parental strain, in absence of mutagenesis, could produce a mixture of both ethyl- and methyl-side-chain anthracyclines (325).

The nogalamycin PKS gene cluster of *S. nogalater* was recently sequenced (276) and also shown to have a structure highly similar to that of the *S. galilaeus* aclacinomycin A PKS gene cluster (Figure 10). This is interesting, considering that nogalamycin biosynthesis is primed with an acetyl moiety, much the same as found in actinorhodin biosynthesis.

Based on the currently available information, Figure 11 shows the hypothetical biosynthesis of aklanonic acid from propionyl-SCoA and malonyl-SCoA. This pathway is modified from the model proposed by Strohl and Connors (247), based on data obtained by Bartel et al. (245) and Rajgarhia and Strohl (310), using as models both tetracenomycin F2 biosynthesis by minimal tetracenomycin PKS genes (126,252–255,324) and aloesaponarin II biosynthesis by actinorhodin biosynthesis genes (245,321).

There are other possible genes that could be involved in polyketide biosynthesis in *Streptomyces* sp. strain C5. In actinorhodin biosynthesis, an extra cyclase encoded by the *act*IV gene is present that is absent from all other PKS gene clusters. The *act*IV gene product is required to obtain the proper cyclization products (endocrocin and aloe-saponarin II) of the minimal, complete PKS gene cluster region (321). Similarly, in the tetracenomycin biosynthesis gene cluster, two cyclases, encoded by *tcm*I and *tcm*N, are required for proper cyclization to obtain tetracenomycin F_2 (257). Thus, there is still the question of what gene encodes the second cyclase in daunorubicin biosynthesis. Or is there a second cyclase? Homologs of *dps*H, the gene that is divergently transcribed from *dps*G (Figure 9), have been found in the PKS gene clusters of *Streptomyces roseofulvus* (frenolicin biosynthesis; 326), *Streptomyces argillaceus* (mithramycin biosynthesis; 327), and *Saccharopolyspora hirsuta* (spore pigment biosynthesis; 328), leading to the suggestion that *dps*H might be the second cyclase (Hutchinson CR, personal communication). A *dps*H homolog, *act*VI–*orf*A (329), also has been found in the actinorhodin biosynthesis pathway and is presumed to be present in both *S. lividans* TK24 and *S. coelicolor* CH999. In our experiments, however, we have not yet found any involvement of DpsH in cyclization of aklanonic acid precursors (310).

Additionally, it has been found in several experiments (e.g., 257,330–332) that the source of ACP is not critical for the activity of type II PKS complexes. This may not hold true for the daunorubicin PKS. In experiments carried out in both *S. lividans* TK24 and *S. coelicolor* CH999, which expressed *dps*ABEF*dau*G and substituted *act*III–*orf*3, the gene encoding actinorhodin ACP for *dps*G (the natural daunorubicin biosynthesis ACP), we observed no production of aklanonic acid. Similarly, Hutchinson (personal communication) reported that substitution of the tetracenomycin ACP for *S. peucetius* DpsG resulted in lack of aklanonic acid formation. Though these experiments are not conclusive, they may indicate a higher specificity for ACP than is observed with other type II PKS multiprotein complexes.

Type II PKS gene clusters typically comprise about five to seven core genes. To synthesize even the most basic polyketide structure, at least three gene products are required: KS_α, KS_β, and ACP. The products of these three genes, in the absence of functional cyclases and/or reductases, are typically strangely folded structures similar to mutactin and SEK4 (257,333).

From extensive mixing and matching experiments using hybrid type II PKS genes, Khosla and colleagues have attempted to describe the functions of the various singular protein components (257,321,330,332). The two most noteworthy of these are the designation "chain length factor" for KS_β (321) and "aromatase" for DpsF (cyclase) homologs (330). It is apparent now, through our studies and those of Hutchinson and his colleagues (310,322,324), that these single-protein/single-function designations may be too simplistic. It is considerably more likely, based on the available evidence, that multiple components of the PKS enzyme complex interact to confer certain functions, particularly chain length, first cyclization bond (i.e., C7–C12 as in actinorhodin and daunorubicin, but C9–C14 in tetracenomycin), choice of starter unit, and cyclization. An example of this complexity is given below.

Meurer and Hutchinson (324) recently carried out experiments in which *S. peucetius dps*A and *dps*B were expressed together with *tcm*MNJ (encoding, respectively, ACP, cyclase, and a putative "helper" protein of tetracenomycin C biosynthesis; 324) to synthesize tetracenomycin F_2, a compound that is initiated with an acetyl moiety, and first cyclized with a C9–C14 bond (324). From this result, they speculated that *dps*A and *dps*B did not contain the information necessary to dictate starter unit specificity or initial cyclization (324). They suggested that *dps*C and *dps*D together were the primary contributing factors for starter unit specificity (324).

Our results indicated that *Streptomyces* sp. strain C5 *dps*CD are not necessary (but are helpful) to specify a propionyl moiety as the starter unit in vivo in either *S. lividans* TK24 or *S. coelicolor* CH999 (310). In light of the results given by Meurer and Hutchinson (324), which indicated that DpsA and DpsB alone did not specify the propionyl starter unit or C7–C12 linkage, we propose that the productive protein–protein interactions of multiple proteins within the homologous PKS, including the KS_α, KS_β, cyclase, and PKR, combined together, specify the propionyl starter unit, chain length, and C7–C12 bond formation.

D.   Conversion of Aklanonic Acid to ε-Rhodomycinone

As mentioned previously, aklanonic acid is the first stable, known intermediate of daunorubicin, doxorubicin, and aclarubicin biosynthesis. Klaus Eckardt and his colleagues isolated aklanonic acid, a metabolite accumulated by *Streptomyces* sp. strain ZIMET 43717 (95,316), chemically synthesized aklanonic acid methyl ester (95), and showed that both compounds could be converted in vivo to aklavinone by blocked mutants of the daunoru- bicin-producing strains *S. griseus* IMET JA5142 (315) and *S. peucetius* (317) and the aclarubicin-producing strain *S. galilaeus* (317). We now know that in daunorubicin and doxorubicin biosynthesis, aklanonic acid is converted to ε-rhodomycinone, the primary aglycone substrate for the glycosyltransferase reaction, in four enzymatically catalyzed steps, as shown in Figure 12. For aclarubicin biosynthesis, aklavinone is the aglycone sub- strate for glycosyltransferase (314).

Through the careful analysis of the accumulated early intermediates, bioconversion of those intermediates to anthracyclinones, and analysis of the mutants producing the accumulated intermediates (68,95,228,315–317), Eckardt and his colleagues at Jena pro- posed a pathway for anthracyclinone formation (227). The pathway for aklanonic acid to ε-rhodomycinone was confirmed by the isolation of single and double mutants of *Strepto- myces* sp. strain C5 blocked in daunorubicin biosynthesis (221), and by in vitro analysis, using both parental and blocked mutant strains, of the conversion of aklanonic acid to its methyl ester, aklaviketone, aklavinone, and ε-rhodomycinone (222).

More recently, Dickens et al. (237,280) and Madduri and Hutchinson (238) showed the genes required for conversion of aklanonic acid to aklaviketone: (a) *dauC/dnrC* encodes aklanonic acid:S-adenosyl-L-methionine methyltransferase, a homodimeric pro- tein (222) of ca. M_r 45,000 (deduced subunit M_r of DauC is 24,319 (237)). These methyl- transferases are small (ca. 220 amino acids) and appear to belong to a new subclass of methyltransferases (237); (b) *dauD/dnrD* encodes aklanonic acid methyl ester cyclase, an unusual protein of ca. M_r 18,500 (for the monomer) that appears unique in the databases (237,238). This protein catalyzes the cyclization of aklanonic acid through what is pre- sumed to be an intramolecular aldol condensation (311), which can occur spontaneously resulting in four possible isomers, leading some to believe previously that an enzyme was not required for this reaction. Isolation of blocked mutants, cloning and sequence analy- sis of the gene, in vitro analysis of the function of the gene product, and recently, purifi- cation of the protein (311) have proved that this is an enzymatically catalyzed reaction (237,238,311); and (c) *dauE* encodes aklaviketone reductase (280), which reduces the 7- oxo moiety of aklaviketone to a hydroxy-group. Interestingly, this enzyme also catalyzes, at somewhat lower efficiency, the reduction of maggiemycin to ε-rhodomycinone, a reac- tion we previously thought not to occur (222), and 7-oxodaumycinone to daunomyci- none (280).

Aklavinone, the product of the DauE reaction (Figure 12), is the major precursor common to all of the anthracyclines of the daunorubicin–aclacinomycin–rhodomycin families, including aclacinomycin, aklavin, daunorubicin, doxorubicin, pyrromycin, carminomycin, rhodomycin, and the cinerubins (124). *S. peucetius dnrF*, which encodes an apparent flavoprotein with a deduced subunit M_r of 52,289, has been characterized by several groups to encode aklavinone 11-hydroxylase (223–226). This gene has been used

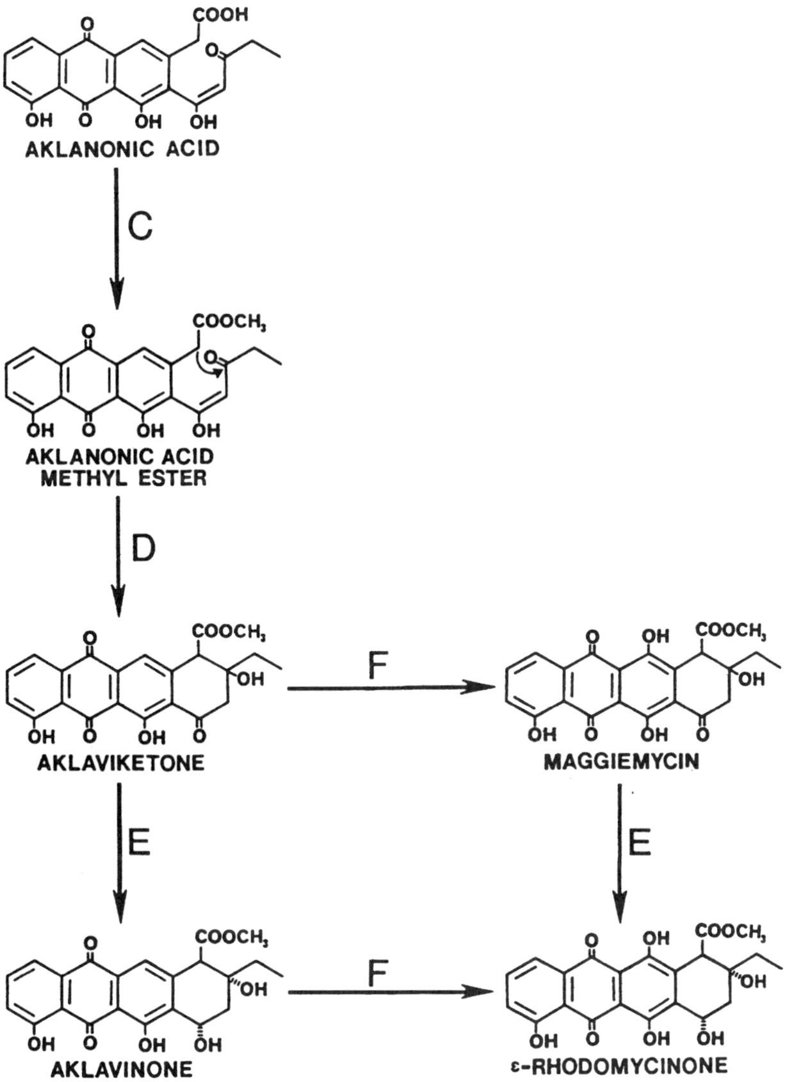

Figure 12 Pathway for the conversion of aklanonic acid to ε-rhodomycinone. DauC/DnrC (aklanonic acid methyltransferase) catalyzes the S-adenosyl-L-methionine-dependent methylation of aklanonic acid to its methyl ester, which undergoes cyclization via intramolecular aldol condensation, catalyzed by DauD/DnrD, to form aklaviketone. Aklaviketone is converted to aklavinone by aklaviketone reductase (DauE/DnrE) and to maggiemycin by aklavinone 11-hydroxylase (DauF/DnrF). Maggiemycin accumulates to significant levels only in *dau*E mutants. Aklavinone is hydroxylated at C11 by DauF/DnrF to form ε-rhodomycinone, which is both accumulated to significant levels by most daunorubicin-producing strains and converted, via glycosylation (Figure 13), to rhodomycin D.

to generate several 11-hydroxy hybrid metabolites in heterologous strains (224,226). The *dau*F gene of *Streptomyces* sp. strain C5, which has been only partly sequenced, is in the same relative position in the gene cluster as *dnr*F (Figure 9). Aclacinomycin-type antibiotics that incorporate aklavinone as their chromophore are produced by strains (e.g., *S. galilaeus*) that do not hydroxylate aklavinone at C11 (25–29). *Streptomyces* sp. strain C5 *dau*F mutants (221), *S. peucetius* subsp. *aureus* (ATCC 31428; 81,334), and a blocked strain of *S. griseus* IMET JA3933 (229), all of which are deficient in 11-hydroxylase activity, accumulate 11-deoxy anthracyclines (81,334).

The anthracycline intermediate ε-rhodomycinone, formed by hydroxylation of aklavinone at position C11 (Figure 12), is actually the major product in many daunorubicin fermentations (4,77,124,335). Whereas most early intermediates in the anthracycline biosynthesis pathway are yellow, ε-rhodomycinone and other compounds containing the 11-hydroxy-group are red or orange. ε-Rhodomycinone has been shown to be converted to daunorubicin and related glycosides by both *Streptomyces* sp. strain C5 (335) and *S. coeruleorubidus* ME130-A4 (270,336), demonstrating that ε-rhodomycinone clearly is an intermediate of daunorubicin biosynthesis, the compelling arguments by Wagner et al. (125) to the contrary notwithstanding.

E. TDP-Daunosamine Biosynthesis

The precise pathway for TDP-daunosamine biosynthesis from TDP-glucose is not known. Nevertheless, based on sequencing of putative TDP-daunosamine biosynthesis genes, a sketchy picture can be assembled. A hypothetical pathway for TDP-daunosamine biosynthesis from TDP-glucose is shown in Figure 13. *S. peucetius* DnmL, encoded by a gene at the "left end" of the biosynthetic gene cluster (Figure 9), is similar in structure to known glucose-1-phosphate:TTP thymidylyltransferases (302) and thus is believed to carry out this reaction. *Streptomyces* sp. strain C5 also has a *dnm*L homolog in the same relative position of the biosynthesis gene cluster.

The product of the thymidylyltransferase reaction, TDP-glucose, is a natural substrate for a well-known reaction catalyzed by TDP-glucose 4,6-dehydratase (306). The TDP-glucose 4,6-dehydratases from both *Streptomyces* sp. strain C5 and *S. peucetius*, purified to homogeneity, were homodimers with subunit values of M_r of 39,000 and 36,000, respectively (306). Although the proteins possessed markedly different N-terminal sequences, their kinetics, inhibition patterns, and pH optima were quite similar (306). An intensive search was made by the Hutchinson laboratory to determine the gene encoding the TDP-glucose 4,6-dehydratase of *S. peucetius* ATCC 29050 (302). What they found was highly interesting, if unexpected. The daunorubicin biosynthesis gene cluster–linked gene encoding TDP-glucose 4,6-dehydratase, *dau*M, contains a natural frameshift mutation—that is, the gene does not produce an active protein. Thus, the TDP-glucose 4,6-dehydratase in *S. peucetius* that is used for TDP-daunosamine biosynthesis is not clustered with the other biosynthesis genes (302). There are two possible implications of these results. First, since ε-rhodomycinone accumulates in several different types of *S. peucetius* fermentations, it is possible that there is a bottleneck at this step, caused by the use of an enzyme that is not "secondary metabolite–specific" in nature. This might be tested by cloning into *S. peucetius* an overexpressed copy of an authentic antibiotic biosynthesis TDP-glucose 4,6-dehydratase. Second, it means that two separate genes (albeit one being nonfunctional) in *S. peucetius* can encode this enzyme (302). Thus, it would be expected that other streptomycetes, such as *S. lividans*, have such a gene for primary metabolite requirements.

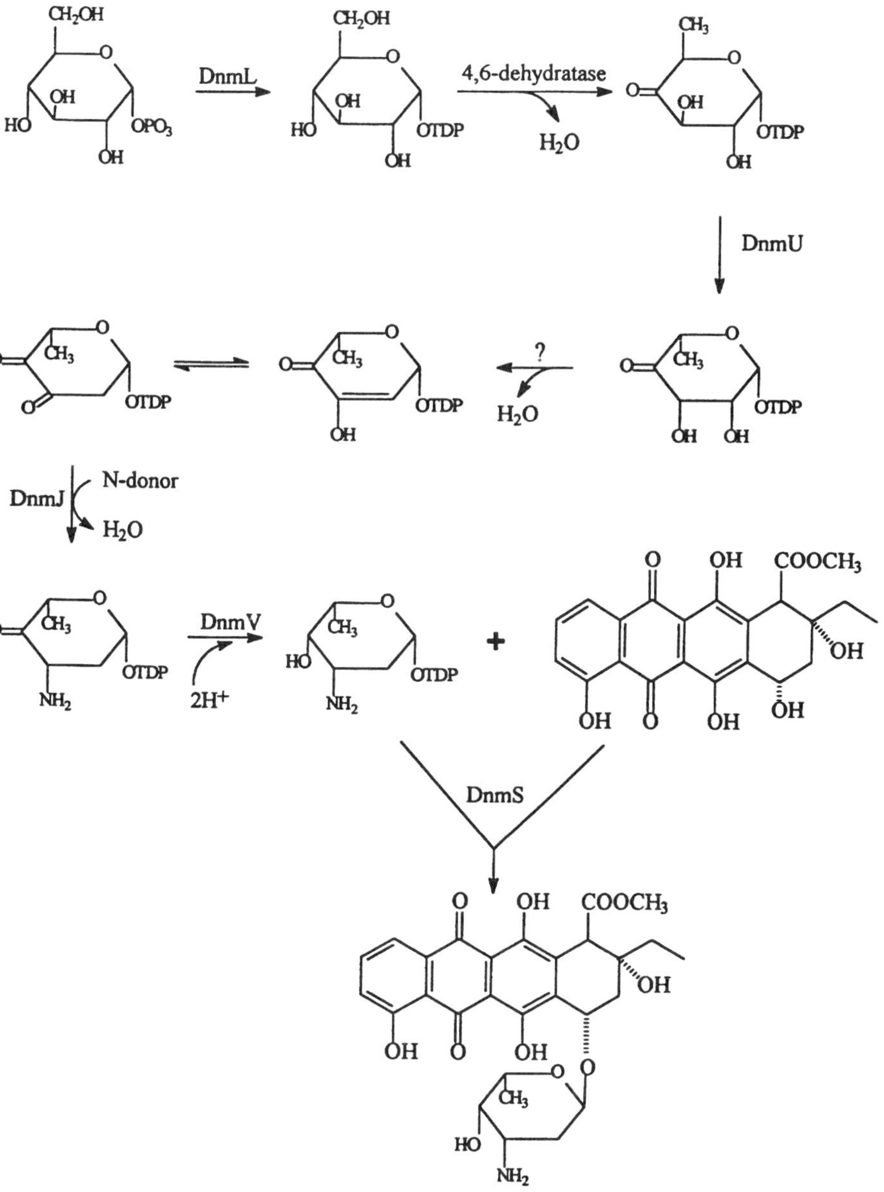

Figure 13 Hypothetical pathway for the biosynthesis of TDP-daunosamine. Glucose-1-phosphate is converted in the presence of TTP to TDP-D-glucose by DnmL. A TDP-glucose 4,6-dehydratase (similar to predicted full-length DnrM) catalyzes the NAD+-dependent conversion of TDP-glucose to TDP-4-keto-6-deoxy-D-glucose, which is converted to TDP-4-keto-L-rhamnose, which is dehydrated by a currently unknown mechanism to form TDP-2,6-deoxy-3,4-ketohexulose, which is hypothesized to be aminated in a pyridoxylamine-dependent manner to TDP-2,6-deoxy-3-amino-4-ketohexulose, which is reduced in an NADPH-dependent reaction by the *dnm*V gene product to form TDP-daunosamine. DnmS catalyzes the transglycosylation reaction of TDP-daunosamine to ε-rhodomycinone to form rhodomycin D, the first intermediate of the glycone portion of the pathway.

The product of the dehydratase reaction mentioned above, TDP-4-keto-6-deoxy-L-glucose, is a known substrate for dNDP-sugar 3,5-epimerase (337). A gene *orf4*, encoding a dNDP-sugar 3,5-epimerase homolog was observed in the small cluster of genes isolated, sequenced, and characterized from the daunorubicin-producing *S. griseus* strain (305). The *dnmU* genes of *S. peucetius* and *Streptomyces* sp. strain C5 are very closely related to both *S. griseus orf4* and other, better characterized 3,5-epimerases (337). Thus, the next hypothesized step in TDP-daunosamine biosynthesis is the conversion of the D-sugar, TDP-4-keto-6-deoxy-D-glucose, to the L-sugar, TDP-4-keto-L-rhamnose (Figure 13). Up to this point, TDP-daunosamine biosynthesis follows that of other, better characterized nucleotide sugars (337). The following steps, however, are less well documented in analogous systems and are, therefore, highly speculative.

The synthesis of TDP-daunosamine from TDP-4-keto-L-rhamnose should require at least three to four enzymes, depending on the ability of certain enzymes to catalyze one or two steps. In the hypothesized scheme proposed by Otten et al. (301), TDP-4-keto-L-rhamnose is dehydrated to give a TDP-2,6-deoxy-3,4-keto-hexulose. There are two possible candidates for this reaction, although neither has been proven to catalyze it. First, there recently has been a realization that there are three possible types of nucleotide-sugar dehydratases (338): (a) those NAD$^+$-requiring enzymes of the class to which TDP-glucose 4,6-dehydratase belongs. These are characterized by having the known GxxGxxG nucleotide binding site required for NAD$^+$ binding (338); (b) those dehydratases belonging to a class of newly discovered enzymes, some members of which are capable of incorporating an N-moiety into the sugar. This group of enzymes, which are known to bind pyridoxylamine phosphate, include DnrJ (307); and (c) a third group of apparent, potential dehydratases has recently surfaced by sequence comparisons. This group, which may include DnmT (338; Hutchinson CR, personal communication), encoded by *dnmT* of both *S. peucetius* and *Streptomyces* sp. strain C5 (Figure 9) ("orf3" of *Streptomyces* sp. C5 in Ref. 280), has no known characteristic sequence signature. It is proposed at this point that DnmT may catalyze the 2-dehydration of TDP-4-keto-L-rhamnose to form the diketo intermediate. An interesting alternative reaction leading to the formation of TDP-2,6-deoxy-3,4-keto-hexulose might be considered. We recently discovered that *Streptomyces* sp. strain C5 DoxA has the ability to hydroxylate at C13, and then to oxidize, through a hypothesized dihydroxy (C13 dihydroxy or 13, 14-dihydroxy) intermediate, followed by dehydration to yield C13 oxo anthracyclines (244). *S. peucetius dnmQ* (301) and its homolog in *Streptomyces* sp. strain C5 (Dickens ML, Woo A, and Strohl WR, unpublished results) encode a cytochrome P450–like protein that lacks the characteristic Cys residue that is involved in the heme-thiol moiety (301; Figure 14). Comparison of the two reactions, namely, that catalyzed in the oxidation of C13 hydroxy to 13-oxo, and 2-dehydration of TDP-4-keto-L-rhamnose, reveals that, except for incorporation of the oxygen by DoxA to give the dihydroxy intermediate, these two reactions are nearly identical (see Figures 13 and 15). Since DnmQ lacks the sequences apparently required for incorporation of oxygen, but retains all other apparent features of cytochrome P450 enzymes, it might be interesting to speculate that its function may be to catalyze the 2-dehydration of TDP-4-keto-L-rhamnose as shown in Figure 13. Elucidation of this critical and interesting biochemical step awaits additional experimentation.

Regardless of the mechanism or gene product that catalyzes the 2-dehydration of TDP-4-keto-L-rhamnose, the resulting product, TDP-2,6-deoxy-3,4-ketohexulose, is expected to be the substrate for the DnmJ-catalyzed transamination reaction (Figure 13) yielding TDP-2,6-deoxy-3-amino-4-ketohexulose. The final step in TDP-daunosamine biosynthesis is thought to be catalyzed by reduction of TDP-2,6-deoxy-3-amino-4-keto-

```
DoxA                     MSGEAPRVA VDPFSCPMMT MQRKPEVHDA FREAGP....  ..........  ..VVEVMAPA GG.PAWVITD DALAREVLAD PRFVKDPDLA
DnmQ            MPT PTSAPPAAPT DSELGRHLLT VRGFHFVFGA LGDPYARRLR GEADHLSLGE LVRDRGPLHG SALGTWVTAD GGISARLLDD PLLGPRHPAS
p450Soy    MTESTTDPAR QNLDPTSPAP ATSFPQDRGC PYHPPAGYAP LREGRP....  ..........  ..LSRVTL.F DGRPVWAVTG HALARRLLAD PRLSTDRSHP
p450ChoP            MTQAA PVTFSTVREN YFGPPAEMQA LRHKAP....  ..........  ..VTRTAF.A DGRPGWLVTG YSAARAVLSD SRFSTA....A
P450Ole         MTD THTGPTPADA VPAYPPFSLPH ALDLDPHYAE LRRDEP....  ..........  ..VSRVRLVTR GEGTAWLVTR MSDARIVLGD SRFSTA....A
p450cam    MTTETIQSN ANLAPLPPHV PERHLVFDFD. MYNPGNLGAG VQEAWA....  ..........  ..V....LQE SNVPDLVWTR CNGGHWIATR GQLIREAYED
Conserved          n..ptp.aa ...f.fd..t mygppavyaa lrea.p....  ..........  ..vsrv.l.a .grpawvvt. ..larrvlad pr.std...a

DoxA       PTAWRGVDDG L....DIPVP ELRPFTLIAV DGEDHRRLRR IHAPAFNPRR LAERTDRIAA IADRLLTELA DSSDRSGEPA ELIGGFPAYHF PLLVICELLG
DnmQ       EGPQEHVLEN VWETWRTCHV TPLGEDLLTP AAADSDRLAA LLGPVLGPRT CTAWQVDAGR AVHRVLDGL.  ......PPHF DVVSDLARPA IAGSLAAVLG
p450Soy    DFP....VPA E....RFAGA QRRRVALLGV DDPEHNTQRR MLIPTFSVKR IGALRPRIQE TVDRLLDAM.  ...EHMGSPA DLVEHFALPV PSMVICALLG
p450ChoP   ............ARG EREHPAVPRA ATLEDERCRR LIAGQFTARR MRQLTGRTER IVREHLDAM.  ...EHMGSPA DLVEHFALPV PSLVIAELLG
P450Ole    ATD....PAT P....RMFPT PPEPDGVLAQ DPPDHTRLRR LVGKAPTARR VEEMRPRVRS LVDSLLDDM.  ...VAHGSPA DLVEFLAVPF VAVICELLG
p450cam    LPEEDIPHLK ....YLTDQM TRPDGSMTFA EAKEA......  ..........  ..LYDYLIP IIEQRRQKPG TDAIS.IVAN GQVNGRPITS DEAKRMCGLL LVGGLDTVVN
Conserved  .tp.....p. ....r.a.g e..pfallav dpp.hrrlrr ll.p.f..rr v..l.priq. .vdrllda.. ...r.g.pa dlvedfAlpf pslvicellG
```

```
DoxA       VPVTDPAMAR EAVGVLKALG LGGPQSAGGD GTDPAGDVPD TSALESLLLE AVHAARREDT RTMTRVLYER AQAEFGSVSD DQLVYMITGL IPAGHDTTG.
DnmQ       LPDEARAELP DLLAACGPVL DSALCPPRLP VARAMTQ..A LRRVRELMAA AVANHLTAPA DGAVSALLAV DPGGGR..DP GDTVTAAVLS TVVGAETAIT
p450Soy    VPYADHAFFE E.....RSQR LLR.GP.GAD DVNRARD... ..ELEEYLGA LVRLRKTEPG DDLLSGLI.. ..AAD.PALTD EELASIAFLL LVAGHGTTAH
p450ChoP   VPPPDREHFQ H.....DTLR WGGFPGR.STE EVTEAFV... ..SLGGGQQR LVRLRRTEPG DGLLDELIHR DHPD.GPVDR EQLVAFAVIL LIAGHETTAH
P450Ole    VPLEDRDLFR T.....FSDA MLSSTRLTAA KIQRVQQ... ..DFMVYMDG LVAQRRDAPT EDLLGALALA TDND.DHLTK GEIVMMGVSL LIAGHETSVH
p450cam    .........LYDYLIP IIEQRRQKPG TDAIS.IVAN GQVNGRPITS DEAKRMCGLL LVGGLDTVVN
Conserved  vP.edrahfr e.......s.r l.g.g...a. e...a...... ..leeyl.a lvaq.rt.pg ddllsaliar dqad..p.td .elv.mavll lvaGheTt.n
                                                                                          L.l.AGHeTt
                                                                                          Oxygen-binding
```

```
DoxA       ..SFLGFLLA EVLAGRLAAD ADGDAISRFV EEALRHHPPV PYTLW.RFAA TEVVIRGVRL PRGAPVLVDI EGTNTDGREH DAPHAFHPDR PSRR...RLT
DnmQ       TVANAVMALL KHDEQWSLLR ADPGRAADAV EETLRWAPPV ..TLRSLITQ GEVQIGGETL EADQHVVVLV DAAQRDPALY EDPDRFRLDR PRSPGFTHMA
p450Soy    MISLGTFTLL SHPEQLAALR AGGTSTAVVV EELLRFLSIA .EG.LQRLAT EDMEVDGATI RKGEGVVFST SLINRDADVF PRAETLDWDR PARH...HLA
p450ChoP   QIALGAFLLL EHPDQLAALR ADPALTESAV EELLRHLSVV HHG.PTRAAL QDADIEGTPV KAGEVVVVSL GAANRDPARF ERPDAVDVTR EDTG...HLA
P450Ole    QITNLVHLLL TERRRYESLV ADPALVPAAC EEMLRYTPLV SAGSFVRVAT EDVELSTVTV RAGEPCVVHF ASANRDEVVF DHADELDFHR ERNP...HIA
p450cam    FLSFSMEFLA KSPEHRQELI ERPERIPAAC EELLRRFSLV ADG...RILT SDYEFHGVQL KKGDQILLPQ MLSGLDEREN ACPMEVDFSR QKVS...HTT
Conserved  qis..vflLl .hpeq.aalr adpa....aav EEllRhl..v ..g...riat edvei.gvtl .agepvvvs. ..anrD..vf .rpda.dfdR prrp...hla
```

```
DoxA       FGDGPHYCIG EQLAQLESRT MIGVLRSRFP QARLAVPVEE LRMCRKGAQT ARLTDLPVWL R*
DnmQ       LAGRDHLGLV APLVRVQCTA VLRALAERLP GLR...AEGE PLRRGRSPVV RAPLSLRLAQ K*
p450Soy    FGFGVHQCLG QHLARAELDI AMRTLFERLP GLRLAVPAHE IRH.KPGDTI QGLLDLPVAW .
p450ChoP   FGHGMHQCLG RQLARIELRV ALTALLERFP HLRLACPAAE IPL.RHDMQV YGADRLPVAN .
P450Ole    FGHGAHHCIG AQLGRLELQE ALSALVRRFP TLDLAEPVAG LRH.KQGMLI RGLERQIVSW *
p450cam    FGHGSHLCLG QHLARREIIV TLKEWLTRIP DFSIA.PGAQ IQ..HKSGIV SGVQALPLVN DPATTKAV*
Conserved  fghg.H.clg .qLarlelrv alralleRfP glrla.paae irw..kgmqv rgll.lpvaw *
           FGhG.H.CiG
           Heme pocket
```

Figure 14 LINE-UP representation of a PILE-UP comparison (GCG package) of the primary amino acid sequences of several related P450 enzymes including DoxA and DnmQ (formerly DnrQ; lacks the active-site Cys residue as indicated at bullet). The consensus sequence was computer generated. Sources of sequences: DoxA (*Streptomyces* sp. strain C5; 244); DnmQ (*S. peucetius*; 301); p450Soy (*S. griseus* CYP105D1, PIR S24750); p450ChoP (*Streptomyces* sp. strain SA-COO; GenBank M31939); p450Ole (*S. antibioticus*; GenBank L37200); and p450cam (*Pseudomonas putida* ATCC 17453; GenBank M12546).

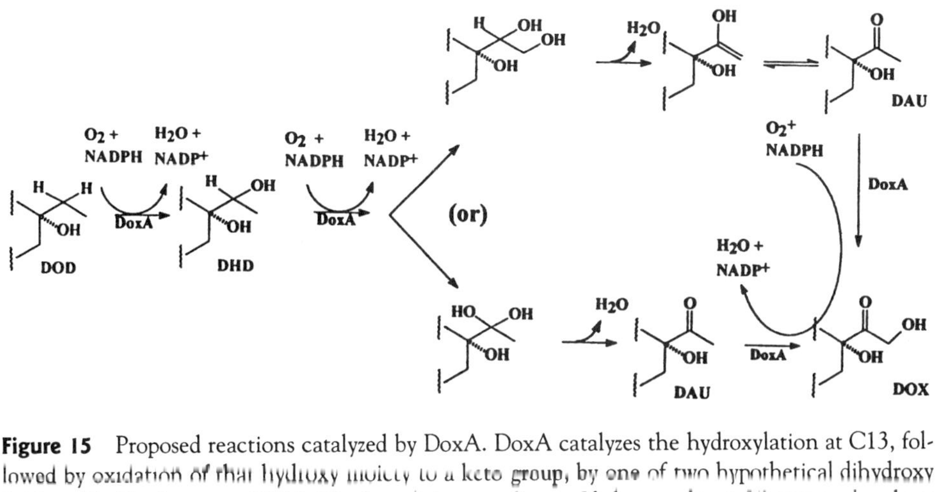

Figure 15 Proposed reactions catalyzed by DoxA. DoxA catalyzes the hydroxylation at C13, followed by oxidation of that hydroxy moiety to a keto group, by one of two hypothetical dihydroxy (either 13-dihydroxy or 13,14-dihydroxy) intermediates. If the resultant 13-oxo molecule is daunorubicin, then it can undergo DoxA-catalyzed hydroxylation at C14.

hexulose to TDP-daunosamine by the *S. griseus orf*5 (305) and *S. peucetius* and *Streptomyces* sp. strain C5 *dnm*V products. These deduced proteins are similar to other 4-epimerases and 4-ketoreductases (339) and contain an obvious NADPH-binding site necessary for the ketoreduction reaction.

Rhodomycin D, is *N*-dimethyldaunosamine (52). In the biosynthesis of TDP-rhodosamine, the sugar moiety found in rhodomycins, aklavin, and the α-sugar of aclarubicin, a pair of *N*-methyltransferase reactions must take place in addition to those reactions mentioned above. Whether the *N*-methyltransferase that catalyzes these methylations functions on the TDP-sugar, or after the sugar is attached to the aglycone, is currently unknown; however, it is likely that it functions on the TDP-sugar, since in aclarubicin biosynthesis additional sugars are added after attachment of the rhodosamine moiety.

F. Glycosyltransferase Reaction

Anthracyclinones, aglycones lacking a sugar moiety, are for the most part biologically inactive. Thus, glycosylation is a key step in the formation of biologically active anthracycline products. Upon discovering oxaunomycin, a potent derivative of daunorubicin isolated from a blocked mutant of *Streptomyces* sp. strain D788, Yoshimoto et al. (189) discovered that 10-carboxy-13-deoxycarminomycin and 13-deoxycarminomycin also were produced, leading them to propose that ε-rhodomycinone was glycosylated to rhodomycin D, which was demethylated and then decarboxylated to form 13-deoxycarminomycin. Based on bioconversion and product formation data from the literature (189,270,336), the production by some strains of ε-rhodomycinone-related glycosides (100), the high frequency of *Streptomyces* sp. strain C5 mutants obtained that accumulated ε-rhodomycinone (indicating multiple mutation targets; 221), our discovery of carminomycin 4-O-methyltransferase (240,241), which only functioned with 4-hydroxyanthracycline glycosides (thus demonstrating that glycosylation had to precede 4-O-methylation) (240,241), and the accumulation in fermentation broths of ε-rhodomycinone by several daunorubicin-producing strains (implying a potential bottleneck reaction; 4,77,335), we concurred with Yoshimoto et al. (189) in proposing that ε-rhodomycinone was in fact the primary aglycone substrate for TDP-daunosamine:anthracyclinone glycosyltransferase in *Streptomyces* sp. strain C5 and *S. peucetius* (124). In the proposed TDP-daunosamine:ε-rhodomycinone glycosyltransferase reaction, TDP-β-L-daunosamine is attached to C7 of the aglycone with the inversion of stereochemistry at the anomeric center (Figure 13). Depending on the strain, the resulting glycoside might be further modified by attachment of additional sugars, either to the 4′-hydroxy-group, or to C10 (if a hydroxy-group is present, as in rhodomycins) (4).

Two open reading frames (ORFs) (*dau*H (280) and *dnm*S (301)) encoding deduced proteins with similarity to known glycosyltransferase enzymes are located within the daunomycin biosynthesis gene cluster (Figures 9 and 16). Both of these enzymes contain the conserved "glycosyltransferase domain" (LPxxAAxxHHGGAGTxxxAxxAGx-PQxxxP; underlined in Figure 16) recently proposed by Cundliffe (340). It is currently hypothesized that one of the genes, *dnm*S, encodes for a glycosyltransferase that produces the first glycone intermediate, ε-rhodomycinone, and the other, *dau*H, may be involved in the formation of higher glycosides of daunomycin, such as baumycins or 4′-daunosaminyldaunorubicin (301). Otten et al. (301) complemented *S. peucetius* mutants that accumulated ε-rhodomycinone with the *dnr*S gene in a high copy number vector

```
C5-DauH              MRV LFATMAARSH VYAQVTLASA LRTAGHEVLV ASQPDVLDDI VRAGLTRVRI GEDLNIEEET REANASFEDD RNLGGLAMSN TKDDPLFWDH
SPE-DnmS             MKV LVTAFAMDAH FNGVVPLAWA LRAAGHDVRV ASQPALTDSI TRAGLTAVPV GTDHQV-QAA MGAMAPGVFA LHLNPDYLEN -RPELLDLEF
gtnodos             MAAGSPAT VFALAPLATA ARNAGHQVVM AANDDMVPVI TASGLPGIAT T--------- ---------D LPIRHFITTD RAGNPEEIPS
gttu22               MRF LFVSGGSAGA VFPITPLALA ARNAGHEVIV GATENVMPLV AATGLPGAPI T--------- ---------S RTMFDFMQRD RHGNPLEIPK
gtantibt    MTTQTTPAHI AMPSIAAHGN VNPSLEVIRE LVARGHRVTY LVARGHRVTY AIPRLLADKV AEAGAEPKLW NSTL----- ---------- ---------- PGPDADPEAW
gtslivdn    MTTRPAHI AMPSIALHGN VNPSLEVIRE LVARGHRVTY AIPRLLADKV AEAGAEPKLW NSTL----- ---------- ---------- PGPDADPEAW
gtpsrham            MHA ILIAIGSAGD VPPPIGLART LKLRGHRVSL CTIPVFRDAV EQHGIAFVPL SDEL----- ---------- ---------- TYRRTWGDPR
gtnogal             MRV MFTVSSWPTH YASLVPLGLA LQAAGHKVRV LCAPSQTDSV AHAGLTFVPV LDGL------ ---------D VPQWLRLQYY EEARQGIWPY
consensus                a..gh v.p..pla.a lraaGH.v.v ........d.v a.aGl..vp. .......... .......... ..........p.
```

```
C5-DauH     ALGMFTAMTA MVFQNVCPEP MVDDLVGLAR DWR---PDLV VHDPLTLAGP VAARLSGAAH ARLLFGPDQM GRNRTAFRAL LDRQRPS--- ----------
SPE-DnmS    LEASTSMLTA AFYAQINNDS MIDEMVDFAL WWR---PDLV VHEPFTFGGA VAAQVTGAAQ ARLLNGPDLF LRVHDRPQQV LHEVPAE--- ----------
gtnodos     DPVEQALFTG RWFARMAASS L-PRMLEFCR AWR---PDLI VGGTMSYVAP LLALHLGVPH VR------- ---------QT WDAIZAD---
gttu22      DPHERNLFNG RGMARLALGS M-EGLVPLVE RWQ---PDVL VAGALSYAAP LVAHRFGLPW VR------- ---------HA LNMGEPS---
gtantibt    ---GSTLLDN R---RTFLND AIQALPQLAD AYADDIPDLV LHDITSYPAR VLARRWGVPA VS--LSPNLV AMKGYEE--- --EVAEPMWR EPRQTER---
gtslivdn    ---GSTLLDN V---EPFLAD AIQSLPQLAQ AYEGDEPDLV LHDIASYTAR VLGRRWEVPV IS--LSPCMV AWEGYEQ--- --EVGEPMWE EPRKTER---
gtpsrham    LWDPKTSFGV L---WQTIAG MIEPVYEYVS AQRHDD-IVV VGSLWALGAR IAHEKYGIPY LSAQVSPSTL LSAHLPPVHP KFNVPEQMPL AMRKLLWRCI
gtnogal     PWLPHPHPVTG EDMAALDEF. ****
consensus        t..t. ...a...... mi..1...a. awr...pdlv v....sy.a. v.a..g.p. .r........ .......... ..........
```

```
C5-DauH     ---CVTTRCA EWLTWTLERW RRQRLD---- ----MSKELV LGQWTIDPTP PSMRIPLDLP CVPVRYVPYN G--PSLLPDW LREPPRHPRR LCLTLGVSLG
SPE-DnmS    ---RRDDALE EWLTWTLE-- -RHGAA---- ----FGPEVI SGHWTIDQMP PSVRFATARP TVPMRFVPYN GPVPAVVPPW LRADPGRPRV L-LTQGITER
gtnodos     ---GIHPGAD AELRPELAEF DLDRLP---- ----LPDVFV ------DICP PSLRPAGAAP AQPMRYVPAN AQRR--LEPW MYRRGERRRV LVTSGSRVAK
gttu22      ---IIDLSAA AELAPELEEM GLSAIP---- ----EPDMYV ------EICP PGARRPDAGP AQFMRYVPFN TQRA--LEPW MYAKGDRPRV LVSAGSRVTA
gtantibt    -----GRAYY ARFEAMLKEN GITEHPDTFA S---HPPRSL V-----LIPK ALQPHADRVD EDVYTFVGAC QGDRAEEGGM QR-PAGAEKV VLVSLGSAFT
gtslivdn    -----GQAYY ARFHAMLKEN GITDHPDPFI G---RPDRSL V-----LIPK ALQPHADRVD ETTYTFVGAC QGDRTAEGDM AR-PEGAEKV VLVSLGSAFT
gtpsrham    ERFKLDRTCA PDINAVRRKV GLETPVKRIP TQWMHSPQGV VCLFPAWFAP PQQDWPQPLH MTGFPLFDGS IPGTPLDDEL QRFLDQGSRP LVFTQGGSTEH
consensus         ..... a.1...1.e. g......... ....p...v ......i.p p..r.a...p ....r.vp.n ..........w .F......rv l...g.....
```

```
C5-DauH     EATGAGTVAA SDVLAAVDGL DVEVVATL-S RNCQELGTLP ANVRAVDFVR LMALLPSCSG IIHHGGSGTF MTALAHATPQ LIVPDMMWDA MEKAHGLARS
SPE-DnmS    STGFTGLPRA GELLASIAEL DAEVVATVKA EEREGLPPLP GNVRVVDSLS LHVVLPSCAA VVEHGGAGTW ATAALHGVPQ LALA-WQWDD VFRAGQLEKL
gtnodos     ESYDKNFEFL RGLAKDVAAM DVELIVAAPE AVADALHDEL PGIRA-GWAP LDVVAPTCDV LVHEHGGAGVST LTGLNAGVPQ LLIPRGA-VL EKPALRVADH
gttu22      ---DYEADAL SALVEKVAGL DVELLIAAPQ EIADALGDLP DNVRA-GCVP LDVVLRTCDL LVHRAGGNTM LHAIVCGVPQ LVIPAMP-KQ VGMSARLAEY
gtantibt    KQPAFYRECV RAF-GNLPGW HL-VLQIGRK VTPAELGELP DNVEVHDMVP QLAILRQADL FVTHAGAGSS QEGLATATPM IAVPQ-AVDQ FGNADMLQGL
gtslivdn    KQPAFYRECV RAF-GELPGW HT-VLQVGRH VDPAELGDVP DNVEVRTWVP QLAILQQADL FVTHAGAGGS QEGLATATPM IAVPQ-AADQ FGNADMLQGL
gtpsrham    LQGDFYAMAL RAL-ERLGAR GLT-FLTGA-- -GQEPLGSLP HEVLQRATAP LGALLPSCAG LVHPGGIGAM SLALAAGVPQ VLLPC-AHDQ FDNAERLVRL
consensus          ..... ral......g. d..v...... ....Lg.1P .nvr......p l.a.lp.c.. .vhhgG.g.. ...ala.gvpq l..p....dq ...a..1..1
                                                                       LP..AA   .HHGGAGT. ..A..AG.PQ ...P
                                                                       **     *****  **    *     **
```

```
C5-DauH     GAGGYV--DA KDVSPDLLRE RVLDLFDDPS YAAGARRVRA EIVGTPSPMD IVPVLERLTA EHQAGGPERS PALKSPSTGG A*
SPE-DnmS    GAGIFLPPHG EGASAGRVRD RLAQVLAEPS FRQGAARIRA EMLRTPAPGA VVPTLEQLTA RHRAPAGQGV RH*
gttu22      GAAITLLPGE DAADA--IAD SCQELLSKDT YGERARELSR EIAAMPSPAS VVDALEPA*
gttu22      GAVXMLTAGQ DD--------- ------SPEW VPRPAGSCWR TRKTRPGPTS *
gtantibt    GVARRL--AT EEATADLLRE TALALVDDPE VARRLRRI-Q AEMAQEGRTR RAADLIEAEL PARHERQEPV GDRPNVGDRP AGVRSDRQRS AL*
gtslivdn    GVARTL--PT EEATAKALRT AALALVDDPE VAARLKEI-Q ARMAQEAGTR GPADLIEAEL AAARG*
gtpsrham    GCGMRL--GV -PLREQELRG ALWRLLEDPA MAAACRRFWE LSQPHSIACG KAAQVVERCH REGDARWLKA AS*
consensus   Gaa..1.... ..a.a..1r. ....1..dp. .a..a..r... .....p.p..
```

Figure 16   LINE-UP representation of a PILE-UP comparison (GCG package) of the primary amino acid sequences of several related glycosyltransferases, most of them involved in antibiotic biosynthesis (or resistance), including *Streptomyces* sp. strain C5 DauH (glycosyltransferase of unknown function) and *S. peucetius* DnmQ (which catalyzes the transfer of daunosamine from TDP-daunosamine to ε-rhodomycinone to form rhodomycin D). The consensus sequence was computer generated. The underlined sequence toward the C-terminal end of the proteins is proposed by Cundliffe (340) to be a "glycosyltransferase signature sequence." Sources of sequences: C5-DauH (*Streptomyces* sp. strain C5; 280); SPE-DnmS (*S. peucetius* ATCC 29050; 301); gtnodos (*S. nodosus*; GenBank A25110); gttu22 (*S. violaceoruber* strain Tü22, granaticin biosynthesis; GenBank L37334); gtantibt (*S. antibioticus*, involved in resistance to macrolides; PIR S33184); gtslivdn (*S. lividans*, involved in macrolide resistance; PIR JS0636); gtpsrham (*Ps. aeruginosa*, involved in rhamnose biosynthesis; PIR B53652); gtnogal (*S. nogalater*, partial sequence of glycosyltransferase from nogalamycin biosynthesis gene cluster; PIR S52405).

and restored daunorubicin production. Substrate specificity for these enzymes in vitro has not been demonstrated, however, primarily because the nucleotide sugars involved in the biosynthesis of these antibiotics are not readily available.

G.   Conversion of Rhodomycin D to Doxorubicin

As shown above, there is now ample evidence indicating that the first glycosylated anthracycline in daunorubicin/doxorubicin biosynthesis pathway is the product of the proposed TDP-daunosamine:ε rhodomycinone glycosyltransferase reaction, 10-carbomethoxy-13-deoxycarminomycin (named herein rhodomycin D; 239). This compound was first isolated and characterized by Yoshimoto and his colleagues as an accumulated intermediate in blocked mutants of *Streptomyces* sp. strain D788 (279,341). The enzymatic conversion of rhodomycin D to doxorubicin requires the following steps (not in any particular order): (a) demethylation of the C16 methoxy residue by a presumed methylesterase; (b) removal of the resultant free carboxyl moiety at C10; (c) hydroxylation at C13; (d) oxidation of the newly formed C13 hydroxy moiety to a keto-group; (e) O-methylation of the C4 hydroxy-group; and (f) hydroxylation at C14 (Figure 17).

Figure 17 shows the proposed pathway for conversion of rhodomycin D to daunorubicin, doxorubicin, and baumycin A_1/A_2. The reactions and genes governing the biosynthesis of daunorubicin and doxorubicin from ε-rhodomycinone have been widely postulated (124–126,176,236,239), but they have not been proven in vitro until very recently (239).

As previously mentioned, Yoshimoto et al. (279) isolated 10-carboxy-13-deoxycarminomycin as a minor product in the fermentation broth of a mutant blocked in daunorubicin biosynthesis. Thus, it has been postulated that rhodomycin D is decarbomethoxylated in two distinct steps, namely, demethylation followed by decarboxylation, to form 13-deoxycarminomycin, which is subsequently converted to carminomycin by a two-step oxidation at position C13 (Figure 17). Yoshimoto et al. (270) demonstrated that *S. coeruleorubidus* ME130-A4 could not glycosylate aglycones that had been methylated at the C4 hydroxy position, leading to the conclusion that glycosylation precedes 4-O-methylation. Similarly, Connors and colleagues (240,241) found that carminomycin 4-O-methyltransferase could not utilize aglycones as substrates, supporting the hypothesis that glycosylation must precede methylation.

Until recently, there was only a single proven reaction within this glycone pathway. The genes encoding carminomycin 4-O-methyltransferase (CMT) have been isolated and sequenced from both *Streptomyces* sp. strain C5 (237) and *S. peucetius* ATCC 29050 (242), and the enzyme has been purified from both organisms (241–243; Walczak R, Dickens ML, and Strohl WR, unpublished data). We have shown previously that CMT activity encoded by *Streptomyces* sp. strain C5 *dau*K enzymatically converted 13-dihydrocarminomycin and carminomycin to 13-dihydrodaunorubicin and daunorubicin, respectively (240,241).

We recently reported the discovery of *dox*A, the gene encoding a cytochrome P450–like enzyme that catalyzed daunorubicin 14-hydroxylase to doxorubicin (244). The gene product of *dox*A, predicted to have an M_r of 46,096, possessed both the highly conserved heme pocket (FGDGPHYCIG) and oxygen-binding (AGHDT) domains characteristic of cytochrome P450s (342) (Figure 14). Neither a ferredoxin nor a NADPH:ferredoxin oxidoreductase gene, encoding expected electron-donating reactions for DoxA, has been found within the *Streptomyces* sp. strain C5 daunorubicin biosynthesis gene cluster that we have sequenced. A similar *dox*A gene has been discovered in *S. peucetius* (Hutchinson CR, personal communication). DoxA showed specificity for only daunorubicin and 13-dihydrodaunorubicin, both of which were converted to doxorubicin (244). Daunomycinone (daunorubicin aglycone), carminomycin, idarubicin, and aklavin were not apparent substrates for DoxA. Unexpectedly, carminomycin was not oxidized to 14-hydroxycarminomycin, even after very long incubations, indicating that it is not a substrate for the C14 hydroxylase reaction. This is surprising, since the C4 and C14 carbons are at opposite ends of the molecule, suggesting that perhaps methylation at C-O-4, which changes a phenol hydroxy-group to a methyl ether, may either significantly increase affinity for the substrate or alter the binding of the molecule to DoxA in the active site to bring about a conformation conducive to C14 hydroxylation.

Additional indirect data were also available that suggested the involvement of another gene product in the biosynthesis of doxorubicin from rhodomycin D. Niemi and

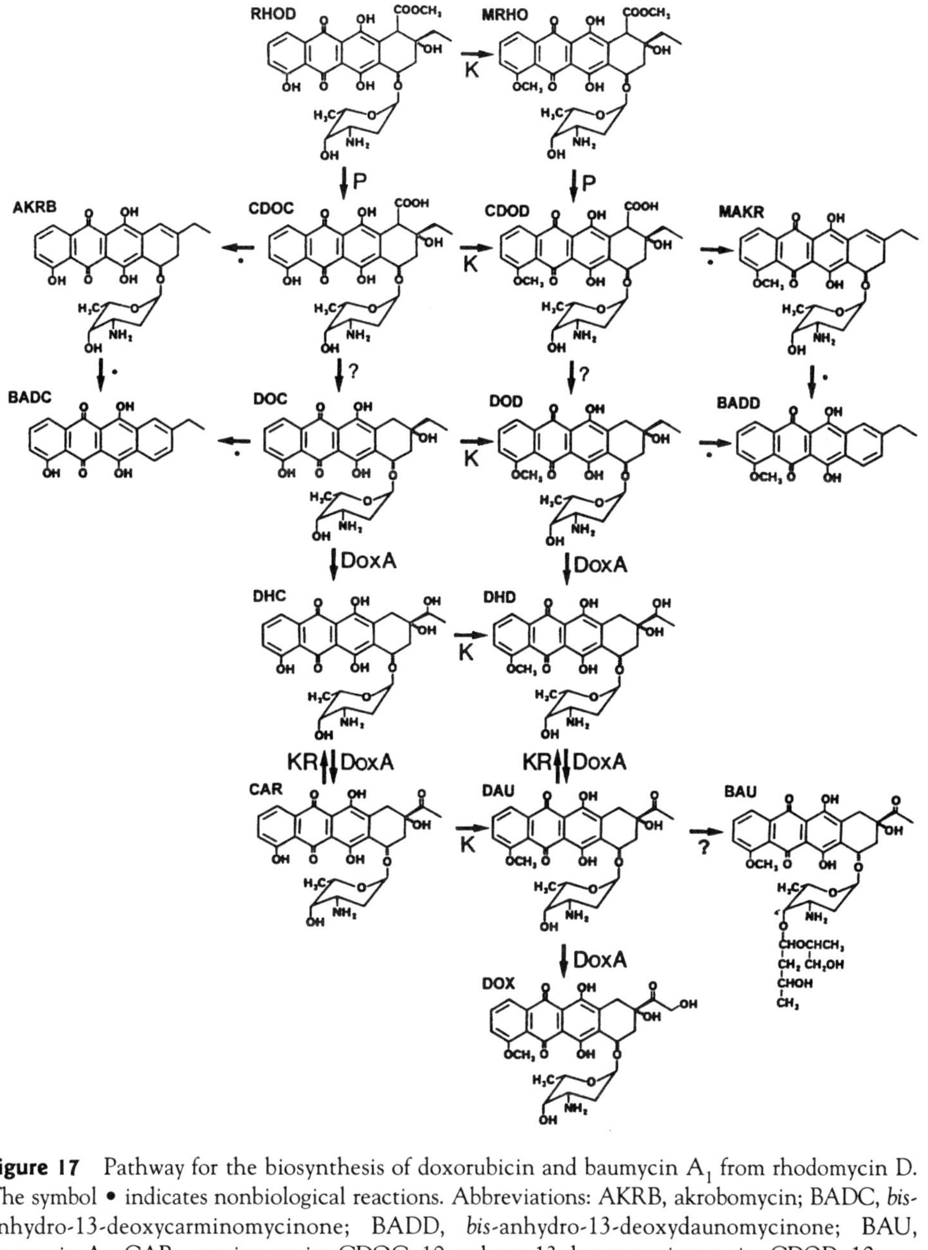

Figure 17 Pathway for the biosynthesis of doxorubicin and baumycin A_1 from rhodomycin D. The symbol • indicates nonbiological reactions. Abbreviations: AKRB, akrobomycin; BADC, *bis*-anhydro-13-deoxycarminomycinone; BADD, *bis*-anhydro-13-deoxydaunomycinone; BAU, baumycin A_1; CAR, carminomycin; CDOC, 10-carboxy-13-deoxycarminomycin; CDOD, 10-carboxy-13-deoxydaunorubicin; DAU, daunorubicin; DHC, 13-dihydrocarminomycin; DHD, 13-dihydrodaunorubicin; DOC, 13-deoxycarminomycin; DOD, 13-deoxydaunorubicin; DOX, doxorubicin; DoxA, 13-deoxyanthracycline 13-hydroxylase, 13-dihydroanthracycline oxidase, and daunorubicin 14-hydroxylase; K, DauK/DnrK, anthracycline 4-O-methyltransferase; MAKR,4-O-methyl-akrobomycin; MRHO,4-O-methyl-rhodomycin D; P, DauP/DnrP, rhodomycin 16-methylesterase; RHOD, rhodomycin D.

his colleagues showed that *Streptomyces purpurascens* RdmC, an apparent esterase homolog, was able to catalyze the in vivo decarbomethoxylation of aclacinomycin and aklavin (65,231). Based on the apparent heterologous functionality of RdmC, they hypothesized that RdmC was the enzyme responsible for demethylation and possibly also decarboxylation of rhodomycin D in rhodomycin biosynthesis (65). Subsequently, homologs of RdmC were found in both *Streptomyces* sp. strain C5 (DauP; 237) and *S. peucetius* (DnrP; 238), both of which have about 55% amino acid sequence identity with RdmC.

We recently proved four new functions that, together, determine the sequence and structure–function relationships among the glycones in doxorubicin biosynthesis, and prove the pathway(s) involved in the biosynthesis of doxorubicin from rhodomycin D (239). The key to our ability to carry out these studies was the availability of 10-carbomethoxy-13-deoxycarminomycin (rhodomycin D) from the National Cancer Institute as compound NSC #263854-H.

First, we showed that *Streptomyces* sp. strain C5 DauK not only could catalyze the methylation of carminomycin and 13-dihydrocarminomycin, but that it also could methylate rhodomycin D, 10-carboxy-13-deoxycarminomycin, and 13-deoxycarminomycin (Figure 17), indicating a much broader substrate specificity for this enzyme than had previously been indicated (240,241). Interestingly, rhodomycin D was readily and completely converted to 4-O-methylrhodomycin D (239), a product that had been previously described as a nonconvertible shunt product of daunorubicin biosynthesis in *Streptomyces* sp. D788 (341). We found, however, that 4-O-methylrhodomycin D was completely converted to other 4-O-methyl anthracyclines. With the expanded substrate range, we propose to rename the products of *dauK* and *dnrK* anthracycline 4-O-methyltransferase (Table 7; Figure 17).

Second, we found that both cultures and extracts of recombinant *S. lividans* TK24, containing the recombinant *dauP* gene from *Streptomyces* sp. strain C5, converted rhodomycin D to 10-carboxy-13-deoxycarminomycin, with trace levels of 13-deoxycarminomycin and the chemical breakdown products, akrobomycin (9,10-anhydro-13-deoxycarminomycin; 33), *bis*-anhydro-13-deoxycarminomycinone (Figure 17). Akrobomycin has been shown to be formed from 10-carboxy-13-deoxycarminomycin by spontaneous decarboxylation and dehydration (33,99), and *bis*-anhydro-13-deoxycarminomycinone is a known chemical breakdown product of both akrobomycin and 13-deoxycarminomycin (82,99). Additionally, both cultures and extracts of *S. lividans* TK24 containing recombinant DauP converted 4-O-methylrhodomycin D to 10-carboxy-13-deoxydaunorubicin, along with trace amounts of 13-deoxydaunorubicin, and the spontaneous breakdown products, 4-O-methyl-akrobomycin and *bis*-anhydro-13-deoxydaunomycinone (239).

Third, we found that while the 10-carboxyl anthracyclines accumulated by DauP-mediated demethylation of the rhodomycin molecules (i.e., 10-carboxy-13-deoxycarminomycin and -daunorubicin), both could be readily decarboxylated in the presence of DauK and DauP, but only marginally decarboxylated by DauP alone. This suggested to us that either the DauKP complex catalyzes this reaction, or that DauK alone can carry out the decarboxylation. 10-Carboxy-13-deoxycarminomycin (product D788-1; 279) has previously been purified from culture broths of a blocked mutant of *Streptomyces* sp. D788 (99,279), indicating that a specific genetically encoded function is required for its metabolism, that is, decarboxylation to 13-deoxycarminomycin.

Fourth, we determined that the recently characterized *dox*A gene from *Streptomyces* sp. strain C5 (244), which encodes a cytochrome P450–like protein that catalyzes the hydroxylation of daunorubicin at C14 to doxorubicin, also conferred two new reactions: (a) the C13 hydroxylation of 13-deoxycarminomycin and 13-deoxydaunorubicin (feudomycin A) to form 13-dihydrocarminomycin and 13-dihydrodaunorubicin, respectively; and (b) oxidation of the 13-hydroxy-group of 13-dihydrocarminomycin and 13-dihydrodaunorubicin to carminomycin and daunorubicin, respectively (239; Figure 17). Several years ago, Oki et al. (343) found that feudomycin A (another name for 13-deoxydaunorubicin) was converted to doxorubicin by blocked mutants of S. *peucetius* subsp. *caesius*, indicating that the oxidation enzymes to carry out this reaction were also present in that strain. Our recent data indicate that this entire oxidation series is catalyzed by one enzyme, DoxA (239). The discovery of a DoxA homolog in S. *peucetius* subsp. *caesius* (Hutchinson CR, personal communication), as would be expected since this strain is the only strain known to produce doxorubicin, indicates that the reactions are the same for that strain as we observed in *Streptomyces* sp. strain C5 (239).

Compounds containing substitutions at the 10-position (aklavin, aclacinomycin A, 10-carboxy-13-deoxycarminomycin, 10-carboxy-13-deoxydaunorubicin, rhodomycin D, and 4-O-methylrhodomycin D) were not substrates for the 13-hydroxylase activity of DoxA, apparently due to steric hindrance (239). Once the 10-carbomethoxy moiety was removed, however, cultures containing DoxA actively oxidized the C13 position from the methylene to hydroxy and from hydroxy to keto moieties, both with the carminomycin (i.e., 4-hydroxy) series and the daunorubicin (i.e., 4-methoxy) series of anthracyclines (Figure 17). The rates of these oxidations were considerably faster (ca. 35-fold) than observed with DoxA-specific hydroxylation of daunorubicin at C14 to form doxorubicin, suggesting that the primary functions of DoxA are indeed the oxidation of 13-deoxy and 13-dihydro species to 13-keto species (239; Dickens ML, Strohl WR, unpublished data).

The C13 hydroxylation of 13-deoxy-anthracyclines is typical of cytochrome P450–like enzymes. The second step, however, oxidation of the C13 hydroxy-group to a keto moiety (Figure 15), is not typical for most cytochrome P450 enzymes. Nevertheless, this reaction also was shown to have an absolute requirement for NADPH and O_2. Thus, we have proposed two possible alternative routes, both invoking a dihydroxy intermediate, for the NADPH- and oxygen-dependent oxidation of 13-dihydrocarminomycin and 13-dihydrodaunorubicin to carminomycin and daunorubicin, respectively (Figure 15).

Yoshimoto et al. (270) proposed that in S. *coeruleorubidus* strain ME130-A4, daunorubicin biosynthesis proceeded via either 13-deoxycarminomycin and 13-dihydrocarminomycin, or alternatively via the methylation of 13-deoxycarminomycin to 13-deoxydaunorubicin, followed by the two-step oxidation at C13. More recently, Yoshimoto et al. (341) proposed, based on the analysis of several blocked mutants, that rhodomycin D is converted to daunorubicin in *Streptomyces* sp. strain D788 by the following route: rhodomycin D → 10-carboxy-13-deoxycarminomycin → 13-deoxycarminomycin → 13-deoxydaunorubicin → 13-dihydrodaunorubicin → daunorubicin. Methylation of 13-deoxycarminomycin was considered the critical step in their proposed pathway. Crespi-Perellino et al. (344) suggested that 13-dihydrodaunorubicin was a degradation product of daunorubicin, leading us to propose, in conjunction with our discovery of CMT (7), that the pathway from rhodomycin D to daunorubicin was via 13-dihydrocarminomycin and carminomycin, and that the methylation step occurred late in the pathway (240,241). Our recent data, which are largely consistent with those of Yoshimoto et al. (341), indicate that several alternative routes may be used to synthesize daunorubicin and doxorubicin. Our evidence for expanded substrate specificity of the anthracycline 4-O-methyltransferase indicates that 4-O-methylation may occur early or late in the glycone pathway. It is also possible that growth and medium conditions resulting in different levels of *dau*P, *dau*K, and *dox*A expression may favor one route over another. Alternatively, the K_m values of the 4-O-methyltransferase for 13-deoxycarminomycin, 13-dihydrocarminomycin, and carminomycin may be different among the various daunorubicin-producing strains.

The results of Crespi-Perellino et al. (344) also now can be explained by the omnipresence of the strong C13 ketoreductase activity in streptomycetes (183,184,239,244,285,287), including both *Streptomyces* sp. strain C5 and *S. peucetius* ATCC 29050, which very likely influenced their results.

If daunorubicin-producing strains such as *S. peucetius* ATCC 29050 and *Streptomyces* sp. strain C5 have *dox*A and the associated physiological capability to convert daunorubicin to doxorubicin, why do they not produce doxorubicin naturally? Why is *S. peucetius* subsp. *caesius*, a mutant, the only strain known to produce doxorubicin? The answers to these questions are not simple. For example, the DNA sequences of *dox*A from wild-type *S. peucetius* ATCC 29050 and *S. peucetius* subsp. *caesius* (ATCC 27952) are identical (Hutchinson CR, personal communication), so that alteration of the protein to favor C14 hydroxylation can be ruled out. In in vivo bioconversion experiments, we observed cultures of *Streptomyces* sp. strain C5 incubated with [³H]daunorubicin produced radioactive baumycins. On the other hand, incubation of [³H]daunorubicin with cultures of *Streptomyces* sp. strain C5 (pANT195), containing an overexpressed, recombinant *dox*A gene, produced radioactive doxorubicin but no radioactive baumycins (239,244; Dickens ML and Strohl WR, unpublished results). Our interpretation of these data, coupled with the biosynthesis data mentioned above and the knowledge that most daunorubicin-producing strains form baumycins as their end products (99,121,323), lead us to propose that the synthesis of baumycins normally outcompetes the synthesis of doxorubicin, especially since the turnover rate for C14 hydroxylase is so low (244). This suggests that mutations affecting the baumycin biosynthesis apparatus, coupled with over-expression of *dox*A, may result in generation of strains capable of doxorubicin overproduction.

H.   Structural Genes Required for Doxorubicin biosynthesis from Primary Metabolites

Based on evidence primarily accumulated using genes and enzymes from *Streptomyces* sp. strain C5, we now can predict the minimal biosynthesis gene products required to synthesize doxorubicin from propionyl-SCoA, malonyl-SCoA, and TDP-daunosamine in a heterologous strain (Table 8). To synthesize aklanonic acid from propionyl-SCoA and malonyl-SCoA, the minimal genes required are *dps*ABEFG*dau*G (*dau*G = *dnr*G in *S. peucetius*). As mentioned earlier in this chapter, *dps*CD ensure that the starter moiety is 100% (or nearly so) propionyl-SCoA, whereas in their absence, a mixture of acetyl-SCoA and propionyl-SCoA are used as starter units. To convert aklanonic acid to ε-rhodomycinone, the products of *dau*CDEF (or the *S. peucetius* homologs *dnr*CDEF) are required. Glycosylation of ε-rhodomycinone with TDP-glucose as the sugar donor requires the *dnm*S product, and conversion of the ε-rhodomycinone glycoside, rhodomycin D, to doxorubicin requires the products of only three genes, *dau*KP*dox*A (Table 8). Obviously, additional gene products encoding proteins such as the ferredoxin and NADPH:ferredoxin oxidoreductase, required for the DoxA reactions, are also

Table 8 Predicted Gene Requirements for Doxorubicin Biosynthesis

Substrates	Products	Genes	ORFs
Genes encoding biosynthetic reactions:			
Propionyl-SCoA + 9 malonyl-SCoA	Aklanonic acid	dpsABEFG, dauG	6
Aklanonic acid	ε-Rhodomycinone	dauCDEF	4
D-Glucose-1-PO$_4$	TDP-Daunosamine	dnmJLM^{a}QTUVZ	8
TDP-Daunosamine + ε-rhodomycinone	Rhodomycin D	dnmS	1
Rhodomycin D	Doxorubicin	dauKP, doxA	3
Nonstructural genes:			
Resistance genes		drrABCD	4
Regulatory genes		dnrNOI	3
Other:			
Genes required to ensure propionyl starter unit		dpsCD	2
Genes of unknown function (baumycin biosynthesis?)		dauHUVXY, dpsH	6
Total:			37

^{a} A structural equivalent of dnmM is required in S. peucetius and perhaps other strains due to a natural frameshift in dnmM (see text for details).

required, but as we have already found, these can be supplied by a heterologous host strain (239,244).

What Table 8 tells us is that of the 37 genes found in the daunorubicin/doxorubicin biosynthesis gene clusters (Figure 9), only 14 gene products of the daunorubicin/doxorubicin gene cluster are required to convert propionyl-SCoA, malonyl-SCoA, and TDP-daunosamine to doxorubicin in a heterologous strain such as S. *lividans* TK24. What about the products of the other 23 genes within the cluster? Of these, we know that dpsCD help to dictate the starter unit in polyketide biosynthesis. Additionally, dnmJLMQTUVZ are hypothesized to be involved in TDP-daunosamine biosynthesis (301,302; Hutchinson CR, personal communication), drrABCD have been shown to be involved in resistance (265,303; Hutchinson CR, personal communication), and dnrNOI have been shown to be regulatory genes (298,300,308,309,345). That leaves the following ORFs with no currently proposed function: dauH (probable glycosyltransferase, but for what reaction?), dauU, dauV, dauX, dauY, dpsH. Though it is possible that some of these genes encode reactions conferring baumycin biosynthesis (see below), proof of such speculation requires additional work.

I. Baumycins and Their Potential Significance

Baumycins (Figure 1) were first described by Hamao Umezawa and his colleagues at the Microbial Chemistry Institute in Tokyo as new members of the daunorubicin group of anthracyclines isolated from culture broths of Streptomyces coeruleorubidus ME130-A4 (30,31,136). Baumycins also have been described as significant products from cultures of Streptomyces sp. strain C5 (121), Streptomyces insignis ATCC 31913, Streptomyces sp. strain D-788 (99), S. peucetius ATCC 29050 (323), and several Actinomadura strains (23,24,32–38; Table 1). McGuire et al. (335) demonstrated that baumycins A$_1$/A$_2$ were one of the major anthracyclines produced during fermentations of Streptomyces sp. C5, with daunomycin produced in much smaller quantities. The fact that baumycins are a major product of this organism leads to speculation that these compounds are the final biosynthetic product of *Streptomyces* sp. C5, not daunomycin. It is in fact highly plausible that all daunorubicin-producing strains actually produce baumycins as the natural pathway end products, which may explain, as described in Sections V.G and V.H, why more strains have not been shown to produce doxorubicin.

Baumycins A_1/A_2 are epimers at C1″ or C3″ that contain an acetal structure thought to be derived by cleavage of a sugar residue (136). In early studies, baumycin A_1 exhibited higher potency and stronger activity and potency against the L1210 leukemia cell line, but because of its instability (i.e., spontaneous chemical degradation to daunorubicin) and poor recovery in fermentation broths, the baumycins as a group were not pursued clinically (136).

Initially, three epimeric pairs of baumycins were identified (A_1/A_2, B_1/B_2, C_1/C_2) (31). Additionally, natural baumycin analogs, such as barminomycins (38), rubeomycins (34,36,37), and other baumycins (35,86,279), have been discovered since the first descriptions of baumycins. The origin of the acetal substituent of baumycins A_1/A_2 is believed to be carbohydrate in nature, suggesting condensation to the 4′-hydroxy position of daunosamine via a glycosyltransferase-mediated reaction (52). To date, however, studies have not proven the carbohydrate derivation of the acetal-group. It is possible that *dau*H (*dnr*H in *S. peucetius*) encodes the glycosyltransferase that couples the baumycin side chain onto the 4′-hydroxy-group of daunosamine.

Interestingly, the nature of the acetal moiety appears to affect the potency of the antibiotic. For instance, baumycins containing a carbinolamine moiety (e.g., barminomycins) generally exhibit a greater cytotoxicity and antitumor activity than the classical anthracyclines (38). In addition, structural variations may occur at C4 or C13 of the anthracyclinone moiety, which may affect the compound's activity (34–37).

Using the concept of biomimicry, Umezawa and colleagues (231) synthesized 4′-O-tetrahydrofuranyl and 4′-O-tetrahydropyranyl derivatives of daunorubicin and doxorubicin to determine the clinical potential of such analogs (136,346). Studies quickly showed that 4′-O-tetrahydropyranyldoxorubicin (THP-doxorubicin, pirarubicin), a structural analog of baumycin A_1 (Figure 1), exhibited excellent activity (231,346). THP-doxorubicin (pirarubicin) was first described in 1979 and is now produced by Meiji Seika (USA) Inc. for clinical trials. Pirarubicin appears to have similar efficacy to doxorubicin with significantly less cardiotoxicity (137).

VI. REGULATION OF DAUNORUBICIN BIOSYNTHESIS

A. Regulatory Genes and Mechanisms in Daunorubicin/Doxorubicin Biosynthesis

There are three known pathway-specific regulatory genes—*dnr*N (300,345), *dnr*O (300), and *dnr*I (298,309)—of the *S. peucetius* daunorubicin/doxorubicin biosynthesis gene cluster. DnrI (originally called part of the $dnrR_1$ locus; 298) was found to be a putative transcriptional activator with moderate similarity to RedD, ActII–Orf4, and AfsR (298). Originally, there was a consideration that *dnr*J also might be involved in regulation (which seemed reasonable considering its location in the same operon as *dnr*I; 298), but *dnr*J (now *dnm*J; Table 7, Figure 9) was later found to encode a TDP-daunosamine biosynthesis gene (307,308). Replacement of DnrI in *S. peucetius* with a Tn5 kanamycin-resistance gene resulted in a mutant that did not produce anthracyclines and that was considerably less resistant to doxorubicin than the wild type (298). Overexpression of DnrI, on the other hand, led to a ca. 10-fold overaccumulation of ε-rhodomycinone (298). Madduri and Hutchinson (308) showed that transcription of both early and late biosynthesis genes depended on the presence of active DnrI. Interestingly, they also showed that the transcript for *dnrJ* overlapped with the converging transcript from *dnmZUV* (308). Considering that *S. peucetius* ATCC 29050 accumulates considerably more ε-rhodomycinone, the compound in the aglycone portion of the pathway, than daunoroubicin (124,308), Hutchinson and Madduri proposed the interesting hypothesis that the overlapped transcripts may act as a natural antisense mechanism limiting transcription of the required sugar biosynthesis genes *dnmZUV* (308). Recently, DnrI was purified and shown to bind to specific sequences upstream of the *dnrGdps*ABCD, *dps*EF, and *dnr*DKPQS operons as well as upstream of the *dnr*C gene, encoded on a monocistronic message. Using footprinting assays, Tang et al. (309) mapped the binding sites in the promoter regions to a set of imperfect inverted repeat sequences of ca. 6 to 10 bp containing a 5′-TCGAG consensus sequence.

A second locus, originally called *dnr*R$_2$ (298), containing the divergently transcribed genes, *dnr*N and *dnr*O (300), was also found to be involved in regulation of the *S. peucetius* daunorubicin/doxorubicin biosynthesis gene cluster. Otten et al. (300) showed that disruption of *dnr*N, the product of which possesses sequence similarity with response regulators such as NarL, DegU, and UvrC (300), resulted in a complete abolition of anthracycline production. Interestingly, however, overexpression of *dnr*I at high copy number suppressed the *dnr*N mutation, but overexpression of *dnr*N did not suppress a *dnr*I knockout mutant. This led to the proposal that *dnr*N regulates expression of *dnr*I in *S. peucetius* (300). Recently, Furuya and Hutchinson (345) confirmed this hypothesis, showing that DnrN, which binds specifically to a sequence in the *dnr*I promoter region, is required for *dnr*I transcription in *S. peucetius*. They also found that daunorubicin inhibited binding of DnrN to the *dnr*I promoter region, leading them to propose that daunorubicin exerts a feed-back inhibition type of regulation by inhibition of DnrN activity (345).

DnrO was found to have sequence similarity with TcmR, the tetracenomycin-resistance gene repressor, as well as with other transcriptional repressors (300). While the role of DnrO has not been fully elucidated, its structure (i.e., it is an apparent repressor), its position, and its divergent transcription from DnrN strongly suggest that it may be involved in DnrN regulation (300). Thus, it appears that a three-membered cascade of regulatory genes—*dnr*O (putative transcriptional repressor possibly active in repressing *dnr*N), *dnr*N (transcriptional activator required for *dnr*I expression), and *dnr*I (transcriptional activator required for activation of structural genes)—are involved in regulation of daunorubicin biosynthesis in *S. peucetius*.

Homologs of *dnr*N, *dnr*O, and *dnr*I are found in the same respective positions in the *Streptomyces* sp. strain C5 (Figure 9). In early studies, we isolated regulatory mutants of *Streptomyces* sp. strain C5 that were unable to synthesize anthracyclines (221). These mutants, named *dau*G mutants, were later found to be complemented (or possibly suppressed, considering the data described above) by overexpression of *dau*I (Li Y and Strohl WR, unpublished data). We also showed that cloning of either *S. peucetius dnr*I or *Streptomyces* sp. strain C5 *dau*I in *S. lividans* caused overproduction of actinorhodin (347), and more recently, we have used *dau*I to promote transcription of daunorubicin PKS genes in the heterologous host, *S. lividans* TK24 (310). Interestingly, *dau*I functions independently of *dau*N to activate both homologous (i.e., *dps*ABCDEFG*dau*G; 310) and heterologous (actinorhodin genes; 347, and Li Y and Strohl WR, unpublished data) gene expression in *S. lividans* TK24, and it appears to require DnrN for transcription in *S. peucetius*

(300,345). Thus, it is possible that a *dnr*N functional homolog is present in *S. lividans*, or alternatively, that *dau*I and *dnr*I are transcribed by *dnr*N-independent mechanisms in *S. lividans* TK24.

B. Resistance Mechanisms

Currently, there are three known resistance genes, *drr*A (265), *drr*B (265), and *drr*C (303), isolated from the daunorubicin producer, *S. peucetius*. Also, Hutchinson (personal communication) has indicated recently that *drr*D appears to be similar to the mitomycin-resistance gene recently characterized by Sherman and colleagues (348). DrrA is a 330 amino acid long, hydrophilic protein found to have strong sequence similarity with ABC (for ATP-binding cassette)-type transporters, whereas DrrB was found to have strong hydrophobic regions typical of transmembrane proteins (265). It appears that these proteins function together to actively export daunorubicin and doxorubicin (265). Recently, Lomovskaya et al. (303) described *S. peucetius drr*C, which encodes a large protein (predicted M_r, 83,386) that possesses strong sequence similarity with *E. coli* UvrA (303). Cloning of *drr*C in *S. lividans* and *E. coli* conferred on the recipient strains resistance to daunorubicin (303). Interestingly, *drr*C could not be deleted in the wild-type strain but could be deleted in a *dnr*J mutant (which accumulates ε-rhodomycinone) (303), indicating that *drr*C is required in the producing strain for resistance to active anthracyclines. By sequence analysis, we have found that homologs of *drr*ABCD are present in the *Streptomyces* sp. strain C5 daunorubicin biosynthesis gene cluster in the same positions as they are found in the *S. peucetius* gene cluster. We have not, however, analyzed the *Streptomyces* sp. strain C5 resistance gene homologs.

VII.   GENE CLONING FOR HYBRID ANTHRACYCLINES

Hybrid antibiotics are new molecules produced by the cloning of genes from one antibiotic-producing strain into another, with the resultant molecules formed being novel to both strains. Strategies for the formation of hybrid antibiotics may include either the mixing and matching of the genes encoding building blocks, that is, polyketide biosynthesis genes, to generate new basic "backbone" structures, or alternatively, the use of genes encoding decoration reactions (i.e., hydroxylases, methyltransferases, oxidases, reductases, and so forth). The first example of hybrid antibiotic production was the formation of dihydrogranatirhodin by the granaticin producer, *Streptomyces violaceoruber* Tü22, transformed with plasmids carrying actinorhodin biosynthesis genes from *S. coelicolor* (349). Similarly, Hopwood et al. (349) also demonstrated that when *Streptomyces* sp. AM-7161 was transformed with certain genes encoding only part of the actinorhodin pathway, the novel hybrid antibiotics mederrhodins A and B were formed. This was an example of the use of decoration reactions to generate novel compounds.

The use of building-block genes, that is, polyketide biosynthesis genes, to generate new backbones was first demonstrated in a seminal study by Bartel et al. (245), who cloned actinorhodin PKS genes into anthracycline-producing *S. galilaeus* strains ATCC 31133 and ATCC 31671 to generate novel structures. The recombinant strains produced aloesaponarin II, an anthraquinone not produced by either of the parental strains (i.e., DNA donor or recipient). In the most minimal gene constructions, genes *actI–orf1* (KS_α) and *actI–orf2* (KS_β) from *S. coelicolor* functioned in *trans* with host ACP, cyclase, and polyketide reductase to produce aloesaponarin II in *S. galilaeus* ATCC 31133 and with host ACP and cyclase (and mutant polyketide reductase) of S. *galilaeus* ATCC 31671 to produce des-oxyerythrolaccin (245). Bartel et al. (245) also found, however, that S. *coelicolor actVI* mutants accumulated aloesaponarin II, showing that the compound could be formed as the result of the products of the *act*I,III,VII,IV loci functioning in the absence of the products from the *act*VI locus. Thus, aloesaponarin II was labeled by the scientific community as a "shunt product" (which it is in S. *coelicolor*). The fundamentally new concept, demon-strated clearly by Bartel et al. (245) and explained in detail by Strohl and Connors (247), that PKS gene products from heterologous strains could *interact* functionally to form new structures not produced by either parent (in the literal sense, aloesaponarin II may be con-sidered a shunt product, but desoxyerythrolaccin is not produced by any mutant of S. *coeli-color* and thus was a true "hybrid" molecule) was not fully appreciated until Khosla and his colleagues published their hybrid PKS experiments in *Science* (321). Since then, anthra-cycline PKS genes (particularly those from the tetracenomycin gene cluster), along with genes from several other type II PKS biosynthesis gene clusters, have been used widely in mix and match experiments to generate both new molecules and an enormous wealth of data on type II PKS function (252,255,257,258,321,322,324,330–332).

In more recent years, efforts to produce hybrid molecules using anthracycline biosynthesis genes and strains have focused more on the use of genes encoding decora-tion reactions. In one case, a gene from S. *purpurascens* ATCC 25489 putatively encod-ing the 10-carbomethoxy esterase (65,235) was cloned into S. *galilaeus* to generate novel decarbomethoxylated aklavinone and 11-deoxy-β-rhodomycinone, both novel anthracy-clines. In another example, S. *peucetius* aklavinone 11-hydroxylase was cloned into S. *galilaeus* to generate 11-hydroxyaclacinomycins (224,226). Using a different approach, the entire gene clusters encoding tetracenomycin and elloramycin were cloned into the urdamycin-producing strain *Streptomyces fradiae* Tü2717, resulting in the production of the novel compounds 6-hydroxytetracenomycin C and 8-olivosyl-8-demethyltetraceno-mycin, the latter a glycosylated tetracenomycin C derivative (350). In this case, the host organism modified the products formed by the recombinant genes (rather than vice versa). Very recently Ylihonko et al. (266) generated interesting hybrid auramycin-like metabolites containing methyl side chains by cloning nogalamycin biosynthesis genes from S. *nogalater* in an aclarubicin-nonproducing mutant of S. *galilaeus* ATCC 31615. The significance of their results, however, still needs to be sorted out, particularly in light of the discussion in Section V.C of this chapter. These examples are probably just the beginning of an entire range of novel anthracyclines that will be generated by mixing and matching various anthracycline biosynthesis genes.

VIII. FUTURE COURSE OF ANTHRACYCLINES

Despite its drawbacks, doxorubicin is still one of the most widely used antitumor drugs available. Can we find a better doxorubicin? This question, posed in the title of a recent paper (1), is paramount in cancer chemotherapy, and certainly to those working in the area of anthracycline biosynthesis. New anticancer drugs with completely different struc-tures, such as taxol, are now being tested for use against many cancers currently treated by anthracyclines. As mentioned earlier in this chapter, out of the thousands of anthra-cycline-based structures tested, the only new anthracyclines showing particular promise are piramycin, which appears to be less cardiotoxic than doxorubicin; epirubicin, which appears to have greater efficacy than daunorubicin in treating leukemia; and idarubicin, which can be given orally. Enough is now known about structure–activity relationships, however, that additional structures, some of which may be synthesized using genetic engineering methods based on knowledge of the biosynthesis of these drugs, should be synthesized and tested in more rational drug design approaches.

Additionally, with the advances in drug delivery methods, which place doxorubicin and its analogs in the direct vicinity of the tumor and which seek to avoid the massive toxicity problems associated with these drugs, doxorubicin itself appears to have been given new life. One of the limitations in doxorubicin production is the availability of stable, overproducing strains. We hope that the knowledge gained about the daunorubicin/doxorubicin biosynthesis genes and their products, the anthracycline-resistance genes, and the regulatory genes will result in the construction of strains able to overproduce doxorubicin and other anthracyclines stably. Someone told one of us (WRS) at a meeting in 1984 that doxorubicin and anthracyclines were "on their way out" in terms of cancer chemotherapy. That statement could not have been more wrong then ... or now.

ACKNOWLEDGMENTS

We sincerely thank Don Ordaz for assistance with the artwork, and C. Richard Hutchinson for several discussions on the biochemistry and molecular biology of anthracycline biosynthesis and for sharing unpublished data and ideas. Work on anthracycline biosynthesis in the Strohl laboratory, including all the unpublished work from the Strohl lab described herein, is funded by a grant (DMB-94-05730) from the National Science Foundation.

REFERENCES

1. Weiss RB. The anthracyclines: Will we ever find a better doxorubicin? Semin Oncol 1992; 19:670–686.
2. Brockmann H, Bauer K. Rhodomycin, ein rotes Antibioticum aus Actinomyceten. Naturwissenschaften 1950; 37:492–493.
3. Brockmann H Anthracyclinone und Anthracycline. (Rhodomycinone, Pyrromycinone und ihre Glykoside). Fortschr Chem Organ Naturst 1963; 121–182.
4. Arcamone F. Doxorubicin: Anticancer Antibiotics. New York: Academic Press, 1981.
5. Brockmann H, Lenk W. Über Actinomycetenfarbstoffe. VI. Pyrromycinone. Chem Ber 1959; 92:1880–1903.
6. Brockmann H, Brockmann H Jr. Rhodomycine, VIII; Antibiotica aus Actinomyceten, L. Chem Ber 1963; 96:1171–1178.
7. Grein A, Spalla C, Di Marco A, Canevazzi G. Descrizione e classificazione di un attinomicette (*Streptomyces peucetius* sp. nova) produttore di Una Sostanza ad attivita antitumorale: La daunocinina. Giorn Microbiol 1963; 11:109–118.
8. Arcamone F, DiMarco A, Gaetani M, Scotti T. Isolamento ed attività antitumorale di un antibiotico da *Streptomyces* sp. Giorn Microbiol 1961; 9:83–90.
9. Cassinelli G, Orezzi P. La daunomicina: Un nuovo antibiotico ad attività citostatica isolamento e proprietà. Giorn Microbiol 1963; 11:167–174.
10. DiMarco A, Gaetani M, Dorigotti L, Soldati M, Bellini O. Studi sperimentali sull "attivita" antineoplastica del nuovo antibiotico daunomicina. Tumori 1963; 49:203–217.
11. DiMarco A, Gaetani M, Orezzi P, Scarpinato BM, Slivestrini R, Soldati M, Dasdia T, Valentini L. "Daunomycin," a new antibiotic of the rhodomycin group. Nature (London) 1964; 201:706–707.

12. DiMarco A, Gaetani M, Dorigotti L, Soldati M, Bellini O. Daunomycin: A new antibiotic with antitumor activity. Cancer Chemother Rep 1964; 38:31–38.

13. Dubost M, Ganter P, Maral R, Ninet L, Pinnert S, Prud'homme J, Werner GH. Un novel antibiotique a properties cytostatique: La rubidomycine. CR Acad Sci 1963; 257:1813–1815.

14. Despois R, Dubost M, Mancy D, Maral R, Ninet L, Pinnert S, Preud'homme J, Charpentie Y, Belloc A, de Chezelles N, Lunel J, Renaut J. Un nouvel antibiotique doué d'activité antitumorale: La rubidomycine (13.057 R.P.). I. Préparation et propriétés. Arzneim Forsch 1967; 17:934–939.

15. Maral R, Bourat G, Fournel J, Ganter P, de Ratuld Y, Werner GH. Un nouvel antibiotique doué d'activité antitumorale: La rubidomycine (13.057 R.P.). II. Activité antitumorale expérimentale. Arzneim Forsch 1967; 17:939–948.

16. Arcamone F, Cassinelli G, Fantini G, Grein A, Orezzi P, Pol C, Spalla C. Adriamycin, 14-hydroxydaunomycin, a new antitumor antibiotic from S. *peucetius* var. *caesius*. Biotechnol Bioeng 1969; 11:1101–1110.

17. Arcamone F, Franceschi G, Penco S. Adriamycin (14-hydroxydaunomycin), a novel antitumor antibiotic. Tetrahedron Lett 1969; 13:1007–1010.

18. Bonadonna G, Monfardini S, de Lena M, Fossati-Bellani F. Clinical evaluation of adriamycin, a new antitumour antibiotic. Brit Med J 1969; 3:503–506.

19. Blum R, Carter S. Adriamycin, a new anticancer drug with significant clinical activity. Ann Intern Med 1974; 80:249–259.

20. Bhuyan BK, Dietz A. Fermentation, taxonomic, and biological studies of nogalamycin. Antimicrob Agents Chemother 1966; 1965:836–844.

21. Bergy ME, Reusser F. A new antibacterial agent (U-20661) isolated from a streptomycete strain. Experientia 1974; 23:254–257.

22. Brodasky TF, Reusser F. Steffimycin B, a new member of the steffimycin family: Isolation and characterization. J Antibiot 1974; 27:809–813.

23. Gauze GF, Sveshikova MA, Ukholina RS, Gavrilina VA, Filicheva VA, Gladkikh EG. Production of antitumor antibiotic carminomycin by *Actinomadura carminata* sp. nov. Antibiotiki 1973; 18:675–678.

24. Brazhnikova MG, Zbarsky VB, Ponomarenko VI, Potapova NP. Physical and chemical characterization and structure of carminomycin, a new antitumor antibiotic. J Antibiot 1974; 27:254–259.

25. Oki T, Matsuzawa Y, Yoshimoto A, Numata K, Kitamura I, Hori S, Takamatsu A, Umezawa H, Ishizuka M, Naganawa H, Suda H, Hamada M, Takeuchi T. New antitumor antibiotics, aclacinomycins A and B. J Antibiot 1975; 28:830–834.

26. Hori S, Shirai M, Hirano S, Oki T, Inui T, Tsukagoshi S, Ishizuka M, Takeuchi T, Umezawa H. Antitumor activity of new anthracycline antibiotics, aclacinomycin-A and its analogs, and their toxicity. Gann 1977; 68:685–690.

27. Oki T, Shibamoto N, Matsuzawa Y, Ogasawara T, Yoshimoto A, Kitamura I, Inui T, Naganawa H, Takeuchi T, Umezawa H. Production of nineteen anthracyclic compounds by *Streptomyces galilaeus* MA 144-M1. J Antibiot 1977; 30:683–687.

28. Oki T, Kitamura I, Yoshimoto A, Matsuzawa Y, Shibamoto N, Ogasawara T, Inui T, Takamatsu A, Takeuchi T, Masuda T, Hamada M, Suda H, Ishizuka M, Sawa T, Umezawa H. Antitumor anthracycline antibiotics, aclacinomycin A and analogues. I. Taxonomy, production, isolation, and physicochemical properties. J Antibiot 1979; 32:791–800.

29. Oki T, Kitamura I, Matsuzawa Y, Shibamoto N, Ogasawara T, Yoshimoto A, Inui T. Antitumor anthracycline antibiotics, aclacinomycin A and analogs. II. Structural determination. J Antibiot 1979; 32:801–819.

30. Komiyama T, Matsuzawa Y, Oki T, Inui T, Takahashi Y, Naganawa H, Takeuchi T, Umezawa H. Baumycins, new antitumor antibiotics related to daunomycin. J Antibiot 1977; 30:619–621.

31. Takahashi Y, Naganawa H, Takeuchi T, Umezawa H, Komiyama T, Oki T, Inui T. The structure of baumycins A1, A2, B1, B2, C1, and C2. J Antibiot 1977; 30:622–624.

32. Nakagawa M, Hayakawa Y, Kawai H, Imamura K, Inoue H, Shimazu A, Seto H, Otake N. A new anthracycline antibiotic, N-formyl-13-dihydrocarminomycin. J Antibiot 1983; 36:457–458.

33. Imamura K, Odagawa A, Tanabe K, Hayakawa Y, Otake N. Akrobomycin, a new anthracycline antibiotic. J Antibiot 1984; 37:83–84.

34. Kimura K, Koyama T, Nakayama S, Tamura K, Miyata N, Kawanishi G. A new anthracycline antibiotic SN-706. J Antibiot 1988; 41:1918–1921.

35. Matsuzawa Y, Yoshimoto A, Kouno K, Oki T. Baumycin analogs isolated from *Actinomadura* sp. J Antibiot 1981; 34:774–776.

36. Ogawa Y, Sugi H, Fujikawa N, Mori H. Rubeomycin, a new anthracycline antibiotic complex. I. Taxonomy of producing organism, isolation, characterization and biological activities of rubeomycin A, A$_1$, B and B$_1$. J Antibiot 1981; 34:938–950.

37. Ogawa Y, Mori H, Yamada N, Kon K. The absolute structures of rubeomycins A and A$_1$ (carminomycins II and III) and rubeomycins B and B$_1$ (4-hydroxybaumycinols A$_1$ and A$_2$). J Antibiot 1984; 37:44–56.

38. Uchida T, Imoto M, Takahashi Y, Odagawa A, Sawa T, Tatsuta K, Naganawa H, Hamada M, Takeuchi T, Umezawa H. New potent anthracyclines, barminomycins I and II. J Antibiot 1988; 41:404–408.

39. Bradner WT, Misiek M. Bohemic acid complex. Biological characterization of the antibiotics, musettamycin and marcellomycin. J Antibiot 1977; 30:519–522.

40. Nettleton DE Jr, Bradner WT, Bush JA, Coon AB, Moseley JE Myllymaki RW, O'Herron FA, Schreiber RH, Vulcano AL. New antitumor antibiotics: Musettamycin and marcellomycin from bohemic acid complex. J Antibiot 1977; 30:525–529.

41. Doyle TW, Nettleton DE Jr, Grulich RE, Balitz DM, Johnson DL, Vulcano AL. Antitumor agent from the bohemic acid complex. 4. Structure of rudolphomycin, minimycin, collinemycin and alcindoromycin. J Am Chem Soc 1979; 101:7041–7049.

42. Nettleton DE Jr, Balitz DM, Doyle TW, Bradner WT, Johnson DL, O'Herron FA, Schreiber RW, Coon AB, Moseley JE, Myllymaki RW. Antitumor agents from bohemic acid complex. III. The isolation of marcellomycin, musettamycin, rudolphomycin, mimimycin, collinemycin, aclindoromycin, and bohemamine. J Nat Prod 1980; 43:242–258.

43. Bush JA, Bradner WT, Tomita K. Production and biological activity of marcellomycin, an antitumor anthracycline antibiotic, and taxonomy of the producing organism. J Antibiot 1982; 35:1174–1183.

44. Hütter K, Baader E, Frobel K, Zeeck A, Bauer K, Gau W, Kurz J, Schröder T, Wünsche C, Karl W, Wendisch D. Viriplanin A, a new anthracycline antibiotic of the nogalamycin group. I. Isolation, characterization, degradation reactions and biological properties. J Antibiot 1986; 39:1193–1204.

45. Bannister B, Zapotocky BA. Protorubradirin, an antibiotic containing a C-nitroso sugar fragment is the true secondary metabolite produced by *Streptomyces achromogenes* var. *rubradiris*. Rubradirin described earlier as its photo-oxidation product. J Antibiot 1992; 45:1313–1324.

46. Cassinelli G, Grein A, Masi P, Suarato A, Bernardi L, Arcamone F, DiMarco A, Casazza AM, Pratesi G, Soranzo C. Preparation and biological evaluation of 4-O-demethyldaunorubicin (carminomycin I) and its 13-dihydro derivative. J Antibiot 1978; 31:178–184.

47. Oki T, Yoshimoto A. Antitumor antibiotics. Ann Rep Ferm Proc 1979; 3:215–251.

48. Aoki M, Shirai H, Nakayama N, Itezono Y, Mori M, Satoh T, Ohshima S, Watanabe J, Yokose K. Structural studies on avidinorubicin, a novel anthracycline with platelet aggregation inhibitory activity. J Antibiot 1991; 44:635–645.

49. Mancy D, Florent J, Preud'homme J. U.S. Patent 3,855,010; 1975.

50. Corbaz R, Ettlinger L, Keller-Schierlein W, Zähner H. Zur Systematik der Actinomyceten. I. Über Streptomyceten mit rhodomycinartigen Pigmenten. Arch Mikrobiol. 1957; 25:325–332.

51. Gonçalves de Lima O, Delle Monache F, D'Albuqueque IL, Marino-Bettoplo GB. The identification of ciclacidine. An antibiotic from *Streptomyces capoamus*. Tetrahedron Lett 1968; 4:471–473.

52. Fujiwara A, Hoshino A. Anthracycline antibiotics. CRC Crit Rev Biotechnol 1986; 3:133–157.
53. Ettlinger L, Gäumann E, Hütter R, Keller-Schierlein W, Fradolfer F, Neipp L, Prelog V, Reusser P, Zähner H. Stoffwechselprodukte von Actinomyceten. XVI. Cinerubine. Chem Ber 1959; 92:1867–1879.
54. Pinnert S, Ninet L. U.S. Patent 3,989,598; 1976.
55. Blumauerová M, Matějů J, Stajner K, Vanek Z. Studies on the production of daunomycinone-derived glycosides and related metabolites in Streptomyces coeruleorubidus and Streptomyces peucetius. Folia Microbiol 1977; 22:275–285.
56. Tsuji T, Takezawa M, Morioka H, Kida T, Horino I, Eto Y, Shibai H. A new anthracycline antibiotic, cosmocarcin A. Agric Biol Chem 1984; 48:3181–3184.
57. Fleck W, Strauss D, Schönfeld C, Jungstand W, Seeber C, Prauser H. Screening, fermentation, isolation, and characterization of trypanomycin, a new antibiotic. Antimicrob Agents Chemother 1972; 1:385–391.
58. Kelly RC, Scletter I, Koert JM, MacKellar FA, Wiley PF. Structures of steffimycin and steffimycin B. J Org Chem 1977; 42:3591–3596.
59. Nakata M, Saito M, Inouye Y, Nakamura S, Hayakawa Y, Seto H. A new anthracycline antibiotic, cinerubin R. Taxonomy, structural elucidation and biological activity. J Antibiot 1992; 45:1599–1608.
60. Fujiwara A, Tazoe M, Hoshino T, Sekine Y, Masuda S, Nomura S. New anthracycline antibiotics, 1-hydroxyauramycins and 1-hydroxysulfurmycins. J Antibiot 1981; 34:912–915.
61. Bradler G, Eckardt K, Fügner R. Zur Characterisierung des Streptomyces-Stammes JA 3043 und Gewinnung von Galirubin und Galirubinon. Zeitschr Allg Mikrobiol 1966; 6:361–365.
62. Královcová E, Blumauerová M, Vaněk Z. Strain improvement in Streptomyces galilaeus, a producer of anthracycline antibiotics galirubins. Folia Microbiol 1977; 22:321–328.
63. Fujiwara A, Hoshino T, Tazoe M, Fujiwara M. Auramycins and sulfurmycins, new anthracycline antibiotics: Characterization of aglycones, auramycinone and sulfurmycinone. J Antibiot 1981; 34:608–610.
64. Fujiwara A, Hoshino T, Tazoe M, Fujiwara M. New anthracycline antibiotics, auramycins and sulfurmycins. I. Characterization of the aglycones and the components A and B. J Antibiot 1982; 35:164–175.
65. Niemi J, Ylihonko K, Hakala J, Pärssinen R, Kopio A, Mäntsälä P. Hybrid anthracycline antibiotics: Production of new anthracyclines by cloned genes from Streptomyces purpurascens in Streptomyces galilaeus. Microbiol (Reading) 1994; 140:1351–1358.
66. Matsuzawa Y, Yoshimoto A, Shibamoto N, Tobe H, Oki T, Naganawa H, Takeuchi T, Umezawa H. New anthracycline metabolites from mutant strains of Streptomyces galilaeus MA144-M1. II. Structure of 2-hydroxyaklavinone and new aklavinone glycosides. J Antibiot 1981; 34:959–964.
67. Oki T, Yoshimoto A, Matsuzawa Y, Takeuchi T, Umezawa H. New anthracycline antibiotic, 2-hydroxyaclacinomycin A. J Antibiot 1981; 34:916–918.
68. Eckardt K, Schumann G, Tresselt D, Ihn W. Biosynthesis of anthracyclinones: Isolation of a new early cyclization product aklaviketone. J Antibiot 1988; 41:788–793.
69. Weber W, Zähner H, Siebers J, Schröder K, Zeeck A. Stoffwechselprodukte von Mikroorganismen. 175. Mitteilung. Tetracenomycin C. Arch Microbiol 1979; 121:111–116.
70. Gauze GF, Brazhnikova MG, Borisova VN, Maksimova TS, Olkhovatova OL, Sveshnikova MA, Federova GB. Production of beromycin and nogalamycin, anthracycline antibiotics, by a new actinomycete species, Streptomyces glomeratus sp. nov. Antibiotiki 1978; 23:483–489.
71. Gauze GF, Maksimova TS, Olkhovatova OL, Terekheva IP, Kochetkova GV, Ilchenko GB. Production of beromycin by Actinomyces griseoruber var. beromycini. Antibiotiki 1972; 17:8–11.
72. Prikrylova V, Podojil M, Sedmera P Vokoun J, Vanek Z, Brazhnikova MG, Kudinova MK. New rhodomycinone from the strain Streptomyces griseoruber 4620. Collect Czech Chem Commun 1980; 45:1991–1995.

73. Higashide E, Hasegawa T, Shibata M, Mizumo K. U.S. Patent 3,655,878; 1972.
74. David L, Duteurtre M, Kergomard A, Kergomard G, Scanzi E. Production of cinerubins by a *Streptomyces griseorubiginosus* strain. J Antibiot 1980; 33:49–53.
75. Strauss D, Fleck WF Leukaemomycin, an antibiotic with antitumor activity. II. Isolation and identification. Zeitschr Allg Mikrobiol 1975; 15:615–623.
76. Mancy D, Ninet L. U.S. Patent 3,997,661; 1976.
77. Kern DL, Bunge RH, French JC, Dixon HW. The identification of ε-rhodomycinone and 7-deoxy-daunorubicinol aglycone in daunorubicin beers. J Antibiot 1977; 30:432–434.
78. Tunac JB, Graham BD, Dobson WE, Lenzini MD. Fermentation by a new daunomycin-producing organism, *Streptomyces insignis* ATCC 31913. Appl Environ Microbiol 1985; 49:265–268.
79. Bieber LW, Da Silva Filho AA, Silva EC, De Méllo JF, Lyra FDA. The anthracycline complex retamycin. 1. Structure determination of the major constituents. J Nat Prod 1989; 52:385–388.
80. Drautz H, Reuschenbach P, Zähner H, Rohr J, Zeeck A. Metabolic products of microorganisms. 225. Elloramycin, a new anthracycline-like antibiotic from *Streptomyces olivaceus*. Isolation, characterization, structure and biological properties. J Antibiot 1985; 38:1291–1301.
81. Arcamone F, Cassinelli G, Dimatteo F, Forenza S, Ripamonti M, Rivola G, Vigevani A, Clardy J, McCabe T. Structures of novel anthracycline antitumor antibiotics from *Micromonospora peucetica*. J Am Chem Soc 1980; 102:1462–1463.
82. Cassinelli G, Forenza S, Rivola G, Arcamone F. 13-Deoxycarminomycin, a new biosynthetic anthracycline. J Nat Prod 1985; 48:435–439.
83. Grein A. Development of biosynthetic anthracyclines of the daunorubicin group by genetic and fermentation studies. Proc Biochem 1981; 16:34–35,46.
84. Cassinelli G, Ballabio M, Grein A, Merli S, Rivola G, Arcamone A, Barbieri B, Bordoni T. A new class of biosynthetic anthracyclines: Anthracyclinone glucuronides. J Antibiot 1987; 40:1071–1074.
85. Ivanitskaya LP, Upiter GD, Sveshnikova MA, Gauze GF. Systematic position, variation and antibiotic properties of tauromycetin producing organism. Antibiotiki 1966; 11:973–976.
86. Nozaki Y, Hida T, Iinuma S, Ishii T, Sudo K, Muroi M, Kanamaru T. TAN-1120, a new anthracycline with potent angiostatic activity. J Antibiot 1993; 46:569–579.
87. Nakagawa M, Furihata K, Furihata K, Adachi K, Seto H, Otake N. The structure of a new anthracycline, cinerubin X, produced by a blocked mutant of *Streptomyces violaceochromogenes*. J Antibiot 1986; 34:1178–1179.
88. Fleck W, Strauss D, Koch A, Prauser H. Fermentation and isolation of new anthracycline antibiotics, violamycin A, BI, BII and their aglycones. Antibiotiki (Moscow) 1975; 20:966–972.
89. Johdo O, Ishikura T, Yoshimoto A, Takeuchi T. Anthracycline metabolites from *Streptomyces violaceus* A262. I. Isolation of antibiotic-blocked mutants from *Streptomyces violaceus* A262. J Antibiot 1991; 44:1110–1120.
90. Kawai H, Hayakawa Y, Nakagawa M, Imamura K, Tanabe K, Shimazu A, Seto H, Otake N. Arugomycin, a new anthracycline antibiotic. J Antibiot 1983; 36:1569–1571.
91. Ishii K, Kondo S, Nishimura Y, Hamada M, Takeuchi T, Umezawa H. Decilorubicin, a new anthracycline antibiotic. J Antibiot 1983; 36:451–453.
92. Ishii K, Nishimura Y, Naganawa H, Kondo S, Umezawa H. The structure of decilorubicin. J Antibiot 1984; 37:344–353.
93. Liu WC, Rao KU. U.S. Patent 3,852,425; 1974.
94. Ubukata M, Uzawa J, Osada H, Isono K. Respinomycin A₁, A₂, B, C and D: A novel group of anthracycline antibiotics. II. Physico-chemical properties and structure elucidation. J Antibiot 1993; 46:942–951.
95. Eckardt K, Tresselt D, Schumann G, Ihn W, Wagner C. Isolation and chemical structure of

aklanonic acid, an early intermediate in the biosynthesis of anthracyclines. J Antibiot 1985; 38:1034–1039.

96. McGuire JC, Thomas MC, Pandey RC, Toussaint M, White RJ. Biosynthesis of daunorubicin glycosides: Analysis with blocked mutants. Moo-Young M, ed. Advances in Biotechnology, Vol 3. New York: Permagon Press, 1980:117–122.

97. Pandey RC, Toussaint MW, McGuire JC, Thomas MC. Maggiemycin and anhydromaggiemycin: Two novel anthracyclinone antitumor antibiotics. J Antibiot 1989; 42:1567–1577.

98. McGuire JC, Glotfelty G, White RJ. Use of cerulenin in strain improvement of the daunorubicin fermentation. FEMS Microbiol Lett 1980; 9:141–143.

99. Fujii S, Kubo K, Johdo O, Yoshimoto A, Ishikura T, Naganawa H, Sawa T, Takeuchi T, Umezawa H. A new anthracycline metabolite D788-1 (10-carboxy-13-deoxocarminomycin) in daunorubicin beer. J Antibiot 1986; 39:473–475.

100. Reddy GCS, Sahai R, Fehlhaber HW, Ganguli BN. Isolation and structure of a new ε-rhodomycin compound produced by a *Streptomyces* species HPL Y-11472. J Antibiot 1985; 38:1423–1425.

101. Hedtman U, Fehlhaber H-W, Sukatsch DA, Weber M, Hoffman D, Kraemer HP. The new cytotoxic antibiotic cytorhodin X, an unusual anthracyclinone-9α-glycoside. J Antibiot 1992; 45:1373–1475.

102. Hegyi JR, Gerber NN. N₁-Pyrromycinone, a new tetracenequinone (anthracyclinone) from *Streptomyces* sp. I-8. Tetrahedron Lett 1968; 13:1587–1589.

103. Kitamura I, Shibamoto N, Oki T, Inui T, Naganawa H, Ishizuka M, Masuda T, Takeuchi T, Umezawa H. New anthracycline antibiotics, rhodirubins. J Antibiot 1977; 30:616–618.

104. Zhang YB, Jin WZ. Isolation and structure determination of minor components of mutactimycins, a group of new anthracycline antibiotics. Chinese J Antibiot 1991; 16:157–164.

105. Xuan L-j, Xu S-h, Zhang H-l, Xu Y-m, Chen M-q. Dutomycin, a new anthracycline antibiotic from *Streptomyces*. J Antibiot 1992; 45:1974–1976.

106. Tulinsky A. The structure of isoquinocycline A. An X-ray crystallographic determination. J Am Chem Soc 1964; 86:5368–5369.

107. Asheshov IN, Gordon JJ. Rutilantin: An antibiotic substance with antiphage activity. Biochem J 1961; 31:101–104.

108. Shan K, Lincoff AM, Young JB. Anthracycline-induced cardiotoxicity. Ann Intern Med 1996; 125:47–58.

109. Doroshow JH. Role of reactive-oxygen metabolism in cardiac toxicity of anthracycline antibiotics. Priebe W, ed. Anthracycline Antibiotics: New Analogues, Methods of Delivery, and Mechanisms of Action. Washington D.C.: American Chemical Society Press, 1995:259–267.

110. Suarato A. Antitumor anthracyclines. Wilman DEV, ed. The Chemistry of Antitumour agents. Glasgow: Blackie and Son, Ltd., 1990:30–62.

111. Weiss RB, Sarosy G, Clagett-Carr K. Russo M, Leyland-Jones B. Anthracycline analogs: The past, present, and future. Cancer Chemother Pharmacol 1986; 18:185–197.

112. U.S. Food and Drug Administration Center for Drug Evaluation and Research Web Site; http://www.fda.gov/cder/drug.htm; downloaded 12/12/96.

113. Fischer DS, Knobf MT, Durivage HJ. The Cancer Chemotherapy Handbook, 4th ed. St. Louis: Mosby, 1993.

114. Kolar C, Bosslet K, Czech J, Gerken M, Hermentin P, Hoffmann D, Sedlacek H-H. Semi-synthetic rhodomycins and anthracycline prodrugs. Priebe W, ed. Anthracycline Antibiotics: New Analogues, Methods of Delivery, and Mechanisms of Action. Washington D.C.: American Chemical Society Press, 1995:59–77.

115. Monneret C, Florent J-C, Gesson J-P, Jacquesy J-C, Tillequin F, Koch M. Synthetic options for reversal of anthracycline resistance and cardiotoxicity. Priebe W, ed. Anthracycline Antibiotics. New Analogues, Methods of Delivery, and Mechanisms of Action. Washington D.C.: American Chemical Society Press, 1995:78–99.

116. Perez-Soler R, Sugarman S, Zou Y, Priebe W. Priebe W, ed. Anthracycline Antibiotics: New Analogues, Methods of Delivery, and Mechanisms of Action. Washington D.C.: American Chemical Society Press, 1995:300–319.

117. Vaněk, Tax J, Komersová, Sedmera P, Vokoun J. Anthracyclines. Folia Microbiol 1977; 22:139–159.

118. White RJ. Anthracyclines. Vining LC, ed. Biochemistry and Genetic Regulation of Commercially Important Antibiotics. Reading, Massachusetts: Addison-Wesley, 1983:277–291.

119. Oki T. Recent developments in the process improvement of production of antitumor anthracycline antibiotics. Adv Biotechnol Proc 1984; 3:163–196.

120. Arcamone F. Antitumor anthracyclines: Recent developments. Med Res Rev 1984; 4:153–188.

121. White RJ, Stroshane RM. Daunorubicin and adriamycin: Properties, biosynthesis, and fermentation. Vandamme EJ, ed. Biotechnology of Industrial Antibiotics. New York: Marcel-Dekker, 1984:569–594.

122. Aubel-Sadron G, Londos-Gagliardi D. Daunorubicin and doxorubicin, anthracycline antibiotics, a physicochemical and biological review. Biochemie 1984; 333–352.

123. Grein A. Antitumor anthracyclines produced by *Streptomyces peucetius*. Adv Appl Microbiol 1987; 32:203–214.

124. Strohl WR, Bartel PL, Connors NC, Zhu C-b, Dosch DC, Beale JM Jr, Floss HG, Stutzman-Engwall K, Otten SL, Hutchinson CR. Biosynthesis of natural and hybrid polyketides by anthracycline-producing streptomycetes. Hershberger CL, Queener SW, Hegeman G, eds. Genetics and Molecular Biology of Industrial Microorganisms. Washington, D.C.: American Society for Microbiology, 1989:68–84.

125. Wagner C, Eckardt K, Ihn W, Schumann G, Stengel C, Fleck WF, Tresselt D. Biosynthese der Anthracycline: eine Neuinterpretation der Ergebnisse zur Daunomycin-Biosynthese. J Basic Microbiol 1991; 3:233–240.

126. Hutchinson CR. Anthracyclines. Vining LC, Stuttard C, eds. Genetics and Biochemistry of Antibiotic Production. Boston: Butterworth-Heinemann, 1995:331–357

127. Crooke ST, Reich SD, eds. Anthracyclines: Current Status and New Developments. New York: Academic Press, 1980.

128. Mathé G, Maral R, De Jager R, eds. Anthracyclines: Current Status and Future Developments. New York: Masson Publishing USA, 1981.

129. El Khadem HS, ed. Anthracycline Antibiotics. New York: Academic Press, 1982.

130. Priebe W, ed. Anthracycline Antibiotics: New Analogues, Methods of Delivery, and Mechanisms of Action. Washington, D.C.: American Chemical Society Press, 1995.

131. Burrill GS. The biotechnology industry. A midyear snapshot. Biopharm 1989; July/August 12,14,16,17.

132. Fukushima M. The overdose of drugs in Japan. Nature 1989; 342:850–851.

133. Scrip's 1995 Yearbook, January 1995, PJB Publications, Ltd., Richmond, UK.

134. Nakashima H, Yamamoto N, Inouye Y, Nakamura S. Inhibition by doxorubicin of human immuno-deficiency virus (HIV) infection and replication *in vitro*. J Antibiot 1987; 40:396–399.

135. Wiley PF. Nogalamycin chemistry and analog synthesis. El Khadem HS, ed. Anthracycline Antibiotics. New York: Academic Press, 1982:97–117.

136. Umezawa H, Yamada K, Oki T. Comparative experimental studies on 4′-O-tetrahydropyranyl-adriamycin and adriamycin. Mathé G, Maral M, De Jager R, eds. Anthracyclines: Current Status and Future Developments. New York: Masson Publishing USA, 1981:183–188.

137. Hirano S, Wakazono K, Agata N, Iguchi H, Tone H. Comparison of cardiotoxicity of pirarubicin, epirubicin, and doxorubicin in the rat. Drugs Exp Clin Res 1994; 20:153–160.

138. Graham MA, Kerr DJ, Workman P. Absorption and distribution of anticancer drugs. Flo-

rence AT, Salole EG, eds. Pharmaceutical Aspects of Cancer Chemotherapy. Oxford: But-terworth-Heinemann, 1993:1–26.

139. Cutts SM, Phillips DR. Use of oligonucleotides to define the site of interstrand cross-links induced by adriamycin. Nucl Acids Res 1995; 23:2450–2456.

140. Cullinane C, van Rosmalen A, Phillips DR. Does adriamycin induce interstrand cross-links in DNA? Biochem 1994; 33:4632–4638.

141. Chen AY, Liu LF. DNA topoisomerases—essential enzymes and lethal targets. Annu Rev Pharmacol Toxicol 1994; 34:191–218.

142. Drlica K, Franco RJ. Inhibitors of DNA topoisomerases. Biochem 1988; 27:2253–2259.

143. Pommier Y. DNA topoisomerases and their inhibition by anthracyclines. Priebe W, ed. Anthracycline Antibiotics: New Analogues, Methods of Delivery, and Mechanisms of Action. Washington D.C.: American Chemical Society Press, 1995:183–203.

144. Taatjes DJ, Gaudiano G, Resing K, Koch TH. Alkylation of DNA by the anthracycline anti-tumor drugs adriamycin and daunomycin. J Med Chem 1996; 39:4135–4138.

145. Mustonen P, Kinnunen PKJ. On the reversal by deoxyribonucleic acid of the binding of adri-amycin to cardiolipin-containing liposomes. J Biol Chem 1993; 268:1074–1080.

146. Wang AH-J, Ughetto G, Quigley GJ, Rich A. Interactions between an anthracycline antibi-otic and DNA: Molecular structure of daunomycin complex to d(CpGpTpApCpG) at 1.2 Å resolution. Biochem 1987; 26:1152–1163.

147. Moore MH, Hunter WN, Langlois d'Estaintot B, Kennard O. DNA-drug interactions. The crystal structure of d(CGATCG) complexed with daunomycin. J Mol Biol 1989; 206:693–705.

148. Wang JY-T, Chao, Wang AH-J. Adducts of DNA and anthracycline antibiotics. Priebe W, ed. Anthracycline Antibiotics. New Analogues, Methods of Delivery, and Mechanisms of Action. Washington D.C.: American Chemical Society Press, 1995:168–182.

149. Chaires JB, Fox KR, Herrera JE, Britt M, Waring MJ. Site and sequence specificity of the daunomycin-DNA interaction. Biochem 1987; 26:8227–8236.

150. Chaires JB, Herrera JE, Waring MJ. Preferential binding of daunomycin to 5′A/TCG and 5′A/TCG sequences revealed by footprinting titration experiments. Biochem 1990; 29:6145–6153.

151. Shelton CJ, Harding MM, Prakash AS. Enzymatic and chemical footprinting of anthracy-cline antitumor antibiotics and related saccharide side chains. Biochem 1996; 35:7974–7982.

152. Wang AH-J, Gao Y-G, Liaw Y-C, Li Y-k. Formaldehyde cross-links daunorubicin and DNA efficiently: HPLC and X-ray diffraction studies. Biochem 1991; 30:3812–3815.

153. van Rosmalen A, Cullinane C, Cutts SM, Phillips DR. Stability of adriamycin-induced DNA adducts and interstrand crosslinks. Nucl Acids Res 1995; 23:42–50.

154. Marchini S, Gonzalez Paz O, Ripamonti M, Geroni C, Bargiotti A, Caruso M, Todeschi S, D'Incalci M, Broggini M. Sequence-specific DNA interactions by novel alkylating anthracy-cline derivatives. Anti-Cancer Drug Design 1995; 10:641–653.

155. Egholm M, Koch TH. Coupling of the anthracycline antitumor drug menogaril to 2′-deoxyguanosine through reductive activation. J Am Chem Soc 1989; 111:8291–8293.

156. Skladanowski A, Konopa J. Relevance of interstrand DNA crosslinking induced by anthra-cyclines for their biological activity. Biochem Pharmacol 1994; 47:2279–2287.

157. Liu LF. DNA topoisomerase poisons as antitumor drugs. Annu Rev Biochem 1989; 58:351–375.

158. Beck WT, Kim R, Chen M. Novel actions of inhibitors of DNA topoisomerase II in drug-resistant tumor cells. Cancer Chemother Pharmacol 1994; 34(Suppl):S14–S18.

159. Roca J, Wang JC. DNA transport by a type II DNA topoisomerase: Evidence in favor of a two-gate mechanism. Cell 1994; 77:609–616.

160. Sehested M, Jensen PB. Mapping of DNA topoisomerase II poisons (etoposide, clerocidin) and catalytic inhibitors (aclarubicin, ICRF-187) to four distinct steps in the topoisomerase II catalytic cycle. Biochem Pharmacol 1996; 51:879–886.

161. Cummings J, Anderson L, Willmott N, Smyth JF. The molecular pharmacology of doxorubicin *in vitro*. Eur J Cancer 1991; 27:532–535.

162. Osheroff N, Corbett AH, Elsea SH, Westergaard M. Defining functional drug-interaction domains on topoisomerase II by exploiting mechanistic differences between drug classes. Cancer Chemother Pharmacol 1994; 34(Suppl):S19–S25.

163. Hickman JA. Apoptosis induced by anticancer drugs. Cancer Metastasis Rev 1992; 11:121–139.

164. Capranico G, Zunino F, Kohn KW, Pommier Y. Sequence-selective topoisomerase II inhibition by anthracycline derivatives in SV40 DNA: Relationship with DNA binding affinity and cytotoxicity. Biochem 1990; 29:562–569.

165. Booser DJ, Hortobagyi GN. Anthracycline antibiotics in cancer therapy. Focus on drug resistance. Drugs 1994; 47:223–258.

166. Jensen PB, Sorensen BS, Sehested M, Demant EJF, Kjeldsen E, Friche E, Hansen HH. Different modes of anthracycline interaction with topoisomerase II. Biochem Pharmacol 1993; 45:2025–2035.

167. Holm B, Jensen PB, Sehested M, Hansen HH. In vivo inhibition of etoposide-mediated apoptosis, toxicity, and antitumor effect by the topoisomerase II–uncoupling anthracycline aclarubicin. Cancer Chemother Pharmacol 1994; 34:503–508.

168. Bachur NR, Johnson R, Yu F, Hickey R, Malkas L. Anthracycline antihelicase action. New mechanism with implications for guanosine-cytidine intercalation specificity. Priebe W, ed. Anthracycline Antibiotics: New Analogues, Methods of Delivery, and Mechanisms of action. Washington, D.C.: American Chemical Society Press, 1995:204–221.

169. Crooke ST, DuVernay VH, Galvan L, Prestayko AW. Structure-activity relationships of anthracyclines relative to effects on macromolecular syntheses. Mol Pharmacol 1978; 14:290–298.

170. DuVernay VH Jr, Essery JM, Eoyle TW, Brander WT, Crooke ST. The antitumor effects of anthracyclines. The importance of the carbomethoxy-group at position-10 of marcellomycin and rudolfomycin. Mol Pharmacol 1979; 15:341–356.

171. DuVernay VH Jr, Pachter JA, Crooke ST. DNA binding studies on several new anthracyclines antitumor antibiotics. II. The importance of the carbomethoxy-group at position-10 of the class II anthracycline molecule. Mol Pharmacol 1979; 16:623–632.

172. DuVernay VH Jr, Crooke ST. Effects of several anthracycline antitumor antibiotics on the transcriptional activity of isolated nuclei. J Antibiot 1980; 33:1048–1053.

173. DuVernay VH, Mong S, Crooke ST. Molecular pharmacology of anthracyclines: Demonstration of multiple mechanistic classes of anthracyclines. Crooke ST, Reich SD, eds. Anthracyclines: Current Status and New Developments. New York: Academic Press, 1980:61–123.

174. DuVernay VH Jr, Eubanks D, Perales R, Prestayko AW, Crooke ST. The antitumor effects of anthracyclines. II. The stereospecificity of the carbomethoxy group at position 10 of the class II anthracycline molecule. Mol Pharmacol 1982; 21:196–203.

175. Arcamone F. Structure-activity relationships. Mathé G, Maral M, De Jager R, eds. Anthracyclines: Current Status and Future Developments. New York: Masson Publishing USA, 1981:79–84.

176. Oki T. Microbial transformations of anthracycline antibiotics and development of new anthracyclines. El Khadem HS, ed. Anthracycline Antibiotics. New York: Academic Press, 1982:75–96.

177. Formelli F, DiMarco A, Casazza AM, Pratesi G, Supino R, Mariani A. Biological properties of 4-demethoxydaunorubicin: In vitro and in vivo studies. Curr Chemother 1978; 2:1240–1242.

178. Supino R, Necco A, Dasdia T, Casazza AM, DiMarco A. Relationship between effects on nucleic acid synthesis in cell cultures and cytotoxicity of 4-demethoxy derivatives of daunorubicin and adriamycin. Cancer Res 1977; 37:4523–4528.

179. Preobrazhenskaya MN, Bakina EV, Povarov LS, Lazhko EI, Aleksandrova LG, Balzarini J, de

Clercq E. Synthesis and cytostatic properties of daunorubicin derivatives, containing *N*-phenylthiourea or *N*-ethylthiourea moieties in the 3'-position. J Antibiot 1991; 44:192–199.

180. Zunino F, Casazza AM, Pratesi G, Formelli F, DiMarco A. Effect of methylation of aglycone hydroxyl groups on the biological and biochemical properties of daunorubicin. Biochem Pharmacol 1981; 30:1856–1858.

181. Matsuzawa Y, Oki T, Takeuchi T, Umezawa H. Structure-activity relationships of anthracyclines relative to cytotoxicity and effects on macromolecular synthesis in L1210 leukemia cells. J Antibiot 1981; 34:1596–1607.

182. DuVernay VH. Molecular pharmacology of anthracycline antitumor antibiotics. Crooke ST, Prestayko AW, eds. Cancer and Chemotherapy, Vol III. Antineoplastic Agents. New York: Academic Press, 1981:233–271.

183. Forrest GL, Akman S, Doroshow J, Rivera H, Kaplan WD. Genomic sequence and expression of a cloned human carbonyl reductase gene with daunorubicin reductase activity. Mol Pharmacol 1991; 40:502–507.

184. Marshall VP, McGovren JP, Richard FA, Richard RE, Wiley PF. Microbial metabolism of anthracycline antibiotics daunomycin and adriamycin. J Antibiot 1978; 31:336–342.

185. Olson RD, Mushlin PS, Brenner DE, Fleischer S, Cusack BJ, Chang BK, Boucek RJ. Doxorubicin cardiotoxicity may be caused by its metabolite doxorubicinol. Proc Natl Acad Sci USA 1988; 85:3585–3589.

186. Horton D, Priebe W. New adriamycin analogs. Synthesis and antitumor activity of 14-substituted 7-O(3,4-di-O-acetyl-2,6-dideoxy-α-L-*lyxo*-hexopyranosyl) daunomycinones. J Antibiot 1981; 34:1019–1025.

187. Tanaka H, Yoshioka T, Shimauchi Y, Matsuzawa Y, Oki T, Inui T. Chemical modification of anthracycline antibiotics. I. Demethoxycarbonylation, 10-epimerization and 4-O-methylation of aclacinomycin A. J Antibiot 1980; 33:1323–1330.

188. Li LH, Kuentzel SL, Murch LL, Pschigoda LM, Krueger WC. Comparative biological and biochemical effects of nogalamycin and its analogs on L1210 leukemia. Cancer Res 1979; 39:4816–4822.

189. Yoshimoto A, Fujii S, Johdo O, Kubo K, Ishikura T, Naganawa H, Sawa T, Takeuchi T, Umezawa H. Intensely potent anthracycline antibiotic oxaunomycin produced by blocked mutant of daunorubicin-producing organism. J Antibiot 1986; 39:902–909.

190. Tsuchiya T, Takagi Y. Synthesis and biological activities of fluorinated daunorubicin and doxorubicin analogues. Priebe W, ed. Anthracycline Antibiotics: New Analogues, Methods of Delivery, and Mechanisms of Action. Washington D.C.: American Chemical Society Press, 1995:100–114.

191. Johdo O, Tone H, Okamoto R, Yoshimoto A. Photochemically obtained *N*-demethyl derivatives of anthracyclines. J Antibiot 1992; 45:1653–1661.

192. Zbinden G, Pfister M, Holderegger C. Cardiotoxicity of N,N-dimethyladriamycin (NSC-261045) in rats. Toxicol Lett 1978; 1:267–274.

193. Zbinden G. Cardiotoxicity models. Mathé G, Maral M, De Jager R, eds. Anthracyclines: Current Status and Future Developments. New York: Masson Publishing USA, 1981:49–53.

194. Arcamone F, Penco S, Vigevani A, Redaelli S, Franchi G, DiMarco A, Casazza AM, Dasdia T, Formelli F, Necco A, Soranzo C. Synthesis and antitumor properties of new glycosides of daunomycinone and adriamycinone. J Med Chem 1975; 18:703–707.

195. Slate DL, Frazer-Smith EB, Rosete JB, Freitas VR, Kim YN, Casey SM. Modulation of doxorubicin efficacy in P388 leukemia following co-administration of verapamil in mini-osmotic pumps. In Vivo 1993; 7:519–524.

196. Giaccone G, Linn SC, Pinedo HM. Multidrug resistance in breast cancer: Mechanisms, strategy. Eur J Cancer 1995; 31A(Suppl 7):S15–S17.

197. Endicott JA, Ling V. The biochemistry of P-glycoprotein-mediated multidrug resistance. Annu Rev Biochem 1989; 58:137–171.

198. Gottesman MM, Pastan I. The multidrug transporter, a double-edged sword. J Biol Chem 1988; 263:12163–12166.

199. Cole SPC, Bhardwaj G, Gerlach JH, Mackie JE, Grant CE, Almquist KC, Stewart AJ, Kurz EU, Duncan AMV, Deeley RG. Overexpression of a transporter gene in a multidrug resistant human lung cancer cell line. Science 1992; 258:1650–1654.

200. Cole SPC, Deeley RG. Multidrug resistance associated with overexpression of MRP. Hait WN, ed. Drug Resistance. Boston: Kluwer Academic Publishers, 1996:39–62.

201. Scheper RJ, Broxterman HJ, Scheffer GL, Kaaijk P, Dalton WS, van Heijningen TH, van Kalken CK, Slovak ML, de Vries EG, van der Valk P. Overexpression of a Mr 110,000 vesicular protein in non P-glycoprotein mediated multidrug resistance. Cancer Res 1993; 53:1475–1479.

202. Doyle LA, Kaufman SH, Fojo AT, Bailey CL, Gazdar AF. A novel 95 kilodalton membrane polypeptide associated with lung cancer drug resistance. Lung Cancer 1993; 9:317–326.

203. Sinha BK. Topoisomerase inhibitors: A review of their therapeutic potential in cancer. Drugs 1995; 49:11–19.

204. Shan K, Lincoff AM, Young JB. Anthracycline-induced cardiotoxicity. Ann Intern Med 1996; 125:47–58.

205. Hale JP, Lewis IJ. Anthracyclines: Cardiotoxicity and its prevention. Arch Dis Childhood 1994; 71:457–462.

206. Keizer HG, Pinedo HM, Schuurhuis GJ, Hoenje H. Doxorubicin (adriamycin): A critical review of free radical–dependent mechanisms of cytotoxicity. Pharm Ther 1990; 47:219–231.

207. Witiak DT, Herman EH. Amelioration of anthracycline-induced cardiotoxicity by organic chemicals. Priebe W, ed. Anthracycline Antibiotics: New Analogues, Methods of Delivery, and Mechanisms of Action. Washington, D.C.: American Chemical Society Press, 1995:268–299.

208. Seifert CF, Nesser ME, Thompson DF. Dexrazoxane in the prevention of doxorubicin-induced cardiotoxicity. Ann Pharmacother 1994; 28:1063–1072.

209. Buss JL, Hasinoff BB. The one-ring open hydrolysis product intermediates of the cardioprotective agent ICRF-187 (dexrazoxane) displace iron from iron-anthracycline complexes. Agents Actions 1993; 40:86–95.

210. Cummings J, Smyth JF. Cytotoxic drug delivery. Florence AT, Salole EG, eds. Pharmaceutical Aspects of Cancer Chemotherapy. Topics in Pharmacy, Vol. 3. Oxford: Butterworth-Heinemann, 1993:27–53.

211. Harrison M, Tomlinson D, Stewart S. Liposome-entrapped doxorubicin: An active agent in AIDS-related Kaposi's sarcoma. J Clin Oncol 1995; 13:914–920.

212. Trail PA, Willner D, Lasch SJ, Henderson AJ, Hofstead S, Casazza AM, Firestone RA, Hellström I, Hellström KE. Cure of xenografted human carcinomas by BR96-doxorubicin immunoconjugates. Science 1993; 261:212–215.

213. Melton RG, Knox RJ, Connors TA. Antibody-directed enzyme prodrug therapy (ADEPT). Drugs Future 1996; 21:167–282.

214. Houba PHJ, Leenders RGG, Boven E, Scheeren JW, Pinedo HM, Haisma HJ. Characterization of novel anthracycline prodrugs activated by human β-glucuronidase for use in antibody-directed enzyme prodrug therapy. Biochem Pharmacol 1996; 52:455–463.

215. Gessen J-P, Jacquesy J-C, Mondon M, Petit P, Renoux B, Andrianomenjanahary S, Dufat-Trinh Van H, Koch M, Bosslet K, Czech J, Hoffman D. Prodrugs of anthracyclines for chemotherapy via enzyme–monoclonal antibody conjugates. Anti-Cancer Drug Design 1994; 9:409–423.

216. Vrudhula VM, Svensson HP, Senter PD. Cephalosporin derivatives of doxorubicin as prodrugs for activation by monoclonal antibody-β-lactamase conjugates. J Med Chem 1995; 38:1380–1385.

217. Andrianomenjanahary S, Dong X, Florent JC, Gaudel G, Gesson J-P, Jacquesy J-C, Koch M, Michel S, Mondon M, Petit P, Renoux B Tillequin F. Synthesis of novel targeted pro-prodrugs of anthracyclines potentially activated by a monoclonal antibody galactosidase conjugate. Bioorg Med Chem Lett 1992; 2:1093–1096.

218. Haisma HJ, Boven E, van Muijen M, Dejong J, Vandervijgh WJF, Pinedo HM. A monoclonal antibody-β-glucuronidase conjugate as activator of the prodrug epirubicin-glucuronide for specific treatment of cancer. Brit J Cancer 1992; 66:474–478.

219. Senter PD. Activation of prodrugs by antibody-enzyme conjugates, a new approach to cancer chemotherapy. FASEB J 1990; 4:188–193.

220. Kerr DE, Senter PD, Burnett WV, Hirschberg DL, Hellstrom I, Hellstrom KE. Antibody–penicillin V–amidase conjugates kill antigen-positive tumor cells when combined with doxorubicin phenoxyacetamide. Cancer Immunol Immunother 1990; 31:202–206.

221. Bartel PL, Connors, NC, Strohl WR. Biosynthesis of anthracyclines: Analysis of mutants of *Streptomyces* sp. strain C5 blocked in daunomycin biosynthesis. J Gen Microbiol 1990; 136:1877–1886.

222. Connors NC, Bartel PL, Strohl WR. Biosynthesis of anthracyclines: Enzymic conversion of aklanonic acid to aklavinone and ε-rhodomycinone by anthracycline-producing streptomycetes. J Gen Microbiol 1990; 136:1887–1894.

223. Hong Y-S, Hwang CK, Hong S-K, Kim YH, Lee JJ. Molecular cloning and characterization of the aklavinone 11-hydroxylase gene of *Streptomyces peucetius* subsp. *caesius* ATCC 27952. J Bacteriol 1994; 176:7096–7101.

224. Hwang CK, Kim HS, Hong Y-S, Kim YH, Hong S-K, Kim S-J, Lee JJ. Expression of *Streptomyces peucetius* genes for doxorubicin resistance and aklavinone 11-hydroxylase in *Streptomyces galilaeus* ATCC 31133 and production of a hybrid aclacinomycin. Antimicrob Agents Chemother 1995; 39:1616–1620.

225. Filippini S, Solinas MM, Breme U, Schlüter MB, Gabellini D, Biamonti G, Colombo AL, Garofano L. *Streptomyces peucetius* daunorubicin biosynthesis gene, *dnrF*: Sequence and heterologous expression. Microbiol 1995; 141:1007–1016.

226. Kim H-S, Hong Y-S, Kim Y-H, Yoo O-J, Lee JJ. New anthracycline metabolites produced by the aklavinone 11-hydroxylase gene in *Streptomyces galilaeus* ATCC 31133. J Antibiot 1996; 49:355–360.

227. Eckardt K, Wagner C. Biosynthesis of anthracyclinones. J Basic Microbiol 1988; 28:137–144.

228. Wagner C, Eckardt K, Tresselt D, Ihn W, Schumann G, Fleck WF. Leukaemomycin-geblockte Mutanten des *Streptomyces griseus* und ihre Pigmente. Zeitschr Allg Mikrobiol 1981; 21:751–760.

229. Wagner C, Stengel C, Eritt I, Schumann G, Fleck WF. Leukaemomycin-geblockte Mutanten des *Streptomyces griseus* und ihre Pigmente. III. 11-Desoxydaunomycinon-derivate aus der Mutante ZIMET 43 699/G44. J Basic Microbiol 1985; 25:687–693.

230. Bonfante V. Toxic and therapeutic activity of 4′-epidoxorubicin. Mathé G, Maral M, De Jager R, eds. Anthracyclines: Current Status and Future Developments. New York: Masson Publishing USA, 1981:149–152.

231. Umezawa H, Takahashi Y, Kinoshita M, Naganawa H, Masuda T, Ishizuka M, Tatsuta K, Takeuchi T. Tetrahydropyranyl derivatives of daunomycin and adriamycin. J Antibiot 1979; 32:1082–1084.

232. Paulick RC, Casey ML, Whitlock HW. A ^{13}C nuclear magnetic resonance study of the biosynthesis of daunomycin from ^{13}CH$_3$^{13}CO$_2$Na. J Am Chem Soc 1976; 98:3370–3371.

233. Casey ML, Paulick RC, Whitlock. Carbon-13 nuclear magnetic resonance study of the biosynthesis of daunomycin and islandicin. J Org Chem 1978; 43:1627–1634.

234. Kitamura I, Tobe H, Yoshimoto A, Oki T, Nagahawa H, Takeuchi T, Umezawa H. Biosynthesis of aklavinone and aclacinomycins. J Antibiot 1981; 34:1498–1500.

235. Niemi J, Mäntsälä P. Nucleotide sequences and expression of genes from *Streptomyces purpurascens* that cause the production of new anthracyclines in *Streptomyces galilaeus*. J Bacteriol 1995; 177:2942–2945.

236. Strohl WR, Ye J, Dickens ML. Daunomycin biosynthesis genes of *Streptomyces* sp. strain C5. Debabov VG, Dudnik YV, Danilenko VN, eds. Proceedings of the Ninth International Symposium on the Biology of the Actinomycetes. Moscow: All-Russia Scientific Research Institute for Genetics and Selection of Industrial Microorganisms, 1995:45–54.

237. Dickens ML, Ye J, Strohl WR. Analysis of clustered genes encoding both early and late steps in daunomycin biosynthesis by *Streptomyces* sp. strain C5. J Bacteriol 1995; 177:536–543.

238. Madduri K, Hutchinson CR. Functional characterization and transcriptional analysis of a gene cluster governing early and late steps in daunorubicin biosynthesis in *Streptomyces peucetius*. J Bacteriol 1995; 177:3879–3884.

239. Dickens ML, Priestley ND, Strohl WR. *In vivo* and *in vitro* bioconversion of ε-rhodomycinone glycoside to doxorubicin: Functions of DauP, DauK, and DoxA. J Bacteriol 1997; 179(8):in press.

240. Connors NC, Bartel PL, Strohl WR. Biosynthesis of anthracyclines: Carminomycin 4-O-methyltransferase, the terminal enzymic step in the formation of daunomycin. J Gen Microbiol 1990; 136:1895–1898.

241. Connors NC, Strohl WR. Partial purification and properties of carminomycin 4-O-methyltransferase from *Streptomyces* sp. strain C5. J Gen Microbiol 1993; 139:1353–1362.

242. Madduri K, Torti F, Colombo AL, Hutchinson CR. Cloning and sequencing of a gene encoding carminomycin 4-O-methyltransferase from *Streptomyces peucetius* and its expression in *Escherichia coli*. J Bacteriol 1993; 175:3900–3904.

243. Scotti C, Hutchinson CR. Immobilization and properties of carminomycin 4-O-methyltransferase, the enzyme which catalyzes the final step in the biosynthesis of daunorubicin in *Streptomyces peucetius*. Biotechnol Bioeng 1995; 48:133–140.

244. Dickens ML, Strohl WR. Isolation and characterization of a gene from *Streptomyces* sp. strain C5 that confers on *Streptomyces lividans* TK24 the ability to convert daunomycin to doxorubicin. J Bacteriol 1996; 178:3389–3395.

245. Bartel PL, Zhu C-b, Lampel JS, Dosch DC, Connors NC, Strohl WR, Beale JM Jr, Floss HG. Biosynthesis of anthraquinones by interspecies cloning of actinorhodin biosynthesis genes in streptomycetes: Clarification of actinorhodin gene functions. J Bacteriol 1990; 172:4816–4826.

246. Tsukamato N, Fujii I, Ebizuka Y, Sankawa U. Nucleotide sequence of the *aknA* region of the aklavinone biosynthetic gene cluster of *Streptomyces galilaeus*. J Bacteriol 1994; 176:2473–2475.

247. Strohl WR, Connors NC Significance of anthraquinone formation resulting from the cloning of actinorhodin genes in heterologous streptomycetes. Mol Microbiol 1992; 6:147–152.

248. Královkova E, Tax J, Blumauerová M, Vanek Z. Bewerlungder Produktion von Glycosiden der ε-Pyrromycinons (Galirubine) bei der Züchtung des Stammes *Streptomyces galilaeus*. Zeitschr Allg Mikrobiol 1977; 17:47–50.

249. Wiley PF, Elrod DW, Marshall VP. Biosynthesis of the anthracycline antibiotics nogalamycin and steffimycin B. J Org Chem 1978; 43:3457–3461.

250. Lasota WS, de Valeriola DL, Piccart MJ. Potential role of oral anthracyclines in older patients with cancer. Drugs Aging 1994; 4:392–402.

251. Rohr J, Zeeck A. Structure-activity relationships of elloramycin and tetracenomycin C. J Antibiot 1990; 43:1169–1178.

252. Hutchinson CR. Antibiotics from genetically engineered microorganisms. Strohl WR, ed. Biotechnology of Industrial Antibiotics, 2nd ed. New York: Marcel Dekker, 1997.

253. Bibb MJ, Biro S, Motamedi H, Collins JF, Hutchinson CR. Analysis of the nucleotide sequence of the *Streptomyces glaucescens tcmI* genes provides key information about the enzymology of polyketide tetracenomycin C antibiotic biosynthesis. EMBO J 1989; 8:2727–2736.

254. Shen B, Hutchinson CR. Enzymatic synthesis of a bacterial polyketide from acetyl and malonyl coenzyme A. Science 1993; 262:1535–1540.

255. Hutchinson CR, Fujii I. Polyketide synthase gene manipulation: A structure-function approach in engineering novel antibiotics. Annu Rev Microbiol 1995; 49:201–238.

256. Summers RG, Wendt-Pienkowski E, Motamedi H, Hutchinson CR Nucleotide sequence of the *tcmII-tcmIV* region of the tetracenomycin C biosynthetic gene cluster of *Streptomyces*

glaucescens and evidence that the *tcmN* gene encodes a multifunctional cyclase-dehydratase-O-methyl transferase. J Bacteriol 1992; 174:1810–1820.

257. McDaniel R, Hutchinson CR, Khosla C. Engineered biosynthesis of novel polyketides: Analysis of TcmN function in tetracenomycin biosynthesis. J Am Chem Soc 1995; 117:6805–6810.

258. Shen B, Hutchinson CR. Deciphering the mechanism for the assembly of aromatic polyketides by a bacterial polyketide synthase. Proc Natl Acad Sci USA 1996; 93:6600–6604.

259. Shen B, Hutchinson CR. Tetracenomycin F1 monooxygenase: Oxidation of a naphthacenone to a naphthacenequinone in the biosynthesis of tetracenomycin C in *Streptomyces glaucescens*. Biochem 1993; 32:6656–6663.

260. Decker H, Rohr J, Motamedi H, Zähner H, Hutchinson CR. Identification of *Streptomyces olivaceus* Tü2353 genes involved in the production of the polyketide elloramycin. Gene 1995; 166:121–126.

261. Dekleva ML, Titus JA, Strohl WR. Nutrient effects on anthracycline production by *Streptomyces peucetius* in a defined medium. Can J Microbiol 1985; 31:287–294.

262. Dekleva ML, Strohl WR. Glucose-mediated acidogenesis by *Streptomyces peucetius*. Can J Microbiol 1987; 33:1129–1132.

263. Hopwood DA, Bibb MJ, Chater KF, Kieser T, Bruton CJ, Kieser HM, Lydiate DJ, Smith CP, Ward JM, Schrempf H. Genetic manipulation of *Streptomyces*: A laboratory manual. Norwich, England: The John Innes Foundation, 1985.

264. Dekleva ML, Strohl WR. Biosynthesis of ε-rhodomycinone from glucose by *Streptomyces* C5. Can J Microbiol 1988; 34:1235–1240.

265. Guilfoile PG, Hutchinson CR. A bacterial analog of the *mdr* gene of mammalian tumor cells is present in *Streptomyces peucetius*, the producer of daunorubicin and doxorubicin. Proc Natl Acad Sci USA 1991; 88:8553–8557.

266. Ylihonko K, Hakala J, Kunnari T, Mäntsälä P. Production of hybrid anthracycline antibiotics by heterologous expression of *Streptomyces nogalater* nogalamycin biosynthesis genes. Microbiol (Reading) 1996; 142:1965–1972.

267. Wiley PF, Koert JM, Elrod DW, Reisender EA, Marshall VP. Bacterial metabolism of anthracycline antibiotics steffimycinone and steffimycinol conversions. J Antibiot 1977; 30:649–654.

268. Marshall VP, Reisender EA, Wiley PF. Bacterial metabolism of daunomycin. J Antibiot 1976; 29:966–968.

269. Shirling EB, Gottlieb D. Cooperative description of type cultures of *Streptomyces*. IV. Species descriptions from the second, third, and fourth studies. Int J Syst Bacteriol 1969; 19:391–512.

270. Yoshimoto A, Oki T, Takeuchi T, Umezawa H. Microbial conversion of anthracyclinones to daunomycin by blocked mutants of *Streptomyces coeruleorubidus*. J Antibiot 1980; 33:1158–1166.

271. McGuire JC, Hamilton BK, White RJ. Approaches to development of the daunorubicin fermentation. Proc Biochem 1979; 14:2–5.

272. Hamilton B, White R, McGuire J, Montgomery P, Stroshane R, Kalita C, Pandey R. Improvement of the daunorubicin fermentation realized at 10,000 liter fermentor scale. Moo-Young M, ed. Advances in Biotechnology, Vol. 3. New York: Permagon Press, 1980:63–68.

273. Nakamura T, Yoshimoto A. Daunomycin fermentation: Enhanced production of daunomycin by iron salt and an approach for its recovery and purification from fermentation broth. J Fac Appl Biol Sci Hiroshima Univ 1995; 34:43–54.

274. Kuhn SP, Lampel JS, Strohl WR. Isolation and characterization of a temperate bacteriophage from *Streptomyces galilaeus*. Appl Environ Microbiol 1987; 53:2708–2713.

275. Lampel JS, Strohl WR. Transformation and transfection of anthracycline-producing streptomycetes. Appl Environ Microbiol 1986; 51:126–131.

276. Ylihonko K, Tuikkanen, Jussila S, Cong L, Mäntsälä P. A gene cluster involved in nogala-mycin biosynthesis from *Streptomyces nogalater:* Sequence analysis and complementation of early-block mutations in the anthracycline pathway. Mol Gen Genet 1996; 251:113–120.

277. Ward JM, Janssen GR, Kieser T, Bibb MJ, Buttner MJ. Construction and characterisation of a series of multi-copy promoter-probe plasmid vectors for *Streptomyces* using the aminogly-coside phosphotransferase gene from Tn5 as indicator. Mol Gen Genet 1986; 203:468–478.

278. Pandey RC, Kalita CC, White RJ, Toussaint MW. Process development in the purification of daunorubicin from fermentation broths. Proc Biochem 1979; 14:6–13.

279. Yoshimoto A, Fuji S, Johdo O, Kubo K, Nishida H, Okamoto R. Anthracycline metabolites from baumycin-producing *Streptomyces* sp. D788. II. New anthracycline metabolites pro-duced by a blocked mutant strain RPM-5. J Antibiot 1993; 46:56–64.

280. Dickens ML, Ye J, Strohl WR. Cloning, sequencing and analysis of aklaviketone reductase from *Streptomyces* sp. strain C5. J Bacteriol 1996; 178:3384–3388.

281. Pandey RC, Toussaint MW. High-performance liquid chromatography and thin-layer chro-matography of anthracycline antibiotics. Separation and identification of components of the daunorubicin complex from fermentation broth. J Chromatogr 1980; 198:407–420.

282. Bachur NR, Gee M. Microsomal reductive glycosidase. J Pharmacol Exp Ther 1976; 197:681–686.

283. Yoshimoto A, Tobe H, Johdo O, Ishikura T, Takeuchi T. Structure sensitivity relationship of anthracycline antibiotics to C7-reduction by redox enzymes. J Antibiot 1991; 44:287–295.

284. Rueckert PW, Wiley PF, McGovern JP, Marshall VP. Mammalian and microbial cell-free conversion of anthracycline antibiotics and analogs. J Antibiot 1979; 32:141–147.

285. Wiley PF, Marshall VP. Microbial conversion of anthracycline antibiotics. J Antibiot 1975; 28:838–840.

286. McCarville M, Marshall V. Partial purification and characterization of a bacterial enzyme catalyzing reductive cleavage of anthracycline glycosides. Biochem Biophys Res Commun 1977; 74:331–335.

287. Marshall VP. Microbial transformations of anthracycline antibiotics and analogs. Dev Industr Microbiol 1985; 26:129–142.

288. Gräfe U, Dornberger K, Wagner C, Eckardt K. Advances in bioconversion of anthracycline antibiotics. Biotech Adv 1989; 7:215–239.

289. Blumauerová M, Královcová E, Matějů J, Jizba J, Vaněk Z. Biotransformations of anthracy-clinones in *Streptomyces coeruleorubidus* and *Streptomyces galilaeus.* Folia Microbiol 1979; 24:117–127.

290. Karnetová J, Matějů J, Sedmera P, Vokoun J, Vaněk Z. Microbial transformation of dauno-mycinone by *Streptomyces aureofaciens* B-96. J Antibiot 1976; 29:1199–1202.

291. Marek M, Valentová O, Demnerová K, Jizba J, Blumauerová M, Kás J. Immobilized prepara-tions for the biotransformation of daunomycinone. Biotechnol Lett 1981; 3:327–330.

292. Aszalos AA, Bachur NR, Hamilton BK, Langlykke AF, Roller PP, Sheikh MY, Sutphin MS, Thomas MC, Wareheim DA, Wright LH. Microbial reduction of the side-chain carbonyl of daunorubicin and N-acetyldaunorubicin. J Antibiot 1977; 30:50–58.

293. Hamilton BK, Sutphin MS, Thomas MC, Wareheim DA, Aszalos AA. Microbial N-acetyla-tion of daunorubicin and daunorubicinol. J Antibiot 1977; 30:425–426.

294. Cassinelli G, Arlandini E, Ballabio M, Bordoni T, Geroni C, Giuliani F, Grein A, Merli S, Rivola G. New biosynthetic anthracyclines related to barminomycins incorporating barbitu-rates in their moiety. J Antibiot 1990; 43:19–28.

295. Stutzman-Engwall KJ, Hutchinson CR. Multigene families for anthracycline antibiotic pro-duction in *Streptomyces peucetius.* Proc Natl Acad Sci USA 1989; 86:3135–3139.

296. Otten SL, Stutzman-Engwall KJ, Hutchinson CR. Cloning and expression of daunorubicin biosynthesis genes from *Streptomyces peucetius* and *S. peucetius* subsp *caesius.* J Bacteriol 1990; 172:3427–3434.

297. Hong Y-S, Hwang CK, Hwang DY, Kim YH, Kim SJ, Lee JJ. Cloning and sequencing of a gene cluster for the resistance to doxorubicin from *Streptomyces peucetius* subsp. *caesius* ATCC 27952. J Microbiol Biotechnol 1992; 2:153–160.

298. Stutzman-Engwall KJ, Otten SL, Hutchinson CR. Regulation of secondary metabolism in *Streptomyces* spp. and overproduction of daunorubicin in *Streptomyces peucetius*. J Bacteriol 1992; 174:144–154.

299. Grimm A, Madduri K, Ali A, Hutchinson CR. Characterization of the *Streptomyces peucetius* ATCC 29050 genes encoding doxorubicin polyketide synthase. Gene 1994; 151:1–10.

300. Otten SL, Ferguson J, Hutchinson CR. Regulation of daunorubicin production in *Streptomyces peucetius* by the $dnrR_2$ locus. J Bacteriol 1995; 177:1216–1224.

301. Otten SL, Liu X, Ferguson J, Hutchinson CR. Cloning and characterization of the *Streptomyces peucetius dnrQS* gene encoding a daunosamine biosynthesis enzyme and a glycosyl transferase involved in daunorubicin biosynthesis. J Bacteriol 1995; 177:6688–6692.

302. Gallo MA, Ward J, Hutchinson CR. The *dnrM* gene in *Streptomyces peucetius* contains a naturally occurring frameshift mutation that is suppressed by another locus outside of the daunorubicin-production gene cluster. Microbiol (Reading) 1996; 142:269–275.

303. Lomovskaya N, Hong S-K, Kim S-U, Fonstein L, Furuya K, Hutchinson CR. The *Streptomyces peucetius drrC* gene encodes a UvrA-like protein involved in daunorubicin resistance and production. J Bacteriol 1996; 178:3238–3245.

304. Ye J, Dickens ML, Plater R, Li Y, Lawrence J, Strohl WR. Isolation and sequence analysis of polyketide synthase genes from the daunomycin-producing *Streptomyces* sp. strain C5. J Bacteriol 1994; 176:6270–6280.

305. Krügel H, Schumann G, Hanel F, Fiedler G. Nucleotide sequence analysis of five putative *Streptomyces griseus* genes, one of which complements an early function in daunorubicin biosynthesis that is linked to a putative gene cluster involved in TDP-daunosamine formation. Mol Gen Genet 1993; 241:193–202.

306. Thompson MW, Strohl WR, Floss HG. Purification and characterization of TDP-D-glucose 4,6-dehydratase from anthracycline-producing streptomycetes. J Gen Microbiol 1992; 138:779–786.

307. Thorson JS, Lo SF, Liu HW, Hutchinson CR. Biosynthesis of 3,6-dideoxyhexoses: New mechanistic reflections upon 2,6-dideoxy, 4,6-dideoxy, and amino sugar construction. J Am Chem Soc 1993; 115:6993–6994.

308. Madduri K, Hutchinson CR. Functional characterization and transcriptional analysis of the $dnrR_1$ locus, which controls daunorubicin biosynthesis in *Streptomyces peucetius*. J Bacteriol 1995; 177:1208–1215.

309. Tang L, Grimm A, Zhang Y-X, Hutchinson CR. Purification and characterization of the DNA-binding protein DnrI, a transcriptional factor of daunorubicin biosynthesis in *Streptomyces peucetius*. Mol Microbiol 1996; 22:801–813.

310. Rajgarhia VB, Strohl WR. Minimal *Streptomyces* sp. strain C5 daunorubicin polyketide biosynthesis genes required for aklanonic acid biosynthesis. J Bacteriol 1997; 179(8):in press.

311. Kendrew SG, Deutsch E, Madduri K, Hutchinson CR. Aklanoic acid methyl ester cyclase: An intramolecular aldol condensation in the biosynthesis of daunorubicin. Bloomington, Indiana Abstracts, Sixth Conference on the Genetics and Molecular Biology of Industrial Microorganisms, 1996:P4.

312. Gibb GD, Dekleva ML, Lampel JS, Strohl WR. Isolation and characterization of a *Streptomyces* C5 mutant strain hyperproductive of extracellular protease. Biotechnol Lett 1987; 9:605–610.

313. Tsukamoto N, Fujii I, Ebizuka Y, Sankawa U. Cloning of aklavinone biosynthesis genes from *Streptomyces galilaeus*. J Antibiot 1992; 45:1286–1294.

314. Ylihonko K, Hakala J, Niemi J, Lundell J, Mäntsälä P. Isolation and characterization of aclacinomycin A–non-producing *Streptomyces galilaeus* (ATCC 31615) mutants. Microbiol (Reading) 1994; 140:1359–1365.

315. Wagner C, Eckardt K, Schumann G, Ihn W, Tresselt D. Microbial transformation of aklanonic acid, a potential early intermediate in the biosynthesis of anthracyclines. J Antibiot 1984; 37:691–692.

316. Eckardt K, Schumann G, Gräfe U, Ihn W, Wagner C, Fleck WF, Thrum H. Preparation of labeled aklanonic acid and its bioconversion to anthracyclinones by mutants of *Streptomyces griseus*. J Antibiot 1985; 38:1096–1097.

317. Schumann G, Stengel C, Eckardt K, Ihn W. Biotransformation of aklanonic acid by blocked mutants of anthracycline-producing strains of *Streptomyces galilaeus* and *Streptomyces peucetius*. J Basic Microbiol 1986; 26:249–255.

318. Dekleva ML, Strohl WR. Activity of phosphoenolpyruvate carboxylase of an anthracycline-producing streptomycete. Can J Microbiol 1988; 34:1241–1246.

319. Tang L, Zhang Y-X, Hutchinson CR. Amino acid catabolism and antibiotic biosynthesis: Valine is a source of precursors for macrolide biosynthesis in *Streptomyces ambofaciens* and *Streptomyces fradiae*. J Bacteriol 1994; 176:6107–6119.

320. Fernández-Moreno MA, Martínez E, Boto L, Hopwood DA, Malpartida F. Nucleotide sequence and deduced functions of a set of cotranscribed genes of *Streptomyces coelicolor* A3(2) including the polyketide synthase for the antibiotic actinorhodin. J Biol Chem 1992; 267:19278–19290.

321. McDaniel R, Ebert-Khosla S, Hopwood DA, Khosla C. Engineered biosynthesis of novel polyketides. Science 1993; 262:1546–1550.

322. Shen B, Summers RG, Wendt-Pienkowski E, Hutchinson CR. The *Streptomyces glaucescens tcmKL* polyketide synthase and *tcmN* polyketide cyclase genes govern the size and shape of aromatic polyketides. J Am Chem Soc 1995; 117:6811–6821.

323. Oki T, Matsuzawa Y, Kiyoshima K, Yoshimoto A. New anthracyclines, feudomycins, produced by the mutant from *Streptomyces coeruleorubidus* ME130-A4. J Antibiot 1981; 34:783–790.

324. Meurer G, Hutchinson CR. Daunorubicin Type II polyketide synthase enzymes DpsA and DpsB determine neither the choice of starter unit nor the cyclization pattern of aromatic polyketides. J Am Chem Soc 1995; 117:5899–5900.

325. Soga K, Furusho H, Mori S, Oki T. New antitumor antibiotics: 13-Methylaclacinomycin A and its derivatives. J Antibiot 1981; 34:770–773.

326. Bibb MJ, Sherman DH, Ōmura S, Hopwood DA. Cloning, sequencing and deduced functions of a cluster of *Streptomyces* genes probably encoding biosynthesis of the polyketide antibiotic frenolicin. Gene 1994; 142:31–39.

327. Lombó F, Blanco G, Fernández E, Méndez C, Salas JA. Characterization of *Streptomyces argillaceus* genes encoding a polyketide synthase involved in the biosynthesis of the antitumor mithramycin. Gene 1996; 172:87–91.

328. Le Gouill C, Desmarais D, Dery CV. *Saccharopolyspora hirsuta* 367 encodes clustered genes similar to ketoacyl synthase, ketoacyl reductase, acyl carrier protein, and biotin carboxyl carrier protein. Mol Gen Genet 1993; 240:146–150.

329. Fernández-Moreno MA, Martínez E, Caballero JL, Ichinose K, Hopwood DA, Malpartida F. DNA sequence and functions of the *actVI* region of the actinorhodin biosynthetic gene cluster of *Streptomyces coelicolor* A3(2). J Biol Chem 1994; 269:24854–24863.

330. McDaniel R, Ebert-Khosla S, Hopwood DA, Khosla C. Engineered biosynthesis of novel polyketides: *actVII* and *actIV* gene encode aromatase and cyclase enzymes respectively. J Am Chem Soc 1994; 116:10855–10859.

331. McDaniel R, Ebert-Khosla S, Hopwood DA, Khosla C. Rational design of aromatic polyketide natural products by recombinant assembly of enzymatic subunits. Nature 1995; 549–554.

332. Khosla C, Zawada RJX. Generation of polyketide libraries via combinatorial biosynthesis. Trends Biotechnol 1996; 14:335–341.

333. Zhang H-I, He X-g, Adefarati A, Gallucci J, Cole SP, Beale JM, Keller PJ, Chang C-j, Floss HG. Mutactin, a novel polyketide from *Streptomyces coelicolor*. Structure and biosynthetic relationship to actinorhodin. J Org Chem 1990; 55:1682–1684.

334. Cassinelli G, Rivola G, Ruggieri D, Arcamone F, Grein A, Merli S, Spalla C, Casazza AM, DiMarco A, Pratesi G. New anthracycline glycosides: 4-O-Demethyl-11-deoxydaunorubicin and analogues from *Streptomyces peucetius* var. *aureus*. J Antibiot 1982; 35:176–183.

335. McGuire JC, Thomas MC, Stroshane RM, Hamilton BK, White RJ. Biosynthesis of daunomycin glycosides: Role of ε-rhodomycinone. Antimicrob Agents Chemother 1980; 18:454–464.

336. Yoshimoto A, Oki T, Umezawa H. Biosynthesis of daunomycinone from aklavinone and ε-rhodomycinone. J Antibiot 1980; 33:1199–1201.

337. Piepersberg W. Molecular biology, biochemistry, and fermentation of aminoglycoside antibiotics. Strohl WR, ed. Biotechnology of Industrial Antibiotics, 2nd ed. New York: Marcel-Dekker, 1997.

338. Summers R. The engineered biosynthesis of novel erythromycins. Bloomington, Indiana: Proceedings, Sixth Conference on the Genetics and Molecular Biology of Industrial Microorganisms, 1996:S20.

339. McPherson DF, Manning PA, Morona R. Characterization of the dTDP-rhamnose biosynthetic genes encoded by the *rfb* locus of *Shigella flexneri*. Mol Microbiol 1994; 11:281–292.

340. Cundliffe E. Glycosyltransfer during tylosin production in *Streptomyces fradiae*. Bloomington, Indiana: Proceedings, Sixth Conference on the Genetics and Molecular Biology of Industrial Microorganisms, 1996:S28.

341. Yoshimoto A, Nakamura T, Kubo K, Johdo O, Tone H. Daunomycin biosynthesis by microbial conversion of precursor metabolites using biosynthetically blocked mutants. J Ferment Bioeng 1995; 79:229–235.

342. Trower MK, Lenstra R, Omer C, Buchholz SE, Sariaslani FS. Cloning, nucleotide sequence determination and expression of the genes encoding cytochrome P-450$_{soy}$ (*soy*C) and ferredoxin$_{soy}$ (*soy*B) from *Streptomyces griseus*. Mol Microbiol 1992; 6:2125–2134.

343. Oki T, Takatsuki Y, Tobe H, Yoshimoto A, Takeuchi T, Umezawa H. Microbial conversion of daunomycin, carminomycin I and feudomycin A to adriamycin. J Antibiot 1981; 34:1229–1231.

344. Crespi-Perellino N, Grein A, Merli S, Minghetti A, Spalla C. Biosynthetic relationships among daunorubicin, doxorubicin, and 13-dihydrodaunorubicin in *Streptomyces peucetius*. Experientia 1982; 38:1455–1456.

345. Furuya K, Hutchinson CR. The DnrN protein of *Streptomyces peucetius*, a pseudo-response regulator, is a DNA-binding protein involved in the regulation of daunorubicin biosynthesis. J Bacteriol 1996; 178:6310–6318.

346. Takeuchi T. Antitumor antibiotics discovered and studied at the Institute of Microbial Chemistry. J Cancer Res Clin Oncol 1995; 121:505–510.

347. Strohl WR, Bartel PL, Li Y, Connors NC, Woodman RH. Expression of polyketide biosynthesis and regulatory genes in heterologous streptomycetes: A review. J Industr Microbiol 1991; 7:163–174.

348. August PR, Flickinger MC, Sherman DH. Cloning and analysis of a locus (*mcr*) involved in mitomycin C resistance in *Streptomyces lavendulae*. J Bacteriol 1994; 176:4448–4454.

349. Hopwood DA, Malpartida F, Kieser HM, Ikeda H, Duncan J, Fujii I, Rudd BAM, Floss HG, Ōmura S. Production of "hybrid" antibiotics by genetic engineering. Nature 1985; 314:642–644.

350. Decker H, Rohr J, Motamedi H, Hutchinson CR, Zähner H. Isolation of hybrid antibiotics from *Streptomyces fradiae* Tü2717. Debabov VG, Dudnik YV, Danilenko VN, eds. Proceedings of the Ninth International Symposium on the Biology of the Actinomycetes. Moscow: All-Russia Scientific Research Institute for Genetics and Selection of Industrial Microorganisms, 1995:68–72.

21

Tetracyclines

Iain S. Hunter
University of Strathclyde, Glasgow, Scotland

Robert A. Hill
University of Glasgow, Glasgow, Scotland

I. INTRODUCTION

Discovered in the early 1950s, the tetracycline family of antibiotics has been in clinical use now for around 40 years. The chemistry and biochemistry of tetracyclines has been reviewed extensively over the years (e.g., 1–4), and the reader is referred to these reviews for excellent coverage of the earlier literature.

The tetracyclines were the first major group of antimicrobial agents for which the term *broad spectrum* was used—namely, they exhibit activity against both gram-positive and gram-negative bacteria. The molecular biochemistry of the mode of action of tetracyclines is not completely understood. They act by arresting translation by the prokaryotic ribosome—at the point where charged tRNAs bind to the "acceptor" site on the ribosome and are then translocated to the site of peptide bond formation. Tetracyclines disrupt the codon–anticodon interactions between tRNA and mRNA, so that binding of aminoacyl-tRNA is prevented. They bind only to prokaryotic (70S) ribosomes, not to the larger (80S) eukaryotic ribosomes.

This specificity (i.e., lack of interference with eukaryotic biology) and broad spectrum activity has led to the widespread use of tetracyclines in fighting infections in humans, animals, fish, and plants. Over 5000 metric tons of antibiotic are estimated to be produced each year (1). Given their long history of extensive clinical use, it is inevitable that many infectious agents have become resistant to tetracyclines (e.g., 5). Prescribing of tetracycline is also contraindicated if the patient is likely to be exposed to strong sunlight (due to an ultraviolet-mediated response), young, or pregnant (the prodigious capacity of tetracyclines to chelate calcium causes problems with development of bone and teeth). Despite this, the tetracyclines continue to enjoy an increasing market.

A. Tetracyclines: New Applications

In human clinical use, the tetracycline family has seen a resurgence of use—as one of the three components (along with bismuth and metronidazole) in a triple formulation for the treatment of stomach ulcers caused by *Helicobacter pylori* (6). Given that *Helicobacter* is attributed as the causative agent in 70% of patients with stomach ulcers, the prospects for large sales of tetracycline to eradicate *Helicobacter* seem particularly promising. The semi-synthetic tetracycline, minocycline, has been shown to be useful in the treatment of rheumatoid arthritis. Minocycline has an anti-inflammatory effect by suppressing T-cell proliferation (7). Minocycline is also growing in importance in the treatment (8) of methicillin-resistant *Staphylococcus aureus* (MRSA)—a multidrug-resistant strain for which vancomycin is the only antibiotic, in current use, to which the infection is sensitive. The inevitability of emergence of resistance to vancomycin means that minocycline is being held in reserve for future use against MRSA. Tetracyclines continue to be the antibiotic of choice for treatment of acne, for which topical application circumvents the problems of systemic absorption of calcium. On a nonroutine basis, its low cost, efficacy, and immediate availability in bulk quantities were the major factors in its selection to treat and to control a recent outbreak of bubonic plague in India.

The agricultural market for tetracyclines, though, far exceeds our use for human health care. This is particularly true in fish farming: in Germany, oxytetracycline and chlortetracycline are the only antibiotics licensed for use in aquaculture (9). Tetracyclines are also the antibiotic of choice to prevent or to treat bacterial infections in U.S. fish farms. The quantities consumed are stunning—a "light user" of tetracyclines will apply 8 kg in a single dose, whereas a "heavy user" will typically apply 168 kg of antibiotic in a single prophylactic dosage (10). A sustained campaign of usage will consume over 0.5 metric ton of antibiotic in 24 days (11). The environmental impact of such a release of biologically active material has, not surprisingly, aroused considerable interest. Detection of the antibiotic is limited to 30 m around the site of application. There also appears to be no correlation between use of the drug and the incidence of drug resistance in the surrounding microbial flora (12), although it is particularly worrying that seafood meat harvested from the aquatic hinterland of such farms contained levels of the antibiotic that exceeded safety limits.

The regulation of the tetracycline resistance factor in Tn*10*, which mediates export of the antibiotic, is well understood (see Section II)—to the extent that the biology of the system is now being exploited biotechnologically to control expression of foreign genes, and as a hybrid system for control of expression in eukaryotic cells. Tetracycline is an excellent effector molecule to use in eukaryotic systems, as it is inert to eukaryotic biology. Gossen and Bujard (13) adapted the regulation of tetracycline resistance in Tn*10* by fusing the Tet repressor with the activating domain of virion protein 16 of *Herpes simplex* virus to generate a tetracycline-controlled transactivator that was expressed constitutively in HeLa cells. The hybrid transactivator stimulated transcription from a minimal promoter sequence derived from the human cytomegalovirus promoter IE combined with *tet* operator sequences. In this way, a bacterial repressor was used as a component to engineer a eukaryotic activator that would respond to tetracyclines.

The system is also being evaluated for gene therapy in transgenic mice models. By hooking up the Cre recombinase of bacteriophage lambda to the tetracycline hybrid system, temporal control by tetracycline was achieved (14). Cre was chosen, as its function in lambda is to excise DNA between 2 "signposts" (the *lox*P sites). Thus, it would appear to be technically feasible to use tetracycline and its biology to carry out some fine genetic needlepoint, targeted to the genes in defined tissues.

The utility of the system has been further enhanced by repositioning one of the *tet* control elements, so that tetracycline can be used either as a positive or negative effector (i.e., for switching on or off) of the gene to be controlled (15). When controlling the expression of SV40 large tumor antigen in pancreatic cells of transgenic mice, tetracycline could be used to inhibit cell proliferation (16). Surprisingly, anhydrotetracycline was 100 times better at mediating this biological response—a result that has now been explained (see Section II) by anhydrotetracycline interacting more productively with the Tet repressor (17).

It would therefore appear that tetracycline could be used as an effector of some quite exotic human biology. However, to adopt these strategies safely, the antibiotic would have to be banned from all other applications, so that there would be no possibility of a patient being exposed to tetracycline from the environment or in food—a tall order viewed from a 1996 perspective.

II. TETRACYCLINE RESISTANCE

Bacterial resistance to tetracyclines was first reported in 1953, very soon after their discovery (18). Tetracycline resistance is often transposon or plasmid borne, which results in horizontal transmission of resistance factors between and among different species. Many nonpathogenic bacteria within the environment carry resistance to tetracyclines, and they are now recognized as an important reservoir in transmission. Resistance factors may reside in this reservoir and then be transferred to pathogenic bacteria, rendering the tetracyclines useless in the control of infection.

There are two main mechanisms (19) by which microbes become resistant: (a) bacterial ribosomes may become resistant to translational arrest by tetracyclines; and (b) tetracyclines may be pumped out of the cell by an energy-consuming efflux mechanism. Neither mechanism involves chemical modification of the drug.

Ohnuki et al. (20) first showed that ribosomes harvested from tetracycline-resistant cultures lost their resistant phenotype when washed in high salt—a property that suggested that the factor (unlike most other ribosomal resistance factors) could modify the ribosomes noncovalently. A combination of molecular genetics and biochemistry has shown that ribosomal resistance to tetracyclines, for which the *tet*M/O system of *Campylobacter* is the paradigm (21), is due to the action of a ribosomal protein with considerable similarity to elongation factor G (EF-G) (22). It had been assumed originally that TetM might act as an alternative EF-G, but this is not the case. Although the two proteins hydrolyze GTP (23) and this GTPase activity depends on contact with the ribosomes, they can be distinguished by sensitivity to fusidic acid: TetM is resistant, whereas EF-G is sensitive. TetM cannot substitute for EF-G (or EF-Tu, to which it also displays similarity) in reconstitution of cell-free translation in vitro. In the presence of TetM, the affinity of tetracycline for ribosomes is decreased, and this is the basis of the resistance phenotype. Resistance is attributed primarily to an increased dissociation of the drug from the ribosome, rather than a decrease in the association of the drug with the protein-synthetic machinery. When TetM is added to ribosomes that have been arrested in translation by tetracycline, bound drug is displaced from the ribosomal complex, allowing translation to proceed (24). The exact molecular details remain to be elucidated.

Bacteroides have a tetracycline resistance factor, which also acts on the ribosomes but is only distantly related to TetM and TetO (less than 40% similarity). It was named TetQ to distinguish it from the others (25). The resistance gene is embedded in a transposon structure (26), which predisposes the resistance factor to be mobilized. Originally, horizontal transfer of TetQ appeared to be confined to Bacteroides (27). However, it was discovered that transfer functions associated with the transposon are unusual in that they are regulated by tetracycline (28) via a complex regulatory network (29,30). These transfer genes can mobilize integrated genetic elements from Bacteroides to *Escherichia coli* (31). Thus, this genetic element, which confers resistance to tetracycline and has a frequency of mobilization and transfer that is enhanced considerably in the presence of low levels of the drug, perhaps suggests a role for antibiotics in the ecosystem that predates human exploitation of the compounds in health care.

The second resistance mechanism is characterized by reduced association of tetracycline with the microbial cell—due to enhanced efflux from the cell rather than reduced uptake of the drug. The *tet*A system of Tn*10*, which is the paradigm for this class of resistance, has been studied intensely (e.g., 32). TetA encodes a membrane protein that contains 12 membrane-spanning segments. Tetracycline is pumped from the cell, while complexed to a metal ion, in exchange for uptake of a proton (thus the exporter is classified as a "tetracycline/H^+ antiporter"). Cells that are expressing TetA have ribosomes that are sensitive to tetracycline, but the drug never reaches its target because it is pumped out of the cell so efficiently. Substantial site-directed mutagenesis of TetA has been undertaken (e.g., 33) with the aim of defining the contacts that tetracycline makes with the efflux protein. With this knowledge, it might then be possible to design a tetracycline that was not a substrate for the efflux protein but was still able to arrest translation. In this way, tetracycline resistance mediated by the TetA exporter would be circumvented. Nelson et al. (34) have adopted another approach to address this problem. They have assayed a large number of tetracycline analogs for their ability to bind to, but not to be transported by, TetA. Such an analog, formulated together with a biologically active tetracycline, would serve to render the cellular route for export inactive, which would trap the active drug inside the cell and allow it to target the ribosome.

TetA has a number of close relatives, which all function as tetracycline exporters and are classified primarily via DNA homology and substrate specificity (35). They are present ubiquitously in both gram-positive and gram-negative bacteria. However, the tetracycline family is also part of a wider grouping of membrane transporters, including the glucose carrier in mammalian systems. Using molecular phylogeny, it has been concluded that these proteins probably did not arise from a single ancestor and that the drug transporters are distributed throughout the phylogeny (36)—indicating that they are not derived from any single strand in the evolutionary tree that might be constructed.

Exporters of the *tet*A family are often found adjacent to a repressor, TetR, which regulates expression of the exporter (37). Expression of the exporter is normally switched off until tetracycline is present in the cell; then, the repressor dissociates from the operator, allowing expression of the resistance factor to proceed and export of the drug from the cell to be achieved. The interaction of a tetracycline with TetR is therefore crucial to the biology of the resistance process. For a tetracycline to be exported normally from the cell, it has to be both a substrate for the TetA exporter and interact with TetR to dissociate the repressor from the DNA. A novel tetracycline that could still be transported out of the cell by the exporter, but that could not act productively with TetR to allow expression of the exporter (and still acted to inhibit translation by the ribosome), would be an effective antibiotic. Knowledge of the interactions between tetracycline and TetR have advanced significantly as a result of elucidating the crystal structure of the complex (38). It came as a surprise to find that the regions of the TetR protein that make contact with the DNA operator of *tet*A are inverted compared with other proteins of similar functionality. Further refinement of the crystal structure and isomorphous replacement with other tetracyclines have enabled the fine details of the molecular interactions to be deduced (39) to the point where it may be possible to enact the rational design of an active tetracycline that will not induce the exporter. This would circumvent this aspect of the resistance problem. Refinement of our understanding of the molecular interactions of a number of tetracyclines with TetR has shown that anhydrotetracycline (which is not particularly effective as an antibiotic) is a much better inducer of expression than is tetracycline itself (17). Thus, anhydrotetracycline is the preferred effector for regulation of expression in eukaryotic cells, as detailed in Section I (16).

Sloan et al. (40) have characterized at the DNA level the unusual *tet*P determinant in Clostridia, which (on biochemical criteria) had been difficult to place into either the ribosomal resistance or exporter categories. They found that it contained genes encoding *both* the ribosomal and efflux mechanisms in overlapping reading frames—an example of the two resistance mechanisms coming together in an efficiently designed and easily transportable unit of DNA.

A novel class of tetracycline resistance, from Bacteroides, came to light in the late 1980s. Unlike the TetM and TetA paradigms of resistance (in which the drug remains chemically unaltered), this resistance factor is responsible for modification of the tetracycline molecule. The resistance factor works only under aerobic conditions, as oxygen is required for its function (41). The gene was designated *tet*X to distinguish it from the other classes. The deduced gene product appears to be an oxidoreductase, from its similarity to other proteins in the database (42). However, chemical identification of the modified tetracycline has remained elusive (43).

III. TETRACYCLINES: ISOLATION AND CHEMISTRY

A. Natural Tetracyclines

Chlortetracycline from *Streptomyces aureofaciens* was the first tetracycline to be isolated, in 1948. Since that time there have been more than 30 new natural tetracyclines, mainly isolated from *Streptomyces* species, including oxytetracycline in 1950 and tetracycline in 1953 (44). Most natural tetracyclines have a common structure (Figure 1) with the β-diketone system in rings B and C essential for antibiotic activity. Some natural tetracyclines such as terramycin X have the acetomido-group at C2 replaced by an acetyl-group, and democycline and demecycline lack the methyl-group at C6 (Table 1).

More recently, the dactylocyclines have been isolated from a *Dactylosporangium* species; these have the opposite stereochemistry at C6 (45). Dactylocyclinone is the parent member of the family that is the 6-epimer of 8-methoxychlorotetracycline from *Actinomadura brunnea* (46). The dactylocyclinones contain unusual sugar moieties, with dactocycline A (Figure 2) being the most active member. A group of tetracyclines including

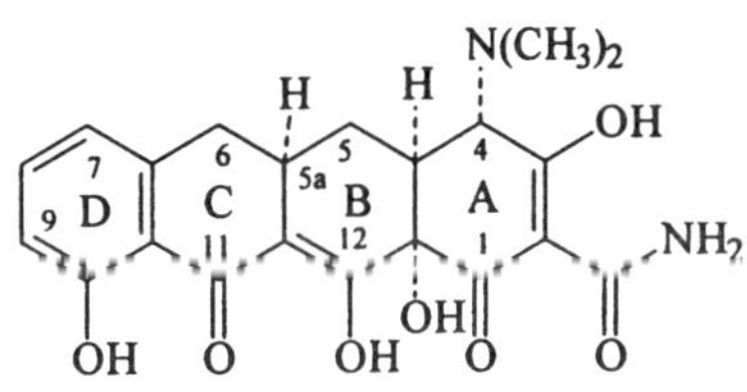

Figure 1   Numbering system for tetracyclines.

Table 1 The Structures of Some Tetracycline Antibiotics

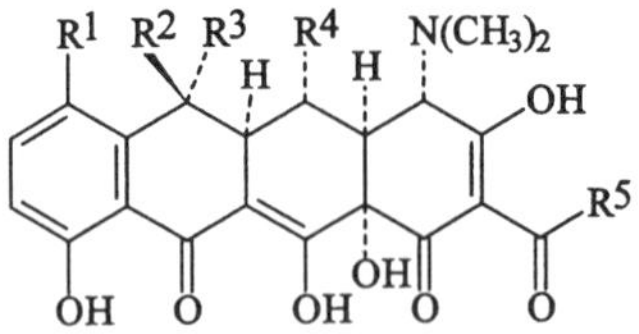

	R1	R2	R3	R4	R5
Tetracycline	H	OH	CH₃	H	NH₂
2-Acetyl-2-decarboxamidotetracycline	H	OH	CH₃	H	CH₃
Terramycin X	H	OH	CH₃	OH	CH₃
2-Acetyl-2-decarboxamido-7-chlorotetracycline	Cl	OH	CH₃	H	CH₃
Chlortetracycline	Cl	OH	CH₃	H	NH₂
Bromotetracycline	Br	OH	CH₃	H	NH₂
Demeclocycline	Cl	OH	H	H	NH₂
6-Demethyltetracycline (Demecycline)	H	OH	H	H	NH₂
Oxytetracycline	H	OH	CH₃	OH	NH₂
6-Deoxytetracycline	H	H	CH₃	H	NH₂
Minocycline	NMe₂	H	H	H	NH₂
Doxycycline	H	H	CH₃	OH	NH₂

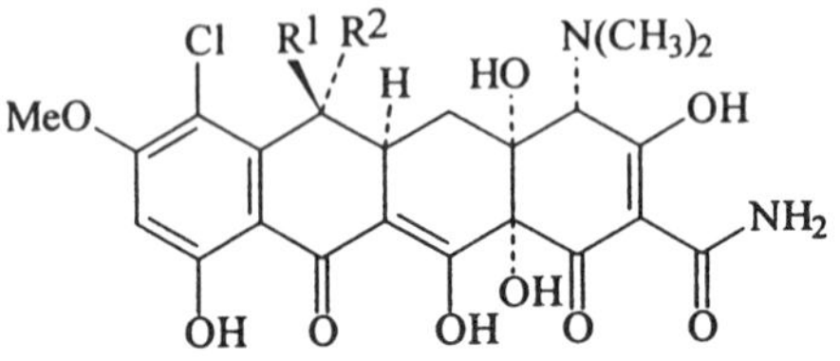

R1 = OH; R2 = CH₃ Dactylocyclinone
R1 = CH₃; R2 = OH 8-Methoxychlorotetracycline
R1 = O ; R2 = CH₃ Dactylocycline A

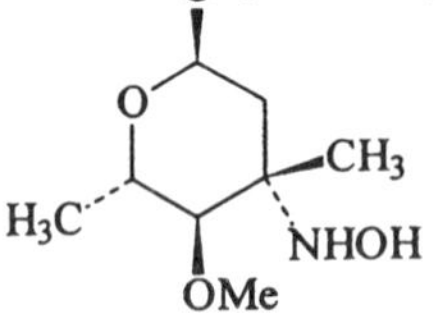

Figure 2 Dactocycline structures.

SF 2575 (Figure 3) have been isolated from *Streptomyces* species that have a C-glycosidic linkage at C9 and a salicyloyl ester at C4 (47,48).

B. Semisynthetic Tetracyclines

Structural modifications in rings C and D have been used to produce a range of semisynthetic tetracyclines with altered antimicrobial activities (49). The aromatic ring D is par-

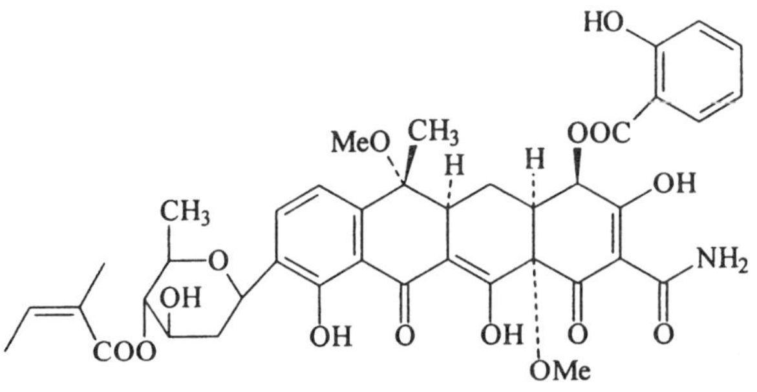

Figure 3   The structure of SF 2575.

ticularly easy to modify to produce useful derivatives. For example, as early as 1953 tetracycline was prepared by dechlorination of chlortetracycline (44). The early work was hampered by the easy epimerization at C4 and by the lability of the benzylic hydroxyl-group at C6. This lability has been used to prepare 6-deoxy derivatives such as 6-deoxytetracycline, doxycycline (Table 1), and methacycline (Figure 4) using dehydration and hydrogenation procedures.

The increased chemical stability of the 6-deoxytetracyclines allows modifications at C7 and C9 by electrophilic substitution. Nitration of 6-demethyl-6-deoxytetracycline (DMDOT) produces a mixture of 7-nitro and 9-nitro derivatives (Figure 5). Reductive methylation of the 7-nitro derivative produces minocycline (MINO) (50). Reduction of the 9-nitro derivative followed by acylation produces *N,N*-dimethylglycylamido-6-demethyl-6-deoxytetracycline (DMG-DMDOT) (51). Minocycline can be similarly modified to produce *N,N*-dimethylglycylamidominocycline (DMG-MINO). These glycylcyclines have interesting biological activities (see Section IV). Replacement of the glycine moiety with other amino acids did not improve activity (52).

8-Methoxychlorotetracycline and the dactylocyclines are the only naturally occurring tetracyclines with a substituent at C8. A synthetic route has been devised to enable substituents to be inserted at C8 in intact tetracyclines (51).

IV.   BIOLOGY OF THE GLYCYLGLYCINE TETRACYCLINES

Without doubt, the most exciting development in the chemotherapeutics of tetracyclines over the last decade has been the synthesis of the class of semisynthetic tetracycline

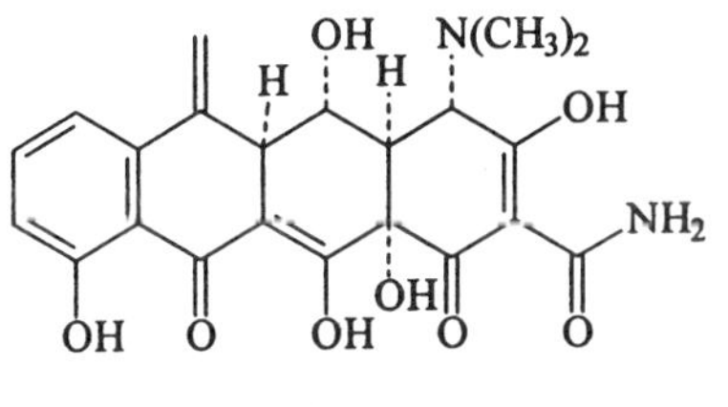

Figure 4   The structure of methacycline.

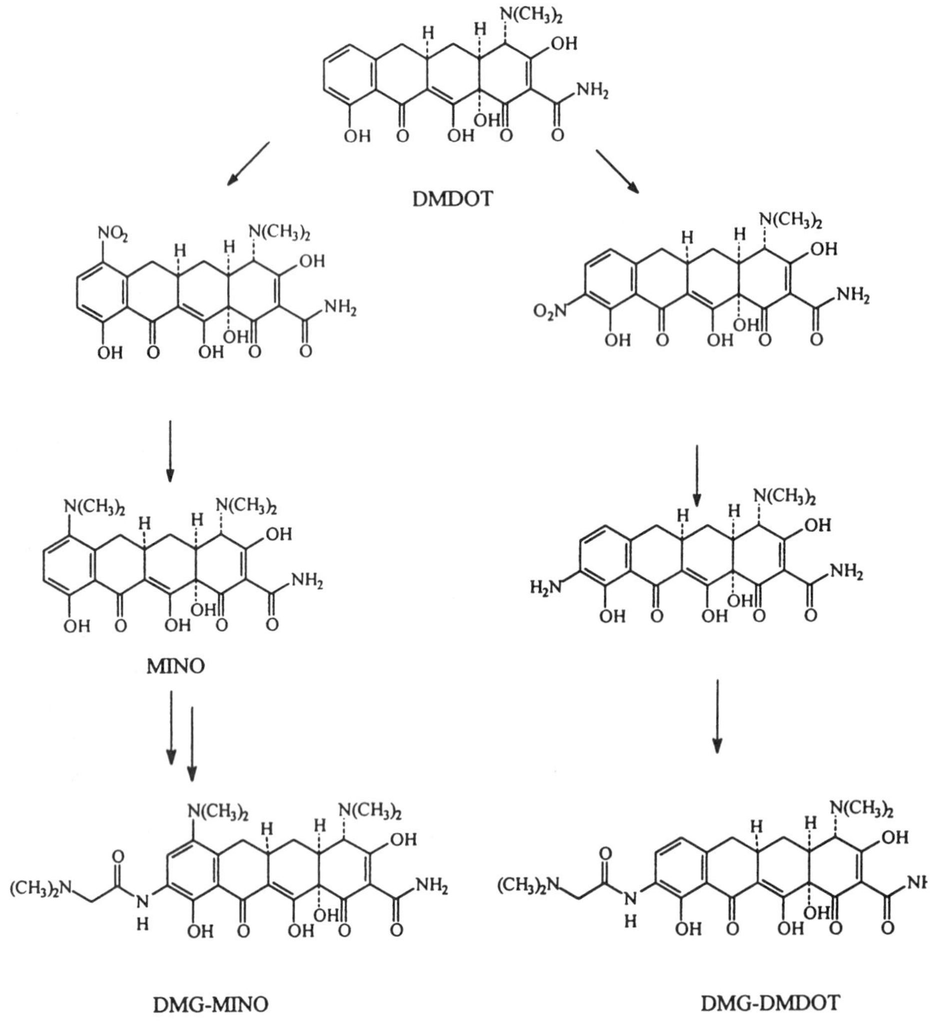

Figure 5 Synthetic transformation of 6-deoxytetracyclines.

derivatives colloquially termed the "glycylglycines" (see Section III.B; 53). These compounds, discovered and patented by the Lederle group in the United States (54), have substituent groups at the 9-position (Figure 1) of the tetracyclic nucleus.

Among the family, the *N,N*-dimethylglycylamido derivative of minocycline (CL 329,998; DMG-MINO (Figure 5)) and that of 6-demethyl-6-deoxytetracycline (CL 331,002; DMG-DMDOT (Figure 5)) proved to have potent biological activity against many pathogenic bacteria (55) and against gram-positive bacteria that were already resistant to tetracycline and to minocycline (56). Of particular note was their efficacy against tetracycline-resistant Mycoplasma (57), Mycobacteria (58), and Neisseria (59).

Like all tetracyclines, the glycylglycines act at the bacterial ribosome to arrest translation (60). Their utility against tetracycline-resistant bacteria is due to their ability to circumvent the two main resistance mechanisms. The glycylglycines bind the ribosome more tightly than previous tetracyclines, so that the TetM resistance factor is unable dis-place them from this site—hence, TetM is unable to protect the ribosomes from the action of these new drugs (61). The TetA-mediated efflux system is ineffective against the glycylglycines, as they are not substrates for the transporter (62). Thus, the cell is unable to prevent the glycylglycines reaching their ribosomal target.

Whereas they are not substrates for the TetA exporter, the glycylglycines do act as effectors of TetR, which means that they induce synthesis of the efflux protein and its insertion in the membrane (albeit the transporter is unable to export the drug). Guay et al. (63) have isolated mutants of the TetA transporter that now confer some resistance to the glycylglycines, and they have characterized them. Two amino acid substitutions were sufficient to confer resistance to the glycylglycines. This observation is a concern, as it may be that resistance to these new compounds, mediated by a mutated TetA, is inevitable. A glycylglycine derivative that does not induce the TetA transporter (i.e., does not interact with TetR) would reduce the selective pressure for such a "second gen-eration" resistance factor to arise.

The glycylglycines have aroused great interest. Some scientists had assumed that all the permutations of chemical adulteration of the tetracycline nucleus must have been attempted and played out in four decades of medicinal chemistry aimed at new chemotherapeutic structures. However, the glycylglycines do illustrate that new discover-ies based on synthetic chemistry are still possible.

V.   GENETICS AND BIOCHEMISTRY

Streptomyces aureofaciens and *Streptomyces rimosus* are used for the production of natural tetracyclines by commercial fermentation. The former produces a mixture of chlortetra-cycline and tetracycline (Table 1)—the proportions of which can be manipulated by including chloride ion (favors chlortetracycline) or bromide (favors tetracycline) in the fermentation (4). Biosynthesis of tetracycline and its chlorinated derivative by *S. aureo-faciens* takes place in parallel: the chloro-group is added midway through the biosynthe-sis. It is therefore impossible to produce chlortetracycline exclusively, as some of the biosynthetic intermediates evade the chlorination step and eventually are biosynthesized to tetracycline. However, it is possible to produce tetracycline exclusively, by mutation of the chlorination gene (64). A similar situation occurs in *S. rimosus*: a mixture of tetracy-cline and oxytetracycline (Table 1) are produced, but in this case the 5-hydroxylase enzyme is extremely active; thus, the equilibrium is far in favor (>95%) of oxytetracy-cline production.

Historically, several research groups have focused on different aspects of the tetra-cyclines. McCormick and workers at Lederle laboratories in the 1960s undertook much of the pioneering chemistry and mutant isolation, wherein many of the intermediates of the biosynthetic pathway were isolated and a scheme for the biosynthetic pathway devised that has stood the test of time (64). They also synthesized many semisynthetic derivatives—presumably with the objective of discovering more potent antibiotics. Then, in the 1970s the Czech group in Prague focused on the microbial physiology of tetracy-cline production by *S. aureofaciens*. These studies led them to investigate the biochem-istry of antibiotic production and of some enzymes of central metabolism, the activity of which was critical to the efficiency of the overall process (e.g., 65,66). The chemistry, biochemistry, and microbial physiology have been undertaken substantially with *S. aureofaciens* and (chlor)tetracycline. By contrast, *S. rimosus* has been the focus of the genetic analysis of oxytetracycline biosynthesis by groups based in Croatia (67) and the United Kingdom (68). These studies have led, in the last 10 years, to an understanding of the molecular genetics of oxytetracycline formation.

A.   Resistance in the Producer

The key to unlocking the molecular genetics of oxytetracycline (OTC) formation was the discovery that the resistance gene for OTC mapped to the same locus (69) as some of the production genes that had been mapped previously (68). It was relatively easy to clone the OTC-resistance gene into an OTC-sensitive mutant of *S. rimosus*, and in fact two separate determinants, *otr*A and *otr*B, were cloned (69). These determinants correspond to the two tetracycline resistance genes, *tet*A and *tet*B, cloned from another strain of *S. rimosus* (20). *otr*A and *otr*B are around 34 kb apart on the chromosome of *S. rimosus*, and between them lie the genes for biosynthesis of the antibiotic (70,71).

*otr*A encodes a polypeptide with substantial similarity to the TetM system (72). It contains a striking GTP-binding motif and substantial similarity to EF-G. It would therefore be surprising if the recent biochemical studies on TetM (24) did not also apply to OtrA, in which case OtrA would appear to function by removing from the producer's ribosomes any newly synthesized OTC that happens to bind. Thus, OtrA acts as a snowplow to keep the ribosomes free of OTC so that protein synthesis may proceed during production of the antibiotic.

*otr*B encodes a hydrophobic protein with some similarity to the TetA exporter of Tn*10*. The DNA sequence of the gene (named *tet*347) from a related *S. rimosus* strain was reported by Reynes et al. (73). Tet347 functions to export the newly synthesized OTC from the cell. A phylogenetic study of *tet*347 with the tetracycline exporters from other organisms concluded that *tet*347 diverged some time ago from the other membrane carriers (74). Cloning of the exporter for chlortetracycline from *S. aureofaciens* has been reported (75), but no further details have emerged. However, a homolog of *tet*347, named *tcr*C, from a high-titer strain derived from the 6-demethylchlortetracycline producer *S. aureofaciens* NRRL3203 has been cloned recently (76). This gene is expressed at high levels during production of the antibiotic. When the chromosomal copy of *tcr*C was disrupted, the resulting recombinant had its resistance to tetracycline reduced, and its capacity to produce the antibiotic dropped to 10% of the control level. This demonstrates the importance of efficient export of antibiotic synthesized *de novo* to the overall productivity of the system.

A third oxytetracycline-resistance factor, *otr*C, was cloned from *S. rimosus* (Hunter, IS, unpublished results). In the wild-type cell, *otr*C probably makes little contribution to the level of resistance to tetracyclines—which exceeds 200 μg/ml. However, when the entire *otc* gene cluster is deleted from the chromosome (77), including both *otr*A and *otr*B, the resistance level decreases to less than 5 μg/ml—probably this low level of resistance is due to *otr*C. Southern blots show that whereas *otr*A and *otr*B are both missing in these strains (71, and see Section V.D), *otr*C is still present and must lie elsewhere on the chromosome. It is only when *otr*C is cloned in a multicopy vector that a true resistance level can be detected. The biochemical mechanism of *otr*C is not yet known.

Using gene probes to *otr*A, *otr*B, and *otr*C from *S. rimosus*, as well as *tet*K and *tet*L from gram-positive transposons, Pang et al. (78) were able to show that clinical isolates of Mycobacteria and Streptomyces that were tetracycline resistant contained genes that were homologous to the tetracycline-resistance probes. The study showed the potential for acquisition of tetracycline resistance within and across the different genera.

B. Enzymes of Tetracycline Biosynthesis

The enzymes of tetracycline biosynthesis have, with few exceptions, proved particularly difficult to study. The substrates for many of the steps are often insoluble or unstable in aqueous solution—hence, there has been a paucity of information on them. The enzymes themselves may also be unstable. However, our knowledge of anhydrotetracycline oxygenase has advanced in recent years. There are several reasons:

1. The substrate for the enzyme (anhydrotetracycline, ATC) is one of the few intermediates in the tetracycline pathway that is stable in aqueous solution.
2. The substrate may be readily prepared by treating tetracycline with strong acid.
3. The oxygenase activity requires NADPH, which is converted to NADP—thus, the reaction can in principle be followed at 340 nm.
4. ATC absorbs strongly at 440 nm, whereas the product of the reaction, dehydrotetracycline (DHTC), has an absorption maximum at 400 nm, which is readily distinguishable from the substrate. Therefore, utilization of the substrate can be monitored by decrease in absorption at 440 nm, while appearance of the product can be monitored at 400 nm. A diode array spectrophotometer, able to monitor absorption at several wavelengths simultaneously, facilitates detection of anhydrotetracycline oxygenase activity.
5. Analytical techniques using high-performance liquid chromatography (HPLC) have been reported that facilitate the separation and quantitation of the reactants and products (79).

Capitalizing on these advantages, Vancurova et al. (80) reported the purification to homogeneity of anhydrotetracycline oxygenase from S. aureofaciens. Almost simultaneously, the purification of the enzyme from S. rimosus was reported (81).

Amino-terminal sequencing of the enzyme from S. rimosus (71) was undertaken as a strategy to clone the gene by "reverse genetics." From the N-terminal residues obtained, it was possible to design oligonucleotides with appropriate redundancies among which, taking advantage of knowledge of the codon usage of Streptomyces, one was likely to contain the DNA sequence encoding the gene product.

Hybridization with the oligonucleotide set showed a clear signal with S. rimosus genomic DNA, and this sequence was cloned. The gene encoding ATC oxygenase (otcC) was contained within the cluster of genes flanked by otrA and otrB (71) in contrast to earlier data (68) where the gene had been mapped (probably erroneously due to the strain being a double mutant (71)) to another part of the chromosome.

Recently, otcC has been sequenced and overexpressed in E. coli (McDowall KJ, Wellinger R, Novotna J, and Hunter IS, unpublished results) using the T7 polymerase expression system (82). The gene product shows high similarity to other hydroxylases involved in antibiotic synthesis, for example, TcmG from Streptomyces glaucescens (83). Using the overexpression system, ATC oxygenase can constitute around 20% of the soluble protein of E. coli.

The homolog of otcC has been cloned and sequenced from a 6-demethylchlortetracycline strain of S. aureofaciens (84). This gene was named cts4 by these authors. Comparison of the deduced amino acid sequence of Cts4 with OtcC shows that the two pro-teins are extremely similar, especially at the deduced flavin-binding site close to the amino-terminus. OtcC is a slightly longer polypeptide, due to having two short tracts of amino acids inserted (Hunter IS, unpublished results). The two enzymes have a subtle difference in enzyme specificity: both use anhydrotetracycline as substrate, whereas only Cts4 can use chloranhydrotetracycline, a difference that must reflect the tertiary struc-ture of the folded polypeptides. The gene cluster for chlortetracycline biosynthesis has been cloned from *S. aureofaciens* ATCC 13899, and an overall restriction map presented (85). Analysis of the restriction sites present in the Cts4 sequence and comparison with the map of the ATCC strain lead to the conclusion that these two strains must be some-what different. It is impossible to superimpose the two maps.

The product of the reaction of ATC oxygenase is DHTC, the last intermediate in the tetracycline biosynthetic pathway before tetracycline dehydrogenase converts it to tetracycline. A coupled enzyme system has been developed to assay conversion of DHTC (produced continuously using ATC oxygenase in vitro) to tetracycline (79,86). The sys-tem has also been used to investigate the role of 5′-deazaflavin—the unusual cofactor involved in electron transfer for this last step in tetracycline biosynthesis (87).

C. Molecular Genetics of Formation of Tetracyclines

The cloning of the entire pathway for oxytetracycline (OTC) biosynthesis (71) and its expression in the naive host, *Streptomyces albus*, which then gained the ability to synthe-size OTC, heralded the beginning of the analysis of the gene cluster. A plausible route for biosynthesis of oxytetracycline had been deduced earlier (Figure 6; 68) from a combined genetic and biochemical investigation. This fitted well with the earlier work (64) on biosynthesis of (chlor)tetracycline.

The biosynthesis can be conveniently broken into constituent parts: synthesis of the polyketide chain, folding of the chain, and subsequent addition of substituent groups. DNA sequencing and analysis of the cluster revealed 23 open reading frames (Figure 7), including the two resistance genes. It should be noted that the DNA segment that con-ferred ability to synthesis OTC on *S. albus* was a 34 kb EcoRI fragment (71), just mar-ginally longer than the DNA depicted in Figure 7. Although it is appealing to perceive the cluster as flanked by the two resistances (and there are very strong transcriptional ter-minators downstream of them), it is conceivable that other genes lie outside the region depicted in Figure 7 but within the EcoRI fragment.

For some of the genes (e.g., the resistances (20), acyl carrier protein (88), and *otc*C (McDowall KJ, Wellinger R, Novotna J, and Hunter IS, unpublished results)), the func-tion has been proven biochemically. For others (e.g., *otc*Y-2 [ketoreductase], *otc*D1 [aro-matase], and *otc*D2 [hydroxylase]), gene function may be inferred from sequence similar-ity to other proteins in the database. However, for others (e.g., *otc*D5, *otc*D4) no function can be deduced readily, although there may be sequences with some similarity in the database.

To describe a plausible relationship between the biochemical pathway (Figure 6) and the architecture of the cluster (Figure 7), the biosynthetic route will be followed, and the likely genes involved will be discussed on that basis.

Synthesis of tetracyclines has been assumed to proceed from a malonamyl-CoA starter unit. There are Streptomyces mutants known to produce tetracycline analogs, for example, 2-acetyl-2-decarboxamide-(oxy)tetracycline (Table 1), in which the 2-carbox-

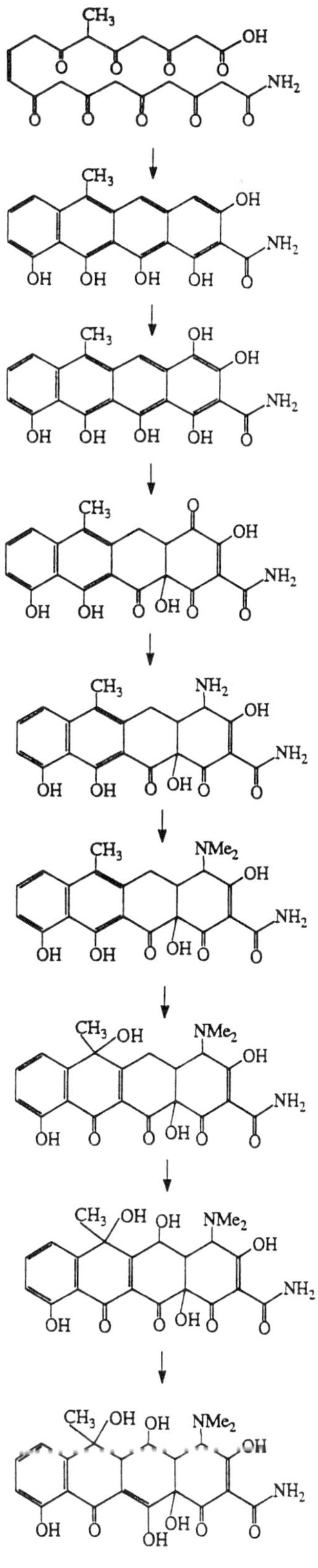

6-Methylpretetramid

4-Hydroxy-6-methylpreteramid

4-Keto-ATC

4-Amino-ATC

Anhydrotetracycline

5a(11a)-Dehydrotetracycline

5a(11a)-Dehydro-OTC

Oxytetracycline

Figure 6 The oxytetracycline pathway.

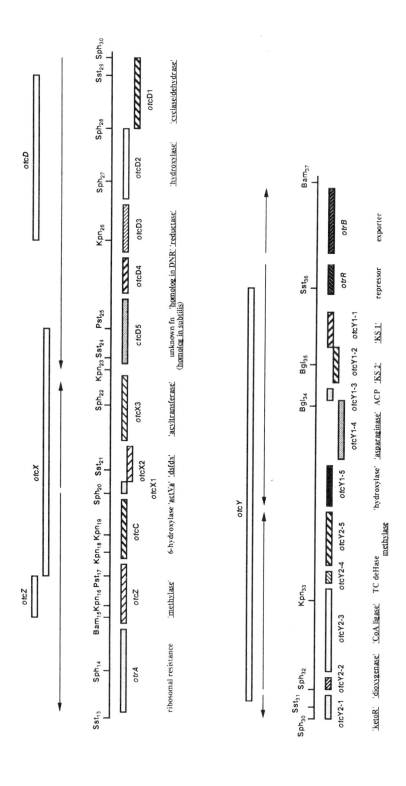

Figure 7 Architecture of the *otc* cluster.

amide-group (R5 in Table 1) is replaced by a 2-acetyl-group (64,89) presumably due to the inability to synthesize the necessary malonamyl-CoA starter unit. The discovery of these end products of the pathway implied that an acetoacetyl-CoA (perhaps available from metabolism of fatty acid) was used as a starter to enable the biosynthesis of the tetracycline analogs, and hence that malonamyl-CoA was the usual starter. However, this has never been proven formally by bio-organic chemistry. The presence of a CoA ligase–like gene product (OtcY2-3) lends credibility to the hypothesis that malonamyl-CoA is the starter unit, rather than malonyl-CoA, which is subsequently converted to the amide. OtcY2-3 has a high degree of similarity to coumarate-CoA ligase, which provides the acylated primer for chalcone synthase (90). The teleological argument here is that if malonyl-CoA were the starter unit, there would be no need for a CoA ligase within the *otc* cluster, as all intermediates are CoA derivatives readily available from cellular metabolism. However, if malonamate were the starting point of the pathway, this would have to be acylated by CoA to act as a primer in the same way as occurs with coumaryl-CoA for chalcone synthase.

In labeling experiments, $[1, 2, 3\text{-}^{13}C_3]$malonate and $[1, 2\text{-}^{13}C_2]$acetate were used as precursors for OTC biosynthesis, and their derived products were determined (91). Only the $[1, 2, 3\text{-}^{13}C_3]$malonate-derived product exhibited significant coupling of carbon-2 with both C1 and the $CONH_2$ substituent (nuclear magnetic resonance in the ^{13}C spectrum), which confirmed that an intact malonate unit was indeed incorporated. The nature of the direct precursor (malonyl-CoA or malonamyl-CoA) remains an open question until either dual labeled (C–N) malonamate is shown to be incorporated intact or gene disruption of the "CoA ligase" is undertaken.

Given that tetracyclines have an unusual starter unit, it is perhaps not surprising that an acyltransferase (*otc*X3) homolog is present in the cluster. Other polyketides derived solely from acetate (i.e., which use acetyl-CoA as the starter unit) do not appear to have such an acyltransferase in their gene clusters. However, daunomycin biosynthesis requires propionyl-CoA as starter, and that gene cluster also contains an acyltransferasae (92). Thus, the acyltransferase for tetracycline biosynthesis would plausibly "load up" the starter unit onto the polyketide synthase complex responsible for synthesis of the backbone.

Irrespective of the nature of the starter unit, sequential condensation of eight malonyl(acetyl)-CoA molecules completes the backbone structure (93). For polyketide antibiotics, such as tetracyclines in which the extension of the polyketide chain is done sequentially by addition of acetate-groups and no further chemistry is performed (so-called type II polyketide synthases; 94,95), three genes are responsible for the condensative synthesis of the backbone (historically named *orf*1,2,3). The DNA sequence of the genes responsible for synthesis of the oxytetracycline backbone and deduced gene products have been described (96). Orf3, the acyl carrier protein (ACP), encodes the small polypeptide to which the growing polyketide chain is attached. The ACP for oxytetracycline biosynthesis has been expressed in *E. coli* and the protein purified (88). Substitution for the ACP gene by that from a heterologous polyketide synthase showed that the ACP does not confer specificity on the length of polyketide chain synthesized (97).

The *orf* 1 and 2 of each type II polyketide synthase are similar to each other, and each *orf*1/2 set from a different microorganism shows considerable similarity to other pair sets (e.g., 95). Orf1 contains the active-site cysteine, to which the growing polyketide chain is assumed to be attached via an ACP intermediate. Thus, *orf*1 has often been named the β-ketoacyl:ACP synthase subunit (abbreviated to KS). Whereas each *orf*2 has striking similarity to the *orf*1 that it is paired with, the various *orf*2 do not possess the catalytic residues. They play an important role in determining the length of the polyketide backbone that is made (98,99) and have been named the chain length factors (CLFs). Each CLF does not specify the length of polyketide on its own—the interaction with KS is also important in determining specificity, as well as interactions with other subunits associated with folding and cyclization of each backbone, in a manner that has yet to be defined fully (100).

When *orf*1,2,3 (i.e., KS, CLF, ACP) from *S. rimosus* were expressed in a *Streptomyces coelicolor* strain engineered to be bereft of synthesis of any other polyketide backbone, a 20-membered carbon skeleton was synthesized (101). This is an extremely interesting result, as oxytetracycline is a 19-carbon structure—made by condensation of the 3-carbon primer with eight iterative additions of 2-carbon units. To make this new structure, the "minimal polyketide synthase" consisting solely of these three *otc* genes must either use a 2-carbon (acetate primer) followed by nine iterative additions of acetate, or an acetoacetate primer followed by eight iterative additions of acetate. Mutants of *S. rimosus* and of *S. aureofaciens* have been described that make 2-acetyl-2-decarboamidotetracyclines (Table 1), using acetoacetyl-CoA as precursor rather than malon(am)yl-CoA (64,89), presumably due to the inability to synthesize the necessary starter unit. One interpretation of these data is that the polyketide synthase "counts" the number of iterative additions of acetate that it makes, rather than the exact number of carbon atoms in the chain—an important point when trying to engineer the synthases to make polyketide chains of different lengths.

The nascent polyketide chain must then be folded into the tetracyclic structure. Again, the exact details of chain folding have not been deduced for any polyketide structure, but a ketoreductase (for which ActIII is the paradigm) and aromatase/cyclase enzyme (or enzymes) are known to be important (102). For oxytetracycline (Figure 7), *otc*Y2-1 (ketoreductase) and *otc*D1 (aromatase) are the likely candidates, although others may also be involved.

Methylation at the 6-position (Figure 1) results in the formation of 6-methylpretetramid—the first isolable biochemical intermediate in the pathway (64). There are two genes the products of which have similarity to methyltransferases (*otc*Y2-5 and *otc*Z). The work conducted earlier in blocked mutants (68) implied that *otc*Z was responsible for methylation at the 6-position. However, Dairi et al. (76) have isolated the homolog of *otc*Z from a 6-demethyl-chlortetracycline-producing strain of *S. aureofaciens* and named it *cts*6. The gene sequence of *cts*6 is uninterrupted. Thus, this strain appears to have a functional methylase, but it does not make a structure that has a methyl at the 6-position. It would appear that either the gene function for *S. rimosus* has been misassigned in the earlier study (68) and *otc*Y2-5 is the 6-methyltransferase, or that the *cts*6 gene is in fact a point mutant impaired in 6-methyltransferase activity. Gene disruption of each *orf* should clarify this apparent paradox.

A hydroxylase is responsible for conversion of 6-methylpretetramid to 4-hydroxy-6-methylpretetramid (Figure 7). The gene cluster contains several genes that by database comparison can be associated with hydroxylation: *otc*C (the proven 6-hydroxylase), *otc*D2, *otc*Y1-5, and *otc*X1. In the original blocked mutant survey, *otc*X was assigned to this biochemical step. OtcX1 is a small polypeptide (quite similar to a polypeptide encoded by the *act*VA region of the actinorhodin cluster of *S. coelicolor* (103)). It is likely to be an ancillary protein in a hydroxylase reaction, rather than the catalyst *per se*. Thus, one is again left to conclude that either *otc*D-2 or *otc*Y1-5 may be responsible for hydroxylation at this step (with the other responsible for the 5-hydroxylation that comes later in the pathway).

The hydroxyl at the 4-position is then reduced to form 4-keto-anhydrotetracycline. A candidate for this step is *otc*D-3, which has similarity with ketoreductases but is more distant from ActIII, mentioned above in the context of chain folding.

Amination at the 4-position results in the formation of anhydrotetracycline. The asparaginase-like gene product encoded by *otc*Y1-4 is an obvious candidate for this function.

4-Keto-anhydrotetracycline is dimethylated at the 4-position to form 4-amino-anhydrotetracycline. The two methylases within the cluster have already been discussed. Whichever (*otc*Z or *otc*Y2-5) is not involved in methylation at the 6-position likely catalyzes this step.

Hydroxylation at the 6-position (by *otc*C) has already been discussed.

In *S. rimosus*, the product of the OtcC reaction, dehydrotetracycline, is hydroxylated at the 5-position to form dehydroxytetracycline. Again, either *otc*Y1-5 or *otc*D-2 (whichever is not involved in the 4-hydroxylation step) would be the favored candidate. This step does not take place in *S. aureofaciens*.

The last step in oxytetracycline biosynthesis is a dehydrogenase step, formally similar to the tetracycline dehydrogenase in *S. aureofaciens*. As detailed in Section V.B, this reaction has received some attention (86)—to the extent that the enzyme complex has been purified substantially. Microsequencing of a polypeptide present in this preparation identified a gene in *S. rimosus*, *otc*Y2-4, the product of which had a striking similarity to the protein from *S. aureofaciens*, but to no other protein in the database. Other proteins are likely involved in this step. However, they may not lie in the *otc* cluster, and the function of *otc*Y2-4 may be to confer specificity on these other proteins to enable the last step in the biosynthetic pathway to proceed.

Although the biochemical pathway ends formally with oxytetracycline, the antibiotic needs to be exported from the cell; this is the true biological role of OtrB—although it also functions in this context as a resistance protein. Just upstream of *otr*B, a gene (named *otr*R) with similarity to some bacterial repressors (but not to TetR; Section II) has been assigned. Whether this gene product is involved solely in the regulation of *otr*B or in the regulation of other genes of the cluster is an open question.

There are a number of other genes present in the cluster (Figure 7), which may or may not play a role in production of oxytetracycline. These are

> *otc*X2, which is a homolog of a gene in *Saccharopolyspora erythraea* located just downstream of the ferredoxin (*fdx*) gene (104). Ferredoxins are usually involved in electron transfer in hydroxylation.
>
> *otc*X3, which has sequence similarity at the peptide level with an open reading frame of unknown function identified by the *Bacillus subtilis* genome sequencing project.
>
> *otc*D5, which has a homolog in the daunorubicin cluster (105) of unknown function.
>
> *otc*Y2-2, which has reasonable similarity with the β-subunit of toluene and benzene dioxygenases. These enzymes confer substrate specificity, whereas the α-subunit does the catalysis.

No gene product similar to ActIIOrf4, the pathway-specific regulator of the actinorhodin pathway (106), has been found (as yet) to be associated with the *otc* cluster: there is certainly no such gene in the DNA segment bounded by the two resistance genes. Almost all gene clusters for biosynthesis of polyketides by the type II route appear to be under the regulation of a homolog of ActIIOrf4, but the gene cluster for biosynthesis of tetracenomycin in *S. glaucescens* is a notable exception. So it remains to be seen just how the regulation of expression of oxytetracycline biosynthesis, which is highly regulated especially by phosphate (4), comes about.

The tetracycline biosynthetic pathway is assumed to parallel that for oxytetracycline, except for the penultimate step (the 5-hydroxylation). The 7-chloro-group in chlortetracycline (Table 1) is added midway through the biosynthetic pathway, certainly before the anhydrotetracycline step (64). The chlorination enzyme has aroused considerable interest, and two haloperoxidase activities have been isolated from *S. aureofaciens* (107). Both have been cloned and analyzed (108,109), but no compelling data have been published to implicate either in the chlorination of tetracycline. Recently (84), the DNA sequence of *cts8* (the gene assigned the chlorination function from the cluster for production of 6-demethyl-chlortetracycline) has been submitted to Genbank. This gene is clearly neither of the two haloperoxidase genes investigated previously.

D.   Genetic Instability of Biosynthesis of Tetracyclines

As *S. rimosus* is well characterized in terms of its genetics and molecular genetics, it is perhaps not surprising that most work on genetic instability has been undertaken on *S. rimosus*—particularly in strain R6, which comes from a commercial lineage used for the production of oxytetracycline in Croatia. This strain degenerates frequently to produce variants that are morphologically distinct, some of which no longer make oxytetracycline. Using pulsed-field gel electrophoresis and molecular genetic probes for genes of the *otc* biosynthetic cluster, it was possible to assign these variants into three classes (110).

Class I variants (which form 99% of those isolated) have parental levels of resistance to tetracyclines, but do not make the antibiotic. No gross DNA rearrangements were detected in primary class I variants, and they may be altered in some aspect of regulation of the gene cluster.

Class II variants of the R6 strain appear at about 1% of the frequency of class I. They have a large deletion (around 750 kb) of the chromosome, including the entire *otc* cluster (110), and are similar to the OTC-sensitive mutants of *S. rimosus* 15883 reported earlier (70). A physical map of *S. rimosus* has now been developed (111). Like *S. coelicolor* (112), *S. rimosus* has a linear chromosome of around 8 Mb. The inverted repeats of *S. rimosus* (550 kb) are the longest yet reported. The *otc* biosynthetic gene cluster is located around 600 kb from one of the chromosome ends, just outside the inverted repeat structure. This location, so close to the linear chromosome end (111), may explain the frequency of deletion of the cluster—although it appears that the deletion in class II variants may not encompass the end of the chromosome.

Class III variants (formed at 0.1% of the frequency of class I) show increased resistance to oxytetracycline, and elevated levels of both a brown pigment and oxytetracycline. The majority of these variants also show a reproducible large-scale DNA rearrangement, which probably included deletion and a low-level reiteration (three or four copies) of a DNA fragment. These class III mutants are relatively unstable: it is not possible to maintain the enhanced level of antibiotic production.

VI.   FINAL PERSPECTIVE

Despite the length of time that they have been used as antibiotics, the tetracyclines seem to have a rosy future in maintaining and enhancing our health care. New developments, such as the glycylglycines, may extend the useful life of tetracyclines in combating resistant infections. The molecular genetics of tetracyclines has advanced significantly in recent years, to the extent that an outline of the architecture of at least the oxytetracycline cluster can be attempted, and comparison with the emerging picture for the chlortetracycline cluster shows some interesting similarities but other differences.

REFERENCES

1. Běhal V, Hunter IS. Tetracyclines. Vining LC, Studdard C, eds. Genetics and Biochemistry of Antibiotic Production. Boston: Butterworth-Heinemann, 1995:359–385.
2. Běhal V. The tetracycline fermentation. Crit Rev Biotechnol 1987; 5:275–317.
3. Běhal V, Bučko M, Hŏstálek Z. Tetracyclines. Vining LC, ed. Biochemistry and Genetic Regulation of Commercially Important Antibiotics. Reading, Massachusetts: Addison Wesley, 1983:255–276.
4. Podojil M, Blumauerová M, Čulík K, Vaněk Z. The tetracyclines. Vandamme EJ, ed. Biotechnology of Industrial Antibiotics. New York: Marcel Dekker, 1984:259–279.
5. Chopra I, Hawket PM, Hinton M. Tetracyclines: Molecular and clinical aspects. J Antibiot Chemother 1992; 29:247–277.
6. Thijs JC, Vanzwet AA, Moolenaar W, Oom JAJ, Dekortes H, Runhaar EATI. Clarithromycin, an alternative to metronidazole in the triple therapy of *Helicobacter pylori* infection. Aliment Pharmacol Therapeut 1994; 8:131–134.
7. Kloppenburg M, Verweij CL, Miltenburg AMM, Verhoeven AJ, Daha MR, Dijkmans BAC, Breedveld FC. The influence of tetracyclines on T-cell activation. Clin Exp Immunol 1995; 102:635–641.
8. Qadri SMH, Halim M, Ueno Y, Saldin H. Susceptibility of methicillin-resistant *Staphylococcus aureus* to minocycline and other antimicrobials. Chemotherapy 1994; 40:26–29.
9. Schlotfeldt HJ, Kleingeld DW. Fifteen years of a fish health-service in Germany—results and implications. Tierarztliche Umschau 1996; 51:694.
10. Capone DG, Weston DP, Miller V, Shoemaker C. Antibacterial residues in marine-sediments and invertebrates following chemotherapy in aquaculture. Aquaculture 1996; 145:55–75.
11. Kerry J, Hiney M, Coyne R, Nicgabhainn S, Gilroy D, Cazabon D, Smith P. Fish feed as a source of oxytetracycline-resistant bacteria in the sediments under fish farms. Aquaculture 1995; 131:101–113.
12. Kerry J, Coyne R, Gilroy D, Hiney M, Smith P. Spatial-distribution of oxytetracycline and elevated frequencies of oxytetracycline resistance in sediments beneath a marine salmon farm following oxytetracycline therapy. Aquaculture 1996; 145:31–39.
13. Gossen M, Bujard H. Tight control of gene-expression in mammalian-cells by tetracycline-responsive promoters. Proc Natl Acad Sci USA 1992; 89:5547–5551.
14. Stonge L, Furth PA, Gruss P. Temporal control of the cre recombinase in transgenic mice by a tetracycline responsive promoter. Nucl Acids Res 1996; 24:3875–3877.
15. Liang X, Hartikka J, Sukhu L, Manthorpe M, Hobart P. Novel, high expressing and antibiotic-controlled plasmid vectors designed for use in gene-therapy. Gene Ther 1996; 3:350–356.
16. Efrat S, Fuscodemane D, Lemberg H, Halemran O, Wang XR. Conditional transformation of a pancreatic beta-cell line derived from transgenic mice expressing a tetracycline-regulated oncogene. Proc Natl Acad Sci USA 1995; 92:3576–3580.
17. Lederer T, Kintrup M, Takahashi M, Sum PE, Ellestad GE, Hillen W. Tetracycline analogs affecting binding to Tn10-encoded Tet repressor trigger the same mechanism of induction. Biochem 1996; 35:7439–7446.

18. Roberts MC. Tetracycline resistance determinants—mechanisms of action, regulation of expression, genetic mobility, and distribution. FEMS Microbiol Rev 1996; 19:1–24.

19. Schnappinger D, Hillen W. Tetracyclines—antibiotic action, uptake, and resistance mechanisms. Arch Microbiol 1996; 165:359–369.

20. Ohnuki T, Katoh T, Imanaka T, Aiba S. Molecular cloning of tetracycline resistance genes from *Streptomyces rimosus* in *Streptomyces griseus* and characterization of the cloned genes. J Bacteriol 1985; 161:1010–1016.

21. Wang Y, Taylor DE. A DNA sequence upstream of the tetO gene is required for full expression of tetracycline resistance. Antimicrob Agents Chemother 1991; 35:2020–2025.

22. Manavathu EK, Hiratsuka K, Taylor DE. Nucleotide sequence analysis and expression of a tetracycline-resistance gene from *Campylobacter jejuni*. Gene 1988; 62:17–26.

23. Taylor DE, Jerome LJ, Grewal J, Chang N. TetO, a protein that mediates ribosomal protection to tetracycline, binds and hydrolyzes GTP. Can J Microbiol 1995; 41:965–970.

24. Burdett V. TetM-promoted release of tetracycline from ribosomes is GTP dependent. J Bacteriol 1996; 178:3246–3251.

25. Nikolich MP, Shoemaker NB, and Salyers AA. A Bacteroides tetracycline resistance gene represents a new class of ribosome protection. Antimicrob Agents Chemother 1992; 36:1005–1012.

26. Nikolich MP, Shoemaker NB, Wang GR, Salyers AA. Characterization of a new-type of Bacteroides conjugative transposon, TCr-EM(7853). J Bacteriol 1994; 176:6606–6612.

27. Nikolich MP, Hong G, Shoemaker NB, Salyer AA. Evidence for natural horizontal transfer of TetQ between bacteria that normally colonize humans and bacteria that normally colonize livestock. Appl Environ Microbiol 1994; 60:3255–3260.

28. Speer BS, Shoemaker NB, Salyers AA. Bacterial resistance to tetracycline—mechanisms, transfer, and clinical significance. Clin Microbiol Rev 1992; 5:387–399.

29. Stevens AM, Shoemaker NB, Li LY, Salyers AA. Tetracycline regulation of genes on Bacteroides conjugative transposons. J Bacteriol 1993; 175:6134–6141.

30. Salyers AA, Shoemaker NB, Li LY. In the drivers seat—the Bacteroides conjugative transposons and the elements they mobilize. J Bacteriol 1995; 177:5727–5731.

31. Shoemaker NB, Wang GR, and Salyers AA. NBU1, a mobilizable site-specific integrated element from *Bacteroides spp.*, can integrate nonspecifically in *Escherichia coli*. J Bacteriol 1996; 178:3601–3607.

32. Aldema ML, McMurry LM, Walmsley AR, Levy SB. Purification of the Tn*10*-specified tetracycline efflux antiporter, TetA, in a native state as a polyhistidine fusion protein. Mol Microbiol 1996; 19:187–195.

33. Fujihira E, Kimura T, Shiina Y, Yamaguchi A. Transmembrane glutamic-acid residues play essential roles in the metal-tetracycline/H+ antiporter of *Staphylococcus aureus*. FEBS Lett 1996; 391:243–246.

34. Nelson ML, Park PH, Levy SB. Molecular requirements for the inhibition of the tetracycline antiport protein and the effect of potent inhibitors on the growth of tetracycline-resistant bacteria. J Med Chem 1994; 37:1355–1361.

35. Levy SB, McMurry LM, Burdett V, Courvalin P, Hillen W, Roberts MC. Nomenclature for tetracycline resistance determinants. Antimicrob Agents Chemother 1989; 33:1373–1374.

36. Parish JH, Bentley J. Relationships between bacterial drug-resistance pumps and other transport proteins. J Mol Evol 1996; 42:281–293.

37. Hillen W, Berens C. Mechanisms underlying expression of Tn*10* encoded tetracycline resistance. Annu Rev Microbiol 1994; 48:345–369.

38. Hinrichs W, Kisker C, Duvel M, Muller A, Tovar K, Hillen W, Saenger W. Structure of the *tet* repressor tetracycline complex and regulation of antibiotic resistance. Science 1994; 264:418–420.

39. Kisker C, Hinrichs W, Tovar K, Hillen W, Saenger W. The complex formed between *tet* repressor and tetracycline-Mg^{2+} reveals mechanism of antibiotic-resistance. J Mol Biol 1995; 247:260–280.

40. Sloan J, McMurry LM, Lyras D, Levy SB, Rood JI. The *Clostridium perfringens* TetP determinant comprises 2 overlapping genes—*tet*A(P), which mediates active tetracycline efflux, and *tet*B(P), which is related to the ribosomal protection family of tetracycline-resistance determinants. Mol Microbiol 1996; 11:403–415.

41. Speer BS, Salyers AA. Characterization of a novel tetracycline resistance that functions only in aerobically grown *Escherichia coli*. J Bacteriol 1988; 170:1423–1429.

42. Speer BS, Bedzyk L, Salyers AA. Evidence that a novel tetracycline resistance gene found on 2 Bacteroides transposons encodes an NADP-requiring oxidoreductase. J Bacteriol 1991; 173:176–183.

43. Speer BS, Salyers AA. Novel aerobic tetracycline resistance gene that chemically modifies tetracycline. J Bacteriol 1989; 171:148–153.

44. Boothe JH, Hlavka JJ. Tetracyclines. In: *Kirk-Othmer Encyclopedia of Chemical Technology*, vol. 3, 4th ed. New York: Wiley, 1992:331.

45. Tymiak AA, Aklonis C, Bolgar MS, Kahle AD, Kirsch DR, OíSullivan J, Porubcan MA, Principe P, Trejo WH, Ax HA, Wells JS, Andersen NH, Devasthale PV, Telikepalli H, Vandervelde D, Zou JY, Mitscher LA. Dactylocyclines—novel tetracycline glycosides active against tetracycline-resistant bacteria. J Org Chem 1993; 58:535–537.

46. Patel M, Gullo VP, Hegde VR, Horan AC, Gentile F, Marquez JA, Miller GH, Puar MS, Waitz J. A novel tetracycline from *Actinomadura brunnea* fermentation, isolation and structure elucidation. J Antibiot 1987; 40:1408–1413.

47. Hatsu M, Sasaki T, Gomi S, Kodama Y, Sezaki M, Inouye S, Kondo S. A new tetracycline antibiotic with antitumor-activity. 2. The structural elucidation of SF2575. J Antibiot 1992; 45:325–330.

48. Horiguchi T, Hayashi K, Tsubotani S, Iinuma S, Harada S, Tanida S. New naphthacenecarboxamide antibiotics, TAN 1518A and TAN 1518B, have inhibitory activity against mammalian DNA topoisomerase-I. J Antibiot 1994; 47:555–556.

49. Rogalski W. Tetracycline. Hlavka JJ, Boothe JH, eds. Handbook of Experimental Pharmacology. 1985:179–316.

50. Church RFR, Schaub RE, Weiss MJ. Synthesis of 7-dimethylamino-6-demethyl-deoxytetracycline (minocycline) via 9-nitro-6-demethyl-6-deoxytetracycline. J Org Chem 1971; 36:723–725.

51. Sum P-E, Lee VJ, Tally FP, Synthesis of novel tetracycline derivatives with substitution at the C-8 position. Tetrahedron Lett 1994; 35:1835–1836.

52. Barden TC, Buckwalter BL, Testa RT, Peterson PJ, Lee VJ. Glycylcyclines. 3. 9-Aminodoxycyclinecarboxamides. J Med Chem 1994; 37:3205–3211.

53. Sum P-E, Lee VJ, Testa RT, Hlavka JJ, Ellestad GA, Bloom JD, Gluzman Y, Tally FP. Glycylcyclines. 1. A generation of potent antibacterial agents through modification of 9-aminotetracyclines. J Med Chem 1994; 37:184–188.

54. European Patent Applications issued to American Cyanomid Company: 0582810; 0582829; 0582788; 0582789; 0582790; 0582791; 1993.

55. Wise R, Andrews JM. In-vitro activities of 2 glycylcyclines. Antimicrob Agents Chemother 1994; 38:1096–1102.

56. Eliopoulos GM, Wennersten CB, Cole G, Moellering RC. In-vitro activities of 2 glycylcyclines against Gram-positive bacteria. Antimicrob Agents Chemother 1994; 38:534–541.

57. Kenny GE, Cartwright FD. Susceptibilities of *Mycoplasma hominis*, *Mycoplasma pneumoniae*, and *Ureaplasma urealyticum* to new glycylcyclines in comparison with those to older tetracyclines. Antimicrob Agents Chemother 1994; 38:2628–2632.

58. Brown BA, Wallace RJ, Onyi G. Activities of the glycylcyclines N,N-dimethylglycylamidominocycline and N,N-dimethylglycylamido-6-demethyl-6-deoxytetracycline against *Nocardia spp.* and tetracycline resistant isolates of rapidly growing Mycobacteria. Antimicrob Agents Chemother 1996; 40:874–878.

59. Whittington WL, Roberts MC, Hale J, Holmes KK. Susceptibilities of *Neisseria gonorrhoeae* to the glycylcyclines. Antimicrob Agents Chemother 1995; 39:1864–1865.

60. Rasmussen BA, Gluzman Y, Tally FP. Inhibition of protein-synthesis occurring on tetracy-cline resistant, TetM-protected ribosomes by a novel class of tetracyclines, the glycylcy-clines. Antimicrob Agents Chemother 1994; 38:1658–1660.

61. Bergeron J, Ammirati M, Danley D, James L, Norci M, Retsema J, Strick CA, Su WG, Sut-cliffe J, Wondrack L. Glycylcyclines bind to the high-affinity tetracycline ribosomal-binding site and evade Tet M–mediated and Tet O–mediated ribosomal protection. Antimicrob Agents Chemother 1996; 40:2226–2228.

62. Someya Y, Yamaguchi A, Sawai T. A novel glycylcycline, 9-(*N,N*-dimethylglycylamido)-6-demethyl-6-deoxytetracycline, is neither transported nor recognized by the transposon Tn*10*-encoded metal-tetracycline/H+ antiporter. Antimicrob Agents Chemother 1995; 39:247–249.

63. Guay GG, Tuckman M, Rothstein DM. Mutations in the TetA(B) gene that cause a change in substrate-specificity of the tetracycline efflux pump. Antimicrob Agents Chemother 1994; 38:857–860.

64. McCormick JRD. Tetracyclines. Gottieb D, Shaw PD, eds. Antibiotics. Vol. II: Biosynthesis. Berlin: Springer-Verlag, 1967:113–122.

65. Hŏstálek Z, Běhal V, Novoná J, Erban V, Čurdová E, Jechnová V. Regulation of expression of chlortetracycline synthesis in *Streptomyces aureofaciens*. Krumphanzl V, Sikyta B, Vaněk Z, eds. Overproduction of Microbial Products. New York: Academic Press, 1982:47–61.

66. Neužil J, Novotná J, Běhal V, Hŏstálek Z. Inhibition studies of glucose 6-phosphate dehy-drogenase from tetracycline-producing *Streptomyces aureofaciens*. Biotechnol Appl Biochem 1986; 8:375–378.

67. Pigac J, Alačević M. Mapping of oxytetracycline genes in *Streptomyces rimosus*. Period Biol 1979; 81:575–582.

68. Rhodes PM, Winskill N, Friend EJ, Warren M. Biochemical and genetic characterization of *Streptomyces rimosus* mutants impaired in oxytetracycline biosynthesis. J Gen Microbiol 1981; 124:329–338.

69. Rhodes PM, Hunter IS, Friend EJ, Warren M. Recombinant DNA methods for the oxytetra-cycline producing *Streptomyces rimosus*. Biochem Soc Trans 1984; 2:586–587.

70. Butler MJ, Friend EJ, Hunter IS, Kaczmarek FS, Sugden DA, Warren M. Molecular cloning of resistance genes and architecture of a linked gene cluster involved in biosynthesis of oxytetracycline by *Streptomyces rimosus*. Mol Gen Genet 1989; 215:231–238.

71. Binnie C, Warren M, Butler MJ. Cloning and heterologous expression in *Streptomyces livi-dans* of *Streptomyces rimosus* genes involved in oxytetracycline biosynthesis. J Bacteriol 1989; 171:887–895.

72. Doyle D, McDowall KJ, Butler MJ, Hunter IS. Characterization of an oxytetracycline resis-tance gene, *otr*A, from *Streptomyces rimosus*. Mol Microbiol 1991; 5:2923–2933.

73. Reynes JP, Calmels T, Drocourt D, Tiraby G. Cloning, expression in *Escherichia coli* and nucleotide sequence of a tetracycline-resistance gene from *Streptomyces rimosus*. J Gen Microbiol 1988; 134:585–598.

74. Sheridan RP, Chopra I. Origin of tetracycline efflux proteins—conclusions from nucleotide-sequence analysis. Mol Microbiol 1991; 5:895–900.

75. Sezonov GV, Isaeva LM, Lomovskaya ND. Molecular cloning of chlortetracycline resistance gene from *Streptomyces aureofaciens* producing strain. Antibiotiki i Khimioterapiya 1990; 35:7–11.

76. Dairi T, Aisaka K, Katsumata R, Hasegawa M. A self-defense gene homologous to tetracy-cline effluxing gene essential for antibiotic production in *Streptomyces aureofaciens*. Biosci Biotech Biochem 1995; 59:1835–1841.

77. Butler MJ, Binnie C, Hunter IS, Sugden DA, Warren M. Genetic manipulation of the oxyte-tracycline biosynthetic pathway genes. Pierce GE, ed. Developments in Industrial Microbi-ology, Vol. 31. Society for Industrial Microbiology, 1990:41–50.

78. Pang Y, Brown BA, Steingrube VA, Wallace RJ, Roberts MC. Tetracycline resistance determinants in Mycobacterium and Streptomyces species. Antimicrob Agents Chemother 1994; 38:1408–1412.

79. Neužil J, Novotná J, Vančurová I, Běhal V, Hŏstálek Z. High performance liquid chromatography of derivatives involved in the terminal steps of tetracycline biosynthesis. Analyst Biochem 1989; 181:125–129.

80. Vančurová I, Volc J, Flieger M, Neužil J, Novotná J, Vlach J, Běhal V. Isolation of pure anhydroteracycline oxygenase from *Streptomyces aureofaciens*. Biochem J 1988; 253:263–267.

81. Butler MJ, Gedge BN. Purification of anhydrotetracycline oxygenase from *Streptomyces rimosus* using fast protein liquid chromatography. Biotechnol Tech 1989; 4:235–238.

82. Tabor S, Richardson CC. A bacteriophage-T7 RNA polymerase promoter system for controlled exclusive expression of specific genes. Proc Natl Acad Sci USA 1985; 82:1074–1078.

83. Decker H, Motamedi H, Hutchinson CR. Nucleotide sequences and heterologous expression of *tcm*G and *tcm*P, biosynthetic genes for tetracenomycin-C in *Streptomyces glaucescens*. J Bacteriol 1993; 75:3876–3886.

84. Genbank Sequence No. 1100765; accession No. D38214; 1994.

85. Ryan MJ, Lotvin JA. European Patent Application 0468217 A2; 1992.

86. Novotná J, Neužil J, Vančurová I, Běhal V, Hŏstálek Z. Enzymes and coenzymes of the terminal part of the antibiotic pathway in Streptomyces producing tetracyclines. Noack D, Krugel H, Baumberg S, eds. Genetics and Product Formation in Streptomyces. New York Plenum Press, 1991; 1991:137–143.

87. Novotná J, Neužil J, Hŏstálek Z. Spectrophotometric identification of 8-hydroxy-5-deazaflavin:NADP oxidoreductase activity in Streptomyces producing tetracyclines. FEMS Microbiol Lett 1990; 59:242–246.

88. Crosby J, Sherman DH, Bibb MJ, Revill P, Hopwood DA, Simpson TJ. Polyketide synthase acyl carrier proteins from *Streptomyces*—expression in *Escherichia coli*, purification and partial characterization. Biochim Biophys Acta: Protein Struct Mol Enzymol 1995; 1251:32–42.

89. Hochstein FA, Schach von Wittenan M, Tanner FW Jr, Murai K. 2-Acetyl-2-decarboxamidooxytetracycline. J Am Chem Soc 1960; 82:5934–5937.

90. Schuz R, Heller W, Hahlbrock K. Substrate specificity of chalcone synthase from *Petroselinum hortense*. J Biol Chem 1983; 258:6730–6734.

91. Thomas R, Williams DJ. Oxytetracycline biosynthesis: Origin of the carboxamide substituent. J Chem Soc Chem Commun 1983; 12:677–679.

92. Ye JS, Dickens ML, Plater R, Li Y, Lawrence J, Strohl WR. Isolation and sequence analysis of polyketide synthase genes from the daunomycin-producing *Streptomyces* sp. strain C5. J Bacteriol 1994; 176:6270–6280.

93. Thomas R, Williams DJ. Oxytetracycline biosynthesis: Mode of incorporation of [1-^{13}C]- and [1,2-^{13}C$_2$]-acetate. J Chem Soc Chem Commun 1983; 12:128–130.

94. Hopwood DA, Sherman DH. Molecular genetics of polyketides and its comparison to fatty acid biosynthesis. Annu Rev Genet 1990; 24:37–66.

95. Hopwood DA, Khosla C. Genes for polyketide secondary metabolic pathways in microorganisms and plants. Chadwick DJ, Whelan J, eds. Secondary Metabolites: Their Function and Evolution, Ciba Foundation Symposium 171. Chichester, England: John Wiley and Sons, 1992:88–112.

96. Kim ES, Bibb MJ, Butler MJ, Hopwood DA, Sherman DH. Sequences of the oxytetracycline polyketide synthase encoding *otc* genes from *Streptomyces rimosus*. Gene 1994; 141:141–142.

97. Khosla C, McDaniel R, Ebert-Khosla S, Sherman DH, Bibb MJ, Hopwood DA. Genetic construction and functional analysis of hybrid polyketide synthases containing heterologous acyl carrier proteins. J Bacteriol 1993; 175:2197–2204.

98. McDaniel R, Ebert-Khosla S, Hopwood DA, Khosla C. Engineered biosynthesis of novel polyketides. Science 1993; 22:1546–1550.

99.   Shen B, Summers RG, Wendt-Pienkowski E, Hutchinson CR. The *Streptomyces glaucescens* *tcmKL* polyketide synthase gene and *tcmN* polyketide cyclase genes govern the size and shape of aromatic polyketides. J Am Chem Soc 1995; 117:6811–6821.

100.   McDaniel R, Ebert-Khosla S, Hong F, Hopwood DA, Khosla C. Engineered biosynthesis of novel polyketides; influence of a downstream enzyme on the catalytic specificity of a minimal aromatic polyketide synthase. Proc Natl Acad Sci USA 1994; 91:11542–11546.

101.   Fu H, Ebert-Khosla S, Hopwood DA, Khosla C. Relaxed specificity of the oxytetracycline polyketide synthase for an acetate primer in the absence of a malonamyl primer. J Am Chem Soc 1994; 116:6443–6444.

102.   Hutchinson CR, Fujii I. Polyketide synthase gene manipulation: A structure-function approach in engineering novel antibiotics. Annu Rev Microbiol 1995; 49:201–238.

103.   Caballero J, Martinez E, Malpartida F, Hopwood DA. Organization and functions of the *actVA* region of the actinorhodin biosynthetic gene cluster of *Streptomyces coelicolor*. Mol Gen Genet 1991; 230:401–412.

104.   Donadio S, Hutchinson CR. Cloning and characterization of the *Saccharopolyspora erythraea* FdxA gene encoding ferredoxin. Gene 1991; 100:231–235.

105.   Krugel H, Schumann G, Hanel F, Fiedler G. Nucleotide-sequence analysis of 5 putative *Streptomyces griseus* genes, one of which complements an early function in daunorubicin biosynthesis that is linked to a putative gene-cluster involved in TDP-daunosamine formation. Mol Gen Genet 1993; 241:193–202.

106.   Gramajo HC, Takano E, Bibb MJ. Stationary-phase production of the antibiotic actinorhodin in *Streptomyces coelicolor* A3(2) is transcriptionally regulated. Mol Microbiol 1993; 7:837–845.

107.   Weng M, Pfeifer O, Krauss S, Lingens F, vanPee KH. Purification, characterization and comparison of 2 nonheme bromoperoxidases from *Streptomyces aureofaciens* ATCC10762. J Gen Microbiol 1991; 137:2539–2546.

108.   Pelletier I, Pfeifer O, Altenbuchner J, vanPee KH. Cloning of a second nonheme bromoperoxidase gene from *Streptomyces aureofaciens* ATCC10762—sequence analysis, expression in *Streptomyces lividans* and enzyme-purification. Microbiol 1994; 140:509–516.

109.   Pfeifer O, Pelletier I, Altenbuchner J, vanPee KH. Molecular cloning and sequencing of a nonheme bromoperoxidase gene from *Streptomyces aureofaciens* ATCC10762. J Gen Microbiol 1992; 38:1123–1131.

110.   Gravius B, Bezmalinovic T, Hranueli D, Cullum J. Genetic instability and strain degeneration in *Streptomyces rimosus*. Appl Environ Microbiol 1993; 59:2220–2228.

111.   Pandža K, Pfalzer G, Cullum J, Hranueli D. Physical mapping shows that the unstable oxytetracycline gene cluster of *Streptomyces rimosus* lies close to one end of the linear chromosome. Microbiol 1997; in press.

112.   Redenbach M, Kieser HM, Deanpaite D, Eichner A, Cullum J, Kinashi H, Hopwood DA. A set of ordered cosmids and a detailed genetic and physical map of the 8 Mb *Streptomyces coelicolor* A3(2) linear chromosome. Mol Microbiol 1996; 21:77–96.

22
Antibiotics from Genetically Engineered Microorganisms

C. Richard Hutchinson
University of Wisconsin, Madison, Wisconsin

I. INTRODUCTION

Antibiotics and many other compounds with useful pharmacological activity have been found by culturing microorganisms isolated from soil samples and elsewhere, beginning with the seminal work of Fleming (1) and Waksmann (2) between 1929 and 1944. Their discoveries of penicillin and streptomycin led to large-scale screening programs in the pharmaceutical industry and thence to many therapeutically important drugs (e.g., antibacterials like the cephalosporins, erythromycins, rifamycins, and tetracyclines; anticancer agents like doxorubicin and the bleomycins; and immunosuppressants like the cyclosporins and rapamycin) during the following four decades. However, since the late 1970s the pace of discovery of new drugs from these sources has slowed considerably, even though microbial metabolites with new types of chemical structures continue to be uncovered regularly. Why has this come about? This question has bedeviled scientists for nearly two decades. In an attempt to offset the decline in discovery rate, the industry has developed more rapid screening methods, resulting in higher-throughput programs for examining culture extracts, and widened the scope of the environmental niches where new microorganisms are sought. Another approach involving the modification of the genes governing secondary metabolism in microorganisms (the theme of this chapter) is being explored in parallel recently. It is hoped that this approach will result in the formation of compounds that are different from the ones being discovered by traditional screening methods and thus complement those efforts.

II. GENETIC ENGINEERING OF BIOSYNTHETIC PATHWAYS

A. Hybrid Antibiotics: Definition and History

If antibiotics are broadly defined as any biologically active product of microbial secondary metabolism, instead of just the compounds with pharmacological activity and potential therapeutic value in animals, then hybrid antibiotics are ones produced by a genetic hybrid, according to the work of Hopwood et al. (3). A hybrid antibiotic may embody structural features found in two different metabolites and thereby represent the formation of a new natural product. The latter feature does not distinguish hybrid antibiotics from older methods for the formation of new antibiotics, such as precursor-directed biosynthesis (4,5), mutasynthesis (6–8), hybrid biosynthesis (9,10), protoplast fusion (11), or intraspecific mating (12), and biotransformation methods in general (13,14), which together have contributed magnificently to antibiotic development. However, I will consider hybrid antibiotics simply as new metabolites resulting from novel combinations of genes, achieved by the introduction of genes from one microorganism into another or the targeted mutation of secondary metabolism genes within the same microorganism.

The first hybrid antibiotics were produced by introducing all the actinorhodin biosynthesis genes from *Streptomyces coelicolor* or just the genes from the *act*VA region into two other *Streptomyces* spp. that also made benzoisochromane quinone antibiotics (3) (Figure 1). Dihydrogranatirhodin [5] has the C3 stereochemistry found in actinorhodin, instead of that present in granaticin [3a] or dihydrogranaticin [3b], and medermrhodin A [4] has an additional hydroxyl compared with medermycin A [2]. The C6 hydroxyl of **4** is a consequence of the presence of the *act*VA region, which is thought to encode the hydroxylase that acts at a comparable position in an actinorhodin precursor (15), whereas the stereochemical change in **5** may have come from use of an intermediate of actinorhodin biosynthesis in the granaticin/dihydrogranaticin pathway. This pioneering discovery was followed by a report (16) that introduction of different combinations of the actinorhodin polyketide synthase genes into several *Streptomyces* spp. resulted in the production of aloesaponarin II [7a] when the *act*I, *act*III, *act*IV, and *act*VII genes were present, but its 2-hydroxy analog [7b; desoxyerythrolaccin] when the *act*III gene was missing from this set (Figure 2). Since aloesaponarin II formation in *Streptomyces galilaeus* ATCC 31133 required only the *act*I genes, this host provided the activities corresponding to the *act*III, *act*IV, and *act*VII gene products. Thus, in this case **7a** is a true hybrid antibiotic, as noted in the 1992 review by Strohl and Connors (17). Actinorhodin [1] was not produced by the recombinant strains, but it was discovered that **7a** and its 2-carboxy analog are normal shunt products of actinorhodin biosynthesis (16, *vide infra*). Similarly, the presence of the *act*III gene caused S. *galilaeus* ATCC 31671 to make **9b,** a precursor of the aclacinomycins, instead of **9a,** which is normally formed because the 31671 strain lacks a functional *act*III homolog. In both cases it is believed that the introduced or native polyketide synthase genes directed the formation of octaketide **6** or decaketide **8,** which the *act*III gene caused to be reduced at the asterisked carbonyls, followed by cyclization to **7a** or **9b.**

B.   Basic Requirements for the Production of Hybrid Antibiotics

Later research on the production of other types of hybrid antibiotics used refinements of the foregoing approach. Before reviewing these achievements, it is useful to summarize the basic requirements for such work. To set the stage, sufficient knowledge has to be acquired in five areas (Figure 3). First, the impetus to attempt hybrid antibiotic production has to come from the availability of two or more known or newly discovered microorganisms that produce antibiotics the biosyntheses of which have a common feature—for instance, derivation of the carbon skeleton by a polyketide pathway or from common carbohydrates or amino acids. (Chapters 5, 8, 9, 13, 17, and 21 provide examples of the typical ways antibiotics are made.) The need for such biosynthetic knowledge may become the second requirement and is met by characterizing the biosynthetic intermediates,

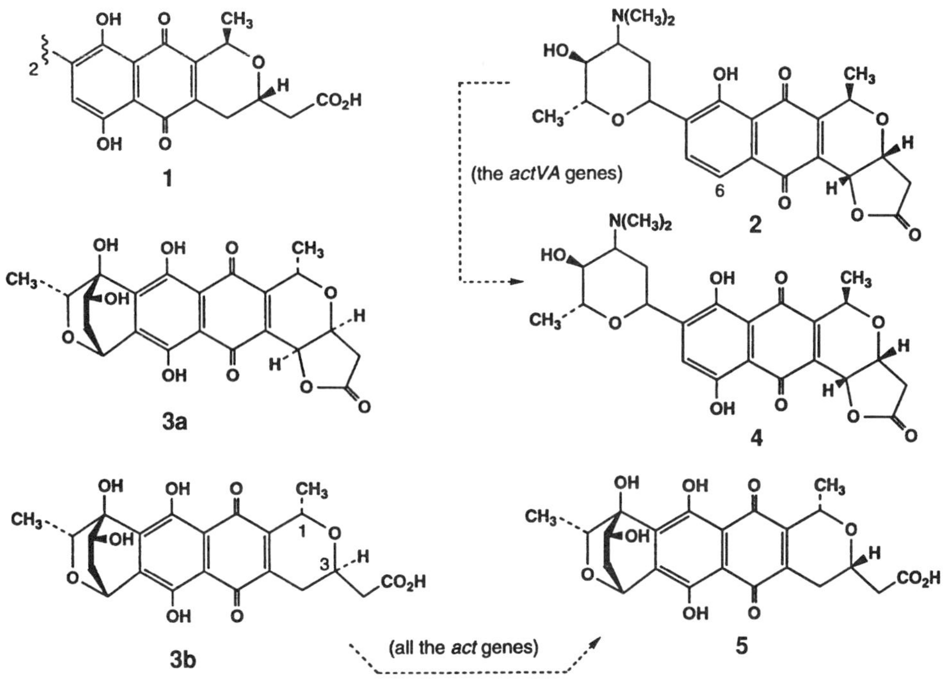

Figure 1 Actinorhodin [1], medermycin A [2], granaticin [3a], dihydrogranaticin [3b], and the hybrid antibiotics mederrhodin A [4] and dihydrogranatirhodin [5] produced by different streptomycetes.

often with the assistance of blocked mutants that accumulate these compounds. Isotope labeling experiments and bioconversion of the putative intermediates can be used to formulate a detailed hypothesis about the sequence of steps in the biosynthetic pathway. Each step then can be confirmed by isolation and characterization of the pathway enzymes using the putative intermediates as substrates.

The third requirement is to establish a gene–enzyme connection, which can be accomplished in several ways. A gene can be found by testing the ability of small segments of DNA, cloned from the producing organism, to restore antibiotic production upon their introduction into a blocked mutant. If the phenotype imparted by the mutation provides a clear picture of the nature of the missing step, the properties of the recombinant strain carrying the cloned DNA result in an immediate assignment of the gene's role. Since the sequence of a large number of antibiotic biosynthesis genes is now available, it may be possible to use a well-characterized gene along with hybridization or polymerase chain reaction (PCR) methods in a search for genes with the same or related function. In either case, once the first gene is found and characterized, the rest of the structural, resistance, and regulatory genes governing the biosynthesis of an antibiotic can usually be found through cloning and characterizing the adjacent DNA, since antibiotic biosynthesis genes have invariably been found to be clustered in one region of the microbial chromosome. (Information about the regulatory and resistance mechanisms can facilitate the construction of hybrid strains.)

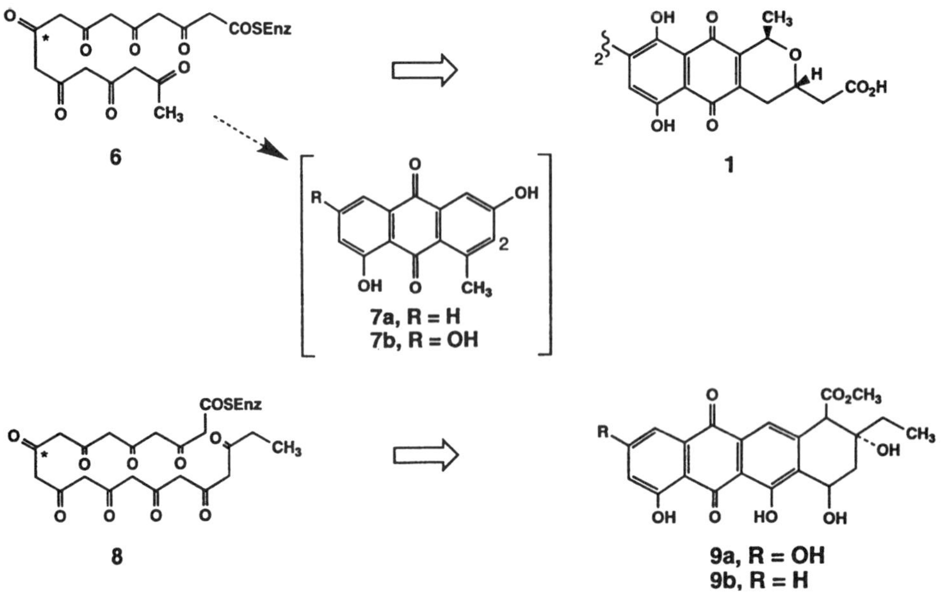

Figure 2 The hybrid antibiotics **7a, 7b,** and **9b** made from octaketide **6,** the precursor of acti-norhodin [1], or decaketide **8,** the precursor of **9a,** by introducing the *act* polyketide synthase genes into different streptomycetes.

1. Organism that produces the parent antibiotics

    a. choose a known microorganism
    b. isolate a new one by a screening program

2. Chemical and biochemical understanding of how the antibiotics are made

    a. determine the simplest biochemical precursors
    b. isolate mutants that do not produce either antibiotic
    c. characterize pathway intermediates
    d. characterize the pathway enzymes

3. Genetic understanding of how the antibiotics are made

    a. find genes that restore antibiotic production to the non-producing mutants
    b. search for genes that produce enzymes with similar structure and function
    c. characterize the cluster of genes for biosynthesis, resistance and regulation of antibiotic production

4. Develop a way to introduce native or modified genes

    a. transformation with plasmid vectors
    b. transfection with phage vectors

5. Determine whether a new antibiotic is produced by the hybrid microorganism

    a. chemical and biochemical assays
    b. pharmacological assays

Figure 3 The basic requirements for manufacturing hybrid antibiotics.

From this point onward, the quest for hybrid antibiotics depends on the ability to introduce one or more genes of interest into a different microorganism from which the gene was cloned or, alternatively, into the same organism if a mutant form of the gene is used. This requirement may become a stumbling block, because finding a suitable vector (plasmid or phage) and a means for its introduction into the host strain (by transformation or transduction) often has to be approached empirically. Fortunately, several of the methods developed for S. coelicolor (18) can be tried with other actinomycetes, or the gene cluster can be moved into a suitable host, such as S. coelicolor or Streptomyces lividans. Filamentous fungi can be manipulated in a similar manner, although the current recombinant DNA methods (19) are less versatile than those developed for bacteria. Finally, the full panoply of chemical and biological assays normally used to screen microorganisms for antibiotic production can be applied to determine whether the recombinant organism produces a new compound with biological activity.

Recent work by the author in collaboration with Abbott laboratories illustrates how these requirements were satisfied in a study of the Streptomyces hygroscopicus ATCC 29253 strain that produces rapamycin, a potentially important immunosuppressive drug. It is desirable to seek analogs of this drug with more potency or less toxicity, and we wished to approach this goal by modifying the rapamycin production genes. Since the carbon skeleton of rapamycin is built by a modular polyketide synthase (Chapter 17), as discussed for erythromycin below, one of the erythromycin polyketide synthase genes was used to clone homologous DNA from S. hygroscopicus by hybridization methods. Two regions containing putative rapamycin production genes were identified by sequence analysis, and transduction with a phage-derived vector was found to be the only means for introducing cloned DNA into the 29253 strain (20). The deletion of genes in each region followed by bioassay of the recombinant strains for the antifungal activity of rapamycin showed that neither set was required for rapamycin production. Although this was an unexpected result (presumably other types of polyketide metabolites are made by these two sets of genes), the correct genes were eventually discovered in the same way (21), and the effect of their deletion or replacement on the production of rapamycin and its hybrid forms could be evaluated (20).

C.   Broader Roles for Genetically Engineered Microorganisms

Although the production of hybrid antibiotics is the theme of this chapter, other commercially important goals can be pursued via the genetic engineering of microorganisms. Once a new antibiotic is discovered, by screening or genetic manipulation, it often is desirable to produce more than the amount made by the naturally occuring or modified strain. This can be done by a number of methods, including the introduction of additional copies of the biosynthetic (22–24) or regulatory (25,26) genes.

In addition to pharmaceuticals, many specialty chemicals such as indigo (27), adipic acid (28), aromatic compounds (29), and semisynthetic opiates (30) can also be made by genetically engineered bacteria. The production of amino acids (31,32), citric acid (33), and biodegradable plastics (34) are other areas where genetically engineered microorganisms play economically important roles. These examples highlight the expanding industrial role of such microorganisms (35,36).

III.   HYBRID ANTIBIOTICS PRODUCED BY GENETICALLY ENGINEERED BACTERIA

A.   Hybrid Antibiotics Produced by Manipulation of Modular (Type I) Polyketide Synthase Genes

Macrolide antibiotics are antibacterial agents used widely in human and veterinary medicine. Erythromycin (ery) was one of the earliest macrolides discovered and is made in *Saccharopolyspora erythraea* by the pathway summarized in Figure 4. This pathway involves a modular, type 1 polyketide synthase consisting of three large multifunctional proteins, DEBS1, -2, and -3, which are encoded by the *ery*A genes (Figure 5) (37,38). The first attempt to produce hybrid erythromycins involved the introduction of randomly cloned DNA from *Streptomyces antibioticus*, which produces oleandomycin, the structure of which is very similar to erythromycin A (Figure 4), into an antibiotic-nonproducing mutant with an 87 bp in-frame deletion in the *ery*AIII gene (38,39). By screening for the restoration of antibiotic production, a recombinant strain was isolated that produced 2-norerythromycin A (Figure 4). Although the absence of the C2 methyl-group cannot be satisfactorily explained, because the cloned DNA could not be isolated from the recombinant for analysis of its function, the result did forecast more interesting achievements made later by using the *ery*A genes.

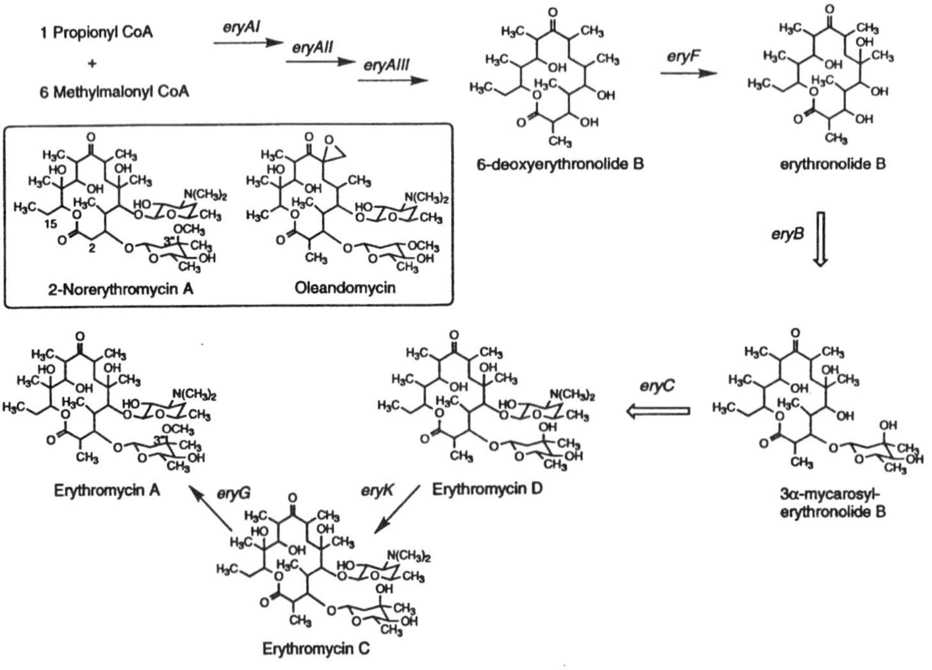

Figure 4   The biosynthesis of erythromycin A in *Saccharopolyspora erythraea*. The names of the principal genes or classes of genes involved are indicated above the thin or thick arrows for single or multiple steps, respectively. The inset shows the hybrid antibiotic 2-norerythromycin A made by introducing DNA from the oleandomycin producer into a blocked mutant of the erythromycin producer.

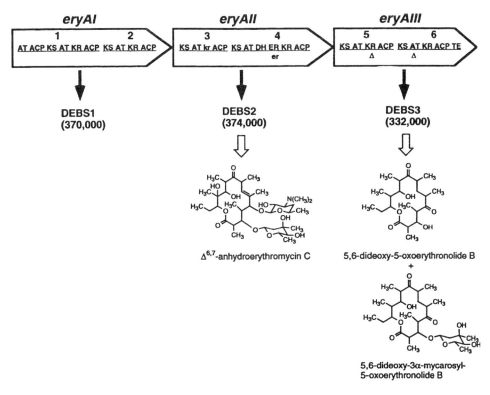

Figure 5   The characteristics of the *ery*A polyketide synthase genes. The three genes are arranged in the order shown by the wedges, and each one produces a DEBS enzyme with two modules (1–6) containing the active-site domains (AT, acyltransferase; ACP, acyl carrier protein; KS, β-ketosynthase; KR, ketoreductase; DH, dehydratase; ER [kr and er indicate an inactive allele], enoyl reductase; TE, thioesterase) arranged in the order shown. The relative molecular weights of each DEBS are shown in parentheses. Hybrid antibiotics produced by an *ery*AII mutant with an inactive ER active site (er) of DEBS2 and by mutant *ery*AIII genes with deleted KR or AT active sites (Δ) are shown below the thick arrows.

The model for the biosynthesis of 6-deoxyerythronolide B, the first macrolactone intermediate of erythromycin biosynthesis (Figure 4), was derived from the predicted amino acid sequences of the DEBS enzymes. Its main feature is a colinearity between the sequence of active sites in DEBS with the steps in the assembly of 6-deoxyerythonolide B. The sites (domains) are arranged in six modules, each of which is responsible for the condensation between the chain starter (propionyl-coenzyme A) and extender (2-methylmalonyl-coenzyme A) units, or the growing carbon chain and each extender unit. Each domain is also responsible for the necessary reductions and dehydrations to achieve the desired oxidation state. This idea was first tested (38) by predicting that a deletion of the first ketoreductase domain in DEBS3 would produce an erythromycin analog with a 5-keto-group, and then showing that the *S. erythraea* AKR5 strain with an 813 bp in-frame deletion in the *ery*AIII gene produced 5,6-dideoxy-5-oxoerythronolide B and its 3α-mycarosyl derivative (Figure 5). This result and the subsequent formation of $\Delta^{6,7}$-anhydroerythromycin C (Figure 5) by the *S. erythraea* EER4S strain (40), in which the

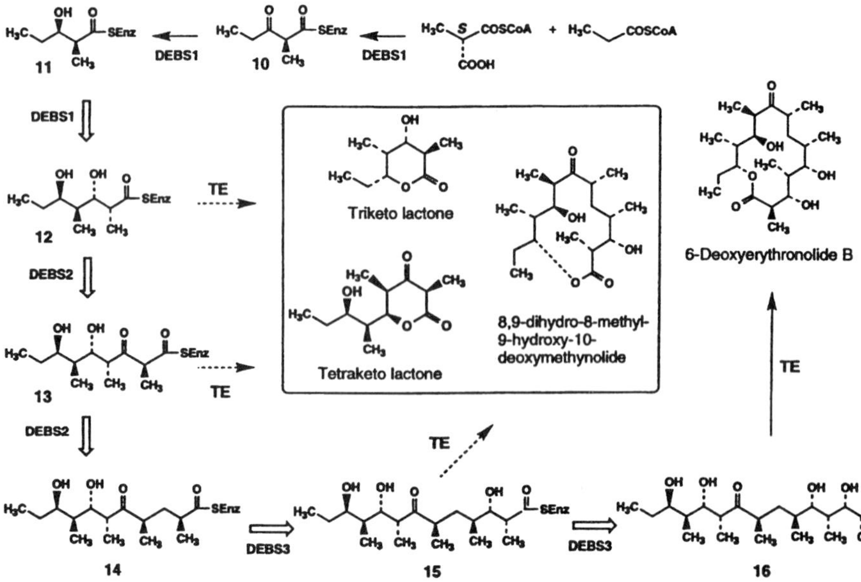

Figure 6 Hypothesis for the processive biosynthesis of 6-deoxyerythronolide B by DEBS1–3. Propionyl-coenzyme A, (2S)-2-methylmalonyl-coenzyme A, and each of the carbon chain assembly intermediates, **10–16,** are attached to thiol-groups of the DEBS proteins. The hybrid antibiotics shown in the inset are produced when the TE (thioesterase) domain is moved from its normal position at the C-terminus of DEBS3 to the ends of specific modules in DEBS2 or DEBS3.

enoylreductase domain of DEBS2 had been inactivated, supported the hypothesis (Figure 6) of processive formation of 6-deoxyerythronolide B by DEBS1–3.

Each module of DEBS1–3 catalyzes the condensation between the two acylthioester substrates and the necessary reduction and dehydration reactions associated with the formation of intermediates **10–16** (Figure 6). Intermediate **16** is then released from DEBS3 and cyclized to 6-deoxyerythronolide B by the action of a thioesterase (TE) domain. All of these reactions take place to produce 6-deoxyerythronolide B in good yield when the *eryAI–III* genes are cloned in plasmid pCK7 in *S. coelicolor* CH999 (41). This heterologous system (42–44) or a specially constructed *S. erythraea eryAI* mutant (45) has been used to show that the TE domain, when moved from its normal position to the end of DEBS1, causes the chimeric enzyme to release and cyclize **12** to a triketo lactone (Figure 6). When the TE domain is placed at the end of the first module of DEBS2, **13** is released and cyclized to a tetraketo lactone (Figure 6) or the hemiketal form of its decarboxylation product (46); and when it is at the end of the first module of DEBS3, **15** is released and cyclized to 8,9-dihydro-8-methyl-9-hydroxy-10-deoxymethynolide (Figure 6) (43). Since only the triketo lactone was made by the *S. erythraea eryAI* mutant even when the *eryAII* and *eryAIII* genes were still present (45), the TE activity not only releases the carbon chain assembly intermediate from DEBS1 or DEBS2, it also prevents the intermediate's transfer to DEBS2 or DEBS3. Moreover, the formation of macrolactone products smaller than 6-deoxyerythronolide B shows that truncation of the DEBS subunits, instead of targeted mutation of their active sites, may be an important way to make hybrid antibiotics. In fact, it should be possible to make a large number of novel compounds in this way because the approach can be extended to rapamycin (21), avermectin (47), soraphen (48), and FR-008 (49), each of which have different chain lengths, as well as the modular polyketide synthase genes governing the biosynthesis of many other macrolide and polyether antibiotics yet to be identified (50). It will be very exciting if novel combinations of such genes can alter the choice of chain extender unit, invert the stereochemistry of the hydroxylated or branched positions, or increase the size of the polyketide chain.

Analogs of the triketo lactone resulting from the utilization of novel starter units or the absence of reduction of **10** to **11** have been made in vitro with cell-free systems (51) and the purified DEBS1:TE hybrid enzyme (52). This method has considerable potential for the synthesis of additional novel natural products if a means can be developed to use the modified DEBS enzymes and their coenzymes on a large scale.

Targeted disruption of the S. *erythraea eryF* gene resulted in the formation of the 6-deoxyerythromycins A–D and their 15-nor analogs (53). Since 6-deoxyerythromycin A is not prone to the acid-catalyzed formation of the antibiotically inactive anhydro-erythromycin A, these novel macrolides may become important anti-infective agents.

Although the erythromycins have been the focal point for the preparation of hybrid macrolide antibiotics, the first hybrid macrolides to be made were novel esters of spiramycin I (Figure 7), resulting from the introduction of the Streptomyces *thermotolerans carE* gene into the spiramycin-producing Streptomyces *ambofaciens* (54) or the Streptomyces *mycarofaciens mdmB* gene into S. *ambofaciens* (55). The 3-O-acetate derivative of tylosin has been made in the same way, using the S. *thermotolerans acyA* gene (56).

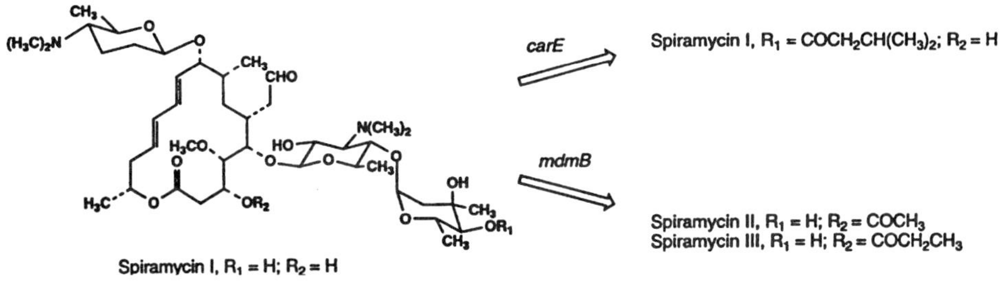

Figure 7 Hybrid 16-membered macrolide antibiotics made by introducing the *carE* or *mdmB* genes into the spiramycin producer.

B. Hybrid Antibiotics Produced by Manipulation of Iterative (Type II) Polyketide Synthase Genes

Antibiotics with aromatic rings in their structures, like oxytetracycline, the anthracycline doxorubicin, and griseofulvin (Figure 8), are also commerically important drugs. The carbon skeleton of such antibiotics is assembled in bacteria by a type II, or iterative, polyketide synthase, the constituents of which are largely monofunctional enzymes, in contrast to the large multifunctional proteins of the type I class (57,58). One of the earliest examples of hybrid antibiotic production (16) involved the use of the actinorhodin (act) polyketide synthase genes, *actI*, -VII, and -IV (59) plus *actIII* (60) to make the anthraquinones **7a** and **7b** (Figure 2).

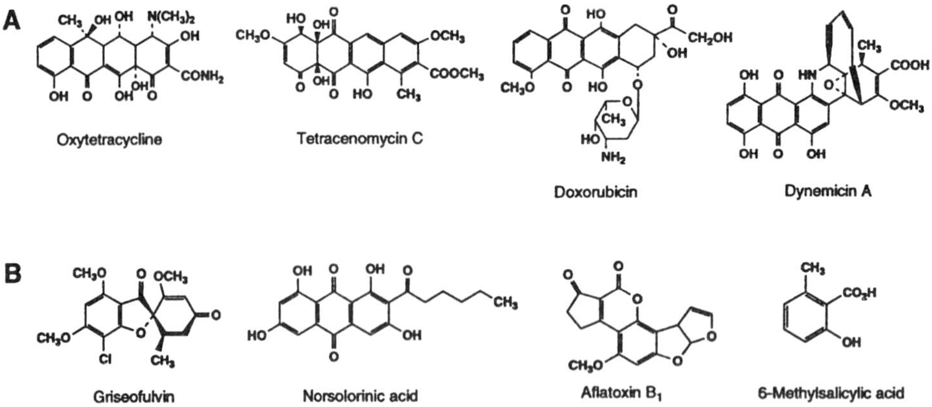

Figure 8   Typical aromatic antibiotics made by (A) bacterial type II iterative polyketide synthases and (B) fungal type I iterative polyketide synthases. Norsolorinic acid is the precursor of aflatoxin B_1.

The quest for hybrid antibiotics of this type has evolved from efforts to elucidate the properties of the three to six enzymes that make up a typical iterative polyketide synthase, as defined by the functions of the polyketide synthases involved in the biosynthesis of actinorhodin and tetracenomycin (tcm) C. Sequence analysis, facilitated by the similarity of the proteins to the well-characterized enzymes of fatty acid biosynthesis, indicated that the *actIORF1*, *actIORF2* (59), and *tcmKL* (61) genes encode the enzyme subunits catalyzing the condensation reaction between the acetate starter unit or the acylthioester intermediates and the malonate extender unit, with the assistance of the acyl carrier proteins (ACPs) encoded by the *actIORF3* and *tcmM* genes. However, it was not clear how enzymes with such similar protein sequences could form two different kinds of aromatic products—the octaketide **17** from the *act* genes or the decaketide TcmF2 from the *tcm* genes (Figure 9)—although it was certain that chain length must be determined by some factor. The ACPs were found not to be determining factors (62), but some insight was provided by discovering that a gene cassette containing the *actIII*, *tcmKL*, *actIORF3*, *actVII*, and *actIV* genes made the decaketide RM20 (Figure 9B, path 2) (63); whereas the the *actIORF1*, *actIORF2*, *tcmM*, and *tcmN* genes made the octaketide UWM1 (Figure 9A, path 4) (64). These results, in comparison with the properties of other gene cassettes (63,64), showed that the size of the acyclic poly-β-ketone intermediates, that is, the number of times the condensation reaction takes place, is dictated by the *actIORF1/actIORF2* or *tcmKL* genes. It is assumed that the homologs of these genes found in many other microorganisms (57,58) have the same role. Consequently, the ActIOrf1 and TcmK enzymes were named the β-ketoacyl:ACP synthases (KSs) because they each have a clearly recognizable active site for the condensation reaction (59,61,65). The ActIOrf2 and TcmL enzymes, the sequences of which are is very similar to that of the KSs but lack the active site, were named chain length factors (CLFs) (63), although the CLFs alone do not determine the chain length (63,64).

Numerous hybrid antibiotics have been made by combinations of the genes encoding the KS, CLF, and ACP proteins, which have been defined as composing the minimal polyketide synthase (66). SEK4 and SEK4b (Figure 9A, path 3) are made by the *actIORF1*, -*ORF2*, and -*ORF3* genes (67,68); SEK15 and SEK15b (Figure 9B, path 3) by

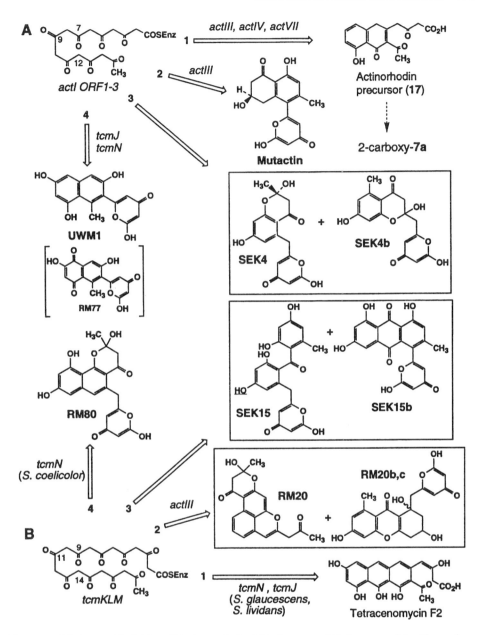

Figure 9 Native and hybrid antibiotics made by (A) the *act* or (B) the *tcm* polyketide synthase genes.

the *tcm*KLM genes (66); and RM20, -20b, and -20c (Figure 9B, path 2) by the *tcm*KL-M*act*III genes (63,66,69). RM18 and RM18b are similar to RM20 but are made from 16C and 18C poly-β-ketones (70). It is not yet clear whether the cyclization patterns reflected in these nine structures are determined enzymatically by the minimal polyketide synthase, spontaneously as a consequence of the inherent chemical reactivity of the poly-β-ketone intermediates, or by a combination of both things.

The act ketoreductase (KR) (60,67), aromatase (ARO), and polyketide cyclase (CYC) enzymes (71) can act on the poly-β-ketone intermediates to form many structurally different fused-ring aromatic compounds. For example, reduction of the C9 carbonyl in an octaketide by the ActIII KR results in the formation of mutactin (Figure 9A, path 2) (72) instead of SEK4 and SEK4b (66). Mutactin can then be spontaneously dehydrated to dehydromuctin with two fused aromatic rings. But if the *act*VII ARO gene is also present, SEK34 (SEK4 without the phenolic hydroxyl) is formed (71). Similarly, the decaketides RM20, -20b, and -20c are formed instead of SEK15 and SEK15b (Figure 9B, path 2 vs. path 3) in the presence of the ActIII KR (66); and SEK43 (SEK15 without the underlined hydroxyl [Figure 9B, path 3]) is formed when the *gris* ARO gene is also present (73). Addition of the *act*VII ARO gene to *tcm*KLM alters the ratio of SEK15 and SEK15b from (1:1) to (16:1) (66); and addition of the *tcm*N CYC gene to *act*IORF1, *act*IORF2, and *tcm*M results in UWM1 (64) or its quinone form RM77 (74) (Figure 9A). Finally, the *whi*EORFVI gene that encodes an ActVII and TcmN homolog acts like *tcm*N when added to the *tcm*KLM genes, but it causes EM18 to be formed along with mutactin and dehydromutactin when added to the *act* minimal polyketide synthase and *act*III KR genes (75). The fused aromatic and reduced rings are switched in EM18 relative to mutactin.

The facts just summarized show how reduction of one of the carbonyls of a poly-β-ketone intermediate or the presence of an ARO or CYC gene can alter the intermediate's subsequent cyclization pattern. In fact, reduction of the decaketide in Figure 9B prevents its cyclization by the TcmN CYC (76), since the *tcm*JKLMN*dps*E cassette (*dps*E is the KR gene from the doxorubicin polyketide synthase; 77) makes a mixture of TcmF2, RM20b, and RM20c (Meurer G, Gerlitz M, Wendt-Pienkowski E, and Hutchinson CR, unpublished results). Conversely, reduction of this decaketide by DpsE is necessary before it can be acted upon by the DpsF (77) or JadOrf4 (78) CYC enzymes, but DpsE is unable to reduce the octaketide made by the Act minimal polyketide synthase. Hence, it would seem that some KR enzymes can distinguish the size of the nascent poly-β-ketone intermediates, even though the information presented in Figure 9 shows that ActIII clearly recognizes octa- and decaketides. Since the decaketide was converted to SEK43 by DpsF or JadOrf4, instead of a product with two or three fused aromatic rings (Meurer G, Gerlitz M, Wendt-Pienkowski E, and Hutchinson CR, unpublished results), additional cyclases must be involved in the formation of the characteristic daunorubicin or angular jadomycin ring systems. Until these additional cyclase genes are identified, the scope for making additional hybrid antibiotics from reduced decaketide precursors appears to be quite limited.

Although the iterative polyketide synthases are quite versatile, as recognized by McDaniel et al. (73) in a paper on the design of aromatic polyketide natural products, it is not known if any of the novel compounds made by these enzymes have valuable biological activity. [The bacterial hosts must not be adversely affected by these novel compounds, as well as by the hybrid antibiotics described in Section III.A, because they can produce them in amounts as high as 0.2 mg/ml. This suggests that as a group they do not have potent antibacterial activity against streptomycetes.] This may require their further metabolism by other enzymes, such as the O-methyltransferases, oxidases, hydroxylases, and glycosyltransferases that typically are part of secondary metabolism. The reactions that elaborate the molecule after carbon chain formation are generally less well studied, even though it is these modifications that define the overall molecular shape and, consequently, are crucial to the molecule's biological properties. Fu et al. (79) have reported that the TcmO O-methyltransferase (76) can convert the 2-carboxy derivative of **7a**

(Figure 10A, **18**), made by the Act minimal polyketide synthase, ActIII KR, ActVII ARO, and ActIV CYC enzymes (63), to its methyl ester. This is understandable because TcmO recognizes similar structural features in its normal substrate, TcmB3 [19]. More remarkable is the formation of novel glycoside **20** (Figure 10B) when a large portion of the elloramycin biosynthesis genes (80) is introduced into the urdamycin-producing *Streptomyces fradiae* (81). The olivose-group of **20** must have been provided by S. *fradiae* genes; the source of the glycosyltransferase that presumably acts on the 8-desmethyltetra-cenomycin substrate is not known, although olivose is attached at the position equiva-lent to the one glycosylated by trimethylrhamnose in elloramycin A (Figure 10B). There-fore, the glycosyltransferase must have recognized either a novel aglycone or thymidine diphospho-2,6-dideoxysugar. Decker et al. (81) have reported that two other novel metabolites, 3,8-didemethyl- and 6-hydroxytetracenomycin C, were made by introducing the *tcm* biosynthesis genes into the urdamycin producer.

Hybrid anthracycline antibiotics related to the aclacinomycins have been made in two ways. The introduction of a region of *Streptomyces purpurascens* DNA containing *actIORF1* homologs into S. *galilaeus* ATCC 31615 (82) resulted in production of the aclacinomycins normally made by S. *galilaeus* plus glycosides of two known S. *purpuras-cens* antibiotics, 10-demethoxycarbonylaklavinone and 11-deoxy-β-rhodomycinone. The authors assumed that the latter two metabolites are hybrid antibiotics. Expression of the

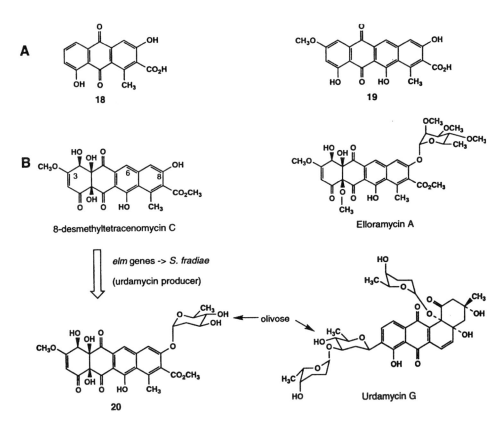

Figure 10 (A) Substrates for methylation by the TcmO O-methyltransferase from *Streptomyces glaucescens*. (B) Native and hybrid antibiotics produced by the tetracenomycin C, elloramycin, and urdamycin G producers.

*Streptomyces peucetius dnr*F aklavinone 11-hydroxylase gene in *S. galilaeus* ATCC 31133 gave rise to the cytotoxic 11-hydroxyaclacinomycin A, B, T, and X antibiotics (83).

The large number of iterative polyketide synthase genes already identified in bacteria (57,58) provides great latitude in exploring the possibility of making additional novel natural products in the way just described. Aromatic polyketides are also made by such enzymes in fungi (Figure 8B) (84–87), which further expands this opportunity if we can learn how the type 1 fungal enzymes (not type II, surprisingly, but still iterative) determine the size and shape of the metabolite produced (58). The successful expression of the gene for the biosynthesis of 6-methylsalicylic acid (Figure 8) in *S. coelicolor* CH999 (88) suggests that fungal polyketide synthase genes may be engineered to produce hybrid antibiotics in bacteria.

C. Hybrid Antibiotics Produced by Manipulation of Oligopeptide Synthetase Genes

Oligopeptide antibiotics are assembled nonribosomally by multifunctional enzymes with domains for amino acid recognition, activation, and ligation (and C2 epimerization or *N*-methylation, if necessary) arranged in the order of each amino acid in the final antibiotic structure (89). Hybrid oligopeptide antibiotics have been made by interchanging the domains among different oligopeptide biosynthesis genes from bacteria and fungi (90,91), as discussed in Chapter 9.

D. Future Prospects

New hybrid antibiotics will continue to be made by manipulation of the polyketide synthase and oligopeptide synthetase genes, since the conceivable permutations of these genes are nearly endless. If the resulting compounds do not have useful antibiotic activity, perhaps because they cannot be converted to their cyclic or glycosidic forms, they still can serve as scaffolds for the combinatorial chemistry programs of industry that are aimed at other drug discovery targets. Carbohydrate-derived antibiotics (see Chapters 21 and 24) may also be amenable to hybrid antibiotic construction if the enzymes that process the biosynthetic intermediates are found to have sufficient flexibility. That this substrate flexibility exists is illustrated by the formation of 8-demethyl-8-O-olivosyltetracenomycin C [20]. Genetically engineered strains have been developed for the production of penicillins (92) and of starting materials for the semisynthesis of cephalosporins (93), although new derivatives of the penicillins are not likely to be found by manipulation of the key enzyme isopenicillin N synthase, according to the work of Huffman et al. (94). Nevertheless, it is only a detailed understanding of how such enzymes function coupled with a knowledge of their kinetic parameters and substrate specificity, and comparisons among different pathways, that will allow them to be used in rational design experiments to produce the hybrid antibiotics with pharmacological activity, the ultimate goal of many researchers in this field.

ACKNOWLEDGMENTS

The work done at the University of Wisconsin described in this chapter was supported in part through grants from the National Institutes of Health (CA35381 and GM46696). I thank Steve Kendrew, Guido Meurer, and Evelyn Wendt-Pienkowski for critical reading of the manuscript.

REFERENCES

1. Fleming A. On the antibacterial action of cultures of a Penicillium, with special reference to their use in the isolation of B. *influenzae*. Br J Exp Pathol 1929; 10:226–236.
2. Schatz A, Bugie E, Waksmann S. Streptomycin, a substance exhibiting antibiotic activity against gram positive and gram negative bacteria. Proc Soc Exp Biol Med 1944; 55:66–69.
3. Hopwood DA, Malpartida F, Kieser HM, Ikeda H, Duncan J, Fujii I, Rudd BAM, Floss HG, Omura S. Production of "hybrid" antibiotics by genetic engineering. Nature 1985; 314:642–644.
4. Behrens OK, Corse J, Edwards JP, Garrison L, Jone RG, Soper QF, van Abeele FR, Whitehead CW Biosynthesis of penicillins. IV. New crystalline biosynthetic penicillins. J Biol Chem 1948; 175:793–809.
5. Thiericke R, Rohr J. Biological variation of microbial metabolites by precursor-directed biosynthesis. Nat Prod Rep 1993; 1993:265–289.
6. Ankenbaur RG, Staley AL, Rinehart KL, Cox CD. Mutasynthesis of siderophore analogues by *Pseudomonas aeruginosa*. Proc Natl Acad Sci USA 1991; 88:1878–1882.
7. Daum SJ, Lemke RJ. Mutational biosynthesis of new antibiotics. Annu Rev Microbiol 1979; 33:241–265.
8. Dutton CJ, Gibson SP, Goudie AC, Holdom KS, Pacey MS, Ruddock JC, Bu'Lock JD, Richards MK. Novel avermectins produced by mutational biosynthesis. J Antibiot 1991; 44:357–364.
9. Omura S, Ikeda H, Matsubara H, Sadakane N. Hybrid biosynthesis and absolute configuration of macrolide antibiotic M-4365 G_1. J Antibiot 1980; 33:1570–1572.
10. Omura S, Sadakane N, Tanaka Y, Matsubara H. Chimeramycins: New macrolide antibiotics produced by hybrid biosynthesis. J Antibiot 1983; 36:927–930.
11. Gomi S, Ikeda D, Nakamura H, Naganawa H, Yamashita F, Hotta K, Kondo S, Okami Y, Umezawa H. Isolation and structure of a new antibiotic, indolizomycin, produced by a strain SK2-52 obtained by interspecies fusion treatment. J Antibiot 1984; 37:1491–1494.
12. Traxler P, Schupp T, Fuhrer H, Richter WJ. 3-Hydroxyrifamycin S and further novel ansamycins from a recombinant strain R-21 of *Nocardia mediterranei*. J Antibiot 1981; 34:971–979.
13. Hardman DJ. Biotransformation of halogenated compounds. Crit Rev Biotechnol 1991; 11:1–14.
14. Rosazza JP. Microbial Transformations of Bioactive Compounds. Boca Raton, Florida: CRC Press, 1982.
15. Caballero JL, Martinez E, Malpartida F, Hopwood DA. Organisation and functions of the *actVA* region of the actinorhodin biosynthetic gene cluster of *Streptomyces coelicolor*. Mol Gen Genet 1991; 230:401–412.
16. Bartel PL, Zhu C-B, Lampel JS, Dosch DC, Connors NC, Strohl WR, Beale JM Jr, Floss HG. Biosynthesis of anthraquinones by interspecies cloning of actinorhodin biosynthesis genes in streptomycetes: Clarification of actinorhodin gene functions. J Bacteriol 1990; 172:4816–4826.
17. Strohl WR, Connors, NC. Significance of anthraquinone formation resulting from the cloning of actinorhodin genes in heterologous streptomycetes. Mol Microbiol 1992; 6:147–152.
18. Hopwood DA, Bibb MJ, Chater KF, Kieser T, Bruton CJ, Kieser HM, Lydiate DJ, Smith CP, Ward JM, Schempf H. Genetic Manipulations of *Streptomyces*: A Laboratory Manual. Norwich, England: The John Innes Foundation, 1985.

19. Timberlake WE. Cloning and analysis of fungal genes. Bennet JW, Lasure, LL, eds. More Gene Manipulations in Fungi. New York: Academic Press, 1991:51–86.

20. Lomovskaya N, Fonstein L, Ruan X, Stassi D, Katz L, Hutchinson CR. Gene disruption and replacement in the rapamycin-producing *Streptomyces hygroscopicus* ATCC 29253 strain, Microbiology, in press.

21. Schwecke T, Aparicio JF, Molnar I, Konig A, Khaw LE, Haydock SF, Oliynyk M, Caffrey P, Cortes J, Lester JB, Bohm GA, Staunton J, Leadlay PF. The biosynthesis gene cluster for the polyketide immunosuppressant rapamycin. Proc Natl Acad Sci USA 1995; 93:7839–7843.

22. Decker H, Summers RG, Hutchinson CR. Overproduction of all of the components of a type II polyketide synthase or only the acyl carrier protein stimulates the production of tetra-cenomycin C biosynthetic intermediates in *Streptomyces glaucescens*. J Antibiot 1994; 47:54–63.

23. Skatrud PL, Tietz AJ, Ingolia TD, Cantwell CA, Fisher DL, Chapman JL, Queener SW. Use of recombinant DNA to improve production of cephalosporin C by *Cephalosporium acremonium*. Bio/Technol 1989; 7:477–485.

24. Malmberg LH, Hu WS, Sherman DH. Precursor flux control through targeted chromosomal insertion of the lyseine ε-aminotransferase (*lat*) gene in cephamycin biosynthesis. J Bacteriol 1993; 175:6916–6924.

25. Fernandez-Moreno MA, Caballero JL, Hopwood DA, Malpartida F. The actinorhodin gene cluster contains regulatory and antibiotic export genes that are direct targets for translational control by the *bldA* tRNA gene of *Streptomyces coelicolor*. Cell 1991; 66:769–780.

26. Stutzman-Engwall KJ, Otten SL, Hutchinson CR. Regulation of secondary metabolism in *Streptomyces* spp. and overproduction of daunorubicin in *Streptomyces peucetius*. J Bacteriol 1992; 174:144–154.

27. Murdock D, Ensley BD, Serdar C, Thalen M. Construction of metabolic operons catalyzing the de novo biosynthesis of indigo in *Escherichia coli*. Bio/Technol 1993; 11:381–386.

28. Frost JW, Draths KM. Environmentally compatible synthesis of adipic acid from glucose. J Am Chem Soc 1994; 116:399–400.

29. Frost JW, Draths KM. Biocatalytic syntheses of aromatics from D-glucose. Annu Rev Microbiol 1995; 49:557–579.

30. French CE, Hailes AM, Rathbone DA, Long MT, Willey DL, Bruce NC. Biological production of semisynthetic opiates using genetically engineered bacteria. Bio/Technol 1995; 13:674–676.

31. Katsumata R, Ikeda, M. Hyperproduction of tryptophan in *Corynebacterium glutamicum* by pathway engineering. Bio/Technol 1993; 11:921–925.

32. Jetten MSM, Sinskey AJ. Recent advances in the physiology and genetics of amino acid producing bacteria. Crit Rev Biotech 1995; 15:73–103.

33. Anderson S, Marks CB, Lazarus R, Miller J, Stafford K, Seymour J, Light D, Rastetter W, Estell D. Production of 2-keto-L-gulonate, an intermediate in L-ascorbate synthesis, by a genetically modified *Erwinia herbicola*. Science 1985; 230:144–149.

34. Poirer Y, Nawrath C, Somerville C. Production of polyhydroxyalkanoates, a family of biodegradable plastics and elastomers, in bacteria and plants. Bio/Technol 1995; 13:142–150.

35. Bailey JE. Toward a science of metabolic engineering. Science 1991; 252:1668–1675.

36. Cameron DC, Tong IT. Cellular and metabolic engineering. Appl Biochem Biotechnol 1993; 38:105–140.

37. Cortes J, Haydock SF, Roberts GA, Bevitt DJ, Leadlay PF. An unusually large multifunctional polypeptide in the erythromycin-producing polyketide synthase of *Saccharopolyspora erythraea*. Nature 1990; 348:176–178.

38. Donadio S, Staver MJ, McAlpine JB, Swanson SJ, Katz L. Modular organization of genes required for complex polyketide biosynthesis. Science 1991; 252:675–679.

39. McAlpine JB, Tuan JS, Brown DP, Grebner, KD, Whittern DN, Buko A, Katz L. New antibiotics from genetically engineerd actinomycetes. I. 2-Norerythromycins, isolation and structural determination. J Antibiot 1987; 40:1115–1122.

40. Donadio S, McAlpine JB, Sheldon PJ, Jackson M, Katz L. An erythromycin analog produced by reprogramming of polyketide synthesis. Proc Natl Acad Sci USA 1993; 90:7119–7123.

41. Kao CM, Katz L, Khosla C. Engineered biosynthesis of a complete macrolactone in a heterologous host. Science 1994; 265:509–512.

42. Kao CM, Luo G, Katz L, Cane DE, Khosla C. Engineered biosynthesis of a triketide lactone from an incomplete modular polyketide synthase. J Am Chem Soc 1994; 116:11612–11613.

43. Kao CM, Luo G, Katz L, Cane DE, Khosla C. Manipulation of macrolide ring size by directed mutagenesis of a modular polyketide synthase. J Am Chem Soc 1995; 117:9105–9106.

44. Brown MJB, Cortes J, Cutter AL, Leadlay PF, Staunton, J. A mutant generated by expression of an engineered DEBS1 protein from the erythromycin-producing polyketide synthase (PKS) in *Streptomyces coelicolor* produces the triketide as a lactone, but the major product is the nor-analogue derived from acetate as starter acid. J Chem Soc Chem Commun 1995; 1995:1517–1518.

45. Cortes J, Wiesmann KEH, Roberts GA, Brown MJB, Staunton J, Leadlay P. Repositioning of a domain in a modular polyketide synthase to promote specific chain cleavage. Science 1995; 268:1487–1489.

46. Kao CM, Luo G, Katz L, Cane DE, Khosla C. Engineered biosynthesis of structurally diverse tetraketides by a trimodular polyketide synthase, J Am Chem Soc 1996; 118:9184–9185.

47. MacNeil DJ, Occi JL, Gewain KM, MacNeil T. Correlation of the avermectin polyketide synthase genes to the avermectin structure: Implications for designing novel avermectins. Ann NY Acad Sci 1994; 721:123–132.

48. Schupp T, Toupet C, Cluzel B, Neff S, Hill S, Beck JJ, Ligon JM. A *Sorangium cellulosum* (Mycobacterium) gene cluster for the biosynthesis of the macrolide antibiotic soraphen A: Cloning, characterization, and homology to polyketide synthase genes from actinomycetes. J Bacteriol 1995; 177:3673–3679.

49. Hu Z, Bao K, Zhou X, Zhou Q, Hopwood DA, Kieser T, Deng Z. Repeated polyketide synthase modules involved in the biosynthesis of a heptaene macrolide by *Streptomyces* sp. FR-008. Mol Microbiol 1994; 14:163–172.

50. O'Hagan D. The Polyketide Metabolites. Chichester: Ellis Horwood, 1991.

51. Pieper R, Luo G, Cane DE, Khosla C. Remarkably broad substrate specificity of a modular polyketide synthase in a cell-free system. J Am Chem Soc 1995; 117:11373–11374.

52. Wiesmann KEH, Cortes J, Brown MJB, Cutter AL, Staunton J, Leadlay PF. Polyketide synthesis in vitro on a modular polyketide synthase. Chem Biol 1995; 2:583–589.

53. Weber JM, Leung JO, Swanson SJ, Idler KB, McAlpine JB. An erythromycin derivative produced by targeted gene disruption in *Saccharopolyspora erythraea*. Science 1991; 252:114–117.

54. Epp J, Huber MLB, Turner JR, Goodson T, Schoner BE. Production of a hybrid macrolide antibiotics in *Streptomyces ambofaciens* and *Streptomyces lividans* by introduction of a cloned carbomycin biosynthetic gene from *Streptomyces thermotolerans*. Gene 1989; 85:293–301.

55. Hara O, Hutchinson CR. A macrolide 3-O-acyltransferase gene from the midecamycin-producing species of *Streptomyces mycarofaciens*. J Bacteriol 1992; 174:5141–5144.

56. Arisawa A, Kawamura N, Takeda K, Tsunekawa H, Okamura K, Okamoto R. Cloning of the macrolide antibiosynthesis gene *acyA*, which encodes 3-O-acyltransferase, from *Streptomyces thermotolerans* and its use for direct fermentative production of a hybrid macrolide antibiotic. Appl Environ Microbiol 1994; 60:2657–2660.

57. Katz L, Donadio S. Polyketide synthesis: Prospects for hybrid antibiotics. Annu Rev Microbiol 1993; 47:875–912.

58. Hutchinson CR, Ikeda I. Polyketide synthase gene manipulation: A structure-function approach in engineering novel antibiotics. Annu Rev Microbiol 1995; 49:201–238.

59. Fernandez-Moreno MA, Martinez E, Boto L, Hopwood DA, Malpartida F. Nucleotide sequence and deduced functions of a set of cotranscribed genes of *Streptomyces coelicolor* A3(2) including the polyketide synthase for the antibiotic actinorhodin. J Biol Chem 1992; 267:19278–12990.

60. Hallam SE, Malpartida F, Hopwood DA. Nucleotide sequence, transcription and deduced function of a gene involved in polyketide antibiotic synthesis in *Streptomyces coelicolor*. Gene 1988; 74:305–320.

61. Bibb MJ, Biro S, Motamedi H, Collins JF, Hutchinson CR. Analysis of the nucleotide sequence of the *Streptomyces glaucescens* tcm1 genes provides key information about the enzymology of tetracenomycin C polyketide antibiotic biosynthesis. EMBO J 1989; 8:2727–2736.

62. Khosla C, McDaniel R, Ebert-Khosla S, Torres R, Sherman D, Bibb MJ, Hopwood DA. Genetic construction and functional analysis of hybrid polyketide synthases containing heterologous acyl carrier proteins. J Bacteriol 1993; 175:2197–2204.

63. McDaniel R, Ebert-Khosla S, Hopwood DA, Khosla C. Engineered biosynthesis of novel polyketides. Science 1993; 262:1546–1550.

64. Shen B, Summers RG, Wendt-Pienkowski E, Hutchinson CR. The *Streptomyces glaucescens* tcmKL polyketide synthase gene and tcmN polyketide cyclase genes govern the size and shape of aromatic polyketides. J Am Chem Soc 1995; 117:6811–6821.

65. Meurer G, Hutchinson CR. Functional analysis of putative β-ketoacyl:acyl carrier protein synthase and acyltransferase active-site-motifs in a type II polyketide synthase of *Streptomyces glaucescens*. J Bacteriol 1995; 177:477–481.

66. McDaniel R, Ebert-Khosla S, Hong F, Hopwood DA, Khosla C. Engineered biosynthesis of novel polyketides: Influence of a downstream enzyme on the catalytic specificity of a minimal aromatic polyketide synthase. Proc Natl Acad Sci USA 1994; 91:11542–11546.

67. Fu H, Ebert-Khosla S, Hopwood DA, Khosla C. Engineered biosynthesis of novel polyketides: Dissection of the catalytic specifity of the *act* ketoreductase. J Am Chem Soc 1994; 116:4166–4170.

68. Fu H, Hopwood DA, Khosla C. Engineered biosynthesis of novel polyketides: Evidence for temporal, but not regiospecific, control of cyclization of an aromatic polyketide precursor. Chem Biol 1994; 1:205–210.

69. Fu H, McDaniel R, Hopwood DA, Khosla C. Engineered biosynthesis of novel polyketides: Stereochemical course of two reactions catalyzed by a polyketide synthase. Biochem 1994; 33:9321–9326.

70. McDaniel R, Ebert-Khosla S., Hopwood DA, Khosla C. Engineered biosynthesis of novel polyketides: Manipulation and analysis of an aromatic polyketide synthase with unproven catalytic specificities. J Am Chem Soc 1993; 115:11671–11675.

71. McDaniel R, Ebert-Khosla S., Hopwood DA, Khosla C. Engineered biosynthesis of novel polyketides: ActVII and ActIV enzymes encode aromatase and cyclase enzymes, respectively. J Am Chem Soc 1994; 116:10855–10859.

72. Zhang HL, He XG, Adefarati A, Gallucci J, Cole SP, Beale JM, Keller PJ, Chang CJ, Floss HG. Mutactin, a novel polyketide from *Streptomyces coelicolor*: Structure and biosynthetic relationship to actinorhodin. J Org Chem 1990; 55:1682–1684.

73. McDaniel R, Ebert-Khosla S, Hopwood DA, Khosla C. Rational design of aromatic polyketide natural products by recombinant assembly of enzymatic subunits. Nature 1995; 375:549–554.

74. McDaniel R, Hutchinson CR, Khosla C. Engineered biosynthesis of novel polyketides: Analysis of tcmN function in tetracenomycin biosynthesis. J Am Chem Soc 1995; 117:6805–6810.

75. Alvarez MA, Fu H, Khosla C, Hopwood DA, Bailey JE. Engineered biosynthesis of novel polyketides: Properties of the *whiE* aromatase/cyclase. Bio/Technol 1996; 14:335–338.

76. Summers RG, Wendt-Pienkowski E, Motamedi H, Hutchinson CR. Nucleotide sequence of the tcmNO region of the tetracenomycin C biosynthetic gene cluster of *Streptomyces glaucescens* and evidence that the tcmN gene encodes a multifunctional cyclase/dehydratase/O-methyltransferase. J Bacteriol 1992; 174:1810–1820.

77. Grimm A, Madduri K, Ali A, Hutchinson CR. Characterization of the *Streptomyces peucetius* ATCC 29050 genes encoding doxorubicin polyketide synthase. Gene 1994; 151:1–10.

78. Han L, Yang K, Ramalingan E, Mosher RH, Vining L. Cloning and characterization of polyketide synthase genes for jadomycin B biosynthesis in *Streptomyces venezuelae* ISP5230. Microbiol 1994; 140:3379–3389.

79. Fu H, Alvarez MA, Khosla C, Bailey JE. Engineered biosynthesis of novel polyketides: Regiospecific methylation of an unnatural substrate by the *tcmO* O-methyltransferase. Biochem 1996; 35:6527–6532.

80. Decker H, Rohr J, Motamedi H, Zahner H, Hutchinson CR. Identification of *Streptomyces olivaceius* Tü 2353 genes involved in the production of the polyketide elloramycin. Gene 1995; 166:121–126.

81. Decker H, Haag S, Udvarnoki G, Rohr J. Novel genetically engineered tetracenomycins. Angew Chem Int Ed Engl 1995; 34:1107–1110.

82. Niemi J, Ylihonko K, Hakala J, Parssinen R, Kopio A, Mantsala P. Hybrid anthracycline antibiotics: Production of new anthracyclines by cloned genes from *Streptomyces purpurascens* in *Streptomyces galilaeus*. Microbiol 1994; 140:1351–1358.

83. Kim HS, Hong YS, Kim YH, Yoo OJ, Lee JJ. New anthracycline metabolites produced by the aklavinone 11-hydroxylase gene in *Streptomyces galilaeus* ATCC 31133. J Antibiot 1996; 49:355–360.

84. Beck J, Ripka S, Siegner A, Schiltz E, Schweizer E. The multifunctional 6-methylsalicylic acid synthase gene of *Penicillium patulum*. Eur J Biochem 1990; 192:487–498.

85. Yu JH, Leonard T. Cloning, sequencing and transcriptional analysis of the polyketide synthase gene for sterigmatocystin biosynthesis in *Aspergillus nidulans*. J Bacteriol 1995; 177:4792–4800.

86. Takano U, Kubo Y, Shimizu K, Mise K, Okuno T, Furusawa I. Structural analysis of PKS1, a polyketide synthase gene involved in melanin biosynthesis in *Colletotrichum lagenarium*. Mol Gen Genet 1995; 249:162–167.

87. Mayorga ME, Timberlake WE. Isolation and molecular characterization of the *Aspergillus nidulans wA* gene. Genetics 1990; 126:73–79.

88. Bedford DJ, Schweizer E, Hopwood DA Khosla C. Expression of a functional polyketide synthase in the bacterium *Streptomyces coelicolor* A3(2). J Bacteriol 1995; 177:4544–4448.

89. Kleinkauf H, von Döhren H. A nonribosomal system of peptide biosynthesis. Eur J Biochem 1996; 236:335–351.

90. Stachless T, Schneider A, Marahiel MA. Rational design of peptide antibiotics by targeted replacement of bacterial and fungal domains. Science 1995; 269:69–72.

91. Stachless T, Schneider A, Marahiel MA. Engineered biosynthesis of peptide antibiotics. Biochem Pharmacol 1996; 51:335–351.

92. Luengo JM. Enzymatic synthesis of hydrophobic penicillins. J Antibiot 1995; 48:1195–1212.

93. Crawford L, Stepan AM, McAda PC, Rambosek JA, Conder MJ, Vinci VA, Reeves CD. Production of cephalosporin intermediates by feeding adipic acid to recombinant *Penicillium chrysogenum* strains expressing ring expansion activity. Bio/Technol 1995; 13:56–62.

94. Huffman GA, Gesellchen PD, Turner JR, Rothenberger RB, Osborne HE, Miller FD, Chapman JL, Queener SW. Substrate specificity of isopenicillin synthase. J Med Chem 1992; 35:1987–2014.

95. Oliynyk M, Brown MJB, Cortes J, Staunton J, Leadlay PF. A hybrid modular polyketide synthase obtained by domain swapping. Chem Biol 1996; 3:833–839.

96. Bedford D, Jacobsen JR, Luo G, Cane DE, Khosla C. A functional chimeric modular polyketide synthase generated via domain replacement. Chem Biol 1996; 3:827–831.

97. Kuhstoss S, Huber M, Turner JR, Paschal JW, Rao RN. Production of a novel polyketide through the construction of a hybrid polyketide synthase. Gene 1996; 183:231–236.

98. Lombo F, Blanco G, Fernandez E, Mendez C, Salas JA. Characterization of *Streptomyces argillaceus* genes encoding a polyketide synthase involved in the biosynthesis of the antitumor mithramycin. Gene 1996; 172:87–91.

ADDENDUM

(III.A) Further reports of hybrid erythromycins have recently appeared. Substitution of the propionyl-coenzyme A specific acyltransferase domain from module 1 of the DEBS1:TE hybrid with one from the rapamycin PKS (21) that specifies malonyl-coenzyme A as the chain extender led to the formation of novel triketo lactones (Figure 6) lacking the methyl group at C-4 (95). Hence, the 2-desmethyl form of intermediate **10** in Figure 6 was formed from malonyl-coenzyme A by the DEBS1:TE hybrid enzyme. Inactivation by random PCR mutagenesis of the module 2 ketoreductase in DEBS1:TE or its replacement with the (normally) inactive ketoreductase domain from module 3 of DEBS2 resulted in the formation of 3-keto forms of the triketo lactone (Figure 6) (96). Successful extension of both of these achievements to the production of desmethyl and deshydroxy analogs of erythromycin A is eagerly awaited.

The carbon skeleton of the spiramycins (Figure 7) and tylosin, a 16-membered macrolide stucturally related to spiramycin I, is made by a modular PKS from acetate, propionate and butyrate-derived precursors. Acetyl-coenzyme A is the starter unit for biosynthesis of platenolide I, the macrolactone product of the spiramycin PKS. Replacement of the starter module of the spiramycin PKS with its tylactone PKS homolog that uses propionyl-coenzyme A as the starter unit, and introduction of this hybrid PKS gene by site-specific integration into a strain of *Streptomyces ambofaciens* in which most of the first gene of the platenolide PKS was deleted and glycosylation of platenolide I was also mutationally blocked resulted in production of 16-methylplatenolide I (97).

(III.B) A putative second and third ring CYC gene has been identified in the cluster of doxorubicin biosynthesis genes in *Streptomyces peucetius*. Addition of the *dpsH* gene, upstream of and transcribed divergently from the *dpsG* ACP gene (77), to a cassette containing the *tcmJ*, *dpsA*, *dpsB*, *tcmM*, *dpsE* and *dpsF* genes resulted in a change from exclusive production of SEK43 to an 11:1 ratio of aklanonic acid to SEK43 in *S. lividans* (G. Meurer, M. Gerlitz, K. Madduri, E. Wendt-Pienkowski and C. R. Hutchinson, unpublished results). Since the *tcmJ*, *dpsA*, *dpsB*, *dpsG*, *dpsE* and *dpsF* genes also produce aklanonic acid and traces of SEK43, *dpsH* both overcomes the negative effect of substituting the *tcmM* ACP gene for *dpsG* and facilitates formation of the second and third rings in aklanonic acid (*tcmJ* has no effect). DpsF appears to catalyze these two cyclizations less efficiently in the absence of DpsH or not at all in the absence of the correct ACP. This observation underscores the belief that the protein:protein interactions are as important as the catalytic activity in type II PKSs; subtle differences in these, as reflected in the effect of *tcmM* and *dpsH*, can lead to aberrrant behavior, such as lack of the complete or normal activity of DpsF. Homologs of *dpsH* are present in at least three other clusters of type II PKS genes (e.g., *mtmX*[98]), but one has not yet been identified in the jadomycin cluster (Leo Vining, personal communication) or the gene clusters governing the biosynthesis of urdamycin and landomycin, two other angucyclines (Andreas Bechthold and Jürgen Rohr, personal communication).

23

Blasticidin S and Related Peptidyl Nucleoside Antibiotics

Steven J. Gould
Oregon State University, Corvallis, Oregon

I. INTRODUCTION

Blasticidin S, **1,** was isolated from *Streptomyces griseochromogenes* (1) as part of a major effort to replace mercury-based compounds for the prevention of *Piricularia oryzae* infection of rice plants in Japan (2). This fungus causes rice blast disease, a major rice pathogen in Japan and other parts of Asia. The structure and absolute stereochemistry of blasticidin S were determined by chemical degradation (3–6), and confirmed by x-ray diffraction (7,8). This work, as well as preliminary studies of blasticidin S biosynthesis, has been reviewed (9).

1

Blasticidin S was first sold in Japan in 1961, and for 20 years it was a major factor in the control of rice blast in that country. In the peak year, 70 tons of blasticidin S were produced by the Kaken Pharmaceutical Company. A number of other chemicals are now used preferentially, including probenazole, isoprothiolane, tricyclazole, and kasugamycin. However, blasticidin S is still used in Japan, as well as in other parts of Asia (e.g., Korea, Taiwan, Thailand) (Miyazaki Y, personal communication). Blasticidin S is still invariably included in reviews of agricultural pesticides (10,11). In addition to its antifungal activity, blasticidin S has been shown to have antibacterial (12), antiviral (13), and antitumor activity (14).

Blasticidin S has been referred to variously as a peptidyl nucleoside, as an aminoacyl nucleoside, and as a 4′-aminoacyl-4′-deoxypyranosylcytosine. In this chapter it will be referred to by the first of these. We will focus on the biosynthesis of blasticidin S and its cometabolites, the mechanism of action of blasticidin S, and resistance exhibited by microorganisms, plants, and animals.

II.   BLASTICIDIN S COMETABOLITES AND OTHER RELATED PEPTIDYL NUCLEOSIDES

A.   Isolation

In the 1970s, Seto et al. isolated a number of new metabolites from *S. griseochromogenes* by screening for compounds with a cytosine-like chromophore (Tables 1 and 2). A number were identified in trace amounts by column and paper chromatography, but amounts adequate for structure elucidation required fractionation of a large quantity of material (500 liters) discarded during commercial production of **1**. These included blasticidin H, **2** (26), and pentopyranic acid, **3** (27), and the pentopyranines A–D (28,29), **4–7** (Tables 2 and 3). Pentopyranic acid was recognized as a possible biosynthetic intermediate to **1**, whereas the others appeared to be products of a number of side pathways.

Efforts during this time to obtain additional intermediates from blocked mutants or by using metabolic inhibitors were largely unsuccessful (16). However, a new compound was observed to accumulate using a chemically defined medium with the pH maintained below 4.0. This proved to be leucylblasticidin S, **8** (16). Another related metabolite, demethylblasticidin S, **9,** was identified and characterized some years later. Inclusion in the fermentation medium of ethionine, a methyltransferase inhibitor, led to a doubling of the accumulation of **9** (15).

Numerous other structurally related microbial metabolites with a broad range of activities have been discovered (Tables 1 and 2). They are produced by various Actinomycetes (*Streptomyces*, *Nocardia*, *Streptoverticillium*) as well as by at least one *Bacillius* sp. Addition of 5-fluorocytosine, **10**, to *S. griseochromogenes* led to accumulation of 5-fluoroblasticidin S, **11**, which had activity similar to **1** (30).

B.   Synthesis

Remarkably little has been done on the synthesis of this family of nucleosides, and the area has been dormant since the 1970s. Between 1969 and 1976 Watanabe's group at the Sloan-Kettering Institute published a series of papers in this area, including total syntheses of gougerotin (31), pentopyranine A (32), and pentopyranine C (33). Others in the series described syntheses of nucleoside derivatives or partial syntheses related to gougerotin and the blasticidins (34–39). A series of gougerotin analogs were synthesized and examined for inhibition of protein biosynthesis (40). A synthesis of cytosinine (41), the nucleoside portion of blasticidin S, and a second synthesis of gougerotin (42) have also been reported.

III.   BIOSYNTHESIS

A.   *Streptomyces griseochromogenes* Whole-Cell Experiments

Biosynthetic studies originally carried out by Seto et al. (43) identified the primary precursors as cytosine (95% incorporation), **12**, D-glucose (4%), **13**, L-α-arginine (30–50%), **14,** and L-methionine (38%), **15** (Figure 1). All of these incorporations were remarkably

Table 1 Blasticidin S and Other Peptidyl Nucleoside Antibiotics with a $\Delta^{2,3}$-Hexenuronic Acid Moiety

	R_1	R_2	R_3	R_4	Ref.
Blasticidin S, **1**	H	H	CO_2H		4
Demethylblasticidin S, **9**	H	H	CO_2H		15
Leucylblasticidin S, **8**	H	H	CO_2H		16
A 83094B	H	CH_2OH	CO_2H		17
Sch 36605	H	CH_2OH	CO_2H		18
Arginomycin	H	H	CO_2H		19
Mildiomycin	H	CH_2OH			20
Mildiomycin D	H	CH_2OH			21
Mildiomycin C	H	H			22

Table 2   Gougerotin and Related Peptidyl Nucleoside Antibiotics with a 3,4-Dideoxy-4-Amino-Pyranose Moiety

	R_1	R_2	R_3	Ref.
Gougerotin		NH_2	OH	23
Bagougeramine A		NH_2	OH	24
Bagougeramine B		HN—$(CH_2)_3$—NH—$(CH_2)_4NH_2$	OH	24
Aspiculamycin		NH_2	OH	25
Blasticidin H, **2**	OH		H	26

Table 3   The Pentopyranines and Cytosylglucuronic Acid

	R_1	R_2	R_3	R_4	R_5	Ref.
Pentopyanine A, **4**	H	OH	H		H	29
Pentopyanine B, **5**	H	H	OH		H	29
Pentopyanine C, **6**	H	OH	H		OH	28
Pentopyanine D, **7**	H	H	OH		OH	28
Pentopyranic acid, **3** (cytosylglucuronic acid)	CO_2H	H	OH	OH	OH	27

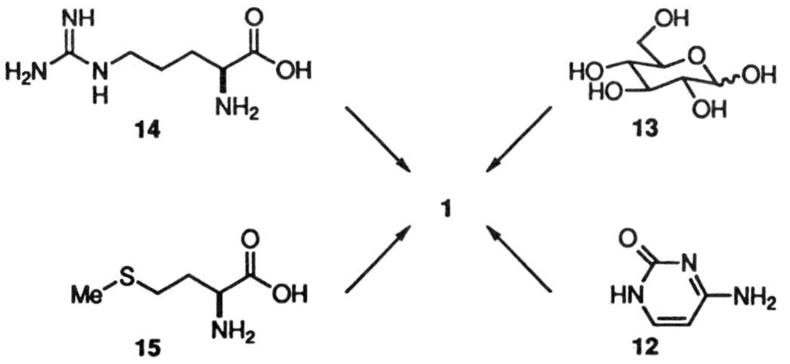

Figure 1 Primary precursors to blasticidin S.

high, especially that of cytosine. We began our investigations by focusing on the conversion of **14** to the L-β-*N*-methylarginine moiety (blastidic acid), **16**, of **1**, and subsequently turned our attention to the formation of the nucleoside portion (cytosinine), **17**, as well, each of which were obtained by acid hydrolysis of **1** (Figure 2).

Naturally occurring β–amino acids are relatively rare and include β-lysine (44,45), β-alanine, β-leucine (46), β-tyrosine (47), and *N*-methyl-β-glutamic acid (48). β-Alanine is known to be formed from degradation of uracil (49,50) or from decarboxylation of aspartic acid (51). β-Tyrosine (found in the peptide antibiotic edeine) is formed from tyrosine by loss of the original α-nitrogen and the *pro-3S* hydrogen, indicative of an ammonia lyase–type process (52). We had shown both with whole cells of *Streptomyces* L-1689-23 (53) and with purified lysine-2,3-aminomutase from *Clostridium subterminale* (54) that β-lysine is formed from L-α-lysine by intramolecular migration of the original α-nitrogen to the β-position accompanied by intermolecular migration of the *pro-3R* hydrogen to the *pro-2S* position.

I. Arginine Metabolism and the Blastidic Acid Moiety

Production of **1** was found to be higher using a complex nutrient medium (55) compared with that using a chemically defined medium (56); in the former case, use of baffled Erlenmeyer flasks (57), rather than the conventional ones, increased the titer from 200 to 1200–1500 mg liter (55). To determine whether β-arginine formation occurred via an aminolyase or aminomutase process, [3-^{13}C, 2-^{15}N]arginine, **14a**, was synthesized and fed with [1-^{14}C]arginine to *S. griseochromogenes*. This resulted in a 30% incorporation of ^{14}C and in retention of both stable isotopes (Figure 3). Heteronuclear spin coupling (J_{CN} = 3.2 Hz) was observed for C3″ in the ^{13}C nuclear magnetic resonance (NMR) spectrum of **1a**. Thus, an aminomutase-catalyzed intramolecular migration, analogous to β-lysine formation, had taken place.

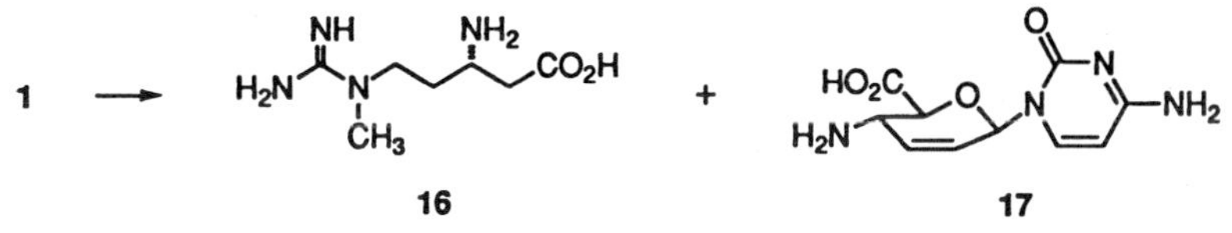

Figure 2 Products of hydrolysis of blasticidin S.

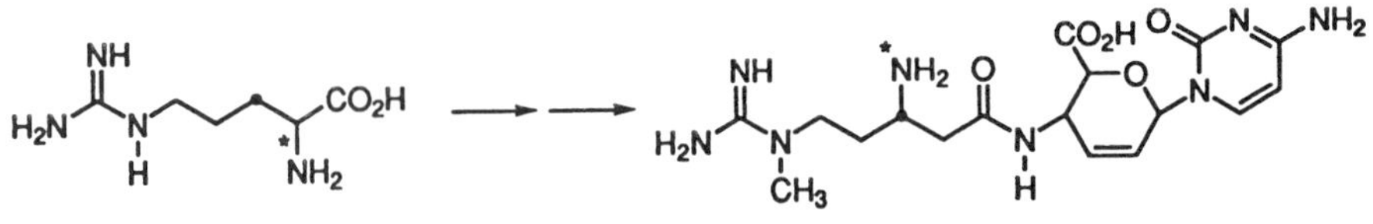

Figure 3   Incorporation of [3-13C, 2-15N]arginine into blasticidin S.

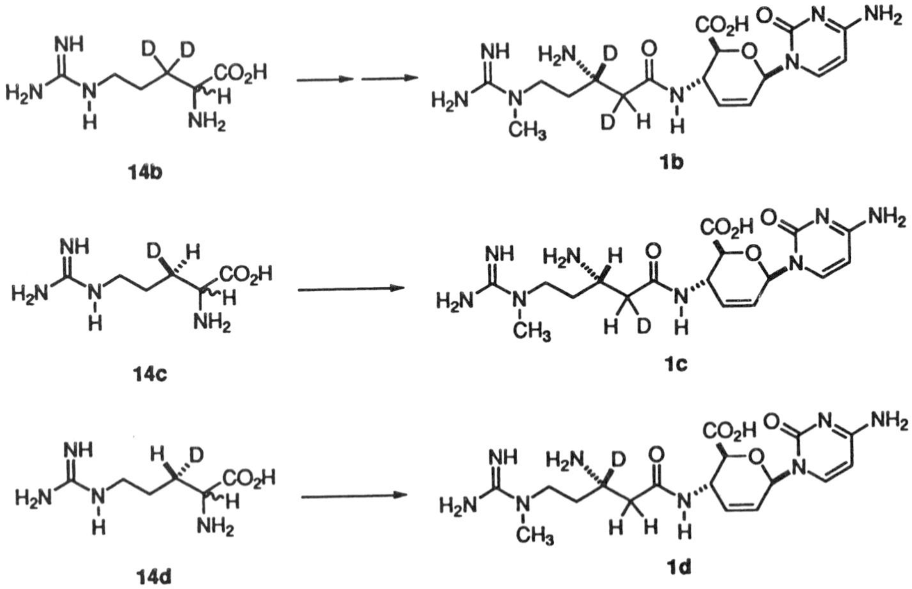

Figure 4   Incorporation of specifically deuterated arginines into blasticidin S.

A variety of deuterated arginines were synthesized and fed to investigate the fates of the hydrogens at C2 and C3, with 2H NMR spectroscopy used to analyze each labeled sample of **1**. These results are summarized in Figure 4, which shows the definitive experiments. Hydrogen had migrated from the β-carbon to the α-carbon (**14b** → **1b**). (3R)-[3-2H]Arginine, **14c**, and (3S)-[3-2H]arginine, **14d**, were used to determine the stereochemistry of hydrogen migration in the arginine aminomutase reaction. Incorporation of each, yielding **1c** and **1d**, respectively, revealed that the *pro-3R* hydrogen had migrated in the aminomutase process, and that the nitrogen migration had occurred with inversion of configuration (55).

The β-argininyl moiety of the blasticidins contains a methyl-group at the δ-nitrogen, whereas antibiotic LL-BM547β (58) contains an unsubstituted β-argininyl moiety. To identify the correct substrate for the arginine-2,3-aminomutase reaction, β-[3-2H₂]arginine, **18**, was synthesized and readily incorporated (48%, based on incorporation of only the 3S isomer) into **1e** (Figure 5). This indicated that N-methylation occurred after the arginine aminomutase reaction (55). δ-N-[13CH₃]Methylarginine, **19,** was also synthesized and fed, but no 13C enrichment was observed in the blasticidin S thus derived, in contrast to a 42% incorporation of radioactivity from co-fed [*guanido*-14C]arginine

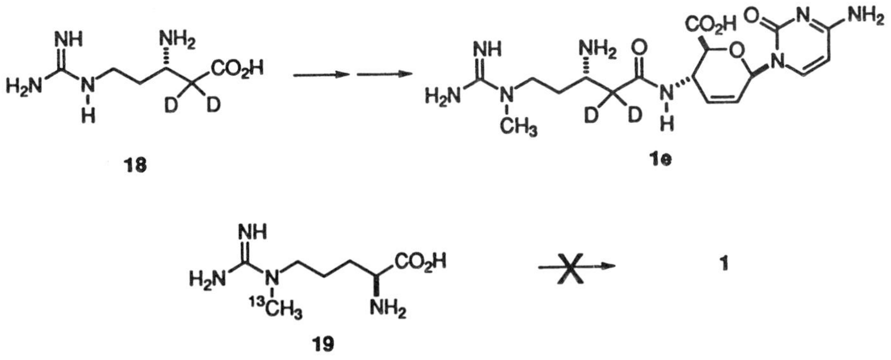

Figure 5 Incorporation of [2, 2-²H₂]-β-arginine into blasticidin S and lack of incorporation of δ-N-[¹³CH₃]methylarginine.

(Figure 5). It was subsequently demonstrated in cell-free studies that *N*-methylation does occur at a late stage in the pathway (59).

2. Glucose Metabolism and the Cytosinine Moiety

Glucose undergoes extensive transformations leading to the hexenuronic acid moiety of **1**. Deuteriated glucoses were fed to determine the fates of the carbinol hydrogens (Figure 6), and these established boundary conditions for plausible biochemical reaction mechanisms. [1-²H]-D-Glucose, **13a**, served as a control, and as expected specifically labeled H1′ of **1f**. Incorporation of [2, 3, 4, 6, 6-²H₅]-D-glucose, **13b**, yielded **1g**, primarily labeled H2′ and H3′. It also labeled H2″ and H4″ of the β-arginine moiety, as well as the *N*-methyl-group (60).

Retention of the original hydrogens at C2 and C3 of glucose revealed that simple dehydrations by β-elimination could not account for the loss of the hydroxyls from these positions. Furthermore, the loss of the C4 hydrogen was presumably related to introduction of the nitrogen, whereas labeling of the *N*-methyl-group and the β-arginine could be

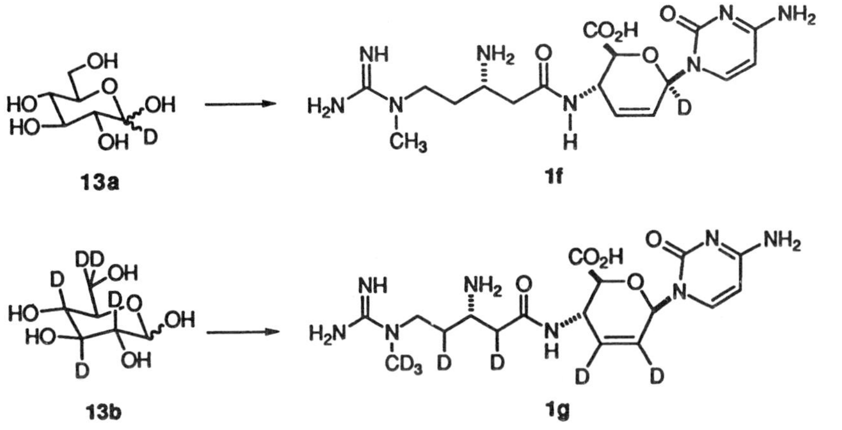

Figure 6 Incorporation of specifically deuterated glucoses into blasticidin S.

readily explained by primary metabolism of glucose generating the *S*-methyl-group of methionine (61) and α-arginine (62).

Fermentation of *S. griseochromogenes* in the presence of [1, 1-²H₂]ethanol, **20**, which acted as a source of in vivo–generated NAD(P)²H (63), led to expected labeling at H2″, H5″, and the *N*-CH₃ (**1h**, Figure 7) (64). Also as expected, no labeling was observed at H2′ or H3′. However, the lack of labeling at H4′, as well, indicated that this hydrogen had been derived from water, which would be consistent with an unusual pyridoxamine phosphate (PMP)–dependent transamination to a 4′-ketosugar intermediate.

Biogenetic analysis suggested that **1** might result from coupling **16** (blastidic acid) and **17** (cytosinine), which had been obtained by hydrolysis of **1**. The reconstitution of **1** from **16** and **17** by a mycelial suspension of *S. griseochromogenes* had been reported (56), but was not reproducible (Seto H, personal communication), and had been tested without the benefit of isotope labels. When the radiolabeled samples **16a** and **17a** were prepared and tested, however, neither was incorporated by *S. griseochromogenes* cultures into **1** (65). These results were inconclusive, however, because in each case most of the radioactivity that had been fed remained in the extracellular broth. [1′-²H]Cytosylglucose, **21**, was synthesized and fed, but it, too, failed to label **1** (Figure 8) (65).

These negative results could be explained by a lack of cell permeability to such putative advanced intermediates. This was circumvented by altering fermentation conditions in order to block potential biosynthetic steps with enzyme inhibitors. These manip-

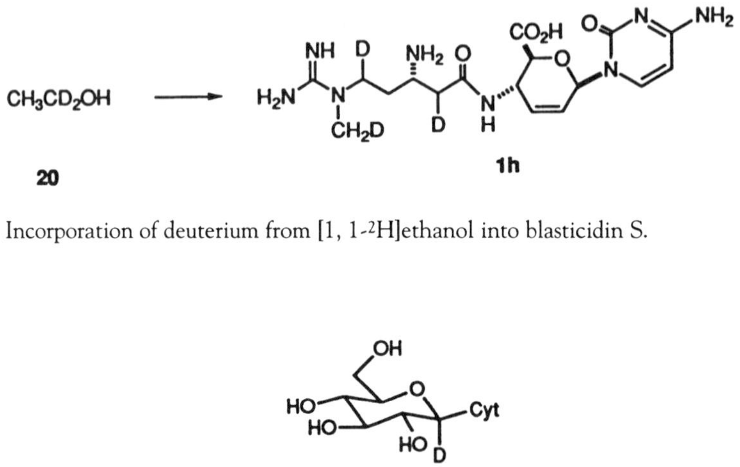

Figure 7   Incorporation of deuterium from [1, 1-²H]ethanol into blasticidin S.

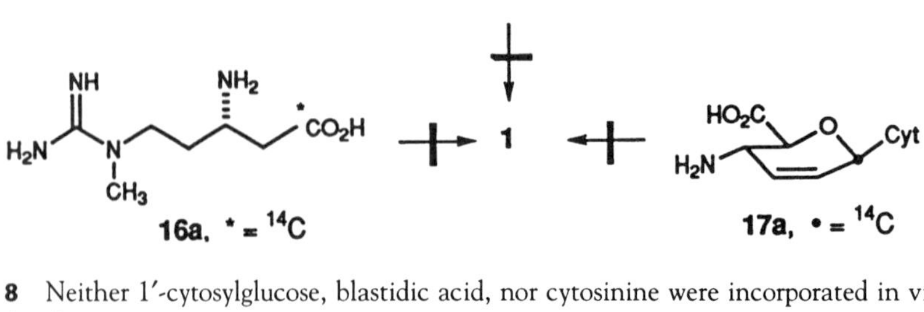

Figure 8   Neither 1′-cytosylglucose, blastidic acid, nor cytosinine were incorporated in vivo into blasticidin S.

ulations were expected to distort the biosynthetic precursor pools and force the accumulation of biosynthetic intermediates or of new metabolites in the fermentation broth. In comparison with attempting to develop blocked mutants, this approach appeared to offer greater flexibility and control in selecting inhibition points. Although such an approach had previously been relatively unsuccessful when homoarginine, 5-bromocytosine, and 5-hydroxymethylcytosine were tested (16), a quite different set of inhibitors subsequently proved to be extremely useful (65). In some cases, large quantities of primary precursors were included.

Numerous permutations on the same types of biochemical reactions were possible, and the selection of inhibitors was based on three assumptions: (a) the 4′-amino-group is introduced after the formation of the cytosine glycosidic bond; (b) the nucleoside portion is coupled to the β–amino acid portion at a relatively late stage; and (c) δ-N-methylation occurs late in the overall pathway. Attention was therefore focused on three potential biosynthetic points: blocking introduction of the 4′-amino-group with transaminase inhibitors [amino-oxyacetic acid (**22**, AOAA) (66–68) and 2-methylglutamic acid (**23**, MeGlu) (69)] or amidotransferase inhibitors [azaserine (**23**) (70) and 6-diazo-5-oxo-L-norleucine (**25**, DON) (71)]; blocking the availability of L-α-arginine with inhibitors of its biosynthesis [L-arginine hydroxamate (**26**, ArgH) (72,73) and MeGlu (69)]; and blocking N-methylation with the methyltransferase inhibitor L-ethionine (**27**, Eth.) (15,74). A synthetic, chemically defined production medium (56) was chosen to simplify interpretation of the results.

High-performance liquid chromatography (HPLC) with photodiode-array detection identified significant accumulations of numerous metabolites with cytosine chromophores. The major compounds that accumulated were isolated and shown to be pentopyranic acid (cytosylglucuronic acid, CGA), **3** (27), pentopyranine C (PPNC), **6** (29), and demethylblasticidin S (DeMeBS), **9** (15). Results from feeding additives at 50 hr and harvesting at 96, 120, and 168 hr are summarized in Tables 4–6, and typical HPLC traces are shown in Figure 9. Cytosine, by itself, proved to be a potent enhancer of CGA and PPNC.

Higher doses of inhibitors were needed to bring about comparable inhibitions using the complex nutrient medium, which by itself yields considerably greater amounts of **1** than does the synthetic medium. Using inhibitors with the complex medium, substantial quantities of **3**, **6**, and **9** were easily purified (e.g., as much as 1.5 g/liter of CGA). Using a combination of 1.0 g/liter of cytosine and 2.0 g/liter of ArgH, five new metabolites were

Table 4 The Effects of Cytosine and of Enzyme Inhibitors on the Production of *S. griseochromogenes* Metabolites at 96 Hours

Additive(s)[a]	CGA[b]	PPNC[b]	DeMeBS[b]	BS[b]
Cytosine	30.5	10.6	1.5	1.1
AOAA	1.9	2.0	0.5	0.6
MeGlu	5.6	2.2	0.6	0.5
ArgH	1.4	11.9	<0.2	0.4
DON	1.2	1.1	0.9	0.8
Azaserine	0.7	1.1	1.0	0.9
Ethionine	4.1	1.5	2.5	0.6
AOAA/MeGlu	2.1	3.1	0.4	0.3
ArgH/MeGlu	3.1	11.0	0.5	0.2

[a] Quantities (mg/100 ml): cytosine, 30; AOAA, 40; MeGlu, 50; ArgH, 200; DON, 30; azaserine, 31; ethionine, 50.
[b] Relative concentration compared with production by a control fermentation to which nothing had been added.
Adapted from Ref. 65.

Table 5 The Effects of Enzyme Inhibitors on the Production of *S. griseochromogenes* Metabolites at 120 Hours

Additive(s)[a]	CGA[b]	PPNC[b]	DeMeBS[b]	BS[b]
AOAA	2.4	2.0	0.7	0.8
MeGlu	7.0	1.8	1.1	0.7
ArgH	1.1	10.1	<0.1	0.5
DON	1.5	1.4	1.0	0.9
Azaserine	0.5	1.3	0.9	0.9
Ethionine	3.1	2.0	0.8	1.0
AOAA/MeGlu	2.8	4.5	0.5	0.5
ArgH/MeGlu	2.2	2.7	0.7	0.3

[a] For amounts fed, see Table 4.
[b] Relative concentration compared with production by a control fermentation to which nothing had been added.
Adapted from Ref. 65.

Table 6   The Effects of Cytosine and of Enzyme Inhibitors on the Production of
S. griseochromogenes Metabolites at 168 Hours

Additive(s)[a]	CGA[b]	PPNC[b]	DeMeBS[b]	BS[b]
Cytosine	70.6	6.4	3.5	1.6
AOAA	3.3	3.2	0.7	0.7
MeGlu	7.5	2.1	1.0	0.6
ArgH	1.6	1.9	0.4	0.6
DON	1.5	1.4	0.0	0.9
Azaserine	0.5	1.2	0.9	0.9
Ethionine	3.4	1.7	1.2	0.7
AOAA/MeGlu	4.5	2.2	0.4	0.6
ArgH/MeGlu	4.1	12.1	0.7	0.4

[a] For amounts fed, see Table 4.
[b] Relative concentration compared with production by a control fermentation to which nothing had been added.
Adapted from Ref. 65.

also isolated (75). One was characterized as pentopyranone, **28,** the presumed intermediate to pentopyranines C and D, another was an isoblasticidin S, **29,** and the remaining three, **30–32,** were adducts derived from **28** and ArgH.

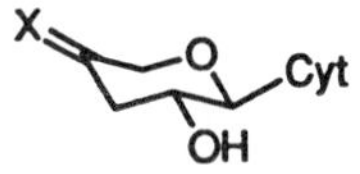

28, X = O
30, X = NOH

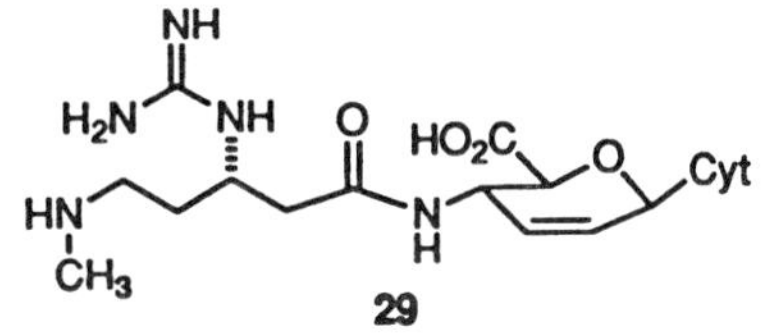

29

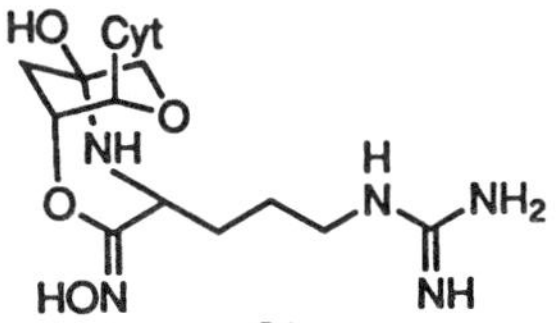

31

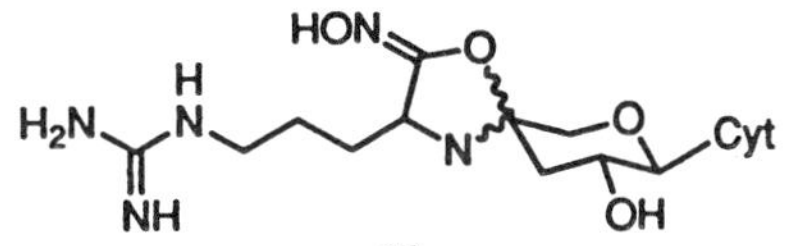

32

The large accumulations of metabolites made possible by these experiments led to the unequivocal identification of a number of intermediates in the blasticidin S pathway, which will be described in the next section. It also led to elucidation of the mechanism of the first sugar deoxygenation in the blasticidin biosynthetic matrix. Thus, the accumulation of pentopyranine C in the presence of either amino-oxyacetic acid or arginine hydroxamate plus cytosine provided conditions in which to explore the C3′ deoxygenation. Using the latter conditions, [3-^{2}H$_2$]-D-glucose, **13c,** was incorporated into CGA (**3a**), pentopyranone (**28a,b**), and pentopyranine C (**6a,b**) (64). In the latter metabolite, the deuterium was distributed 85:15 at H3′$_{axial}$:H3′$_{equatorial}$, whereas in pentopyranone it was approximately evenly distributed at the two sites (54:46). The hydrogens at C3′ of pentopyranone were shown to readily exchange in D$_2$O at pD 9.3, indicating that the 15% label at H3′$_{equatorial}$ of **6b** was due to nonenzymatic epimerization of the

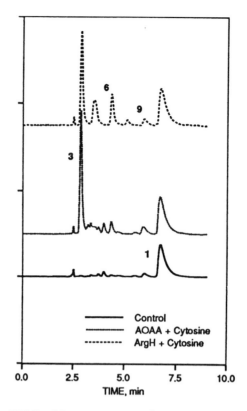

Figure 9 Representative HPLCs of *Streptomyces griseochromogenes* fermentations in the presence of enzyme inhibitors. Bottom trace: no inhibitors added; middle trace: amino-oxyacetic acid and cytosine added; top trace: arginine hydroxamate and cytosine added. Compounds identified are blasticidin S (1), cytosylglucuronic acid (3), pentopyranine C (4), and demethylblasticidin S (9). (Adapted from Ref. 65.)

pentopyranone prior to enzymatic reduction (Figure 10). Thus, the replacement of oxygen by hydrogen occured with retention of configuration.

A decrease in blasticidin S accumulation accompanied by an increase in CGA accumulation in the presence of amino-oxyacetic acid, with a contrasting lack of any significant effect from either azaserine or DON, was consistent with involvement of a PMP-dependent transaminase, rather than a glutamine amidotransferase, to generate the 4'-deoxy-4'-aminosugar moiety. The only prior example of such a biochemical process is C3' deoxygenation in the biosynthesis of 3',6'-dideoxycarbohydrates found in the lipopolysaccharide components of a number of Gram-negative bacterial cell envelopes (76). In the one example studied (CDP-ascarylose, 33), this deoxygenation is a PMP-dependent (77) 1,4-elimination (78,79) involving loss of the *pro-R* hydrogen of PMP (Figure 11). Since this is followed by a conjugate reduction involving an NAD+-dependent electron transfer, there is no net transamination in this pathway.

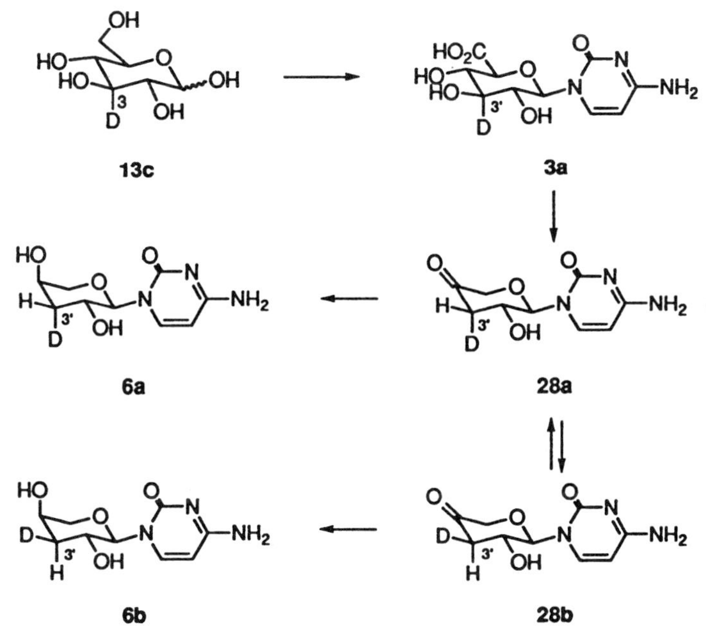

Figure 10 Stereochemistry of C3′ deoxygenation in the biosynthesis of pentopyranine C from [3-²H]-D-glucose.

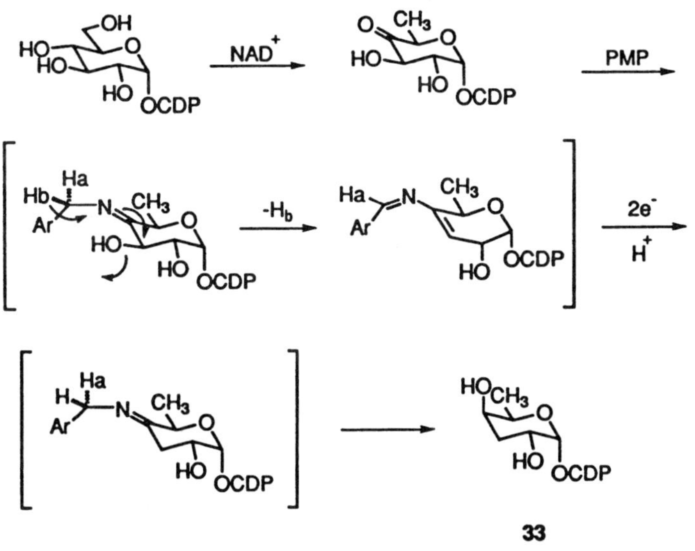

Figure 11 Stereochemistry and mechanism of formation of CDP-ascarylose from CDP-glucose.

B.   Streptoverticillium rimofaciens Whole-Cell Studies

Except for one paper on mildiomycin biosynthesis (22), no other in vivo studies have been reported for this class of peptidyl nucleosides. Addition of 5-hydroxymethylcytosine (**34,** HMC) to fermentations of *Streptoverticillium rimofaciens* increased production of mildiomycin, **35,** by 50% (Figure 12). Replacement of **34** by cytosine, **12,** yielded a new mildiomycin (C), **36,** now containing a cytosine moiety. When both bases were provided, cytosine was used to the exclusion of HMC (see Section III.D.1 for a possible explanation). 5-Methyl-, 5-bromo-, 5-iodo-, and 5-fluorocytosyl mildiomycins were also obtained by adding the appropriate base to the fermentation medium. All showed strong inhibitory activity against powdery mildew. A cytidine 5′-monophosphate 5-hydroxymethylase was subsequently isolated from this organism (see Section III.D).

C.   Streptomyces griseochromogenes Cell-Free Studies

The in vivo studies with *S. griseochromogenes* revealed a number of probable intermediates in the pathway leading directly to blasticidin S. They also revealed a number of apparent shunt pathways. Some of the key points have been confirmed by cell-free studies, including clarifying the identity of the first step in the nucleoside subpathway and that of the final intermediate in the blasticidin S pathway. Cell-free studies have also been carried out for part of the mildiomycin pathway.

1.   Demethylblasticidin S N-Methyltransferase

Leucylblasticidin S, **8** (Table 1), had been reported to accumulate when fermentations of *S. griseochromogenes* were kept below pH 4.0. When washed cells were presented with **8,** it disappeared and blasticidin S appeared in a time-dependent manner (16). However, it was subsequently shown that washed mycelia produced a measurable amount of **1,** even without the addition of **8** (59). Although it is probable that **8** can be converted to **1,** it may be the result of a nonspecific leucylaminopeptidase (80).

The discovery of demethylblasticidin S, **9,** was reported nine years after the discovery of **8** and presented an alternative biosynthetic possibility in which *N*-methylation would be the last step to **1.** As described in the previous section, fermentation of *S. griseochromagenes* in the presence of added cytosine and ethionine resulted in a significant increase in the titer of **9** with a concomitant decrease in that of **1.** An even larger effect

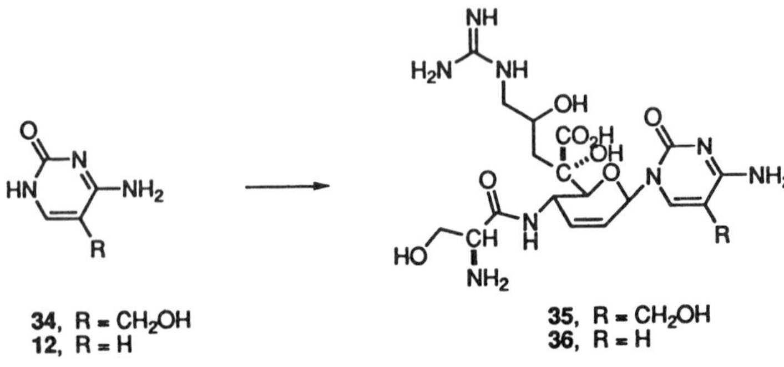

Figure 12   Formation of mildiomycin and mildiomycin C from 5-hydroxymethylcytosine and from cytosine, respectively, by *Streptoverticillium rimofaciens*.

was obtained when nonphysiological concentrations of both cytosine (0.30 g/liter) and arginine (2.0 g/liter) were used in the fermentation medium. A five- to seven-fold increase in **9** and a twofold increase in **1** were observed, suggesting that the methyltransferase had become the rate-limiting step.

A cell-free extract (CFE) of *S. griseochromogenes* converted mixtures of **9** and *S*-adenosyl-L-[$^{14}CH_3$]methionine ([$^{14}CH_3$]SAM) to **1i** (HPLC with radiochemical detection) (59). Incorporations of 0.85–1.20% were obtained. Hydrolysis to cytosinine and [^{14}C]blastidic acid (**16b**) showed that >97% of the radioactivity was retained in the blastidic acid (Figure 13). Thus, methylation is the last step in the biosynthesis of blasticidin S.

2. Cytosylglucuronic Acid Synthase

Based on the lack of incorporation of [1'-^{2}H]-cytosylglucose into **1**, and the extraordinary titers of cytosylglucuronic acid, **3**, that were obtained with the enzyme inhibitors, the latter was tested as a blasticidin intermediate. Uptake of unlabeled **3** by *S. griseochromogenes* mycelia was not detectable (HPLC analysis), and efforts to prepare a cell-free extract or protoplasts that could metabolize **3** to **1** were unsuccessful. However, cell-free extracts could make **3b** from [2-^{14}C]cytosine, **12a**, and UDP-glucuronic acid, **37** (Figure 14). Neither UDP-glucose, UDP-galactose, nor UDP-galacturonic acid could substitute for **37** (81).

[5-^{3}H-1', 2', 3', 4', 5', 6'-^{14}C]CGA, **3c**, prepared enzymatically from [5-^{3}H]cytosine and UDP[U-^{14}C]-D-glucuronic acid, yielded labeled blasticidin S **1j** when a portion was fed to *S. griseochromogenes* (Figure 15). Most of the original **3c** was recovered unchanged.

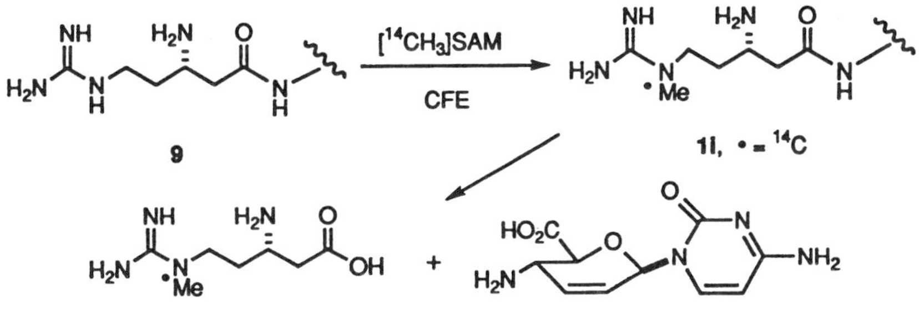

Figure 13 Demonstration of demethylblasticidin S *N*-methyltransferase activity in cell-free extracts of *S. griseochromogenes*.

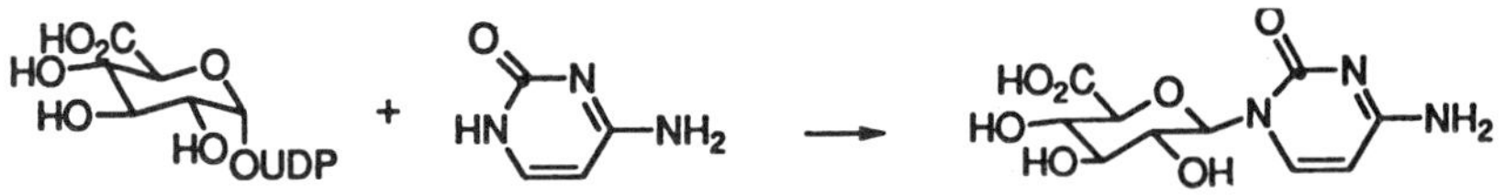

Figure 14 Formation of cytosylglucuronic acid from cytosine and UDP-glucuronic acid by cell-free extracts of *S. griseochromogenes*.

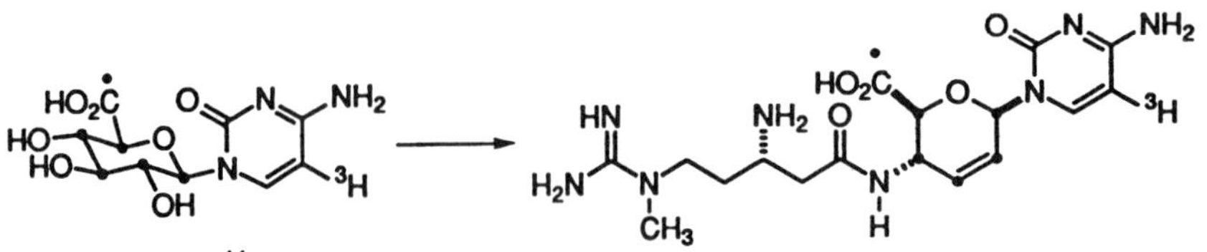

Figure 15   Incorporation of [5-³H-1′, 2′, 3′, 4′, 5′, 6′-¹⁴C]cytosylglucuronic acid into blastici-din S.

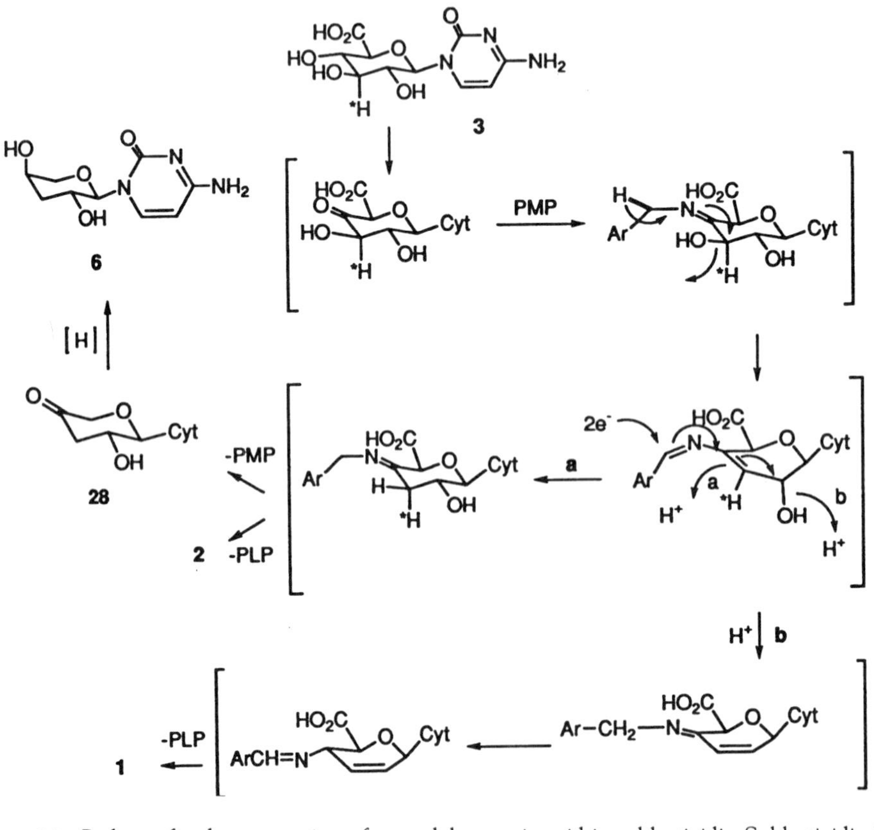

Figure 16   Pathway for the conversion of cytosylglucuronic acid into blasticidin S, blasticidin H, and pentopyranine C.

Thus, the first committed step in the nucleoside branch of the blasticidin pathway is formation of **3**. The subsequent deoxygenations and transaminations leading to blasticidins S and H and to pentopyranine C are summarized in Figure 16.

CGA synthase has been purified ~900-fold by a six-step procedure that yielded a single, monomeric peptide of M_r 43,000 (82). Activity is optimum pH 8.4–8.6, with an apparent K_m of 6.0 μM for UDP-glucuronic acid and 243 μM for cytosine, and with a V_{max} of 14.6 μmol/mg · min. CGA synthase is a soluble protein and does not appear to require any external cofactors or metal ions for catalysis. The activity was slightly stimu-

Table 7   Relative Rates of 5-X-Cytosines as Substrates for CGA Synthase

X =	H	F	I	HOCH$_2$	CH$_3$
Rate (%) =	100	130	110	95	65

lated by Mg^{2+} and Ca^{2+}, and it was inhibited by Fe^{2+}, Co^{2+}, and Zn^{2+}. Activity was neither inhibited nor enhanced by EDTA or by phospholipid (phosphatidylcholine), but it was inhibited by UDP, one of the reaction products.

CGA synthase is specific for UDP-glucuronic acid and for either cytosine or 5-substituted cytosines; neither uracil nor adenine were competent acceptors. The relative rates of cytosine derivatives as acceptors in the CGA synthase reaction are given in Table 7 (Guo J and Gould SJ, unpublished results). The suitability of 5-fluorocytosine, **10,** as a substrate readily explains the production of 5-fluoroblasticidin S, **11,** when **10** was fed to *S. griseochromogenes* (22). The formation of 5-hydroxyCGA from 5-hydroxycytosine (83,84) may be relevant to mildiomycin biosynthesis (85) (see Section III.D).

Functionally, CGA synthase belongs to the family of UDP-glucuronosyltransferases (UDP-GTs). Though these are common in mammalian metabolism and at least two have been reported from fungi (86,87), CGA synthase is the first such enzyme reported from a prokaryote. The eukaryotic UDP-GTs are membrane associated in vivo (88) and require added phospholipid (e.g., phosphatidylcholine) when purified (89,90). They catalyze glucuronidation of a wide variety of lipophilic endogenous metabolites and xenobiotics (89). CGA synthase may also be involved in the biosynthesis of other peptidyl nucleoside antibiotics (17–19,23,24,85,90,91).

3.   Cytosinine:Pyridoxal Phosphate Tautomerase

Evidence that cytosinine, **17,** is produced by *S. griseochromogenes* and, therefore, should be a true blasticidin intermediate, has recently been obtained (92). If the second sugar deoxygenation in the blasticidin S pathway followed as a consequence of the PMP-assisted first deoxygenation (Figure 16), subsequent tautomerization of **38** to **39** and hydrolysis should yield cytosinine (Figure 17). This was demonstrated by incubating cytosinine and pyridoxal phosphate (PLP) with a cell-free extract from *S. griseochromogenes* in a D$_2$O-enriched buffer. In three separate experiments, the recovered cytosinine was found to contain deuterium at C4' (**17b**) and at C2' (**17c**), 5–36% and 1–5% enriched, respectively, based on the deuterium enrichment in each incubation medium (67–80%). The exchange at C2' follows as a logical outcome of the mechanism. No exchange at either site was observed when boiled extract was used or when cytosinine and PLP were incubated alone.

4.   UDP-Glucose 4'-Epimerase and 6'-Oxidoreductase

In early experiments, [1-^{14}C]-D-glucose had been incorporated 1.8%, whereas [1-^{14}C]-D-galactose was incorporated 15.2% (81). This disparity was reconciled with the recognition of the role of 3 in blasticidin biosynthesis and the characterization of CGA synthase. Although neither UDP-glucose nor UDP-galactose could serve directly as the donor, CGA was formed when NAD$^+$ was added to incubations containing either of these nucleosides. These results revealed the presence of UDP-glucose 6'-oxidoreductase, necessary

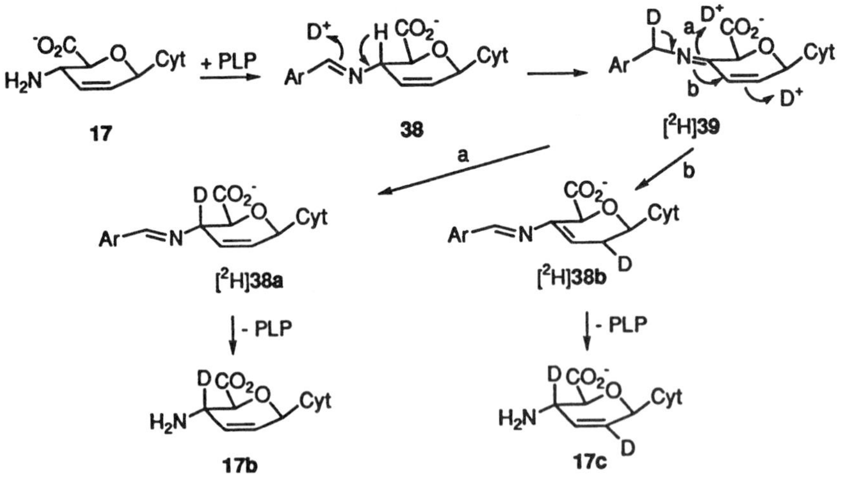

Figure 17   Demonstration of cytosinine:pyridoxal phosphate tautomerase activity in cell-free extracts of S. *griseochromogenes*.

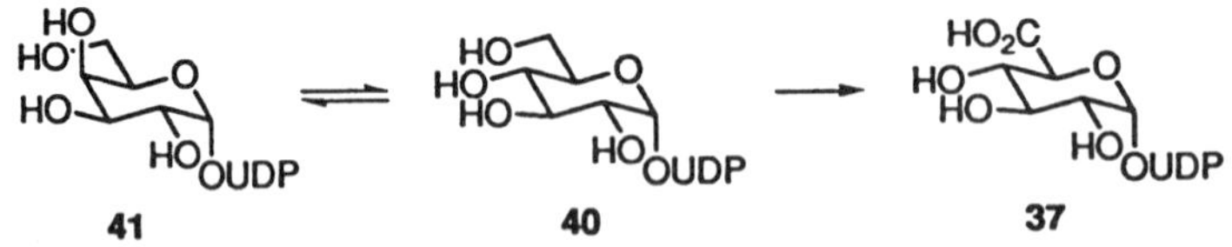

Figure 18   Interconversion of UDP-galactose and UDP-glucose, and oxidation of UDP-glucose to UDP-glucuronic acid.

for oxidation of UDP-glucose, **40,** to **37,** as well as the presence of UDP-glucose 4'-epimerase, which interconverts UDP-galactose, **41,** and **40** (Figure 18) (93). The eight-fold greater incorporation of labeled galactose compared with that of labeled glucose presumably simply reflects the lesser role played by the former sugar in general metabolism.

5.   Pentopyranone Oxidoreductase-1

Blasticidin H, gougerotin, the bagougeramines, and aspiculamycin contain a 3,4-dideoxy-4-aminoglucuronic acid residue (Table 2) in place of the hexenulosonic acid moiety of blasticidin S. S. *griseochromogenes* also produces pentopyranines C and D, **6** and **7,** respectively (Table 3). In vivo experiments (Section III.A.2) defined the metabolism of CGA for both loss of the C3 and C4 hydroxyl-groups and introduction of the C4 amino-group. These experiments established the relationships of the $\Delta^{2,3}$-nucleoside sugar residues and the 3-deoxynucleoside sugar residues. While none of the enzyme affecting deoxygenations of CGA have as yet been detected, one of the tailoring enzymes from the pentopyranine shunt has been identified.

The detection of pentopyranone, **28,** in cultures of S. *griseochromogenes* grown in the presence of arginine hydroxamate and cytosine provided a source for this apparent precursor to pentopyranines C and D. Pentopyranone was tested as an oxidoreductase substrate with cell-free extracts of S. *griseochromogenes*. NAD+ and NADP+ were each tested with this extract, but only the former was found to be a competent coenzyme, and

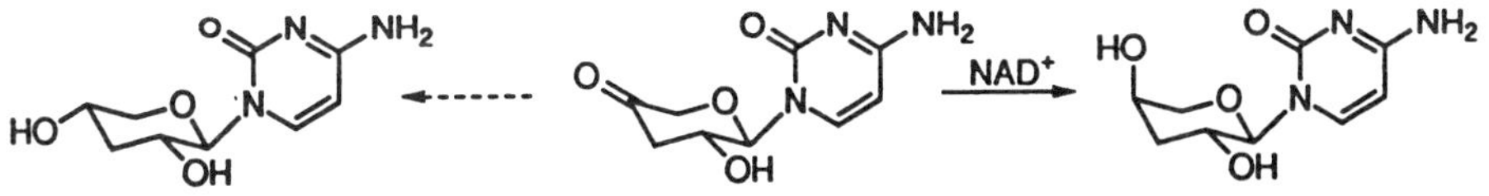

Figure 19 Demonstration of pentopyranone oxidoreductase-1 activity in cell-free extracts of *S. griseochromogenes*.

only reduction to **6** was observed (Figure 19) (Gould SJ and Klumpp M, unpublished results). Presumably a different enzyme, not expressed under these culture conditions, is needed to produce **7**.

D. *Streptoverticillium rimofaciens* Cell-Free Studies

1. CMP 5-Hydroxymethylase

Mildiomycin (20,94) and mildiomycin D (21), differ from blasticidin S in the array of substituents on the dihydropyran ring and by the presence of 5-hydroxymethylcytosine in place of cytosine (Table 1). Just as addition of cytosine to *S. griseochromogenes* fermentations increased blasticidin S production (65), addition of **34** to *S. rimofaciens* increased mildiomycin accumulation (22). However, directed biosynthesis experiments with cultures of *S. rimofaciens* yielded the cytosine-containing mildiomycin C in preference to mildiomycin when cytosine was made available (Section III.B). This may indicate that the competent enzyme originally evolved as a CGA synthase, with *S. rimofaciens* now lacking the ability to produce free cytosine but able to produce and use 5-hydroxymethylcytosine in its place.

A cell-free extract of *S. rimofaciens* converted cytosine monophosphate (**42**, CMP) and formaldehyde to **34** in the presence of tetrahydrofolic acid (THFA) and Fe^{2+} (83). 2-Mercaptoethanol stimulated this activity, and Mg^{2+} could replace iron, albeit at a somewhat reduced activity. The product of a large-scale incubation that included [$^{13}CH_3$]paraformaldehyde was unequivocally characterized by ultraviolet/visible (UV/vis) and ^{13}C nuclear magnetic resonance (NMR) spectroscopies.

The *S. rimofaciens* hydroxymethylase was specific for the C_1 acceptor. Neither cytidine, cytosine, dCMP, nor UMP could replace CMP. Thus, this activity is different from the enzyme previously reported from *Escherichia coli* infected with T-even bacteriophages (95), which hydroxymethylated only dCMP. The crude *S. rimofaciens* preparation could use either formaldehyde or serine for the C_1 donor, presumably via an intermediate such as [5, 10-methylene]THFA.

2. Hydroxymethyl CMP N-Ribotidase

The crude *S. rimofaciens* CFE only yielded **34,** indicating the presence of an enzyme that could cleave the presumed initial product, 5-hydroxymethyl CMP, **43.** This latter activity was subsequently detected, and the two activities were separated by standard procedures (84). Thus, biosynthesis of mildiomycin apparently begins with CMP hydroxymethylase followed by hydroxymethyl N-ribotidase to yield **34,** which is then presumably converted to 5-hydroxymethyl CGA, **44,** by CGA synthase (Figure 20). Two

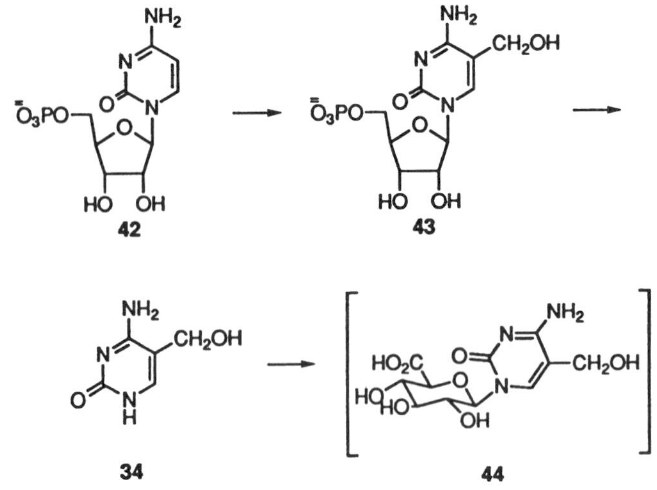

Figure 20 Apparent formation of 5-hydroxymethylcytosylglucuronic acid from cytosine monophosphate in the biosynthesis of mildiomycin by *S. rimofaciens*.

close analogs of blasticidin S, antibiotics A 83094B (17) and Sch36605 (18), also contain 5-hydroxymethylcytosine in place of cytosine, and presumably have the same enzymatic capabilities.

E. Summary

At present, there are nearly two dozen peptidyl nucleosides containing a cytosine or hydroxymethyl cytosine base that have been isolated from various Gram-positive bacteria. It is likely that different forms of the same enzyme, CGA synthase, are responsible for formation of the initial nucleoside intermediate to each of these metabolites. The chemistry used for deoxygenations at C2′ and C3′ and for introduction of the C4′ amino-group is apparently also conserved, although some pathways use only the first of the two deoxygenation steps. The major variations within each of these pathways occur in generating the starting pyrimidine base and in the formation and coupling of the amino acid residues subsequently attached to the sugar moiety. Indeed, though the origin has been established for free 5-hydroxymethylcytosine needed for pathways such as the one for mildiomycin, the source of free cytosine for blasticidins and most of the other pathways is unknown. The hydroxymethyl *N*-ribotidase of *S. rimofaciens* was not active with cytidine itself. So far, only the amino acid subpathway of the blasticidins (arginine-2,3-aminomutase) has been studied. Clearly, much new biochemistry remains to be learned from these pathways.

IV. MECHANISM OF ACTION

The mechanism of action of blasticidin S has been studied for more than 20 years. In the 1960s, it was recognized that blasticidin S stimulates T-factor-dependent binding of phenylalanine tRNA to ribosomes (96), and that it inhibited the effects of puromycin in a manner similar to chloramphenicol (97). Blasticidin S binds strongly to the 50S subunit in a manner noncompetitive with puromycin (98). These properties were generally found for related antibiotics such as gougerotin, bamicetin, and amicetin. In studies with an *E. coli* B ribosomal system, blasticidin S was the most effective of these at inhibiting the puromycin reaction (premature termination of peptide synthesis) (99).

Blasticidin S increased binding of the donor substrate to the ribosomal donor site and decreased binding of the acceptor to the acceptor site (99), possibly by binding to the aminoacyl and cytosyl recognition regions for the CCA terminus of tRNAs (100,101). More recently, the kinetics of blasticidin S inhibition of peptide bond formation in the *E. coli* ribosomal system were examined (102). It was found to be a slow-binding inhibitor, and at low concentrations blasticidin S was a competitive inhibitor of puromycin, with a $K_i = 0.2$ μM. At higher concentrations the inhibition was found to be mixed noncompetitive, which suggested that it induces a conformational change that prevents the puromycin reaction and slows peptide bond formation.

V. BLASTICIDIN RESISTANCE

A. Microbial Resistance

Only one biochemically defined mechanism of antibiotic deactivation has so far been identified in a blasticidin S producer (*Streptoverticillium* sp. JCM 4673) (103). This organism produces an acetyltransferase that acetylates **1**, although the precise site of acetylation has not been identified. The enzyme has an M_r of 15 kDa and K_m of 2 and 3 mM for blasticidin S and acetyl-CoA, respectively. Acetylation is a self-resistance mechanism for a number of antibiotic types (104–106), and this appears to be true for blasticidin S as well. Since leucylblasticidin S is inactive as an antibiotic and is cleaved enzymatically to blasticidin S (16), this, too, may represent a self-resistance mechanism. Two genes from *S. griseochromogenes* have been cloned into *Streptomyces lividans* that confer resistance to **1** (Gould SJ, Petrich A, and Fuller G, unpublished results). They are currently being subcloned for sequencing and analysis.

The best-characterized blasticidin S resistance mechanism in nonproducers is cytosyl deamination, which yields the uracil analog of blasticidin S with ~1% of the original antibiotic activity against *P. oryzae* (107). Deaminase activity has been detected in *Aspergillus fumigatus* (107), and deaminases have been isolated from *Aspergillus terreus* (108) and *Bacillus cereus* (109). The *A. terreus* enzyme was purified by conventional chromatographies (110) and by affinity chromatography (111), and found to have an M_r of 30 kDa (110) and K_m of 21.2 μM (111). Its substrate specificity was confined to blasticidin S and a limited number of derivatives, whereas the methyl ester, cytosinine, and gougerotin were only slightly active. Two deaminase genes, *bsr* (112) and *BSD* (113), have been cloned and sequenced.

Two classes of blasticidin S–resistant mutants of *Saccharomyces cerevisiae* have been isolated (114). Neither phenotype is associated with ribosomes, which are the target of blasticidin S action. Both genes for this resistance were found to be recessive, indicating that they were unlikely to be responsible for inactivation of **1**. It was suggested that they most likely affect permeability of **1** to the cells.

B. Animal Resistance

Numerous antibiotics that inhibit protein synthesis in bacteria have been shown to also inhibit eukaryotic cells in tissue culture (115). Blasticidin S is one of a variety of such antibiotics that have been used to study ribosome function in eukaryotes (116). Mouse leukemias (e.g., FM3a mammary carcinoma) sensitive to blasticidin S have been mutated with nitrosoguanidine, and blasticidin-resistant cell lines isolated (117). One of these was shown to be altered in the 60S ribosomal subunit, most likely at the aminoacyl tRNA acceptor site (116). This mutant, and a spontaneous mutant with very similar properties, showed cross-resistance with gougerotin, puromycin, and sparsomycin.

C. Plant Resistance

Although blasticidin S has played a major role in the control of *P. oryzae* infections of rice, it is toxic to this plant at higher concentrations (118). Blasticidin S has been used to study plant protein synthesis under a variety of stress conditions. Examples include effects on the production of the phytoalexin glyceollin, and related compounds, in soybean (119,120), of furanoterpenes in sweet potato (121), and of avenalumin in oats (122).

VI. GENETICS OF MICROBIAL RESISTANCE

Three blasticidin S resistance genes have been cloned and sequenced. An acetyltransferase gene, *bls*, from a blasticidin S producer, *S. rimofaciens* (123), was cloned into *S. lividans* as a 1129 bp *BclI–PstI* fragment using pIJ702. The acetyltransferase was coded on a 408 bp open reading frame (ORF), and the apparent promoter was located upstream in a 185 bp *HincII* DNA fragment that overlapped 10 base pairs with the ORF. The sequence of the expected protein product, BAC, had no significant homology to other antibiotic-modifying acetyltransferases (e.g., puromycin or streptothricin (124–126)).

The *B. cereus* K55-S1 blasticidin S deaminase gene, *bsr*, was found on a native 10.5 kbp plasmid, pBSR8 (127,128), which could confer blasticidin S resistance on *Bacillus subtilis* and *E. coli*. The gene was subcloned into *E. coli* on a 1.5 kbp *EcoRI/BamHI* DNA fragment, and *bsr* was apparently contained in a 420 bp ORF (112). Sequencing the deaminase from *E. coli* provided the first 46 amino acids from the N-terminus, and these match exactly with those predicted from *bsr*. A deaminase gene from *A. terreus*, *BSD*, has also been cloned into *E. coli* and sequenced to reveal a 393 bp ORF (113). Not surprisingly, there was no homology to the DNA sequence of *bsr*. Comparison of the predicted amino acid sequences derived from *BSD* and *bsr* indicated 27.2% identity and another 25% of similar nature. A significant local homology over an 11 bp segment corresponded to a portion of the cytidine/deoxycytidine deaminase of *B. subtilis* (129). However, neither of the two blasticidin S deaminases deaminated cytosine or cytidine.

Two apparent blasticidin S resistance genes have been cloned from *S. griseochromogenes*. One is contained on a 2.6 kb *BamHI* fragment and the other on a 5.0 kb *BamHI* fragment (Gould SJ, Petrich A, and Fuller G, unpublished results). The latter has been sequenced and contains a 1.7 kb ORF that appears to contain sequences for an ATP binding motif as well as homology to a number of resistance genes involved in small-molecule transport. It therefore appears to represent a third mechanism for blasticidin S resistance, and a new mechanism for nucleoside antibiotics.

The *bsr* gene has been used as a selectable marker to develop a plant transformation system for tobacco (130,131). *BSD* and *bsr* have also been used as selectable markers for transformation of fungi such as *Schizosaccharomyces pombe* (*BSD* (113,132)), *P. oryzae*

(*BSD* (113,132) and *bsr* (133)), and *Rhizopus niveus* (*bsr* (134)), as well as the slime mold *Dictyostelium discoideum* (*bsr* (135)). The gene *bsr* has also been used as a selection marker for *B. subtilis* (136) and for mammalian (HeLa) cells (137).

REFERENCES

1. Takeuchi S, Hirayama K, Ueda K, Sakai H, Yonehara H. Blasticidin S, a new antibiotic. J Antibiot Ser A 1958; 11:1–5.
2. Misato T, Ishii I, Asakawa M, Okimoto Y, Fukunaga K. Ann Phytopathol Soc Jpn 1959; 24:302–306.
3. Otake N, Takeuchi S, Endo T, Yonehara H. Chemical studies on blasticidin S. II. The structure of cytosinine and uracinine. Agric Biol Chem 1966; 30:126–131.
4. Otake N, Takeuchi S, Endo T, Yonehara H. The structure of blasticidin S. Tetrahedron Lett 1965; 1411–1419.
5. Fox JJ, Watanabe KA. Nucleosides. XXXII. On the structure of blasticidin S, a nucleoside antibiotic (1). Tetrahedron Lett 1966; 897–903.
6. Yonehara H, Otake N. Absolute configuration of blasticidin S. Tetrahedron Lett 1966; 3785–3791.
7. Onuma S, Nawata Y, Saito Y. An X-ray analysis of blasticidin S monohydrobromide. Bull Chem Soc Jpn 1966; 39:1091.
8. Swaminathan V, Smith JL, Sundaralingam M, Coutsogeorgopoulos C, Kartha G. Crystal and molecular structure of the antibiotic blasticidin S hydrochloride pentahydrate. Biochim Biophys Acta 1981; 655:335–341.
9. Yonehara H. Blasticidin S: Properties, biosynthesis, and fermentation. Vandamme EJ, ed. Biotechnology of Industrial Antibiotics. New York: Marcel Dekker, 1984:651–663.
10. Isono K. Antibiotics as non-polluting agricultural pesticides. Comment Agric Food Chem 1990; 2:123–142.
11. Tanaka Y, Omura S. Agroactive compounds of microbial origin. Annu Rev Microbiol 1993; 47:57–87.
12. Shomura T, Inoue M, Niida T, Hara T. The improved assay method of blasticidin S. J Antibiot 1964; 17:253–261.
13. Hirai A, Wildman SG, Hirai T. Specific inhibition of TMV-RNA synthesis by blasticidin S. Virology 1968; 36:646–651.
14. Tanaka N, Sakagami Y, Nishimura T, Yamaki H, Umezawa H. Activity of cytomycin and blasticidin S against transplantable animal tumors. J Antibiot 1961; 14:123–126.
15. Seto H, Yonehara H. Studies on the biosynthesis of blasticidin S. VII. Isolation of demethyl-blasticidin S. J Antibiot 1977; 30:1022–1024.
16. Seto H, Otake N, Yonehara H. Studies on the biosynthesis of blasticidin S. II. Leucylblasticidin S, a metabolic intermediate of blasticidin S biosynthesis. Agric Biol Chem 1968; 32:1299–1305.
17. Larsen SH, Berry DM, Paschal JW, Gilliam JM. 5-Hydroxymethylblasticidin S and blasticidin S from *Streptomyces setonii* culture A83094. J Antibiot 1989; 42:470–471.
18. Cooper R, Conover M, Patel M. Sch 36605, structure of a novel nucleoside. J Antibiot 1988; 41:123–125.
19. Argoudelis AD, Baczynskyj L, Kuo MT, Laborde AL, Sebek OK, Truesdell SE, Shilliday FB. Arginomycin: Production, isolation, characterization and structure. J Antibiot 1987; 40:750–760.
20. Harada S, Mizuta E, Kishi T. Structure of mildiomycin, a new antifungal nucleoside antibiotic. J Am Chem Soc 1978; 100:4895–4897.
21. Tashiro S, Sugita N, Iwasa T, Sawada H. Structure of mildiomycin D. Agric Biol Chem 1984; 48:881–885.

22. Sawada H, Katamoto K, Suzuki T, Akiyama S-i, Nakao Y. Microbial production of mildiomycin analogues by the addition of cytosine analogues. J Ferment Technol 1984; 62:537–543.

23. Kanzaki T, Higashide E, Yamamoto H, Shibata M, Nakazawa K, Iwasaki H, Takewaka T, Miyake A. Gougerotin, a new antibacterial antibiotic. J Antibiot (Ser A) 1962; 15:93–98.

24. Takahashi A, Ikeda D, Naganawa H, Okami Y, Umezawa H. Bagougeramines A and B, new nucleoside antibiotics produced by a strain of *Bacillus circulans*. II. Physico-chemical properties and structure determination. J Antibiot 1986; 39:1041–1046.

25. Haneishi T, Terahara A, Arai M. Aspiculamycin, a new cytosine nucleoside antibiotic. II. Physico-chemical properties and structural elucidation. J Antibiot 1974; 27:334–338.

26. Seto H, Yonehara H. Studies on the biosynthesis of blasticidin S. IV. The isolation and structure of blasticidin H. J Antibiot 1977; 30:1019–1021.

27. Seto H, Furihata K, Yonehara H. Studies on the biosynthesis of blasticidin S. V. Isolation and structure of pentopyranic acid. J Antibiot 1976; 29:595–596.

28. Seto H. Isolation of pentopyranines A, B, C and D. Agric Biol Chem 1973; 37:2415–2419.

29. Seto H, Otake N, Yonehara H. The structures of pentopyranines A and C, two cytosine nucleosides with α-L-configuration. Agric Biol Chem 1973; 37:2421–2426.

30. Kawashima A, Seto H, Ishiyama T, Kato M, Uchida K, Otake N. Fluorinated blasticidin S. Agric Biol Chem 1987; 51:1183–1184.

31. Watanabe KA, Falco EA, Fox JJ. Total synthesis of gougerotin. J Am Chem Soc 1972; 94:3272–3274.

32. Watanabe KA, Chiu TMK, Hollenberg DH, Fox JJ. Nucleosides. LXXXVII. Total synthesis of pentopyranine A, an α-L-cytosine nucleoside elaborated by *Streptomyces griseochromogenes*. J Org Chem 1974; 39:2484–2486.

33. Chiu TMK, Ohrui H, Watanabe KA, Fox JJ. Nucleosides. LXXXIV. Total synthesis of pentopyranine C, a nucleoside elaborated by *Streptomyces griseochromogenes*. J Org Chem 1973; 38:3622–3624.

34. Watanabe KA, Chiu TMK, Reichman U, Chu CK, Fox JJ. Nucleosides. XCV. Total synthesis of pentopyranamine D, the nucleoside moiety of blasticidin H. Tetrahedron 1976; 32:1493–1495.

35. Chiu TMK, Watanabe KA, Fox JJ. Nucleosides LXXXIII. Synthetic studies on nucleoside antibiotics. 11. Synthesis of methyl 4-amino-3,4-dideoxy-β-D-*ribo*-hexopyranoside and -hexopyranosiduronic acid (derivatives related to the carbohydrate moiety of gougerotin). Carbohydr Res 1974; 32:211–216.

36. Watanabe KA, Wempen IM, Fox JJ. Nucleosides. LXXII. Synthetic studies on nucleoside antibiotics. 7. An improved synthesis of C-substance. Carbohydr Res 1972; 21:148–153.

37. Watanabe KA, Kotick MP, Fox JJ. Nucleosides. LXIII. Synthetic studies on nucleoside antibiotics. 3. Total synthesis of 1-(4-amino-4-deoxy-β-D-glucopyranosyluronic acid)cytosine, the nucleoside moiety of gougerotin. J Org Chem 1970; 35:231–236.

38. Watanabe KA, Goody RS, Fox JJ. Nucleosides LXVIII. Synthetic studies on nucleoside antibiotics. 5. 4-Amino-2,3-unsaturated sugars related to the carbohydrate moiety of blasticidin S. Tetrahedron 1970; 26:3883–3903.

39. Kotick MP, Klein RS, Watanabe KA, Fox JJ. Nucleosides. LXII. Synthetic studies on nucleoside antibiotics. 2. Synthesis of methyl 4-amino-4-deoxy-D-glucosiduronic acid derivatives related to the carbohydrate moiety of gougerotin. Carbohydr Res 1969; 11:369–377.

40. Coutsogeorgopoulos C, Bloch A, Watanabe KA, Fox JJ. Inhibitors of protein synthesis. 4. Studies of the structure-activity relationship of gougerotin and some of its analogs. J Med Chem 1975; 18:771–776.

41. Kondo T, Nakai H, Goto T. Synthesis of cytosinine, the nucleoside component of antibiotic blasticidin S. Tetrahedron 1973; 29:1801–1806.

42. Lichtenthaler FW, Morino T, Winterfeldt W, Sanemitsu Y. Nucleosides. XXVI. An alternate synthetic approach to gougerotin. Tetrahedron Lett 1975; 41:3527–3530.

43. Seto H, Yamaguchi I, Otake N, Yonehara H. Studies on the biosynthesis of blasticidin S. I. Precursors of blasticidin S biosynthesis. Agric Biol Chem 1968; 32:1292–1298.

44. Stadtman TC. Lysine metabolism by Clostridia. Meister A, ed. Advances in Enzymology and Related Areas of Molecular Biology Vol. 38. New York: John Wiley and Sons, 1973:413–448.

45. Ohsugi M, Kahn J, Hensley C, Chew S, Barker HA. Metabolism of L-β-lysine by a *Pseudomonas*. Purification and properties of a deacetylase-thiolesterase utilizing 4-acetamidobutyryl CoA and related compounds. J Biol Chem 1981; 256:7642–7651.

46. Poston JM. Coenzyme B12-dependent enzymes in potatoes: Leucine 2,3-aminomutase and methylmalonyl-CoA mutase. Phytochem 1978; 17:401–402.

47. Kurylo-Borowska Z, Abramsky T. Biosynthesis of β-tyrosine. Biochim Biophys Acta 1972; 264:1–10.

48. Summons RE. Occurrence, structure and synthesis of 3-(N-methylamino)glutaric acid, an amino acid from *Prochloron didemnii*. Phytochem 1981; 20:1125–1127.

49. Smith EL, Hill RL, Lehman IR, Lefkowitz RJ, Handler P, White A. Principles of Biochemistry: General Aspects, 7th ed. New York: McGraw-Hill, 1983:638.

50. Williamson JM, Brown GM. Purification and properties of L-aspartate-α-decarboxylase, an enzyme that catalyzes the formation of β-alanine in *Escherichia coli*. J Biol Chem 1979; 254:8074–8082.

51. Walsh C. Flavin- and pterin-dependent monooxygenases. In: Enzymatic Reaction Mechanisms. San Francisco: W. H. Freeman, 1979:Chapter 12.

52. Parry RJ, Kurylo-Borowska ZK. Biosynthesis of amino acids. Investigation of the mechanism of β-tyrosine formation. J Am Chem Soc 1980; 102:836–837.

53. Thiruvengadam TK, Gould SJ, Aberhart DJ, Lin H-J. Biosynthesis of streptothricin F. 5. Formation of β-lysine by *Streptomyces* L-1689-23. J Am Chem Soc 1983; 105:5470–5476.

54. Aberhart DJ, Gould SJ, Lin H-J, Thiruvengadam TK, Weiller BJ. Stereochemistry of lysine 2,3-aminomutase isolated from *Clostridium subterminale* strain SB4. J Am Chem Soc 1983; 105:5461–5470.

55. Prabhakaran PC, Woo NT, Yorgey P, Gould SJ. Biosynthesis of blasticidin S from L-α-arginine. Stereochemistry in the arginine-2,3-aminomutase reaction. J Am Chem Soc 1988; 110:5785–5791.

56. Yonehara H, Otake N. Biological and chemical reconstruction of blasticidin S. Antimicrob Agents Chemother 1965:855–857.

57. Bellco. Bellco Glass Inc., Vineland, New Jersey. Stock No. 2547.

58. McGahren WJ, Morton GO, Kuntsmann MP, Ellestad GA. Carbon-13 nuclear magnetic resonance studies on a new antitubercular peptide antibiotic LL-BM547β. J Org Chem 1977; 42:1282–1286.

59. Guo J, Gould SJ. Biosynthesis of blasticidin S. Cell-free demonstration of N-methylation as the last step. Bioorg Med Chem Lett 1991; 1:497–500.

60. Gould SJ, Tann CH, Prabhakaran PC, Hillis LR. [2,3,4,6,6-^{2}H$_5$]-D-Glucose as a general probe for sugar transformations in microbial metabolism: Application to the biosynthesis of sarubicin A, blasticidin S, and streptothricin F. Bioorg Chem 1988; 16:258–271.

61. Smith EL, Hill RL, Lehman IR, Lefkowitz RJ, Handler P, White A. Principles of Biochemistry: General Aspects, 7th ed. New York: McGraw-Hill, 1983:403–404, 583, 607–611.

62. Smith EL, Hill RL, Lehman IR, Lefkowitz RJ, Handler P, White A. Principles of Biochemistry: General Aspects, 7th ed. New York: McGraw-Hill, 1983:584–585, 617.

63. Schneider MJ, Ungemach FS, Broquist HP, Harris TM. Biosynthesis of swainsonine in *Rhizoctonia leguminicola*. Epimerization at the ring fusion. J Am Chem Soc 1982; 104:6863–6865.

64. Gould SJ, Guo J. Stereochemistry of C-3 deoxygenation of sugar nucleosides: Formation of pentopyranine C from [3-^{2}H]-D-glucose by *Streptomyces griseochromogenes*. J Am Chem Soc 1992; 114:10176–10181.

65. Gould SJ, Guo J, DeJesus K, Geitmann A. Nucleoside intermediates in blasticidin S biosynthesis identified by the *in vivo* use of enzyme inhibitors. Can J Chem 1994; 72:6–11.

66. Wallach DP, Crittenden NJ. Studies on the GABA pathway. I: The inhibition of γ-aminobu-tyric acid-α-ketoglutaric acid transaminase *in vitro* and *in vivo* by U-7524 (amino-oxyacetic acid). Biochem Pharmacol 1961; 5:323–331.

67. Brunk DG, Rhodes D. Amino acid metabolism of *Lemna minor* L. III. Responses to aminooxyacetate. Plant Physiol 1988; 87:447–453.

68. Khomutov AR, Gabibov AG, Khurs EN, Tolosa EA, Shuster AM, Goryachenkova EV, Khomutov RM. Biochemistry of vitamin B6. Korpela T, Christen P, eds. Proceedings of the Seventh International Union of Biochemistry Symposium. Basel, Boston: Birkhauser Verlag, 1987:317–320.

69. Sukhareva BS, Dunathan HC, Braunstein AE. The stereochemistry of the abortive trans-amination shown by glutamate decarboxylase. FEBS Lett 1971; 15:241–244.

70. Kurashashi O, Noda-Watanabe M, Toride Y, Takenouchi T, Akashi K, Morinaga Y, Enei H. Production of L-tryptophan by azaserine-, 6-diazo-5-oxo-L-norleucine- and cinnamate-resis-tant mutants of *Bacillus subtilis* K. Agric Biol Chem 1987; 51:1791–1797.

71. Kida T, Shibai H. Inhibition by hadacidin, duazomycin A, and other amino acid derivatives of *de novo* starch synthesis. Agric Biol Chem 1985; 49:3231–3237.

72. Nakayama K, Yoshida H. Fermentative production of L-arginine. Agric Biol Chem 1972; 36:1675–1684.

73. Baumberg S, Mountain A. *Bacillus subtilis* 168 mutants resistant to arginine hydroxamate in the presence of ornithine or citrulline. J Gen Microbiol 1984; 130:1247–1252.

74. Neidleman SL, Bienstock E, Bennett RE. Biosynthesis of 7-chloro-6-demethyltetracycline in the presence of aminopterin and ethionine. Biochim Biophys Acta 1963; 71:199–201.

75. Guo J, Gould SJ. Cytosine glycosides from *Streptomyces griseochromogenes*. Phytochem 1993; 32:535–41.

76. Williams NR, Wander JD. In: Pigman W, Horton D, eds. The Carbohydrates: Chemistry and Biochemistry. Orlando, Florida: Academic Press, 1980; 1B:761.

77. Rubenstein PA, Strominger JL. Enzymatic synthesis of cytidine diphosphate 3,6-dideoxyhex-oses. VII. Mechanistic roles of enzyme E1 and pyridoxamine 5'-phosphate in the formation of cytidine diphosphate-4-keto-3,6-dideoxy-D-glucose from cytidine diphosphate-4-keto-6-deoxy-D-glucose. J Biol Chem 1974; 249:3776–3781.

78. Shih Y, Yang D-y, Weigel TM, Liu H-w. Biosynthesis of 3,6-dideoxyhexoses: Stereochemical analysis of the deprotonation catalyzed by the pyridoxamine 5'-phosphate dependent enzyme CDP-4-keto-6-deoxy-D-glucose-3-dehydrase isolated from *Yersinia pseudotuberculosis*. J Am Chem Soc 1990; 112:9652–9624.

79. Han O, Miller VP, Liu H-w. Mechanistic studies of the biosynthesis of 3,6-dideoxyhexoses in *Yersinia pseudotuberculosis*: Purification and characterization of CDP-6-deoxy-$\Delta^{3,4}$-glucoseen reductase based on its NADH:dichlorophenolindolphenol oxidoreductase activity. J Biol Chem 1990; 265:8033–8041.

80. Bhowmik T, Marth EH. Protease and peptidase activity of *Micrococcus* species. J Dairy Sci 1988; 71:2358–2365.

81. Guo J, Gould SJ. Biosynthesis of blasticidin S from cytosylglucuronic acid (CGA). Isolation of cytosine/UDP-glucuronosyltransferase and incorporation of CGA by *Streptomyces griseochromogenes*. J Am Chem Soc 1991; 113:5898–5899.

82. Gould SJ, Guo J. Cytosylglucuronic acid synthase (cytosine: UDP-glucuronosyltransferase) from *Streptomyces griseochromogenes*, the first prokaryotic UDP-glucuronosyltransferase. J Bacteriol 1994; 176:1282–1286.

83. Sawada H, Suzuki T, Akiyama S-i, Nakao Y. Formation of 5-hydroxymethylcytosine from cytidine 5'-mono-phosphate by *Streptoverticilium rimofaciens*. J Ferment Technol 1985; 63:17–21.

84. Sawada H, Suzuki T, Akiyama S-i, Nakao Y. Biosynthetic pathway of 5-hydroxymethylcyto-sine by *Streptoverticilium rimofaciens*. J Ferment Technol 1985; 63:23–27.

85. Harada S, Kishi T. Isolation and characterization of mildiomycin, a new nucleoside antibi-otic. J Antibiot 1978; 31:519–524.

86. Flores-Carreon A, Balcazar A, Ruiz-Herrera J. Characterization of glucuronosyl transferase from *Mucor rouxii*: Requirement for polyuronide acceptors. Exp Mycol 1985; 9:294–301.

87. Wachett LP, Gibson DT. Metabolism of xenobiotic compounds by enzymes in cell extracts of the fungus *Cunninghamella elegans*. Biochem J 1982; 205:117–122.

88. Siest G, Antoine B, Fournel S, Magdalou J, Thomassin J. The glucuronosyltransferases: What progress can pharmacologists expect from molecular biology and cellular enzymology? Biochem Pharmacol 1987; 36:983–989.

89. Bock KW. Roles of UDP-glucuronosyltransferases in chemical carcinogenesis. CRC Critic Rev Biochem Mol Biol 1991; 26:129–150.

90. Hochman Y, Zakim D, Vessey DA. A kinetic mechanism for modulation of the activity of microsomal UDP-glucuronyltransferase by phospholipids: Effects of lysophosphatidylcholines. J Biol Chem 1981; 256:4783–4788.

91. Takahashi A, Saito N, Hotta K, Okami Y, Umezawa H. Bagougeramines A and B, new nucleoside antibiotics produced by a strain of *Bacillus circulans*. I. Taxonomy of the producing organism and isolation and biological properties of the antibiotics. J Antibiot 1986; 39:1033–1040.

92. Gould SJ, Zhang Q. Cytosinine:Pyridoxal phosphate tautomerase, a new enzyme in the blasticidin S biosynthetic pathway. J Antibiot 1995; 48:652–656.

93. Smith EL, Hill RL, Lehman IR, Lefkowitz RJ, Handler P, White A. Principles of Biochemistry: General Aspects, 7th ed. New York: McGraw-Hill, 1983:450.

94. Kamiya K, Wada Y, Takamoto M. Crystal and molecular structure of mildiomycin monobenzoate heptahydrate. Tetrahedron Lett 1978; 44:4277–4280.

95. Flaks JG, Cohen SS. Virus-induced acquisition of metabolic function. I. Enzymatic formation of 5-hydroxymethyldeoxycytidylate. J Biol Chem 1959; 234:1501–1506.

96. Yukioka M, Morisawa S. Studies on the mechanism of action of gougerotin. (I) Enhancement of polyphenylalanine synthesis by gougerotin. J Biochem 1969; 66:225–232.

97. Coutsogeorgopoulos C. Inhibitors of the reaction between puromycin and polylysyl-RNA in the presence of ribosomes. Biochem Biophys Res Commun 1967; 27:46–52.

98. Kinoshita T, Tanaka N, Umezawa H. Binding of blasticidin S to ribosomes. J Antibiot 1970; 23:288–290.

99. Cerna J, Rychlik I, Lichtenthaler FW. The effect of the amino acyl-4-aminohexosyl-cytosine group of antibiotics on ribosomal peptidyl transferase. FEBS Lett 1973; 30:147–150.

100. Lichtenthaler FW, Trummlitz G. Structural basis for inhibition of protein synthesis by the aminoacyl-aminohexosyl-cytosine group of antibiotics. FEBS Lett 1974; 38:237–242.

101. Pestka S. Studies on the formation of transfer ribonucleic acid-ribosome complexes. VIII. Survey of the effect of antibiotics on N-acetyl-phenylalanyl-puromycin formation: Possible mechanism of chloramphenicol action. Arch Biochem Biophys 1970; 136:80–88.

102. Theocharis DA, Synetos D, Kalpaxis DL, Drainas D, Coutsogeorgopoulos C. Kinetics of inhibition of peptide bond formation on bacterial ribosomes. Arch Biochem Biophys 1992; 292:266–272.

103. Sugiyama M, Takeda A, Paik S-Y, Nimi O. Isolation and properties of a blasticidin S acetylating enzyme from a producer organism. J Antibiot 1989; 42:135–137.

104. Shaw WV, Hopwood DA. Chloramphenicol in acetylation in *Streptomyces*. J Gen Microbiol 1976; 94:159–166.

105. Keeratipibul S, Sugiyama M, Nomi R. Mechanism of resistance to streptothricin of a producing microorganism. Bio/Technol 1983; 5:441–446.

106. Sugiyama M, Paik S-Y, Nomi R. Mechanism of self-protection in a puromycin producing microorganism. J Gen Microbiol 1985; 131:1999–2005.

107. Seto H, Otake N, Yonehara H. Biological transformation of blasticidin S by *Aspergillus fumigatus* sp. 1. Isolation, characterization and structures of transformed products and their biological properties. Agric Biol Chem 1966; 30:877–886.

108. Yamaguchi I, Seto H, Misato T. Substrate binding by blasticidin S deaminase, an aminohydrolase for novel 4-aminopyrimidine nucleosides. Pestic Biochem Physiol 1986; 25:54–62.

109. Endo T, Furuta K, Kaneko A, Katsuki T, Kobayashi K, Azuma A, Watanabe A, Shimazu A. Inactivation of blasticidin S by *Bacillus cereus*. I. Inactivation mechanism. J Antibiot 1987; 40:1791–1793.

110. Yamaguchi I, Shibata H, Seto H, Misato T. Isolation and purification of blasticidin S deaminase from *Aspergillus terreus*. J Antibiot 1975; 28:7–14.

111. Yamaguchi I, Misato T. Active center and mode of reaction of blasticidin S deaminase. Agric Biol Chem 1985; 49:3355–3361.

112. Kobayashi K, Kamakura T, Tanaka T, Yamaguchi I, Endo T. Nucleotide sequence of the *bsr* gene and N-terminal amino acid sequence of blasticidin S deaminase from blasticidin S resistant *Escherichia coli* TK121. Agric Biol Chem 1991; 55:3155–3157.

113. Kimura M, Kamakura T, Tao QZ, Kaneko I, Yamaguchi I. Cloning of the blasticidin S deaminase gene (*BSD*) from *Aspergillus terreus* and its use as a selectable marker for *Schizosaccharomyces pombe* and *Pyricularia oryzae*. Mol Gen Genet 1994; 242:121–129.

114. Ishiguro J, Miyazaki M. Characterization of blasticidin S–resistant mutants of *Saccharomyces cerevisiae*. Curr Genet 1985; 9:179–181.

115. Contreras A, Vazquez D, Carrasco L. Inhibition, by selected antibiotics, of protein synthesis in cells growing in tissue cultures. J Antibiot 1978; 31:598–602.

116. Kuwano M, Takenaka K, Ono M. The cross-resistance of mouse blasticidin S–resistant cell lines to puromycin and sparsomycin, inhibitors of ribosome function. Biochim Biophys Acta 1979; 563:479–489.

117. Kuwano M, Matsui K, Takenaka K, Akiyama S-i, Endo H. A mouse leukemia cell mutant resistant to blasticidin S. Int J Cancer 1977; 20:296–302.

118. Misato T. Mode of action of agricultural antibiotics developed in Japan. Residue Rev 1969; 25:93–106.

119. Yoshikawa M, Yamaguchi K, Masago H. *De novo* messenger RNA and protein synthesis are required for phytoalexin-mediated disease resistance in soybean hypocotyls. Plant Physiol 1978; 61:314–317.

120. Holliday MJ, Keen NT, Long M. Cell death patterns and accumulation of fluorescent material in the hypersensitive response of soybean leaves to *Pseudomonas syringae* pv. *glycinea*. Physiol Plant Path 1981; 18:279–287.

121. Oba K, Uritani I. Mechanism of furano-terpene production in sweet potato root tissue injured by chemical agents. Agric Biol Chem 1981; 45:1635–1639.

122. Mayama S, Tani T, Ueno T, Midland SL, Sims JJ, Keen NT. The purification of victorin and its phytoalexin elicitor activity in oat leaves. Physiol Mol Plant Path 1986; 29:1–18.

123. Perez-Gonzalez JA, Ruiz D, Esteban JA, Jiménez A. Cloning and characterization of the gene encoding a blasticidin S acetyltransferase from *Streptoverticillum* sp. Gene 1990; 86:129–134.

124. Vara J, Malpartida F, Hopwood DA, Jimenéz A. Cloning and expression of a puromycin *N*-acetyl transferase from *Streptomyces alboniger* in *Streptomyces lividans* and *Escherichia coli*. Gene 1985; 33:197–206.

125. Lacalle RA, Pulido D, Vara J, Zalacain M, Jimenéz A. Molecular analysis of the *pac* gene encoding a puromycin *N*-acetyltransferase gene from *Streptomyces alboniger*. Gene 1989; 79:375–380.

126. Horinouchi S, Furaya K, Nishiyama M, Suzuki H, Beppu T. Nucleotide sequence of the streptothricin acetyltransferase gene from *Streptomyces lavendulae* and its expression in heterologous hosts. J Bacteriol 1987; 169:1929–1937.

127. Kamakura T, Kobayashi K, Tanaka T, Yamaguchi I, Endo T. Cloning and expression of a new structural gene for blasticidin S deaminase, a nucleoside aminohydrolase. Agric Biol Chem 1987; 51:3165–3168.

128. Endo T, Kobayashi K, Nakayama N, Tanaka T, Kamakura T, Yamaguchi I. Inactivation of blasticidin S by *Bacillus cereus*. II. Isolation of a plasmid, pBSR8, from *Bacillus cereus*. J Antibiot 1988; 41:271–273.

129. Song BH, Neuhard J. Chromosomal location, cloning and nucleotide sequence of the *Bacillus subtillus cdd* gene encoding cytidine/deoxycytidine deaminase. Mol Gen Genet 1989; 216:462–468.

130. Kamakura T, Yoneyama K, Yamaguchi I. Expression of the blasticidin S deaminase gene (*bsr*) in tobacco: Fungicide tolerance and a new selective marker for transgenic plants. Mol Gen Genet 1990; 223:332–334.

131. Yamaguchi I, Yoneyama K, Anzai H, Kamakura T. Transgenic plants engineered for the detoxification of a pathogenic toxin and a fungicide. Frehse H, ed. Pesticide Chemistry Advances International Research, Development, Legislation, Proceedings International Congress Pesticide Chemistry 7th, 1990; 1991:615–625.

132. Yamaguchi I, Kimura M, Kamakura T. Molecular cloning of cDNA for blasticidin S deaminase of *Aspergillus terreus*. Jpn Kokai Tokkyo Koho JP 06 70,768 [94 70,768] 1994 Mar 15; 121:490.

133. Tao QZ, Kimura M, Yamaguchi I. A novel dominant drug resistance marker for transformation of *Pyricularia oryzae*. You C, Chen Z, Ding Y, eds. Biotechnology in Agriculture: Proceedings of the First Asia-Pacific Conference on Agricultural Biotechnology, Beijing, China, August 20–24, 1992. Netherlands: Kluwer Academic Publishers, 1993:457–461.

134. Yanai K, Horiuchi H, Takagi M, Yano K. Transformation of *Rhizopus niveus* using a bacterial blasticidin S resistance gene as a dominant selectable marker. Curr Genet 1991; 19:221–226.

135. Sutoh K. A Transformation vector for *Dictyostelium discoideum* with a new selectable marker *bsr*. Plasmid 1993; 30:150–154.

136. Itaya M, Yamaguchi I, Kobayashi K, Endo T, Tanada T. The blasticidin S resistance gene (*bsr*) selectable in a single copy state in the *Bacillus subtilis* chromosome. J Biochem 1990; 107:799–801.

137. Izumi M, Miyazawa H, Kamakura T, Yamaguchi I, Endo T, Hanaoka F. Blasticidin S–resistance gene (*bsr*): A novel selectable marker for mammalian cells. Exp Cell Res 1991; 197:229–233.

24

New Processes for Production of 7-Aminocephalosporanic Acid from Cephalosporin

Takao Isogai

Fujisawa Pharmaceutical Co., Ltd., Tokodai, Tsukuba, Ibaraki, Japan

I. INTRODUCTION

Cephem antibiotics have been the world's most frequently used antibiotics in the treatment of a variety of bacterial infections. They have a broader antimicrobial spectrum and are more resistant to β-lactamases than penicillin. In addition, people with allergies to penicillin are usually not sensitive to cephem antibiotics (1,2).

Acremonium chrysogenum (formerly named *Cephalosporium acremonium*) is the sole fungus used industrially for the production of cephalosporin C. 7-Aminocephalosporanic acid (7-ACA), the starting material for the production of a number of clinically important cephem antibiotics (1–3) such as cefazolin and ceftizoxime, is derived industrially from cephalosporin C by either complex chemical methods (1) or a two-step procedure consisting of chemical and enzymatic steps (4). 7-Aminodeacetylcephalosporanic acid (7-ADACA) is also the starting material for the production of clinically important oral cephem antibiotics (3,5), such as cefixime (FK027) and cefdinir (FK482), and is derived from 7-ACA by hydrolysis with sodium hydroxide. Establishment of an efficient process for an enzymatic or microbial production of 7-ACA and 7-ADACA has been an important priority for the cephem antibiotic production industry.

In this chapter, I describe enzymes converting cephalosporin C to 7-ACA, and the construction of a novel strain for the direct production of 7-ACA and 7-ADACA by metabolic pathway engineering (6,7).

II. ENZYMES CONVERTING CEPHALOSPORIN C TO 7-ACA

A. Enzymatic Conversion of Cephalosporin C to 7-ACA

Cephalosporin acylases include two types of enzymes: cephalosporin C acylase (CC acylase), which can hydrolyze cephalosporin C and 7-β-(4-carboxybutanamido)cephalosporanic acid (GL-7-ACA) to 7-ACA; and GL-7-ACA acylase, which can hydrolyze GL-7-ACA to 7-ACA (Figure 1). GL-7-ACA is generated from cephalosporin C by the action of D–amino acid oxidase (DAO) or by a chemical method. Thus, two methods are utilized for enzymatic synthesis of 7-ACA from cephalosporin C, one using two enzymes, DAO and GL-7-ACA acylase, and the other using CC acylase only.

The reaction scheme for enzymatic synthesis of 7-ACA from cephalosporin C is shown in Figure 1. The pathway involves the oxidative deamination of cephalosporin C into 7-β-(5-carboxy-5-oxopentanamido)cephalosporanic acid (keto-AD-7-ACA) by DAO. A portion of the product further reacts nonenzymatically with hydrogen peroxide, which is formed as a by-product in the above reaction, to give GL-7-ACA. GL-7-ACA is hydrolyzed by GL-7-ACA acylase to 7-ACA. C7 side chains of cephalosporin C, keto-AD-7-ACA, and GL-7-ACA are hydrolyzed by CC acylase to 7-ACA. However, the CC acylase activity for cephalosporin C is low compared with that for GL-7-ACA.

B.   D–Amino Acid Oxidases Active Against Cephalosporin C

DAO is a flavoenzyme, containing flavin adenine dinucleotide (FAD) as the prosthetic group, that catalyzes oxidation of D–amino acids to their corresponding keto acids. DAOs have been found widely in microorganisms as well as in the tissues of animals (8). On the other hand, the cultured cells of DAO-producing strains, *Fusarium solani* M-0718 (FERM P-2688) and *Trigonopsis variabilis* CBS4095 (ATCC58536), or their processed materials effectively convert cephalosporin C into GL-7-ACA via keto-AD-7-ACA (9,10). Deduced amino acid sequences of DAOs from *F. solani* M-0718 and *T. variabilis* CBS4095 are shown in Figure 2 (11,12).

I.   DAO of F. solani M-0718

We isolated a DAO active against cephalosporin C from cultured mycelia of *F. solani* M-0718, and we determined 98 amino acid residues of it (11). This isolated DAO gave a single band with a relative molecular mass (M_r) of 40 kDa on sodium lauryl sulfate polyacrylamide gel electrophoresis (SDS-PAGE). The K_m and V_{max} values for cephalosporin C were 3.55 mM and 33.8 μmol/min/mg protein, respectively, and the pH optimum was 7.0–7.5.

We also cloned *F. solani* DAO cDNA using oligonucleotide probes corresponding to the partial amino acid sequences (11). Analysis of the nucleotide sequences of the clones revealed an open reading frame of 1083 nucleotides that encoded 361 amino acids

---

Abbreviations: 7-ACA, 7-Aminocephalosporanic acid; 7-ADACA, 7-Aminodeacetylcephalosporanic acid; 7-ADOCA, 7-aminodeacetoxycephalosporanic acid; Ap^R, ampicillin resistance; 6-BH-7-ACA, 7-β-(6-bromohexanoylamido)cephalosporanic acid; CC acylase, cephalosporin C acylase; CAE, cephalosporin C acetylesterase; DAC, deacetylcephalosporin C; DAO, D–amino acid oxidase; D-H-AD-7-ACA, 7-β-(D-5-carboxy-5-hydroxypentanamido) cephalosporanic acid; D-H-AD-7-ADACA, 7-β-(D-5-carboxy-5-hydroxypentanamido)deacetylcephalosporanic acid; DL-H-AD-7-ACA, 7-β-(DL-5-carboxy-5-hydroxypentanamido)cephalosporanic acid; DL-H-AD-7-ADACA, 7-β-(DL-5-carboxy-5-hydroxypentanamido)deacetylcephalosporanic acid; GL-7-ACA, 7-β-(4-carboxybutanamido)cephalosporanic acid; GL-7-ADACA, 7-β-(4-carboxybutanamido)deacetylcephalosporanic acid; keto-AD-7-ACA, 7-β-(5-carboxy-5-oxopentanamido) cephalosporanic acid; keto-AD-7-ADACA, 7-β-(5-carboxy-5-oxopentanamido)deacetylcephalosporanic acid; Hm^R, hygromycin B resistance; LLD-ACV, δ-(L-α-aminoadipyl)-L-cysteinyl-D-valine; PAC, penicillin G acylase; SDS-PAGE, sodium lauryl sulfate polyacrylamide gel electrophoresis.

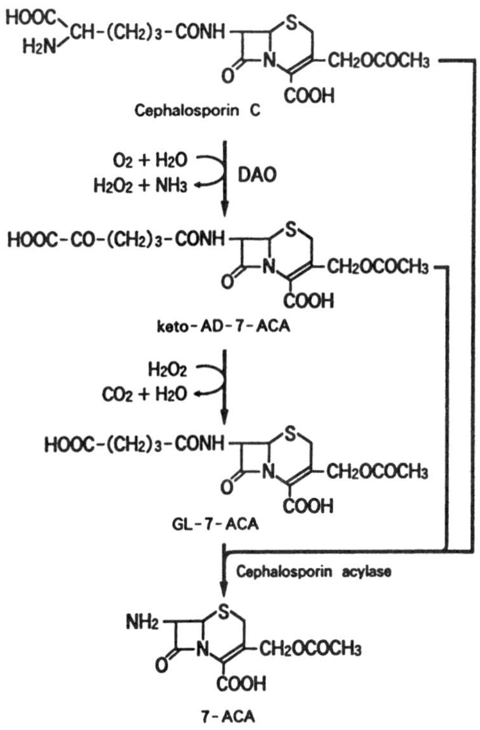

Figure 1   The reaction scheme for enzymatic synthesis of 7-ACA from cephalosporin C. The substrate specificities of cephalosporin acylases are described in the text.

(molecular weight 39,696). The genomic DNA of *F. solani* DAO was cloned using the DAO cDNA as a probe, and it had three introns (53, 50, and 54 bp) near the ATG codon in the coding region. A high-level expression plasmid carrying the *F. solani* DAO cDNA was constructed, and this was used to overproduce DAO in *Escherichia coli*. The recombinant DAO had almost the same molecular activity as the native DAO against cephalosporin C, and the N-terminal amino acid sequence of it was identical to that predicted from the cDNA (11,15).

2.   DAO of T. variabilis CBS4095

Szwajcer and Mosbach (10) isolated DAO active against cephalosporin C from cultured cells of *T. variabilis* CBS4095. The isolated DAO gave a single band with a molecular size of 43 kDa on SDS-PAGE. The K_m values for cephalosporin C, D-phenylalanine, D-alanine, D-methionine, and D-leucine were 13, 10, 76, 0.76, and 0.12 mM, respectively.

Komatsu et al. (12) determined the N-terminal amino acid sequence (41 residues) of the *T. variabilis* DAO, and they cloned the DAO genomic DNA using oligonucleotide probes corresponding to the amino acid sequence. From analysis of the nucleotide sequence of the clone, they found that the DAO genomic DNA has an open reading frame that encoded 355 amino acids and one intron (36 bp) near the ATG codon in the coding region. An expression plasmid carrying the *T. variabilis* DAO genomic DNA without the intron was constructed, and this was used to overproduce the DAO active on cephalosporin C in *E. coli*.

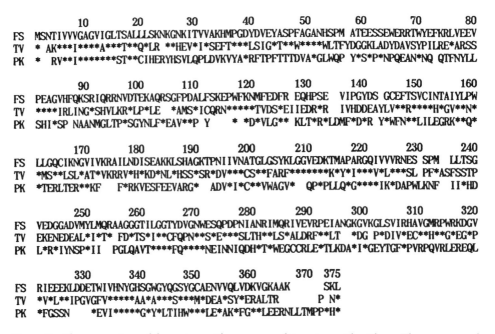

Figure 2 The comparison of the amino acid sequences of D–amino acid oxidases. The sequence of *F. solani* DAO (FS) (11) is shown compared with those of the DAOs from *T. variabilis* (TV) (12) and porcine kidney (PK) (13,14). Amino acids of DAOs identical with *F. solani* DAO are shown as *.

Vicenzi and Hansen (16) have developed an economical process for the enzymatic oxidation of cephalosporin C to GL-7-ACA at a pilot plant scale utilizing nonviable whole cells of *T. variabilis* containing high levels of DAO. Prior to use, the whole cells were permeabilized with a 25% acetone–water solution and then incubated at pH 11, which served to selectively deactivate catalase. The treated cells were utilized within a "cross-flow filter-reactor" that allowed easy and economical recycling of the cells for repeated use. The overall yield of GL-7-ACA from cephalosporin C was 90–95% (16).

3. Comparison of the Amino Acid Sequences of DAOs

The amino acid sequence of the *F. solani* DAO (11) shows 37% identity to that of *T. variabilis* DAO (12) and 25% identity to that of porcine kidney DAO [EC 1.4.3.3] (13,14), which has a weak oxidative activity against cephalosporin C (Figure 2). The amino acid sequence of *T. variabilis* DAO also shows relatively low identity (20%) to that of porcine kidney DAO. The *T. variabilis* and *F. solani* DAOs have the same approximate oxidative deamination rate against cephalosporin C, in spite of the amino acid sequence identity being relatively low.

Watanabe et al. (17) and Miyano et al. (18) reported that Tyr-228 (250 in Figure 2) and His-307 (335 in Figure 2) of porcine kidney DAO play important roles in enzymatic properties. These two residues are conserved among all three DAOs. An amino acid sequence of Gly–X–Gly–X–X–Gly, which may be the binding site of the adenine of FAD (19), is conserved near the *N*-terminus of all three DAOs (11). DAO is one of the principal and characteristic enzymes of the peroxisomes of porcine kidney (14). The *F.*

solani DAO at the C-terminus has the highly conserved peroxisome targeting signal sequence, –SKL (20). The *F. solani* DAO also may be a peroxisomal enzyme.

C. Cephalosporin Acylases

An immobilized GL-7-ACA acylase of *Pseudomonas* sp. GK16 has been utilized for industrial production of 7-ACA by the chemical and enzymatic method from cephalosporin C via GL-7-ACA by the Asahi Chemical Company (4,21). Several additional cephalosporin acylase genes have been reported (22–28). Enzymatic properties of various cephalosporin acylases are summarized in Table 1, and amino acid sequences of these are shown in Figure 3.

1. GL-7-ACA Acylases

Matsuda and Komatsu (22) cloned the GL-7-ACA acylase gene from *Pseudomonas* sp. GK16, and they analyzed the gene products by maxicell analysis. From the results (22), they proposed a possible process for formation of the active GL-7-ACA acylase as (a) synthesis of a polypeptide containing sequences for the signal peptide and the small and large subunits as the translation product from the GL-7-ACA acylase gene; (b) translocation of the product into periplasm and processing of the signal sequence to give rise to the 70 kDa polypeptide; and (c) processing of the 70 kDa polypeptide to the small and large subunits, and formation of an active enzyme complex by association of both the subunits.

We also cloned the GL-7-ACA acylase gene from *Pseudomonas* sp. C427 (23). The DNA sequence revealed an open reading frame of 2154 bp coding for 718 amino acid

Table I   Enzymatic Properties of Cephalosporin Acylases

Enzyme	Molecular size[a] (kDa)		Optimum[b]pH	K_m[b] (mM)	V_{max}[b] (μmol/min/mg protein)	Ref.
	SDS-PAGE	Sequence				
GK16 GL-7-ACA acylase	α: 16	n.p.[c]	7–8	0.16	4.9	21, 22
	β: 54	n.p.				
C427 GL-7-ACA acylase	α: 18	17.9	7–8	0.36	6.1	23
	β: 60	57.9				
SE83 CC acylase (acylase II)	α: 26	25.4	9	n.p.[c]	n.p.[c]	25, 26
	β: 57	58.2				
N176 CC acylase	α: 26	25.4	9	2.6	100	28, 29
	β: 58	58.2				
V22 CC acylase	α:26	25.4	9	2.2	132	27, 28
	β: 56	58.3				
J1 GL-7-ACA acylase	70	69.2	8	3.2	5.3	24, 29

[a] Molecular sizes of enzymes were determined by SDS-PAGE or amino acid sequences deduced from DNA sequences, and the subunit structures were designated as α (small subunit) and β (large subunit). However, J1 GL-7-ACA acylase is a single polypeptide.
[b] Optimum pH, K_m, and V_{max} were determined against GL-7-ACA.
[c] n.p.: not published.

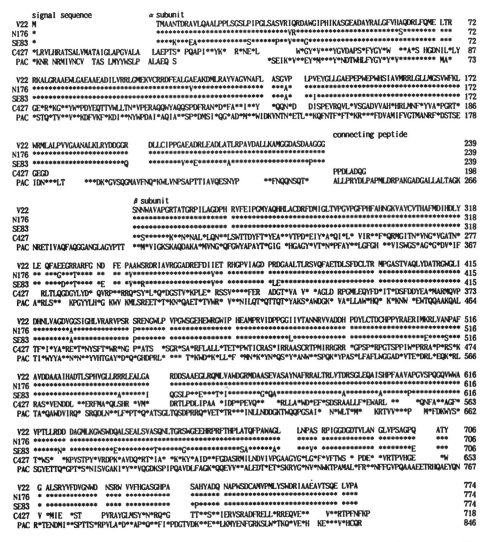

Figure 3 Comparison of the amino acid sequences of cephalosporin and penicillin acylases. The sequence of CC acylase from *Pseudomonas diminuta* V22 (V22) (27) is shown compared with those of CC acylase from *P. diminuta* N176 (N176) (28), CC acylase from *Pseudomonas* sp. SE83 (SE83) (26), GL-7-ACA acylase from *Pseudomonas* sp. C427 (C427) (23), and penicillin G acylase from *E. coli* ATCC11105 (PAC) (30). Amino acids of cephalosporin and penicillin acylases identical with CC acylase from *P. diminuta* V22 are shown as *.

residues. The nucleotide and amino acid sequences of the C427 GL-7-ACA acylase show high identities (97%) with those of the GK16 GL-7-ACA acylase, for which only partial nucleotide (1041 bp) and amino acid (311 residues) sequences have been elucidated (22). The GK16 and C427 GL-7-ACA acylases could not hydrolyze cephalosporin C to 7-ACA, but they had a low deacylating activity for keto-AD-7-ACA compared with that for GL-7-ACA.

A high level of active enzyme production was achieved with a plasmid coding for the C427 GL-7-ACA acylase in which the amino terminal sequence (positions 1–32) of native acylase was replaced by the sequence MFPTT (23). The productivity was approximately 2 g/liter in flask fermentation, which is not a high cell density fermentation. The result also indicates that the signal sequence of the native acylase is not necessary for the processing of the C427 GL-7-ACA acylase.

Aramori et al. (24) cloned an another type of GL-7-ACA acylase gene from *Bacillus laterosporus* J1. The DNA sequence revealed an open reading frame of 1902 bp coding for 634 amino acid residues, and the acylase was composed of a single polypeptide with the molecular size of 70 kDa analyzed by SDS-PAGE. This acylase has a unique molecular structure compared with those of cephalosporin acylases of *Pseudomonas*. The J1 GL-7-ACA acylase hydrolyzed GL-7-ACA to 7-ACA, but it could not hydrolyze cephalosporin C and keto-AD-7-ACA (24).

2. Cephalosporin C Acylases

Matsuda et al. (25,26) cloned a CC acylase gene, *acyII*, from *Pseudomonas* sp. SE83. The DNA sequence contained a single open reading frame (2322 bp) for two nonidentical subunits (25.4 and 58.2 kDa), predicting a common precursor (83.6 kDa). The CC acylase hydrolyzed cephalosporin C directly to 7-ACA, and the CC acylase activity for cephalosporin C was low (5%) compared with that for GL-7-ACA (100%).

We also cloned CC acylase genes from *Pseudomonas diminuta* V22 and N176 (27,28). The CC acylases were able to directly convert cephalosporin C into 7-ACA, and they were shown to be composed of two nonidentical subunits with molecular sizes of 26 and 56–58 kDa when analyzed by SDS-PAGE. The deduced amino acid sequences of the V22, N176, and SE83 CC acylases were compared with each other (Figure 3). The number of amino acid residues was 774, the same as among the CC acylases. The numbers of nonidentical amino acid residues between V22 and SE83, between N176 and SE83, and between V22 and N176 were 53, 50, and 11, respectively.

Substrate specificities of N176 and V22 CC acylases are shown in Table 2. The K_m and k_{cat} values of N176 CC acylase for cephalosporin C at pH 8.7 were 21.5 mM and 5.93 sec^{-1}, respectively. N176 CC acylase activity for keto-AD-7-ACA was relatively high compared with that for GL-7-ACA. It appears that keto-AD-7-ACA may be hydrolyzed by V22 and SE83 CC acylases at the same approximate rates.

Table 2   Substrate Specificities of N176 and V22 CC Acylases

Substrate	Substrate specificity[a] (units/mg protein)	
	N176 CC acylase	V22 CC acylase
GL-7-ACA (pH 7.5)	26.8	23.5
GL-7-ACA (pH 8.7)	46.3	37.4
keto-AD-7-ACA (pH 7.5)	23.4	n.t.[b]
Cephalosporin C (pH 8.7)	1.55	1.74

[a] Substrate specificities were determined from reactions in 0.1 M Tris-HCl (each pH) at 37°C for 10 min with 10 mg/ml of each substrate.
[b] n.t.: not tested.

3. *Protein Engineering of Cephalosporin Acylase*

Comparison of the amino acid sequences of CC acylases and GL-7-ACA acylases from *Pseudomonas* (21,23,25,28) and penicillin G acylase (PAC) from *E. coli* ATCC11105 (30) are shown in Figure 3. These enzymes consist of two nonidentical subunits processed from a common precursor polypeptide encoded by a single open reading frame. PAC and C427 acylase have *N*-terminal signal sequences, but this sequence is not found in CC acylases, which are cytoplasmic enzymes. The similarities between V22 CC acylase, C427 GL-7-ACA acylase, and PAC are approximately 20%. However, several clusters of high similarity are observed both in the α and β subunits. Conserved amino acids within these identical regions may play an important role in the enzyme reaction.

Ishii et al. (31) determined an affinity-labeled residue, Tyr-270, of N176 CC acylase with a substrate analog, 7-β-(6-bromohexanoylamido)cephalosporanic acid (6-BH-7-ACA). The enzyme was inactivated by incubation with 6-BH-7-ACA. Tyr-270 is perfectly conserved between cephalosporin acylases and PAC (Figure 3). However, replacement of Tyr-270 with a Phe residue by site-directed mutagenesis of N176 CC acylase resulted in a K_m value of the mutant acylase that was increased slightly, and a k_{cat} value that was decreased to about 50% of that of the wild type (31). The role of Tyr-270 may be to assist other residues that are involved in the stabilization of the transition state.

The *N*-terminal Ser of the β subunit is also perfectly conserved between cephalosporin acylases and PAC (Figure 3) (31). Slade et al. (32) and Martin et al. (33) have reported that the *N*-terminal Ser of the β subunit of penicillin acylase acts a nucleophile in the catalysis. Ishii et al. (34) mutated Ser-239 of N176 CC acylase to Cys by site-directed mutagenesis, and the mutated acylase caused a major decrease in catalytic activity. The residue, Ser-239, may play a role as an active residue in N176 CC acylase.

Nobbs et al. (35) reported chemical modification of N176 CC acylase with tetranitromethane and site-directed mutagenesis of tyrosine residues in the enzyme. The chemical modification of N176 CC acylase with tetranitromethane caused complete loss of activity. The modified tyrosine residues of the enzyme were analyzed. Tyr-270 was completely modified and Tyr-52 was partially modified. They altered each of the 15 tyrosines in the N176 CC acylase to Leu by site-directed mutagenesis (35). The mutated acylase, in which Tyr at position 270 is changed to Leu, showed GL-7-ACA and CC acylase activities reduced to 28.0 and 32.2% of native acylase, respectively, at pH 8.7. A similar reduction in the activities was also observed in the case of a Tyr-491 mutant, although nitration of this residue was not confirmed by chemical modification. However, mutation of Tyr-52 to Leu produced little change in acylase activity. The mutated acylase, in which Tyr-705 was changed to Leu, had a lowered pH optimum for GL-7-ACA. This mutation may be useful for further improvement of CC acylases. These results indicate that Tyr-270 and Tyr-491 probably exist near the active site of the N176 CC acylase but are not essential for activity, as well as identifying a residue, Tyr-705, that influences the pH optimum of the enzyme.

Ishii et al. (34) and Saito et al. (36) mutated Met-269 and Ala-271 neighboring Tyr-270 of N176 CC acylase to various amino acids by site-directed mutagenesis, and they determined those specific activities against cephalosporin C. They found that mutations of Met-269 to Tyr and Phe caused 1.5- and 1.7-fold, respectively, increases of specific activities over wild-type acylase against cephalosporin C. Kinetic studies of these mutants, designated as M269Y and M269F, revealed the K_m values against cephalosporin C were not changed, but their k_{cat} values increased 1.6- and 1.7-fold, respectively, when compared with that of the wild type. These results indicate that the mutation of Met-269 to aromatic amino acids may be responsible for stabilizing the activated complex of the N176 CC acylase with cephalosporin C. Moreover, they found that M269Y was more efficient at converting cephalosporin C to 7-ACA than the wild type in conditions similar to a bioreactor system (34).

III. DIRECT PRODUCTION OF 7-ACA AND 7-ADACA BY METABOLIC PATHWAY ENGINEERING IN *ACREMONIUM CHRYSOGENUM*

Establishment of a process for the microbial production of 7-ACA and 7-ADACA had been sought, but a 7-ACA- or 7-ADACA-producing strain had not yet been reported. Though native antibiotic biosynthetic gene clusters had been cloned and expressed in heterologous hosts (37–40), the expression of an "artificial" antibiotic biosynthetic gene cluster was also unreported. To establish a 7-ACA- or 7-ADACA-producing strain, a novel 7-ACA biosynthetic gene cluster was constructed from fungal and bacterial genes and then introduced into *Acremonium chrysogenum* (6,7,27).

A. Construction of a Novel Strain for the Production of 7-ACA and 7-ADACA

1. Direct Production of 7-ACA in A. chrysogenum

Although the CC acylase can directly convert cephalosporin C into 7-ACA, microbial production of 7-ACA using the CC acylase as a sole converting enzyme is not expected to be very efficient for the following reasons. The CC acylase is about 20- to 30-fold less active in converting cephalosporin C than it is with GL-7-ACA. The pH of the cultured broth of a cephalosporin C fermentation is 5.5 to 6.5 and rises to about 7 at the end of the fermentation, whereas the CC acylase has a pH optimum of 9 and is only about 25% active at pH 7. Thus we adopted the 7-ACA biosynthetic pathway outlined in Figure 1 for construction of a novel 7-ACA-producing strain. In the pathway, cephalosporin C is converted to keto-AD-7-ACA and GL-7-ACA by *F. solani* DAO (11,12); then keto-AD-7-ACA, GL-7-ACA, and cephalosporin C are hydrolyzed to 7-ACA by *P. diminuta* V22 CC acylase (6,25–28).

A plasmid, pHDV11 (18.9 kbp) (Figure 4), containing the 7-ACA biosynthetic gene cluster was constructed using the DAO gene from *F. solani* M-0718 and the CC acylase gene from *P. diminuta* V22 (6). Since an out-of-frame ATG exists just upstream of the translation start codon in the V22 CC acylase gene, the gene deleted for that ATG was used for construction of pHDV11. We also constructed a plasmid, pHBV1, containing only the V22 CC acylase gene, and we expected the plasmid to be able to direct the synthesis of 7-ACA, although at lower levels than pHDV11. The hygromycin B resistance gene (HmR) (41) was chosen as a selection marker in *A. chrysogenum*. The promoter and regulatory elements of an alkaline protease gene from *A. chrysogenum* (6,42) were utilized for expression of DAO, CC acylase, and HmR genes in *A. chrysogenum*.

A. chrysogenum BC2116 (FERM BP-2707), a relatively high producing strain of cephalosporin C, was transformed with pHDV11 and pHBV1. The HmR transformants were cultured in a complex medium, and their production of antibiotics was assayed by high-performance liquid chromatography (HPLC). The pHDV11 transformants (Hm165 and Hm178) produced about 150 µg/ml of 7-ACA. The pHBV1 transformants (Hm155 and Hm172) produced about 50 µg/ml of 7-ACA (6). 7-ACA isolated from the cultured broth of Hm178 had ^{1}H nuclear magnetic resonance (NMR) and infrared spectra that

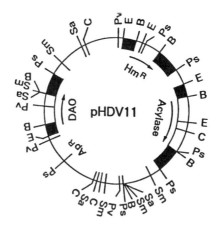

Figure 4   The schematic representation of plasmid pHDV11 (18.9 kbp). The DNA sequences are denoted as follows: thin line, vector DNA and HmR (hygromycin B resistance) gene (41); solid boxes, the regulatory elements of the alkaline protease gene from A. *chrysogenum* ATCC11550 (6,42); open boxes, DAO cDNA of *F. solani* (11) and CC acylase (Acylase) genomic DNA of *P. diminuta* V22 (6,27). Restriction enzyme sites: B, *Bam*HI; C, *Cla*I; E, *Eco*RI; Ps, *Pst*I; Pv, *Pvu*II; Sa, *Sac*I; Sm, *Sma*I.

were essentially identical to those of an authentic sample of 7-ACA (6). Transformants that had only DAO and HmR genes, however, did not produce 7-ACA. These results indicate that the constructed 7-ACA biosynthetic gene cluster in pHDV11 functioned in A. *chrysogenum,* and 7-ACA-producing strains were established.

2.   Direct Production of 7-ADACA by Recombinant A. chrysogenum

A monocell isolated strain of A. *chrysogenum* Hm178, the pHDV11 transformant, was used for further studies. We analyzed time course productions of cephalosporins by Hm178 fermentation in complex media (7). Hm178 produced 282 µg/ml 7-ADACA, 183 µg/ml 7-ACA, and 70 µg/ml 7-aminodeacetoxycephalosporanic acid (7-ADOCA) in the cultured broth. GL-7-ACA, keto-AD-7-ACA, and 7-β-(5-carboxy-5-oxopentanamido)deacetylcephalosporanic acid (keto-AD-7-ADACA) were undetectable in the cultured broth. There is a possibility that a 3-hydroxymethyl of deacetylcephalosporins lactonizes with the 4-carboxyl to form the lactones at low pH (43). However, 7-ADACA lactone was not detected in the cultured broth of Hm178. Moreover, production of 7-ADACA and 7-ACA by Hm178 were correlated to those of DAC (deacetylcephalosporin C) and cephalosporin C, respectively. The production of 7-ADOCA by Hm178 was detected later in the fermentation than was 7-ADACA. The 7-ADACA isolated from the cultured broth had ^{1}H NMR spectra essentially identical with that of an authentic sample of 7-ADACA.

However, a monocell isolated strain of A. *chrysogenum* Hm172, the transformant of pHBV1, produced low levels of 7-ADACA (23 µg/ml) and 7-ACA (32 µg/ml), and no detectable amount of 7-ADOCA (7). Furthermore, 7-ADACA, 7-ACA, and 7-ADOCA were not detected in the cultured broth of the host strain, A. *chrysogenum* BC2116.

Thus, A. *chrysogenum* Hm178 containing pHDV11, which was constructed from enzyme genes of both DAO and CC acylase, was confirmed to synthesize and secrete not only 7-ACA but 7-ADACA, although the production amounts of 7-ACA and 7-

ADACA were not yet commercially significant. Nevertheless, for the first time, we demonstrated the feasibility of introducing new biosynthetic capabilities into industrial microorganisms by combination of fungal and bacterial genes.

B. Biosynthetic Pathways of 7-ACA and 7-ADACA in Recombinant *A. chrysogenum*

1. Analysis of DAO and CC Acylase Expressed in *A. chrysogenum*

Neither DAO nor CC acylase has a leader sequence, suggesting that both enzymes should be produced cytoplasmically. The cultured mycelia of Hm178 in complex medium were disrupted to produce a crude enzyme extract, with which cephalosporin C and DAC were incubated for in vitro bioconversion analysis (7). 7-ACA, keto-AD-7-ACA, and GL-7-ACA were detected from cephalosporin C as substrate, and 7-ADACA, keto-AD-7-ADACA, and 7-β-(4-carboxybutanamido)deacetylcephalosporanic acid (GL-7-ADACA) were also detected from DAC as substrate. The substrate specificities of DAO and CC acylase in the crude enzyme solution from Hm178 were analyzed using cephalosporin C, DAC, GL-7-ACA, and GL-7-ADACA. No significant difference in substrate specificities was observed between the two enzymes expressed in *A. chrysogenum* and native DAO from *F. solani* M-0718 or V22 CC acylase expressed in *E. coli* (7). In addition, recombinant CC acylase had a relatively high deacylating activity for not only keto-AD-7-ACA, but keto-AD-7-ADACA. However, those enzyme activities were not detected in an enzyme solution from the host strain, *A. chrysogenum* BC2116.

Cephalosporin acylase genes from *Pseudomonas* strains are expressed as a single precursor protein, which is an inactive form, and then posttranslationally cleaved at a specific site to give the active heterodimer enzyme. The CC acylase activity against GL-7-ACA of the crude enzyme solution from Hm178 was relatively high (about 55%) compared with the DAO activity (100%) against cephalosporin C of the crude enzyme solution from the strain (7). Western blot analysis indicated that the V22 CC acylase protein of Hm178 was processed correctly (7).

These results indicate that the genes encoding both DAO and CC acylase were expressed in Hm178, and 7-ACA and 7-ADACA were biosynthesized. Furthermore, the enzymatic activity capable of producing of 7-ADACA from DAC via keto-AD-7-ADACA and GL-7-ADACA exists in the crude enzyme solution of Hm178, along with the enzymatic activity that can produce 7-ACA from cephalosporin C via keto-AD-7-ACA and GL-7-ACA.

2. Possible Biosynthetic Pathways of 7-ADACA in *A. chrysogenum* Hm178

Biosynthetic pathways of 7-ACA and 7-ADACA in *A. chrysogenum* Hm178 are shown in Figure 5 (27). 7-ACA is synthesized from cephalosporin C by DAO and CC acylase produced in Hm178, and 7-ADACA is probably also synthesized from DAC by those enzymes produced in Hm178. This possibility of 7-ADACA production is supported by the following results: (a) the enzymatic activities required to produce 7-ADACA from DAC via keto-AD-7-ADACA and GL-7-ADACA exist in the recombinant strain Hm178 (7,27); (b) cephalosporin C is produced from DAC by acetyltransferase (*cef*G) in *A. chrysogenum* (44–46); and (c) the production of 7-ADACA by Hm178 correlated with that of DAC (7).

7-ADOCA production by Hm178 also was observed (7), and 7-ADOCA possibly was synthesized by DAO and CC acylase from deacetoxycephalosporin C, which is a precursor of DAC in cephalosporin C biosynthesis (44,47–49) (Figure 5).

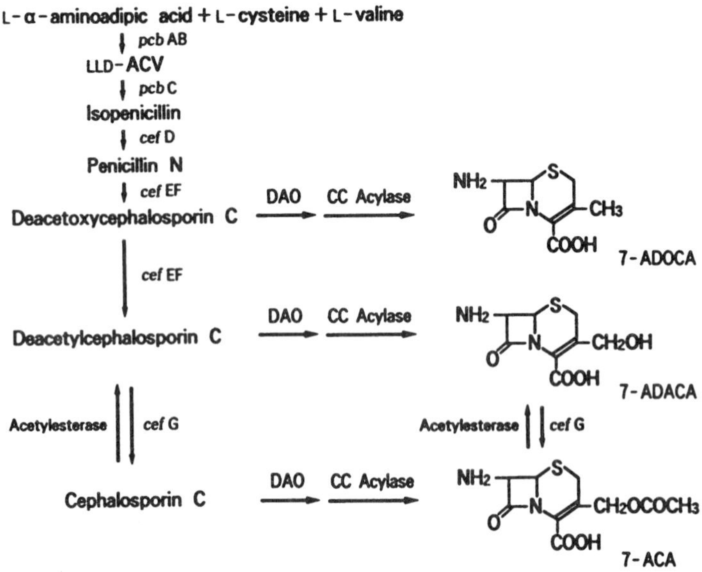

Figure 5   The biosynthetic pathways of 7-ACA and 7-ADACA in recombinant *A. chrysogenum*. LLD-ACV is δ-(L-α-aminoadipyl)-L-cysteinyl-D-valine.

Hinnen and Nüesch (50) reported the enzymatic hydrolysis of cephalosporin C by an extracellular cephalosporin C acetylesterase (CAE) of *A. chrysogenum*. 7-ACA is also hydrolyzed by this enzyme (51). However, the CAE has a pH optimum of 7.6 and is only 25% active at pH 6.5 (50). In addition, CAE is produced at the end of the cephalosporin C fermentation by *A. chrysogenum* (50). Therefore, a large amount of 7-ADACA is likely to be synthesized from DAC in Hm178.

In either case, 7-ADACA and 7-ACA are synthesized from L-α-aminoadipic acid, L-cysteine, and L-valine by participating cephalosporin C biosynthetic genes and newly introduced DAO and CC acylase genes in *A. chrysogenum* Hm178 (Figure 5).

3.   New Biosynthetic Possibility for 7-ACA and 7-ADACA Production by *A. chrysogenum* Hm178

We reported that HmR transformants of *A. chrysogenum* expressing only the DAO gene, as well as some transformants of pHDV11 having DAO and weak acylase activities, produced GL-7-ACA and GL-7-ADACA (6,7). However, those products were detected as products of different retention times compared with those of standard samples under a newly developed analysis condition of HPLC.* Those products were isolated and analyzed by ^{1}H NMR and fast atom bombardment mass spectroscopy (FAB-MS). Additionally, the α-hydroxyadipyl side chains of those products were analyzed by an isomer

---

*The newly developed HPLC analytical condition for cephalosporins: LiChrospher 100 RP-18(e) (5 μm, 4 × 250 mm); elution, 5 mM 1-heptanesulfonic acid sodium salt, 5 mM 18-Crown-6, 100 mM citric acid monohydrate, and 3.9 mM trisodium citrate with 16% methanol and 0.5% tetrahydrofuran; column temperature, 40°C; flow rate, 1 ml/min; detection, UV at 254 nm.

analytical HPLC method.[†] The products originally thought to be GL-7-ACA and GL-7-ADACA were determined to be 7-β-(D-5-carboxy-5-hydroxypentanamido)cephalosporanic acid (D-H-AD-7-ACA) and 7-β-(D-5-carboxy-5-hydroxypentanamido)deacetylcephalosporanic acid (D-H-AD-7-ADACA), respectively (Figure 6) (M. Fukagawa, H. Sasaki, Y. Saito, M. Yamashita and T.I., *manuscript in preparation*). D-H-AD-7-ACA and D-H-AD-7-ADACA were stable in the culture broth of *A. chrysogenum*.

Relative enzyme activities of crude V22 CC acylase from *A. chrysogenum* Hm178 and purified N176 CC acylase are given in Table 3 (M. Fukagawa, H. Sasaki, Y. Saito, M. Yamashita and T.I., *manuscript in preparation*). 7-β-(DL-5-Carboxy-5-hydroxypentanamido)cephalosporanic acid (DL-H-AD-7-ACA), reported on in Table 3, was chemically synthesized from keto-AD-7-ACA by reducing it with $NaBH_4$, and then 7-β-(DL-5-carboxy-5-hydroxypentanamido)deacetylcephalosporanic acid (DL-H-AD-7-ADACA) was enzymatically synthesized from DL-H-AD-7-ACA by converting it with CAE from *Aureobasidium pullulans* IFO4466 (52). V22 CC acylase from Hm178 and N176 CC acylase had notably high deacylating activities against keto-AD-7-ACA and D-H-AD-7-ACA compared with that against cephalosporin C. A deacylating activity of N176 CC acylase from keto-AD-7-ADACA to 7-ADACA was almost the same as that from keto-AD-7-ACA to 7-ACA. The enzyme activity against DL-H-AD-7-ACA was about twice that against DL-H-AD-7-ADACA. V22 CC acylase of Hm178 and N176 CC acylase had almost the same deacylating activities against keto-AD-7-ACA and D-H-AD-7-ACA. From these results, deacylating activities against D-H-AD-7-ADACA of those acylases are estimated to be about half of those against D-H-AD-7-ACA (M. Fukagawa, H. Sasaki, Y. Saito, M. Yamashita and T.I., *manuscript in preparation*).

Moreover, no D-H-AD-7-ACA and only a small amount of D-H-AD-7-ADACA were detected in the cultured broth of Hm178. The amount of 7-ACA produced by Hm178 corresponded to the sum of D-H-AD-7-ACA produced by transformants expressing only the DAO gene and 7-ACA produced by transformants expressing only the CC acylase gene (6).

Biosynthesis from keto-AD-7-ACA and keto-AD-7-ADACA to D-H-AD-7-ACA and D-H-AD-7-ADACA, respectively, may be catalyzed by a D-specific α-keto acid dehydrogenase of the host strain, *A. chrysogenum*, in a manner similar to the enzyme mechanism of VanH of *Enterococcus faecium* BM 4147 and D-lactate dehydrogenases of *Lactobacillus* and *Leuconostoc* (53). When cephalosporin C was incubated with toluene-treated resting mycelia of recombinant strains expressing only the DAO gene, D-H-AD-7-ACA was not detected, but keto-AD-7-ACA and GL-7-ACA were produced by that reaction. In control assays, 7-ACA was produced by incubating cephalosporin C with toluene-treated resting mycelia of recombinant strain Hm178, which expressed both enzyme genes, DAO and CC acylase.

These results indicate that the biosynthetic pathways of 7-ACA and 7-ADACA from cephalosporin C and DAC via keto-AD-7-ACA and keto-AD-7-ADACA, and D-H-AD-7-ACA and D-H-AD-7-ADACA, respectively, may exist in Hm178. A large amount of 7-ACA and 7-ADACA may be synthesized from cephalosporin C and DAC via those products in *A. chrysogenum* Hm178.

[†]The isomer HPLC analytical condition: Cosmosil $5C_{18}$ (4.6 × 150 mm); elution, 2 mM L-phenylalanine and 1 mM $(CH_3COO)_2Cu$ with 10% methanol (pH 4.5 with CH_3COOH); column temperature, 40°C; flow rate, 1 ml/min; detection, UV at 280 nm.

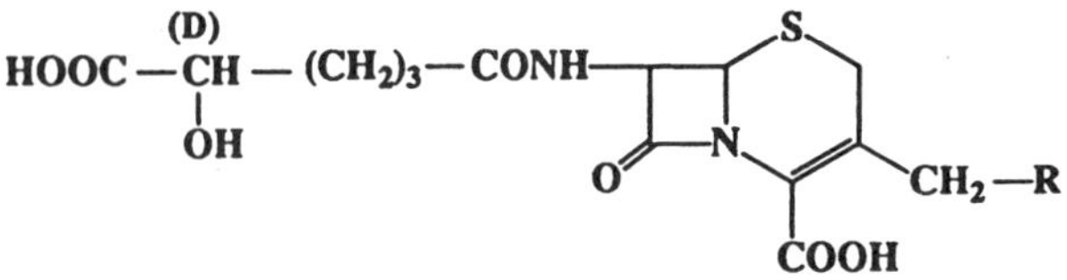

Figure 6   Structures of D-H-AD-7-ACA and D-H-AD-7-ADACA. R: —OCOCH₃, D-H-AD-7-ACA; —OH, D-H-AD-7-ADACA.

Table 3   Relative Enzyme Activities of Purified N176 CC Acylase and Crude V22 CC Acylase from A. *chrysogenum* Hm178

Enzyme	Substrate	Relative enzyme activity[a](%)
Purified N176 CC acylase	GL-7-ACA	100
	D-H-AD-7ACA	46
	DL-H-AD-7-ACA	24
	keto-AD-7-ACA	53
	Cephalosporin C	1.2
	GL-7-ADACA	155
	DL-H-AD-7-ADACA	11
	DAC	1.0
Crude V22 CC acylase of A. *chrysogenum* Hm178	GL-7-ACA	100
	D-H-AD-7-ACA	42
	DL-H-AD-7-ACA	17
	keto-AD-7-ACA	56
	GL-7-ACA	100*
	GL-7ADACA	255*

[a] Relative enzyme activities were determined from reactions in 0.1 M phosphate buffer (pH 7.5) at 30°C for 10 min with about 2 mg/ml of each substrate. However, incubations for * reactions were performed for 30 min.

C.   Stability of Transformants and Improvement of 7-ADACA Production

I.   Stability of Transformants

We have detailed data about one transformant, which was obtained by transformation of an industrially used high-producing strain of cephalosporin C, A. *chrysogenum* 3112, with pHDV11. The selection of the 7-ADACA high-producing A. *chrysogenum* A10 and the stability of the strain are shown in Figure 7.

A. *chrysogenum* 3112 was transformed with pHDV11. Several relatively high 7-ADACA- and 7-ACA-producing Hm[R] transformants were selected, and monocell isolations were performed on plates containing no hygromycin B. From these transformants, a 7-ADACA and 7-ACA high-producing strain, A. *chrysogenum* A10, was selected. In the monocell isolation of A10, 98% of colonies were Hm[R] strains (127 Hm[R]/130 strains), and a 7-ADACA and 7-ACA high-producing Hm[R] strain, A. *chrysogenum* A10-14, was selected. A monocell isolation of A10-14 on plates containing no hygromycin B was

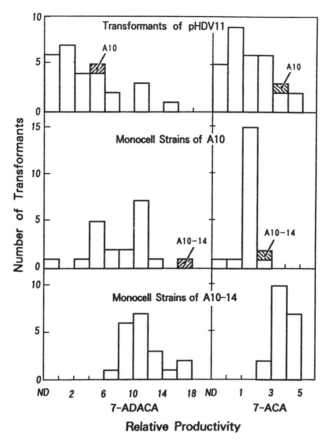

Figure 7   The selection of A. *chrysogenum* A10, a 7-ADACA high-producing pHDV11 transformant, and the stability of the strain. Production of 7-ADACA and 7-ACA are shown as relative productivity. ND, not detected.

then carried out. Resultant strains were Hm^R (25 Hm^R/25 strains) and produced relatively high amounts of 7-ADACA and 7-ACA. We obtained a stable 7-ADACA and 7-ACA high-producing strain by two cycles of monocell isolations. However, transformants of pHBV1 containing CC acylase alone to A. *chrysogenum* 3112 produced only low levels of 7-ACA and 7-ADACA.

To clarify whether this stability was due to integrative transformation, we examined the cellular DNA of A10-14 by Southern blot analysis. The result indicated that most of the DNA of pHDV11, with the exception of a small deleted region of the Ap^R (ampicillin resistance) gene, was integrated as a single copy in the chromosome.

2.   Improvement of 7-ADACA Production

We obtained the 7-ADACA and 7-ACA high-producing strain, A. *chrysogenum* A10-14, as described above. The productivity of 7-ADACA and 7-ACA by A10-14 was increased severalfold depending on the cephalosporin C producing level of the host strain when compared with that of *A. chrysogenum* Hm178. The strain, A10-14, was selected as a parent strain for improvement of productivity. No detectable amount of 7-ADOCA was produced by this strain.

7-ADACA was considerably more stable than 7-ACA in the culture broth. In addition, DAC was effectively produced by fermentation of cephalosporin C–producing *A. chrysogenum* in the presence of CAE-producing strains such as *Aureobasidium pullulans* IFO4466 (52) and *Rhodosporidium toruloides* CBS349 (54) or processed extracts of these strains. *A. chrysogenum* has CAE, but this activity was not sufficient for 7-ADACA fermentation. Therefore, A10-14 was cultured with small amounts of *A. pullulans* IFO4466 or *R. toruloides* CBS349 in the complex medium, and it effectively produced 7-ADACA in the cultured broth as a one-step fermentation of 7-ADACA. In the mixed fermentations, 7-ACA produced by recombinant *A. chrysogenum* was effectively converted to stable 7-ADACA by CAE of *A. pullulans* or *R. toruloides*, and the productivity was improved.

One possibility for the improvement of 7-ADACA production is the complete conversion of the remaining DAC by improvement of the production of both enzymes, DAO and CC acylase. A plasmid was constructed using improved 5′-noncoding regions of both the DAO gene and site-directed mutagenized (M269Y) CC acylase gene for improvement of 7-ADACA production. The constructed plasmid was introduced into *A. chrysogenum* 3112 by transformation, and 7-ADACA productivity of the transformants increased about twofold compared with that of A10-14, likely due to the improvements in DAO and CC acylase production and activities. As the result of these modifications, 7-ADACA productivity was improved, and 7-ADACA was detected as a major product in the culture broths of these improved strains.

REFERENCES

1. Queener SF, Webber JA, Queener SW, eds. Beta-Lactam Antibiotics for Clinical Use. New York: Marcel Dekker, 1986.
2. Sakane K, Inamoto Y, Takaya T. A new oral cephem, cefdinir: Its structure-activity relationships and biological profile. J Antibiot 1992; 45:909–925.
3. Yamanaka H, Chiba T, Kawabata K, Takasugi H, Masugi T, Takaya T. Studies on β-lactam antibiotics. IX. Synthesis and biological activity of a new orally active cephalosporin, cefixime (FK027). J Antibiot 1985; 38:1738–1751.
4. Tsuzuki K, Komatsu K-I, Ichikawa S, Shibuya Y. Enzymatic synthesis of 7-aminocephalosporanic acid (7-ACA). Nippon Nogeikagaku Kaishi 1989; 63:1847–1853.
5. Inamoto Y, Chiba T, Kaminura T, Takaya T. FK482, a new orally active cephalosporin synthesis and biological properties. J Antibiot 1988; 41:828–830.
6. Isogai T, Fukagawa M, Aramori I, Iwami M, Kojo H, Ono T, Ueda Y, Kohsaka M, Imanaka H. Construction of 7-aminocephalosporanic acid (7ACA) biosynthetic operon and direct production of 7ACA in *Acremonium chrysogenum*. Bio/Technol 1991; 9:188–191.
7. Fukagawa M, Isogai T, Aramori I, Iwami M, Kojo H, Ono T, Kohsaka M, Imanaka H. Direct production of 7-aminodeacetylcephalosporanic acid by *Acremonium chrysogenum* Hm178. Agric Biol Chem 1991; 55:2163–2165.
8. Matsumoto K. Cephalosporin acylase. Hakko to Kogyo 1980; 38:216–237.
9. Fujii T, Yamamoto K, Yamamoto S, Matsumoto K, Mizuno M. Cephalosporin compound preparation—by reaction of cephalosporin C with D–amino acid oxidase producing fungus. Jpn Kokai Tokkyo Koho (Jpn Patent Application) JP 51044695; 1976.

10. Szwajcer E, Mosbach K. Isolation and partial characterization of a D–amino acid oxidase active against cephalosporin C from the yeast *Trigonopsis variabilis*. Biotechnol Lett 1985; 7:1–7.

11. Isogai T, Ono H, Ishitani Y, Kojo H, Ueda Y, Kohsaka M. Structure and expression of cDNA for D–amino acid oxidase active against cephalosporin C from *Fusarium solani*. J Biochem (Tokyo) 1990; 108:1063–1069.

12. Komatsu K, Matsuda A, Sugiura K. DNA fragment encoding D–amino acid oxidase. Jpn Kokai Tokkyo Koho (Jpn Patent Application) JP 62262994; 1987.

13. Ronchi S, Minchiotti L, Galliano M, Curti B. The primary structure of D–amino acid oxidase from pig kidney. J Biol Chem 1982; 257:8824–8834.

14. Fukui K, Watanabe F, Shibata T, Miyake Y. Molecular cloning and sequence analysis of cDNA encoding porcine kidney D–amino acid oxidase. Biochem 1987; 26:3612–3618.

15. Isogai T, Ono H, Kojo H. D–Amino acid oxidase, production—by culture of *E. coli* transformants containing expression vectors originated from *Fusarium solani* M-0718. Eur Patent Application EP 364275 A; 1990.

16. Vicenzi JT, Hansen GJ. Enzymatic oxidation of cephalosporin C using whole cells of the yeast *Trigonopsis variabilis* within a "cross-flow filter-reactor." Enzyme Microb Technol 1993; 15:281–285.

17. Watanabe F, Fukui K, Momoi K, Miyake Y. Site-specific mutagenesis of lysine-204, tyrosine-224, tyrosine-228, and histidine-307 of porcine kidney D–amino acid oxidase and the implications as to its catalytic function. J Biochem (Tokyo) 1989; 105:1024–1029.

18. Miyano M, Fukui K, Watanabe F, Takahashi S, Tada M, Kanashiro M, Miyake Y. Studies on Phe-228 and Leu-307 recombinant mutants of porcine kidney D–amino acid oxidase: Expression, purification, and characterization. J Biochem (Tokyo) 1991; 109:171–177.

19. Wierenga RK, Hol WGJ. Predicted nucleotide-binding properties of p21 protein and its cancer-associated variant. Nature 1983; 302:842–844.

20. Miyazawa S, Osumi T, Hashimoto T, Ohno K, Miura S, Fujiki Y. Peroxisome targeting signal of rat liver acyl-coenzyme A oxidase resides at the carboxy terminus. Mol Cell Biol 1989; 9:83–91.

21. Ichikawa S, Shibuya Y, Matsumoto K, Fujii T, Kodaira R. Purification and properties of 7β-(4-carboxybutanamido)cephalosporanic acid acylase produced by mutants derived from *Pseudomonas*. Agric Biol Chem 1981; 45:2231–2236.

22. Matsuda A, Komatsu K-I. Molecular cloning and structure of the gene for 7β-(4-carboxybutanamido)cephalosporanic acid acylase from a *Pseudomonas* strain. J Bacteriol 1985; 163:1222–1228.

23. Ishii Y, Saito Y, Fujimura T, Isogai T, Kojo H, Yamashita M, Niwa M, Kohsaka M. A novel 7-β-(4-carboxybutanamido)cephalosporanic acid acylase isolated from *Pseudomonas* strain C427 and its high-level production in *Escherichia coli*. J Ferment Bioeng 1994; 77:591–597.

24. Aramori I, Fukagawa M, Tsumura M, Iwami M, Ono H, Kojo H, Kohsaka M, Ueda Y, Imanaka H. Cloning and nucleotide sequencing of a novel 7β-(4-carboxybutanamido)-cephalosporanic acid acylase gene of *Bacillus laterosporus* and its expression in *Escherichia coli* and *Bacillus subtilis*. J Bacteriol 1991; 173:7848–7855.

25. Matsuda A, Matsuyama K, Yamamoto K, Ichikawa S, Komatsu K-I. Cloning and characterization of the genes for two distinct cephalosporin acylases from a *Pseudomonas* strain. J Bacteriol 1987; 169:5815–5820.

26. Matsuda A, Toma K, Komatsu K-I. Nucleotide sequences of the genes for two distinct cephalosporin acylases from a *Pseudomonas* strain. J Bacteriol 1987; 169:5821–5826.

27. Isogai T, Fukagawa M. Direct production of 7-aminocephalosporanic acid and 7-aminodeacetylcephalosporanic acid by recombinant *Acremonium chrysogenum*. Actinomycetol 1991; 5:102–111.

28. Aramori I, Fukagawa M, Tsumura M, Iwami M, Isogai T, Ono H, Ishitani Y, Kojo H, Kohsaka M, Ueda Y, Imanaka H. Cloning and nucleotide sequencing of new glutaryl 7-ACA and

cephalosporin C acylase genes from *Pseudomonas* strains. J Ferment Bioeng 1991; 72:232–243.

29. Aramori I, Fukagawa M, Tsumura M, Iwami M, Ono H, Ishitani Y, Kojo H, Kohsaka M, Ueda Y, Imanaka H. Comparative characterization of new glutaryl 7-ACA and cephalosporin C acylases. J Ferment Bioeng 1992; 73:185–192.

30. Schumacher G, Sizmann D, Haug H, Buckel P, Bock A. Penicillin acylase from *E. coli:* Unique gene-protein relation. Nucl Acids Res 1986; 14:5713–5727.

31. Ishii Y, Saito Y, Sasaki H, Uchiyama F, Hayashi M, Nakamura S, Niwa M. Affinity labelling of cephalosporin C acylase from *Pseudomonas* sp. N176 with a substrate analogue, 7β-(6-bromohexanoylamido)cephalosporanic acid. J Ferment Bioeng 1994; 77:598–603.

32. Slade A, Horrocks AJ, Lindsay CD, Dunbar B, Virden R. Site-directed chemical conversion of serine to cysteine in penicillin acylase from *Escherichia coli* ATCC11105. Effect on conformation and catalytic activity. Eur J Biochem 1991; 197:75–80.

33. Martin J, Slade A, Aitken A, Arche R, Virden R. Chemical modification of serine at the active site of penicillin acylase from *Kluyvera citrophila*. Biochem J 1991; 280:659–662.

34. Ishii Y, Saito Y, Fujimura T, Noguchi Y, Sasaki H, Niwa M, Shimomura K. High-level production, chemical modification and site-directed mutagenesis of cephalosporin C acylase from *Pseudomonas* sp. N176. Eur J Biochem 1995; 230:773–778.

35. Nobbs TJ, Ishii Y, Fujimura T, Saito Y, Niwa M. Chemical modification and site-directed mutagenesis of tyrosine residues in cephalosporin C acylase from *Pseudomonas* strain N176. J Ferment Bioeng 1994; 77:604–609.

36. Saito Y, Ishii Y, Fujimura T, Sasaki H, Noguchi Y, Yamada H, Niwa M, Shimomura K. Protein engineering of a cephalosporin C acylase from *Pseudomonas* strain N176. Ann NY Acad Sci 1996; 782:226–241.

37. Malpartida F, Hopwood DA. Molecular cloning of the whole biosynthetic pathway of a *Streptomyces* antibiotic and its expression in heterologous host. Nature 1984; 309:462–464.

38. Chen CW, Lin H-F, Kuo CL, Tsai H-L, Tsai JF-Y. Cloning and expression of a DNA sequence conferring cephamycin C production. Bio/Technol 1988; 6:1222–1224.

39. Smith DJ, Burnham MKR, Edward J, Earl AJ, Turner G. Cloning and heterologous expression of the penicillin biosynthetic gene cluster from *Penicillium chrysogenum*. Bio/Technol 1990; 8:39–41.

40. Gutiérrez S, Diez B, Alverez E, Barredo JL, Martin JF. Expression of the *pen*DE gene of *Penicillium chrysogenum* encoding isopenicillin N acetyltransferase in *Cephalosporium acremonium*: Production of benzylpenicillin by the transformants. Mol Gen Genet 1991; 225:56–64.

41. Gritz L, Davies J. Plasmid-encoded hygromycin B resistance: The sequence of hygromycin B phosphotransferase gene and its expression in *Escherichia coli* and *Saccharomyces cerevisiae*. Gene 1983; 25:179–188.

42. Isogai T, Fukagawa M, Kojo H, Kohsaka M, Aoki H, Imanaka H. Cloning and nucleotide sequence of the complementary and genomic DNAs for the alkaline protease from *Acremonium chrysogenum*. Agric Biol Chem 1991; 55:471–477.

43. Wildfeuer ME. Aqueous acetylation of desacetyl glutaryl 7-amino-cephalosporanic acid (7ACA) and speculation on the origin of desacetyl cephalosporin C in fermentation broth. J Antibiot 1994; 47:64–71.

44. Ingolia TD, Queener SW. Beta-lactam biosynthetic genes. Med Res Rev 1989; 9:245–264.

45. Matsuda A, Sugiura H, Matsuyama K, Matsumoto H, Ichikawa S, Komatsu K-I. Molecular cloning of acetyl coenzyme A: deacetylcephalosporin C O-acetyltransferase cDNA from *Acremonium chrysogenum*: Sequence and expression of catalytic activity in yeast. Biochem Biophys Res Commun 1992; 182:995–1001.

46. Matsuda A, Sugiura H, Matsuyama K, Matsumoto H, Ichikawa S, Komatsu K-I. Cloning and disruption of the *cef*G gene encoding acetyl coenzyme A: deacetylcephalosporin C O-acetyltransferase from *Acremonium chrysogenum*. Biochem Biophys Res Commun 1992; 186:40–46.

47. Gutierrez S, Diez B, Montenegro E, Martin JF. Characterization of the *Cephalosporium acremonium pcb*AB gene encoding α-aminoadipyl-cysteinyl-valine synthetase, a large multido-

main peptide synthetase: Linkage to the *pcbC* gene as a cluster of early cephalosporin biosynthetic genes and evidence of multiple functional domains. J Bacteriol 1991; 173:2354–2365.

48. Samson SM, Belagaje R, Blankenship DT, Chapman JL, Perry D, Skatrud PL, VanFrank RM, Abraham EP, Baldwin JE, Queener SW, Ingolia TD. Isolation, sequence determination and expression in *Escherichia coli* of the isopenicillin N synthetase gene from *Cephalosporium acremonium*. Nature 1985; 318:191–194.

49. Samson SM, Dotzlaf JE, Slisz ML, Becker GW, Van Frank RM, Veal LE, Yeh W-K, Miller JR, Queener SW, Ingolia TD. Cloning and expression of the fungal expandase/hydroxylase gene involved in cephalosporin biosynthesis. Bio/Technol 1987; 5:1207–1214.

50. Hinnen A, Nüesch J. Enzymatic hydrolysis of cephalosporin C by an extracellular acetylhydrolase of *Cephalosporium acremonium*. Antimicrob Agents Chemother 1976; 9:824–830.

51. Gutiérrez S, Velasco J, Fernandez FJ, Martin JF. The *cef*G gene of *Cephalosporium acremonium* is linked to the *cef*EF gene and encodes a deacetylcephalosporin C acetyltransferase closely related to homoserine O-acetyltransferase. J Bacteriol 1992; 174:3056–3064.

52. Imanaka H, Miyoshi T, Konomi T, Kubochi Y, Hattori S, Kawakita T. High yield preparation of de-acetylcephalosporin C by treating cephalosporin C with acetylesterase obtained from *Aureobasidium* strain. Eur Patent Application EP 44736 A; 1982.

53. Bugg TDH, Wright GD, Dutka-Malen S, Arthur M, Courvalin P, Walsh CT. Molecular basis for vancomycin resistance in *Enterococcus faecium* BM4147: Biosynthesis of a depsipeptide peptidoglycan precursor by vancomycin resistance proteins VanH and VanA. Biochem 1991; 30:10408–10415.

54. Smith A, Bailey PJ. Antibiotic desacetyl-cephalosporin C production by fermentation of cephalosporin C producing microorganisms e.g. *Acremonium chrysogenum* in the presence of acetylesterase enzyme. U.S. Patent 4,533,632; 1985.

25

Chemoenzymatic Production of the Antiviral Agent Epivir™

Mahmoud Mahmoudian and Michael J. Dawson
Glaxo Wellcome Research and Development, Stevenage, Herts, England

I. INTRODUCTION

A. Anti–Human Immunodeficiency Virus Agents

Human immunodeficiency virus (HIV) is the causative agent of acquired immunodeficiency syndrome (AIDS), which is characterized by a chronic suppression of many immune functions and a concomitant increase in susceptibility to opportunistic infections (1,2). In the search for selective antiretroviral drugs, much work has focused on the HIV-encoded RNA-dependent DNA polymerase (reverse transcriptase, RT) as the target. This enzyme is required for the replication of the HIV genome, catalyzing the conversion of the HIV RNA to a double-stranded DNA copy. Among the most promising inhibitors of HIV replication that are targeted at the virus-encoded RT are the 2',3'-dideoxynucleosides zidovudine (AZT, also known as Retrovir), didanosine (ddI), and zalcitabine (ddC). These compounds, which are activated intracellularly to their corresponding 5'-triphosphates, act as inhibitors and chain terminators of HIV-RT (3). Other anti-HIV agents include carbocyclic analogs of 2',3'-dideoxynucleosides and 2',3'-didehydro-2',3'-dideoxynucleosides such as carbovir (c-d4G) (4,5), the four-membered oxetanocins and carbocyclic oxetanocins (6,7), 4-hydroxy-1,2-butadienyl derivatives of adenine (adenallene) and cytosine (cytallene) (8,9), stavudine (d4T) (10,11), 4-amino-1-(2R-hydroxymethyl-[1,3]oxathiolan-5S-yl)-1H-pyrimidin-2-one (3TC, also known as Epivir) (12), (−)-2',3'-dideoxy-5-fluoro-3'-thiacytidine (FTC) (13), and the acyclic nucleoside phosphonate 9-(2-phosphonylmethoxyethyl)adenine (PMEA) (14).

As of mid 1995, four nucleoside analogs (Retrovir, ddI, ddC, d4T) had been approved for clinical use for the treatment of HIV infection. These compounds are, however, associated with significant toxic side effects [e.g., bone marrow suppression (Retrovir), peripheral neuropathy (ddI, ddC)], and taken together with the emergence of drug-resistant virus strains, this limits their efficacy as single therapeutic agents for the treatment of AIDS (15).

Epivir™ is a registered trademark of the Glaxo Wellcome group of companies.

Together with the advent of the protease inhibitors, Saquinavir, Indinavir, and Ritonavir, the recent approval of Epivir for use in combination with Retrovir marks a new way forward in AIDS therapy.

B. Carbocyclic Nucleosides

Prior to our involvement with Epivir at Glaxo Wellcome, we had spent a number of years investigating the potential of carbocyclic nucleosides as antiviral agents. Carbocyclic analogs of purine and pyrimidine nucleosides have generated a great deal of interest as anti-HIV and antiherpetic agents (16–18). Carbocyclic nucleosides, in which a methylene-group replaces the oxygen atom of the ribose ring, generally benefit from greater metabolic stability than their furanose counterparts (17). Traditionally, in most cases, these compounds have been synthesized and tested initially in racemic form. Where the enantiomers have been examined, biological activity shown by the racemate has been found to reside primarily in the "natural" enantiomer, whereas the corresponding "unnatural" optical form has been found to be inactive or shows substantially reduced potency (18–21). Enzymes have frequently been used to resolve the enantiomers of carbocyclic and 2′,3′-dideoxynucleoside analogs for further biological testing (19,22–27). For example, adenosine deaminase has been used to prepare the optical antipodes of a wide range of carbocyclic analogs of purine nucleosides (19,23,24), whereas other carbocyclic nucleosides have been resolved by enantiospecific hydrolysis of their monophosphates (18).

Despite several synthetic approaches to the "cyclopentane" moiety of carbocyclic nucleosides, starting from noncarbohydrate synthons or readily available meso intermediates, no universally applicable methodology is yet available for the asymmetric synthesis of these compounds (28–31). An efficient access to chirality is via enantioselective resolution of a prochiral or a meso intermediate prior to the addition of the purine or pyrimidine base. For example, pig liver esterase (PLE) has been used in a chemoenzymatic approach to the synthesis of optically active (–)-aristeromycin and (–)-neplanocin (32), whereas cyclic γ-acetamido esters were resolved to obtain (–)-4-*cis*-amino-2,3-*trans*-dihydroxy hydroxymethyl cyclopentane as a key intermediate in the synthesis of carbocyclic nucleosides (33). Although hydrolytic enzymes often display a limited degree of enantiospecificity with such unnatural substrates, reaction conditions can in many cases be optimized to improve the enantioselectivity (34).

1. Carbovir (c-d4G)

The 2′,3′-didehydro-2′,3′-dideoxycarbocyclic nucleoside, (±)-carbovir (Figure 1), is a potent and selective inhibitor of HIV in vitro (35). Its hydrolytic stability and ability to inhibit infection and replication of the virus in human T-cell lines at concentrations 200- to 400-fold below toxic levels has made carbovir a potentially useful antiretroviral agent. In whole cell assays using MT-4 cells, (–)-carbovir [(–)-3, Figure 1] has similar activity against HIV (RF strain) to Retrovir (IC_{50}, 0.0015 and 0.001 μg/ml, respectively) (36). (–)-Carbovir is approximately 2-fold more active than the corresponding racemate, whereas the (+)-enantiomer is at least 75-fold less active than (–)-carbovir (5). One of the routes to (–)-carbovir considered at Glaxo Wellcome was synthesis from the chiral natural product (–)-aristeromycin (–)-1 (Figure 1). (–)-Aristeromycin was a very attractive starting material because it was readily available as a secondary metabolite of *Streptomyces citrocolor* and would afford (–)-carbovir without the need to resort to an optical resolution. Synthesis of (–)-carbovir from (–)-aristeromycin involved nine steps requiring

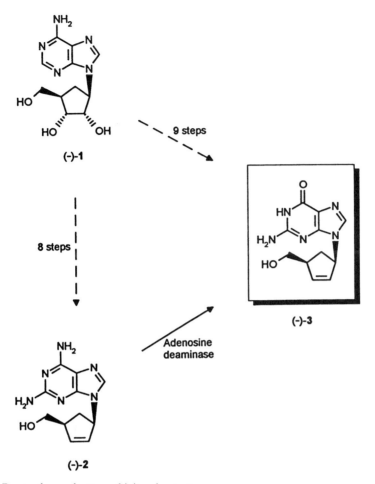

Figure 1 Routes for production of (–)-carbovir, 3.

two distinct transformations: an adenine to guanine base interconversion and introduction of the 2′,3′-double bond from the 2′,3′-diol (37). One approach for the base conversion involved the hydrolytic deamination of *cis*-4-[2,6-diamino-9*H*-purin-9-yl]-2-cyclopentenemethanol dihydrochloride, (–)-2, using adenosine deaminase (Figure 1). (–)-2 was prepared from aristeromycin in eight steps (37). To obtain sufficient material for further biological evaluation, the chemoenzymatic route was investigated and a process developed to produce (–)-carbovir on a kilogram scale (38).

Adenosine deaminase (EC 3.5.4.4) is commercially available from mammalian (calf intestinal mucosa) and microbial (*Aspergillus* sp.) sources with moderate activity (0.5–1.5 units/mg protein). Although this enzyme is widespread in animal tissue, its concentration in most cases is low (39). Using standard purification techniques, the enzyme was adsorbed directly onto an anion exchanger to provide a rapid method for its recovery (50–340 units/mg protein). Bioconversions with the partially purified enzyme were carried out at pH 7.5 in fermentors (up to 70 liter working volume). At 20 g/liter input of (–)-2, the product (–)-carbovir (Figure 1) was much less soluble, crystallizing during the course of reaction, and was subsequently recovered by filtration (>90% theoretical yield). To allow enzyme reuse, adenosine deaminase was immobilized onto Eupergit-C (Rhom

Pharma, Darmstadt, Germany) to give a stable enzyme preparation. Given the low solubility of (–)-carbovir, the concentration of (–)-**2** was reduced to 2.5 g/liter in bioconversions with immobilized enzyme so that the beads could easily be recovered from the reaction mixture without interference from the product. The enzyme was reused for up to 10 cycles without any significant loss of activity. This work demonstrated the potential of adenosine deaminase as a catalyst for large-scale production of optically pure (–)-carbovir. More recently, alternative routes to gain access to either enantiomer of carbovir have also been reported (40,41).

2. *c-BVdU* and *c-dG*

Two other potent antiviral agents of interest at Glaxo Wellcome were (+)-carbocyclic 2′-deoxy-5-[(E)-2-bromovinyl]uridine, **5** (*c*-BVdU), and (+)-carbocyclic 2′-deoxyguanosine, **8** (*c*-dG), Figure 2. (+)-**5** possesses activity against *Herpes simplex* virus 1 (HSV-1) and *Varicella zoster* virus (chicken pox and shingles) in vitro and in vivo, and (+)-**8** is active against HSV-2, human cytomegalovirus, and hepatitis B virus (42,43). As an alternative to total asymmetric synthesis of **5** and **8**, and to avoid late-stage resolution, we envisaged the introduction of an enzymatic or microbial step, to obtain key homochiral synthons, at an early stage in the synthetic strategy. One approach considered was the enzymatic resolution of ester intermediates, prior to the addition of the base, that could be used in the synthesis of **5** (27). Among the hydrolytic enzymes screened, PLE gave the highest enantioselectivity with 4-(benzoylamino)-2-cyclopentenecarboxylic acid, methyl ester (±)-**4**. The residual ester, which was of the correct absolute stereochemistry [(+) 1S, 4R] for synthesis of (+)-**5** (eight steps), could be obtained in high optical purity after optimization of the reaction conditions (Figure 2). In an attempt to shorten synthetic routes to **5** and **8**, we also investigated an alternative method using the stereoselective reduction of **6** by growing cells of *Mucor circinelloides* (44). Asymmetric reduction of carbonyl compounds with microorganisms is recognized as a valuable approach to organic synthesis (45,46). Optimization of fermentation conditions, pH, and temperature resulted

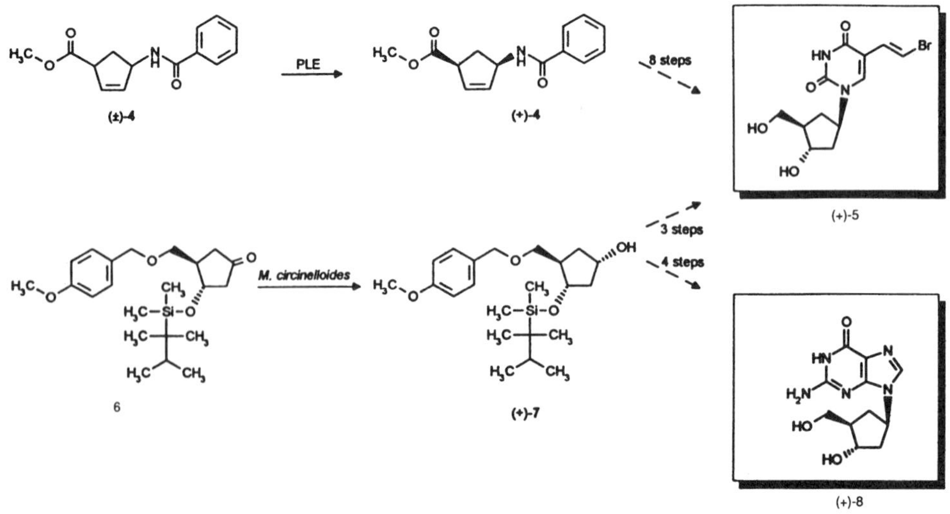

Figure 2   Chemoenzymatic synthesis of (+)-*c*-BVdU, **5,** and (+)-*c*-dG, **8**.

in the production of the desired intermediate (+)-7, in an optically pure form (enantiomeric excess, ee > 98%; yield, 62%), which was used for the convergent syntheses of (+)-5 (three steps) and (+)-8 (four steps) (Figure 2). Furthermore, the α-hydroxy (+)-7 has been shown to be a versatile intermediate that can be used for the convergent synthesis of a variety of chiral purine and pyrimidine carbocyclic nucleoside analogs (44).

II. EPIVIR

Racemic 4-amino-1-(2-hydroxymethyl-[1,3]oxathiolan-5-yl)-1H-pyrimidin-2-one, 10 (BCH189), in which the 3′-carbon in the β-ribose ring of 2′,3′-dideoxycytidine has been replaced by a sulfur atom (1,3-oxathiolane), was originally synthesized by BioChem Pharma Inc., Laval, Quebec, Canada (Figure 3). This potent and selective anti-HIV agent has been shown to be less cytotoxic than Retrovir in vitro (15). In contrast to the majority of nucleoside analogs that display antiviral activity primarily or exclusively residing in the "natural" β-D-isomer, work at Glaxo Wellcome has demonstrated that the enantiomers of 10 are equipotent in vitro against HIV-1 and HIV-2, but the "unnatural" β-L-(−)-isomer Epivir [(−)-10, Figure 3] is substantially less cytotoxic than its corresponding "natural" β-D-(+)-isomer (12,47). As expected, the α-L-(+)- and α-D-(−)-enantiomers appear to be less effective than the corresponding β-isomers (48).

Epivir is activated intracellularly to its 5′-triphosphate derivative (Epivir-TP) (49), which is a weak inhibitor of the HIV-1 reverse transcriptase in vitro; its main mode of action is via chain termination of reverse transcription (50). In vitro studies against HIV-1 clinical and laboratory strains in several cell lines have shown activity with an IC_{50} of 0.003–1.14 μM (12). In vitro activity has also been demonstrated against Retrovir-resistant isolates (51), and in comparison with Retrovir, Epivir displays lower toxicity against normal and HIV-infected peripheral blood lymphocytes (12).

The intracellular half-life of Epivir-TP in peripheral blood lymphocytes is 10.5–15.5 hr (49), and in vivo Epivir is primarily excreted unchanged by the renal route (52). The 5′-triphosphate of the (+)-enantiomer has a fivefold greater activity against purified HIV-1 reverse transcriptase than Epivir-TP, but it also has a much shorter half-life than Epivir-TP (3.5–7 hr), (49). These data may explain the comparable antiviral potency of the two enantiomers. Clinical studies have shown Epivir to be well tolerated at high doses, with a good bioavailability and pharmacokinetic profile compared with other nucleoside analogs, and it does not appear to cause bone marrow toxicities in vitro (51,53).

The use of drug combinations is a powerful approach to anti-HIV chemotherapy, which may give rise to an equivalent antiviral effect with reduced toxicity, or an increase in drug efficacy if synergy between the two compounds occurs. In the latter case, if lower overall drug doses can be used, it follows that toxicity may also be reduced. Many combinations of Epivir and Retrovir exhibit synergistic antiviral effects against a range of HIV-1 clinical isolates with no evidence of gross antagonistic effects (54). Additive effects were evident in combinations with ddC or ddI (54,55). Epivir also synergistically inhibits the replication of a laboratory strain of HIV-1 (RF strain) in MT-4 cells in vitro in combination with R82150, a nonnucleoside reverse transcriptase inhibitor, and the protease inhibitor Saquinavir.

The Food and Drug Administration (FDA) recently granted Glaxo Wellcome permission to market Epivir (3TC), 150–300 mg dose, for use in combination with Retrovir (AZT) for the treatment of people with HIV infection. The advisory committee of the

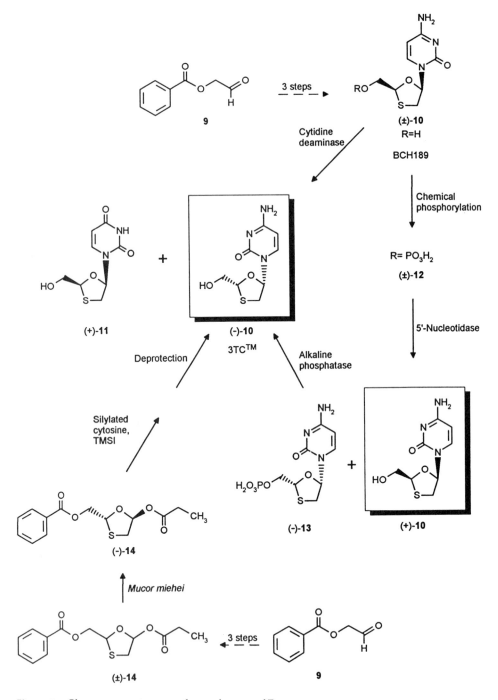

Figure 3   Chemoenzymatic routes for production of Epivir.

FDA considered the findings of several clinical trials before recommending approval of Epivir. These showed that

1. The combination therapy with Retrovir is more effective than other licensed treatments in maintaining the immune system and reducing the amount of HIV in people with HIV infection.
2. The use of Epivir and Retrovir in combination delays the emergence of variants of HIV that are resistant to Retrovir.
3. The addition of Epivir to Retrovir therapy does not induce any additional side effects—Epivir is well tolerated.

The combination of Epivir and Retrovir is the first two-drug treatment for "first-line" use, that is, in individuals who have not previously been given an anti-HIV drug. This marks a significant advance in the treatment of HIV infection, and it is anticipated that this combination will become a cornerstone of HIV treatment.

III.   DEVELOPMENT OF A PROCESS FOR PRODUCTION OF OPTICALLY PURE EPIVIR

Initially, chiral high-performance liquid chromatography (HPLC) was used to separate the (+) and (−)-enantiomers of 10 (BCH189, Figure 3); this enabled the anti-HIV activity and cytotoxicity in vitro of each isomer to be determined (12,47). This method was, however, not amenable to scale-up to provide the larger quantities of Epivir required for further evaluation. One of the initial routes considered was the enzymatic resolution using 5′-nucleotidase and alkaline phosphatase that would allow access to both enantiomers of 10 (Figure 3). This approach had been applied previously at Glaxo Wellcome to the enantiospecific hydrolysis of 5′-monophosphate derivatives of racemic carbocyclic nucleoside analogs (18) and was extended to resolve the enantiomers of BCH189 (56). The chemically synthesized monophosphate derivative (±)-12 was resolved using 5′-nucleotidase from *Crotalus atrox* venom (EC 3.1.3.5), and the resulting mixture was separated by chromatography and purified on silica gel, to give (+)-10 (ee > 99%, Figure 3). Hydrolysis of the remaining monophosphate (−)-13 with alkaline phosphatase from *Escherichia coli* (EC 3.1.3.1) afforded the corresponding (−)-enantiomer (Epivir) in an optically pure form (Figure 3). It was, however, imperative to determine the absolute stereochemistry of (+)- and (−)-10 prior to establishing a chiral synthesis of the preferred (−)-enantiomer. Based on the precedent discussed earlier, it was expected that (+)-10 should have the "natural" absolute stereochemistry. To prove this, (−)-10 (Epivir, Figure 3) was treated with 4-bromobenzoyl chloride to afford the corresponding N^4-amide. The presence of the heavy bromine atom allowed the absolute stereochemistry of this material to be determined by x-ray crystallography, confirming the "unnatural" configuration of Epivir (56).

To produce larger quantities of Epivir, the 5′-nucleotidase route was inefficient, and other approaches were investigated. One such route considered was the enantioselective deamination of (±)-10 with cytidine deaminase (EC 3.5.4.5) (Figure 3) (57). Because of earlier work with adenosine deaminase to obtain optically pure carbovir at the kilogram scale, we envisaged that the resolution of (±)-10 may also be amenable to further scale-up. However, unlike adenosine deaminase, cytidine deaminase was not commercially available and had not been widely used for preparative transformations. Initially, cytidine deaminase was partially purified by ammonium sulfate fractionation (55–75% saturation) from a clarified cell extract of a wild-type *E. coli* B. Enzyme (0.3 units) was incubated with (±)-**10**, 0.33 mg in a 1 ml reaction volume, for 24 hr. After this time, chiral HPLC analysis indicated that the (+)-**10** had been deaminated to give the uridine analog (+)-**11**, leaving Epivir, essentially optically pure (Figure 3). We considered this to form the basis of a process for large-scale preparation of Epivir and, hence, embarked on a program to optimize the fermentation of cytidine deaminase, to immobilize the enzyme for reuse, to optimize the reaction conditions, and to develop an efficient isolation process for the product. An outline of this process is shown in Figure 4.

A.   Fermentation of *E. coli* for the Production of Cytidine Deaminase

Cytidine deaminase is widely distributed among microorganisms, where its physiological role is to scavenge exogenous and endogenous cytidine (58,59). In enteric bacteria such as *E. coli* and *Salmonella typhimurium*, the enzyme is inducible to high levels, allowing these organisms to grow rapidly with cytidine as sole nitrogen source (60). We, therefore, chose to investigate *E. coli* as a source of large quantities of enzyme for use in production of Epivir.

Table 1 shows cytidine deaminase production by *E. coli* strains JM103 and B, with and without cytidine. As expected, production was approximately 10 times as great in the presence of cytidine. To obviate the need to add cytidine to the fermentation, a constitutive mutant was sought. In *E. coli*, cytidine deaminase and uridine phosphorylase are coordinately expressed under the control of the CytR repressor (61). Expression of both genes is induced by cytidine, but not by uridine. Consequently, mutants that can grow well on uridine are likely to have a defective *cytR* gene and will express both enzymes constitutively. The mutant strain 3732E (uridine⁺) was obtained by selecting for rapid growth on uridine as described by Munch-Petersen et al. (61). Cytidine deaminase production by 3732E was shown to be independent of cytidine (Table 1). Furthermore, specific activity was significantly higher than for JM103 even when the latter strain was grown in the presence of cytidine.

Enzyme production by the constitutive mutant was sufficient to support biotransformation work at a substantial scale, but for production scale, a still better source of enzyme was required. This was achieved by cloning the cytidine deaminase gene (*cdd*) onto a multicopy plasmid under the control of the λP$_L$ promotor (57). The resulting plasmid pPLcddE was introduced into *E. coli* TG1 (Amersham) by transformation, conferring resistance to tetracycline (Figure 5). The recombinant strain (*E. coli* TG1[pPLcddE], 3804E) supported an extremely high level of cytidine deaminase production; the specific activity was up to 80 times that achieved with the constitutive mutant (Table 1).

The time course of cytidine deaminase production, by the constitutive mutant and recombinant strain, was examined in 5 liter fermentors. The specific activity of cytidine deaminase in the mutant strain 3732E continued to increase after the culture had stopped growing (Figure 6A). With the clone, 3804E, very little enzyme was expressed at 30°C. After increasing the temperature to 42°C, to induce the λP$_L$ promoter, the cytidine deaminase activity rose to 40 units/mg protein over the next 3 hr of culture (Figure 6B). Similarly, production of enzyme by both strains was scaled up in 450 liter fermentors to obtain the larger quantities of cytidine deaminase required for further work (Table 1).

B.   Isolation and Immobilization of Cytidine Deaminase

After the initial demonstration of activity in a clarified cell extract from *E. coli* B (Table 1), we turned our attention to developing a robust procedure for isolation and immobi-

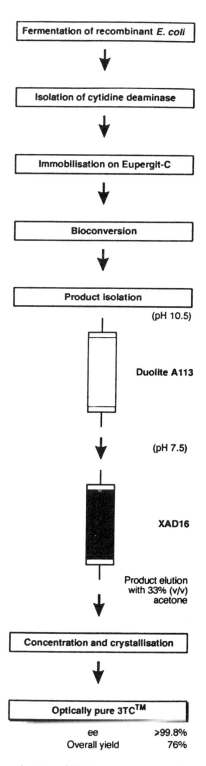

Figure 4   The process for production of Epivir.

Table I   Cytidine Deaminase Production by Various *E. coli* Strains[a]

Strain	Scale	− Cytidine	+ Cytidine[b]
B	50 ml	0.01	0.13
JM103	50 ml	0.02	0.21
	4 liters	0.08	0.11
3732E	50 ml	0.23–0.73	0.33
	4 liters	0.51–0.75	0.44
	450 liters	0.71	nd
3804E	50 ml	40–60	nd
	5 liters	40	nd
	450 liters	57	nd

[a] Various *E. coli* strains were grown with and without cytidine (5 mM). The growth medium was LPSG1 except for *E. coli* B (CDD medium). LPSG1 contained (per liter of distilled water) Lab Lemco, 40 g; peptone, 40 g; NaCl, 5 g; glycerol, 50 g. CDD medium contained (per liter of distilled water) glutamic acid, 3 g; $MgSO_4$, 0.2 g; K_2SO_4, 2.5 g; NaCl, 2.3 g; $Na_2HPO_4 \cdot 2H_2O$, 1.1 g; $NaH_2PO_4 \cdot 2H_2O$, 0.6 g. All strains were grown at 37°C except for 3804E, which was grown in a modified LPSG1 (containing tetracycline, 5 mg/liter; Lab Lemco 35 g/liter) at 28–30°C; then the enzyme production was induced by increasing the temperature to 40°C in early exponential growth. After approximately 24 hr growth, cells were harvested and cell-free extracts were assayed for cytidine deaminase activity. The inoculum (0.3% v/v) for growth of 3804E at 450 liters consisted of a 16-hr-old 5 liter fermentation grown in the presence of tetracycline (5 mg/liter). Strains were stored as lyophylizates for long-term storage, but for routine use they were maintained at 4°C on nutrient agar plates. Strain 3804E was maintained on nutrient agar plates containing tetracycline (5 mg/liter). The figures in the table are specific activities expressed in units/mg protein. One unit of activity was defined as the amount of enzyme required to deaminate 1 μmol of cytidine per minute at 25°C.
[b] nd: not determined.

lization of the enzyme. Cytidine deaminase was partially purified by column chromatography at a small scale; a 20-fold purification, with good recovery of the enzyme, was obtained by ion-exchange and hydrophobic interaction chromatography followed by ammonium sulfate precipitation. As the scale of operation was increased, the procedure was modified to include a batch adsorption step rather than column chromatography; after cell disruption, the clarified lysate was adsorbed onto cellulose DE52 and the enzyme was eluted with 0.3–0.5 M NaCl (50–70% recovery).

The significant improvement in the production of cytidine deaminase with the constitutive mutant and especially the recombinant strain prompted us to investigate the possibility of simplifying enzyme preparation further by using crude extracts without enzyme purification. The batch adsorption step was, therefore, omitted from the isolation procedure. The cell extracts were found to be satisfactory for use in the biotransformation. There was no evidence of competing side reactions, and the enzyme activity was found to be remarkably stable. Typically, 4 kg (wet weight) of *E. coli* 3732E cell paste was suspended in 20 liters of lysis buffer (KH_2PO_4, 50 mM; EDTA, 1 mM; DTT, 1 mM; ρ-hydroxybenzoic acid ethyl ester, 500 ppm; pH 7.5) and disrupted by three passages through a Manton–Gaulin homogenizer. The extract was clarified using continuous centrifugation and/or microfiltration and concentrated approximately 5-fold. The solution was further clarified by centrifugation (20,000 × g for 60 min) prior to immobilization. A

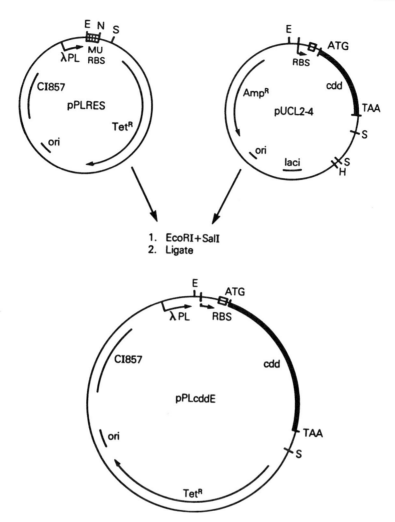

Figure 5 Construction of plasmid pPLcddE. The *Eco*RI to *Sal*I(S) *cdd* gene fragment from pUCL2-4 was ligated between the corresponding sites in expression plasmid pPLRES to create plasmid pPLcddE (steps 1 and 2). The *cdd* gene fragment (in bold) contains part of the *cdd* promoter (small arrow), the ribosome binding site (RBS), and initiation (ATG) and termination (TAA) codons. The positions of the λ leftward promoter (P_L), the gene encoding the temperature-sensitive λ repressor protein (CI857), the origin of replication (*ori*), and the tetracycline resistance gene (Tet^R) are as indicated. Other notation indicates the ampicillin resistance gene (Amp^R), the lac repressor gene (*lac*I), and restriction enzyme sites *Nco*I (N) and *Hind*III (H). (Reproduced from Ref. 57 with the permission of Butterworth-Heinemann.)

4 kg batch of the mutant strain (3732E) typically yielded 150,000 units of cytidine deaminase, whereas 15,000,000 units could be obtained from 4 kg of the clone (3804E). For larger-scale operations, even the clarification step could be omitted, and the crude extract was directly immobilized, without centrifugation, to give a stable enzyme preparation.

Due to previous work with immobilized adenosine deaminase, we chose to use Eupergit-C (Rhom Pharma) as a stable, robust support for immobilization of cytidine

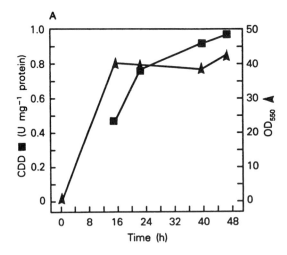

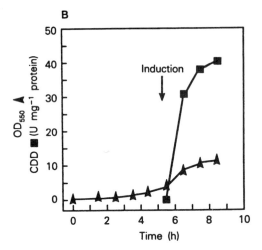

Figure 6   Fermentation time course. *E. coli* 3732E (A) and *E. coli* 3804E (B) were grown in 5 liter fermentations in LPSG1 medium. The inoculum consisted of 16- to 24-hr-old shake-flask culture (1.25% v/v). The optical density and cytidine deaminase activity were measured at intervals during the fermentation. The enzyme production by 3804E was induced by a temperature shift from 30 to 42°C, as shown by the arrow. (Reproduced from Ref. 57 with the permission of Butterworth-Heinemann.)

deaminase. Eupergit-C beads (150 μm) are hydrophilic and contain reactive epoxide groups that bind covalently to the enzyme. Typically, the extract was added to dry Eupergit-C (100 mg protein/g beads), and the mixture was left to stand at room temperature with occasional mixing to ensure adequate infiltration. The extent of immobilization was monitored by the loss of protein and cytidine deaminase activity from the supernatant. Within the first 48 hr, most of the immobilization had occurred, but it was allowed to

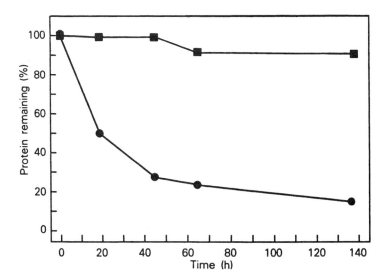

Figure 7 Time course of immobilization of cytidine deaminase on Eupergit-C. Clarified lysate from *E. coli* 3732E was incubated at room temperature with occasional stirring either with (●) or without (■) Eupergit-C beads (100 mg protein/g dry beads). Immobilization was carried out at pH 7.5. At intervals, the protein remaining in solution was measured (see Ref. 62) and expressed as a percentage of the initial protein concentration. Upon completion of immobilization, beads were washed with a buffer (Tris-HCl, 100 mM; EDTA, 1 mM; DTT, 1 mM; p-hydroxybenzoic acid ethyl ester, 500 ppm; pH 7.0) containing 0.5 M NaCl to remove unbound or loosely bound protein. Washing was continued until the absorbance of the supernatant at 280 nm was less than 0.1. The beads were stored at 4°C in the above buffer, without the addition of NaCl. (Reproduced from Ref. 57 with the permission of Butterworth-Heinemann.)

proceed up to 150 hr so that the reaction neared completion (Figure 7). To optimize the binding capacity of the beads, the effect of varying the protein-to-bead ratio on the immobilization procedure was investigated using cytidine deaminase from the overexpressing clone (3804E). With protein concentrations ranging from 10 to 200 mg/g beads, the activity was proportional to the relative amounts of protein used, indicating that the binding capacity had not been exceeded. As expected from the increased specific activity versus cytidine, immobilized preparations from the cloned strain were several fold more active against (±)-10 (Figure 3) when compared with preparations from the constitutive mutant (3732E) under similar conditions.

C.   Scale-Up of Production of Epivir

As the development of Epivir progressed, multikilogram quantities of optically pure material were required for toxicological studies. Initially, free cytidine deaminase from *E. coli* 3732E was used to produce Epivir in gram quantities (Figure 8). The enzyme showed a high degree of specificity for (+)-10. Chiral HPLC analysis of the deaminated products showed that only 1–2% of Epivir was hydrolyzed over the course of the reaction. The reaction was allowed to proceed to 51–52% conversion, at which time all the (+)-10 had been deaminated (Figure 9).

For further scale-up, the use of immobilized enzyme was highly desirable. The potential for reuse of immobilized cytidine deaminase was shown by a series of small-scale

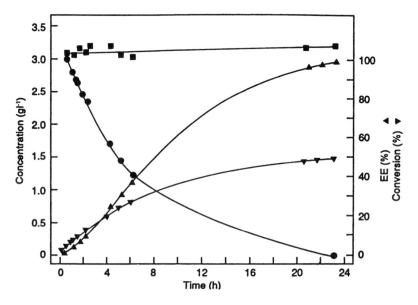

Figure 8   Enzymatic resolution of (±)-**10** (BCH189) at 90 g scale using free cytidine deaminase. Ninety grams of racemic **10** was incubated at 32°C with 1800 units of cytidine deaminase in a 15 liter volume in a 20 liter fermentor. The pH was adjusted to 7.0 with concentrated ammonia solution and maintained constant by the addition of 20% (v/v) acetic acid. At intervals, samples were analyzed by chiral HPLC [column, Cyclobond I acetyl (250 × 0.46 mm); mobile phase, triethylammonium acetate (0.2% v/v), pH 5.5; flow rate, 1 ml/min; detection wavelength, 270 nm]. (■) Epivir, g/liter; (●) (+)-**10**, g/liter; (▲) ee (Epivir); (▼) conversion (% deamination of racemic **10**). (Reproduced from Ref. 57 with the permission of Butterworth-Heinemann.)

reactions (5 ml, 5 mg substrate input). Beads were washed with distilled water after completion of each cycle. The same batch of enzyme was used for 16 cycles; the increase in reaction time observed was thought to be due mainly to physical loss of the beads during the washing step (Figure 10).

A 20 kg campaign was carried out as a series of 3 kg (500 liter working volume) batches of racemic **10** (Figure 3) using immobilized cytidine deaminase from the constitutive mutant 3732E. Deamination of (+)-**10** was initially rapid, but approached completion via a very gentle asymptote. Careful chiral HPLC was needed to judge when the residual Epivir had reached sufficiently high optical purity (ee > 99.5%). In practice, cessation of alkalinization of the medium by ammonia release was a particularly useful indicator that the reaction was "completed" (Figure 11). The same batch of enzyme was used for at least 15 cycles. Although the reaction time increased from 35 to more than 70 hr, this was attributed primarily to physical loss of the beads during collection and washing. To improve volumetric productivity, the effect of increased substrate concentration was investigated; no inhibition was noted up to 30 g/liter input. These higher concentrations were, therefore, used when the process was transferred to the factory.

D.   Product Isolation

Having successfully scaled up the bioconversion stage of the process, we focused on developing a simple, efficient strategy for isolation of Epivir. Initial work involved small-scale

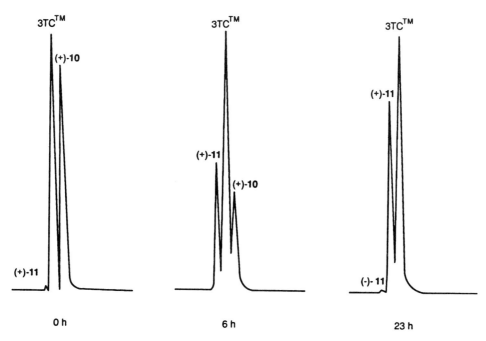

Figure 9   Resolution of (±)-**10** by chiral HPLC. Reaction conditions are as stated in the legend to Figure 8. Chemical structures are as shown in Figure 3.

isolation procedures using ion-exchange chromatography (QAE Sephadex), followed by desalting of Epivir on a polystyrene divinyl benzene resin (XAD16) column and recovery by freeze-drying. Neither the ion-exchange step, due to poor flow characteristics of the column, nor freeze-drying were suitable for operation at larger scale. A series of resins were, therefore, tested, and Duolite A113, a strongly basic polystyrene quaternary ammonium resin, which had a good capacity for the uridine analog [(+)-**11**, Figure 3], was selected and used for larger-scale operations. The freeze-drying step was also replaced by direct crystallization of product from the concentrated solution.

At the completion of each cycle of reaction (500 liter, 3 kg substrate input), the pH was adjusted to 10.5 with concentrated ammonia solution and the mixture was applied to a column of Duolite A113 super resin in the OH⁻ cycle (Figure 4). The uridine analog (+)-**11** adsorbed to the resin, whereas Epivir was not retained. The column was washed with 0.04% ammonia solution. This wash and the column spent, which contained the Epivir solution, were combined, the pH adjusted to 7.5 with concentrated H_2SO_4, and the mixture applied to an XAD16 resin column. The column was washed with distilled water, and Epivir was eluted with 33% (v/v) acetone in water. Fractions containing Epivir were combined and concentrated approximately four-fold on a Balfour wiped film evaporator. The concentrate was warmed to 50°C to dissolve any crystals, and the solution was vacuum-filtered through Whatman 54 filter paper before further concentration to a slurry (3 liter) using a rotary evaporator. After cooling, the crystalline product was recovered by filtration. Typically, 1.15 kg of highly pure Epivir (average recovery 76%) was recovered from each 3 kg batch. Purity was better than 97% by HPLC, and the enantiomeric excess (ee) was at least 99.8%.

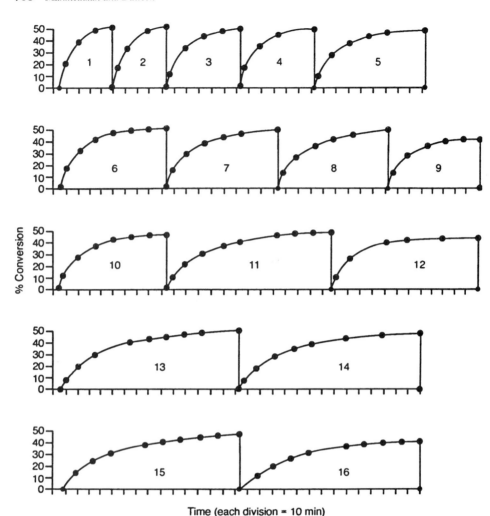

Figure 10 Multiple reuse of immobilized cytidine deaminase at analytical scale. Five milligrams of racemic **10** was incubated with 40 units of enzyme in a 5 ml buffer (100 mM Tris-HCl, pH 7.0) at 20°C. At intervals, samples were removed, cleared of enzyme beads, and analyzed by reverse phase HPLC [column, Spherisorb ODS-2 (150 × 0.48 mm); mobile phase, 50 mM $NH_4H_2PO_4$ (pH 2.5) containing 5% (v/v) acetonitrile; flow rate, 1.5 ml/min; detection wavelength, 270 nm]. The beads were washed with distilled water prior to use. Numbers 1–16 are cycles of reuse for the same batch of enzyme. (●) conversion (% deamination of racemic **10**).

Using this approach, 20 kg of optically pure Epivir was isolated to support the development program. For further scale-up, the process was transferred to our production site at Ulverston, Cumbria, where several tons of Epivir were produced using immobilized cytidine deaminase from the recombinant strain.

IV. ALTERNATIVE ROUTES TO EPIVIR

One major drawback with the routes discussed earlier, (a) enzymatic resolution of (±)-**12** using 5′-nucleotidase and alkaline phosphatase and (b) enantioselective deamination of

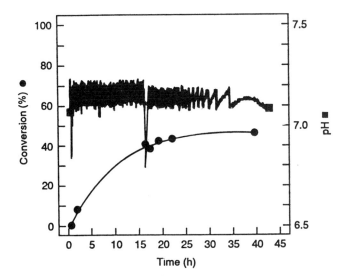

Figure 11 Enzymatic resolution of (±)-**10** at 3 kg scale using immobilized cytidine deaminase. Three kilograms of racemic **10** was incubated at 32°C with 30,000 units of immobilized cytidine deaminase in a 500 liter volume in a 780 liter fermentor. The pH was adjusted to 7.0 and maintained constant by the addition of 20% (v/v) acetic acid. Upon completion of the reaction, the mixture was pumped out through a 0.1 mm steel mesh, and the retained beads were stored at 4°C. (■) pH; (●) conversion (% deamination of racemic **10**). (Reproduced from Ref. 57 with the permission of Butterworth-Heinemann.)

(±)-**10** (BCH189) with cytidine deaminase, is late-stage resolution of the racemic drug (Figure 3). In practice, 50% of the valuable starting material was unused, and as the scale of operation increased, alternative routes for the manufacture of Epivir were sought. Nevertheless, resolution using immobilized cytidine deaminase was the only scalable route *initially* available that enabled us to rapidly produce multiton quantities of optically pure Epivir for clinical trials.

Epivir presented a significant challenge to our synthetic chemists, requiring control of stereochemistry of the two potentially epimerizable acetal centers. Despite the considerable progress made in developing conditions for β-stereoselectivity in glycosylation reactions (63,64), the maintenance of optical purity in synthesis of homochiral Epivir required that no epimerization of the O,S-acetals occur during coupling. The recent reports of the syntheses of (+)-**10** from D-mannose (65), 21 steps, and D-galactose (66), 18 steps, and of the corresponding (−)-enantiomer from L-gulose (67), 16 steps, prompted us to disclose our own efforts in the synthesis of Epivir (51,68). Two approaches were considered.

    1.   Condensation of the homochiral starting material, (+)-thiolactic acid, **15**, with 2-benzoylacetaldehyde gives a 1:2 mixture of the diastereomeric oxathiolane acids, **16**, **17**. After chromatographic separation, **17** may be treated with lead tetraacetate to furnish an anomeric mixture of the anti and syn acetates, **18**. After direct coupling with silylated cytosine, in the presence of trimethylsilylated (TMS)-iodide, separation of the pure β-anomer and deprotection affords Epivir (four steps, Figure 12a). The enantiomeric purity was judged to be at least 96% as determined by nuclear magnetic resonance (NMR) spectrometry using the chiral shift reagent (−)-R-2,2,2-trifluoro-1-(9-anthryl)ethanol (68).

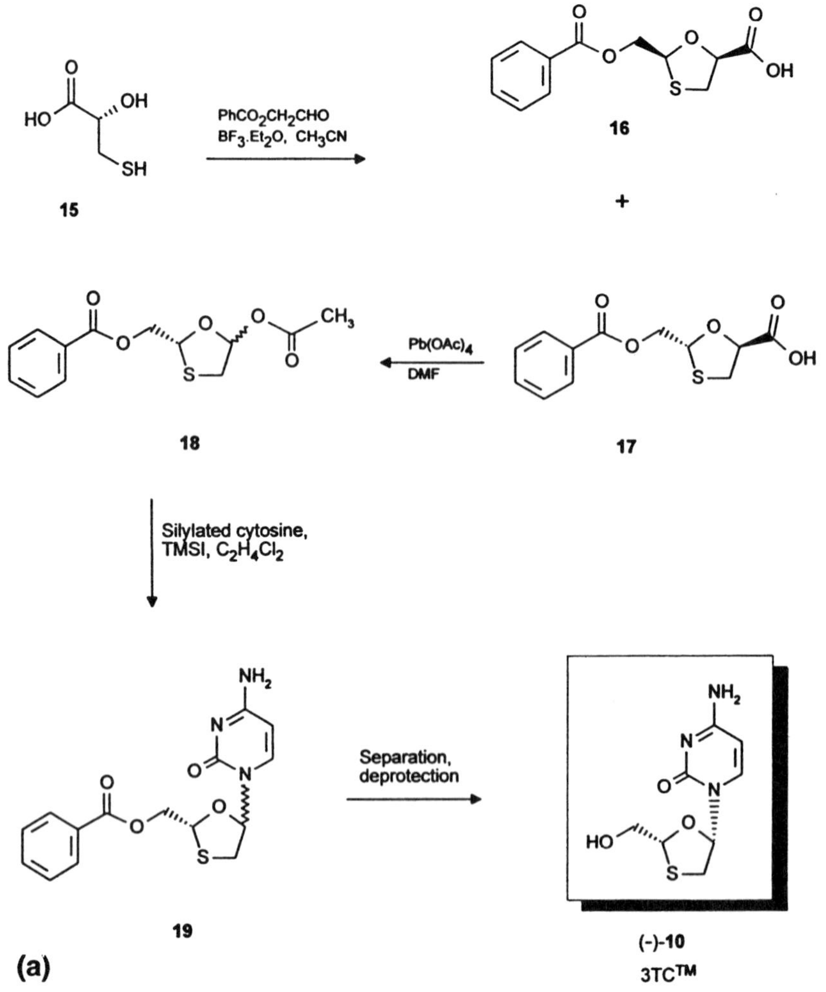

Figure 12 Two approaches to the synthesis of Epivir.

2. Alternatively, racemic acid, **21**, may be prepared by condensation of glyoxylic acid, **20**, and dithianediol (Figure 12b). Resolution and coupling with cytosine may be achieved in a number of ways. For example, acetylation with acetic anhydride gives a mixture of the racemic cis/trans acetoxy acids, **22**. Partial resolution of **22** can be achieved with (+)-norephedrine, but better purity is achieved by crystallization of the menthyl ester (–)-**23**. Coupling with silylated cytosine and final reduction yields Epivir (six steps, Figure 12b) (51).

Due to our earlier work with the carbocyclic nucleosides (+)-**5** and (+)-**8** (Figure 2), we also investigated enzymatic methods to effect resolution prior to the addition of the cytosine base. One such route considered was the enantioselective hydrolysis of racemic *trans*-5-propionyloxy-1,3-oxathiolane-2-methanol benzoate, **14**, to obtain the key intermediate (–)-**14** (69) (Figure 3). The *trans*-oxathiolane benzoate, **14**, synthesized from benzoyloxyacetaldehyde, **9** (three steps), was an attractive substrate because it could

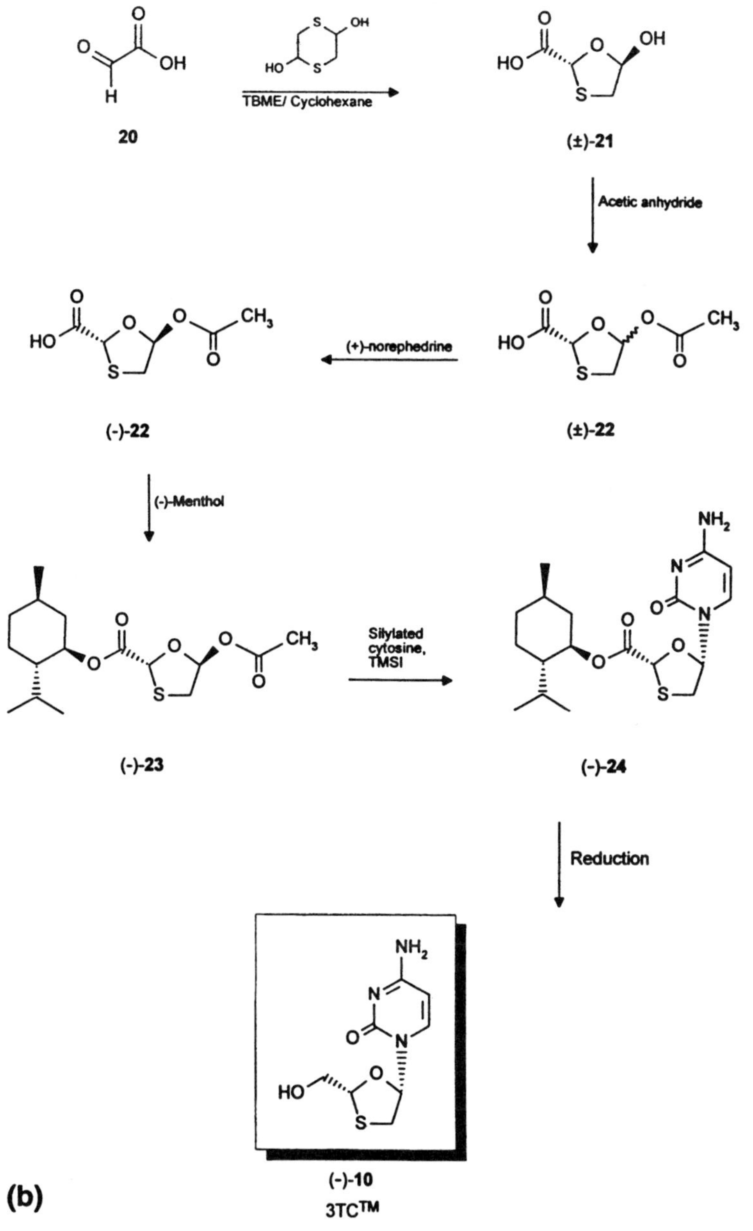

(b)

Figure 12b

easily be accommodated into the existing synthetic route. Interestingly, 9 was also a common starting material for the synthesis of (±)-10 (three steps, Figure 3). Several commercially available lipases and proteases were screened for the ability to hydrolyze racemic oxathiolane, 14, enantioselectively. *Mucor miehei* lipase was identified as the most efficient biocatalyst. All other enzymes tested were less enantioselective than *M. miehei* lipase, but it is interesting to note that *Candida cylindracae (rugosa)* and *Chromobacterium viscosum* lipases and subtilisin showed the opposite enantioselectivity to M. *miehei* lipase, albeit in very low ee (69). Bioconversion of **14** with M. *miehei* lipase afforded enantiomerically enriched residual ester of the correct absolute stereochemistry, (−)-2R, for the subsequent synthesis of Epivir (two steps, Figure 3). However, these enzymatic approaches were considered to offer no advantage over the conventional resolutions described in Figure 12b).

V. SUMMARY

Cytidine deaminase from E. *coli* has a relatively broad specificity. The enzyme has been shown to be tolerant to changes in the base (e.g., 5-fluoro, 5-methyl) and in the sugar (arabinose, 2'-deoxyribose) (22,70). Our finding that E. *coli* cytidine deaminase can deaminate racemic **10** (BCH189, Figure 3) enantioselectively extends the understanding of the specificity of this enzyme. This also suggests that, by analogy with adenosine deaminase (19,23,24), cytidine deaminase will become a generally useful reagent for the resolution of unnatural cytidine nucleosides. Interestingly, the mammalian enzyme also appears to deaminate (±)-**10** enantioselectively (48,49,71).

Although there are many reports in the literature of enzyme-catalyzed resolutions at laboratory scale (72,73), there are still few examples of processes operating at pilot and production scale (40,57,74–76). The cloning and overexpression of the enzyme, under the control of a high-level inducible promoter, was essential to the development of a scalable process. Cytidine deaminase has been cloned from both *Bacillus* (77,78) and E. *coli* (79), but only the B. *subtilis* enzyme had previously been overexpressed (from the *lac* promotor) in a high copy number plasmid (78).

Also crucial for developing a large-scale process was the demonstration that cytidine deaminase can be immobilized to give a stable enzyme preparation that can be reused many times in the reaction. The absence of substrate inhibition allowed high volumetric productivities to be achieved and assisted downstream processing. A robust scalable product isolation process was developed to yield crystalline Epivir (3TC). Here a simple two-column process, with adsorption–desorption rather than chromatographic steps, was used. Overall, yields through the resolution process of 76% were obtained. The overall process proved remarkably robust in a factory setting, with batches of enzyme surviving entire production campaigns.

The resolution with cytidine deaminase was the only scalable route available to us for the synthesis of Epivir through much of the preclinical and clinical development of the drug. However, end-stage resolution was never likely to be the optimal economic route in the longer term, and chemical resolution of an early-stage intermediate (cf. Figure 12b) now forms the basis of the manufacturing process for Epivir.

ACKNOWLEDGMENTS

This chapter represents contributions from a large team of scientists at Glaxo Wellcome Research and Development. The authors gratefully acknowledge the contributions of colleagues from Glaxo Wellcome Operations for the scale-up of this process. The support of and valuable discussions with G. C. Lawrence and his team, and B. S. Baines are also gratefully acknowledged.

REFERENCES

1. Gallo RC, Sarin PS, Gelman EP, Robert-Gurott M, Richardson E, Kalyanaraman VS, Mann D, Sidhu GD, Stahl RE, Zolla-Pazner S, Leibowich J, Popvic M. Isolation of a human T-cell leukemia virus in AIDS. Science 1983; 220:865–867.

2. Fauchi AS, Masur H, Gelman EP, Markham PD, Hahn BH, Lane HC. NIH conference. The AIDS update. Ann Intern Med 1985; 102:800–813.

3. Hao Z, Cooney DA, Hartman NR, Perno CF, Fridland A, de Vico AL, Sarngadharan MG, Johns DG. Factors determining the activity of 2′,3′-dideoxynucleotides in suppressing human immunodeficiency virus in vitro. Mol Phamacol 1988; 34:431–435.

4. Vince R, Hua M, Brownell J, Daluge S, Lee F, Shannon W, Lavelle G, Qualls J, Weislow O, Kiser R, Canonico P, Schultz R, Narayanan V, Mayo J, Shoemaker R, Boyd M. Potent and selective activity of a new carbocyclic nucleoside analogue (carbovir NSC 615846) against HIV in vitro. Biochem Biophys Res Commun 1988; 156:1046–1053.

5. Carter SG, Kessler JA, Rankin CD. Activities of (–)-carbovir and 3′-azido-3′-deoxythymidine against human immunodeficiency virus in vitro. Antimicrob Agents Chemother 1990; 34:1297–1300.

6. Seki JI, Shimada N, Takahashi K, Takita T, Takeuchi T, Hoshino H. Inhibition of infectivity of HIV by a novel nucleoside, oxetanocin, and related compounds. Antimicrob Agents Chemother 1989; 33:773–775.

7. Tseng CKH, Marquez VE, Milne GWA, Wysocki RJ, Mitsuya H, Shirasaki T, Driscoll JS. A ring-enlarged oxetanocin-A analogue as a inhibitor of HIV infectivity. J Med Chem 1991; 34:343–349.

8. Hayashi S, Phadtare S, Zemlica J, Matsukura M, Mitsuya H, Broder S. Adenallene and cytallene; acyclic nucleoside analogues that inhibit replication and cytopathic effect of HIV in vitro. Proc Natl Acad Sci USA 1988; 85:6127–6131.

9. Hayashi S, Norbec DW, Rosenbrook W, Fine RL, Matsukura M, Plattner JJ, Broder S, Mitsuya H. Cyclobut-A and cyclobut-G, carbocyclic oxetanocin analogues that inhibit the replication of HIV in T-cells and monocytes and macrophages in vitro. Antimicrob Agents Chemother 1990; 34:287–294.

10. Mansuri MM, Starrett JE, Ghazzouli I, Hitchcock MJM, Sterzycki RZ, Brankovan V, Lin TS, August EM, Prusoff WH, Sommadossi JP. 1-(2,3-dideoxy-β-D-glycero-pent-2-enofuranosyl)thymine (d4T). A highly potent and selective anti-HIV agent. J Med Chem 1989; 32:461–466.

11. Mansuri MM, Farina V, Starrett JE, Benigni DA, Brankovan V, Martin JC. Preparation of the isomers of ddC, ddA, d4C and d4T as potential retroviral agents. Bioorg Med Chem Lett 1991; 1:65–68.

12. Coates JAV, Cammack N, Jenkinson HJ, Jowett MI, Pearson BA, Penn CR, Rouse PL, Viner KC, Cameron JM. (–)-2′-Deoxy-3′-thiacytidine is a potent, highly selective inhibitor of human immunodeficiency virus Type 1 and Type 2 replication in vitro. Antimicrob Agents Chemother 1992; 36:733–739.

13. Schinazi RF, McMillan A, Cannon D, Mathis R, Lloyd RM, Peck A, Sommadossi JP, St. Clair M, Wilson J, Furman PA, Painter G, Choi WB, Liotta DC. Selective inhibition of human immunodeficiency viruses by racemates and enantiomers of cis-5-fluoro-1-[2-(hydroxymethyl)-1,3-oxathiolan-5-yl]cytosine. Antimicrob Agents Chemother 1992; 36:2423–2431.

14. Naesen L, Balzarini J, de Clercq EA. Single-dose administration of 9-(2-phosphonylmethoxyethyl)adenine (PMEA) and 9-(2-phosphonylmethoxyethyl)-2,6-diaminopurine (PMEDAP) in the prophylaxis of retrovirus infection in vivo. Antiviral Res 1991; 16:53–64.

15. Soudeyns H, Yao XJ, Gao Q, Belleau B, Kraus JL, Nguyen-Ba N, Spira B, Wainberg M. Anti-human immunodeficiency virus Type 1 activity and in vitro toxicity of 2′-deoxy-3′-thiacytidine (BCH189), a novel heterocyclic nucleoside analogue. Antimicrob Agents Chemother 1991; 35:1386–1390.

16. Cermak RC, Vince R. (±)-4β-Amino-2α,3α-dihydroxy-1β-cyclopentanemethanol hydrochloride. Carbocyclic ribofuranosylamine for the synthesis of carbocyclic nucleosides. Tetrahedron Lett 1981; 22:2331–2332.

17. Marquez VE, Lim M. Carbocyclic nucleosides. Med Res Rev 1986; 6:1–40.

18. Borthwick AD, Butt S, Biggadike K, Exall AM, Roberts SM, Youds PM, Kirk BE, Booth BR, Cameron JM, Cox SW, Marr CL, Shill MD. Synthesis and enzymatic resolution of carbocyclic 2′-*ara*-fluoro-guanosine: A potent new anti-herpetic agent. J Chem Soc Chem Commun 1988; 656–658.

19. Vince R, Brownell J. Resolution of racemic carbovir and selective inhibition of human immunodeficiency virus by the (−)-enantiomer. Biochem Biophys Res Commun 1990; 168:912–916.

20. Balzarini J, Baumgartner H, Bodenteich M, de Clercq EA, Griengl H. Synthesis and antiviral activity of the enantiomeric forms of carba-5-iodo-2′-deoxyuridine and carba-(*E*)-5-(2-bromovinyl)-2′deoxyuridine. J Med Chem 1989; 32:1861–1865.

21. Balzarini J. Metabolism and mechanism of anti-retroviral action of purine and pyrimidine derivatives. Pharm World Sci 1994; 16:113–126.

22. Krenitsky TA, Koszalka GW, Tuttle JV, Rideout JL, Elion GB. An enzymatic synthesis of purine D-arabinonucleosides. Carbohydr Res 1981; 97:139–146.

23. Herdewijn P, Balzarini J, de Clercq EA, van der Harghe H. Resolution of aristeromycin enantiomers. J Med Chem 1985; 28:1385–1386.

24. Secrist JA, Montgomery JA, Shealy YF, O'Dell A, Clayton SJ. Resolution of racemic carbocyclic analogues of purine nucleosides through the action of adenosine deaminase. Antiviral activity of the carbocyclic 2′-deoxyguanosine enantiomers. J Med Chem 1987; 30:746–749.

25. Hutchinson DW. New approaches to the synthesis of anti-viral nucleosides. TIBTECH 1990; 8:348–353.

26. Hoong LK, Strange LE, Liotta DC, Koszalka GW, Burns CL, Schinazi RF. Enzyme-mediated enantioselective preparation of pure enantiomers of the anti-viral agent 2′,3′-dideoxy-5-fluoro-3′-thiacytidine (FTC) and related compounds. J Org Chem 1992; 57:5563–5565.

27. Mahmoudian M, Baines BS, Dawson MJ, Lawrence GC. Resolution of 4-amino-cyclopentanecarboxylic acid methyl esters using hydrolytic enzymes. Enzyme Microb Technol 1992; 14:911–916.

28. Noyori R, Sato T, Hayawa Y. A stereocontrolled general synthesis of *c*-nucleosides. J Am Chem Soc 1978; 102:2561–2563.

29. Schmidt RR, Lieberknecht A. Functional derivatives of D-ribose by optical resolution with recycling. Angew Chem Int Ed Engl 1978; 17:769–770.

30. Just G, Liak TJ, Lim M, Potvin P, Tsantrizos YS. *c*-Nucleosides and related compounds. The synthesis of D,L-2′-*epi*-showdomycin and D,L-showdomycin. Can J Chem 1980; 58:2024–2033.

31. Kozikowski AP, Ames A. Total synthesis of the *c*-nucleoside *dl*-showdomycin by a Diels-Alder, retrograde Dieckmann strategy. J Am Chem Soc 1981; 103:3923–3924.

32. Arita M, Adachi K, Ito Y, Sawai H, Ohno M. Enantioselective synthesis of the carbocyclic nucleosides (−)-aristeromycin and (−)-neplanocin-A by a chemicoenzymatic approach. J Am Chem Soc 1983; 105:4049–4055.

33. Sicsic S, Ikbal M, Le Goffic F. Chemoenzymatic approach to carbocyclic analogues of ribonucleotides and nicotinamide ribose. Tetrahedron Lett 1987; 28:1887–1888.

34. Laane C, Boeven S, Hilhorst R, Veeger C. Optimisation of biocatalysis in organic media. Laane C, Tramper J, Lilly MD, eds. Biocatalysis in Organic Media. Amsterdam: Elsevier Science Publishers BV, 1987:65–84.

35. White EL, Parker WB, Macy LJ, Chaddix SC, McCaleb G, Secrist JA, Vince R, Shannon WM. Comparison of the effect of carbovir, AZT, and dideoxynucleoside triphosphates on the activity of human immunodeficiency virus reverse transcriptase and selected human polymerases. Biochem Biophys Res Commun 1989; 161:393–398.

36. Coates JAV, Inggall HJ, Pearson BA, Penn CR, Storer R, Williamson C, Cameron JM. Carbovir; the (−)-enantiomer is a potent and selective anti-viral agent against human immunodeficiency virus *in vitro*. Antiviral Res 1991; 15:161–168.

37. Exall AM, Jones MF, Mo CL, Myers PL, Paternoster IL, Singh H, Storer R, Weingarten GG, Williamson C, Brodie AC, Cook J, Lake DE, Meerholz CA, Turnbull PJ, Highcock RM. Synthesis of (−)-aristeromycin and X-ray structure of (−)-carbovir. J Chem Soc Perkin Trans (I) 1991; 2467–2477.

38. Pun KT, Baines BS, Lawrence GC. Isolation, immobilisation and use of adenosine deaminase in the synthesis of (−)-carbovir, a purine nucleoside analogue. Fifth European Congress on Biotechnology, Copenhagen, 1990: Abstract TUP 111, p. 292.

39. Brady TG, O'Connell W. A purification of adenosine deaminase from the superficial mucosa of calf intestine. Biochem Biophys Acta 1962; 62:216–229.

40. Taylor SJC, Sutherland AG, Lee C, Wisdom R, Thomas S, Roberts SM, Evans CT. Chemoenzymatic synthesis of (−)-carbovir utilising a whole cell–catalysed resolution of 2-azabicyclo[2.2.1]hept-5-en-one. J Chem Soc Chem Commun 1990; 1120–1121.

41. Evans CT, Roberts SM, Shoberu KA, Sutherland AG. Potential use of carbocyclic nucleosides for the treatment of AIDS: Chemoenzymatic synthesis of the enantiomers of carbovir. J Chem Soc Perkin Trans (I) 1992; 589–592.

42. Cameron JM. New anti-herpes drugs in development. Rev Med Virol 1993; 3:225–236.

43. Boehme RE, Bereford A, Hart GJ, Angier SJ, Thompson G, van Wely G, Huang JL, Mack P, Soike KF. GR95168X (chiral carbocyclic BVdU) is highly effective against simian *Varicella* virus infections of African green monkeys. Antiviral Res 1994; 23:97–98.

44. Borthwick AD, Crame AJ, Exall AM, Weingarten GG, Mahmoudian M. A short, convergent synthesis of two chiral anti-viral agents (+)-carbocyclic 2'-deoxy-5-[(E)-2-bromovinyl]uridine and (+)-carbocyclic 2'-deoxyguanosine. Tetrahedron Lett 1995; 36: 6929–6932.

45. Sato T, Fujisawa T. Stereocontrol in bakers' yeast reduction leading to natural product synthesis. Biocatalysis 1990; 3:1–15.

46. Ward OP, Young CS. Reductive biotransformations of organic compounds by cells or enzymes of yeast. Enzyme Microb Technol 1990; 12:482–493.

47. Coates JAV, Cammack N, Jenkinson HJ, Mutton IM, Pearson BA, Storer R, Cameron JM, Penn CR. The separated enantiomers of 2'-deoxy-3'-thiacytidine (BCH189) both inhibit human immunodeficiency virus replication *in vitro*. Antimicrob Agents Chemother 1992; 36:202–205.

48. Schinazi RF, Chu CK, Peck A, McMillan A, Mathis R, Cannon D, Jeong LS, Beach JW, Choi WB, Yeola S, Liotta DC. Activities of the four optical isomers of 2',3'-dideoxy-3'-thiacytidine (BCH189) against human immunodeficiency virus Type 1 in human lymphocytes. Antimicrob Agents Chemother 1992; 36:672–676.

49. Cammack N, Rouse P, Marr CLP, Reid PJ, Boehme RE, Coates JAV, Penn CR, Cameron JM. Cellular metabolism of (−)-enantiomeric 2'-deoxy-3'-thiacytidine. Biochem Pharmacol 1992; 43:2059–2064.

50. Gray NM, Marr CL, Penn CR, Cameron JM, Bethell RC. The intracellular phosphorylation of (−)-2'-deoxy-3'-thiacytidine and the incorporation of 3TC™ 5'-monophosphate into DNA by HIV-1 reverse transcriptase and human DNA polymerase γ. Biochem Pharmacol 1995; 50:1043–1051.

51. Cameron JM, Collis P, Daniel M, Storer R, Wilcox P. Lamivudine. Drugs Future 1993; 18:319–323.

52. Pluda J, Ruedy J, Levitt N, Cooley T, Berard P, Rubin M, Yarchoan R. A phase I/II study of 3TC™. Thirty-second Interscience Conference on Antimicrobial Agents and Chemotherapy, Anaheim, California, 1992: Abstract 560.

53. Francis CE, Hunter Λ, Berney JJ, Cameron JM. *In vitro* myelotoxicity studies with 3TC™. Eighth International Conference on AIDS and Third STD World Congress, Amsterdam, 1992: Abstract PuA 6027.

54. Viner KC, Cammack N, Coates JAV, Hooker EU, Penn CR, Rouse P, Cameron JM. 3TC™: Combination studies with AZT and other inhibitors of HIV-1 replication *in vitro*. Ninth International Conference on AIDS, Berlin, 1993: Abstract PoA-25.

55. Cameron JM, Cammack N. Anti-viral combinations containing nucleoside analogues. Eur Pat Appl 0 513 917 A1; 1992.

56. Storer R, Clemens IR, Lamont B, Noble SA, Williamson C, Belleau B. The resolution and absolute stereochemistry of the enantiomers of *cis*-1[2-(hydroxymethyl)-1,3-oxathiolan-5-yl]cytosine (BCH189): Equipotent anti-HIV agents. Nucleosides Nucleotides 1993; 12:225–236.

57. Mahmoudian M, Baines BS, Drake CS, Hale RS, Jones P, Piercey JE, Montgomery DS, Purvis IJ, Storer R, Dawson MJ, Lawrence GC. Enzymatic production of optically pure 3TC™ (Lamivudine): A potent anti-HIV agent. Enzyme Microb Technol 1993; 15:749–755.

58. Sakai T, Yu T, Omata S. Distribution of enzymes related to cytidine degradation in bacteria. Agric Biol Chem 1976; 9:1893–1895.

59. Neuhard J. Utilisation of preformed pyrimidine bases and nucleosides. Munch-Petersen A, ed. Metabolism of Nucleotides, Nucleosides, and Nucleobases in Microorganisms. London: Academic Press, 1983:95–148.

60. Hammer-Jespersen K. Nucleoside metabolism. Munch-Petersen A, ed. Metabolism of Nucleotides, Nucleosides, and Nucleobases in Microorganisms. London: Academic Press, 1983:203–258.

61. Munch-Petersen A, Nygaard P, Hammer-Jespersen K, Fiil N. Mutants constitutive for nucleoside-catabolising enzymes in *Escherichia coli* K12. Isolation, characterisation and mapping. Eur J Biochem 1972; 27:208–215.

62. Bradford MM. A rapid and sensitive method for the quantitation of microgram quantities of protein utilising the principle of protein-dye binding. Analyt Biochem 1976; 72:248–254.

63. Chu CK, Babu JR, Beach JW, Ahn SK, Huang H, Jeong LS, Lee SJ. A highly stereoselective glycosylation of 2-(phenylselenenyl)-2,3-dideoxyribose derivative with thymine; synthesis of 3′-deoxy-2′,3′-didehydrothymidine and 3′-deoxythymidine. J Org Chem 1990; 55: 1418–1420.

64. Wilson LJ, Liotta DC. A general method for controlling glycosylation stereochemistry in the synthesis of 2′-deoxyribose nucleosides. Tetrahedron Lett 1990; 31:1815–1818.

65. Chu CK, Beach JW, Jeong LS, Choi WB, Cormer FI, Alves AJ, Schinazi RF. Enantiomeric synthesis of (+)-BCH189, (+)-(2S, 5R)-1-[2-hydroxymethyl]-1,3-oxathiolan-5-yl]cytosine from D-mannose and its anti-HIV activity. J Org Chem 1991; 56:6503–6505.

66. Jeong LS, Alves AJ, Carrigan SW, Kim HO, Beach JW, Chu CK. An efficient synthesis of enantiomerically pure (+)-(2S, 5R)-1-[2-(hydroxymethyl)-1,3-oxathiolan-5-yl]cytosine, (+)-BCH189, from D-galactose. Tetrahedron Lett 1992; 35:595–598.

67. Beach JW, Jeong LS, Alves AJ, Pohl D, Kim HO, Chang CN, Doong SL, Schinazi RF, Cheng YC, Chu CK. Synthesis of enantiomerically pure (−)-(2R, 5S)-1-[2-(hydroxymethyl)-1,3-oxathiolan-5-yl]cytosine as a potent anti-viral agent against hepatitis B virus (HBV) and human immunodeficiency virus (HIV). J Org Chem 1992; 57:2217–2219.

68. Humber DC, Jones MF, Payne JJ, Ramsay MVJ, Zacharie B, Jin H, Siddiqui A, Evans CA, Tse HLA, Mansour TS. Expeditious preparation of (−)-2′-deoxy-3′-thiacytidine. Tetrahedron Lett 1992; 33:4625–4628.

69. Cousins RPC, Mahmoudian M, Youds PM. Enzymatic resolution of oxathiolane intermediates; an alternative approach to the anti-viral agent lamivudine (3TC™). Tetrahedron Asymm 1995; 6:393–396.

70. Hosono H, Kuno S. The purification and properties of cytidine deaminase from *E. coli*. J Biochem 1973; 74:797–803.

71. Chang CN, Doong SL, Zhou JH, Beach JW, Jeong LS, Chu CK, Tsai CH, Cheng YC. Deoxycytidine deaminase–resistant stereoisomer is the active form of racemic 2′,3′-thiacytidine in the inhibition of hepatitis B virus replication. J Biol Chem 1992; 267:13938–13942.

72. Jones JB. Enzymes in organic synthesis. Tetrahedron 1986; 42:3351–3403.

73. Davies HG, Green RH, Kelly DR, Roberts SM. Recent advances in the generation of chiral intermediates using enzymes. Crit Rev Biotechnol 1990; 10:129–153.

74. Lowe DA. Industrial importance of biotransformations of β-lactam antibiotics. Dev Ind Microbiol 1983; 26:143–155.

75. Walts AE, Fox EM, Jackson CB. R-Glycidyl butyrate, evolution of a laboratory procedure to an industrial process: Optimization and scale up. Biotech USA 1987; 91–98.

76. Battistel E, Bianchi D, Cesti P, Pina C. Enzymatic resolution of S-(+)-naproxen in a continuous reactor. Biotechnol Bioeng 1991; 38:659–664.

77. Chang JS, Song BH, Kim JG, Hong SD. Molecular cloning of *Bacillus stearothermophilus cdd* gene encoding thermostable cytidine, deoxycytidine deaminase. Kor J Appl Microbiol Bioeng 1989; 17:334–342.

78. Song BH, Neuhard J. Chromosomal location, cloning and nucleotide sequence of the *Bacillus subtilis cdd* gene encoding cytidine, deoxycytidine deaminase. Mol Gen Genet 1989; 216:462–468.

79. Albrechtsen B. CRP-, cAMP- and cyt R-regulated promotors in *E. coli* K12; the *cdd* promotor. Mol Microbiol 1989; 3:1385–1390.

26

Biochemical and Fermentation Technological Approaches to Production of Pravastatin, a HMG-CoA Reductase Inhibitor

Nobufusa Serizawa, Masahiko Hosobuchi, and Hiroji Yoshikawa
Sankyo Company, Ltd., Tokyo, Japan

I. INTRODUCTION

Coronary heart disease (CHD) is one of the major causes of death in Western countries and Japan. Among CHDs, ischemic heart disease (IHD) leads to the highest mortality rate. The number of patients suffering from IHD in Japan is gradually increasing. This trend is attributable, in part, to a growing elderly population and westernized food intake. It is well known that the three major risk factors for IHD are hypercholesterolemia, hypertension, and smoking. Hypercholesterolemia has long been considered to be the most important of these factors (1). Several epidemiological studies, such as the Framingham Heart Study (2), the Pooling Project (3), and the Multiple Risk Factor Intervention Trial (MRFIT) (4), have demonstrated the relationship between plasma cholesterol levels and the development of IHD. Two trials have indicated that reduction of plasma cholesterol levels in hypercholesterolemic patients by drug treatment decreases the incidence of CHD: the U.S. Lipid Research Clinics Coronary Primary Prevention Trial (LRC-CPPT) (5,6) using a bile acid sequestrant, cholestyramine, and the Helsinki Heart Study (7) using gemfibrozil. To reduce the risk associated with high serum cholesterol levels, the development of several hypolipidemic drugs and therapies has been explored in many countries.

Cholesterol is supplied by absorption from diet (0.3–0.5 g/day in human) and biosynthesis (1.0–1.2 g/day) and is excreted mainly as bile acids into feces (0.8–1.3 g/day) (8). To reduce body cholesterol, three major strategies can be considered: (a) inhibition of cholesterol absorption by a compound such as β-sitosterol, (b) inhibition of bile acid reabsorption by a compound such as cholestyramine, and (c) inhibition of cholesterol biosynthesis. Since more than 70% of the total input of body cholesterol in humans is derived from *de novo* synthesis, it is expected that plasma cholesterol levels can be reduced by inhibition of cholesterol biosynthesis.

As shown in Figure 1, cholesterol is synthesized from acetyl–coenzyme A (CoA) in a process that includes more than 20 enzymatic steps. The rate-limiting enzyme of this pathway is 3-hydroxy-3-methylgultaryl (HMG)-CoA reductase [mevalonate: NADP+

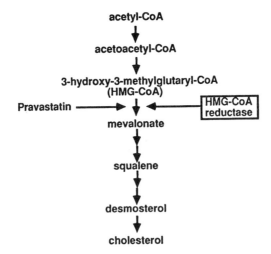

acetyl-CoA

acetoacetyl-CoA

3-hydroxy-3-methylglutaryl-CoA
(HMG-CoA)

Pravastatin ────────▶   ◀──── | **HMG-CoA**
reductase |

mevalonate

squalene

desmosterol

cholesterol

Figure 1   Pathway of cholesterol biosynthesis, showing the reaction that pravastatin inhibits.

oxidoreductase (CoA-acylating), EC 1.1.1.34], which catalyzes the reduction of HMG-CoA to mevalonate. In general, the later steps of biosynthesis, those close to the target substances, are most suitable for inhibition because the production of other substances is minimally disturbed. Hydrophobic substances such as cholesterol have been shown to be an exception to this concept, due to the accumulation of hydrophobic intermediates.

In 1971, we started screening for inhibitors of cholesterol synthesis from culture broth of microorganisms using a cell-free enzyme system from rat liver. After screening the microorganisms, ML-236B (mevastatin, Figure 2) was discovered in the culture broth of *Penicillium citrinum* in 1975 (9). It is noteworthy that compactin, a compound identical to ML-236B, was independently isolated by Beecham Pharmaceuticals as a weak antifungal antibiotic (10) two years after Sankyo's patent filing.

As shown in Figure 2, a portion of the ML-236B structure resembles that of HMG (3-hydroxy-3-methylglutarate); this is the part of HMG-CoA that serves as the substrate of HMG-CoA reductase. Accordingly, ML-236B and the related compounds shown in Figure 2 inhibit the enzyme in a competitive manner with respect to HMG-CoA. Despite having a marked inhibitory activity on cholesterol synthesis in vitro and in vivo, ML-236B did not show hypocholesterolemic activity in rats or mice, commonly used in the initial stage of evaluation of efficacy in animals. Almost three years passed before we found that ML-236B showed strict species specificity.

It is well known that the liver and intestine are the major organs involved in *de novo* cholesterogenesis. We focused on finding a drug having enhanced target-organ-directed characteristics, because a target-organ-directed inhibitor would be expected to minimally disturb cholesterol metabolism in other organs, including hormone-producing organs. After screening microbial products as well as chemically and biologically modified derivatives of ML-236B, pravastatin was finally chosen as the candidate for development. Pravastatin has stronger and more tissue-selective inhibition of cholesterol synthesis than ML-236B (11).

Pravastatin contains a hydroxyl-group at the 6β-position of its decaline structure (Figure 2). This drug was first found as a minor urinary metabolite of ML-236B in dogs in 1979. For the industrial hydroxylation of ML-236B, chemical syntheses were initially

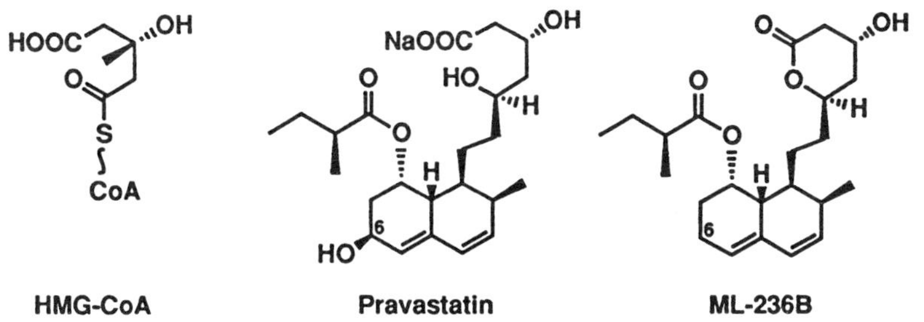

Figure 2 Structures of pravastatin and related compounds.

attempted, but high costs made this method unfeasible. For this reason, microbial hydroxylation was chosen for the production of pravastatin. After screening for microorganisms capable of converting ML-236B to pravastatin, *Streptomyces carbophilus* was selected for the second step of the fermentation process (12,13).

In 1981, pravastatin was chosen for development as a hypolipidemic drug, and clinical trials began in 1984. Pravastatin was approved for production in 1989 and launched in the same year as "Mevalotin" in Japan. The drug was licensed to Bristol-Myers Squibb Company and has been developed worldwide. Pravastatin has already been sold commercially in 47 countries including Japan.

This chapter focuses on the production of pravastatin. Pravastatin is produced by a two-step fermentation; the first step is production of ML-236B, and the second is hydroxylation of ML-236B. The mechanism of microbial hydroxylation of ML-236B and industrialization of the production of pravastatin are described here in detail.

II. PRODUCTION BY TWO-STEP FERMENTATION

A. ML-236B Production by *Penicillium citrinum*

1. Biosynthesis of ML-236B

ML-236B is thought to be derived from polyketide chains, one 18-carbon and one 4-carbon, formed from acetate units in the normal head-to-tail fashion. This putative biosynthetic route is similar to the route reported for lovastatin biosynthesis (Figure 3) (14).

2. Strain Improvement of P. citrinum for Enhanced Productivity

The amount of ML-236B produced by the original strain was too small for industrial production. Strain improvement of *P. citrinum* for enhanced productivity included mutagenesis of spore suspension by ultraviolet (UV) irradiation and NTG (15,16). We selected high ML-236B producing strains still capable of morphological development using nystatin-containing agar plates. Nystatin inhibits synthesis of the cell wall. Analysis of fat concentration in the cell membrane indicated that nystatin-resistant strains contain less ergosterol in the cell membrane.

Generally, strain improvement has the potential to increase yield dramatically. Traditional methods, such as random screening or resistant isolation after mutagenesis, can likely provide high-yield strains. For improvement of the ML-236B-producing strain, *P.*

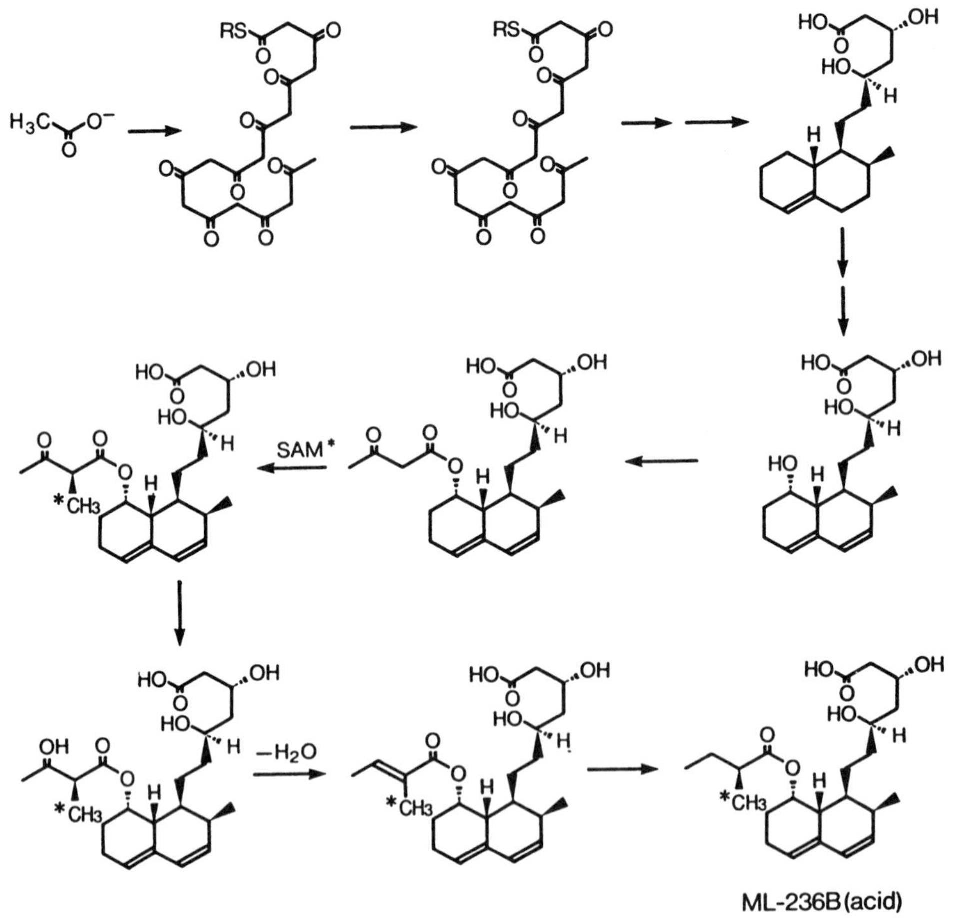

Figure 3   A proposed biosynthesis of ML-236B.

citrinum, traditional screening methods were applied. Recently, several modern techniques, such as protoplast fusion and gene manipulation, also have been introduced for strain improvement. The availability of a suitable transformation system for *P. citrinum* is an essential prerequisite.

The most straightforward and industrially available approach for the transformation was to develop a dominant selective strategy. Transformation systems based on resistance to the aminocyclitol antibiotic hygromycin B (HmB) have been described for several filamentous fungi, including *Cephalosporium acremonium* (17), *Aspergillus nidulans* (18), and *Aspergillus niger* (18), *Penicillium roqueforti* (19), and a few plant pathogenic species (20–22). The transformation of *P. citrinum* to HmB resistance was accomplished by vectors pDF333 and pDF345 (Figure 4). The recombinant strain contains the *Escherichia coli* HmB phosphotransferase (*hpt*) gene under control of the *A. nidulans* 3-phosphoglycerate kinase (*pgk*) gene promoter (23) and the cloned *P. citrinum pgk* promoter and terminator (15).

After transformation, colonies were randomly selected and screened for the presence of vectors pDF333 and pDF345 by Southern hybridization experiments. Integration of pDF333 or pDF345 into the *P. citrinum* chromosomal DNA was observed, confirming

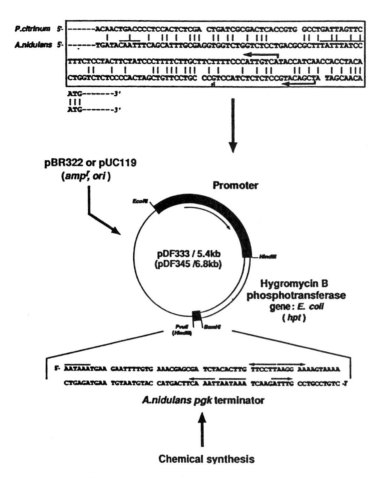

Figure 4   Construction of the transformation vectors. The structure maps of plasmids pDF333 and pDF345.

that the strain had been introduced into *P. citrinum* HmB^r by transformation. Tandem integrations seem to be a common feature of transformation systems in filamentous fungi. The most plausible explanation for this pattern is that a second copy of the plasmid is inserted into the first integrated plasmid via homologous recombination by a single crossover. Whether the recombinations are produced during integration or following growth on a selective medium remains to be determined. By analogy with other systems, heterologous integration most likely involves multiple integration. Thus, in all transformants so far analyzed, we have found that integration occurred in tandem at different sites in the chromosomal DNA.

The stability of some primary transformants was evaluated by repeated vegetative transfer from a selective to a nonselective medium. All the transformants conserved their resistance to HmB after passage through the nonselective medium. The hybridization patterns and intensities obtained from a probe that contained the *hpt* gene were identical in all cases. These observations agree with the high degree of stability reported for transformants of various filamentous ascomycetes. Such a system should be useful in producing *P. citrinum* transformants with useful characteristics, particularly transformants that carry extra copies of *P. citrinum* genes to increase ML-236B production and transformants that carry heterologous genes to allow *in situ* modification of ML-236B. Improvement of ML-236B productivity in *P. citrinum* is possible using this transformation system.

B. Microbial Hydroxylation

The discovery of penicillin, streptomycin, and other antibiotics led to the development of microbial chemistry for both academic and industrial applications. In 1952, Peterson and Murray (24) discovered that *Rhizopus nigricans* could oxygenate steroids at C11. This finding represented the first successful microbial transformation of an exogenous compound. Since then, numerous types of reactions have been performed by means of microbial transformation. It is well known that microorganisms can synthesize, transform, and degrade substances such as secondary metabolites that possess complicated structures. Microorganisms can produce active enzyme systems that can catalyze chemical reactions with foreign substances that are added to the culture medium of the microorganisms. In contrast with chemical reagents, the reactions employing microbial enzymes are highly selective and stereospecific. Thus, production strategies frequently employ microorganisms in place of one-step organic syntheses. Pravastatin, first isolated as a minor urinary metabolite of ML-236B, was found to inhibit cholesterol synthesis more potently in vitro than its parent compound. The hydroxylation reaction by which pravastatin is formed could not be performed easily through conventional synthetic methods, and so we set out to isolate microorganisms capable of hydroxylating ML-236B at the 6β-position to form pravastatin. This section focuses on the production of pravastatin by microbial hydroxylation, and we also discuss the mechanism by which ML-236B is hydroxylated to pravastatin by a novel actinomycete cytochrome P-450.

1. Discovery of Microorganisms Capable of Hydroxylating ML-236B to Pravastatin

Various microorganisms were tested for the ability to hydroxylate ML-236B at the 6β-position (25). Resulting from an extensive screening program, *Mucor hiemalis* SANK 36372 was found to be one of the most effective microorganisms for that hydroxylation. *M. hiemalis* SANK 36372 converted ML-236B mainly to pravastatin. Neither this nor any of the other fungi, however, tolerated high concentrations of ML-236B in the culture broth, probably because of the antifungal activity of the substrate.

ML-236B does not have antibiotic activity on many strains of actinomycetes and bacteria. Therefore, identified cultures and isolates of these unaffected strains from soil samples were tested for their ability to hydroxylate ML-236B.

The microflora in soil are greatly affected by environmental conditions such as climate, vegetation, and mineralogical properties. We collected soil samples from several areas of Australia, which has different environmental conditions from those of Japan. In general, the pH values of Australian soils are higher, and the contents of organic matter and moisture are lower than in Japanese soils. These characteristics of Australian soils are not favorable for microorganisms, particularly actinomycetes. Thus, actinomycetes found in such conditions would be expected to possess unusual characteristics.

Isolates from soil samples collected in Australia had potent hydroxylating abilities on ML-236B at the 6β-position. The strains were identified as *Amycolata* (formerly *Nocardia*). Because of the identification of these soil isolates as *Amycolata*, some strains of this genus from the stock culture were tested for hydroxylating activity. It was found that *Amycolata autotrophica* could hydroxylate ML-236B to pravastatin.

Strain SANK 62781 was identified as a strain of A. *autotrophica*. Strains SANK 62881 and SANK 62981 were identified as new subspecies of A. *autotrophica* for which the name A. *autotrophica* subsp. *canberrica* and A. *autotrophica* subsp. *amethystina* have been proposed, respectively (26,27). All A. *autotrophica* strains were found to tolerate ML-236B and to have strong transformation activities, and all produced dihydroxylated by-product. The supply of pravastatin produced by bioconversion using these strains was sufficient for pharmacological tests and developmental studies.

2.   *Streptomyces carbophilus* as a Potent Converter of ML-236B

To produce pravastatin on an industrial scale, we screened for microorganisms having strong hydroxylating activity and that produced few by-products (12,13,28). A. *autotrophica* strains grew well on D-trehalose media. After further screening for fresh isolates of actinomycetes that grew on D-trehalose, strain SANK 62585, isolated from Australian soil, was discovered as a potent converter producing only limited by-products. The morphological and physiological characteristics suggested that strain SANK 62585 belonged to the genus *Streptomyces*. Among known species of *Streptomyces*, *Streptomyces regenesis* shared the most similarities with strain SANK 62585. Strain SANK 62585 differed from S. *regensis* in four main points: spore chain form, spore chain length, melanoid pigment, and soluble pigment. These differences suggested that strain SANK 62585 should be classified as a new species of the genus *Streptomyces*, to which the name *Streptomyces carbophilus* was given.

C.   Hydroxylation Mechanism of ML-236B to Pravastatin by a Novel Actinomycete Cytochrome P-450

A most noteworthy finding was the discovery of S. *carbophilus* as a potent converter. This permitted the production of pravastatin on an industrial scale. An understanding of the hydroxylation mechanism of ML-236B to pravastatin is requisite for industrial-scale production.

As mentioned previously, pravastatin was first found as a minor urinary metabolite of ML-236B in dogs, suggesting the participation of hepatic cytochromes P-450. When pravastatin was later obtained from microbes, a microbial counterpart to cytochrome P-450 was anticipated to play a role in this hydroxylation.

For the last two decades, microbial cytochrome P-450 has been studied as a model system of those in higher animals. In prokaryotes, the most extensive studies have been carried out on the camphor hydroxylation system in *Pseudomonas putida* (29–33). Other well-studied bacterial cytochrome P-450 proteins are the fatty acid hydroxylation system in *Bacillus megaterium* ATCC 14581 (34–38), the steroid hydroxylation system in B. *megaterium* ATCC 13368 (39), and cytochrome P-450c in *Rhizobium japonicum* (40). The cytochrome P-450 proteins that catalyze the hydroxylation of 6-deoxyerythronolide B, an intermediate of erythromycin A biosynthesis in *Saccharopolyspora erythraea* (formerly *Streptomyces erythraeus*), have been characterized (41). In actinomycetes, cytochrome P-450–dependent monooxygenase systems were found to participate in the detoxification of xenobiotics; the induction of cytochrome P-450s was also observed (42,43).

1.   Purification and Characterization of Cytochrome P-450sca from S. carbophilus

The soluble cytochrome P-450 induced by ML-236B • Na was detected in the cell-free extract prepared from sonically disrupted S. *carbophilus*. The soluble cytochrome P-450 was induced by ML-236B • Na in *S. carbophilus* as detected in its cell-free extract. A characteristic absorption maximum at 451 nm corresponding to cytochrome *P*-450 appeared only when ML-236B • Na was added to the medium, demonstrating the induction of cytochrome *P*-450 by ML-236B • Na. Because it originates from *S. carbophilus*, we named it cytochrome *P*-450sca. Cytochrome *P*-450sca has two isomers (12). The specific activities of cytochromes *P*-450sca-1 and *P*-450sca-2 were 17.63 and 19.62 nmol/mg protein, respectively. Electrophoresis of cytochrome *P*-450sca-1 and *P*-450sca-2 revealed a single protein band of 46 + 1 kDa, suggesting that cytochromes *P*-450sca-1 and *P*-450sca-2 might be identical. However, the amino acid compositions of cytochromes *P*-450sca-1 and *P*-450sca-2 differed. The differing compositions, and thus differing molecular masses, of these enzymes should result in two distinct bands upon electrophoresis. At the present time, we cannot determine why these peptides are not separated by electrophoresis. Identical bands were obtained when electrophoresis was performed without addition of 2-mercaptoethanol. In Western blot analysis of cytochromes *P*-450sca-1 and cytochrome *P*-450sca-2, both proteins reacted similarly to the anti-(cytochrome *P*-450sca-2) antibody.

The reduced-CO versus reduced difference spectra both of purified cytochromes *P*-450sca-1 and *P*-450sca-2 showed absorbance maxima at 448 nm. The addition of ML-236B • Na to a cytochromes *P*-450sca-1 or *P*-450sca-2 solution caused an immediate shift to the high-spin form with the Soret peak appearing at 386 nm. K_s values obtained by the substrate difference spectra were 179 mM for cytochrome *P*-450sca-1 and 229 mM for cytochrome *P*-450sca-2. The absorption spectra of the oxidized cytochromes *P*-450sca-1 and *P*-450sca-2 had absorption maxima at 417, 537, and 573 nm, and those for both proteins reduced by dithionite had absorption maxima at 413 and 544 nm. The CO-bound reduced forms of both proteins had absorption maxima at 420, 447, and 549 nm.

Amino acid analysis showed that the composition of cytochromes *P*-450sca-1 and *P*-450sca-2 are closely related to other bacterial cytochromes *P*-450 (Table 1) (12,44). Cytochromes *P*-450sca-1 and *P*-450sca-2 contained hydrophobic residues in relatively high percentages (46 and 47%, respectively), as is generally observed in other cytochromes *P*-450. To gain additional insights into *P*-450sca and the *P*-450sca gene, the use of recombinant techniques will be required.

2. A Two-Component-Type Cytochrome P-450 in Prokaryotes that Catalyzes Hydroxylation of ML-236B • Na to Pravatstatin

This section describes resolution of the cytochrome *P*-450 monooxygenase system of *S. carbophilus*, purification of the NADH-cytochrome *P*-450 reductase, and reconstitution of the hydroxylation activity by endogenous components (13).

Incubation of the cell-free extracts from *S. carbophilus* with pyridine nucleotides and ML-236B • Na indicated that the cytochrome *P*-450sca monooxygenase system required NADH as an electron donor. We used NADH as electron donor and DCIP as an artificial electron acceptor for assay of electron transfer in the cytochrome *P*-450sca monooxygenase system. In general, actinomycetous cytochrome *P*-450 systems require NADH. This is in contrast with mammalian cytochrome *P*-450 systems, in which NADH is not required (13).

NADH-cytochrome *P*-450 reductase was purified as a single polypeptide chain with a molecular weight of 51 kDa. The absorption spectrum of the purified protein showed typical flavoprotein absorption maxima at 370 and 446 nm, and a shoulder at 475 nm. Consistent with the detection of the flavin prosthetic group, the purified NADH-

Table 1 Amino Acid Composition[a] of Bacterial and Mammalian Cytochrome P-450 Proteins

Amino acid	P-450$_{sca-1}$	P-450$_{sca-2}$	P-450I	P-450$_{cam}$	RLM (rat liver)
Asx	39	37	45	35	42
Thr	31	30	22	19	23
Ser	22	21	17	24	26
Glx	42	40	48	56	42
Pro	27	27	31	30	24
Gly	29	26	36	25	35
Ala	48	45	41	31	23
Cys	3	2	n.d.[b]	8	4
Val	31	30	30	25	28
Met	8	8	7	10	8
Ile	18	18	18	26	29
Leu	50	49	53	42	53
Tyr	5	5	6	9	16
Phe	15	15	19	18	28
His	14	14	5	13	14
Lys	9	8	9	12	29
Arg	34	34	35	27	17
Trp	1	1	n.d.	4	4
Total	426	410	n.d.	414	445

Source: Ref. 12.

[a] The composition of cytochromes P-450$_{cam}$ and P-450$_{sca-2}$ were obtained from nucleotide sequencing data. The composition of cytochrome P-450I, rat liver cytochrome P-450, and cytochrome P-450$_{sca-1}$ were determined by amino acid analysis.

[b] n.d., not determined

cytochrome P-450 reductase protein contained FAD and FMN molecules. The FMN molecule was easily dissociated from the reductase ($K_d = 5 \times 10^{-5}$ M).

NADH-dependent reductase catalyzed the hydroxylation of ML-236B • Na to pravastatin in the presence of a purified cytochrome P-450sca (13). Elimination of cytochrome P-450sca or reductase from this assay system abolished all hydroxylating activity. These two proteins were essential for the reconstitution of hydroxylation. The addition of iron–sulfur protein or phosphatidylcholine to this system did not enhance activity. Neither did the addition to this system of phosphatidylethanolamine, which is a component of the membrane in streptomycetes, or total lipid extracted from S. *carbophilus* stimulate hydroxylating activity. A production mechanism for the synthesis of pravastatin in S. *carbophilus* is proposed in Figure 5 based on these findings.

Cytochrome P-450 monooxygenase systems can be classified as of either two- or three-component type (43). Three-component-type systems are composed of cytochrome P-450 reductase, cytochrome P-450, and an iron–sulfur protein, whereas two-component-type systems are composed of cytochrome P-450 reductase and cytochrome P-450. The results of many previous works have shown that almost all prokaryotes have three-component (mitochondrial) type cytochrome P-450 systems (29,45,46), and those of eukaryotes, such as yeast, are of the two-component (microsomal) type (47). Cytochrome

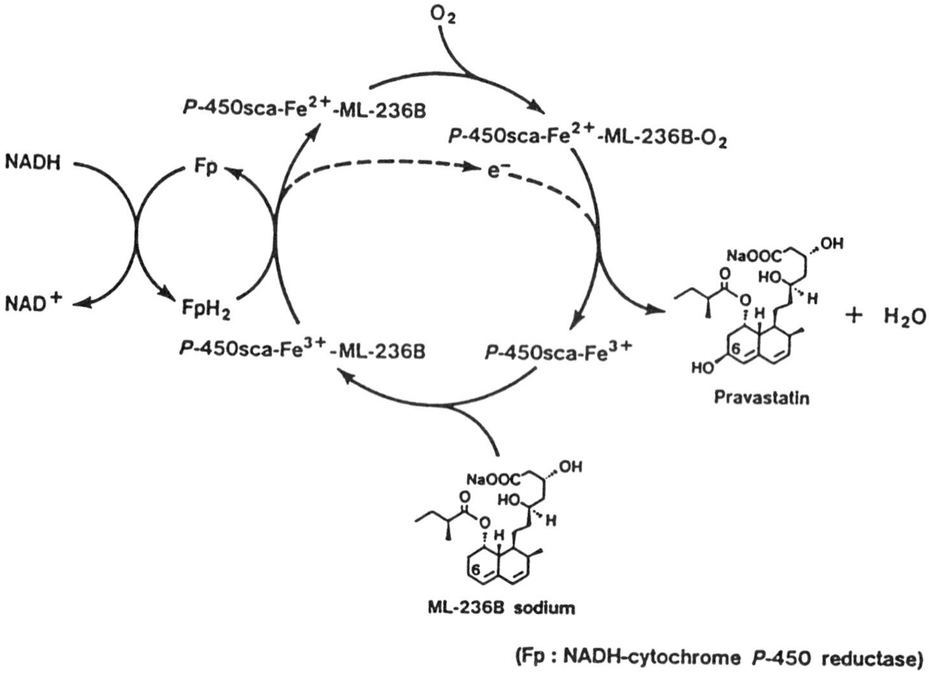

Figure 5　A proposed mechanism for the synthesis of pravastatin in *S. carbophilus*.

P-450BM-3, from *B. megaterium*, exists as a single polypeptide that is capable of catalyzing the entire monooxygenase reaction of a substrate with the addition of only NADPH and O_2 (34).

However, a two-component-type cytochrome P-450 monooxygenase system has not been reported for prokaryotes. The cytochrome P-450sca monooxygenase system is composed of P-450 and flavoprotein, and the addition of ferredoxin did not stimulate any hydroxylation activity. NADH-cytochrome P-450 reductase from *S. carbophilus* contained both FAD and FMN. Therefore, the cytochrome P-450sca monooxygenase system should be classified as a two-component-type system. Many previous studies have indicated that all two-component-type cytochrome P-450 systems require phospholipid. However, phosphatidylcholine, phosphatidylethanolamine, and total lipid fraction from *S. carbophilus* do not enhance the enzyme activity of the P-450 system. The cytochrome P-450sca monooxygenase system may exist in the soluble fraction, whereas all previously described two-component-type cytochrome P-450 systems are membrane bound. Thus, the presence of a two-component-type system in a prokaryote is novel.

The prokaryotic nature of actinomycetes has been confirmed by determination of their fine structure and chemical composition; however, they have also been regarded as a group of organisms with affinities to both bacteria and fungi. Considered together, the intermediate character of the cytochrome P-450sca monooxygenase system, with features between those of prokaryotes and eukaryotes, may reflect the position of actinomycetes in evolution.

III. FERMENTATION TECHNOLOGICAL APPROACH

To produce microbial products in an industrial-scale fermentation, several kinds of techniques are required. Strain and medium improvements are very effective in increasing the yield of fermentation products. However, as the yield increases, problems often arise, such as product inhibition or limitation of dissolved oxygen (DO). To overcome these problems, it is important to study the characteristics of the strains and determine which biochemical engineering approaches are effective. In this section, we describe mainly a mycelial morphology control and computer application for both two-step fermentations.

A. Fermentative Production of ML-236B by *P. citrinum*

To produce a consistantly high yield of ML-236B, we carried out the following research (48):

1. Increase in the rate of oxygen uptake by addition of a surfactant
2. Effect of morphology on ML-236B production
3. Computer control of ML-236B production based on fuzzy logic

1. Increase in the Rate of Oxygen Uptake by Addition of a Surfactant

As the ML-236B production increased by strain improvement, oily and waxy precipitates were liberated by the strain, and ML-236B production stopped. Microscopic observation showed that the oily substance easily attached to the mycelial surface. To dissolve this oily substance, addition of a surfactant was investigated. The effect of addition of a surfactant on ML-236B production in a 30 liter fermentor is shown in Figure 6. ML-236B production in the cultivation with added surfactant was 30% higher than that of control culture without added surfactant. A flask culture study confirmed that this oily substance was removed by the addition of surfactant and that the rate of oxygen uptake increased (49).

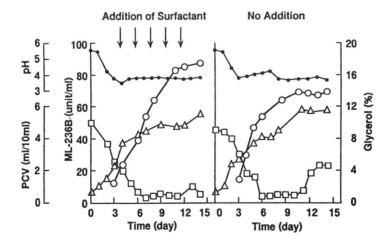

Figure 6   Effect of surfactant addition on ML-236B production. △, PCV (paced cell volume); □, glycerol concentration; ●, pH; ○, ML-236B production (units/ml); ↓, addition of 0.5% of surfactant.

2. Effect of Morphology on ML-236B Production

In submerged cultures, filamentous microorganisms exhibit two types of morphology, the filamentous and the pellet forms. Mycelial morphology often affects culture rheology (50) and production of secondary metabolites. Pellet growth is known to be favorable for citric acid production by *A. niger* (51) and itaconic acid production by *A. erreus* (52), whereas filamentous growth is favorable for penicillin production by *Penicillium chrysogenum* (53) or fumaric acid production by *Rhizopus arrhizus* (54).

In the case of *P. citrinum*, pellet growth is favorable for ML-236B production (55). Figure 7 shows the time courses of ML-236B production cultures containing either the pellet or the filamentous form. In the culture with pellet form, the culture broth had a low viscosity and DO could be readily maintained at more than 3 ppm, and ML-236B production increased to 76 units/ml. On the other hand, in the culture with filamentous form, the viscosity of the culture broth became very high and DO decreased to 0 ppm at the maximum agitation speed. Under these conditions, ML-236B production was less than 10 units/ml.

Table 2 shows the effect of the number of free mycelia inoculated into the flask culture on ML-236B production. As the number of free mycelia inoculated into the production culture increased, the number of pellets increased and the diameters decreased. When more than 3×10^6 free mycelia were inoculated, the morphology of the production culture broth changed to the filamentous form. From this result, the optimum pellet diameter for producing ML-236B was estimated to be as small as possible, if the pellet forms were maintained.

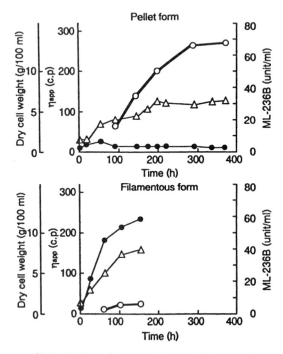

Figure 7 Time courses of ML-236B production culture exhibiting pellet and filamentous forms. ○, ML-236B production (units/ml); △, dry cell weight (g/100 ml); ●, apparent viscosity at a shear rate of 125/sec.

Table 2 Effect of the Number of Free Mycelia on ML-236B Production in S-5808[a]

No. of inoculated free mycelia (ml^{-1})	No. of pellets formed (ml^{-1})	Diameter of pellet[b] (μm)	ML-236B production[b] (units/ml)
9.2×10^6	3.3×10^6 [c]	Filamentous	32
3.1×10^6	2.8×10^6 [c]	Filamentous	37
9.2×10^5	9.0×10^4	60–100	47
3.1×10^5	1.8×10^4	150–300	44
9.2×10^4	6.6×10^3	300–400	40
3.1×10^4	1.3×10^3	400–800	42
9.2×10^3	2.0×10^2	600–1000	32
3.1×10^3	2.0×10^2	1000–1200	6
9.2×10^2	7.5×10	1200–1600	2
3.1×10^2	1.3×10	1000–1800	0.5

[a] Preculture (MBG3-4 medium) was carried out for 4 days, following which the preculture broth was inoculated into a flask containing the production culture medium (MBG3-8 medium).
[b] Pellet diameter and ML-236B production were measured after 9 days of cultivation.
[c] Number of free mycelia was measured by spreading the diluted culture broth on MBG3-4 agar plates and counting the colonies that grew on the plates.

In large-scale fermentation processes, several seed culture steps are required to increase the cell mass for proper inoculum size. Figure 8 shows the changes in pellet size and the number of pellets and free mycelia during four successive seed cultures. There was a tendency for the diameter of the original pellets to increase and the number of pellets to decrease. However, many small pellets, which were clearly distinguishable from the original pellets, appeared in the third seed culture. Taking into consideration the existence of free mycelia in the seed cultures, it is believed that the new pellets were formed by agglomeration of the free mycelia.

From these results, we considered that in order to produce small pellets in great numbers in the main culture, the number of free mycelia in the final seed culture should be more than 10^6/ml. However, after four successive seed cultures, it was impossible to increase free mycelia to more than 10^4 or 10^5 with pellet growth. We considered that the number of free mycelia in seed cultures could be increased by changing the morphology in the seed culture from the pellet form to the filamentous form.

Metz (56,57) reported that the following factors affect mycelial morphology: agitation (mechanical shearing) (58,59), medium concentration, aeration (60), pH, inoculation amount, surfactant addition, and growth rate. A high concentration medium (HCP medium) was the most effective for changing the mycelial morphology from pellet to filamentous in *P. citrinum*.

A seed strain in which the fourth seed culture was used to inoculate the production fermentor was very important for obtaining a constant number of free mycelia. Figure 9 shows the relationship between agitation speed and the number of free mycelia during the fourth seed culture, and between ML-236B production in the production fermentor and free mycelia in the fourth seed culture. DO concentration in the fourth seed culture was controlled at more than 3 ppm by changing the agitation speed. Agitation speed increased as the cell mass and number of free mycelia increased. The number of free mycelia was proportional to the agitation speed when the fourth preculture broth was inoculated into the production culture. Maximum ML-236B production was obtained

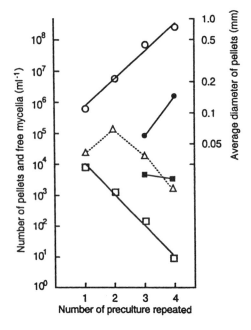

Figure 8 Effect of repeating preculture on morphology. ○, average diameter of original pellets; □, number of original pellets; ●, average diameter of new pellets; ■, number of new pellets; △, number of free mycelia.

when a culture containing 2 to 4×10^6/ML-236B of free mycelia was used to inoculate the production fermentor.

These results suggest that inoculation of the production fermentor from a fourth seed culture broth is the most suitable for ML-236B production when the agitation speed in the fourth seed culture is increased to about 450 to 550 rpm.

Figure 10 shows the time course data for the ML-236B production culture. In the new process, the growth rate is faster and pellet size smaller than those in the conventional process. In the new process, pH of the culture broth decreased to 4, which is the optimum for ML-236B production, after 50 hr of cultivation. In the conventional process, on the other hand, pH did not decrease to 4 until 150 hr. ML-236B production in the new process is 50% higher than that in the conventional process.

To examine the consistency of ML-236B production with the new process, 10 fermentation runs were conducted under identical culture and preculture conditions; we ensured that the number of free mycelia in the fourth seed culture was virtually constant in all 10 runs. We found the morphology controlling method enabled us to form small pellets in great numbers in the production culture, and to produce a consistently high yield of ML-236B.

3. Computer Control of ML-236B Production Based on Fuzzy Logic

ML-236B production culture by *P. citrinum* depended strictly on the culture broth pH, which was regulated by the sugar feed rate (61). In the past, skilled operators regulated pH by manually controlling the rate of sugar feeding. Although relatively effective, this process is highly laborious, as it requires constant monitoring and adjustment throughout

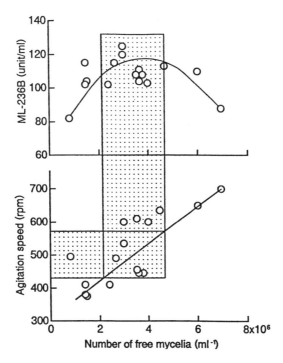

Figure 9 Relationship between agitation speed and number of free mycelia in the fourth preculture, and between ML-236B production in production culture and free mycelia in the fourth preculture. The boxed area indicates the optimum region of agitation speed and the number of free mycelia for ML-236B production.

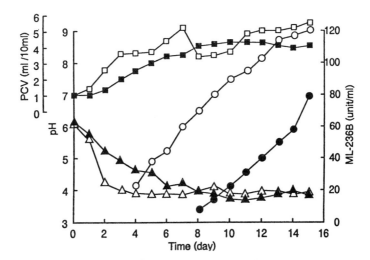

Figure 10 Time courses of ML-236B production culture using the new (open symbols) and conventional (filled symbols) preculture processes. ○, ML-236B production (units/ml); △, pH; □, PCV; ◇, maltose concentration (g/liter).

cultivation. Thus, we have attempted to develop an automatic system for controlling the rate of sugar feeding. Recently, fuzzy control methods were applied to the system based on the intuition and experience of experts and skilled operators. In the fermentation processes, fuzzy logic has been applied to baker's yeast production (62), the moromi process for Japanese sake production (63–65), and glutamic acid production (66,67), to name a few examples.

To construct software for fuzzy control, it is necessary to design membership functions and fuzzy rules. The rules for the production culture are given in Table 3. In these, sugar concentration in the culture broth is an important variable for controlling pH, and so we attempted to estimate the sugar consumption from the CO_2 evolution rate. Figure 11 shows the relationship between total CO_2 evolved and the amount of sugar consumed. The correlation coefficient for the regression line was calculated to be 0.91. We decided that total CO_2 evolution should be adopted as a parameter for fuzzy control since it showed a good linear relationship with sugar consumption.

Figure 12 shows the typical time course of ML-236B production culture with manual control of the sugar feeding rate. We determined that cultivation could be divided into five clusterized phases. The feeding control strategy was altered for each phase; phase 1 is "before feeding," phase 2 is "feeding start," phase 3 is "adjust pH according to pH value," phase 4 is "adjust pH by pH value and pH slope," and phase 5 is "stable control phase."

Figure 13 shows the membership function for each state variable and the method of control in each phase. All the rules and classifications are those described in Table 3. We used the total CO_2 evolved, pH, and pH slope as measurement variables for control. S,

Table 3   Rules for Culture Phase Identification and Selection of Sugar Feeding

1. If the concentration of the reducing sugar is more than 1%, then the culture is in phase 1, and no sugar is to be fed.

2. If the concentration of the reducing sugar is less than 1% during the period from 30 to 50 hr after starting the cultivation, then the culture is in phase 2, and the sugar feeding is to be maintained at a constant feed rate.

3 If the pH value is less than 4.3, then the culture is in phase 3, and the feed rate is to be gradually reduced.

4. If the pH value is less than 4.0 and the slope of the pH begins to rise, then the culture is in phase 4, and the feed rate should be gradually increased.

5 If the pH value is around the set point, then the feed rate should be decided on according to the following relationship:

pH value	Sugar feed rate
High	Increase
Low	Decrease
Slope of pH	Sugar feed rate
Up	Increase
Down	Decrease

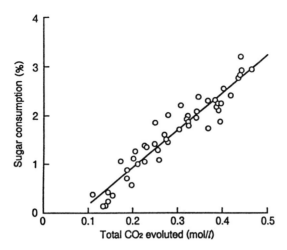

Figure 11 Relationship between sugar consumption and total CO$_2$ evolved.

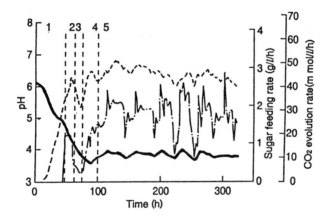

Figure 12 Time courses of CO$_2$ evolution, sugar feeding, and pH in ML-236B production culture under manual control of the sugar feed rate. -----, CO$_2$ evolution rate (mmol/liter/hr); ---, sugar feeding rate (g/liter/hr); ——, pH. Cultivation was divided into five phases, where the feeding strategy was as described in Section III. A.3, Figure 14, and Table 3.

M, and B are abbreviations for small, medium, and big, respectively. We used the phase clusterization method reported by Konstantin (68) and Kishimoto (66). First, the phase of culture growth was determined from the pattern of the state variable classified by each membership function. Second, the probability that the measured state falls into the phase was calculated. Third, the value of the operative variable was calculated for each situation. Sugeno's third inference method (69) was used for defuzzification.

A schematic diagram of the instruments used in the fuzzy control experiments is given in Figure 14. Data on exhaust CO$_2$, pH, DO, and agitation speed were collected by the system controller, and these were sent to the control computer. Feeding rates were calculated using fuzzy theory. Figure 15 shows the time course of ML-236B production

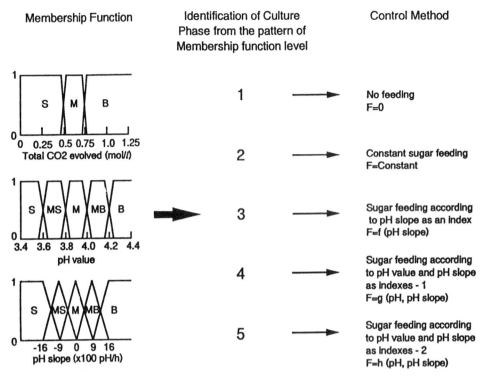

Figure 13 The membership function for each state variable and the method of control in each phase, referring to the rules and classification shown in Table 3.

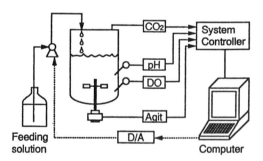

Figure 14 Schematic diagram of computer control system using fuzzy theory.

culture under fuzzy control. The time course of probability of the classified culture phases inferred by fuzzy rules are shown in the upper portion. Sugar feeding began when the maltose concentration was about 10 g/liter. The pH value decreased gradually and was controlled to 3.8 to 4.0 after 80 hr of cultivation. By using the fuzzy control system, the pH value could be accurately maintained. We could therefore examine the effect of pH on ML-236B production. We found that the optimum pH range for ML-236B production was from 3.7 to 3.9. ML-236B production under fuzzy control was 10% higher than that

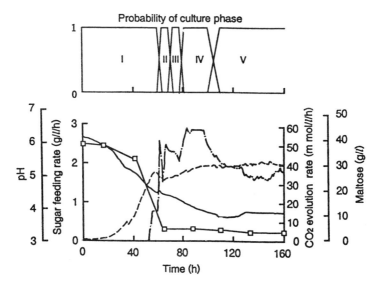

Figure 15   Time courses of probability of culture phases in ML-236B production culture with fuzzy control of sugar feed rate. -----, CO_2 evolution rate (mmol/liter/hr); — sugar feeding rate (g/liter); ——, pH. □, maltose concentration (g/liter).

under manual control. We believe that precise control of the pH value by fuzzy logic yielded the high ML-236B production.

B.   Control of Microbial Hydroxylation

Many studies have been made of computer control of the fermentation process. One of the limitations in computer control of fermentation is the difficulty in monitoring the factors affecting the production yield (70,71). In recent years, many investigators have reported that the components of fermentation broth, such as key nutrients and metabolites, may be analyzed on-line by using a combined system of continuous filtration module and high-performance liquid chromatography (HPLC) (72,73). We tried to apply this system to large-scale pravastatin fermentation (74). Of the several strains (28) that converted ML-236B into pravastatin, *S. carbophilus* was the best considering conversion ratio, conversion rate, and total amount of substrate fed in one batch of culture. Matsuoka et al. (12) found that the enzyme for hydroxylation was cytochrome *P-450*. However, in fed-batch culture of this strain, when ML-236B • Na was fed too quickly in manual control, the hydroxylation reaction was inhibited, causing ML-236B to accumulate in the broth.

Figure 16 shows the time courses of the *P-450* concentration, conversion rate, and ML-236B • Na concentration during the conversion culture with manual control of the feed rate. As the ML-236B • Na concentration increased, the *P-450* concentration and the conversion rate also increased. It appears that the amount of *P-450* induced is directly proportional to the concentration of ML-236B • Na, unless the ML-236B • Na concentration is high enough to be inhibitory. From this, we hypothesized that a higher conversion rate could be obtained by keeping ML-236B • Na concentration at an optimum level. Figure 17 shows the schematic diagram of the computer control system for regulat-

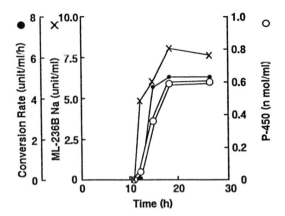

Figure 16   Time course of concentration of cytochrome *P*-450 induced by ML-236B•Na. ×, ML-236B•Na concentration (units/ml); ○, cytochrome *P*-450 concentration (nmol/ml); ●, conversion rate (units/ml/hr).

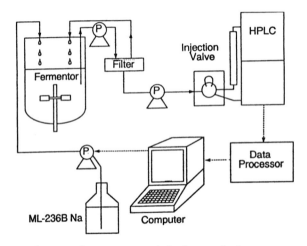

Figure 17   Schematic diagram of computer coupled substrate feeding system.

ing ML-236B • Na concentration in the fermentor. The fermentation broth was filtered through a flow filtration module. A fixed amount of filtrate was transferred to HPLC at certain intervals. ML-236B • Na concentration data measured by HPLC were transmitted to the control computer. The computer analyzed the data and calculated the feed rate of ML-236B • Na to keep the ML-236B • Na concentration in the culture broth.

The block diagram for the control system of ML-236B • Na concentration in the broth is shown in Figure 18. The feed rate was calculated by using the estimated conversion rate (CVR_{ES}), and the data on ML-236B • Na concentration was analyzed by the automatic monitoring system. The conversion rate was calculated using the following equation. As the difference between V_1 and V_2 is very small,

$$CVR = \frac{F}{V} + ML_1 - ML_2 \tag{1}$$

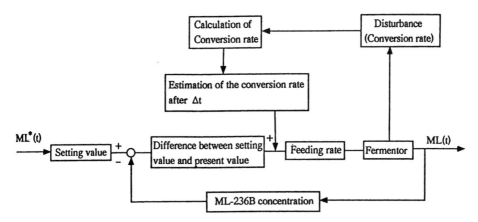

Figure 18 Block diagram of software of control system.

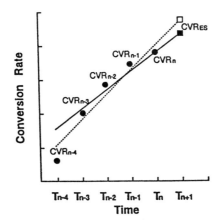

Figure 19 Estimation of conversion rate. Conversion rate at T_{n+1} is estimated using five data sets of conversion rate (CVR_{n-4} to CVR_n; conversion rate at T_{n-4} to T_n). ●, conversion rate obtained; ■, estimated conversion rate using regression analysis with weight on conversion rate that is heavier near T_n; □, estimated conversion rate using regression analysis without weight. ——, regression analysis with weight; ·····, regression analysis without weight.

Figure 19 shows the estimation method for the conversion rate (30). The estimated conversion rate (CVR_{ES}) at the time ($T_n + 1$) after Δt from the last sampling time (T_n) was determined by using regression analysis of the latest five conversion rates by adding the weight of CVR_{n-4} to CVR_n. Using CVR_{ES} and ML_n, the feeding rate was defined by the following equation, where ML_{st} is the set point for the concentration of ML-236B • Na.

$$\frac{F}{V} = \frac{CVR_{ES}\,\Delta t - (ML_{st} - ML_n)}{\Delta t} \tag{2}$$

We applied these feed-back and feed-forward control methods to this system. The relationship between ML-236B • Na concentration and conversion rate was investigated using a 30 liter fermentor (Figure 20). ML-236B • Na concentration was kept at 0, 2.5,

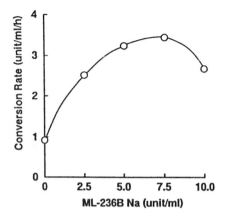

Figure 20   Relationship between ML-236B•Na concentration and the average conversion rate.

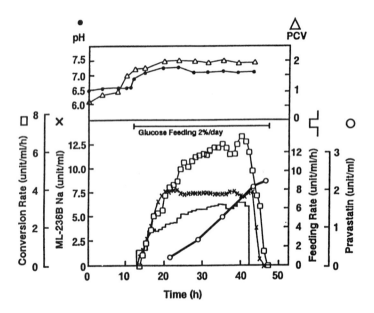

Figure 21   Time course of cultivation in pilot-scale fermentor (6000 liters) under computer control of ML-236B•Na concentration. ×, ML-236B•Na concentration (units/ml); ○, pravastatin concentration (units/ml); □, conversion rate (units/ml/hr); ⌐⌐, feeding rate (units/ml/hr); ●, pH; △, packed cell volume (ml/10 ml broth)

5.0, 7.5, or 10.0 units/ML-236B using the computer control system. The highest average conversion rate was obtained between 5.0 and 7.5 units/ML-236B.

The microbial conversion culture with computer-coupled substrate feeding system was scaled up from the 30 liter fermentor to a 6000 liter fermentor (Figure 21). This is one example of the time course of pravastatin production in the 6000 liter fermentor under computer control. When glucose was consumed completely and pH value increased sharply at about 12 hr after inoculation, feeding of ML-236B • Na and glucose was begun.

ML-236B • Na concentration increased to the optimum level (7.5 ± 0.2 units/ML-236B) and was maintained at this level for over 20 hr. Using this computer-coupled system, volumetric productivity of pravastatin was increased threefold over that of manual control. To increase pravastatin production to an industrial scale, several biochemical technology techniques are applied. In particular, the mycelial morphology control method and application of computer control were consistently effective in increasing ML-236B and pravastatin production. We have already used all these techniques in an industrial-scale fermentor.

IV. CONCLUSION

More than 20 years have passed since we started screening culture broths for inhibitors of cholesterol biosynthesis. As a result of our efforts, ML-236B was discovered in Japan as the first potent and specific inhibitor of HMG-CoA reductase. This compound contributed to the Nobel Prize–winning work of Goldstein and Brown in which they elucidated the mechanism of the low-density lipoprotein (LDL) receptor pathway. After the discovery of ML-236B, many attempts were made to find other HMG-CoA reductase inhibitors, and some potent inhibitors including pravastatin have already been commercialized. The HMG-CoA reductase inhibitors currently available share several characteristics: (a) clear mechanism of cholesterol-lowering effects, (b) potent activity for lowering LDL cholesterol levels, (c) predictable responsiveness for efficacy, and (d) high tolerability. Because of these characteristics, HMG-CoA reductase inhibitors are in clinical use worldwide and play a pivotal role in the therapy of hyperlipidemic patients.

Pravastatin is produced by a two-step fermentation: first, ML-236B is produced by *P. citrinum*, followed by the hydroxylation of ML-236B by *S. carbophilus* to form pravastatin. In an effort to increase the productivity of these fermentation processes, new technologies have been developed, and the mechanism of hydroxylation has been extensively investigated.

REFERENCES

1. Page HI, Berrettoni JN, Butkus A, Sones FM Jr. Prediction of coronary heart disearse based on clinical suspicion, age, total cholesterol, and triglyceride. Circulation 1970; 42:625.
2. Kannel WB, Castelli W, Gordon T, McNamara PM. Serum cholesterol, lipoproteins, and the risk of coronary heart disease. Ann Intern Med 1971; 74:1–12.
3. The Pooling Project Research Group (Cook L). Relationship of blood pressure serum cholesterol, smoking habit, relative weight and ecg abnormalities to incidence of major coronary events. Final report of the pooling project. J Chron Dis 1978; 31:201.
4. Stamler J, Wentworth D, Neaton J. Is relationship between risk of premature death from coronary heart disease continuous and graded? Findings in 356,666 primary screenees of the Multiple Risk Factor Intervention Trial. J Am Med Assoc 1986; 256:2823–2828.
5. Lipid Research Clinics Program. The lipid research clinics coronary primary prevention trial results. I. Production in incidence of coronary heart disease. J Am Med Assoc 1984; 251:351–364.
6. Lipid Research Clinics Program. The lipid research clinics coronary primary prevention trial results. II. The relationship of reduction in incidence of coronary heart disease to cholesterol lowering. J Am Med Assoc 1984; 251:365–374.

7. Frick MH, Elo O, Haapa K, Heinonen OP, Heinsalmi P, Helo P, et al. Helsinki Heart Study: Primary-prevention trial with gemfibrozil in middle-aged men with dyslipidmia. Safety of treatment, changes in risk factors, and incidence of coronary heart disease. N Engl J Med 1987; 317:1237–1245.

8. Dietschy JM, Wilson JD. Regulation of cholesterol metabolism. N Engl J Med 1970; 282:1179–1183.

9. Endo A, Kuroda M, Tsujita Y, Terahara A, Tamura C. Jap. Pat., Kokai, 50-155690; 1975.

10. Brown AG, Smale TC, King TJ, Hasenkam R, Thompson RH. Crystal and molecular structure of compactin, a new antifungal metabolite from *Penicilliun brevicompactum*. J Chem Soc Perkin Trans 1976; 1:1165.

11. Tsujita Y, Kuroda M, Shimada Y, Tanzawa K, Arai M, et al. CS-514, a competitive inhibitor of 3-hydroxy-3-methylglutaryl coenzyme A reductase: Tissue-selective inhibition of sterol synthesis and hypolipidemic effect on various animal species. Biochim Biophys Acta 1986; 877:50–60.

12. Matsuoka T, Miyakoshi S, Tanzawa K, Nakahara K, Hosobuchi M, Serizawa N. Purification and characterization of cytochrome P-450sca from *Streptomyces carbophilus*. Eur J Biochem 1989; 184:707.

13. Serizawa N, Matsuoka T. A two component-type cytochrome P-450 monooxygenase system in a prokaryote that catalyzes hydroxylation of ML-236B to pravastatin, a tissue-selective inhibitor of 3-hydroxy-3-methylglutaryl coenzyme A reductase. Biochim Biophys Acta 1991; 1084:35–40.

14. Shiao M-S, Don H-S. Biosynthesis of mevinolin, a hypocholestrolemic fungal metabolite, in *Aspergillus terreus*. Proc Natl Sci Counc B 1987; Rec. 11:223–231.

15. Nara F, Watanabe I, Serizawa N. Development of a transformation system for filamentous, ML-236B (compactin)-producing fungus *Penicillium citrinum*. Curr Genet 1993; 23:28–32.

16. Nara F, Watanabe I, Serizawa N. Cloning and sequencing of the 3-phosphoglycerate kinase (PGK) gene from *Penicillium citrinum* and its application to heterologous gene expression. Curr Genet 1993; 23:134–140.

17. Queener SW, Ignolia TD, Skatrud PL, Chapman JL, Kaster KR. A system for genetic transformation of *Cephalosporium acremonium*. Schlessinger D, ed. Microbiology. Am. Soc. Microbiol., 1985:467.

18. Punt PJ, Oliver RP, Dingemanse MA, Pouwels PH, van der Hondel CAMJJ. Transformation of *Aspergillus* based on the hygromycin B resistance marker from *Escherichia coli*. Gene 1989; 56:117–124.

19. Durand N, Reymond P, Fevre M. Transformation of *Penicillium roqueforti* to phleomycin- and to hygromycin B-resistance. Curr Genet 1991; 19:149.

20. Oliver RP, Roberts IN, Harling R, Kenyon R, Punt PJ, Dingemanse MA, van der Hondel CAMJJ. Transformation of *Fulvia fulva*, a fungal pathogen of tomato, to hygromycin B resistance. Curr Genet 1987; 12:231–233.

21. Kistler HC, Benny UK. Genetic transformation of the fungal wilt pathogen *Fusarium oxysporum*. Curr Genet 1988; 13:145.

22. Hunag D, Bhairi S, Staples RC. A transformation procedure for *Botryotinia squamosa*. Curr Genet 1989; 15:411.

23. Clements JM, Roberts CF. Transcription and processing signals in the 3-phosphoglycerate kinase (PGK) gene *Aspergillus nidulans*. Gene 1986; 44:97–105.

24. Peterson H, Murray HC. Microbiological oxygenation of steroids at carbon 11. J Am Chem Soc 1952; 74:1871.

25. Serizawa N, Nakagawa K, Hamano K, Tsujita Y, Terahara A, Kuwano H. Microbial hydroxylation of ML-236B (compactin) and monacolin K. J Antibiot 1983; 36:604–607.

26. Serizawa N, Serizawa S, Nakagawa K, Furuya K, Okazaki T, Terahara A. Microbial hydroxylation of ML-236B (compactin): Studies on microorganisms capable of 3β-hydroxylation of ML-236B. J Antibiot 1983; 36:887–891.

27. Okazaki T, Serizawa N, Enokita R, Torikata A, Terahara A. Taxonomy of actinomycetes capable of hydroxylation of ML-236B (compactin). J Antibiot 1983; 36:1176–1183.

28. Okazaki T, Enokita R, Miyaoka H, Otani H, Torikata A. *Streptomyces darwinensis* sp. nov., *S. cactaceus* sp. nov., and *S. carbophilus* sp. nov. isolated from Australian soils. Annu Rep Sankyo Res Lab 1989; 41:123.

29. Katagiri M, Ganguli BN, Gunsalus IC. A soluble cytochrome *P*-450 functional in methylene hydroxylation. J Biol Chem 1968; 243:3543–3546.

30. Peterson J. Camphor binding by *Pseudomonas putida* cytochrome P-450. Arch Biochem Biophys 1971; 144:678–693.

31. Poulos TL, Finzel BC, Gunsalus IC, Wagner GC, Kraut J. The 2.6-Å crystal structure of *Pseudomonas putida* cytochrome *P*-450. J Biol Chem 1985; 260:16122–16130.

32. Unger BP, Gunsalus IC, Sliger SG. Nucleotide sequence of the *Pseudomonas putida* cytochrome *P*-450cam gene and its expression in *Escherichia coli*. J Biol Chem 1986; 261:1158–1163.

33. Koga H, Aramaki H, Yamaguchi E, Takeuchi K, Horiuchi T, Gunsalus IC. camR, a negative regulator locus of the cytochrome *P*-450cam hydroxylase operon. J Bacteriol 1986; 166:1089–1095.

34. Narhi LO, Fulco AJ. Phenobarbital induction of a soluble cytochrome *P*-450-dependent fatty acid monooxygenase in *Bacillus megaterium*. J Biol Chem 1982; 257:2147–2150.

35. Schwalb J, Narhi LO, Fulco AJ. Purification and characterization of pentobarbital-induced cytochrome *P*-450BM-1 from *Bacillus megaterium* ATCC 14581. Biochim Biophys Acta 1985; 838:302–311.

36. Narhi LO, Fulco AJ. Characterization of a catalytically self-sufficient 119,000 dalton cytochrome *P*-450 monooxygenase induced by barbiturates in *Bacillus megaterium*. J Biol Chem 1986; 261:7160–7169.

37. Wen LO, Fulco AJ. Cloning of the gene encoding a catalytically self-sufficient cytochrome *P*-450 fatty acid monooxygenase induced by barbiturates in *Bacillus megaterium* and its functional expression and regulation in heterologous (*Escherichia coli*) and homologous (*Bacillus megaterium*) hosts. J Biol Chem 1987; 262:6676–6682.

38. Narhi LO, Fulco AJ. Identification and characterization of two functional domains in cytochrome *P*-450BM-3, a catalytically self-sufficient monooxygenase induced by barbiturates in *Bacillus megaterium*. J Biol Chem 1987; 262:6683.

39. Berg A, Ingelman-Sundberg M, Gustafsson J-A. Purification and characterization of cytochrome *P*-450meg. J Biol Chem 179; 254:5264–5271.

40. Goewert DK, Weaver CC, Carey D, Appleby CA. P-450 hemeproteins of *Rhizobium japonicum*: Purification by affinity chromatography and relationship to P-450cam and P-450$_{LM-2}$. Biochem Biophys Res Commun 1976; 69:437.

41. Shafiee A, Hutchinson R. Macrolide antibiotic biosynthesis: Isolation and properties of two forms of 6-deoxyerythronolide B hydroxylase from *Saccharopolyspora erythraea* (*Streptomyces erythreus*). Biochem 1987; 26:6204–6210.

42. Romesser J, O'Keefe DP. Induction of cytochrome *P*-450-dependent sulfonylurea etabolism in *Streptomyces griseolus*. Biochem Biophys Res Commun 1986; 140:650–659.

43. Sariaslani FS, Kunt DA. Induction of cytochrome *P*-450 in *Streptomyces griseus* by soybean flour. Biochem Biophys Res Commun 1986; 141:405–410.

44. Watanabe I, Nara F, Serizawa N. Cloning, characterization and expression of the gene encoding cytochrome *P*-450$_{sca-2}$ from *Streptomyces carbophilus* involved in production of Pravastatin, a specific HMG-CoA reductase inhibitor. Gene 1995; 163:81–85.

45. Serizawa N. Cytochrome *P*-450 of actinomycetes [in Japanese]. Nippon Nogeikagaku Kaishi 1992; 66:149–153.

46. Sariaslani FS, Trower MK, Buchholz SE. Xenobiotic transformations by *Streptomyces griseus*. Dev Ind Microbiol 1989; 30:161–171.

47. Aoyama Y, Kubota S, Kumaoka H, Furumichi A. NADPH-cytochrome P-450 reductase of yeast microsomes. Arch Biochem Biophys 1978; 185:362.

48. Hosobuchi M, Shioiri T, Ohyama J, Arai M, Iwado S, Yoshikawa H. Production of ML-236B, an inhibitor of 3-hydroxy-3-methylglutaryl CoA reductase, by *Penicillium citrinum*: Improvement of strain and culture conditions. Biosci Biotech Biochem 1993; 57:1414.

49. Ngian KF, Lin SH. Diffusion coefficient of oxygen in microbial aggregates. Biotechnol Bioeng 1976; 18:1623.

50. Kim JH, Lebeault JM, Reuss M. Comparative study on rheological properties of mycelial broth in filamentous and pelleted form. Appl Microb Biotechnol 1983; 18:11.

51. Whitaker A, Long PA. Fungal pelleting. Proc Biochem 1973; 11:27.

52. Clark DS. Submerged citric acid fermentation of ferrocyanide treated beet molasses: Morphology of pellets of *Aspergillus niger*. Can J Microbiol 1962; 8:133.

53. Smith JJ, Lilly MD, Fox RI. The effect of agitation on the morphology and penicillin production of *Penicillium chrysogenum*. Biotechnol Bioeng 1990; 35:1011.

54. Byrne GS, Ward OP. Effect of nutrition on pellet formation by *Rhizopus arrhizus*. Biotechnol Bioeng 1989; 33:912.

55. Hosobuchi M, Ogawa K, Yoshikawa H. Morphology study in production of ML-236B, a precursor of pravastatin sodium, by *Penicillium citrinum*. J Ferment Bioeng 1993; 76:470.

56. Metz B, Kossen NWF. The growth of mold in the form of pellet. Biotechnol Bioeng 1977; 19:781.

57. Metz B, Kossen NWF, Van Suizdum JC. The rheology of mold suspensions. Adv Biochem Eng 1979; 11:103.

58. Bandyopadhyay B, Humphrey AE, Taguchi H. Dynamic measurement of the volumetric oxygen transfer coefficient in fermentation system. Biotechnol Bioeng 1967; 9:533.

59. Mitard A, Riba JP. Morphology and growth of *Aspergillus niger* ATCC 26036 cultivated at several shear rates. Biotechnol Bioeng 1988; 32:835.

60. Wittler R, Baumgartl H, Lubber DW, Schngerl K. Investigation of oxygen transfer into *Penicillium chrysogenum* pellets by microprobe measurement. Biotechnol Bioeng 1986; 28:1024.

61. Hosobuchi M, Fukui F, Suzuki T, Yoshikawa H. Fuzzy control in microbial production of ML-236B, a precusor of pravastatin sodium. J Ferment Bioeng 1993; 76:482.

62. Filev DP, Kishimoto M, Sengupta S, Yoshida T, Taguchi H. Application of fuzzy theory to simulation of batch fermentation J Ferment Technol 1985; 63:545.

63. Oishi K, Tominaga M, Kawato A, Abe Y, Imayasu S, Nanba A. Application of fuzzy control theory to the sake brewing process. J Ferment Technol 1991; 72:115.

64. Tsuchiya Y, Koizumi J, Suenari K, Teshima Y, Nagai S. Construction of fuzzy rules and fuzzy simulator based on the control techniques of Hiroshima Toji (experts) [in Japanese]. Hakko Kogaku 1990; 68:123.

65. Suenari K, Tsuchiya Y, Teshima Y, Koizumi J, Nagai, S., Performance of sake mash brewing with fuzzy control [in Japanese]. Hakko Kogaku 1990; 68:131.

66. Kishimoto M, Yoshida T. Application of fuzzy theory on fermentation process. Hakko Kogaku 1991; 69:107.

67. Nakamura T, Kuratani T, Morita Y. Fuzzy control application to glutamic acid fermentation. Proc. of IFAC Modeling and Control of Biotechnology Process, 1985:211.

68. Konstantin K, Yoshida T. Physiological state control of fermentation processes. Biotechnol Bioeng 1988; 16:1145.

69. Sugeno M. Fuzzy seigyo, 1st ed. Tokyo; Nikkan Kogyo Shinbunsha, 1988:88–90.

70. Dairaku K, Yamane T. Use of the porous teflon tubing method to measure gaseous or volatile substances dissolved in fermentation liquids. Biotechnol Bioeng 1979; 21:1671.

71. Yamane T, Matsuda M, Sada E. Application of porous teflon tubing method to automatic fed-batch culture of microorganisms. II. Automatic constant-value control to fed substrate (ethanol) concentration in semibatch culture yeast. Biotechnol Bioeng 1981; 23:2509.

72. Dincer AK, Kalyanpur M, Skea W, Ryan M, Kierstead T. Continuous on-line monitoring of fermentation processes. Dev Ind Microbiol 1984; 25:603.

73. Bayer T, Herold T, Hiddessen R, Schgerl K. On-line monitoring of media composition during the production of cephalosporin C. Anal Chim Acta 1986; 190:213.

74. Hosobuchi M, Kurosawa K, Yoshikawa H. Application of computer to monitoring and control of fermentation process: Microbial conversion of ML-236B Na to pravastatin. Biotech Bioeng 1993; 42:815.

Index

ABC-transporter (*see* ATP-binding cassette transporter)
absA gene, 57
Acarbose (*see also* Amylostatins), 89
Acetyl-CoA carboxylase, 565
   acc genes encoding, 565
Aclarubicin (Aclacinomycin A) (*see* Anthracyclines) 577, 580, 584, 587, 590-592, 595, 604, 606,   612, 620, 622, 633
Acquired immunodeficiency syndrome (AIDS), 2, 8, 19, 455, 545, 585
Acremonium chrysogenum (*see also* *Cephalosporium acremonium*), 733, 741-748
   cephalosporin C acetylesterase (CAE) of, 744
   strain 3112, 746
   strain A10, 746-747
      A10-14 overproducing derivative, 746-748
      stability of, 746-747
   strain BC2116 (FERM BP-2707), 741
      transformed with plasmids pHBV1 and pHDV11, 741
      transformed with plasmid pHDV11 alone (strain Hm178), 742-748
      production of 7-aminocephalo-sporanic acid (7-ACA) by, 741-748
      production of 7-aminodeacetyl-cephalosporanic acid (7-ADACA) by, 742-748
      recombinant D-amino acid oxidase in, 743-745
      recombinant cephalosporin C acylase in, 743-746
Acremonium luzulae, 309
Acremonium species, 309
Actinomadura, 635
   A. carminata, 580-581, 603
   strain 1029-AV1, 581, 603

[*Actinomadura*]
   A. roseoviolacea, 603
      var. *miuraensis* strain 07, 581, 603
   A. sp. strain D326, 581, 603
   A. sp. strain MG465-yF4, 581, 603
Actinomycetes, 2, 55, 785
Actinomycins, 199, 335-356
   biosynthesis of, 199, 335-356
      amino acid activation in, 337
      catabolite repression in, 350
      elongation in, 345-347
      epimerization in, 337, 346-347
      ester bond formation in, 337
      hydroxykynureninase in, 338, 351
      initiation reactions in, 343-345
      kynureninase in, 338, 349-351
      kynurenine formamidase in, 338, 349-351
      mutants blocked in, 347-350
      N-methylation in, 230, 337, 343
      peptide synthetases in, 336-337, 419
      regulation of, 350-356
         guanosine pentaphosphate (pppGpp) synthetase I in, 355
         guanosine tetraphosphate (ppGpp) in, 354-355
         termination in, 347
      tryptophan pyrrolase in, 349
   C1-C3, 336
   catabolism of tryptophan and, 337
   D, 335, 337, 346
   half molecule of (monocyclic acylpenta-peptide lactones), 341
   3-hydroxyanthranilic acid precursor (3-HA) of, 338
      methylation of, 338
   D-methylamino acids of, 335
   N-methylamino acids of, 335, 342
   4-methyl-3-hydroxyanthranilic acid (4-MHA) precursor of, 337-349
   natural analogs of, 336

[Actinomycins]
  phenoxazinone carboxylic acid (actinocin)
      chromophore of, 337-338
  synthetase of, 338-339, 349-351
      phsA gene forpromotor or regulation
          of, 351-354
      phsB silent gene and, 353
      purification of, 338
      regulation of, 350-352
  strains producing, 336
  synthetase of, 199, 228, 289
      actinomycin synthetase I (ASMS I),
          339, 343, 347-349
          inhibition of, 341
          kinetics of, 340-341
          regulation of, 350
          substrates for, 340
      actinomycin synthetase II (ASMS II),
          342-349
          elongation reactions of, 345-348
          epimerization reactions of, 346-348
          initiation of 4-MHA peptide
              formation by, 344-345
          4'-phosphopantetheine of, 343, 345
      actinomycin synthetase III (ASMS III),
          342-349
          N-methyltransferase domain of, 343
          4'-phosphopantetheine of, 343
Actinoplanes, 375
  A. teichomyceticus, 367-368
  A. utahensis, 319, 415, 419-420
      A21978C lipopeptide complex
          deacylation by, 415, 419-420
      echinocandin deacylase from, 319
  A. spp., 420, 441
      A21978C lipopeptide complex deacyla-
          tion by, 420
      actagardine (lantibiotic) production by,
          441
      strain N902-109 (rapamycin producer),
          498
Actinorhodin, 17, 563, 615, 618, 620, 674,
      684-685, 691-695
  biosynthesis of, 618, 620, 684
      polyketide synthase genes for, 618,
          638-639, 691-695
  production of hybrid antibiotics using,
      17-18, 620, 638-639, 684-686,
      691-695
      aloesaponarin II, 17-18, 620, 638-639,
          684, 686, 691-694
      desoxyerythrolaccin, 684, 686, 691
      dihydrogranatirhodin, 684-685

[Actinorhodin]
    mederrhodin A, 638, 684-685
    structure of, 685
Actinospectacin (*see* Spectinomycin)
Actinospectose, 106
Actinosporangium
    A. bohemicum C-36145 (ATCC 31127),
        605
    A. brunnea, 663
    A. sp., 552
Acyclovir, 2
Aculeacin Aγ (*see* Echinocandins)
Acyl carrier protein (ACP), 227
N-Acyl-homoserine lactone (*see also* Auto-
        regulators), 77, 139
Acylpeptide lactones (*see* Actinomycin)
Adenomycin, 113
Adenosine deaminase, 755
    immobilization of, 755-756
    synthesis of (—)-carbovir with, 756
Adipic acid, 687
Adipyl-6-aminopenicillanic acid (adipyl-6-
        APA), 267
ADP-ribosylation, 137, 140
Aeromonas hydrophila, 612
A factor (*see also* Autoregulators), 65,
        135-137
AIDS (*see* Acquired immunodeficiency
        syndrome)
Alamethicin, 485
Alarmones, 138
Alicyclobacillus acidocaldarius, 508-509
Allosamidins, 91, 115, 116, 141
    chitinase inhibition by, 91
    structures of, 101
Aloesaponarin II, 17-18, 620, 638-639, 684,
        686, 691-694
    biosynthesis of, 17-18, 620, 638-639
Amidinotransferases
    in aminoglycoside biosynthesis, 125-126,
        146-147
Amikacin, 95, 149, 420
    structure of, 102
Amino acids, 687
δ-(α-Aminoadipyl)-cysteinyl-D-valine (ACV)
        synthetase (*see* β-lactams)
7-Aminocephalosporanic acid (7-ACA)
        (*see also* Cephems), 267, 733-748
    enzymatic synthesis of, 733-748
        D-amino acid oxidase (DAO) in,
            734-736, 741-745, 748
            characteristics of, 734-735
            sequence of, 736-737

[7-Aminocephalosporanic acid]
    7-β-(4-carboxybutanamido)cephalo-
        sporanic acid (GL-7-ACA)
        precursor of, 733
        acylase for, 733, 737-741
    7-β-(5-carboxy-5-oxopentanamido)-
        cephalosporanic acid (keto-AD-7-
        ACA) precursor of, 733-734
    cephalosporin C acylase (CC acylase)
        for, 733-734, 737-748
    from cephalosporin C, 733-742
    recombinant strain for production of, 733,
        741-745
    structure of, 735, 744
7-Aminodeacetoxycephalosporanic acid (7-
        ADOCA), 742, 744
7-Aminodeacetylcephalosporanic acid (7-
        ADACA), 733, 741-748
    enzymatic synthesis of, 733-748
        7-β-(4-carboxybutanamido)deacetyl-
        cephalosporanic acid (GL-7-
        ADACA) precursor of, 743-744
        7-β-(5-carboxy-5-oxopentanamido)de-
        acetylcephalosporanic acid (keto-
        AD-7-ADACA) precursor of,
        743-744
    from deacetylcephalosporin C (DAC),
        742-743
    recombinant strain for production of, 733,
        742-747
    improvement of, 747-748
    structure of, 735, 744
Aminocyclitol-aminoglycoside antibiotics
        (ACAGAs) (see also Aminoglyco-
        sides), 81-150
    formation of, 114-129
    glycosidase inhibition by, 82
    hypersensitive mutants of, 82
    pathway formulae for biosynthesis of, 85
    resistance mechanisms for, 94, 130-133
Aminodisaccharide antibiotics, 101
Aminoglycosides, 5, 8, 14, 81-150
    AC4437, 84
    acetyltransferases for, 111
    biosynthesis of, 81-129
        ammonium repression of, 138
        decision phase model for, 135
        feedback repression of, 138
        regulatory mechanisms for, 134-140
    chronology for discovery of, 83

[Aminoglycosides]
    cyclitol formation in, 113-116
        alternative pathways for, 116
    definition of, 84
    2-deoxystreptamine (2-DOS) containing,
        82, 85
        pathway design for, 95
    export of, 129-130
    genetics of, 100-112
    genomic instability and, 146
    "molecular fossils," 142, 147
    mechanisms for self-resistance against, 110,
        130-133
    monosaccharide aminosugar derivatives
        of, 100
    pathway design for biosynthesis of, 92
    pseudodisaccharide 2-deoxystreptamine-
        containing, 94
    resistance genes for, 109-112, 130
    semisynthetic, 94, 95, 98, 101
        structures of, 102
    subunits for, 112
        biosynthesis of, 112-127
Aminotransferases
    in aminoglycoside biosynthesis, 103,
        117-120
    pyridoxal-phosphate (PLP)-dependent,
        114, 117
        secondary metabolic aminotransferase
        (SMAT) subfamily of, 117-120,
        145
        mechanism of action in, 118
        conserved structure of, 118
Amphotericin B (see also Polyenes), 128, 315,
        322-324, 330, 551, 562
    combination therapy with 5′-
        fluorocytosine, 315
    gene cluster in producing strain, 145
    minimal inhibitory concentrations of,
        321
    toxicity of, 315, 324
Ampicillin, 241, 425
Amsacrine, 590, 598
Amycolata (previously Nocardia), 784
    A. autotrophica strain SANK 62781,
        784
        hydroxylation of ML-236B to
        pravastatin by, 784
        subsp. amethystina SANK 62981, 785
        subsp. canberrica SANK 62881, 785

Amycolatopsis, 375
  A. mediterranei ATCC 13685 (ISP 5501),
        521, 523-528, 533-537
    B factor autoregulator in, 533-534
    blocked mutant strain T 104 from,
        534-535
    fermentation for production of rifa-
        mycins by, 525-526, 537-540
    immobilization of, 538
    linkage map for, 526
    mutagenesis of, 526
    overproducing strains of, 534-536
    phage susceptibility of, 525, 536
    strain improvement of, 535-536
  A. sp., 91, 100
Amylostatins, 89, 99, 113, 128, 141
Amythiamycins (see also Thiopeptides),
        393
Anabaena sp., 565
Ansamycins (*see also* Rifamycins), 521
  geldanamycin, 521
  mycotrienin, 521
  streptovaricins, 521
Anthracyclines (*see also* Daunorubicin,
        Doxorubicin), 107, 111, 129,
        563, 577-640
  aclarubicin (aclacinomycin A), 577, 580,
        584, 587, 590-592, 595, 604, 606,
        612, 620, 622, 633, 695-696
    biosynthesis of, 618, 620
    structure of, 579
    topoisomerase II binding by, 590-592
  aklavin, 593, 595, 622, 630, 633
  antibody-directed enzyme prodrug
        therapy (ADEPT) strategies
        for, 601-602
  antitumor activities of, 577, 584-585,
        639-640
  auramycin, 594, 604, 639
    methyl side chain of, 594
  baumycins, 577-578, 580, 603, 610-611,
        630-631, 634-636
    oxalic acid hydrolysis of, 610
    structure of, 578
  betaclamycin A, 596
  biosynthesis of, 614, 616-617
    aglycones in, 595, 610, 622, 635
    aklanonic acid in, 615, 618-623
      methyl-side-chain derivative of,
        619-620
    aklavinone in, 603-604, 622-623
    anthracycline 4-O-methyltransferase
      in, 604, 613, 628, 630-633

[Anthracyclines]
  carminomycin 4-O-methyltransferase
        (*see* anthracycline 4-O-
        methyltransferase)
  cyclases in, 619-623, 693-694
  dauK (*dnrK*) product (anthracycline
        4-O-methyltransferase) in, 604,
        617, 630-633
  dauP (*dnrP*) product (rhodomycin D
        esterase) in, 604, 617, 631-633
  dauF (*dnrF*) product (aklavinone 11-
        hydroxylase) in, 604, 616, 622-624,
        639, 696
  13-dihydrocarminomycin in, 603,
        630-633
  13-dihydrodaunorubicin in, 603,
        630-633
  doxA gene product (13, 14-hydroxylase)
        in, 604, 614, 616, 627, 630-633
  dps (polyketide synthase) genes,
        614-622, 694, 702
  dpsC (*E. coli* KAS III homolog) product
        in, 618-620
  dpsD (acyltransferase) product in,
        618-620
  dpsE (*aknA*) product (anthracycline
        polyketide reductase) in, 604,
        617-618
  dpsG product (acyl carrier protein) in,
        616, 618-621, 702
  genes encoding, 614-617, 634-635
    promoters of, 637-638
    transcriptional regulators of,
        637-638
  glycosyltransferase in, 128, 628-630
  ketosugar aminotransferase (SMAT)
        enzymes in, 117
  polyketide synthase (type II) for, 606,
        614-621
  propionyl starter unit for, 618-620
  regulation of, 636-638
  rhodomycin D in, 579, 614, 625,
        628-633
  ε-rhodomycinone in, 577, 579, 603,
        622-625, 628-631, 634-637
  TDP-daunosamine pathway in, 614,
        624-628, 635
  C9-side chain of, 594, 619
  C13-reduction of, 594
  cardiotoxicity of, 580, 598-600
    acute, 599
    chronic, 599
    cumulative, 580, 598-600

[Anthracyclines]
dexazoxane (Zinecard) treatment for, 600
free-radical cause of, 599
late-onset, 599
carminomycin, 577-578, 580, 584, 591-594, 598, 603, 611-612, 622, 630-633
cinerubins, 605, 622
classes I and II of, 591-592
cytotoxic activity of, 586, 595, 605, 613
on HeLa cells, 595
on L1210 leukemia cells, 595, 605
on P388 murine leukemia cells, 605, 613
daunorubicin (daunomycin), 577-578, 580, 584-600, 603-606, 610-622, 630-639
biosynthesis of, 615-635
DaunoXome (liposomal), 585, 601
purification of, 609-611
structure of, 578
daunosamine moiety of, 596
13-dihydrodoxorubicin, 603
ditrirubicin B, 587
DNA interaction with
affinity for, 596, 597
alkylation of, 589
crosslinkage of, 588-589
intercalation of, 586-589, 593
doxorubicin (adriamycin), 577-578, 580, 583-600, 603-604, 611-613, 629-640
biosynthesis of, 629-635
genes encoding, 635
pathway for, 631
BR96-DOX, 601
Doxil (liposomal), 585, 601
structure of, 578
elloramycin, 150, 606, 639, 695
epirubicin (4'-epidoxorubicin), 578, 580, 584, 586, 596, 600, 604
esorubicin, 596
extraction of, 609-612
fermentation for, 606-608
feudomycin C
methyl side chain of, 594, 619
free radical generation by, 586, 599-600
helicase inhibition by, 587, 591
hybrid forms of, 638-639, 695-696
10-demethoxycarbonylaklavinone, 695
8-demethyl-8-O-olivosyltetracenomycin C, 696

[Anthracyclines]
11-deoxy-β-rhodomycinone, 695
11-hydroxyaclacinomycins, 696
idarubicin, 577-580, 584-586, 593-594, 604-605, 612, 630
leukaemomycins, 603
lipophilicity of, 593, 597
liposomal preparations of, 585, 601
marcellomycin, 579, 591-592, 595
market for, 583
media for growth and production in, 606-608
menogaril, 577, 579, 580, 584, 586, 604-605
monoclonal antibody conjugation with, 601
multidrug resistance (MDR) (see also Multidrug resistance), 583, 590, 597, 600
induction by anthracyclines, 590, 597-598
lung resistance protein (LRP)-mediated, 597-598
multidrug resistance protein (MRP)-mediated, 597
P95-mediated, 598
P170 protein (Pgp, gp170)-mediated, 597-598
topoisomerase II (atMDR)-mediated, 597
verapamil antagonism of, 598
mussettamycin, 591, 595
nogalamycin, 579-580, 591, 595, 605, 612, 639
biosynthesis of, 618, 620
purification of, 611
structure of, 579
oxaunomycin, 595
pirarubicin (tetrahydropyranyldoxo-rubicin), 577-580, 584, 586, 596, 604, 612, 636
polyketide synthases of, 614-621, 691-695
purification of, 609-612
pyrromycin, 578, 622
resistance genes for, 635, 638
rhodomycins, 578, 605, 622
rudolfomycin, 591-592, 595
semisynthetic analogs, 594
steffimycins, 577, 579-580, 605, 612
purification of, 611
structure of, 579

[Anthracyclines]
structure-activity relationships (SARs) of, 593, 597
sulfurmycinone, 604
tetracenomycin C, 577, 579, 606, 618, 620-621, 637, 639, 692-695
biosynthesis of, 618, 620-621, 637, 694-695
polyketide synthase genes for, 618, 620, 692-695
hybrid metabolites from, 692-696
topoisomerase II with
aclarubicin interaction with, 590-591, 595
altered topoisomerase II-multidrug resistance (at-MDR) induced by, 590-591, 597
cleavable complex formed by, 590-592, 595
interactions of, 586-587, 589-591
model for interaction of, 589-590
poisons of, 590-591, 597-598
transformation of, 612-613
13-oxo reduction in, 612-613
NADPH-dependent reductive deglycosylation in, 612
zorubicin (rubidazone), 580, 584, 594
Antibiotic paradox, 9, 10
Antibiotics
antifungal, 2, 5
antiviral, 2
bacteriocidal, 1, 13, 14, 141
bacteriostatic, 1, 13, 14, 141
biosynthesis of, 56-57
definition of, 1
development of, 1-19
discovery of, 2, 684
expanded sources for, 15
Golden Era of, 3
hybrid, 17, 18, 620, 638-639, 683-697
definition of, 683-684
history of, 683-684
requirements for production of, 684-687
important in 1996, 20-43
induction of, 65-77
markets for, 2, 5, 8
new era of, 9, 11-15
paradigms for, 441-444
promising, 12
rediscovery of, 5
resistance to, 8-11
semisynthetic, 2, 11
synergistic effects of, 14

[Antibiotics]
targets, 7
Anthelminthic agents, 3
Antiinfectives (*see also* Antibiotics), 2, 8, 13
Antiviral agents (*see* Antibiotics, antiviral)
Apis mellifera (honeybee)
cationic peptides from, 475
Apramycins, 85, 96, 111, 125
Arbekacin, 14, 95, 102, 149
Archaea, 82, 141
glucosaminyl archaetidyl-*myo*-inositols of, 82
Aridicin (*see* Glycopeptides)
Aristeromycin, 113, 115, 116
Aromatase, 17
Arthrobacter sp., 188
Ascidians, 552
Ascomycins (*see also* FK506 and FK523), 16, 497-516
ascomycin (immunomycin, FK520), 16, 498
biosynthesis of, 498-502
butyryl-CoA formation in, 501-502
(1*R*, 3*R*, 4*R*)-dihydroxycyclohexane-carboxylic acid (DHCHC) precursor of, 506-509
incorporation of precursors in, 500-501
macrolide ring of, 498-502
methyltransferase reactions in, 506
pipecolate-derived moiety in, 503-505
shikimic acid precursor of, 506-509
prolyl analog of, 505
structure of, 500
Ashimycins, 84, 128
Aspartate aminotransferase family, 111
Aspergillosis (disseminated), 324
Aspergillus, 241
adenosine deaminase from, 755
A. *aculeatus*, 319
A. *erreus*, 790
itaconic acid production by, 790
A. *fumigatus*, 322-325, 329, 723
activity of LY303366 against, 322-325
activity of pneumocandins against, 329
A. *nidulans*, 222, 233, 242, 246-249, 255, 260, 261, 318, 782
echinocandin production by, 222
transformation of, 782
A. *niger*, 782
citric acid production by, 790
transformation of, 782
A. *parasiticus*, 503
A. *rugulosis*, 318
A. *sydowi*, 319

[*Aspergillus*]
  A. *terreus*, 723
    blasticidin S deaminase from, 723
  A. species, 315, 317, 331
Astromycin (*see* Fortimycin)
ATP-binding cassette (ABC)-transporters,
    111, 129, 448, 598, 638
Augmentin, 262
Aureobasidium pullulans IFO4466
  cephalosporin C acetylesterase from, 748
Autoregulators, 65-77, 135-139
  A-factor, 65, 68, 72, 135-139
    binding protein (receptor), 74, 76
    receptor protein (ArpA), 139
    stimulation of membrane-bound
        GTPases by, 139
  B-factor, 533-534
  binding proteins, 74
  butanolides IM, 139
  butyrolactone-type, 65-77, 139
  factor C, 136, 140
  Factor I, 65, 68
  IM2, 65-66, 72, 74
    binding protein (receptor) for, 74
  N-Acyl-homoserine lactone, 77, 139
  virginiae butanolides (VB), 67-77
    binding protein (receptor) for, 71-74
Avermectin, 403, 405, 510, 691
  biosynthesis of, 509
    genes encoding, 403, 510
    type I polyketide synthase of, 403,
        509-510, 563
Averufin, 503
Avoparcin, 363, 373
Azoles, 6
AZT (Retrovir) (*see* Human immunodefi-
    ciency virus)

Bacillus
  aminoglycoside-producing, 82
  B. *brevis*, 188, 197, 202-203, 207, 227,
      245
    strain ATCC 8185, 227
  B. *cereus*, 723-724
    blasticidin S deaminase from, 723-724
  B. *circulans* NRRL B3312
    autoresistance in, 129-130
    ButB protein of, 129
    butirosin production by, 129-130, 149
  B. *licheniformis*, 189, 203
  B. *megaterium*, 397, 427

[*Bacillus*]
  strain ATCC 13368
    P450 steroid hydroxylation system
        of, 785
  strain ATCC 14581
    P450 fatty acid hydroxylation
        system of, 785
  thiopeptide-resistant mutants of,
      397
  B. *pumilus*, 91
  B. *stearothermophilus*
    DegT protein of, 117
  B. *subtilis*, 117, 137, 189, 192, 201-208,
      450-451, 459-461, 675, 724-725,
      772
    p-aminobenzoic acid (PABA) synthase
        from, 558-560
    cytidine deaminase from, 772
    production of extracellular hydrolases
        by, 117
    production of recombinant lantibiotics
        by, 459-461
    production of subtilin by, 459-461
    strain 168, 459-461
    strain ATCC 6633, 460-461
    surfactin-nonproducing mutants of,
        196-197, 204-207
  B. spp., 393, 397
    thiocillins produced by, 393
Bacitracin, 189, 350, 393
Bacteria
  drug-resistant, 8, 15, 19, 363
  Gram-negative, 11, 13, 142-143, 363
    antibiotic-resistant, 11, 363
  Gram-positive, 13, 142
    antibiotic-resistant, 13, 363, 420
    antibiotics against, 165, 415, 420
    production of lantibiotics by, 440
    vancomycin-resistant, 13, 420
  nosocomial pathogens of, 94
Bacteriocins, 457
Bacteriophages, 50-52
  att sites for, 53-54
  φC31, 53, 609
  plaque formation on streptomycetes by,
      51
Bacteroides sp., tetracycline resistance
    mechanisms of, 661-663
Balhimycin (*see* Glycopeptides)
BarA (butyrolactone autoregulator
    receptor), 74

barA gene, 74-76
Benanomycins, 316
Beauveria
    nivea (*see Tolypocladium inflatum*)
    species, 309
Berninamycin (*see also* Thiopeptides), 393,
        398
Biomimicry, 19
Blasticidins (*see* Peptidyl Nucleosides)
bldA (bald) gene, 140
Bleomycin, 393
Bluensidine, 84, 115-120
Bluensomycin, 100, 125, 146
    biosynthesis gene cluster for, 104
    producing strain for, 117
Boholmycin, 85, 89, 126, 132, 149
Bombina variegata (frog), 473
    bombinin cationic peptide from, 473
Bortrytis cinerea, 231
Burkholderia cepacia
    natural resistance to cationic peptides
        by, 477
Butirosins, 85, 91, 95, 111, 217

Calcineurin (protein phosphatase), 279,
        497-499
    biological response to inhibition of,
        497-499
Campylobacter
    C. coli acquired aminoglycoside resistance
        in, 131
    *tet*M/O tetracycline resistance system of,
        661
Carminomycin (*see also* Anthracyclines),
        577-578, 580, 584, 591-594,
        598, 603, 611-612, 622,
        630-633
Cancer, 455
    breast, 15
    chemotherapy for, 557, 585, 639
    Kaposi's sarcoma
        treatment of, 585, 601
    ovarian, 15
    taxol for treatment of, 15
Candicidin (*see also* Polyenes), 553, 558-564,
        569-570
    p-aminobenzoic acid (PABA) precursor of,
        558-562
        PABA synthase for, 558-562,
            569-570
        pabAB genes for, 558, 569-570
    biosynthesis of, 560-564
        polyketide synthase for, 561-564

[Candicidin]
    regulation of, 569-570
Candida
    C. albicans, 315, 320-323, 329, 479, 552,
            557
        cell membranes of, 557
        cell walls of, 315-316
        fluconazole-resistant, 323, 325
        killed by defensins, 479
    C. cylindraceae (*rugosa*), 771
        lipase from, 771-772
    C. glabrata, 321
    C. krusei, 321
    esophagitis caused by, 320
    fluconazole-resistant, 315
    species, 315, 317, 321, 331
Candidiasis
    disseminated, 322
    murine model for, 322-327, 329-330
    treatment of, 322
Carbamoyltransferases
    in aminoglycoside biosynthesis, 125-126
Carbapenems, 11, 77
    inducer for production of, 77
Carbocyclic nucleosides, 753-757, 770
    antiviral activities of, 754
    (—)-aristeromycin, 754
        produced by Streptomyces coelicolor,
            754
    (+)-carbocyclic 2'-deoxy-5-[(*E*)-2-bromo-
            vinyl]uridine (c-BVdU), 756
    (+)-carbocyclic 2'-deoxyguanosine (c-dG),
            756
    carbovir (c-d4G), 753-756
        in vitro inhibition of HIV by, 754
        synthesis of, 755
    (—)-neplanocin, 754
Carcinoscorpius rotundicauda
    tachyplesin cationic peptides from, 475
Cationic peptides, 14, 438, 471-489
    antibiotic activities of
        antibacterial, 471-472, 476-478,
            485-487
        anticancer, 471
        antiendotoxin, 471, 478-479, 486-487
        antifungal, 471-472, 479
        antiviral, 471-472, 479
    as enhancers, 14
    bacteriocidal activity of, 477-478
    cathelicidin family of, 472
        homologous proregion sequences of,
            472-473
    cecropin-melittin hybrid of, 477, 481

[Cationic peptides]
convergent evolution of, 471, 480
crystallization of, 480
defense mechanisms against microbes, 471
immunogenicity of, 479-480
mechanisms of action of, 457-458, 483
    channel formation in membranes by, 483-486
    detergent-like effect of, 483
preprodefensins, 472
recombinant biosynthesis of, 488-489
stability of, 480
structural classes of, 474
    β-defensins, 472-474
        from bovine neutrophil (BNBD5), 472
        tracheal antimicrobial peptide (TAP), 472
    α-helical cationic peptides, 472-474
        bombinin, 473
        brevinins, 473
        cecropin A, 472-474
        dermaseptin, 473
        magainins, 438, 458, 473-474, 476, 480
        PGLa, 473
        PGO, 473
        xenopsin, 473
    histidine-rich, 472-474
        histadin 2, 472
    insect defensins, 472-474
        charybdotoxin of scorpion, 474
        phormicin, 473-474
        royalism from bees, 474
        sapaecin (sapecin), 472-474, 480
    loops, 472-474
    mammalian defensins, 472-474, 481, 483
        human defensins (HD-5, 6), 472
        human neutrophil peptides (HNP-1, 2, 3, 4), 472, 479, 480
        model for structure of, 482
        mouse defensins (cryptidins), 472, 479
    proline-rich, 472-475
        abaecin, 474-475
        apidaecin, 474-475
        bactenecin 5 (bac5), 472-474, 480
        hymenoptaecin, 475

[Cationic peptides]
    tachyplesins, 472-474
        antifungal activities of, 479
        polyphemusins I, II, 475
        tachyplesins I, II, III, 475
    thionins, 472-476, 480
        Ac-AMP, 476
        BTH6, 475
        Mj-AMP, 476
    tryptophan-rich, 472-474, 479, 481
        indolicidin, 472, 479, 481
    structure-activity relationships (SARs) of, 482
    ubiquity of, 471
Cecropins (see also Cationic peptides), 438, 458, 472-474, 476, 480, 483-484
    absence of cysteine residues in, 473
    cecropin P1 from pig intestine, 474
    collapse of membrane potential by, 456-458, 473
    model for membrane interaction of, 484
    production by moths, 456
Cefpirome
    synergism with magainin, 478
Cell walls (see also Peptidoglycan)
Centers for Disease Control and Prevention (CDC), 9
Cephabacin, 251
    stability against β-lactamases by, 251
Cephadroxil, 266
Cephalexin, 266
Cephaloglycine, 267
Cephalosporins (see also β-Lactams), 2, 242, 248, 251, 363, 733
    7-aminodeacetoxycephalosporanic acid (7-ADCA) as precursor for, 266
    biosynthetic precursor for, 56
    cephalosporin C, 251, 266, 733-736
        acetylesterase (CAE) of, 744
        acylases of (see also 7-Aminocephalo-sporanic acid [7-ACA]), 733-734, 737-748
        bottlenecks in the biosynthesis of, 265-266
        deamination of, 734-736
        late genes in the biosynthesis of, 251
    market for, 2, 5
    7-α-methoxycephalosporin C, 251

[Cephalosporins]
  pathway for biosynthesis of, 243
  scale-up of recombinant, 265
Cephalosporium, 241
  C. acremonium, 199, 244, 246-250, 257,
      258, 260-262, 265-267, 733,
      741, 782
    7-aminocephalosporanic acid (7-ACA)
        producing strain of, 741
    recombinant strain improvement of,
        265-266
    transformation of, 782
  ACV synthetase of, 199
Cephalothin, 267
Cephamycins (*see also* β-Lactams), 242, 251
  A, 251
  B, 251
  C, 251, 254-255, 267
  pathway for biosynthesis of, 243
Cephems, 267
  cefazolin, 733
  cefdinir (FK482), 733
  cefixime (FK027), 733
  ceftizoxime, 733
  properties of, 733
  synthesis of
    7-aminocephalosporanic acid (7-ACA)
        as precursor for, 267, 733
    7-aminodeacetylcephalosporanic acid
        (7-ADACA) as precursor for,
        733
Cephradine, 266
Cerulenin, 562
Chain length factor (CLF), 17, 621, 673, 692
Chainia sp., 552
Chalcone (polyketide) synthase, 562, 672
Chaunopycnis species, 309
Chitin (*see* Fungi, cell walls in)
Chloramphenicol, 401, 457, 722-723
  inhibition of ribosomal protein synthesis
      by, 401, 722-723
Chloro-orienticin (*see* Glycopeptides)
Chlortetracycline (*see also* Tetracyclines),
      663-664, 668-671, 675
Chromobacterium viscosum, 771-772
  lipase from, 771-772
Cilofungin (LY121019; *see* Echinocandins)
Ciprofloxacin, 2
Clavams, 262-264
Clavulanic acid, 252, 262-265
  biosynthesis of, 262-265
  clavaminate synthase (CAS) in,
      263-264
  genes for, 253, 263-264

[Clavulanic acid]
  proclavaminate amidinohydrolase
      (PAH) in, 264
  market for, 262
  oxazolidine ring of, 262-264
Clerocidin, 590
Clindamycin (*see also* Lincomycin), 165
Cloning vectors (*see* Plasmids)
Clostridium
  C. difficile, 363, 373
    pseudomembranous colitis caused by,
        363, 373, 423
      daptomycin treatment of, 423
      vancomycin treatment of, 363,
        373
  C. subterminale
    β-lysine formation in, 707
Cnidarians, 552
Crotalus atrox, 759
Cryptococcus neoformans, 315
Cryptosporiopsis sp.
  production of sporiofungins by, 319
Cochliobolus carbonum, 188
Coleophoma empetri, 319
  production of WF11899 (lipopeptide anti-
      fungal agent) by, 319
Colicin, 456, 475
Combinatorial chemistry, 18, 19
Compounds, semisynthetic (*see* antibiotics,
      semisynthetic)
Coronary heart disease (CHD), 779
  hypercholesterolemia in, 779, 801
  ischemic heart disease (IHD), 779
Coronatine (phytotoxin), 198
Cyclic AMP (cAMP), 135, 137, 356
  in oleandomycin biosynthesis, 137
Cyclitol, 81
  mechanisms for formation of, 81
Cyclophilin, 232, 279
  complexation with cyclosporin, 279,
      497-499
    binding of complex to calcineurin, 279,
        497-499
D-Cycloserine, 65
Cyclosporin(s), 1, 3, 16, 188, 217
  A, 189, 279
    modifications from, 281-283
    (2S, 3R, 4R, 6E)-2-amino-3-hydroxy-4-
        methyloct-6-enoic acid (*see also*
        bmt) in, 280, 281
    analogs of, 281-283, 299-303
    antifungal activity of, 279
    anti-inflammatory activity of, 279
    antiparasitic activity of, 279

[Cyclosporin(s)]
    assay for, 281
    biosynthesis of, 279-309, 401
        alanine racemase activity in, 285, 288,
            309
        aminoacyl adenylates in, 289
        L-2-aminobutyric acid in, 285
        chain elongation reactions in,
            291-292
        in vitro, 297, 299-308
        origin of amino acids in, 286
        precursor-directed, 286-287
        reaction scheme in, 293
        thiotemplate mechanism for, 289, 294
        L-threonine dehydratase in, 288
        bmt {(4R)-4-[(E)-2-butenyl]-4-methyl-
            L-threonine} (see also [2S, 3R,
            4R, 6E]-2-amino-3-hydroxy-4-
            methyloct-6-enoic acid) in,
            280-285, 299
        elongation of, 285
        polyketide synthase for, 285, 309
        thioester of, 285
    C$_9$ unsaturated β-hydroxy-a-amino acid
        of (see bmt)
    ^{13}C-incorporation into, 286
    clinical activities of, 279
    cyclophilin-binding of, 279, 497-499
    fermentation conditions for production
        of, 281
    immunosuppressive activity of, 279, 299,
        307
    incorporation of amino acids into,
        299-308
    linear precursor peptides of, 292
    N-methylation of amino acids in, 281,
        286, 288, 343
    mode of action of, 499
    natural variants of, 281-283
    non-immunosuppressive analog, 232
    nonproteinogenic amino acids in, 285
    positions in, 299-308
    structure of, 280
    suppression of T-lymphocyte proliferation
        by, 279
    synthetase, 192, 231, 232, 245, 288,
        289-309
        amino acid activation domains of, 294
        ATP-pyrophosphate exchange assays
            for, 191, 196, 225
        diketopiperazine cyclo-(D-Ala-Leu)

[Cyclosporin(s)]
        synthesis by, 291
        diketopiperazine cyclo-(D-Ala-MeLeu)
            synthesis by, 288, 291-294
        inhibition of, 290
        methyltransferase domains in, 196
        modules of, 292
        gene for, 289
        N-methylation reactions of, 223, 230,
            288, 290
        4'-phosphopantetheine moieties of,
            291-292, 294
        proteolytic digestion of, 292
        substrate specificity of, 299-308
    use in organ and bone marrow
        transplantations, 279
Cyclothiazomycin (see also Thiopeptides),
    393
Cylindrocarpon lucidum Booth NRRL 5760,
    280-281, 308
Cylindrotrichum oligospermum (Corda)
    Bonorden, 295-296, 309
Cystic fibrosis, 8
Cytidine deaminase, 758, 760-762, 772
    Epivir (3TC) synthesis using, 758, 760,
        762-769
    immobilization of, 760, 762-769, 772
    isolation of, 760, 762-763
    production of, 762-764, 772
    regulation of, 760, 766
Cytochrome P450s, 513, 626-627, 630-633
    DoxA (daunorubicin 13, 14-hydroxyl-
        ase) in, 604, 614, 616, 627,
        630-633
    electron donors for, 786-787
    hydroxylases, 604, 614, 616, 626-627,
        630-633, 785
    mechanism of activity for, 788
    metyrapone as inhibitor of, 513
    NADH-cytochrome P-450 reductase of,
        786-787
    P450cam, 785, 787
    P-450sca (see also Pravastatin), 785-788
    P-450I, 787
    RLM (rat liver P450), 787
    types (1-, 2-, or 3-component) of, 787

Dactimicin, 88, 126, 127
Dactylosporangium
    D. matsuzakiense ATCC 31570, 107,
        111, 132

[*Dactylosporangium*]
   D. sp., 88, 663
Dalbaheptide (*see also* Vancomycin and
      Glycopeptides), 364
Dalfopristin (*see also* Synercid), 13
Daptomycin (LY146032) (*see also* Lipo-
      peptides), 217, 364, 415-431
   bacteriocidal activity of, 420, 426-429
   biosynthesis of, 416-417, 430
      peptide synthetase genes for, 430
   calcium-dependent insertion into
      membranes by, 428-429
   clinical studies on, 423-426
   improvement in production, 57, 416
   in vitro activity of, 420-421
   in vivo activity of, 421-426
   lipopeptide nature of, 364, 415-416
   N-methylation of, 230
      novel mechanism(s) of action of, 420,
        426-429
      dissipation of membrane potential,
        426-429
      inhibition of peptidoglycan synthesis,
        426-429
   protection against aminoglycoside renal
      toxicity by, 420
   structure of, 417
   synergy with antibiotics by, 420
Daunorubicin (daunomycin) (*see also*
      Anthracyclines), 128, 577-578,
      580, 584-600, 603-606, 610-622,
      630-639, 673, 675
ddl gene product (*d*-alanine-*d*-alanine ligase),
      372
Defense peptides (*see* Defensins)
Defensins (*see also* Cationic peptides), 438,
      455-458, 472-476
   collapse of membrane potential by,
      456-458
   pre-immune system immunity of, 458
Dehydroquinate pathway, 115-116
   3-dehydroquinate synthases of, 115
6-Deoxyhexoses, 81, 565-567
   l-dihydrostroptose pathway in formation
      of, 122-124
      GalE-family of oxidoreductases in,
        122-124
   formation of D- and L- forms of, 120-121
      hexose-1-phosphate nucleotidyltrans-
        ferase in, 121
      NDP-hexose 4, 6-dehydratase in, 121
      NDP-4-keto-6-deoxyhexose 3, 5-epimerase
        in, 121

[6-Deoxyhexoses]
   general pathways for biosynthesis of,
      120-125, 565-566
   genes encoding, 103-104, 121, 565-567
   hexosamine pathway in formation of,
      122
   N-methyl-L-glucosamine (NMGLA)
      biosynthesis in, 122-124
1-Deoxynojirimycin (enzyme inhibitor), 91,
      125, 126
2-Deoxystreptamine (2-DOS) (*see*
      Aminoglycosides)
Depsipeptide synthetase, 289
Destomycins, 86, 96
Dibekacin, 94, 149
Dictyostelium discoideum, 725
Didemnins, 15
Dihydrofolate synthase, 16
Dihydropteroate synthase, 16
Dihydrostreptose, 112
Dihydrostreptosylstreptidine (AC-4437),
      106
Directed biosynthesis, 4
Directed evolution, 18
Diseases (*see* Infectious diseases)
DNA integration into chromosome, 54
DNA gyrase, 5
Doxorubicin (Adriamycin) (*see also* Anthra-
      cyclines), 577-578, 580, 583-600,
      603-604, 611-613, 629-640, 691
Drosophila
   cecropins (cationic peptides) from,
      473

Ebola virus (*see also* Viruses), 8
Echinocandins, 217, 315-331
   aculeacin Aγ, 317
   administration of, 330
   analogs of, 316-317
   B, 317-320
   C, 317
   D, 317
   inhibition of fungal cell wall biosynthesis
      by, 316-318
   inhibition of glucan synthase by, 329,
      331
   in vitro antifungal efficacies of, 321, 328
   mulundocandin, 317
   nucleus of, 316
   orally-active, 319
   pneumocandin (*see also* Pneumocandins)
      A$_O$, 317, 327
      B$_O$, 327

[Echinocandins]
pharmacokinetic properties of, 330
semisynthetic analogs of, 316-320
L-671, 329, 327
L-693, 989, 327
L-705, 589, 328
L-731, 373, 328
L-733, 560, 328, 331
semisynthetic analogs of, 316-320
LY121019 (cilofungin), 320, 327, 331
minimal inhibitory concentrations of, 321-322
LY225489, 320
LY280949, 320
LY303366, 320-322, 327, 331
sporiofungin A, 317, 319
structure-activity studies of, 320
WF11899A, 317, 319
Efflux pumps, 16, 661-663
Elongation factors (EF)
EF-G, 394, 405-406
EF-Tu, 63, 141, 394-395, 405-406
GTP-hydrolysis by, 394-395
Embden-Meyerhof-Parnas pathway, 113
Endonucleases (see Restriction endonucleases)
Endotoxin (see also Lipopolysaccharide), 478-479
induction of interleukins 1 and 8 and tumor necrosis factor by, 478
Enniatins, 188-189, 222, 227, 343, 350
synthetase, 196, 199-201, 231, 233, 289, 292
methylation domains in, 196
N-methylation reactions of, 223, 229
Entamoeba histolytica
inhibition by magainin B, 480
Enterobacter
E. aerogenes, 558
E. cloacea, 477
Enterobacteria, 82, 144
common antigen-ECA of, 82
Enterobactin, 188
Enterococcal infections, 13
Enterococci
hospital acquired infections of, 9
multidrug resistant, 9, 10
pathogenic, 363
transfer of aminoglycoside resistance by, 131
vancomycin resistant, 9, 13, 14, 364, 376, 379-382

[Enterococci]
antibiotics effective against, 364, 376, 379-382, 415, 430
emergence of, 371
VanA-type, 371-374, 379-382
cross-resistant to all natural glycopeptides by, 371
molecular basis of, 372-374
van genes encoding, 372-373
VanB-type, 371, 373-374, 379
Enterococcus
E. casseliflavus
intrinsic vancomycin resistance in, 374
E. faecalis, 9, 11, 371, 420-425
penicillin-resistant, 425
teichoplanin-resistant, 385
vancomycin-resistant, 371
antibiotics effective against, 371, 420-423
E. faecium, 9, 371, 420-422, 426-428
antibiotic-resistant, 14
vancomycin-resistant, 371, 426
antibiotics effective against, 371, 420-423
strain BM 4147, 745
VanH from, 745
E. flavescens
intrinsic vancomycin resistance in, 374
E. gallinarum
intrinsic vancomycin resistance in, 374
E. hirae, 252, 428-429
E. raffinosus, 425
Epipodophyllotoxins, 598
Epivir (3TC) (see also Human immuno-deficiency virus), 753, 757-772
chemical name for, 753
chiral HPLC for isolation of, 759, 765-767
biosynthesis of, 758-772
adenosine deaminase in, 759, 763
immobilization of, 759
alkaline phosphatase in, 758-759, 768
BCH189 in, 757-758, 766, 769
758, 766, 769
cytidine deaminase in, 758-765, 772
immobilization of, 760-769, 772
5'-nucleotidase in, 759, 768
Crotalus atrox venum as source of, 759
scale-up of, 765-766
large scale preparation of, 760-761,

[Epivir (3TC)]
765-766
purification of, 766-768
synthesis of, 769-772
Eremomycin (*see* Glycopeptides)
Erwinia carotovora, 77
Erythromycin, 128, 363, 457, 498, 688-691
$\Delta^{6,7}$-anhydroerythromycin C, 689
biosynthesis of, 315, 688-691
genes for, 510, 688-691
eryA, 510, 563-564, 688-691
eryF, 691
extender units for, 689
pathway for, 688
starter unit for, 689
6-deoxyerythronolide B (DEB), 688-690
processive biosynthesis of, 690
6-deoxyerythronolide B synthase (DEBS),
509, 563-564, 688-691, 702
eryA encoding, 510, 563-564, 688-691
domains of, 689-690
modules of, 689-690
type I polyketide synthase structure of,
509, 563-564, 688-691
hybrid products of, 688-691, 702
5, 6-dideoxy-5-oxoerythronolide B,
689
8, 9-dihydro-8-methyl-9-hydroxy-10-
deoxymethynolide, 690
2-norerythromycin A in, 688
tetraketo lactone, 690
triketo lactone, 690-691, 702
sugar biosynthesis in, 567
Escherichia coli, 8, 53, 55, 76, 191, 197, 249,
258, 405-406, 429-430, 527,
558-560, 662, 721, 724, 735,
759-765
acetyl-CoA carboxylase genes (*acc*) of,
565
acyl carrier protein of, 227
alkaline phosphatase from, 759, 768
p-aminobenzoic acid (PABA) synthase
from, 558
pabAB genes for, 558
pabC gene for, 559
aminoglycoside resistance in, 131
bacteriocidal activity against, 382
colicin production by, 456
conjugation with streptomycetes, 429
consensus promoter sequences of, 259
cytidine deaminase from, 760-762, 772
Epivir (3TC) synthesis using, 758, 760,
762-769

[*Escherichia coli*]
immobilization of, 760, 762-769, 772
isolation of, 760, 762-763
production of, 760, 762-764, 766, 772
expression in, 670, 735, 743, 761, 763-764,
772
fermentation of, 764, 772
ketoacylsynthase III (KAS III) of, 618
NusG protein of, 71
RelA of, 355
RNA polymerase β' subunit (*rpoC*-
encoded) of, 405-406
plasmid-encoded TEM β-lactamases of,
477
polynucleotide phosphorylase (PNPase)
of, 355
ribosomal protein biosynthesis in, 723-724
inhibition by antibiotics of, 723
S10 operon of, 403, 405-406
spc operon of, 403, 405-406
SpoT of, 355
streptomycete conjugation with, 53, 55
stringent response in, 354-355
relA locus of, 354
spoI locus of, 354
spoT locus of, 354
strain O157:H7, 8
tetracycline efflux mechanism of, 477,
662
transfer of tetracycline resistance to, 662
UvrA of, 638
Ethyl methanesulfonate EMS), 49, 50
Etoposide, 590
Eupergit-C (Rhom Pharma) beads
immobilization of enzymes with, 755, 759,
761, 763-765

Factor I (*see* Autoregulators)
Fatty acid synthases
Type I (vertebrate), 562
Type II (bacterial and plant), 562
Fermentation processes
anthracycline produced by, 606-608
computer control of, 792-801
fuzzy logic in, 792-797
feed control strategies for, 794-797
FK506 (tacrolimus) produced by,
513-516
hydroxylation of ML-236B (mevastatin) to
pravastatin in, 797-801
computer control of, 797-801
scale-up of, 800-801
lincomycin production in, 167-169

[Fermentation processes]
  ML-236B (mevastatin) production in,
      789-797
    optimization of, 789-797
  polyenes produced in, 568-569
  rapamycin produced in, 513-516
  recombinant *E. coli*
    production of cytidine deaminase in,
        762-764, 772
  rifamycin production in, 525-526, 537-538
  tetracyclines produced in, 668
Fibronectin, 16
FK506 (Tacrolimus), 1, 16, 217, 497-516
  approval for use in liver transplants, 497
  biosynthesis of, 498-502
    genes encoding, 513
      fkbA (encoding polyketide synthase),
          513
      fkbD (encoding methyltransferase),
          513
    methyltransferases in, 506
  fermentation optimization of, 513-516
  mode of action of, 499
  structure of, 500
  type I polyketide synthase for, 513
FK506 binding protein 12 (FKBP12), 497
  binding of FK506 to, 497
  binding of FK506-FKBP12 complex to
      calcineurin, 497-499
  binding of rapamycin to, 497
    binding of rapamycin-FKBP12 to FRAP,
        497
FK520 (*see* Ascomycins)
FK523 (L-683, 795) (*see also* Ascomycins), 498
  structure of, 500
FKBP12-rapamycin associated protein
      (FRAP), 497-499
  phosphatidylinositol kinase activity of,
      497
Flavobacterium, 241, 249, 255, 256
  F. saccharophilum
    D-glucoside 3-dehydrogenase from, 98
  β-lactam production by, 241, 256
Fluconozole, 315, 321
  minimal inhibitory concentrations of, 322
  resistance to, 315, 321, 330
Fluoroquinolones, 2, 10
FR901459, 309
Food and Drug Administration (FDA), 3,
      443-444, 584, 757

[Food and Drug Administration (FDA)]
  generally recognized as safe (GRAS) status
      by, 437, 444
  ban of antibiotic residues in food by,
      443
Fortimycins, 82, 87, 92, 95, 107, 113, 121,
      124, 126, 141
  biosynthesis gene cluster for, 107
  genes for biosynthesis of, 107-109
  pathway design for, 98
  pathway for biosynthesis of, 109
  resistance mechanisms for, 110
  modifications of, 107
  structures of, 97
Fosfomycin, 420
Frankia sp., 148
Frenolicin, 621
FtsZ, 16
Fungi
  cell walls of, 316-318
    chitin in, 316
      synthesis of, 316
      UDP-N-acetyl-D-glucosamine pre-
          cursor of, 316
    glucan polymers in, 316
      1,3-β-linked D-glucose of, 316
      1,3-β-linked D-glucose of, synthesis of,
          318, 331
    α-mannans of, 316
  filamentous, 687, 790-792
  infections by, 315, 330
Fungistatic agents, 315
Fungicidal, 315, 330
Fusarium
  F. scirpi, 188, 222, 227
  F. solani, 267
    production of ramihyphin A by, 309
    strain M-0718 (FERM P-2688), 734
      D-amino acid oxidase (DAO) of, 267,
          734-736, 741-745, 748
  species, 308

GalE family (*see also* 6-Deoxyhexoses), 122-124
GE2270 A (*see also* Thiopeptides), 393
Genetic recombination, 50
Gentamycin(s), 85, 93, 116, 121, 125, 133,
      420, 425-426
Giardia lamblia, 479
Glucose kinase
  repression by, 137

Glycocinnamoylspermidines (aminoglycoside antibiotics), 128
    LL-BM123α, 85, 126, 133
    LL-BM123β, 85
    LL-BM123γ1 (gamma), 85
    LL-BM123γ2 (gamma), 85
    structures of, 88
Glycopeptides (*see also* Vancomycin), 5, 363-385
    A47934 (sulfonated glycopeptide), 55, 368
        blocked mutants of, 368
        production of, 55
    A80407, 376
    A82850, 376
    A84575, 376
    affinity for D-alanyl-D-alanine by, 368-370
    aridicin aglycone, 367
        mannosylation of, 367
    biosynthesis of, 367
        assembly of amino acids for, 367
        formation of ether or C-C bonds in, 367
        glycosylation in, 367
        synthesis of atypical amino acids for, 367
    dalbaheptide structure of, 364
        modification of aglycones of, 383
    discovery of, 374-376
        target based screens for, 375-376
    generalized structure of, 366
    group I (vancomycin-type), 364
        A82846 (*see also* eremomycin), 364, 376
            LY264826 complex, 376
        balhimycin, 364
        chloro-orienticin, 364
        eremomycin (A82846A), 364, 377-378
            N-alkyl derivatives of, 377-379
            N-alkyl derivatives of, biological activity of, 378-379
        halogenation of, 364
        vancomycin (*see* Vancomycin)
    group II (actinoidin-type), 364
        actinoidin, 364
        avoparcin, 364, 366
        synmonicin, 364
    group III (ristocetin-type), 364
        A41030, 364
        actaplanin, 364
        ristocetin, 364, 376
        structures of, 367
        teichoplanin subgroup of (*see also* Teichoplanin), 365
            A84575, 365

[Glycopeptides]
    ardacin, 365, 375
    kibdelin, 365, 375
    parvodicin, 365, 375
    teichoplanin (*see* Teichoplanin)
    inhibition of peptidoglycan synthesis by, 368-371, 375
    semisynthetic, 376-385
        N-alkyl derivatives, 376-380
        carboxamide derivatives, 376
        core modifications of, 384-385
        LY307599 (biphenyl), 380
        LY333328 (chlorobiphenyl), 14, 380
    strains producing, 375
    structure-activity relationships (SARs) of, 376-385
Glycosidase inhibitors, 89-91, 148
Glycosyltransferases
    in aminoglycoside biosynthesis, 127-129
    in anthracycline biosynthesis, 628-629
    macrolide (MGT), 128, 133, 629
    reactions of, 125, 628-629
    signature sequence of, 628-629
Glycothiohexide α (*see also* Thiopeptides), 393
Glycylglycines (*see also* Tetracyclines), 666-668, 676
Gramicidin S, 188-189, 217, 222
    grs operon for biosynthesis of, 201-202, 207-208
    synthetase of, 191-197, 223, 226, 233, 244, 289, 346
Granaticin, 638, 684-685
Griseofulvin, 691
Growth promotants, 3
Guanosine pentaphosphate, 355
    synthetase I (pppGpp synthetase I) for, 355
Guanosine tetraphosphate (ppGpp), 135, 138, 354-355

Habekacin (*see* Arbekacin)
Haemophilus influenzae, 557
Hantavirus, 8
HC toxin, 188-189
    synthetase for, 198, 231
HeLa cells, 595, 725
Helicobacter pylori
    stomach ulcers caused by, 659
Hepatitis B virus, 75

Herbicides, 3
Herpes simplex virus (HSV), 756

Hexosemonophosphate shunt pathway, 113

Histoplasma capsulatum, 315

HIV (*see* Human immunodeficiency virus)

Homologous recombination, 53-55
  by neutral insertion, 55
  Campbell-like insertions in, 53
  chromosomal integration and, 54
  double crossovers, 55

Hospital-acquired infections, 8, 9, 374

Human cytomegalovirus, 756

Human immunodeficiency virus (HIV), 2, 15, 16, 585, 753-754, 757, 759
  approved drugs for treatment of, 753
  aspartyl proteinase of, 16
  drugs for treatment of, 2, 753
    adenallene, 753
    carbovir (c-d4G) (*see also* Carbocyclic nucleosides), 753-754
    cyclosporin, 279
    cytallene, 753
    didanosine (ddI), 753, 757
      peripheral neuropathy caused by, 753
    (—)-2', 3'-dideoxy-5-fluoro-3'-thiacytidine (FTC), 753
    Epivir (3TC) (*see also* Epivir), 753, 757-772
      biosynthesis of, 758-772
      cytidine deaminase in, 758-765, 772
      chemical name for, 753
      chiral HPLC for isolation and scale-up of, 759, 765-767
      immobilization of, 760-769, 772
      large scale preparation of, 760-761, 765-766
      purification of, 766-768
      synthesis of, 769-772
    epivir-5'-triphosphate (epivir-TP), 757
    oxetanocins, 753
    9-(2)-phosphonylmethoxyethyl)adenine (PMEA), 753
    proteinase inhibitors, 19
      Indinavir, 753
      Ritonavir, 753
      Saquinavir, 753
    Retrovir (AZT), 753, 759
      bone marrow suppression caused by, 753

RF strain of, 754

[Human immunodeficiency virus (HIV)]
    stavudine (d4T), 753
    zalcitabine (ddC), 753, 757
      peripheral neuropathy casued by, 753
  maturation of, 16
  retrovir-resistant isolates of, 757
  reverse transcriptase of, 753, 757, 759
  RNA of, 397, 753
    TAR region of, 397
    TRP-185 and, 397

Humicola sp. ATCC 20620
  biotransformation of rifamycin B by, 542-543

Hyalophora cecropia (silk moth), production of cecropins by, 473

Hybrid antibiotics (*see* Antibiotics, hybrid)

5'-Hydroxy-2''-N-demethylstreptomycin, 84

5'-Hydroxystreptomycin, 102

Hydroxylamine (HA), 49

3-Hydroxy-3-methylglutaryl (HMG)-CoA reductase, 779-780, 801
  3-hydroxy-3-methylglutaryl (HMG)-CoA substrate of, 779-781
  inhibitors of, 780
    lovastatin, 781
    mevastatin (ML-236B, compactin) (*see also* Pravastatin, biosynthesis of), 780-782, 784-797
      biosynthesis of, 781-782
      fermentation production and optimization of, 789-797
      hydroxylation of, cytochrome P450sca for, 785-788
      hydroxylation of, fermentation process for, 797-801
      structure of, 781
    pravastatin (Mevalotin) (*see also* Pravastatin), 779-801
      biosynthesis of, 779-801
      market for, 781
      structure of, 781

3-Hydroxypicolinic acid, 407

Hygromycin
  A, 90, 100, 128
  B, 86, 90, 96, 141

Hypoderma eucalyptii (*Leptostroma* anamorph), 309

Imipenem, 4, 11, 420
Immobilization of enzymes, 755, 759, 761,
     763-765
Immunocompromised hosts, 315
     AIDS patients, 315
     azole-resistant *Candida* sp. in, 315
     treatment of secondary infections in,
         545
     cancer patients, 315
     transplant patients, 315
Immunomycin (*see* Ascomycins)
Immunophilins (Rotomases) (*see also* Cyclo-
         philin and FK506 binding protein
         12), 497
Immunosuppressive agent, 1, 16
Indigo, 687
Inducing material (IM) (*see* Autoregulators)
Infections
     bacterial, 14
     enterococcal, 13
     lantibiotic treatment of, 455
     nosocomial, 9
Infectious diseases, 8
     newly emerging, 8, 9, 11, 13, 19
     reemerging, 8, 11, 19
     rifamycins in treatment of, 523
     under control, 8
Inosamycins, 86, 111, 128
Interleukin
     endotoxin induction of, 478
     IL1, 478
     IL2, 497-498
     IL8, 478
Introns
     self-splicing group I, 142-143
         inhibition of activity by aminoglyco-
             sides, 142-143
Invertase inhibitor, 98
Isoniazid, 11
Isepamicin, 95, 102
Isoprothiolane, 703
Istamycin group, 87, 89, 92, 113, 126

Jadomycin, 694, 702
     type II polyketide biosynthesis genes for,
         694
Jaspis sp. (marine sponge), 552
     antifungal compounds from, 552
     ergosterol antagonism of, 552

Kanamycins, 85, 92, 125, 149, 703
Kaposi's sarcoma (*see* Cancer)
Kasugamycins, 85, 88, 110, 115, 133, 141, 149

Ketosugar (or ketocyclitol) aminotransferases
     (SMAT family) (*see* aminotransfer-
         ases)
Klebsiella pneumoniae
     aminoglycoside-hypersensitive strain of,
         91
     labelled shikimic acid from auxotrophic
         mutant of, 506

β-Lactamases, 10, 16, 252
     evolution of, 10
     inhibitors of, 252
     plasmid-borne, 10
     types of, 10
β-Lactams (antibiotics), 5, 56, 188, 217,
         241-268
     α-aminoadipate biosynthesis for, 242, 244
         bacterial pathway, 242, 244
             lysine e-aminotransferase (LAT) of,
                 242, 244, 254-255
         fungal pathway, 242, 244
     bacteriocidal activity of, 241
     biosynthesis of, 188, 191
         ACV synthetase in, 188, 192-195, 199,
             219, 223, 226, 228, 231-233,
             242-245
             conserved 4'-phosphopantetheine
                 site in, 245
             conserved thioesterase domain of,
                 245
             pcbAB gene for, 244-245
         acyl-CoA-isopenicillin acyltransferase,
             248
             acyl-CoA-isopenicillin N
                 acyltransferase (IAT) activity of,
                 249
             acyl-CoA:6-APA acyltransferase
                 (AAT) activity of, 249
             analysis of mutants of, 249
             isopenicillin N amidohydrolase
                 activity of, 249
             penicillin amidase activity of, 249
             site-directed mutational analysis of,
                 249
         branchpoints in, 256
         cephalosporin 7-α-hydroxylase, 251
         deacetoxycephalosporin C (DAC)
             carbamoyltransferase (OCT), 251
         deacetoxycephalosporin C synthase
             (DAOCS) in, 249-250
         deacetylcephalosporin C (DAC)
             acetyltransferase (DACAT) in,
             251

[β-Lactams (antibiotics)]
  deacetylcephalosporin C synthase
      (DACS) in, 249-250
  horizontal gene transfer in, 257
  isopenicillin N epimerase in, 250
      pyridoxal 5'-phosphate cofactor of,
          250
  isopenicillin N synthetase (IPNS) in,
      192, 242, 245-248, 257, 696
      active site of, 248
      conserved structures of, 245-247
      crystal structure of, 246
      evolutionary relatedness of, 257
      multiple alignment of sequences of,
          247
      pcbC gene for, 245-247
  biosynthesis genes for, 253-255
      eukaryotic (fungal) gene clusters, 253,
          255-256
      introns in, 257
      regulation of, 260-262
      transcriptional analysis of, 260-262
      prokaryotic gene clusters, 253-255
      regulation of, 259-260
  clavam biosynthesis and (see also
      Clavulanic acid), 262-265
  inhibition of cell wall biosynthesis by, 241
  metabolic intermediates of
      α-aminoadipate, 242, 244
      δ-(α-aminoadipyl)-cysteinyl-D-valine
          (ACV) precursor, 219, 222, 223,
          241
      6-aminopenicillanic acid (6-APA), 243,
          248
      o-carbamoyl-deacetoxycephalosporin C
          (OCDAC), 243, 255
      deacetoxycephalosporin C (DAOC),
          243, 250, 255, 743-744
      deacetylcephalosporin C (DAC), 243,
          250, 255, 256, 742-744
      isopenicillin N, 242, 245, 255, 256
      penicillin N, 250
      thiazolidine ring of, 250
  pathway for, 243
  penicillin-binding proteins (PBPs) and,
      252
  resistance to, 10
  self-resistance to, 251-252
Lactobacilli
  D-alanyl-D-lactate in cell walls of, 374

[Lactobacilli]
  intrinsic resistance to glycopeptides
      (vancomycin) of, 374
Lactobacillus sp., 188, 745
  D-lactate dehydrogenase from, 745
Lactocin S (see also Lantibiotics), 439
Lactococcin A, 456
Lactococcus lactis, 437, 458-460, 475, 487
  food-grade lactic acid bacterium, 437
  nisin from, 458-460, 475, 487
  strain ATCC 11454, 459
Landomycin, 702
Lanthionine antibiotics (see Lantibiotics)
Lantibiotics (see also Nisin), 187, 217, 393,
      437-461
  analogs (lantibodies) of, 455
  antimicrobial action of, 455-458
  ATP-binding cassette (ABC)-transporters
      of, 448
  collapse of membrane potential by,
      455-458
  covalent modification by, 456-457
  currently known, 440
  dehydroalanine (Dha) residues of, 439,
      453-455
  dehydrobutyrine in, 475
  engineering of, 450-453
  genes encoding, 444-448
      immunity (self-resistance), 446
      LanA (encoding prelantibiotic
          polypeptides), 445-446
  immunogenic properties of, 452-453
  inhibition of spore outgrowth by, 457
  lanthionine bridge in, 440, 475
  lantibodies, 455
  β-methyllanthionine bridge in, 440, 475
  posttranslational modifications of, 448
  prelantibiotic polypeptide (LanA product),
      439, 447-448
      processing of, 438-439, 447-448
  proteolytic cleavage of, 452
      resistance to, 452
  two-component regulators of, 448
  type A (nisin-like), 440
      cytolysin, 440, 447
          genes encoding, 444-445
      epidermin, 440-441, 444-450
          gene cluster for, 444-446, 448, 452
          treatment of skin infections with,
              441

[Lantibiotics]
    epilancin K7, 440, 447
    gallidermin, 440-441, 447, 450
    lacticins, 439-440, 444-447
    nisin, 438-461, 475
        chimeras of, 449
        genes encoding, 444-449, 452
        production of, 458-461
        structure of, 442
    nisin A, 450
    nisin Z, 447
    pep5, 440, 444-445, 447, 450, 475
        genes encoding, 444-445, 452
    salivaricin, 440, 447
    streptococcin, 440, 447
    subtilin, 440-442, 444-452, 458-461
        chimeras of, 449
        genes encoding, 444-449, 452
        structure of, 442
    type B (duramycin-like)
        ancovenin, 440-441
            inhibition of angiotensin-converting
                enzyme by, 441
        cinnamycin (lanthiopeptin, Ro 09-0198),
            440-441
            anti-herpes simplex virus (HSV1)
                activity of, 441
            structure of, 442
        duramycin A, 440-441
            lysinoalanine bridge of, 441
        duramycin B, 440-441
        duramycin C, 440-441
        production by *Streptomyces* spp., 441
    type C
        actagardine, 440-441
            inhibition of peptidoglycan
                biosynthesis by, 441
        mersacidin, 440-441
            immunosuppressive activity of,
                441
            structure of, 442
        voltage-dependent membrane pore
            formation by, 455-456, 475
Leader peptidases, 16
Legionnaires disease, 8, 11
Leprosy, 523, 543
Leuconostoc sp.
    D-lactate dehydrogenase from, 745
Limulus polyphemus
    polyphemusin (tacheplesin analogs)
        cationic peptides from, 475
Lincomycin, 136, 165
    assay for, 170

[Lincomycin]
    biosynthesis of, 171-178
        N-demethyllincomycin (NDL)
            synthetase in, 176
        methyltransferase in, 177-178, 181
    biosynthetic gene cluster for, 174-175,
        178-181
    chloro-derivative of, 165
    chromosomal instability and, 181-182
    commercial production by Upjohn of, 165
    cosynthetic factor (7, 8-didemethyl-8-
        hydroxy-5-deazariboflavin) for,
        173-174
    L-dihydroxyphenylalanine (DOPA) as a
        precursor for, 170-174
    ethylhygric acid (EHA), 170-174
    fermentation for production of, 167-169
        determination of diaminopimelic acid
            (DAP) in, 166-169
    lincomycin A, 169-172
        propylproline precursor of, 165, 170-174
    lincomycin B (side product), 165, 166,
        169-172
        ethylproline precursor of, 170-174
    melanin biosynthesis and, 172
    methylthiolincosamide (MTL) of, 165, 171
        biosynthesis of, 174-178
    peptide bond in, 217
    production in defined medium, 170
    propylhygric acid (PHA) of, 165, 170-174
    propylproline addition to fermentations
        of, 170
    scale-up of process for production of,
        167-169
    L-tyrosine labelling of, 171-174
Lincosamides, 111, 129
Lipopeptides, 415-431
    A21978C complex of, 415-416, 419-431
        alkyl fatty acid side chains of, 415
        analogs of, 420
        cyclic depsipeptide moiety of, 415-416
        N-decanoyl analog of (*see* Daptomycin)
        factors (C_0, C_1, C_2, C_3, C_4, C_5) of, 416
        in vitro activities of, 420-421
        in vivo activity of, 421-426
        L-kynurenine in, 416
        membrane interactions with, 428
        removal of fatty acyl side chains of,
        415
    A54145 complex of, 415-423, 430
        biosynthesis of, 418
            thiotemplate peptide synthetase of,
                418-419

[Lipopeptides]
   factors (A, A₁, B, B₁, C, D, E, F) of, 415-418
      fermentation feeding affecting production of, 419
      in vitro activities of, 420-422
      removal of side chains of, 415
      structure of, 417
   daptomycin (LY146032) (*see also* Daptomycin), 57, 217, 230, 364, 415-431
Lipopolysaccharides (LPS) (*see also* Endotoxin), 82, 144, 478-479
   binding of cationic peptides to, 479
   O-chains of, 144
Liposodomycin B, 16
Lividomycin, 110
LL-BM123 antibiotics (*see* Glycocinnamoylspermidines)
Luciferase (firefly), 229
   adenylate-forming reaction of, 223
   crystal structure of, 223
Lyme disease, 8, 11
D-Lysergic acid, 407
Lysine e-aminotransferase, 56
   lat gene for, 56
Lysinomycin
   inhibition of group I self-splicing introns by, 142
Lysobacter, 241
   L. lactamgenes, 249-252, 256
      cephabacin production by, 251
      β-Lactam production by, 241
Lysobactin, 231
Lysteria monocytogenes, 13
LY333328 (*see* Glycopeptides)

Macrocin, 56
   intermediate in tylosin biosynthesis, 56
Macrolide-lincosamide-streptogramin (MLS) resistance, 7, 14, 179
Macrolides, 1, 2, 5, 129
   actinomycete that produces, 56
   biosynthesis
      SMAT enzymes of, 117
      glycosyltransferase for, 128
      production of A83543, 55
   resistance to, 7, 14, 128, 133, 179, 629
Magainins (*see also* Cationic peptides), 438, 458, 473-474, 476, 480

[Magainins]
   analogs of, 480
   anticancer activities of, 480
   B, 480
   collapse of membrane potential by, 456-458
   production by frogs, 456, 473
   synergism with cefpirome, 478
Magic bullet(s), 9, 441, 442
Mannonojirimycin, 125, 126
6'''-O-α-Mannopyranosylaminosidostreptomycin, 84
Marine bacteria, antibiotic production by, 15
Medicinal chemists, 19
Meningitis, 10
Merepenem, 4
Methanesulfonate (MMS), 49
Methicillin, 363
3-Methyl-4-hydroxyanthranilic acid, 407
Methylmalonyl-CoA mutase, 564
N-Methyl-N'-nitro-N-nitrosoguanidine (MNNG), 49
6-Methylsalicylic acid, 696
N-Methyl-*scyllo*-inoamine (rhizopine), 82, 148
Methylthiolincosamide (*see* Lincomycin)
Methyltransferases, 124, 177-178, 181, 196, 229-231, 506, 512
   S-adenosyl-L-methionine-dependent, 124
Metronidazole, 659
Metyrapone (cytochrome P450 inhibitor), 513
Mevalotin (*see* Pravastatin)
Micamycins, 63
Microcin B17, 393, 475
Micrococcin(s) (*see also* Thiopeptides), 393-394
   stimulation of GTP hydrolysis by, 394
Micrococcus
   M. luteus, 405-406
   M. spp., 393, 397
Micromonospora
   M. chalcea strain 69-683, 111
   M. halophytica, 166
   M. olivasterospora (ATCC 21819), 88, 107, 111, 126, 127
      aminoglycoside resistance genes of, 111, 132
      fortimycin blocked mutants of, 107
      fortimycin biosynthesis genes of, 107-109

[*Micromonospora*]
    M. *pilosospora*, 88
    M. *purpurea*, 116
    M. sp. SF-2089, 107, 111, 132
    M. sp., 88, 91, 124
Mideplanin (*see* Teichoplanin)
Mikamycin, 230
Minimycin, 66
Minosaminomycin, 85
Mistranslation, 141, 142
Mithramycin, 621, 702
    polyketide biosynthesis gene cluster for,
        621
Mitomycin C, 3, 638
Mitoxantrone, 590
Monensin, 3
Monocillium sp. ATCC 20621
    biotransformation of rifamycins by, 542
mTOR (mammalian target of rapamycin)
        (*see* FKBP12-rapamycin binding
        protein)
Mucor
    M. *circinelloides*, 756
        stereoseletive reduction by, 756
    M. *heimalis*, 784
        hydroxylation of ML-236B by, 784
    M. *miehei*, 758, 771-772
        lipase from, 771-772
Multidrug resistance (MDR), 7-8, 448, 583,
        590, 597, 600
    exporter proteins, 7
    lung resistance protein (LRP)-mediated,
        597-598
    multidrug resistance protein (MRP)-
        mediated, 597
    P95-mediated, 598
    P170 protein (Pgp, gp170)-mediated,
        597-598
    pathogens with, 8
    proteins conferring, 7-8
    topoisomerase II (atMDR)-mediated,
        597
    verapamil antagonism of, 598
Multienzyme complexes, 289
Multifunctional polypeptides, 289
Mulundocandin (*see* Echinocandins)
Mureidomycin A, 16
Mutagenesis, 49-52, 429
Mutasynthesis, 4
Mutations, 50, 57
Mycobacterium, 667, 669
    acquisition of tetracycline resistance by,
        669
    M. *avium*, 545

[*Mycobacterium*]
    M. *leprae*, 405-406
    M. *tuberculosis*, 11
    isoniazid- and rifamycin-resistant, 11
    multidrug resistant, 11, 14, 667
Mycoplasma
    M. *capricolum*, 405-406
    tetracycline-resistant strains of, 667
Mycothiol, 144
D-*Myo*-inositol-3-phosphate synthase, 113-115
Myomycins, 85, 89, 115, 126, 133
Myxobacteria
    antibiotic production by, 15

Nalidixic acid, 3, 471
Natural products, 2, 3, 8, 12, 20-43
Nebramycin complex, 111, 121
Neisseria, 667
    N. *gonorrhoeae*, 557
    N. *meningitidis*, 557
Nemadectin, 54
Neocosmospora species, 309
    production of cyclosporin A by, 309
Neomycins, 85, 112, 136, 175
    producer of, 111
    resistance genes for, 110
    structures of, 90
3, 3'-Neotrehalosadiamine (a, β-gycosidic
        antibiotic), 91
Nephrotoxicity, 82, 142
Neplanocins, 113, 115-116
Netilmicin, 95, 102, 420
Neurospora crassa
    p-aminobenzoic acid (PABA) synthase
        from, 558
Nikkomycins, 316
Nisin (*see also* Lantibiotics), 437-461
    assays for, 459
    bacteriocidal activity of, 438
    biosynthesis of, 438-440
        genes encoding, 444-448
            chimeras of, 449
            mutagenesis of, 438, 452
            regulation of, 448
    collapse of membrane potential by,
        455-458
    conversion of prenisin to, 439
    covalent modification by, 455-457
    dehydroalanine (Dha) residue of, 439,
        453-455
    generally regarded as safe (GRAS) status
        of, 437
    lanthionine bridge of, 440
    leader peptide (region) of, 439, 448

[Nisin]
    nontoxic nature of, 437
    paradigm, 441-444
    posttranslational modification of, 439-440,
        445, 448
    prenisin (prelantibiotic) precursor of, 439,
        445
    production of, 458-461
    products from, 459
        Ambicin N, 459
        Nisaplin, 459
    ribosomally-synthesized peptide of, 438
    structure of, 442
    transport of, 448
    uses for
        food preservative, 437-438
        prevention of bovine mastitis, 437
        prevention of oral plaque and gingivitis,
            437
4-Nitroquinoline-1-oxide (NQO), 49, 50
Nocardia
    N. lactamdurans, 242, 244, 246, 249-252,
        254-255
        cephamycin biosynthesis genes of,
            253-255
        LAT of, 242
    N. mediterranea (Streptomyces mediterranei)
        (see Amycolatopsis mediterranei)
        production of aminocyclitol-aminoglyco-
            side by, 85
    species, 704
Nodulation (Nod) factors, 82, 148
    hexosamine-based lipooligosaccharide, 82
Nojirimycin, 126
Norerythromycins (see Erythromycin)
Nosiheptide (see also Thiopeptides), 230,
        393-409
    indolic acid moiety of, 398-402
        3, 4-dimethyl-2-indole-carboxylate
            (DMI) intermediate of, 399-400
            activating enzyme for, 407-409
            ATP-dependent activation of, 407
    peptide synthetase genes for biosynthesis
        of, 408
    pyridine group of, 398
    resistance gene (nshR), 396
    thiazole formation in, 393, 401
Novobiocin, 350
Nucleotide-diphosphate (NDP)-hexose 3, 5-
        epimerases, 124

Nucleotide-diphosphate (NDP)-hexose oxido-
        reductases, 119
Nucleotide-diphosphate (NDP)-hexose synthe-
        tases, 119
Nucleotide-diphosphate (NDP)-4-ketohexose
        isomerases, 119
NusG, 71

Oleandomycin, 133, 688
ORF1590, 140
Ostreogrycins, 63
Otitis media, 10
Ototoxicity, 82, 143
Outer membrane protein permeability, 11
Oxazolidones, 14
Oxytetracycline (OTC) (see also Tetra-
        cyclines), 663-664, 670-676, 691

P26k gene, 76
Paclitaxel (see Taxol)
Papulacandin glycolipids, 316
Paromomycin, 110
Pathogens (see Bacteria)
PCR (see polymerase chain reaction)
Penicillin(s) (see also β-Lactams), 2, 241-256,
        265-266, 438-445, 733
    biosynthetic precursors of, 56
    discovery of, 442, 683
    G, 241, 248, 266
        chemical ring expansion of, 266
    hydrophobic
        late genes for synthesis of, 248-249
        recombinant improvement in production
            of, 265-266
    market, 2, 5
    paradigm, 441-443, 457
    resistance to, 363
    structural analogs (10, 000) of, 444
    V, 266
Penicillin binding proteins (PBPs) (see also
        β-Lactams), 10, 11, 252
Penicillium, 241
    P. citrinum, 780-784, 789-797, 801
        mevastatin (ML-236B) produced by,
            780, 789-797, 801
            fermentation optimization of, 789-797
            plasmid transformation of, 782-783
            strain improvement of, 781-784
    P. chrysogenum, 192, 242, 244-249, 255, 260-
        262, 266-267

[*Penicillium*]
    lysine auxotroph of, 242
    filamentous growth of, 790
    recombinant strain improvement of, 266
    P. roqueforti, 782
Pentosephosphate cycle, 112, 135
Peptide antibiotics
    cyclizations of, 218
    epimerization of residues in, 218
    non-ribosomal synthesis of, 217
    rational design of, 198, 201-202
    thioether crosslinks in, 218
Peptide synthetases, 187-208, 217-234, 289
    N-acylation reactions of, 230, 231
    adenylate formation reaction, 222, 223, 231
    amino acid activating domains of, 193-194
    amino acid (substrate) selection by, 219, 222
    aminoacyl adenylates in, 191, 193, 222, 226
    aminoacylation reaction of, 222, 227
    ATP-pyrophosphate exchange assays for, 191, 196, 225
    consensus sequences of motifs in, 225
    current status of research on, 220-221
    domain organization of, 192-197
    elongation reactions of, 228-229
    epimerase/racemase domains of, 198-200, 228-229
    epimerization reaction, 222, 228
    interdomain ("spacer") regions of, 197-198
    methyltransferase domains in, 196, 229-231
    module sizes of, 219
    modules of, 226
    multienzyme thiotemplate model for, 187-191, 198-201
    peptide bond formation reaction, 222
    peptide chain elongation in, 198
    4'-phosphopantetheine cofactor of, 191, 194-197, 218, 222-227, 231-232
    targeted domain replacements of, 201-203
    thioesterase domain of, 198
    type I (amino acid activating) domains in, 194
    type II (N-methyl-amino acid-activating) domains in, 196
    Walker A box in, 193
Peptidoglycan, 368-369
    biosynthesis of, 368-369
        D-alanyl-D-alanine moiety in, 368-373, 385
        assembly of precursors for, 368
        inhibition of, 368-369, 375

[Peptidoglycan]
    screens for inhibition of, 375
    affinity methods for, 375-376
    glycopeptide antibiotic inhibition by, 368
Peptidolide SDZ compounds
    SDZ 90-215, 289
    SDZ 104-125, 232
    SDZ 214-103, 295-308
        analogs of, 298-308
        biosynthesis of, 296
        in vitro, 297
        minor metabolites in, 296-298
        structure of, 296
        synthetase of, 289, 295-297, 299
Peptidyl nucleosides, 703-725
Peptidyl nucleosides, blasticidins, 703-725
    A 83094B, 706, 722
    blasticidin S, 703-705, 707-725
        acetylation of, 723
        biosynthesis of, 704, 707-722
            blastidic acid in, 710
            cytosinine moiety of, 709-710, 719
            cytosinine:pyridoxal phosphate tautomerase, 719
            cytosylglucuronic acid (CGA) precursor of, 711-714, 717-720
            cytosylglucuronic acid (CGA) synthase, 717-719
            demethylblasticidin S in, 704-705, 711-714
            demethylblasticidin S N-methyltransferase in, 716-717
            effects of inhibitors on, 711-713
            L-β-N-methylarginine (blastidic acid) moiety of, 707-708
            pentapyranone precursor of, 720-721
            pentapyranone oxidoreductase-I, 720-721
            precursors for, 707
            UDP-glucose 4'-epimerase, 719-720
            UDP-glucose 6'-oxidoreductase, 719-720
        market for, 703
        mechanism of action of, 722-723
        resistance against
            animal, 723-724
            genetics of, 724-725
            microbial, 723-725
            plant, 724
    isoblasticidin S, 713
    leucylblasticidin S, 704-705
    mildiomycins, 705, 716, 721

[Peptidyl nucleosides, blasticidins]
    biosynthesis of, 721-722
    CMP 5-hydroxymethylase in, 721
    hydroxymethyl CMP N-ribotidase,
        721-722
    Sch 36605, 706, 722
Peptidyl nucleosides, gougerotins, 704, 706,
        720
    aspiculamycin, 706, 720
    bagougeramines, 706, 720
    blasticidin H, 703-705, 718, 720
    gougerotin, 704, 706, 720, 723
Peptidyl nucleosides, pentopyranines, 704,
        706
    pentopyranine A, 704, 706
    pentopyranine C, 704, 706, 711-715, 718
    pentopyranine D, 706, 713
Petaiboles (antifungal), 231
Phaseolotoxin, 188
Phospho-N-acetylmuramylpentapeptide
        translocase, 16
1-Phosphoryl-6-glucosaminyl myo-inositol, 84
Phyllomedusa sauvagii (frog), dermaseptin
        cationic peptide from, 473
Pig liver esterase (PLE), 754, 756
Piricularia oryzae, 703, 724
Planobispora rosea, 393
Plasmids, 50
    conjugal vector, 56
    cosmid pOJ436, 54-56
    broad host range, 50
    integrative cloning vectors, 55
    DNA of, 53
    inhibition of secondary metabolism by
        freely replicating, 54
    nonreplicating forms of, 55
    pA387, 527
    pCK7, 690
    pDF333, 782-783
    pDF345, 782-783
    pDM10, 527
    pHBV1, 741
    pHDV11, 741-747
    pHJL401, 57
    pIJ61, 609
    pIJ702, 53, 56, 609
    pIJ922, 609
    pJLA503, 201
    pKC505, 609
    pKC796, 56

[Plasmids]
    pMEA100, 527
    pMEA123, 527
    pPLcddE, 763
    pPLRES, 763
    pSAM2-based vectors, 54
    self-replicating, 53
Plastics (biodegradable), 687
Platenolide I, 702
    mutants blocked in biosynthesis of, 702
    polyketide synthase for, 702
Pneumocandins, 188, 319
    A_O, 317, 327
    B_O, 327
    pharmacokinetic properties of, 330
    semisynthetic analogs of, 316-320
        L-671, 329, 327
        L-693, 989, 327
        L-705, 589, 328
        L-731, 373, 328
        L-733, 560, 328
Pneumocystis carinii, 315, 317, 326, 330, 331
Pneumococci, 379
Poisson distribution model for mutagenesis,
        49
Polyenes, 6, 551-570
    activity of, 551-552
        antibacterial, 551-552
        antifungal, 551-552
            ergosterol antagonism of, 552
        delay of Creutzfeldt-Jacob disease by,
            557
        immunostimmulatory, 552, 557
        insecticidal, 552
        inhibition of HIV replication by, 557
    amphotericin B, 551-552, 554-557, 562
        stimulation of macrophage tumor
            necrosis factor production by, 557
        structure of, 554
    aureofungin, 556
    axenomycins, 552
    biosynthesis of, 557-567
    biosynthesis of, aromatic moiety of,
        558-562
        p-aminobenzoic acid (PABA) precursor
          of, 558-562
          ligase, 562
          synthase for, 558-562
          synthase for, genes encoding,
            559-560

[Polyenes]
    macrocyclic lactone rings of, 552, 557
    methylmalonyl-CoA mutase in, 564
    pathway for, 561
    polyketide synthase for, 561-564
      genes encoding, 563-564, 570
      regulation by phosphate, 569-570
    candicidin, 553, 556-564, 569-570
    candidinin, 555
    6-deoxysugars of, 553, 555-556
    dermostatin A, 554
    faeriefungin (pentaene macrolide), 551,
      554-555, 557
      bacteriocidal activity of, 551-552
      mosquito lavaecidal activity of, 552
      nematodicidal activity of, 552
    fermentation of, 568-569
    filipin, 554
    FR-008 (heptaene aromatic polyene), 563,
      691
    fungimycin (perimycin), 555, 560, 562
      N-methyl-PAAP of, 560
    hepaene subgroup, 556
      aromatic moieties of, 556
        p-aminoacetophenone (PAAP), 556,
        563
        p-N-methylacetophenone (N-methyl-
        PAAP), 556
    levorin, 562
    lucensomycin, 562
    nystatin, 551, 554-557, 562
      aglycone of, 562
    pimaricin, 554
    polyfungin B, 555
    pore formation in membranes by, 557
    tetrafungin, 552, 555
    trichomycin, 555
Polyenzyme systems, 218-219
Polyketides
    aromatic, 17-18, 687
    hybrid, 17-18, 620
Polyketide synthases (PKSs),
    conserved 4'-phosphopantetheine binding
      domains of, 194
    type I, 17, 509-513, 561-564
      iterative forms of, 692, 696
        6-methylsalicylic acid synthesized by,
        696
      modules of, 510-511, 563-564, 688-691
      processive forms of, 688-691
    type II, 17, 563, 606, 615-621, 638-639,
      671-674
      acyl carrier proteins (ACPs) of, 692

[Polyketide synthases (PKSs)]
    chain length factors of, 17, 621, 673,
      692
    cyclases of, 691-695
    iterative function of, 692
    ketoreductases (KR) of, 691-695
    ketosynthases (KS) of, 691-695
    recombinant, 18, 619-621, 638-639, 673,
      684, 686, 691-694
    recombinant, hybrid molecules pro-
      duced by
      aloesaponarin II, 17-18, 620, 638-639,
        684, 686, 691-694
      2-carboxy-aloesaponarin II
        (endocrocin), 684, 686, 693
      dehydromutactin, 694
      desoxyerythrolaccin, 684, 686, 691
      EM18, 694
      mutactin, 693-694
      RM18, 693
      RM18b, 693
      RM20, 692-693
      RM20b, 693
      RM20c, 693
      RM77, 693-694
      RM80, 693
      SEK4, 692-694
      SEK4b, 692-694
      SEK15, 692-694
      SEK15b, 692-694
      SEK34, 694
      SEK43, 694
      tetracenomycin (tcm) F2, 693-694
      UWM1, 692-694
Polymerase chain reaction (PCR), 18, 193,
    201-202, 353, 685
Polymyxin, 230
Polyoxins, 316
Postantibiotic era, 9
Pradimicins, 316
Pravastatin (Mevalotin) (*see also* Pravastatin),
    779-801
Pravastatin (Mevalotin), biosynthesis of,
    779-801
    mevastatin (ML-236B, compactin) in,
      780-782, 784-797
      biosynthesis of, 781-782
      fermentation production of, 789-797
        optimization of, 789-797
      hydroxylation to pravastatin of,
        784-788
        cytochrome P450sca for, 785-788
        fermentation process for, 797-801

Pravastatin (Mevalotin), market for, 781
Pravastatin (Mevalotin), structure of, 781
Precursor flux, 56-57
Pristinamycins, 13, 63, 230
    I$_A$, 13
    IB, 63
    IC, 63
    II$_A$, 13, 63
    IIB, 63
Probenazole, 703
Promoter sequences, 57
Propylhygric acid (PHA) (*see* Lincomycin)
Protein kinases, 140
Protein-protein interactions, 458
Protoplast transformation, 50, 52
Pseudomembranous colitis, 363
Pseudomonads
    aminoglycoside production by, 82
    phytopathogenic, 198, 230
    sorbistin production by, 82, 148
Pseudomonas
    Ps. aeruginosa, 8, 9, 629
        cecropin-melittin hybrid cationic
            peptide killing of, 477
        meropenem-resistant, 11
        aminoglycoside resistance in, 131
        antibiotic activity against, 16
        intrinsic antibiotic resistance of, 11, 477,
            489
        opportunistic pathogen, 11
        pipecolate pathway in, 503
        pyocyanin biosynthesis in, 559
    Ps. cepacia, 557
    Ps. diminuta, 267
        strain N176
            cephalosporin C acylase (CC acylase)
                from, 737-740
        strain V22
            cephalosporin C acylase (CC acylase)
                from, 737-748
    Ps. putida, 627
        camphor hydroxylase of, 785
    Ps. syringae, 77, 188
        var. *phaseolica*, 188
    Ps. tolaasi, 188
    Ps. sp. strain C427
        7-β-(4-carboxybutanamido)cephalo-
            sporanic acid (GL-7-ACA) acylase
            of, 737-740
    Ps. sp. strain GK16

7-β-(4-carboxybutanamido)cephalo-
        sporanic acid (GL-7-ACA) acylase
        of, 737-738
Puromycin
    SMAT enzymes in biosynthesis of, 117
    inhibition of ribosomes protein synthesis
        by, 722-723
Purpurosamine, 124-125
Pyoverdin, 188

Quinolones (*see also* Fluoroquinolones),
        2, 3, 5, 471
Quinoxaline-2-carboxylic acid, 407
Quinupristin (*see also* Synercid), 13

Ramihyphin A, 309
Ramoplanin, 364
Rana (frog)
    cationic peptides from, 473
    R. brevipoda, 473
    R. esculenta, 473
Rapamycin, 1, 16, 217, 497-516, 687, 691,
        702
    antifungal activity of, 498
    antitumor activity of, 498
    biosynthesis of, 498-502
        cytochrome P450 in, 513
        (1R, 3R, 4R)-dihydroxycyclohexane-
            carboxylic acid (DHCHC) pre-
            cursor of, 506-509
        genes encoding, 509-513
            disruption of, 509-510
            rapA (encoding Raps1 polyketide
                synthase component), 509-511
            rapB (Raps2 polyketide synthase
                component), 509-511
            rapC (Raps3 polyketide synthase
                component), 509-511
        incorporation of precursors into, 499-
            500
        macrolide ring of, 498-501
        methyltransferases in, 506, 512-513
        pipecolate-derived moiety in, 503-505
            adenylation of, 504-505
        shikimic acid precursor of, 506-509,
            515-516
        type I polyketide synthase for, 509-512,
            702
            modules of, 510-512
    fermentation optimization of, 513-516

[Rapamycin]
 immunosuppressive activity of, 497-499
 mode of action of, 499
 structure of, 499
Rational drug design, 19
Regulatory genes in antibiotic biosynthesis,
  57-58
relC mutation, 138
Replication fork, 49
Restriction endonucleases, 50
Restriction/modification, 50-53
Resveratrol (polyketide) synthase, 562
Rheumatoid arthritis, 660
Rhizobia, *N*-Methyl-*scyllo*-inoamine
  production by, 82, 148
Rhizobium
 R. *japonicum*, 785
  P-450c in, 785
 R. *meliloti*
  MosB protein of, 117
Rhizomucor pusillus
 sillucin (cationic peptide) from, 475
Rhizopus
 R. *arrhizus*
  fumaric acid production by, 790
 R. *nigricans*, 784
  oxygenation of steroids by, 784
 R. *niveus*, 725
Rhizopine (*see N*-Methyl-*scyllo*-inoamine)
Rhodosporidium toruloides CBS349
 cephalosporin C acetylesterase from,
  748
Ribosomes
 50S subunit of, 394-395
  GTPase center of, 394-395
 ribosomal proteins of
  L11, 394
   complex formation with thiopeptide
    antibiotics, 394
 ribosomal RNA (rRNA) of
  16S ribosomal RNA (rRNA), 111
   interaction of aminoglycosides with,
    141
   methylation of, 131
   methyltransferases for, 111, 132
   spectinomycin interaction with, 141
  12S mitochondiral rRNA, 143
  23S ribosomal RNA (rRNA)
   complexation of thiopeptides with,
    394, 405
   methylases, 395-396
   methylation of, 165, 179, 395-396
Ribostamycins, 85, 111
Rifampicin (*see* Rifamycins)

Rifamycins, 11, 521-545, 558
 analysis of, 540-541
 biosynthesis of, 527-531
  3-amino-5-hydroxybenzoate intermediate (AHBA) of, 529, 533-534, 558
  synthase for, 534
  B-factor regulation in, 533-534
 biotransformation of, 542-543
 demethyl-desacetyl-rifamycin SV,
  530-531
 fermentation of, 525-526
 halomicin B, 523-524
 30-hydroxyrifamycin SV, 532
 incorporation of precursors into, 528,
  533
 3-methylthio-rifamycin SV, 523-524
 oxidase for, 542
 protorifamycin I, 530-531
 purification of, 541-543
 rifampicin, 536, 543
  pharmacokinetic properties of, 543
  treatment of infectious diseases with,
   543
  treatment of intracellular infections
   with, 543
 rifamycin B, 521-524, 528-536, 540-543
  biosynthesis pathway for, 531
  conversion of, 522
  fermentation of, 521
   diethylbarbituarate (barbital) added
    to medium for, 521, 532-533
  structure of, 522
 rifamycin complex (A, B, C, D), 530,
  532-533
 rifamycin G, 523, 530, 532, 533
 rifamycin O, 521-524, 540-542
 rifamycins Q, P, R, Verde, 532
 rifamycin S, 521-524, 528, 530-534,
  540-543
  chemical synthesis of, 544
  transformation of, 530-534, 540-543
 rifamycin SV, 521-524, 530-534, 537,
  540-543
  barbital inhibition of conversion of,
   533
 rifamycin W, 528, 530-532, 534-535
 rifamycin Y, 524, 530-532
 rifamycin Z, 530
 semisynthetic, 523
  rifabutin, 523, 545
  rifamide, 523
  rifapentine, 523, 545
  rifaximin, 523, 545
  structure-activity relationships

[Rifamycins]
  (SARs) of, 544-545
  thiazorifamycins P, Q, Verde, 532
  tolypomycin Y, 523-524
Rifomycins A, B, C, D, E (see Rifamycins)
RNA polymerase sigma factors, 140, 353

Saccharomyces cerevisiae, 258, 315, 559
  blastimycin S-resistance strains of,
      723
  cell walls of, 315
  pab gene from, 559
Saccharopolyspora
  Sa. erythraea (formerly Streptomyces erythrae-
      us), 509, 563, 567, 675, 688
    eryA genes of, 510, 563, 688-691
    mutants of, 689
    P450 hydroxylation system in, 785
  Sa. hirsuta ATCC 20501, 86, 107, 111,
      132, 621
  Sa. spinosa, 53
  Sa. sp., 89, 345
Sacrophaga peregrina (flesh fly)
  sarcotoxin I (cationic peptide) from,
      473-475
Salmonella, 565, 567
  S. enterica type B, 145
    O-chain biosynthesis of, 145
  S. typhimurium, 760
    cytidine deaminase from, 760
Sandimmun/Neoral (see Cyclosporin)
Sannamycins (see Istamycin group)
Schizosaccharomyces pombe, 724
Screening
  broad-based, 5, 15
  high-throughput, 4, 16, 17, 19
  mechanism based, 375
  programs, 15, 19
  serendipity in, 4
  target-based, 2, 13, 16
    affinity methods for, 375-376
SDZ compounds (see Peptidolide SDZ
      compounds)
Secondary metabolic aminotransferase
      (SMAT) (see Aminotransferases)
Seldomycins, 85, 94, 125, 149
Semisynthetic drugs (see antibiotics, semi-
      synthetic)
Serratia
  S. marcesens, 232, 288
  S. sp., 188

Shigella
  multidrug resistant, 9
  S. flexneri, 9
  S. sp., 9, 10
Showdomycin, 66
Sisomycins, 107
Soraphen, 691
Sorbistins, 82, 148
  structures of, 99
Spectinomycins, 87, 133, 149
  bacteriostatic action of, 141
  biosynthesis gene cluster for, 104
  6-deoxyhexose sugars of, 121
  genes for biosynthesis of, 106, 121
  pathway design for, 87
  producing strain for, 116
  resistance against, 120, 131
Spenolimycin, 85, 106, 107
Spiramycin biosynthesis, 57, 691
  spiramycin I, 691, 702
    hybrid antibiotics of, 691, 702
    novel esters of, 691
  srmR activator gene in, 57
Sporaricins, 89
Spore pigment, 621
  polyketide biosynthesis gene cluster for,
      621
  whiE genes, 694
Sporiofungin A (see Echinocandins)
Sponges, 552
Stachybotrys chartarum, 309
Staphylococci, 14, 363
  coagulase-negative, 374, 380
    glycopeptide resistance in, 374
    S. haemolyticus, 374
  glycopeptide-resistant, 374
  methicillin-resistant, 9, 11, 363, 372, 543
  multidrug resistant, 9
  penicillin-resistant, 9
  vancomycin resistant, 9, 11
Staphylococcus
  S. aureus, 9, 10, 11, 63, 363, 379-380, 415,
      420-427, 430, 541, 579
    aminoglycoside-resistant, 14
    cloxacillin-tolerant strain of, 426
    endocarditis caused by
      daptomycin treatment of, 423-426,
          430
    methicillin-resistant (MSRA), 10, 14,
        379-380, 415, 430, 476, 489, 660
      antibiotics effective against, 379-380,

[*Staphylococcus*]
 415, 420-424, 430, 660
 Oxford strain of, 10
  transfer of vancomycin resistance to, 11
  vancomycin-resistant, 11
 S. epidermidis, 363, 379, 415, 420-422
  methicillin-resistant (MSRE), 379, 415
  antibiotics effective against, 379, 415,
   420-422
  pep5 (cationic peptide) from, 475
  recognition as a pathogen, 363
 S. haemolyticus, 374
  coagulase-negative nature of, 374
Staphylomycin, 63
str/sts (streptomycin biosynthesis) genes,
  100-112, 117
Strain development, 49-58
Streptidine, 84, 112, 115
 biosynthesis of, 116-120, 131
Streptococci, 363, 380
Streptococcus
 S. cremoris
  nisin-sensitive, 459
 S. pneumoniae, 9
  penicillin-resistant, 10, 415, 430
   antibiotics effective against, 415,
    420-422, 430
 S. pyogenes, 420-423
  antibiotics effective against, 420-423
Streptogramins, 13, 14, 63
Streptomyces
 consensus promoter sequences of, 259
 hormones, 71, 135
 linear chromosomes of, 146
 molecular genetics of, 49-58
 S. acrimycini JI2239 (candicidin producer),
  560
 S. actuosus, 393, 396-397, 401-402, 405-409
  biosynthesis gene cluster of, 406
  defined medium for, 397
  nosiheptide resistance (*nshR*) of, 396
  orf699 of, 405
  orfC of, 405-406
   similarity to *entD* and *sfp* products,
    405
  peptide synthetase genes in, 408
 S. albus
  strain G, 50
  tetracycline producer, 671
 S. ambofaciens, 57, 691
 S. antibioticus, 128, 132, 137, 262, 336-341,
  347-355, 393, 627, 629, 688
  blocked mutants of, 347-349
  giant linear plasmid in, 350

[*Streptomyces*]
 s^E gene (*sigE*) of, 354
 strain NF-18, 67, 70
 S. argillaceus, 621
 S. aureofaciens, 173, 668-670, 673-675
  strain B-96, 612
  strain NRRL 3203, 669
 S. avermitilis, 403, 509
  avermectin biosynthesis gene cluster of,
   403, 509
 S. azureus, 393-397, 401-402, 405-406,
  409
  thiostrepton biosynthesis by, 393
  thiostrepton resistance gene (*tsr*) of,
   394-396
 S. bifurcus strain 23219, 581, 603
 S. bikiniensis, 65
 S. bluensis DSM40564, 105, 125, 145
 S. carbophilus, 781
  strain SANK 62585, 785, 797-801
   hydroxylation of ML-236B (meva-
    statin) to pravastatin by and
    fermentation optimization of, 781,
    785, 797-801
   NADH-cytochrome P-450 reductase
    of, 786-787
   P450sca of, 785-788
   P450sca-1 and -2 of, 786
 S. cattleya, 251
 S. cellulosae ATCC 12625 (fungichromin
  producer), 568
 S. chrysomallus, 199, 336, 339-342, 348-349,
  354, 419
  blocked mutants of, 348-349
  production of actinomycin C by, 336,
   339
 S. cinnamonensis, 502, 564
  production of monensin A by, 502
 S. citricolor, 115
 S. clavuligerus, 56, 138, 242, 244, 249-252,
  254-255, 259-264, 267
  cephamycin biosynthesis genes of,
   253-255, 259-260
  clavulanic acid production by, 262-264
 S. coelicolor, 17, 347, 350, 395, 526, 615,
  618-619, 638, 673-674, 684, 687,
  754
  methylenomycin production by, 350
  rel mutants of, 395
  strain A3(2), 74, 615
  strain CH999, 619, 621, 690, 696
  var. *aminophilus* (fungimycin producer),
   560, 567
 S. coeruleorubidus, 580-581, 603, 605, 607,

[*Streptomyces*]
608, 609, 612, 614, 620, 624, 630
strain 8899, 581, 603
strain 31723, 581, 603
strain JA10092, 581, 603
strain ME130-A4 (ATCC 31276),
580-581, 602-603, 614, 620, 630,
633, 635
S. collinus, 502, 508-509
S. cucumerosporus, 342
S. cyaneofuscatus, 65
S. elgretius UC-5453, 581, 605
S. erythreae (see also *Saccharopolyspora*
erythrea), 227
S. espinosus, 166, 172, 178
S. flavopersicus NRRL 2820, 106, 120, 131,
139
S. fradiae, 49, 50, 55, 115, 124, 132, 144,
145, 178, 407, 415-419, 429-430
strain A54145 (NRRL 18158), 415-419
cyclic lipopeptides produced by,
415-419, 429-430
strain ATCC 10745, 111
strain Tü2717, 639
S. galilaeus, 17, 581, 604, 607-609, 615, 618,
620, 639
mutants of, 604
strain ATCC 31615, 607, 639, 695
strain MA-144-M1 (ATCC 31133),
580-581, 602, 604, 607-609, 615,
618, 620, 638-639, 684
S. gilvospiralis, 107
S. glaucescens
strain GLA.O (ETH 22794), 102,
104-106, 122-125, 128-132, 136-
139, 145-146, 606, 618, 670, 675
S. griseochromogenes, 703-704, 707, 710,
712-714, 716-721, 723-724
S. griseoruber, 603
S. griseus, 53, 65, 104-106, 115, 124, 125,
128-140, 145-146, 559-560, 563,
567, 603, 613-614, 624, 626-628
candicidin production by, 567
cephamycin-producing strain, 255
strain 45H, 140
strain DSM 40236, 102
strain IFO, 74
strain IMRU 3570 (candicidin
producer), 559
strain JA5142 (anthracycline producer),
582, 602-603, 614-615

[*Streptomyces*]
strain N2-3-11, 102, 117, 137
strain S104, 137
var. *autotrophicus*, 551
S. hawaiiensis, 393
S. hygroscopicus, 86, 111, 563, 567, 687
strain ATCC 29253 (rapamycin producer), 687
strain AY B-994 (ATCC 29253, NRRL
5491), 498, 500, 509, 514
fermentation optimization of, 514-516
rapamycin biosynthetic gene cluster
of, 509
strain AY B-1206, 503, 514
subsp. *ascomyceticus* (ATCC 14891,
MA6475), 498-507, 516
ascomycin (FK520, immunomycin)
production by, 498
butyryl-CoA formation in, 501-502
subsp. *glebosus* DSM40823, 105, 117,
125
subsp. *limoneus*, 89
subsp. *yakushiaensis* strain 7238 (FERM
BP-928, MA6531), 498, 516
ascomycin (FK520, immunomycin)
production by, 498
S. insignis ATCC 31913, 603, 606, 610,
614, 635
S. jumonjinensis, 262, 264
S. kanamyceticus, 112, 132, 137, 149
S. kasugaensis MB273, 110, 132
S. katsuharamanus, 262, 264
S. laurentii, 393, 396-397, 401-403, 405-409
fermentation of, 397
peptide synthetase genes in, 408
resistance gene (*tsnR*) of, 396, 403,
405-406
S. lincolnensis, 145
blocked mutants of, 178
lincomycin biosynthesis genes of,
178-182
strain 78-11 (lincomycin production
strain), 182
strain LM4344, 181-182
strain NRRL 2936 (wild-type), 182
var. *lincolnensis*, 165-172, 174-175,
178-182
S. lipmanii, 52, 249, 251, 262
S. lividans, 120, 128-130, 139, 178, 250-251,
264, 395, 609, 612, 619, 621, 629,
632, 687, 723

[*Streptomyces*]
strain JG10, 559
strain TK21, 74
strain TK24, 609, 612, 619, 621, 638
S. *mediterranei* (*see Amycolatopsis mediter- ranei*)
S. *mycarofaciens*, 691
mdmB gene from, 691
S. *nodosus*, 145, 567, 629
S. *nogalater* UC-2783 (ATCC 27451), 580, 582, 602, 605-609, 615, 618, 620, 629, 639
protoplast transformation of, 609
S. *noursei* (nystatin producer), 567
S. *olivaceus* straun Tü2353, 606
S. *parvulus*, 338, 349-351, 354
S. *pseudogriseolus*, 166, 172
S. *peucetius*, 608
antifungal polyene produced by, 609
protoplast transformation of, 609
strain ATCC 29050, 579-580, 582, 602-609, 612-629, 635-638, 696, 702
subsp. *aureus* (ATCC 31428), 624
subsp. *caesius* (ATCC 27952), 580, 582, 608, 633
subsp. *carminatus*, 582, 603
S. *purpurascens* ATCC 25489, 578, 582, 605, 607, 615, 632, 639, 695
S. *regenesis*, 785
S. *rimosus*, 111, 565, 668-670, 673-676
chromosome of, 676
forma *paromomycinus*, 111
OTC-sensitive strain 15883, 676
S. *roseofulvus*, 621
S. *roseosporus*, 57, 415-416, 419, 429-430
lipopeptide biosynthesis genes of, 430
strain A21978.65, 416
strain NRRL 11379, 415-416, 419
transposon insertional mutagenesis of, 429
S. *sannanensis* IFO 14239, 107, 109, 111, 132
S. *steffisbergensis* UC-5044 (ATCC 27466), 580, 582, 605-609
protoplast transformation of, 609
S. *subrutilus*, 91, 125
S. *tenebrarius*, 111
S. *tenjimariensis* ATCC 31603, 88, 107, 109, 111, 127, 132
S. *thermotolerans*, 691
acyA gene from, 691
carE gene from, 691
S. *toyocaensis*, 55

[*Streptomyces*]
S. *triangulatus* subsp. *angiostaticus*, 603
S. *tsukabaensis*, 498
S. *validensis*, 115
S. *variabilis*, 166
S. *vellosus*, 166
S. *violaceoruber* Tü22, 629, 638
S. *virginiae*, 63, 65, 71-76, 139, 503
S. *viridochromogenes*, 65, 603
S. sp. 5541 (nemadectin producer), 54
S. sp. AC4437, 128
S. sp. AM-7161, 638
S. sp. C5 (ATCC 49111) (daunorubicin producer), 577, 582, 602-604, 606-607, 612-635, 638
protoplast transformation of, 609
S. sp. D788, 602-603, 614, 628-629, 632, 635
S. sp. DOA 1205, 578
S. sp. FRI-5, 65, 139
S. sp. L-1689-23, 707
β-lysine formation in, 707
S. sp. MA6548 (rapamycin producer), 513
S. sp. MA6858 (ATCC 55098), 506
S. sp. SA-COO, 627
S. species, 2, 100, 116, 441, 669, 704
ancovenin (lantibiotic) production by, 441
Streptomycin (*see also* Aminoglycosides), 82, 86, 133, 420, 457, 683
biosynthesis gene cluster for, 104
biosynthesis of, 103-106
genes encoding, 103
pathway design for, 87, 92
pathway for, 103-105
export of, 106
oxidation of, 106
phosphotransferases for, 105
regulation of, 134-140
resistance mechanisms for, 106
amino acid-mediated stimulation of production of, 138
strains producing, 102
scyllo-inositol-derived aminocyclitols of, 84
Streptosporangium roseum, deacylation of lipo- peptide complex A21978C by, 420
Streptoverticillium
S. *rimofaciens*, 716, 721-722, 724
S. sp. strain JCM 4673, 723
S. sp., 100, 552, 704
Stringent response (*see also* Guanosine tetraphosphate (ppGpp)), 135, 138, 354-355, 395
Subtilin (*see also* Lantibiotics), 440-442
Sulfa drugs, 442

Superoxide, 143
Surfactin, 189, 217, 430
    biosynthesis of, 195-197
        N-acylation in, 230
        regulation of, 203-207
            pheromone-like peptides in, 205-206
            phosphorelay model in, 204-206
            srfA operon for, 194-195, 201-205
        competence and, 204-207
        4'-phosphopantetheine cofactor of, 195-197
        sfp gene of, 203, 405
        synthase, 192, 195-197, 231
            mutagenesis of, 196-197
            targeted domain replacement of (*see also*
                Peptide synthetase), 201-203, 430
            novel lipopeptides produced by, 201
Synercid, 9, 13, 19
Synergistins, 63
Syringolide, 77
Syringomycin, 188
Syringopeptins, 231
Syringotoxin, 188

Tachypleus (horseshoe crabs)
    tachyplesin cationic peptides from, 475
    T. gigas, 475
    T. tridentatus, 475
Tacolimus (*see* FK506)
Taxanes, 15
Taxol, 15, 577, 639
T cells, 497-499
    activation of, 498
    antigen presentation by, 497-499
        inhibition of calcineurin-caused block-
            age of, 497-499
Teichoic acid synthesis, 218
Teichoplanin, 9, 363-365, 368, 370-375,
        380-383, 425
    A40926, 381
        MDL 63, 042 from, 381
        MDL 63, 246 from, 381
    discovery of, 375
    screens for, 375
    semisynthetic derivatives of, 380-383
        mideplanin, 380-383
        MDL 62, 600, 381
        sodium borohydride reduction of,
            383-384
    structure of, 365
Teniposide, 590

Tetracenomycin (*see also* Anthracyclines),
        577, 579, 606, 618, 620-621,
        637, 639, 675, 692-695
    glycosylation of, 150, 639, 695
    polyketide biosynthesis genes for, 618,
        620, 692-695
        hybrid metabolites from, 692-696
            8-demethyl-8-O-
                olivosyltetracenomycin C, 696
    regulation of, 637
    structure of, 579, 695
Tetracyclines, 2, 111, 363, 563, 659-676
    biosynthesis of, 669-675
        acyl carrier protein in, 671
        acyltransferase in, 673
        anhydrotetracycline (ATC) in, 661, 669,
            674
        anhydrotetracycline oxygenase in, 670
        dehydrotetracycline (DHTC) in, 670,
            674
        dehydroxytetracycline in, 674
        4-keto-anhydrotetracycline (ATC) in,
            674
        malonamyl-CoA starter unit for,
            672-673
        6-methylpretetramide in, 674
        mutants blocked in, 674-675
        pathway for, 671
        tetracycline dehydrogenase in, 670-671,
            674
        type II polyketide synthase in, 671-674
    broad spectrum activity of, 659
    chlortetracycline, 663-664, 668-671, 675
    dactylocyclines, 663-664, 666
        dactocycline A, 663
        dactylocyclinone, 663
        structures of, 664
    demecycline, 663
    democycline, 663
    6-deoxytetracycline, 666
    doxycycline, 666
    fermentation processes for, 668
    genes encoding, 667-675
    genetic instability in production of, 675-
        676
        classes of variants, 676
    glycylglycines, 666-668, 676
        efficacy of, 667
        ineffectiveness of tetracycline resistance
            mechanisms against, 667-668
        N, N-dimethylglycylamido-6-demethyl-

[Tetracyclines]
6-deoxytetracycline (DMG-DMDOT), 666-667
N, N-dimethylglycylamidominocycline (DMG-MINO), 666-667
semisynthesis of, 666-667
interactions with ribosome of, 659
market for, 659
methacycline, 666
8-methoxychlorotetracycline, 666
minocycline, 660
T-cell suppressive activity of, 660
oxytetracycline (OTC), 663-664, 670-676
resistance mechanisms against, 660-663
Clostridial TetP system for, 663
in production strains, 668-669
plasmid-mediated, 661
regulation of, 660
ribosomal resistance, 661
*Campylobacter tet*M/O system, 661
Bacteroides TetQ system, 661
Tn*10*-mediated efflux mechanism for, 660-663
E. coli TetA system, 662
TetR-mediated regulation of, 662-663
TetR-mediated regulation of, induction by anhydrotetracycline, 663
TetX system, 663
oxidoreductase activity of, 663
transposon-mediated, 661-663
SF 2575, 663, 665
structures of, 664-666
tetracycline, 659-664, 668-669
terramycin X, 663
uses for, 659
acne, 660
eukaryotic controllable-expression systems, 660
fish farming, 660
Helicobacter pylori, 659-660
methicillin-resistant *Staphylococcus aureus* (MSRA), 660
rheumatoid arthritis, 660
Thiocillins (*see also* Thiopeptides), 393
Thioesterases, 198
Thiopeptin(s) (*see also* Thiopeptides), 393, 395
Thiopeptides (thiopeptide antibiotics), 217, 393-409
amythiamycins, 393, 395
berninamycin, 393
biosynthesis of, 393-409
macrocyclic ring system (macrocycle) in,

[Thiopeptides]
393, 401
thiotemplate mechanism for, 401-409
peptide synthetase in, 401-404
cyclothiazomycin, 393
inhibition of renin by, 394
inhibition of bacterial protein synthesis by, 394
micrococcins, 393-395
self-resistance to, 397
structure of, 394
GE2270 A, 393-395
structure of, 394
glycothiohexide a, 393
structure of, 394
nosiheptide, 393-409
nosiheptide, indolic acid moiety of, 398-402
3,4-dimethyl-2-indole-carboxylate (DMI) intermediate of, 399-400
activating enzyme for, 407-409
ATP-dependent activation of, 407
nosiheptide, peptide synthetase genes for biosynthesis of, 408
nosiheptide, pyridine group of, 398
nosiheptide, resistance gene (*nshR*), 396
nosiheptide, structure of, 394
nosiheptide, thiazole formation in, 393, 401
resistance genes, 394-396
similarity with TRP-185, 396
resistance mechanisms, 394-397
siomycins, 393
thiocillins, 393
thiopeptins, 393, 395
thiostrepton, 393-409
Thiostrepton (*see also* Thiopeptides), 230, 393-409
dihydrothioazole formation in, 393, 401
high yields of, 397
quinaldic acid moiety of, 393, 398-399, 402
4-(1-hydroxyethyl)-2-quinolinecarboxylate (HEQ) intermediate of, 398-399
activating enzyme for, 407-409
ATP-dependent activation of, 407
peptide synthetase genes for biosynthesis of, 408
reactions required to assemble, 403-404
resistance to, 394
resistance genes (*tsr, tsnR*), 396, 403
tetrahydropyridine group of, 398
Thiostrepton-induced proteins (Tip), 395
Thiostreptone (*see* thiostrepton)
TipA (*see* Thiostrepton-induced proteins)

Tobramycin, 111, 121, 149, 420
Tolaasin (pseudomonad toxin), 188
Tolypocladium
    species, 309
    T. inflatum, 16, 280, 308-309, 497
        Gams strain NRRL 8044, 280-281, 288
            alternative names for, 280
            blocked mutants of, 288
            cyclosporin production by, 280
            defined medium for, 281
            immobilization of, 281
            mutants of, 281
            taxonomy of, 280
        strain 7939/45, 292, 296-297
    T. niveum, 188, 280
    T. terricola, 309
Topoisomerase II, 586
    aclarubicin interaction with, 590-591, 595
    altered multidrug resistance (at-MDR) of,
        590-591, 597-598
    drug-related cleavable complex formed by,
        590-591, 595
    anthracycline interactions with, 586-587,
        589-591
    doxorubicin interaction with, 590-591
    isozymes of, 589
    model for activity of, 589-590
    poisons of, 590-591, 597-598
Transducing lysates, 53
Transduction, 53
Translation, 141-142
Transposons,
    exchange, 55, 56
    IS*112*, 106
    IS*493*, 57
    mutagenesis, 57, 192, 196
    Tn*3*, 372
    Tn*10*, 660
    Tn*917*, 196, 204
    Tn*1546*, 372-373
        VanA-resistance genes on, 372-374
    Tn*4560*, 179-181
    Tn*5096*, 55, 57
    Tn*5099*, 55, 57, 58, 429-430
    Tn*5099-10*, 55, 57
    Tn*5100*, 55
    Tn*5100-4*, 57
Trehazolin (trehalostatin), 91, 102, 115, 116
Trichoderma
    T. harzianum, 231

[*Trichoderma*]
    T. polysporum NRRL 8044 (*see Tolypocladi-
        um inflatum*)
    T. viride, 308
Tricyclazole, 703
Trigonopsis variabilis CBS4095 (ATCC 58536),
        734-736
    D-amino acid oxidase (DAO) of,
        734-736
Triostin, 230
Trypanosoma cruzi
    inhibition by magainin B, 480
Tuberculosis, 11, 523, 543
    reemergence of, 11
    rifamycins for treatment of, 523, 543
Tumor necrosis factor, 478
Tylosin, 55-57, 128, 498, 691, 702
    3-O-acetate derivative of, 691
    biosynthesis of, 55, 56
        anabolic glycosyltransferase in, 128
        genes encoding, 49-50, 55
        macrocin O-methyltransferase in, 56
        rate-limiting step in, 55-57
    producing strain of, 50, 55
Tyrocidine, 188-189, 217, 227
    synthetase of, 193, 244, 289
    tyc operon for, 197, 207-208

UDP-glucose 4-epimerase (GalE) (*see also*
        6-Deoxyhexoses), 124
Ultraviolet light (UV), 49
Urdamycin, 639, 695, 702

Vaccines, 13
Validamycins, 89, 112, 113, 128, 135, 175
Validoxylamines, 89
Valiols, 82
Valiolamine, 89, 115
Vancomycin(s) (*see also* Glycopeptides), 9,
        10, 14, 217, 363-385, 425, 660
    affinity for D-alanyl-D-alanine by,
        368-371
    biosynthesis of, 367
    dalbaheptide structure of, 364
    inhibition of peptidoglycan biosynthesis
        by, 368-371
    resistance to, 9-14, 364, 371
        delayed emergence of, 364
        plasmid-borne, 364
        trends in emergence of, 373

[Vancomycin(s)]
    VanA-type (*see also* Enterococci), 371
    VanB-type, 371
  resurgence of, 363
  semisynthetic derivatives of, 377-379
  structure-activity relationships (SARs) of,
    377-383
  structure of, 365, 369
Varicella zoster virus, 756
VbrA, 71
Vector (*see* Plasmids)
Vernamycins, 63
Virginiae butanolides (VB) (*see also* Auto-
    regulators), 67-77, 139
  binding activity, 74
  receptor protein for, 71, 74
Virginiamycins, 63-66, 71, 217
Viruses, 753-756
  drugs for treatment of, 753-756
  Ebola, 8
  hantavirus, 8

[Viruses]
  hepatitis B virus, 756
  herpes simplex virus (HSV), 441
    HSV-1, 441, 756
    HSV-2, 756
  human cytomegalovirus, 756
  human immunodeficiency virus (HIV), 2,
    15, 16, 585, 753-754, 757, 759
  Varicella zoster, 756

WF11899A (*see* Echinocandins)

Xenopus laevis (African clawed frog)
  magainin cationic peptides from, 473

Yersinia enterocolitica, 120
Yogurt, 437

Zalerion arboricola, 188, 222
  echinocandin production by, 222
  pneumocandin production by, 319